Case-Based Geriatrics:
A Global Approach

Case-Based Geriatrics:
A Global Approach

Victor Hirth, MD, MHA, AGSF
Professor of Clinical Internal Medicine
University of South Carolina School of Medicine
Medical Director, Geriatric Services
Palmetto Health Richland
Columbia, South Carolina

Darryl Wieland, PhD, MPH, AGSF
Professor of Medicine
University of South Carolina School of Medicine
Research Director, Division of Geriatric Services
Palmetto Health Richland
Columbia, South Carolina

Maureen Dever-Bumba, FNP, DrPH (c)
Associate Director, Geriatric Education
Associate Director, Palmetto State Geriatric Education Center
University of South Carolina School of Medicine
Columbia, South Carolina

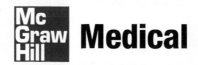

New York   Chicago   San Francisco   Lisbon   London   Madrid   Mexico City   Milan
New Delhi   San Juan   Seoul   Singapore   Sydney   Toronto

Case-Based Geriatrics: A Global Approach, First Edition

1 2 3 4 5 6 7 8 9 0   CTP/CTP   14 13 12 11 10

ISBN: 978-0-07-162239-4
MHID: 0-07-162239-X

This book was set in Goudy by Glyph International.
The editors were Jim Shanahan and Karen G. Edmonson.
The production supervisor was Catherine Saggese.
Project management was provided by Tania Andrabi, Glyph International.
The designer was Mary McKeon; the cover designer was Barsoom Design.
China Translation & Printing Services, Ltd. was printer and binder.

This book is printed on acid-free paper.

Library of Congress Cataloging-in-Publication Data

Case-based geriatrics : a global approach / [edited by] Victor Hirth, Darryl
        Wieland, Maureen Dever-Bumba.
            p. ; cm.
        Includes bibliographical references and index.
        ISBN-13: 978-0-07-162239-4 (pbk. : alk. paper)
        ISBN-10: 0-07-162239-X (pbk. : alk. paper)   1. Geriatrics—Examinations, questions, etc.
    2. Geriatrics—Case studies.
        I. Hirth, Victor.   II. Wieland, Darryl.   III. Dever-Bumba, Maureen.
        [DNLM: 1. Examination Questions—Case Reports.   2. Geriatrics—Case
    Reports.   3. Aging—Case Reports.   WT 18.2]
        RC952.6.C37 2011
        618.970076—dc22
                                                                            2010035826

McGraw-Hill books are available at special quantity discounts to use as premiums and sales promotions, or for use in corporate training programs. To contact a representative, please e-mail us at bulksales@mcgraw-hill.com.

Contents

Contributors

Mel L. Anderson III, MD
Associate Professor
Chief, Hospital Medicine
Denver VA Medical Center
Denver, Colorado
Chapter 44/Stroke

Gaurav Arora, MD, MS
Fellow in Gastroenterology
University of Texas Medical School at Houston and
MD Anderson Cancer Center
Houston, Texas
Chapter 39/Common Gastrointestinal Problems

Carol W. Babcock, MFT
Manager, The Center for Palliative Care/Transitions
The Medical Center of Central Georgia
Macon, Georgia
Chapter 19/Multi-Professional Team Care

Karlene Ball, PhD
Professor and Interim Chair
Department of Psychology
University of Alabama at Birmingham
Birmingham, Alabama
*Chapter 15/Older Drivers: Safe Mobility
in the Later Years*

Sandra Bellantonio, MD
Assistant Professor of Medicine
Tufts University School of Medicine
Chief, Geriatrics Section
Baystate Medical Center
Springfield, Massachusetts
Chapter 43/Congestive Heart Failure

Rachel Benz, RN, BSN
Research Nurse
University of Alabama at Birmingham
School of Nursing
Birmingham, Alabama
*Chapter 15/Older Drivers: Safe Mobility
in the Later Years* .

James T. Birch, Jr., MD, MSPH
Assistant Professor
Medicine and Palliative Care
Division of Geriatric Medicine and Palliative Care
Department of Family Medicine
University of Kansas School of Medicine
Kansas City, Kansas
Chapter 21/Perioperative Care of the Older Adult

Patricia Lanoie Blanchette, MD, MPH
Professor
Department of Geriatric Medicine
John A. Burns School of Medicine
University of Hawaii
Honolulu, Hawaii
Chapter 10/Assessing Decisional Capacity in Older Adults

Peter Boling, MD
Professor of Medicine
Director of Geriatrics
Virginia Commonwealth University
Richmond, Virginia
Chapter 24/Home Care

Maura Brennan, MD
Associate Professor of Medicine
Division of General Medicine and Geriatrics
Department of Medicine
Tuft University School of Medicine
Baystate Medical Center
Springfield, Massachusetts
Chapter 23/Advanced Illness Care and Elders at the End of Life

Allan S. Brett, MD
Professor of Medicine
Director, Division of General Internal Medicine
Department of Medicine
University of South Carolina, School of Medicine
Columbia, South Carolina
Chapter 12/Approach to Laboratory Testing and Imaging in Aging

Diane Chau, MD, FACP
Chief, Division of Geriatric Medicine
Department of Internal Medicine
University of Nevada School of Medicine, Reno
Veterans Affairs Medical Center
Reno, Nevada
Chapter 10/Assessing Decisional Capacity in Older Adults

Elizabeth Cogbill, MD
Fellow in Geriatrics
Department of Geriatrics
Medical College of Wisconsin
Milwaukee, Wisconsin
Chapter 13/Considerations Prior to Drug Prescribing in the Elderly

Erin L. Cooper, MD
Fellow in Geriatrics
Section of Geriatrics and Gerontology
Department of Internal Medicine
University of Nebraska Medical Center
Omaha, Nebraska
Chapter 22/Discharge Planning and Transitional Care

Carolyn Crane Cutilli, MSN, RN, ONC, CRRN
Doctoral Student, PhD Nursing
Mortality Clinical Nurse Reviewer, Clinical Effectiveness
and Quality Improvement
U of P Health System
Phildelphia, Pennsylvania
Duquesne University
Pittsburgh, Pennsylvania
Chapter 11/Health Literacy Assessment and Practice

Kathryn M. Denson, MD
Assistant Professor of Medicine
Division of Geriatrics
Medical College of Wisconsin
Zablocki VAMC
Froedtert Memorial Lutherian Hospital
Milwaukee, Wisconsin
*Chapter 13/Considerations Prior to Drug Prescribing
in the Elderly*

Maureen Dever-Bumba, FNP, DrPh (c)
Associate Director, Geriatric Education
Associate Director, Palmetto State GEC
University of South Carolina School of Medicine
Columbia, South Carolina
Chapter 1/Why Geriatrics and Gerontology?

Sreekanth Donepudi, MD, MPH
Fellow, Division of Geriatric Medicine
University of Nevada School of Medicine, Reno
Reno, Nevada
*Chapter 10/Assessing Decisional Capacity
in Older Adults*

Jonathan W Donley, PT, DPT, MEd, ATC
Director, Geriatric Mobility Clinic
Palmetto Health Richland
University of South Carolina School of Medicine
Columbia, South Carolina
*Chapter 26/An Approach to Assessing and Ordering
Physical Therapy*

Reed Dopf, MD
Fellow, Division of Geriatric Medicine
University of Nevada School of Medicine, Reno
Reno, Nevada
*Chapter 10/Assessing Decisional Capacity
in Older Adults*

Edmund H. Duthie, Jr., MD
Professor of Medicine
Medical College of Wisconsin
Chief, Geriatrics/Gerontology
Froedtert Memorial Lutherian Hospital
Milwaukee, Wisconsin
*Chapter 13/Considerations Prior to Drug Prescribing
in the Elderly*

Gilles O. Einstein, PhD
Professor
Department of Psychology
Furman University
Greenville, South Carolina
Chapter 3/Physical and Cognitive Function

Gladys L. Fernandez, MD
Assistant Professor of Surgery
Department of Surgery
Baystate Medical Center
Springfield, Massachusetts
*Chapter 28/Interprofessional Management of the Complex
Acute Surgical Patient*

Susan M. Friedman, MD, MPH
Associate Professor
University of Rochester School of Medicine and Dentistry
Attending Physician
Highland Hospital
Rochester, New York
Chapter 40/Hip Factures

David A. Ganz, MD, PhD
Assistant Professor of Medicine
VA Greater Los Angeles Healthcare System
Health Services Research and Development Center
of Excellence
UCLA Multicampus Program in Geriatric Medicine
and Gerontology
Los Angeles, California
Chapter 34/ Falls and Mobility Disorders

Angela Gentili, MD
Associate Professor of Internal Medicine
Director, Geriatrics Fellowship Program
Virginia Commonwealth University Health System
McGuire VA Medical Center
Richmond, Virginia
Chapter 18/Sexuality

Claudene J. George MD, RPh
Assistant Professor of Medicine
Albert Einstein College of Medicine
Division of Geriatrics
Montefiore Medical Center
Bronx, New York
Chapter 32/Polypharmacy

Michael Godschalk, MD
Professor of Internal Medicine
Virginia Commonwealth University School of Medicine
Director, Geriatric Health Care Center
McGuire VA Medical Center
Richmond, Virginia
Chapter 18/Sexuality

Adam Golden, MD
Assistant Professor of Clinical Medicine
Geriatrics Institute
University of Miami Miller School of Medicine
Geriatric Research, Education, and Clinical Center
and Research Service
Bruce W. Carter VA Medical Center
Miami, Florida
Chapter 2/The Biology of Aging and Emerging Interventions

Loren S. Greenberg, MD, MS
Assistant Professor of Medicine
Albert Einstein College of Medicine
Division of Geriatrics
Montefiore Medical Center
Bronx, New York
Chapter 31/Dementia

David Haber, PhD
Associate Director of the Fisher Institute for Wellness and Gerontology
John and Janice Fisher Distinguished Professor of Wellness and Gerontology
Ball State University
Muncie, Indiana
Chapter 14/Health Promotion and Disease Prevention

Ihab Hajjar, MD, MS
Assistant Professor of Medicine
Harvard Medical School
Institute for Aging Research
Hebrew Senior Life
Division of Gerontology
Beth Israel Deaconess Medical Center
Boston, Massachusetts
Chapter 45/Management of Hypertension in the Elderly

Anne L. Harrison, PT, PhD
Director of Professional Studies
Associate Professor
Division of Physical Therapy
College of Health Sciences
University of Kentucky
Lexington, Kentucky
Chapter 8/Aging and Sensory Loss: Vision, Hearing, Somatosensory, and Vestibular

Anna M. Hicks, MD
Fellow in Geriatrics
Department of General Medicine, Geriatrics and Palliative Medicine
University of Virginia School of Medicine
Charlottesville, Virginia
Chapter 5/The Medical Evaluation
Chapter 6/Medical Evaluation of the Older Person

Victor Hirth, MD, MHA
Professor of Medicine
University of South Carolina School of Medicine
Medical Director, Geriatric Services
Palmetto Health Richland
Columbia, South Carolina
Chapter 1/Why Geriatrics and Gerontology?

Michelle Horhota, PhD
Assistant Professor
Department of Psychology
Furman University
Greenville, South Carolina
Chapter 3/Physical and Cognitive Function

Margo-Lea Hurwicz, PhD
Associate Professor
Departments of Anthropology and Gerontology Program
University of Missouri—St. Louis
St. Louis, Missouri
Chapter 4/The Global Demography of Aging
Chapter 5/Cultural Competence in Geriatric Care

Kathryn Hyer, MPP, PhD
Director, Florida Policy Exchange Center on Aging, School of Aging Studies, University of South Florida
Tampa, Florida
Chapter 19/Multi-Professional Team Care

Lee A. Hyer, PhD, ABPP
Professor of Psychiatry and Health Behavior
Mercer School of Medicine, Georgia Neurosurgical Institute
Macon, Georgia
Chapter 19/Multi-Professional Team Care

Theodore M. Johnson, II, MD, MPH
Professor and Chief, Division of Geriatric Medicine and Gerontology
Emory University School of Medicine
Birmingham/Atlanta VA Geriatric Research, Education, and Clinical Center
Decatur, Georgia
Chapter 33/Urinary Incontinence

Stephen L. Kates, MD
Associate Professor
Department of Orthopaedics and Rehabilitation
University of Rochester, School of Medicine and Dentistry
Director Geriatric Fracture Center
Highland Hospital
Rochester, New York
Chapter 40/Hip Fractures

Peter Khang, MD
Program Director, Geriatrics Fellowship
University of California Los Angeles
Chapter 36/The Frailty Syndrome

Dae Hyun Kim, MD, MPH
Instructor in Medicine, Harvard Medical School
Division of Gerontology, Beth Israel Deaconess Medical Center
Boston, Massachusetts
Chapter 45/Management of Hypertension in the Elderly

Wessam Labib, MD, MPH
Assistant Professor
Director of Medical Student Education
Department of Family Medicine/Geriatric Medicine
Loma Linda University
Loma Linda, California
Chapter 34/Falls and Mobility Disorders

Kuo-Wei Lee, MD
Clinical Instructor
Kaiser Permanente Los Angeles Medical Center
Chapter 36/The Frailty Syndrome

Alexandra E. Leigh, MD
Assistant Professor of Medicine
University of Alabama at Birmingham
Center for Palliative and Supportive Care
Birmingham, Alabama
Chapter 35/Weight Loss

Brian Leo, MD
Fellow in Geriatrics
Geriatric Department
Kaiser Permanente
Livermore, California
Chapter 21/Perioperative Care of the Older Adult

Allison Lindauer, RN, FNP
Assistant Professor
Oregon Health and Science University
Internal Medicine and Geriatrics
Portland, Oregon
Chapter 17/Family Caregiving

William Logan, MD
Associate Professor
University of South Carolina—School
of Medicine
Department of Geriatrics
Senior Primary Care/Palmetto Health
Columbia, South Carolina
Chapter 14/Health Promotion and Disease Prevention

Amanda H. Lucas, MSN, RN, ACNS-BC, CCRN
Clinical Nurse Specialist
The Center for Palliative Care/Transitions
The Medical Center of Central Georgia
Macon, Georgia
Chapter 19/Multi-Professional Team Care

William L. Lyons, MD
Associate Professor
Section of Geriatrics and Gerontology
Department of Internal Medicine
University of Nebraska Medical Center
Omaha, Nebraska
Chapter 22/Discharge Planning and Transitional Care

Maria Maiaroto, GNP, BC
Clinical Nurse Instructor
Yale University School of Nursing
Geriatric Nurse Practitioner
Geriatric Consult Service
VA Connecticut Healthcare System
West Haven, Connecticut
Chapter 20/Geriatric Consultation Services

Jeffrey De Castro Mariano, MD
Attending Physician and Clinical Instructor
Department of Continuing Care
Kaiser Permanente Los Angeles Medical Center
Assistant Clinical Professor
Division of Geriatric Medicine
David Geffen School of Medicine at UCLA
Chapter 7/Functional Assessment

Robert M. McCann, MD, FACP
Professor of Medicine
University of Rochester School of Medicine and Dentistry
Chair of Medicine, Highland Hospital
Rochester, New York
Chapter 25/Long-Term Care

Mark A. McDaniel, PhD
Professor
Department of Psychology
Washington University
St. Louis, Missouri
Chapter 3/Physical and Cognitive Function

Daniel Ari Mendelson, MS, MD, FACP
Associate Professor of Medicine, Division of Geriatrics
University of Rochester School of Medicine and Dentistry
Director of Consultative Services
Department of Medicine, Highland Hospital
Rochester, New York
Chapter 25/Long-Term Care
Chapter 40/Hip Fractures

Deborah C. Messecar, PhD, MPH, RN, GCNS-BC
Associate Professor
Oregon Health and Science University School of Nursing
Portland, Oregon
Chapter 17/Family Caregiving

Eun-Shim Nahm, PhD, RN
Associate Professor
University of Maryland School of Nursing
Baltimore, Maryland
Chapter 27/Integrating Technology into Older Adult Living

Anne Olson, PhD, CCC-A
Associate Professor
Division of Communication Sciences and Disorder
College of Health Sciences
University of Kentucky
Lexington, Kentucky
Chapter 8/Aging and Sensory Loss: Vision, Hearing, Somatosensory, and Vestibular

Susan Ott, MD
Professor of Medicine
Department of Medicine
University of Washington
Seattle, Washington
Chapter 41/Osteoporosis

Julie McCole Phillips, MD
Assistant Professor of Clinical Medicine
Albany Medical College
Stratton VA Medical Center
Albany, New York
Chapter 23/Advanced Illness Care and Elders at the End of Life

Caroline Powell, MD
Assistant Professor
University of South Carolina School of Medicine
Attending Physician
Palmetto Health Richland Hospital
Columbia, South Carolina
Chapter 12/Approach to Laboratory Testing and Imaging in Aging

Barbara Resnick, PhD, CRNP, FAAN
Professor
University of Maryland School of Nursing
Baltimore, Maryland
Chapter 27/Integrating Technology into Older Adult Living

David B. Reuben, MD
Director, Multicampus Program in
Geriatric Medicine and Gerontology
Chief, Division of Geriatrics
Archstone Professor of Medicine
David Geffen School of Medicine at UCLA
UCLA Med-Geriatrics
Los Angeles, California
Chapter 7/Functional Assessment

Heather Riggs, MD
Hematology-Oncology/Geriatrics Fellow
Indiana University Simon Cancer Center
Hematology-Oncology Fellowship Program
Indianapolis, Indiana
Chapter 39/Interdisciplinary Team Care of the Older Adult with Cancer

Christine S. Ritchie, MD, MSPH
Associate Professor of Medicine
University of Alabama at Birmingham
Director, University of Alabama Center
for Palliative and Supportive Care
Birmingham, Alabama
Chapter 35/Weight Loss

Larry E. Robinson, D. Min, MFT
Professor Emeritus
Mercer University
Life Choices Coordinator
The Center for Palliative Care/Transitions
The Medical Center of Central Georgia
Macon, Georgia
Chapter 19/Multi-Professional Team Care

Susan Rodiek, PhD, NCARB
Associate Professor
The Ronald L. Skaggs Endowed Professor in Health Facilities
Design
Center for Health Systems and Design, College of
Architecture
Texas A&M University
College Station, Texas
*Chapter 16/Changing Living Environments for Older Adults:
Environmental Supports for Aging in Place*

Laurence Z. Rubenstein, MD, MPH
Reynolds Professor and Chairman
Reynolds Department of Geriatric Medicine
The University of Oklahoma College of Medicine
Oklahoma City, Oklahoma
Chapter 34/Falls and Mobility Disorders

Fadi Saab, MD
Cardiology Fellow
Baystate Medical Center
Tufts University SOM
Springfield, Massachusetts
Chapter 43/Congestive Heart Failure

Cynthia T. Schaefer, RN, MSN
Assistant Professor of Nursing
Doctoral Student, School of Nursing
Dequesne University, Pittsburgh
University of Evansville
Evansville, Indiana
Chapter 11/Health Literacy Assessment and Practice

Cathy C. Schubert, MD
Associate Professor of Clinical Medicine
Department of Medicine and Geriatrics
Indiana University
Indianapolis, Indiana
*Chapter 29/Interdisciplinary Team Care of the Older Adult
with Cancer*

Sarah Schumacher, DO
Clinical Assistant Professor
University of South Carolina—School of Medicine
Department of Geriatrics
Senior Primary Care/Palmetto Health
Columbia, South Carolina
Chapter 14/Health Promotion and Disease Prevention

Mayu Sekiguchi Runge, MD, MPH
Harvard Palliative Medicine Fellow
Massachusetts General Hospital
Boston, Massachusetts
*Chapter 23/Advanced Illness Care and Elders at the
End of Life*

Rachel Selby-Penczak, MD
Assistant Professor of Medicine
Virginia Commonwealth University Health Systems
Richmond, Virginia
Chapter 24/Home Care

Scott Shaffer, PT, PhD, ECS, OCS
Assistant Professor
Lieutenant Colonel, US Army
Doctoral Program in Physical Therapy
US Army-Baylor University
Fort Sam Houston, Texas
*Chapter 8/Aging and Sensory Loss: Vision, Hearing,
Somatosensory, and Vestibular*

Keerti Sharma, MB, BS
Assistant Professor of Clinical Medicine
Division of Geriatrics, Department of Medicine
Albert Einstein College of Medicine
Montefiore Medical Center
Bronx, New York
*Chapter 9/Atypical Presentation of Diseases
in the Older Adult*

Mara Slawsky, MD
Assistant Professor of Medicine
Tufts University
Director, Heart Failure Program
Director, Cardiovascular Fellowship Program
Baystate Medical Center
Springfield, Massachusetts
Chapter 43/Congestive Heart Failure

Mihaela S. Stefan, MD
Assistant Professor of Medicine
Division of General Medicine and Geriatrics
Department of Medicine
Baystate Medical Center
Springfield, Massachusetts
*Chapter 28/Interprofessional Management of the Complex
Acute Surgical Patient*

Daniel Swagerty, MD, MPH
Professor of Family Medicine and Internal Medicine
Associate Chair for Geriatrics and Palliative Care
Department of Family Medicine
Associate Director, Landon Center on Aging
University of Kansas School of Medicine
Kansas City, Kansas
Chapter 21/Perioperative Care of the Older Adult

Stephen Thielke, MD, MSPH, MA
Assistant Professor
University of Washington, Psychiatry and Behavioral Sciences
Geriatric Research, Education and Clinical Center
Seattle VA Medical Center
Seattle, Washington
Chapter 37/Evaluating and Treating Depression in Older Adults

David R. Thomas, MD
Professor of Medicine
St. Louis University Health Sciences Center
St. Louis, Missouri
Chapter 38/Pressure Ulcers

George Triadafilopoulos, MD, DSc
Clinical Professor of Medicine
Division of Gastroenterology and Hepatology
Stanford University School of Medicine
Stanford, California
Chapter 39/Common Gastrointestinal Problems

Bruce R. Troen, MD
Professor of Medicine
Director, Molecular Gerontology Program
Division of Gerontology and Geriatric Medicine
University of Miami Miller School of Medicine
Geriatric Research, Education, and Clinical Center and
Research Service
Bruce W. Carter VA Medical Center
Miami, Florida
Chapter 2/The Biology of Aging and Emerging Interventions

Nina Tumosa, PhD
Associate Director for Education
St. Louis Veterans Administration Medical Center
Professor of Internal Medicine
St. Louis University
St. Louis, Missouri
Chapter 4/The Global Demography of Aging
Chapter 5/Cultural Competence in Geriatric Care

Greg Valania, DO
Fellow in Cardiology
Tufts University
Baystate Medical Center
Springfield, Massachusetts
Chapter 43/Congestive Heart Failure

Steven D. Vannoy, PhD, MPH
Assistant Professor
Psychiatry and Behavioral Sciences
University of Washington Medical Center
Seattle, Washington
Chapter 37/Evaluating and Treating Depression in Older Adults

Camille P. Vaughan, MD, MS
Assistant Professor, Division of Geriatric Medicine
and Gerontology
Emory University School of Medicine
Birmingham/Atlanta VA Geriatric Research, Education,
and Clinical Center
Decatur, Georgia
Chapter 33/Urinary Incontinence

Lisa M. Walke, MD
Assistant Professor
Section of Geriatrics
Department of Medicine
Yale University School of Medicine
Chief, Geriatrics Consult Service
VA Connecticut Healthcare System
New Haven, Connecticut
Chapter 20/Geriatric Consultation Services

Jeffrey I. Wallace, MD, MPH
Associate Professor
Division of Geriatric Medicine
Department of Medicine
University of Colorado Denver
Aurora, Colorodo
Chapter 44/Stroke

Carol Parker Walsh, JD, PhD
Assistant Professor
School of Nursing
Oregon Health and Science University
Portland, Oregon
Chapter 17/Family Caregiving

Judith L. Warren, PhD
Professor, Special Initiatives Coordinator
Texas AgriLIFE Extension Service, Texas A&M University
System
Texas A&M University
College Station, Texas
Chapter 16/Changing Living Environments for Older Adults:
Environmental Supports for Aging in Place

Franklin S. Watkins, MD
Instructor, Internal Medicine and Geriatrics
J. Paul Sticht Center on Aging
Wake Forest University School of Medicine
North Carolina Baptist Hospital
Winston-Salem, North Carolina
Chapter 30/Delirium

Stephen G. Weber, MD, MS
Associate Professor, Section of Infectious Diseases
and Global Health
Chief Healthcare Epidemiologist
University of Chicago Medical Center
Chapter 42/Approach to Common Infections
in Older Adults

Darryl Wieland, MPH, PhD
Research Director, Division of Geriatrics Services
Palmetto Health Richland
Professor of Medicine
University of South Carolina School of Medicine
Columbia, South Carolina
Chapter 1/Why Geriatrics and Gerontology?

Mark E. Williams, MD
Professor of Medicine
Ward K. Ensminger Distinguished Professor
of Geriatric Medicine
Department of General Medicine, Geriatrics
and Palliative Medicine
University of Virginia School of Medicine
Charlottesville, Virginia
Chapter 6/Medical Evaluation of the Older Person

Jeff D. Williamson, MD, MHS
Professor of Internal Medicine
Chief, Geriatric Medicine
Wake Forest University School of Medicine
Director, J. Paul Sticht Center on Aging
North Carolina Baptist Hospital
Winston-Salem, North Carolina
Chapter 30/Delirium

Preface

We have designed *Case-Based Geriatrics: A Global Approach* to be a resource useful for geriatrics educators in the training of medical students in their clerkship years, family and internal medicine residents, geriatrics fellows, nurse practitioners, physician assistants, as well as students in nursing, pharmacy, social work, dentistry, dietary, and rehabilitation disciplines. The three main sections are *Issues in Aging*, which consists of foundational chapters for the geriatrics practitioner and other clinicians treating aging patients; *Interprofessional Geriatrics*, which exemplifies the great extent to which geriatrics is "a team sport"; and *Geriatric Syndromes and Important Issues*, which brings a problem-based focus to the student or trainee.

Unlike a traditional medical textbook, most of the chapters here are built around case descriptions. These chapters use case descriptions as an integral part of the content and as a learning tool. The cases are directed toward the learning objectives that the authors have for the learner. In geriatrics, cases may be "infinitely complex," involving multiple health domains, associated impairments and disabilities, common comorbid conditions, caregiver and home environments as resources or issues, and health care system issues. Here, however, we have aimed to introduce cases with more common levels of complexity as experienced in clinical practice, and we trust that the iteration of case descriptions and related content across chapters will help instructors and learners make cognitive and practical connections among larger "lumps" of complexity encountered in older patients and geriatric care.

Finally, the "global" theme introduced in our subtitle can be understood in several ways: in terms of the multiple domains of health and health threats (biomedical, functional, psychosocial, economic, and environmental) in aging people; and in the corresponding need for comprehensiveness of assessment, planning, and care. Of course, "global" also recognizes the ubiquity of aging in the world. Thus, geriatrics is of universal relevance. Further, in the developed world, aging is accompanied by growing diversity. Thus, there is an increasing need for understanding and navigation and cultural contexts and systems of care on the part of geriatric physicians and care providers. We hope that our textbook will make some small contribution to the worldwide improvement of geriatric care.

The Editors

Acknowledgments

We would like to acknowledge the hard work and dedication of all the team members who helped with the many aspects of organizing this book. Lynn Betterley for her superior organizing skills and leading the support team; Joyce Gossard and Austin Beasley for obtaining copyright permissions; Kimberly Hollins and Shawn Fagan for formatting and labeling all images, tables, and illustrations; Melissa Lewie for helping with the multitude of computer issues ranging from network drives to log-in permissions and software updates; and Donna Simon, the geriatrics practice manager, for making sure that the staff had the time and resources to perform their jobs efficiently. All in all, putting together a geriatrics textbook is not unlike providing good geriatric care. It requires a team, each member knowing and understanding his or her responsibilities and communicating effectively with other team members so that they function as one unit. We would also like to thank Judy Baskins, the Director of Geriatric Services at Palmetto Health, and Paul Eleazer, Division Director for Geriatrics at the University of South Carolina; without their support this project would not have been possible.

We hope you enjoy this book which comes from the tremendous efforts of over 90 authors and co-authors who donated their time to contribute to this work. We enjoyed the process of putting this book together and hope that it will yield much useful information and knowledge for you.

PART

I

Issues in Aging

1

Why Geriatrics and Gerontology?

Victor Hirth, MD, MHA

Darryl Wieland, PhD, MPH

Maureen Dever-Bumba, FNP, DrPhD (c)

● **LEARNING OBJECTIVES**

1. Define "geriatrics" and describe its approach to care of older adults.
2. Compare and contrast conventional and geriatric standards of care.
3. Explain threats to the provision of care to older adults.

CASE PRESENTATION: THE STANDARD OF CARE

Ms. Shin is a 78-year-old Chinese-American female who has been widowed for the past 22 years. Her underlying hypertension has been under variable to poor control for the past 5 years. She has degenerative arthritis affecting both knees and shoulders, sometimes limiting her mobility. She was recently diagnosed with type 2 diabetes but has no known complications. She was started on Cardizem (diltiazem) CD 240 mg once a day for her elevated blood pressure. On Friday afternoon, she calls her primary care provider, because for the past 72 hours she has been short of breath and having difficulty walking more than 15 feet (4.6 meters) without having to rest. A nurse tells her, "It sounds like you should be seen, but we don't have any appointments this afternoon. I suggest you go to the emergency room at the hospital. I'll call ahead so they know you are coming."

Every day, cases like this occur all over the world. What are our expectations in offering treatment to this patient? Are there processes or systems of care that might anticipate and prevent potential complications? Why might the outcome for this person be different in one setting than in another? Worldwide, the aging population is profoundly changing many aspects of societies and economies, including the demands placed on health care professionals, health care financing and systems, and the network of formal and informal caregivers to older people.

Geriatrics is defined as the branch of medicine that deals with the problems and diseases of old age and aging people.[1] Although correct as far as it goes, this definition misses the larger picture. Geriatrics in its broadest sense is the field of medicine that strives to provide patient care in the most comprehensive way. It considers not just diagnosis and treatment, but also the patient's preferences for care; the cultural and ethnic background that affects how the patient receives, interprets, and contextualizes his or her illness; and consequently how this affects the patient's decision-making and interaction with the health care system. Geriatrics also weighs the risks and benefits of treatment in the balance of the patient's physical function, living situation, and health care priorities (comfort, cure, palliation, etc.), as well as weighing how strong or weak the evidence base may be for a particular treatment or intervention. As such, geriatrics differs from the predominant, Western, Oslerian teaching of "Occam's razor," in which physicians are taught to distill a single diagnosis to explain disease presentation. While such focus on disease- and organ-based problems has proven extraordinarily useful in understanding and treating much acute illness and disability, it can lead to unfortunate outcomes, particularly in older adults with chronic, multi-morbid conditions and deficits in other dimensions of health and well-being.

CASE PRESENTATION (continued)

Ms. Shin arrives in the emergency room and is told to fill out a stack of papers "for insurance purposes." She is sent to the waiting room. After 45 minutes, she is called back by the triage nurse. When she is asked, "What brings you in today?" Ms. Shin explains that in the past 3 days she has had a sudden onset and rapid progression of shortness of breath. She had to sit up much of the night, because when she lay down, she felt "like I was smothering." The nurse obtains her vital signs: heart rate 104, respirations 28, temperature 98.4°F (37°C), blood pressure 165/92, weight 105 lbs (47.7 kg), and pulse oximetry on room air of 84%. Ms. Shin is started on oxygen and brought back to an exam room. Thirty minutes later, a physician enters, introduces herself, and asks a few questions before starting her exam. During the physical examination, she notes the patient's shortness of breath as well as wet-sounding crackles at both lung bases extending to the mid-lung zone. She listens to the heart, examines the abdomen and legs, and then states, "Ms. Shin, I'm pretty sure you have congestive heart failure. I'm going to order a few tests, including an x-ray, and give you a diuretic to get rid of some of this fluid. I'll be back once these tests are complete." She turns and leaves. Ms. Shin sits there dumbfounded, wondering what happened and why she was not given an opportunity to ask questions. Five minutes later, a nurse comes by to start an IV and administer a medication. "What is this?" Ms. Shin asks. The nurse says, "It's Lasix (furosemide), it will make you urinate and get the water off your lungs. The doctor also ordered a Foley catheter, so you won't have to run to the bathroom after I give you this medicine." "I'm not sure I want that, I've never had a catheter," replies Ms. Shin. "Don't worry," says the nurse, you'll be glad you have it once it's in."

What has been described so far is "the standard of care" that would be recognized in emergency departments any-where. Yet this scenario is one of an incipient disaster unless action is taken quickly, as experienced geriatricians would attest. In patients like Ms. Shin, the "standard of care" can easily result in untoward outcomes that, once realized, may

look to unschooled clinicians to have been inevitable and attributable to "age" or "poor health"—that is, to causes other than the care itself. The emergency room, by its design, is where assessment and care are rapidly provided. Yet this very setting increases the risk to vulnerable older adults who may be unfamiliar and unprepared for the organized chaos sur-rounding them. Unfortunately, this same approach to care can also be found in the typical outpatient medical office and other settings where environment, practice style, and other factors are not conducive to the needs and desires of the older adult.[2]

In our case, factors intrinsic to older adults and factors in the environment can have a substantial role in the potential for adverse outcomes. Intrinsic risk factors for Ms. Shin include:

- Underlying hypertension
- Degenerative arthritis
- Type 2 diabetes mellitus
- New-onset shortness of breath
- Any allergies or medication side effects she has had in the past
- Any unknown past medical history

Other risk factors that would not be evident to the emergency room physician include:

- Living alone with unknown social support network
- Her level of physical function (in terms of basic and instrumental activities of daily living)
- Whether she has any cognitive impairment or depression
- What medications and over-the-counter remedies she has been taking

Other consideration important in clinical decision-making:

- Her preferences for care (treatments, hospitalization, code status, end-of-life care)
- Her health literacy
- Whether she has a health care proxy if she is unable to make decisions
- Her financial situation (health insurance, income, expenses, etc.)
- Cultural or social aspects of her care that are important to her
- Whether anyone is dependent on her care for their well-being (ie, is *she* a caregiver?)

Ultimately, this process of assessment should include as many aspects of Ms. Shin's social, internal, and external environ-mental considerations as is feasible to render a treatment plan most consistent with her wishes, understanding, and medical situation.[3] This is why systems of care geared toward older adults are very important in optimizing care and reducing risks. Such systems include dedicated geriatric practices, in which every patient receives a comprehensive assessment at intake and annually to assess health, function, environment, finances, and health care preferences. They also include home visit programs and practices, where geriatric physicians or nurse practitioners provide care in the older adult's own home without the chaos of a busy medical system; such services are valued and highly rated by older adults. There are also guided care programs, in which the care team operates by standard-ized protocols optimized to minimize the risks of medical treatment to vulnerable older adults, and in which patients and their caregivers receive effective education and support to manage their medical conditions. There are other models of care, such as the program of all-inclusive care for the elderly (PACE), which use a day health care model and an interdisciplinary team management approach to successfully care for frail and disabled older adults who otherwise would be consigned to nursing homes.[4]

The paucity of effective, high-quality systems of geriatric care is manifestly linked to the lack of geriatrics expertise in clinical and academic training institutions. The full spectrum of health care professionals—from physicians to nurses, therapists, pharmacists, and others—requires at least some familiarity and basic competence in caring for an aging patient population, but few receive training of any depth or breadth. One broad strategy to increase geriatrics training would be for Medicare, which supports residency training in the United States, to require core content in aging and geriatrics for each specialty. Such a requirement would not only affect residency training but also help transform undergraduate medical education toward attention to the needs of an aging population.

More narrowly, the lack of trainees considering careers in geriatrics is attributable to perceived lack of "prestige" in such careers, societal bias against aging and the aged, poor reimbursement by Medicare and insurance companies for nonprocedural cognitive skills provided in geriatrics, and perhaps a feeling from governmental stakeholders that the problem will "take care of itself."[5,6] How are we to increase the number of providers who are specially trained in geriatrics? Some promising approaches include scholarships for students willing to enter a field of geriatric specialty, student debt loan forgiveness for those who commit to serve the older adult population, and academic career awards for physicians who train physicians and those from other disciplines in geriatric care. Some have argued that the root problem is poor reimbursement for geriatric care, and thus that reimbursement for geriatrics should be increased. While seemingly the simplest solution, increasing reimbursement is also the most challenging. Debates concerning the "relative values" of different aspects of health care generally become zero-sum arguments, wherein (for example) increased payments for "cognitive" specialists or primary care are seen to be at the expense of procedural care. Such debates only intensify in an environment of uncontrolled, escalating health care expenditure and increasingly desperate cost-containment efforts. Pressing such arguments may be counterproductive, since Medicare and private insurance do not pay well for most older adult care, and our ultimate objective is the preparation and positive engagement of all health care providers in caring for aging patients.

CASE PRESENTATION (continued)

Four hours later, Ms. Chin has orders written for admission to the hospital. Her admitting diagnosis is congestive heart failure. She is written for 40 mg of IV furosemide, continuous oxygen by nasal cannula with oximetry, a subcutaneous anticoagulant for DVT prophylaxis, diphenhydramine as needed for sleep, and her Foley catheter to be continued with monitoring of her intake and output as well as daily weights. When she gets to her room, she is pleased to see that it is a private room so she will not have to share it with someone else. She is moved from the gurney to the hospital bed, is shown the bed controls and the nurse call light, and is then asked if she has any questions. She replies, "I have a bunch of questions, but I think they're all for the doctor, thank you."

During the night, her continuous pulse oximeter alarms regularly, disturbing what little sleep she is getting between the nurse aides checking her vital signs and the noise from the hallway. At 3 AM, she gets up to go to the bathroom. She is very groggy from all the noise and does not remember that she is in the hospital, or that she has a Foley catheter in place. Unbeknownst to her, when she got out of bed she caught her IV on the bed sheets and it was pulled out and is pouring blood down her arm. Then, when she is about 3 feet from her bed, she feels very light-headed, and feels a pull from her between her legs. The Foley catheter tubing and bag attached to her bed stretches but does not yield. In an instant, she falls to the floor, which is accompanied by a loud pop from her right hip. She moans in pain as an aide who was walking by her room finds her on the floor and calls for help.

The care that Ms. Shin received up to this point certainly looks reasonable to the untrained eye; however, there are a number of "missed opportunities" that might have provided Ms. Shin with a safer environment and a lower likelihood of suffering a complication from this hospitalization. For the older patient, it is usually not one factor that leads to an untoward outcome, but the interplay of multiple factors.[7] Developing a list of possible contributors and ways to moderate the contributors is not difficult, but it does depend on trained providers who will recognize and mitigate the risk factors.

Possible Contributor	Proposed Solution
Excessively high dose of diuretic	Start at lowest dose and add more if needed
Dosing diuretic at night	Dose during daytime only
Foley catheter	Provide bedside commode
Beeping oximeter	Check oximetry with vital signs rather than continuously
Getting out of bed without help	Find room near nursing station, employ bed alarm

In Ms. Shin's case, a much better idea might have been to manage her on an outpatient basis only, with regularly scheduled follow-up in the office, or better yet with regular home visits, until she is over the acute phase of her congestive heart failure. Nonetheless, recognizing that the emergency department is a high-risk environment for older adults and that typical acute hospitalization also provides a number of pitfalls for older adults, numerous opportunities exist for improving systems and procedures of care for older adults.

Though underappreciated by many hospital systems, geriatrics has developed and is uniquely positioned to provide enhanced care for older adults. So why should older adults require care that is different from what is provided to younger adults? Just as children are different from adults, older persons are similarly and perhaps in more ways different from their chronologically (and sometimes but not always physiologically) younger counterparts. Just a few of the differences that result in an increased heterogeneity of older adults include cohort effects of the older generation growing up in a different place and time; survivor effects related to genetics; environmental exposures; diet; the accumulation of age-related diseases and conditions such as stroke, Alzheimer disease, arthritis, and others; as well as the effects of education, social status, financial situation, housing, and social support networks. Not only are the effects of all these factors different on each individual as he or she ages, but the magnitude and type of effect may vary from one individual to another.

When these factors converge in an older adult, it is easy to see that there are a number of reasons why (1) each older individual is uniquely different from another; (2) chronologic age might not be a very good indicator of a person's "physiologic age"; and consequently (3) good geriatric care requires an understanding of these factors and their effect on what geriatricians and patients ultimately care about, the older adult's overall function and quality of life irrespective of the number of diseases or conditions. This comes to the principal point of geriatrics: to optimize the overall function and quality of life for the older adult so that he or she can remain at the highest level of independent living for as long as possible.

Ultimately, geriatric care is not always about trying to have older adults live as long as possible, but to live as full a life as possible for the time they have. There are certainly many older patients who would elect to defer life-prolonging therapy when the risks and side effects of treatment outweigh the benefit of longer life, as can sometimes be the case for cancer chemotherapy or treatments that require hospitalization or surgery. However, the provider must keep in mind that for any given set of clinical circumstances or conditions, two "identical" patients might choose completely different options based on what they value, and the clinician must be prepared to handle both situations in a professional and non-judgmental way.

The field of geriatrics is just now entering the time of its greatest demand. The worldwide aging of the population, and the need for expertly trained providers in geriatrics, will create a tremendous demand for health care professionals for the next several decades irrespective of discipline. This change in the population will also shift the types of care provided from what historically has been predominantly acute care to chronic care, with an emphasis on function and independence. Only if health care policy leaders and health care providers understand and provide care with these considerations in mind will the care of older and medically complex adults be optimized to provide the highest quality of life for people in their waning years.

References

1. *Merriam-Webster's Online Dictionary*. Accessed May 5, 2010.

2. Fitzgerald R. The future of geriatric care in our nation's emergency departments: Impact and implications report. *Am Coll Emerg Phys.* 2008. Available at http://www.acep.org/WorkArea/DownloadAsset.aspx?id=43376.

3. Wieland D, Hirth V. Comprehensive geriatric assessment. *Cancer Control.* 2003;10:454-462.

4. Hirth V, Baskins J, Dever-Bumba M. Program of all-inclusive care (PACE): Past, present, and future. *J Am Med Dir Assoc.* 2009;10:155-160.

5. Hirth V, Eleazer GP, Dever-Bumba M. A step toward solving the geriatrician shortage. *Am J Med.* 2008;121:247-251.

6. Besdine R, Boult C, Brangman S. Task Force on the Future of Geriatric Medicine. Caring for older Americans: The future of geriatric medicine. *J Am Geriatr Soc.* 2005;53(suppl):S245-S256.

7. Wang L, van Belle G, Kukull WB, Larson EB. Predictors of functional changes: A longitudinal study of nondemented people aged 65 or older. *J Am Geriatr Soc.* 2002;50:1525-1534.

2

The Biology of Aging and Emerging Interventions

Bruce R. Troen, MD

Adam Golden, MD

● **LEARNING OBJECTIVES**

1. Describe the characteristics of an aging organism.
2. Compare and contrast models of aging and evidence that supports each theory.
3. Describe interventions associated with longevity including vitamin use, exercise, and dietary manipulation.
4. Discuss commonly used over-the-counter remedies thought to promote health and longevity, and their effectiveness.

PRE-TEST

1. **Which of the following is NOT a characteristic of aging organisms?**

   A. Reduced ability to respond adaptively to environmental stimuli

   B. Increased susceptibility and vulnerability to disease

   C. Increased mortality with age after maturation

   D. Increased efficiency of physiologic organ capacity

2. **Which of the following is TRUE regarding the role of genetics in aging?**

   A. Human aging is a tightly controlled genetically programmed event.

   B. Traits that have a role in improving reproductive fitness always improve longevity.

   C. Accelerated aging syndromes can result from single-gene mutations.

   D. All species have common aging mechanisms.

3. **Telomere length has been correlated with all of the following EXCEPT:**

   A. Frailty

   B. Survival in elderly twins

   C. Better health in centenarians

   D. Physical activity

● INTRODUCTION

The question as to why people age has plagued humankind throughout history. Aging (senescence) can be described as a constellation of deteriorative changes in structure and function, which result in a loss of homeostasis and an increase in the probability of death. There are at least five characteristics of an aging organism, described in the next sections.

Increased Mortality with Age after Maturation

The average life span of humans has increased dramatically over time, yet the maximum life span potential (MLSP) has remained approximately constant (Figure 2–1).[1] Gompertz first described the exponential increase in mortality with aging due to various causes, a phenomenon that still pertains today.[2] A greater than 130-fold increase in death rates is seen from young adults to the oldest group.[3] Table 2–1 shows the death rate for all causes in 2005.

A Variety of Poorly Understood Biochemical Changes in Cells and Tissues

Notably, lean body mass and total bone mass decrease with age.[4,5] Total body fat (subcutaneous plus visceral) remains the same, and consequently the percentage of adipose tissue increases with age. Many markers at the cellular level have been described in various tissues[6]; two of the first to be described were increases in lipofuscin[7] and increased cross-linking in extracellular matrix molecules such as collagen.[8,9] Recent studies have shown that DNA damage markers such as gamma-H2AX and 53BP1 are up-regulated in primates and presumably arise from DNA double-strand breaks (DSB) and/or dysfunctional chromosome ends called telomeres.[10,11] Additional examples include age-related changes in both the rates of transcription of specific genes and the rate of protein synthesis and numerous age-related alterations in post-translational protein modifications, such as glycation and oxidation.[12,13]

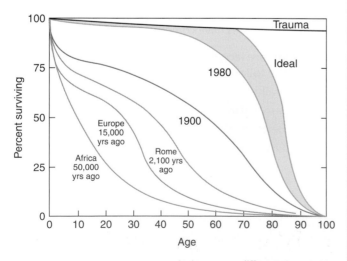

FIGURE 2–1. Percent survival curve for humans at different times in history with varying environments, nutrition, and medical care. The 50% survival values have improved but maximum life span potential has remained the same.

● TABLE 2–1 2005 Death Rate from All Causes	
Age	Death Rate per 100,000 population
25-34	104.4
35-44	193.3
65-74	2,137.1
75-84	5,260.0
85+	13,798.6

Progressive Decrease in Physiologic Organ Capacity with Age

Both cross-sectional and longitudinal studies have documented physiologic declines, such as those in glomerular filtration rate, maximal heart rate, and vital capacity.[14] These decreases occur linearly from about the age of 30; however, the rate of decline is quite heterogeneous from organ to organ and individual to individual.[15,16]

Reduced Ability to Respond Adaptively to Environmental Stimuli with Age

The diminished ability to maintain homeostasis is manifested not primarily by changes in resting or basal parameters but in the altered response to an external stimulus such as exercise or fasting.[17] The loss of "reserve" results in blunted maximum responses as well as delays in reaching peak levels and returning to basal levels. For example, the immune response appears to be impaired in older individuals, leading to reduced ability to fight infections, less protection from vaccinations, higher incidences of autoimmunity, and impaired antigen affinity and class-switching by lymphocytes.[18]

Increased Susceptibility and Vulnerability to Disease

The incidence and mortality rates for many diseases increase with age and parallel the exponential increase in mortality.[19] For the five leading causes of death for people over 65, the relative increase in death rates compared to people aged 25 to 44 is:

- Heart disease: 92-fold
- Cancer: 43-fold
- Stroke: > 100-fold
- Chronic lung disease: > 100-fold
- Pneumonia and influenza: 89-fold[20]

The basis for these dramatic rises in mortality is incompletely understood, but presumably involves changes in the function of many types of cells that lead to tissue/organ dysfunction and systemic illness. Interestingly, centenarians live 90% to 95% of their lives in very good health,[21] which despite a very high annual mortality at the end of their lives, represents a marked compression of morbidity towards the end of life and is close to the idealized survival curve in Figure 2-1.

An appreciation of these concepts is important, as the goal of geroscience, which explores relationships between aging and age-related diseases, is not just to increase life span but to find interventions that can potentially slow the body's age-related changes and enhance health span. Patients will often spend an enormous amount of time and money to find anything that can retard or reverse the aging process. Many will look to their doctor for advice, while others will be drawn to a variety of alternative medicine sources. In this chapter we will provide an overview of some of the current models of aging. We will then review the evidence-based literature for potential interventions that may positively impact the aging process.

CASE PRESENTATION 1: MODELS OF AGING

A 39-year-old man comes to your office as follow-up for a concussion that he received 1 week earlier. He is a famous heavyweight boxer who recently lost his heavyweight title fight in an 11th-round knockout. He has mild hypertension, but has refused to take medications, because the drugs "make him feel funny" and interfere with his training. He currently has no changes in vision or headaches and his neurologic exam is normal. Although he feels fine, he is fearful that he is now "over the hill."

● BRIEF OVERVIEW OF MODELS OF AGING

Case 1 highlights the fact that the molecular mechanisms responsible for aging begin to work decades before the person appears old and frail. From about the age of 30, the functional capacity of organs and tissues slowly begins to decline. Science is just beginning to unravel the mystery of the mechanisms that cause the cells, tissues, and organs to decline in function and that ultimately result in death. While research has yielded some exciting insights into the underlying mechanisms, it is important to note that no one theory can neatly explain the aging process.

Normal aging increases the susceptibility to diseases such as diabetes and pneumonia. To make matters more complicated, it appears that certain diseases, such as diabetes, may accelerate age-related changes to the body. Consequently, a deleterious positive feedback can ensue. However, public health initiatives and treatments for once commonly fatal diseases have led to a dramatic increase in the average life expectancy in developed nations during the 20th and 21st centuries. Modern medicine has also allowed millions of people to live functionally active lives to more advanced ages. Finding cures to common diseases would lead to further increases in the average life span, but would likely have a limited effect on lengthening the MLSP.[22]

● THE ROLE OF GENETICS

The MSLP appears to have a genetic component. Early studies have shown a linear relationship between the maximum number of fibroblast doublings and the maximum life span of a given species. In humans, there is a correlation between life expectancy among monozygotic twins. Epidemiologic studies have also shown that the children of centenarians are more likely to live to advanced ages.[23] Another study has also found that exceptional longevity and healthy aging represent an inherited phenotype across three generations.[24]

Despite these observations, the notion that human aging is a tightly controlled genetically programmed event is not supported by modern research studies. Similarly, no longevity genes that modulate normal aging have been identified in humans. However, a variety of polymorphisms in genes implicated in metabolic signaling, inflammation, and stress response pathways may play a role in both aging and longevity in humans.[25] There are a number of accelerated aging syndromes that result from single gene mutations, the most notable of which is Hutchinson-Gilford syndrome (progeria), which is caused by a mutation in the lamin A gene.

Part of the problem in the study of the genetics of aging is that there is no obvious selective pressure for all species to have common aging mechanisms. Evolution selects for those features that improve reproductive fitness at relatively early stages in life. Furthermore, for most of human history, the average life span has been less than 30 years. Consequently, evolutionary pressures would be unable to act upon elderly individuals. Indeed, features that improve reproductive fitness can exert positive, neutral, or even negative effects on longevity.[26] Some genetic traits may allow an organism to live longer as they represent the optimization of early fitness. Other traits may improve the organism's reproductive fitness, but may have a negative effect on longevity, which is known as antagonistic pleiotropy. Still other traits may have a role in improving reproductive fitness, but have no role in longevity. Furthermore, genetic mechanisms that have been recognized to play a role in improving longevity in fruit flies or mice may not necessarily play a similar role in humans. We will give a brief overview of several molecular models of aging.

● TELOMERE LENGTH

Much research has focused on the length of the telomeres. Telomeres are found at the end of chromosomes, and function to protect the genetic code from degradation and abnormal fusions with other chromosomes. Telomere shortening with progressive mitotic divisions may represent a counting mechanism for senescence.[27] Normal somatic cells have no telomerase activity. Therefore, with repeated cell divisions, telomeres progressively shorten until they reach a critical length, at which time the cell is no longer able to divide (senescence). The average telomere length of chromosomes decreases with both in vitro and in vivo aging of fibroblasts[28] and peripheral blood lymphocytes.[29] Indeed, telomere length in lymphocytes progressively declines as a function of donor age from newborn to great-grandparents in their 80s.[30] Over the age of 60, those with shorter telomeres exhibited poorer survival, in part due to increased mortality secondary to heart and infectious diseases.[31] Telomere length has been correlated with survival in elderly twins,[32] better health in centenarians,[33] and physical activity[34]; however, in one elderly cohort no correlation was found between telomere length and frailty.[35] A more recent study found no association between telomere length and survival or specific causes of death, but reported a correlation between telomere length and self-reported health and greater years of healthy life.[36] Telomeric shortening may be related to oxidative damage in cells, since improvement of mitochondrial function, the major determinant of cellular reactive oxygen species production, slows telomere shortening.[37] Telomeres may be the missing link between DNA damage and oxidative stress and therefore represent at least part of the mechanism behind the internal "clock" that governs cellular life span.

FREE RADICAL THEORY/OXIDATIVE STRESS

Aerobic metabolism generates several reactive oxygen species that are commonly referred to as "free radicals," although this is misleading since one of the major intermediates is hydrogen peroxide, which contains no unpaired electrons and is therefore not a radical. These reactive oxygen species (ROS) can react with macromolecules in a self-perpetuating manner; they create free radicals out of subsequently attacked molecules, which in turn create free radicals out of other molecules, thereby amplifying the effect of the initial free radical attack. ROS appear to play a role in regulating differential gene expression, cell replication, differentiation, and apoptotic cell death (in part by acting as second messengers in signal transduction pathways).[38] In many lower organisms such as worms and flies, there is a complex and inconsistent correlation between levels of reactive oxygen species and senescence. However, production of ROS in the heart, kidney, and liver of a group of mammals was found to be inversely proportional to the maximum life span.[39] However, overexpression of catalase, an antioxidant enzyme, targeted to the mitochondria does increase life span and improve functional health of mice as they age.[40] Transgenic mice that overexpress thioredoxin, another antioxidant protein, also exhibit about a 30% improvement in mean life span.[41] A series of studies has demonstrated that oxidative stress resistance of dermal fibroblasts correlates with the longevity of the species.[42-44] The mechanisms by which these oxygen intermediates lead to cellular senescence are still incompletely understood.[45] In addition, there are models where this correlation does not appear. Antioxidants, in general, only appear to have a significant effect on life span extension if their levels/function are limiting or under conditions of stress. Thus, overexpression of enzymes that are already present at robust levels are not likely to increase life span because increasing expression does not enhance catalytic efficiency of these enzymes, which are already operating at near optimal rates. Furthermore, given the importance of antioxidant enzymes to survival of aerobically respiring organisms, there is a certain amount of redundancy between different antioxidants, and different tissues require their individual actions to different extents.

MITOCHONDRIAL DYSFUNCTION THEORY

The accumulation of reactive oxygen species leads to the accumulation of somatic mitochondrial DNA mutations. As the damage to the DNA increases, the metabolic function of the mitochondria decreases. Mitochondrial DNA (mtDNA) undergoes a progressive age-related increase in oxygen free radical damage in skeletal muscle, the diaphragm, cardiac muscle, and the brain. This exponential increase in damage correlates with the increase in both point and deletional somatic mtDNA mutations seen with age. Interestingly, extrapolation of the curve to the point where 100% of cardiac mtDNA exhibits deletion mutations gives an age of 129.[46] Defects in mitochondrial respiration with age are found in normal tissues and also in a number of age-related diseases such as Parkinson's disease, Alzheimer's disease, Huntington's chorea, and other movement disorders.[25] Mutations in mtDNA that have been found include Alzheimer's, Parkinson's, and a large number of skeletal and cardiac myopathies. While age-related mitochondrial DNA damage is seen in a variety of human tissues, it is not clear that such damage directly contributes to normal human aging or susceptibility to diseases of aging.

Mitochondrial biogenesis and efficiency also appear to play an important role in cellular fitness and organismal longevity.[47] Maintenance of energy production and prevention and/or amelioration of oxidative stress by mitochondria are key to healthy aging. Caloric restriction is the most reliable intervention to extend life span in a number of species, including mammals such as rodents, dogs, and rhesus monkeys.[48] Multiple signals modulate PGC1-alpha activity and subsequent mitochondrial production and efficiency, such as AMP kinase, sirtuins, and nitric oxide, all of which can be increased by caloric restriction. Furthermore, caloric restriction increases mitochondrial biogenesis in healthy humans.[49] Perhaps the best intervention to enhance mitochondrial production and function is exercise, which can at least partly normalize age-related mitochondrial dysfunction[50] and can significantly reverse age-related transcriptional alterations.[51]

DNA DAMAGE THEORY

This theory holds that DNA accumulates damage from environmental agents and errors in replication. As the damage increases, the ability of the cell to carry out its cellular functions begins to decline, and impairment of genomic maintenance has been implicated in aging.[52] Defects in DNA repair mechanisms form the basis of a majority of human progeroid syndromes.[25] The ability to repair ultraviolet radiation-induced DNA damage in cell cultures derived from various species is directly correlated with the maximum life span potential,[53] and repair of double strand breaks is also diminished in fibroblasts and lymphocytes from older humans.[54] However, there is not enough experimental support to conclude that these differences between species are a causative factor in aging.

ACCELERATED AGING SYNDROMES IN HUMANS

No disease exists that is an exact phenocopy of normal aging. However, several human genetic diseases, including Hutchinson-Guilford syndrome (the "classic" early-onset progeria seen in children), Werner syndrome ("adult" progeria), Cockayne syndrome or NFE syndrome (another childhood-onset progeroid disease), and Down syndrome exhibit features of accelerated aging.[25] Consistent with the classic theories of aging, the human progeroid syndromes suggest that the critical determinants of aging are likely to be oxidative stress levels, accumulation of DNA damage/chromosomal instability, and nonfunctional or reduced DNA repair mechanisms.

HEALTH SPAN

Despite extensive research on longevity, we still know relatively little about the underlying molecular mechanisms. The goal of increasing maximum life span may never be within our reach. An acceptance of our limited knowledge regarding this extraordinarily complicated process makes us inherently cautious about endorsing any interventions that claim to retard the aging process or extend longevity. However, as noted earlier, centenarians spend a great majority of their life in good health. Recent investigations have explored the contributors to health span, the period of a person's life that is generally free from serious disease, chronic illness, or disability. Are there physiologic and genetic markers that are predictive of adding "life" to our years, rather than years to our life? Conversely, can frailty be avoided? A generally accepted definition of frailty includes three or more of the following criteria: unintentional weight loss (10 lbs [4.5 kg] in past year), self-reported exhaustion, weakness (grip strength), slow walking speed, and low physical activity.[55] Additional indicators of frailty have included poor balance and impaired cognition.[56] Frailty has been found to predict fractures, falls, physical disability, hospitalization, and death. Frailty is associated with inflammation,[57] lower levels of anabolic hormones,[58] and metabolic impairments.[59] In the Cardiovascular Health Study, inflammation was found to be associated with multiple causes of death, permitting the investigators to conclude that inflammatory processes may represent a common pathophysiological pathway to all causes of mortality in the elderly.[60] Recent studies have explored the predictive value of physiologic indices and allostatic load, which can be thought of as multiplex integrated indicators of physiological dysregulation in response to internal and external stresses over time.[61] Increased allostatic load is correlated with greatly frailty[62] and predicts future frailty over a 3-year period.[61] (For more on frailty, see Chapter 36.) Newman and associates found that a physiologic index consisting of carotid ultrasound, pulmonary function testing, brain magnetic resonance scan, serum cystatin-C, and fasting glucose was correlated with limitation in mobility, difficulty in performing activities of daily living, and mortality.[63] Additional research will likely permit practitioners to utilize a variety of physiologic and biochemical indices to predict risk and tailor interventions to maintain and prolong health span.

CASE PRESENTATION 2: HORMONE REPLACEMENT THERAPY

A 62-year-old father of one of your colleagues comes to see you in clinic as a new patient. He has not seen a doctor in almost 5 years. He has no medical complaints and is a successful businessman who has been in relatively good health his entire life. Past medical history reveals no chronic illnesses and his past surgical history is significant only for an appendectomy in his 30s. He takes no prescription medications.

His social history reveals that he recently got married for the second time to a woman in her mid-30s. He also tells you that he quit smoking 3 months ago. Prior to that time, he used to smoke half a pack of cigarettes per day. He consumes 1 or 2 drinks of whisky every evening. He exercises by playing golf two times a week. He does not follow any particular diet. A review of systems is unremarkable.

On physical exam he is 5'11" (180 cm) and weighs 210 lbs (95.5 kg). His blood pressure is 118/74 with a pulse of 78. Physical examination of his head, neck, lungs, heart, abdomen, extremities, and skin was unremarkable.

You discuss the current guidelines for preventive health and order a screening colonoscopy and lipid profile. He mentions a few of his friends have started taking some anti-aging hormones. He asks you for your opinion. What can you recommend for this man?

Physicians must be aware that interventions that address frailty may be different from those that address longevity. It is important to educate this patient that there is no "anti-aging" hormone. When most people hear the term "anti-aging" they envision a possible fountain of youth that will rejuvenate them. In reality, most products do not address longevity, but instead make one or more of the following claims, which typically fall within the realm of health span:

- Increased energy and strength
- Reduced body fat
- Increased lean muscle mass
- Enhanced virility
- Enhanced immune response
- Increased hair growth
- Reversal of heart disease
- Elimination of arthritis pain

To date there are no randomized controlled trials that demonstrate a pharmacologic or supplement intervention to increase longevity.

GROWTH HORMONE

Many men are enticed to take growth hormone based on testimonials and pictures from magazines and the Internet. With aging, there is a gradual decrease in both growth hormone and the levels of IGF-1, which is the main mediator of growth hormone action.[64] Declining levels of growth hormone along with estrogen deficiency in women and testosterone deficiency in men may be associated with muscle weakness, decreased virility, decreased concentration, and increased fatigue.[65]

Use of Recombinant Human Growth Hormone in the Elderly

As an anti-aging treatment, the goal is in theory to restore IGF-1 levels to those of a normal young adult. Athletes and body builders who abuse growth hormone already have normal growth hormone levels and are trying to achieve supraphysiological levels. Initial studies in healthy aged men showed administration of growth hormone could increase lean body mass and decrease body fat.[66] These men also reported having more energy and more interest in sex. However, there was no increase in physical performance independent of exercise. A more recent study showed a similar effect in healthy elderly men and woman given an oral ghrelin mimetic (a compound that stimulates the release of growth hormone).[67]

Despite these results, no functional benefits or life extension have ever been shown with recombinant growth hormone, recombinant IGF-1, growth hormone-releasing molecules, or orally active synthetic growth hormone-secretagogues.[68] Furthermore, there is no evidence of significant improvements in frailty with the restoration of growth hormone and IGF-I levels to within the young adult range.[65,69]

The adverse effects of growth hormone supplementation include carpal tunnel syndrome, edema, arthralgias, gynecomastia, and glucose intolerance. In addition there may be an increased cancer risk with the use of growth hormone. A recent meta-analysis found that the greater the IGF-1 concentration, the greater the risk of prostate cancer with an odds ratio of 1.38 (95% CI, 1.19 to 1.60; $p < 0.001$).[70]

In summary, growth hormone repletion may make older adults look better but will not improve functional performance. It is also associated with a variety of potentially serious side effects. The other question is whether hormone replacement will improve life expectancy. There is much basic science research suggesting that the opposite is true: higher levels of growth hormone may be associated with an increase in mortality. Indeed, mouse models of aging suggest that diminished IGF-1 expression and function are correlated with increased life span.

There is even some epidemiological evidence that supports an inverse relationship between growth hormone levels and life expectancy. A study of 864 middle-aged policemen in Paris found that men with higher growth hormone levels had increased mortality.[71] Other studies have found that polymorphisms in the IGF-1 receptor that reduced activity were more commonly seen in subjects living to an extreme old age[72] and that polymorphisms in the signaling pathways downstream of insulin/IGF-1 were also reported to be associated with human longevity.[73]

● TESTOSTERONE

Low testosterone levels in men (as measured by a morning free testosterone level) may be associated with a decrease in muscle strength and libido and an increase in body fat.[74,75] Symptomatic androgen deficiency has been noted to be prevalent among older men in multiple longitudinal studies.[76] While testosterone replacement therapy may increase lean muscle mass and decrease bone resorption in older men, its effect on functional status, insulin resistance, and cognition remain unproven.[75,77] Testosterone replacement therapy may in theory increase the risk of prostate cancer and/or benign prostatic hyperplasia; however, with careful follow-up, this risk does not appear to be significant.[76]

● DEHYDROEPIANDROSTERONE

Dehydroepiandrosterone (DHEA) is a steroid hormone produced by the adrenal gland. Its exact physiologic role remains unclear. DHEA is secreted in short bursts, which are normally larger and occur with increasing frequency at night. At the present time, the clinical benefits of DHEA supplementation in older adults remain unknown.

DHEA is sold as a food supplement at health food stores. No one knows if DHEA supplements are safe for older adults. There is some concern that DHEA can get converted to testosterone in men or estrogen in women. In addition, there is no clear consensus regarding the correct dose to take, or the length of time that this hormone can be used safely.

CASE PRESENTATION 3: VITAMINS AND OTHER NUTRITIONAL PRODUCTS

An 82-year-old man comes to your office as a new patient. His past medical history is significant for mild hypertension. An ophthalmologist recently told him that he has early macular degeneration. When you ask about medications that he is taking, he pulls out a sheet of paper with a long list. The list consists of:

- Metoprolol: 25 mg twice daily
- Aspirin: 325 mg daily
- Multivitamin: 1 tablet twice daily
- Vitamin C: 500 mg 2 tablets twice daily
- Vitamin E: 1000 mg twice daily
- Vitamin D: 2000 IU daily
- Beta-carotene: 25,000 IU daily
- Selenium: 200 µg daily
- Co-enzyme Q10: 300 mg daily
- Glucosamine: 4 tablets daily
- Fish oil: 1 tablet daily
- Folate: 1 mg daily

As you are writing this list down, he remarks, "Most doctors don't know anything about vitamins." What advice can you give him regarding the potential benefits and harms of the nutritional supplements that he is taking?

POTENTIAL BENEFITS OF VITAMINS

In an attempt to slow the effects of aging and to prevent age-related co-morbidities, many seniors use one or more nutritional supplements. A recent nationwide study found that almost 50% of seniors use vitamin or mineral supplements.[78] Baby boomers and seniors are barraged with numerous radio, television, Internet, and print media advertisements touting the anti-aging benefits of vitamin and mineral supplements. As geriatricians, what can we tell our patients about the effectiveness and safety of these nutritional supplements?

Research involving the use of vitamins in older adults is often difficult to conduct and interpret for a variety of reasons. Vitamin users often have healthier diets, higher incomes, and better access to health care than non-vitamin users. Another issue is that Western diets are already fortified with many vitamins and minerals. Many of the interventional studies involving the use of vitamin supplements excluded frail elderly patients.

Clinical studies involving nutritional supplements use pharmaceutical-grade preparations, but what patients buy over the counter is generally not pharmaceutical grade. Because these supplements are regulated as food products, not as drugs, the Food and Drug Administration (FDA) does not monitor or regulate the purity or dosing of nutritional supplements.

ANTIOXIDANT VITAMINS

Antioxidant vitamins are cofactors that allow specific enzymes to more effectively metabolize the free radical by-products of oxidative metabolism. By equating oxidative metabolism with the cause of aging, antioxidant vitamins are widely promoted in the lay media as an anti-aging therapy.

In a large, multi-centered, randomized placebo-controlled trial, patients with dry age-related macular degeneration (ARMD) were randomized to an antioxidant vitamin supplement versus a placebo.[79] Patients receiving the supplement had a 25% lower risk of progression to wet ARMD. While this formulation may slow down the progression of macular degeneration, concern has arisen following the results of randomized control trials with the antioxidant β-carotene. Several studies have shown an increased incidence of cancer and some have shown an increase in mortality.[80] No studies have shown a benefit of β-carotene on mortality.

Initial studies with vitamin E suggested that this antioxidant vitamin may play a role in the tertiary prevention of coronary artery disease and dementia. Subsequent studies failed to confirm these benefits.[80,81]

Several randomized controlled trials have demonstrated that the use of antioxidant vitamins by cancer patients may reduce the side effects of chemotherapy and/or radiation therapy. This information, however, must be weighed against the concern that these the vitamins may serve to protect tumor cells as well as healthy cells from oxidative damage generated by radiation therapy and some chemotherapeutic agents.[82] Therefore, many oncologists and radiation oncologists currently recommend against the use of supplemental antioxidants during chemotherapy and radiation therapy out of a concern that the vitamins may lead to tumor protection and reduced survival.

SO WHAT ABOUT A MULTIVITAMIN?

While we often recommend that our older patients take a multivitamin, what does the evidence show? There is no benefit with regards to mortality, cancer, or heart disease. Nursing home residents who took a multivitamin had a better antibody response to the flu shot. However, the residents who took the vitamin did not have a lower risk of infections or an improvement in mortality.[83]

FOLATE

In recent years, elevated levels of homocysteine have been shown to be a risk factor for atherosclerotic disease. Elevated homocysteine may also have a role in the development of vascular dementia. Folic acid supplementation decreases homocysteine levels, but randomized controlled studies have failed to show an improvement in cognition or in the incidence of strokes.[80,84]

GLUCOSAMINE

Many people are currently using glucosamine as a treatment for painful joints. While initial studies demonstrated a decrease in joint space narrowing, more recent studies have failed to show any clinically significant benefits.[85-87] Glucosamine is commercially available often in combination with oral chondroitin sulfate. Chondroitin sulfate either alone or in combination with glucosamine has not been shown to be beneficial in the treatment of osteoarthritis.[87] Fortunately, both glucosamine and chondroitin sulfate appear to have a low risk of serious side effects.

VITAMIN D

A meta-analysis of 18 independent, randomized controlled trials involving over 57,000 patients found that the relative risk for mortality among vitamin D users was 0.93 (0.87-0.99).[88] Other randomized controlled trials suggest that the use of vitamin D may be associated with a lower risk of cancer.[89]

Multiple studies have shown that vitamin D supplements may also have a role in the prevention of falls.[90,91] Two important points need to be made about these data. One is that these studies used doses of vitamin D that ranged from 800 to 2000 IU per day. The second point is that the potential benefit of vitamin D is not related just to its effect on maintaining bone strength. Rather, it is believed that vitamin D may have a role in retarding the natural muscle wasting that occurs with aging (sarcopenia). Vitamin D insufficiency is widespread, regardless of geographical location. It is particularly prevalent in the elderly and has far-ranging health consequences including osteoporosis, falls, increased risk of cancer, and altered glucose and lipid metabolism.[92] Increasing evidence strongly supports the benefits of vitamin D supplementation and also reveals that present recommendations are inadequate, especially for older individuals. Although additional studies are still needed to further optimize diagnostic and therapeutic approaches, physicians should consider prescribing cholecalciferol—as much as 2000 IU per day—to all elderly patients. Oral cholecalciferol supplementation at that level is inexpensive, safe, and effective, and has great potential to improve the quality of life of the elderly.

● OMEGA-3 FATTY ACIDS

The omega-3 fatty acid pathway involves the conversion of alpha-linolenic acid (ALA) into eicosapentaenoic acid (EPA) and docosahexaenoic acid (DHA) through a pathway that involves three different steps. EPA and DHA are then converted into anti-inflammatory prostaglandins and anti-inflammatory leukotrienes.[93]

Sources high in ALA include flax seeds and walnuts. EPA and DHA are the omega-3 fatty acids found in fish oils. This distinction is important because the three-step conversion of ALA into EPA and DHA appears to be impaired in men, but not women.[94]

The American Heart Association has endorsed use of omega-3 fatty acids for the secondary cardiovascular events in patients with coronary artery disease. This is the first time that this organization has endorsed the use of a nutritional supplement.[95] The American Heart Association recommends 1 g/d of EPA and DHA for coronary artery disease patients. A word of caution: over-the-counter fish oil products may contain 1 g of fish oil. However, the amount of EPA and DHA may be far less.

In theory, fish oil may affect platelet aggregation. This effect should be considered in patients who are already on blood thinners (warfarin, clopidogrel, aspirin, enoxaparin) and in the preoperative assessment of older adults.[95]

● CO-ENZYME Q10

Co-enzyme Q10 (ubiquinone) is an essential cofactor that functions as an electron carrier of the mitochondrial respiratory chain. Clinical studies involving co-enzyme Q10 suggest that it may improve the ejection fraction among patients with congestive heart failure.[96] Co-enzyme Q10 is currently being studied for its potential role in the treatment of a variety of neurodegenerative disorders. In recent years, the use of this nutritional supplement has increased dramatically when it was shown that patients who take HMG-CoA reductase inhibitors (statins) have much lower levels of co-enzyme Q10.[97] However, supplementation with co-enzyme Q10 does not appear to lower the prevalence or severity of statin-induced myalgia.[98]

● GREEN TEA

In vitro studies have shown that green tea contains compounds that have strong antioxidant effects.[99] Animal studies suggest that a protective effect against the development of cancer, coronary artery disease, and diabetes. Human studies

have shown an association between the drinking of green tea and a wide variety of health benefits, including a lower mortality rate.[99] Clinical interventional studies are currently under way.

> ## CASE PRESENTATION 4: EXERCISE AND DIETARY INTERVENTIONS
>
> A 76-year-old woman comes to see you 8 weeks after she was hospitalized with chest pain. She was ruled out for a myocardial infarction and had a negative stress thallium examination. She has a history of hypertension and osteoarthritis. She used to play tennis up until 4 years ago, but stopped due to lower back pain. She was walking in the mall 3 times a week until 6 months ago, when her exercise partner had a stroke. In the past 6 months she has not exercised and has not been watching what she eats. She has gained 11 lbs. She comes to you for exercise and dietary advice. What are you going to tell her?

● THE EXERCISE PRESCRIPTION

Exercise has been shown to be associated with a variety of beneficial effects including:

- Lower risk for falls
- Improved glucose homeostasis
- Improved cardiovascular function
- Improved flexibility
- Better quality sleep
- Fewer symptoms of depression
- Less arthritis pain of hips and knees

Developing an effective individualized exercise program can be very challenging. The proper exercise prescription must address strength, endurance, and flexibility.[100] Lifting weights alone is often not helpful. An analysis of 121 controlled trials showed in 73 trials that resistance exercise in older adults was associated with an improvement in muscle strength and a small reduction in functional disability.[101] It is important to note that resistance training may also increase the risk of musculoskeletal injuries in older adults.

Aerobic and endurance exercise may improve cardiovascular function, but patients and physicians need to be careful. An older adult who has not exercised for years should be assessed for coronary artery disease before beginning an exercise routine. Fortunately, the woman in the case above had a recent negative stress thallium examination. Musculoskeletal injuries involving the feet, knees, hips, or lower back may limit a patient's participation in an endurance exercise program. Further caution is required for patients taking medications that may impair cardiovascular response. Those who cannot exercise for a full 30 minutes will benefit just as well from 2 daily 15-minute blocks.

Potential exercises to recommend to older patients include walking, pool exercises, Tai Chi, and an elder-specific yoga program. The specific recommendations made will depend on the patient's medical conditions, motivation, financial resources, and local access to exercise programs.

DIET

The Healthy Ageing Longitudinal study in Europe (HALE) found that a Mediterranean diet, moderate alcohol use, physical activity, and nonsmoking were associated with a greater than 50 percent decrease in the rate of mortality in healthy 70- to 90-year-olds.[102] The Physicians' Health Study showed that regular exercise, smoking abstinence, weight management, and blood pressure control increased longevity and improved functional status among elderly men.[103] It is also important to note that a diet high in fruits and vegetables is associated with lower risk for CV disease but not for cancer.[104]

Several studies have compared a Mediterranean diet to a cardiac-prudent diet. In these studies, the Mediterranean diet was associated with lower plasma glucose levels and a lower risk of metabolic syndrome.[105-108] Patients with metabolic syndrome who consumed a Mediterranean diet also had lower levels of CRP, IL-6, IL-7, and IL-18.[106]

CALORIE RESTRICTION

The concept of calorie restriction (CR) as an anti-aging intervention traces its roots to a Venetian nobleman named Luigi Cornaro who was born in 1464. Faced with poor health, he began a lifestyle of temperance at age 40. One important component of his new lifestyle was limiting his diet to 12 ounces of food and 14 ounces of wine per day. He noticed a dramatic improvement in his health and at age 83 began writing the details about his diet and lifestyle in a book entitled *La Vita Sobria*. Luigi Cornaro lived to be 102 years old.

It was not until the 1950s that researchers actually began to scientifically study the potential benefits of calorie restriction. These early studies found that calorie-restricted mice and fruit flies had a significantly longer mean and maximum life span. The improvement in longevity is even seen when the calories are restricted later in the life of the organism.

A 30% calorie restriction in rhesus monkeys has no effect on the long-term metabolic rate, but leads to increases in time to sexual maturity, proliferative capacity of fibroblasts, and HDL.[109] Concomitantly, decreases are observed in oxidative damage to muscles, glycation end products, serum IL-6, body temperature, LDL, fasting glucose and insulin, and fat and lean body mass. Longer-term follow-up has demonstrated that calorie restriction has reduced the incidence of death and age-related diseases such as diabetes, cancer, cardiovascular disease, and brain atrophy.[110] There are several important caveats to calorie-restricted diets. It appears that that there is a diminishing benefit if CR is started later in life. However, significant CR started early leads to a much smaller adult size. It is important to note that in studies involving calorie-restricted diets, intakes of vitamins and minerals are optimized and not restricted.

A notable connection between single-gene effects upon aging in yeast and higher eukaryotes was revealed by the finding that overexpression of the SIR2 gene and its homolog SIRT1 (sirtuin 1) extend life span in yeast and nematodes, respectively.[111] Aging and DNA damage induce SIR protein complexes to localize to sites of genomic instability, resulting in de-silencing of genes. Sirtuin genes can function as anti-aging genes in yeast, worms, and flies.[112] There are seven mammalian sirtuin genes whose protein products function as histone deacetylases (SIRT1, 2, 3, 5, 6, 7) and/or ADP-ribosyltransferases (SIRT4, 6). The actions of sirtuins link metabolism and mitochondrial biogenesis and efficiency to aging.[111,113] SIRT1 modulates the activity of multiple critical transcriptional regulators of metabolism, including FOXO1, FOXO3a, PPARα, PPARγ, and PGC-1α, which in turn impacts fatty acid oxidation, gluconeogenesis and glycolysis, oxidative capacity, fat mobilization and adipogenesis, and insulin secretion. Calorie restriction increases SIRT1 expression in muscle.[49] Transgenic mice that overexpress SIRT1 exhibit a phenotype that resembles calorie restriction; they are leaner, more metabolically active, have improved glucose homeostasis, and perform better upon physical challenge.[114] Furthermore, SIRT1 transgenic mice exhibit lower activation of proinflammatory cytokines when exposed to a high-fat diet.[115] Polymorphisms in the human SIRT1 gene correlate with energy expenditure[116] and with BMI and the risk of obesity,[117] but do not appear to associate with longevity.[118,119] However, a SIRT3 polymorphism was found to be correlated with survival in the very old.[120]

Calorie Restriction in Humans

Studying calorie restriction in humans is difficult because of our long life span. Several short-term studies have shown that calorie restriction in humans is associated with lower insulin levels, body temperature, and blood pressure.[121,122]

What is the mechanism for caloric restriction? Ostensibly, it could be hypothesized that fewer calories results in less oxidative metabolism, which would lead to the formation of fewer free radicals. However, this model is apparently too simplistic. Additional factors likely involve up-regulation of mitochondrial function and activity, possibly mediated through sirtuin gene function (SIRT 1, 3, 4, and 5).[49,123]

SIRTUINS AND RESVERATROL

While calorie restriction is a powerful intervention for increasing longevity in lower organisms and may enhance health span in humans, in a nation plagued by obesity, compliance with highly restrictive diets is not feasible. Therefore, active investigation is under way to develop agents that can mimic the beneficial effects of a calorie-restricted diet. One promising candidate is resveratrol, a compound found in the skin of red grapes and consequently in wine. Resveratrol is notable for its ability to activate sirtuins and to increase maximum life span in lower organisms, such as yeast, worms, and flies.[124] Resveratrol treatment improves the exercise capacity, insulin sensitivity, mitochondrial biogenesis, and survival of mice on a high-fat, high-calorie diet.[125] Resveratrol can prevent diet-induced obesity concurrently with improved mitochondrial production, insulin sensitivity, and exercise endurance by activating SIRT1 and PGC-1α.[116] Resveratrol treatment of mice can also delay age-related changes in physical performance, bone mineral density, inflammation, and vasculature,[126] and concomitantly induces transcriptional profiles in a variety of tissues similar to those seen with dietary restriction.[126,127] Consequently, there has been much interest in resveratrol as a supplement to enhance health and increase life span in humans. However, resveratrol does not appear to extend the maximum life span of mice, but can increase the mean life span of mice with cardiovascular- and obesity-related pathology that would otherwise die earlier. In other words, resveratrol may very well act to enhance life span, particularly in those with underlying pathologies such as diabetes and cardiovascular disease.

Before you start recommending red wine to all of your patients, be aware that the amount of resveratrol in red wine varies widely, and the half-life in humans is on the order of minutes. In addition, to consume the amount of resveratrol that is effective in animal studies may require the consumption of scores or even hundreds of bottles of red wine! There is also much hyperbole on the Internet concerning resveratrol. Furthermore, since it is sold as a nutraceutical, it is not regulated by the FDA. A number of trials with resveratrol are underway, and at least one pharmaceutical company has begun trials on a proprietary formulation.

CONCLUSION

Despite the claims made in the media, there are currently no simple anti-aging therapies for geriatricians to recommend to their patients. As our understanding of the biology of aging and its impact upon the susceptibility to and manifestation of disease continues to deepen and expand, we can look forward to the development of interventions that can prevent and reduce frailty and age-related diseases and syndromes, thereby enhancing the health span and quality of life of the elderly.

References

1. Cutler RG. Evolutonary perspective of human longevity. In: Hazzard WR, Andres R, Bierman EL, et al., eds. *Principles of Geriatric Medicine and Gerontology.* 2nd ed. New York: McGraw-Hill; 1985:16.

2. Gompertz B. On the nature of the function expressive of the law of human mortality and on a new mode of determining life contingencies. *Philos Trans R Soc Lond.* 1825;115:513.

3. Kung HC, Hoyert DL, Xu JQ, Murphy SL. *Deaths: Final Data for 2005.* Hyattsville, MD: National Center for Health Statistics; 2008.

4. Shock NW, Greulich RC, Andres R, et al., eds. *Normal Human Aging: The Baltimore Longitudinal Study of Aging.* Washington, DC: US Department of Health and Human Services; 1984.

5. Riggs BL, Melton LJ. Involutional osteoporosis. *N Engl J Med.* 1986;314:1676-1686.

6. Florini JR. Composition and function of cells and tissues. *Handbook of Biolochemistry in Aging.* Boca Raton: CRC Press; 1981.

7. Strehler BL. *Time, Cells, and Aging.* 2nd ed. New York: Academic Press; 1977.

8. Dialauta J. Cross linkage and the aging process. In: Rothstein M, ed. *Theoretical Aspects of Aging.* New York: Academic Press; 1974:43.

9. Kohn RR. Aging of animals: Possible mechanisms. *Principles of Mammalian Aging.* 2nd ed. Englewood Cliffs, NJ: Prentice-Hall; 1978.

10. Herbig U, Ferreira M, Condel L, et al. Cellular senescence in aging primates. *Science.* 2006;311:1257.

11. Jeyapalan JC, Ferreira M, Sedivy JM, Herbig U. Accumulation of senescent cells in mitotic tissue of aging primates. *Mech Ageing Dev.* 2007;128:36-44.

12. Finch CE. Introduction: Definitions and concepts. *Longevity, Senescence, and the Genome.* Chicago: University of Chicago Press; 1990.

13. Schneider EL, Rowe JW, eds. *Handbook of the Biology of Aging.* 4th ed. San Diego: Academic Press; 1996.

14. Shock NW. Longitudinal studies of aging in humans. In: Finch CE, Schneider EL, eds. *Handbook of the Biology of Aging.* 2nd ed. New York: Van Nostrand Reinhold; 1985:721.

15. Lakatta EG. Changes in cardiovascular function with aging. *Eur Heart J.* 1990;11(suppl C):22-29.

16. Lindeman RD, Tobin J, Shock NW. Longitudinal studies on the rate of decline in renal function with age. *J Am Geriatr Soc.* 1985;33:278-285.

17. Adelman RC, Britton GW, Rotenberg S, et al. Endocrine regulation of gene activity in aging animals of different genotypes. In: Bergsma D, Harrison DE, eds. *Genetic Effects on Aging.* New York: Alan R. Liss; 1978:355.

18. Dorshkind K, Montecino-Rodriguez E, Signer RAJ. The ageing immune system: Is it ever too old to become young again? *Nat Rev Immunol.* 2009;9:57-62.

19. Brody JA, Brock DB. Epidemiological and statistical characteristics of the United States elderly population. In: Finch CE, Schneider EL, eds. *Handbook of the Biology of Aging.* 2nd ed. New York: Van Nostrand Reinhold; 1985:3.

20. Rosenberg HM, Ventura SJ, Maurer JD, et al. Births and deaths: United States, 1995. *Mon Vital Stat Rep.* 1996;45:31-33.

21. Hitt R, Young-Xu Y, Silver M, Perls T. Centenarians: The older you get, the healthier you have been. *Lancet.* 1999;354:652.

22. Olshansky SJ, Carnes BA, Cassel C. In search of Methuselah: Estimating the upper limits to human longevity. *Science.* 1990;250:634-640.

23. Adams ER, Nolan VG, Andersen SL, Perls TT. Centenarian offspring: Start healthier and stay healthier. *J Am Geriatr Soc.* 2008;56:2089-2092.

24. Atzmon G, Rincon M, Rabizadeh P, Barzilai N. Biological evidence for inheritance of exceptional longevity. *Mech Ageing Dev.* 2005;126:341-345.

25. Rai P, Troen BR. Cell and molecular aging. In: Rosenthal RA, Zenilman ME, Katlic MR, eds. *Principles and Practice of Geriatric Surgery.* 2nd ed. New York: Springer-Verlag, in press.

26. Kirkwood TB. Human senescence. *Bioessays.* 1996;18;1009-1016.

27. Harley CB. Telomere loss: Mitotic clock or genetic time bomb? *Mutat Res.* 1991;256:271-282.

28. Lindsey J, McGill NI, Lindsey LA, et al. In vivo loss of telomeric repeats with age in humans. *Mutat Res.* 1991;256:45-48.

29. Vaziri H, Schachter F, Uchida I, et al. Loss of telomeric DNA during aging of normal and trisomy 21 human lymphocytes. *Am J Hum Genet.* 1993;52:661-667.

30. Frenck RW Jr., Blackburn EH, Shannon KM. The rate of telomere sequence loss in human leukocytes varies with age. *Proc Natl Acad Sci USA.* 1998;95:5607-5610.

31. Cawthon RM, Smith KR, O'Brien E, et al. Association between telomere length in blood and mortality in people aged 60 years or older. *Lancet.* 2003;361:393-395.

32. Kimura M, Hjelmborg JV, Gardner JP, et al. Telomere length and mortality: A study of leukocytes in elderly Danish twins. *Am J Epidemiol.* 2008;167:799-806.

33. Terry DF, Nolan VG, Andersen SL, et al. Association of longer telomeres with better health in centenarians. *J Gerontol A Biol Sci Med Sci.* 2008;63:809-812.

34. Ludlow AT, Zimmerman JB, Witkowski S, et al. Relationship between physical activity level, telomere length, and telomerase activity. *Med Sci Sports Exerc.* 2008;40:1764-1761.

35. Woo J, Tang NL, Suen E, et al. Telomeres and frailty. *Mech Ageing Dev.* 2008;129:642-648.

36. Njajou OT, Hsueh WC, Blackburn EH, et al. Association between telomere length, specific causes of death, and years of healthy life in health, aging, and body composition, a population-based cohort study. *J Gerontol A Biol Sci Med Sci.* 2009;64:860-864.

37. Passos JF, Saretzki G, von Zglinicki T. DNA damage in telomeres and mitochondria during cellular senescence: Is there a connection? *Nucleic Acids Res.* 2007;35:7505-7513.

38. Finkel T. Oxidant signals and oxidative stress. *Curr Opin Cell Biol.* 2003;15:247-254.

39. Sohal RS, Svensson I, Sohal BH, Brunk UT. Superoxide anion radical production in different animal species. *Mech Ageing Dev.* 1989; 49:129-135.

40. Schriner SE, Linford NJ, Martin GM, et al. Extension of murine life span by overexpression of catalase targeted to mitochondria. *Science.* 2005;308:1909-1911.

41. Mitsui A, Hamuro J, Nakamura H, et al. Overexpression of human thioredoxin in transgenic mice controls oxidative stress and life span. *Antioxid Redox Signal.* 2002;4:693-696.

42. Salmon AB, Murakami S, Bartke A, et al. Fibroblast cell lines from young adult mice of long-lived mutant strains are resistant to multiple forms of stress. *Am J Physiol Endocrinol Metab.* 2005;289: E23-E29.

43. Maynard SP, Miller RA. Fibroblasts from long-lived Snell dwarf mice are resistant to oxygen-induced in vitro growth arrest. *Aging Cell.* 2006;5:89-96.

44. Harper JM, Salmon AB, Leiser SF, et al. Skin-derived fibroblasts from long-lived species are resistant to some, but not all, lethal stresses and to the mitochondrial inhibitor rotenone. *Aging Cell.* 2007;6:1-13.

45. Lu T, Finkel T. Free radicals and senescence. *Exp Cell Res.* 2008;10:1918-1922.

46. Ozawa T. Genetic and functional changes in mitochondria associated with aging. *Physiol Rev.* 1997;77:425-464.

47. Lopez-Lluch G, Irusta PM, Navas P, de Cabo R. Mitochondrial biogenesis and healthy aging. *Exp Gerontol.* 2008;43:813-819.

48. Mair W, Dillin A. Aging and survival: The genetics of life span extension by dietary restriction. *Annu Rev Biochem.* 2008;77:727-754.

49. Civitarese AE, Carlin S, Heilbronn LK, et al. Calorie restriction increases muscle mitochondrial biogenesis in healthy humans. *PLoS Med.* 2007;4:e76.

50. Lanza IR, Short DK, Short KR, et al. Endurance exercise as a countermeasure for aging. *Diabetes.* 2008;57:2933-2942.

51. Melov S, Tarnopolsky MA, Beckman K, et al. Resistance exercise reverses aging in human skeletal muscle. *PLoS One.* 2007;2:e465.

52. Garinis GA, van der Horst GT, Vijg J, Hoeijmakers JH. DNA damage and ageing: New-age ideas for an age-old problem. *Nat Cell Biol.* 2008;10:1241-1247.

53. Hart RW, Setlow RB. Correlation between deoxyribonucleic acid excision-repair and life-span in a number of mammalian species. *Proc Natl Acad Sci USA.* 1974;71:2169-2173.

54. Sedelnikova OA, Horikawa I, Redon C, et al. Delayed kinetics of DNA double-strand break processing in normal and pathological aging. *Aging Cell.* 2008;7:89-100.

55. Fried LP, Tangen CM, Walston J, et al. Frailty in older adults: Evidence for a phenotype. *J Gerontol A Biol Sci Med Sci.* 2001;56:M146-M156.

56. Rockwood K, Mitnitski A. Frailty in relation to the accumulation of deficits. *J Gerontol A Biol Sci Med Sci.* 2007;62:722-727.

57. Leng SX, Xue QL, Tian J, et al. Inflammation and frailty in older women. *J Am Geriatr Soc.* 2007;55:864-871.

58. Leng SX, Cappola AR, Andersen RE, et al. Serum levels of insulin-like growth factor-I (IGF-I) and dehydroepiandrosterone sulfate (DHEA-S), and their relationships with serum interleukin-6, in the geriatric syndrome of frailty. *Aging Clin Exp Res.* 2004;16:153-157.

59. Walston J, McBurnie MA, Newman A, et al. Frailty and activation of the inflammation and coagulation systems with and without clinical comorbidities: Results from the Cardiovascular Health Study. *Arch Intern Med.* 2002;162:2333-2341.

60. Newman AB, Sachs MC, Arnold AM, et al. Total and cause-specific mortality in the cardiovascular health study. *J Gerontol A Biol Sci Med Sci.* 2009;64:1251-1261.

61. Gruenewald TL, Seeman TE, Karlamangla AS, Sarkisian CA. Allostatic load and frailty in older adults. *J Am Geriatr Soc.* 2009;57:1525-1531.

62. Szanton SL, Allen JK, Seplaki CL, et al. Allostatic load and frailty in the women's health and aging studies. *Biol Res Nurs.* 2009;10:248-256.

63. Newman AB, Boudreau RM, Naydeck BL, et al. A physiologic index of comorbidity: Relationship to mortality and disability. *J Gerontol A Biol Sci Med Sci.* 2008;63:603-609.

64. Corpas E, Harman SM, Blackman MR. Human growth hormone and human aging. *Endocr Rev.* 1993;14:20-39.

65. Blackman MR. Use of growth hormone secretagogues to prevent or treat the effects of aging: Not yet ready for prime time. *Ann Intern Med.* 2008;149:677-679.

66. Rudman D, Feller AG, Cohn L, et al. Effects of human growth hormone in men over 60 years old. *N Engl J Med.* 1990;323:1-6.

67. Nass R, Pezzoli SS, Oliveri MC, et al. Effects of an oral ghrelin mimetic on body composition and clinical outcomes in healthy older adults: A randomized trial. *Ann Intern Med.* 2008;149:601-611.

68. Lanfranco F, Gianotti L, Giordano R, et al. Ageing, growth hormone and physical performance. *J Endocrinol Invest.* 2003;26:861-872.

69. Harman SM, Blackman MR. Use of growth hormone for prevention or treatment of effects of aging. *J Gerontol A Biol Sci Med Sci.* 2004;59:652-658.

70. Roddam AW, Allen NE, Appleby P, et al. Insulin-like growth factors, their binding proteins, and prostate cancer risk: Analysis of individual patient data from 12 prospective studies. *Ann Intern Med.* 2008;149:461-471.

71. Maison P, Balkau B, Simon D, et al. Growth hormone as a risk for premature mortality in healthy subjects: Data from the Paris prospective study. *BMJ.* 1998;316:1132-1133.

72. Suh Y, Atzmon G, Cho MO, et al. Functionally significant insulin-like growth factor 1 receptor mutations in centenarians. *Proc Natl Acad Sci USA*. 2008;105:3438-3442.

73. Pawlikowska L, Huntsman S, Sung A, et al. Association of common genetic variation in the insulin/IGF1 signaling pathway with human longevity. *Aging Cell*. 2009;8:460-472.

74. Kazi M, Geraci SA, Koch CA. Considerations for the diagnosis and treatment of testosterone deficiency in elderly men. *Am J Med*. 2007;120:835-840.

75. Miner MM, Seftel AD. Testosterone and ageing: What have we learned since the Institute of Medicine report and what lies ahead? *Int J Clin Pract*. 2007;61:622-632.

76. Lakshman KM, Basaria S. Safety and efficacy of testosterone gel in the treatment of male hypogonadism. *Clin Interv Aging*. 2009;4:397-412.

77. Kane RL, Ouslander JG, Abrass IB, Resnick B. Decreased vitality. In: *Essentials of Clinical Geriatrics*. 6th ed. New York: McGraw-Hill; 2009:363-399.

78. Qato DM, Alexander GC, Conti RM, et al. Use of prescription and over-the-counter medications and dietary supplements among older adults in the United States. JAMA. 2008;300:2867-2878.

79. Age-Related Eye Disease Study Group. A randomized, placebo-controlled, clinical trial of high-dose supplementation with vitamins C, and E, beta carotene, and zinc for age-related macular degeneration and vision loss: AREDS report no. 8. *Arch Ophthalmol*. 2001;119:1417-1436.

80. NIH State-of-the-Science Panel. National Institutes of Health state-of-the-science conference statement: Multivitamin/mineral supplements and chronic disease prevention. *Ann Intern Med*. 2006;45:364-371.

81. Sesso HD, Buring JE, Christen WG, et al. Vitamins E and C in the prevention of cardiovascular disease in men: The physicians' health study II randomized controlled trial. JAMA. 2008; 300:2123-2133.

82. Lawenda BD, Kelly KM, Ladas EJ, et al. Should supplemental antioxidant administration be avoided during chemotherapy and radiation therapy? *J Natl Cancer Inst*. 2008;100:773-783.

83. Liu BA, McGeer A, McArthur MA, et al. Effect of multivitamin and mineral supplementation on episodes of infection in nursing home residents: A randomized, placebo-controlled study. *J Am Geriatr Soc*. 2007;55:35-42.

84. Aisen PS, Schneider LS, Sano M, et al. High-dose B vitamin supplementation and cognitive decline in Alzheimer disease: A randomized controlled trial. JAMA. 2008;300:1774-1783.

85. Agency for Healthcare Research and Quality. *Treatment of Primary and Secondary Osteoarthritis of the Knee*. Structured abstract. October 2007. Available at: http://www.ahrq.gov/clinic/tp/oakneetp.htm.

86. Rozendaal RM, Koes BW, van Osch GJVM, et al. Effect of glucosamine sulfate on hip osteoarthritis: A randomized trial. *Ann Intern Med*. 2008;148:268-277.

87. Sawitzke AD, Shi H, Finco MF, et al. The effect of glucosamine and/or chondroitin sulfate on the progression of knee osteoarthritis: A report from the glucosamine/chondroitin arthritis intervention trial. *Arthritis Rheum*. 2008;58:3183-3191.

88. Autier P, Gandini S. Vitamin D supplementation decreases all-cause mortality in adults and older individuals. *Arch Intern Med*. 2007;167:1730-1737.

89. Lappe JM, Travers-Gustafson D, Davies KM, et al. Vitamin D and calcium supplementation reduces cancer risk: Results of a randomized trial. *Am J Clin Nutr*. 2007;85:1586-1591.

90. Bischoff-Ferrari HA, Dawson-Hughes B, Willett WC, et al. Effect of vitamin D on falls: A meta-analysis. JAMA. 2004;291: 1999-2006.

91. Flicker L, MacInnis RJ, Stein MS, et al. Should older people in residential care receive vitamin D to prevent falls? Results of a randomized trial. *J Am Geriatr Soc*. 2005;53:1881-1888.

92. Cherniack EP, Levis S, Troen BR. Hypovitaminosis D: A widespread epidemic. *Geriatrics*. 2008;63:24-30.

93. Ausman, JI. Why omega-2 fatty acids are important to neurosurgeons. *Surg Neurol*. 2006;65:325.

94. Williams CM, Burdge G. Long-chain n-3 PUFA: Plant v. marine sources. *Proc Nutr Soc*. 2006;65:42-50.

95. Lee JH, O'Keefe JH, Lavie CJ, et al. Omega-3 fatty acids for cardioprotection. *Mayo Clin Proc*. 2008;83:324-332.

96. Sander S, Coleman CI, Patel AA, et al. The impact of coenzyme Q10 on systolic function in patients with chronic heart failure. *J Card Fail*. 2006;12:464-472.

97. Young JM, Florkowski CM, Molyneux SL, et al. Effect of coenzyme Q10 supplementation on simvastatin-induced myalgia. *Am J Cardiol*. 2007;100:1400-1403.

98. Schaars CF, Stalenhoef AF. Effects of ubiquinone (coenzyme Q10) on myopathy in statin users. *Curr Opin Lipidol*. 2008;19:553-557.

99. Khan N, Mukhtar H. Tea polyphenols for health promotion. *Life Sci*. 2007;81:519-533.

100. Signorile JE. Translational training: Turning fitness gains into functional fitness. *J Active Aging*. 2005;4:46-57.

101. Liu CJ, Latham NK. Progressive resistance strength training for improving physical function in older adults. *Cochrane Database Syst Rev*. 2009;3:CD002759.

102. Knoops KTB, de Groot LCPG, Kromhout D, et al. Mediterranean diet, lifestyle factors, and 10-year mortality in elderly European men and women. JAMA. 2004;292:1433-1439.

103. Yates LB, Djoussé L, Kurth T, et al. Exceptional longevity in men: Modifiable factors associated with survival and function to age 90 years. *Arch Intern Med*. 2008;168:284-290.

104. Hung H-C, Joshipura KJ, Jiang R, et al. Fruit and vegetable intake and risk of major chronic disease. *J Natl Cancer Inst*. 2004; 96:1577-1584.

105. Estruch R, Martinez-Gonzalez MA, Corella D, et al. Effects of a Mediterranean-style diet on cardiovascular risk factors. *Ann Intern Med*. 2006;145:1-11.

106. Esposito K, Marfella R, Ciotola M, Di Palo C. Effect of a Mediterranean-style diet on endothelial dysfunction and markers of vascular inflammation in the metabolic syndrome: A randomized trial. JAMA. 2004;292:1440-1446.

107. Salas-Salvadó J, Fernández-Ballart J, Ros E, Martínez-González MA, et al. Effect of a Mediterranean diet supplemented with nuts on metabolic syndrome status: One-year results of the PREDIMED randomized trial. *Arch Intern Med*. 2008;168:2449-2458.

108. Shai I, Schwarzfuchs D, Henkin Y, et al. Weight loss with a low-carbohydrate, Mediterranean, or low-fat diet. *N Engl J Med*. 2008;359:229-241.

109. Mattison JA, Lane MA, Roth GS, Ingram DK. Calorie restriction in rhesus monkeys. *Exp Gerontol*. 2003;38:35-46.

110. Colman RJ, Anderson RM, Johnson SC, et al. Caloric restriction delays disease onset and mortality in rhesus monkeys. *Science*. 2009;325:201-204.

111. Kaeberlein M, McVey M, Guarente L. Using yeast to discover the fountain of youth. *Sci Aging Knowledge Environ*. 2001;1:pe1.

112. Guarente L. Sirtuins in aging and disease. *Cold Spring Harb Symp Quant Biol*. 2007;72:483-488.

113. Schwer B, Verdin E. Conserved metabolic regulatory functions of sirtuins. *Cell Metab*. 2008;7:104-112.

114. Bordone L, Cohen D, Robinson A, et al. SIRT1 transgenic mice show phenotypes resembling calorie restriction. *Aging Cell*. 2007;6:759-767.

115. Pfluger PT, Herranz D, Velasco-Miguel S, et al. Sirt1 protects against high-fat diet-induced metabolic damage. *Proc Natl Acad Sci USA*. 2008;105:9793-9798.

116. Lagouge M, Argmann C, Gerhart-Hines Z, et al. Resveratrol improves mitochondrial function and protects against metabolic disease by activating SIRT1 and PGC-1alpha. *Cell*. 2006;127:1109-1122.

117. Zillikens MC, van Meurs JB, Rivadeneira F, et al. SIRT1 genetic variation is related to BMI and risk of obesity. *Diabetes*. 2009;58:2828-2834.

118. Flachsbart F, Croucher PJ, Nikolaus S, et al. Sirtuin 1 (SIRT1) sequence variation is not associated with exceptional human longevity. *Exp Gerontol*. 2006;41:98-102.

119. Kuningas M, Putters M, Westendorp RG, et al. SIRT1 gene, age-related diseases, and mortality: the Leiden 85-plus study. *J Gerontol A Biol Sci Med Sci*. 2007;62:960-965.

120. Bellizzi D, Rose G, Cavalcante P, et al. A novel VNTR enhancer within the SIRT3 gene, a human homologue of SIR2, is associated with survival at oldest ages. *Genomics*. 2005;85:258-263.

121. Everitt AV, LeCouteur DG. Life extension by calorie restriction in humans. *Ann NY Acad Sci*. 2007;1114:428-433.

122. Heilbronn LK, de Jonge L, Frisard MI, DeLany JP. Effect of 6-mointh calorie restriction on biomarkers of longevity, metabolic adaptation, and oxidative stress in overweight individuals: A randomized controlled trial. JAMA. 2006;295:1539-1548.

123. Guarente L. Mitochondria—a nexus for aging, calorie restriction, and sirtuins? *Cell*. 2008;32:171-175.

124. Allard JS, Perez E, Zou S, de Cabo R. Dietary activators of Sirt1. *Mol Cell Endocrinol*. 2009;299:58-63.

125. Baur JA, Pearson KJ, Price NL, et al. Resveratrol improves health and survival of mice on a high-calorie diet. *Nature*. 2006;444:337-342.

126. Pearson KJ, Baur JA, Lewis KN, et al. Resveratrol delays age-related deterioration and mimics transcriptional aspects of dietary restriction without extending life span. *Cell Metab*. 2008;8:157-168.

127. Barger JL, Kayo T, Vann JM, et al. A low dose of dietary resveratrol partially mimics caloric restriction and retards aging parameters in mice. *PLoS One*. 2008;3:e2264.

POST-TEST

1. Which of the following is TRUE regarding growth hormone use?
   A. Adverse effects of growth hormone supplementation include myocardial infarction.
   B. Growth hormone decline is not a consequence of aging, but rather of disease.
   C. Restoring growth hormone levels to the young adult range increases vitality.

2. Potential benefits of vitamin use are complicated/clouded by all of the following EXCEPT:
   A. Vitamin users often have healthier diets, higher incomes, and better access to health care than non-vitamin users.
   B. Western diets are already fortified with many vitamins and minerals.
   C. Nutritional supplements use pharmaceutical-grade preparations.
   D. Interventional studies involving the use of vitamin supplements excluded frail elderly patients.

3. Taking a multivitamin as an older adult has been shown to:
   A. Increase mortality
   B. Reduce cancer risk
   C. Lower the risk of infection
   D. Improve antibody response to flu vaccination

4. Which of the following is TRUE?
   A. Glucosamine is beneficial in the treatment of osteoarthritis.
   B. Vitamin D supplements may have a role in the prevention of falls.
   C. Omega-3 fatty acids are often taken for an improvement in cognition.
   D. The drinking of green tea has no identifiable health benefits.

ANSWERS TO PRE-TEST
1. D
2. C
3. A

ANSWERS TO POST-TEST
1. B
2. C
3. D
4. B

3

Physical and Cognitive Function

Gilles O. Einstein, PhD
Michelle Horhota, PhD
Mark McDaniel, PhD

● LEARNING OBJECTIVES

1. Describe the physical and cognitive abilities that are most affected by normal aging and then explain the impact of these changes on normal functioning.
2. Differentiate between different types of memory and how these types of memory are uniquely affected by aging.
3. Explain lifestyle factors that promote positive cognitive abilities in the older years.
4. Discuss the relationship of physical problems (eg, hearing problems) to cognitive abilities (eg, memory).
5. Appreciate how the attitudes of others and an older person's personal attitudes about aging and memory ability affect actual cognitive performance and health.

PRE-TEST

1. **Which of the following best characterizes cognitive changes with age?**
   A. Most people show no cognitive decline until the age of 65, and then the decline is precipitous.
   B. Most people show very little change in their cognitive abilities as they age.
   C. All people show large declines as they age.
   D. There are very large individual differences between people in the amount of cognitive decline that occurs with age.

2. **Which of the following statements is TRUE with respect to physical changes with age?**
   A. Changes in an older adult's vision or hearing have no impact on their cognitive abilities.
   B. Women are more likely to report deficits in hearing as they age.

   C. Older adults experience a reduction in their useful field of view, which can have an impact on one's driving abilities.
   D. Most changes in vision are severe and have a great impact on the daily lives of older adults.

3. **The type of memory that is associated with facts and general knowledge is:**
   A. Semantic memory
   B. Episodic memory
   C. Prospective memory
   D. Working memory

If you were asked to describe a typical older adult, what would be the first words that come to your mind? Would it be wise, interesting, and active? Or perhaps frail, slow, and difficult? Research suggests that people hold a range of age stereotypes that reflect both positive and negative characteristics.[1] These stereotypes reflect the large variability that is seen within older adults. You can probably think of older adults who suffer from hearing loss or cognitive decline, and yet you can probably also think of others who remains highly functioning. Why is this? Unfortunately there is no single easy explanation for why one individual ages successfully and another ages more poorly. Adopting a lifespan developmental perspective highlights that aging is associated with both gains and losses, and that the variability between people is largely due to differing contextual factors between individuals.[2] Genetics and intrinsic factors (eg, motivations) impact both physical and cognitive development, further increasing the variability among individuals.

This chapter will discuss literature on normative physical and cognitive changes in older adulthood, keeping in mind that individual variability due to genetic, contextual, and intrinsic factors will exist around these norms. In particular we will point out the contextual and intrinsic factors that older adults have some control over in the sections on minimizing declines in cognition. Although there is a growing body of literature focusing on genetics, most of this research focuses on non-normative aging processes, such as determining genetic predispositions to Alzheimer disease. Non-normative aging is out of the scope of this chapter and thus will not be discussed here. We will organize our discussion by following the hypothetical progression of changes exhibited by an individual throughout his later adult years.

CASE PRESENTATION 1: NORMAL AGING?

Frank is 56 years old. He is out for dinner with his family to celebrate his youngest daughter's graduation from college. Recently he has started to wear reading glasses, and he finds it difficult to read the menu in the dim lighting of the restaurant. As individuals around the table break into multiple conversations, Frank notices that he has difficulty hearing the conversations over the background noise of the busy restaurant. The next day he asks his wife if he should visit his doctor to see if these changes in his vision and hearing are normal or if they reflect something more serious.

● NORMATIVE PERCEPTUAL CHANGES WITH AGE

What Frank is experiencing in this example is very typical of aging individuals. The older people are, the more likely they will experience changes in their vision and hearing, however, people age differently and therefore some 80-year-olds will maintain good vision and hearing whereas some 50-year-olds will have vision and hearing problems. This section presents findings from the literature on normative changes in vision and hearing. Although other senses (taste, smell, and touch) also experience change, less research has been conducted in those areas.[3,4]

Vision

One of the first normative changes in vision that many individuals notice is presbyopia, that is, the difficulty seeing close objects clearly. This is evident if you look around a restaurant filled with middle-aged patrons; many will hold the menus farther away from them if they do not have reading glasses. Presbyopia occurs because of a structural change; the inner layers of the lens of the eye stiffen, and this causes the lens to lose its ability to adjust and focus.[5] A person's ability to see details gradually begins to decline before age 60 and declines more rapidly after age 60.

A second normative change is the amount of time it takes older adults to adapt to changes in lighting. Older adults take longer to adjust to changes in brightness.[6] This change is more likely due to neural changes in the brain, and this change is observed for both dark adaptation (eg, moving from outside where it is bright and sunny into a dark gardening shed) and light adaptation (moving from a dark gardening shed back outdoors to the garden on a sunny day).

One final normative change that aging individuals experience is a reduction in their useful field of view (UFOV).[7] The UFOV represents the information that can be visually processed without turning the head or moving the eyes. These normative changes all can have an impact on aspects of daily life; however, most individuals are able to manage these changes without severe impact on their abilities.

It is estimated that about 20% of individuals over the age of 65 suffer severe vision loss,[8] and research shows that this interferes with activity levels. To assess a person's everyday functions, researchers typically use the Activities of Daily Living (ADL) measure[9] (see Chapter 7 for further details on functional assessments such as the ADL). The ADL assesses a person's ability to complete basic activities on one's own such as eating, bathing, dressing, toileting, moving in and out of bed, and continence. A second measure, the Instrumental Activities of Daily Living (IADL), assesses more complex activities such as preparing a meal, shopping, using the telephone, mode of transportation, housekeeping, laundry, handling finances, and managing one's own medication.[10] Individuals with severe vision loss show declines in their abilities to complete both basic and complex activities.[11,12] Thus, it is not surprising that individuals who suffer from vision loss report that maintenance of their independence is one of their most important concerns.[13] Among individuals with normative vision loss, an awareness of the difficulties that they may be experiencing is a first step toward being sensitive to their needs.

Hearing

Thinking back to Frank's situation in the restaurant, how common is hearing loss for middle-aged and older adults? The most common hearing problem that is reported is presbycusis, a reduced sensitivity to high-pitched tones.[14] Hearing loss is gradual and accelerates in later years; some research suggests that about 30% of all Americans over 70 report having some hearing difficulty.[15] Typically, males report greater deficits in the high-pitched range.[16] There are several different types of presbycusis that have varying implications: some individuals report hearing loss across all pitches, others show loss that is greatest in certain ranges of pitches, and another subset of individuals with neural presbycusis report difficulty understanding speech.[17]

Clearly, the loss of hearing is detrimental for older adults' communication abilities, and therefore much of the research on hearing loss has focused on changes in language comprehension. Healthy older adults often report difficulty understanding very rapid speech.[18] Further, declines in hearing are greater when the language task is increased in difficulty, such as when sentences are syntactically complex.[19] Thus, some issues with hearing that older adults report do not appear to stem solely from their hearing abilities; rather, some problems also relate to changes in one's processing abilities. Changes in processing abilities will be discussed in the next section.

Additionally, difficulties that older adults have with hearing can be mitigated or exacerbated by changes already discussed concerning visual processing. Vision is commonly used to help individuals in situations where it is hard to hear. Listeners can watch facial movements (eg, watching a person's mouth movements) in addition to paying attention to gestures that help convey a speaker's meaning. The limitation to reading visual cues is that low-frequency speech sounds such as vowels and voicing are necessary complements to the visual cues in order to decipher them.[20] But because typical age-related hearing loss is in the high-frequency range, conversational skills are not necessarily impaired in individuals experiencing typical mild hearing loss that comes with normative aging. This explains why many older individuals who show signs of hearing loss in medical tests do not report limitations in their conversational abilities. Individuals with low frequency loss show decreases in conversational fluency and acknowledge conversational problems such as misunderstandings. We will also discuss additional issues with communication later in the chapter.

Taste, Smell, and Touch

Taste, smell, and touch also experience change with age; however, less research has been conducted in these areas.[21] The ability to discriminate among tastes declines with age, but there is evidence that the number of taste buds and receptor cells does not change.[22] In fact, changes in taste sensitivity are typically modest. This is in contrast to olfactory changes, which tend to show significant declines.[23] Older adults typically show impairments in memory for smells and odor recognition.[24] With respect to the sense of touch, older adults show a decline in spatial acuity in touch. That is, when asked to touch two small probes, the probes have to be farther apart for an older person to recognize that there is not just one probe but two. Young adults can tell the difference with a much smaller distance between the probes.[25] Despite having little impact on general measures of cognition in nonclinical older adult samples, smell, taste, and touch can have a significant impact on quality of life. In particular, declines in the ability

to smell and taste have been shown to impact the nutritional states of older adults through their food selection.[26,27]

Although little research has been conducted in the area of normative sensory change in olfaction, more research has been conducted on olfaction in Alzheimer patients. Individuals with Alzheimer disease experience greater declines in their sense of smell than are found in normative samples of older adults.[28,29] In fact, many researchers argue that olfactory tests should be used as a clinical marker of Alzheimer disease[30] and can be used to discriminate Alzheimer disease from vascular dementia.[31]

CASE PRESENTATION 2: CHANGES IN MEMORY

Frank is now 67 years old. He corrected his vision using bifocals and still has difficulty hearing in noisy environments; however, his sensory abilities have not declined much since he first started noticing some decline about 10 years earlier. In fact things have been going quite well. Recently, he and his wife Betty attended their 50th high school reunion. They were amazed at how many events they remembered from high school and yet, when they were introduced to an old classmate's wife, Frank could not remember her name 5 minutes later! Frank's wife made a point to repeat the woman's name when she realized that Frank had forgotten it. How typical are Frank's experiences?

● NORMATIVE COGNITIVE CHANGES WITH AGE

There are many normative cognitive changes that occur with age. As with sensory changes, there are large individual differences between people in the amount of decline that they experience. Some individuals decline rapidly whereas others function well into their 80s. What parts of the cognitive system decline and what parts remain relatively stable? To discuss this issue, we first have to explain a little bit about the cognitive system. Psychologists used to think that memory was a single storage unit. Now, it is believed that information is processed by different types of memory systems. Table 3–1 and Figures 3–1 through 3–4 provide a summary of how several memory processes change with age.

Working Memory

Working memory is the type of memory that a person uses when he or she is actively processing information.[32] You can think of it as your mental sketchpad. You can also think of it as your mental capacity or "fuel" for performing the mental tasks at hand. There are storage components of working memory, where you hold the information that you are processing, as well as the executive control functions that process and operate on mental representations. For example, you are using working memory when you calculate a tip on your restaurant bill in your head, using the storage components to hold the

● **TABLE 3–1** Summary of Important Processes and Resources for Memory and How They Are Affected by Aging

Process/Resource	Definition	Examples	Affected by Aging?
Working memory	Mental resources used for manipulating, storing, and evaluating the current contents of consciousness	Reading and thinking about a newspaper article, multiplying numbers in your head thinking about the best solution to a problem	Yes
Attention or selective Attention	The process of focusing or concentrating your mental processes on relevant information information and ignoring distraction	Focusing attention on a speaker and ignoring background noises, focusing on reading an article and ignoring other concerns in your life (like weekend plans)	Yes
Processing speed	The speed of a mental process	The speed with which you can make a mental comparison	Yes
Long-term memory— Episodic memory	Memory for the episodes in your life	Memory for breakfast this morning, of your dad scolding you as a child, the instructions your doctor just gave you concerning your medication	Yes
Long-term memory— Semantic memory	Memory for knowledge	Knowing the current president, the meaning of a word, the combatants in World War II	No

numbers and the executive control components when you process the numbers to calculate the tip amount. As you can see in Figure 3–1, working memory capacity or "mental fuel" tends to decline with age. This change is driven by changes in the executive functions, rather than the storage span, which shows minimal age differences.[33,34] This change occurs because several processes that are related to the processing of information in working memory decrease with age.

First, the ability to selectively attend to information declines with age. Selective attention is the ability to focus one's attention on something while ignoring background distractions. An example is if you are in the middle of reading a very good book you may fail to hear the timer go off for the cup of tea you are brewing. In the example, when Frank attended his reunion, his ability to pay attention to one conversation in the midst of people around him engaging in secondary conversations involved selective attention. Older adults

have more difficulty filtering out irrelevant information.[36] Therefore, in situations where there are multiple conversations or a lot of background noise, it is common for older adults to experience difficulty.

A second process that declines in older adulthood is the ability to process information quickly. Studies that have examined cognitive slowing show that this process begins to decline when a person reaches the early 30s (Figure 3–2). As with the other findings reported in this chapter, there are large individual differences between people. Thus, it is possible to find an individual who is 65 who performs equivalently to a person who is 40 on speeded tasks. However, on the whole, individuals can expect to experience some declines in their processing speed. These declines have been linked to many cognitive outcomes. In particular, there is a strong relationship between working memory abilities and a person's processing speed abilities, suggesting that at least some of the declines we find in working memory may be due to changes in speed.[37]

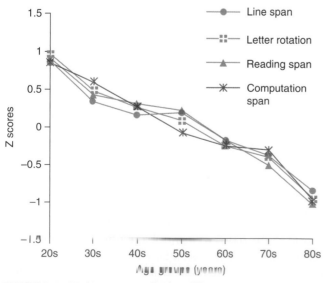

FIGURE 3–1. Working memory. (*Park et al.*[35])

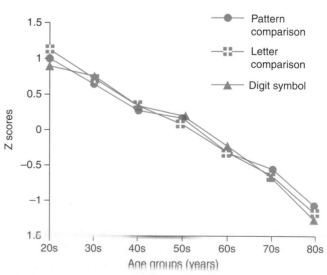

FIGURE 3–2. Perceptual speed. (*Park et al.*[35])

Long-Term Memory

A second memory system is what people typically think of when they think about memory. Think back to Frank's experience at the high school reunion. He was able to recall stories from the good old days rather easily. This type of memory is called long-term memory. As far as we know, long-term memory is unlimited in size, and individuals can continue to add information to it. In fact, the more you know about a particular topic, the easier it is to remember information related to it. One way to think about memory is that it is like an interconnected network of information. Stories that have been repeated many times, such as exploits from high school, become easy to recall because they are well practiced. The more one practices something, the stronger the link in the network becomes. Similarly, if you are knowledgeable in a certain topic, you may have noticed that it is easy to learn new information about that topic. This is because you have a strong network of information stored away that allows you to easily make connections to the new information. When you think about one part of the network, all of the connected areas also come to mind more easily. For example, if you are a football fan, you may learn new statistics about your favorite team easily. If you are not a football fan, learning that same new information is very difficult. Learning something brand new is more difficult as we age because we have to create the connections and links to remember from scratch.

Memory researchers have observed that there are different types of long-term memory, and that these different types of memory decline in different ways with age. Memories about personally experienced events are called episodic memories, referring to "episodes" from your life. These types of memories can include stories from one's distant past but could also include what you ate for breakfast this morning or all the nuances of a conversation that you had recently with your physician. Older adults tend to have difficulty with episodic memories that are from the recent past (Figure 3–3). In the example, Frank had difficulty remembering the name of a

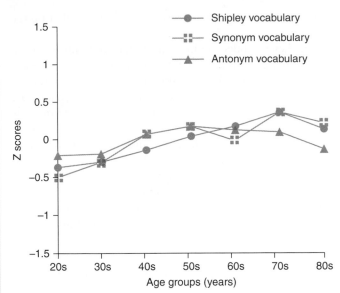

FIGURE 3–4. Semantic memory. (*Park et al.*[35])

classmate's wife to whom he was just introduced. Names are particularly difficult to remember because they are arbitrary; there is not any information that you can use in your existing knowledge base to help you figure out whether a woman's name is Carol or Susan. In order to commit this type of information to memory you need to invest substantial effort. Older adults may also want to take good notes to help them remember this kind of information.

A second type of long-term memory is semantic memory, which is memory for facts and general knowledge. This includes information such as vocabulary words, general facts, and capital cities of countries around the world. These memories typically are well practiced and are easy to retrieve from memory because they are well connected to other information. Thus, research does not find that older adults do more poorly on this type of memory (Figure 3–4).[38]

CASE PRESENTATION 3: MEMORY LAPSES

On the way home from the high school reunion, Frank realized that he had forgotten to tell his friend Dave that they had to reschedule their golf game for the weekend. Frank made a note to call Dave in the morning so he wouldn't forget to give him the message again.

Prospective Memory

Another kind of memory demand that we often face is prospective memory, which is remembering to perform actions in the future. From carrying out the basic tasks of life (eg, remembering to turn off the oven) to taking care of health needs (eg, remembering to take one's medication) to maintaining good social relations (eg, remembering a lunch engagement or to reschedule your golf game), our lives are full of prospective memory demands. A striking feature of the research examining how aging effects prospective memory is the variability in the findings.[39] Whereas some studies

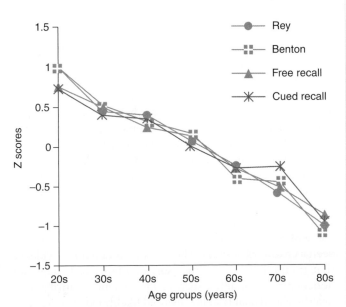

FIGURE 3–3. Visuospatial and episodic memory. (*Park et al.*[35])

show very large age differences, others show small or no age differences.

The key to understanding this pattern of results seems to be whether there is a good external cue that can be used to help remembering.[40] In those situations in which there are no cues, it is very easy to get distracted and especially so for older adults. Thus, these kinds of situations seem to be particularly difficult for older adults. For example, if Frank needs to remember to pay his bills sometime during the day and simply forms a general intention to do so, he is very likely to forget. On the other hand, if when forming the intention, Frank establishes a good cue like taking his checkbook and putting it in a prominent location that he will see at the appropriate time, he is very likely to remember to pay his bills. Having good external cues is a general remedy for age-related memory difficulties, and we will revisit this theme shortly.

The research on memory we have just reviewed suggests that older adults' memory performance is mixed. On some tasks they do poorly and yet on others they do well. An easy way to differentiate tasks that an older adult continues to perform well compared to tasks for which an older adult has difficulty is to think about whether the task requires controlled or automatic processing. A controlled process is a task that requires mental effort to complete. This means that it requires both working memory and processing speed to get the job done. Automatic processing occurs for tasks that can be completed quickly and efficiently with minimal use of resources. Trying to commit a person's name to memory is effortful, and therefore individuals have difficulty with it, whereas remembering stories that have been told many times before is much easier to do. Older adults typically have much more difficulty with tasks that are not well practiced and require more effortful processing.

Techniques for Improving Older Adults' Cognition

CASE PRESENTATION 4: STAYING SHARP

Frank and his friend Dave met up to play golf and the topic of their reunion came up. They were pleased at how many of their friends still seemed cognitively sharp but they also noted that it was a bit scary that others were clearly starting to show some cognitive changes. Frank wondered what the differences were between those who changed more and those who didn't. Some of their old friends talked about taking in lectures at the local university while others swore that completing a crossword puzzle a day was their secret to staying sharp. Others seemed to stay physically fit but didn't appear to really challenge their brains, whereas others were physically unwell but played bridge three times a week. It was hard for Frank and Dave to figure out whether any of these techniques consistently worked

Given that there are well-documented declines in some aspects of older adults' cognitive functioning, researchers have searched for way to improve older adults' abilities. This section will provide examples of some effective methods that have been shown to help older adults. As mentioned, older adults experience difficulty with tasks that require effortful processing. One way to improve their performance is therefore to reduce the amount of effort that is required. When it comes to memory, an effective way to make the process easier is to provide older adults with cues. Research shows that individuals who use cues are much more likely to remember information than those who do not use cues. For example, imagine that Frank took a 1-week vacation in Italy and then later tried to recall his experiences to a group of friends. If he relied solely on his memory, then it is very likely that his recollections would be sparse and very general in nature. If, however, Frank had kept a diary during his trip and had taken photographs, and if he used these to prompt his memory, then his recollections would be much richer (and probably a lot more accurate). Research has shown that older adults remember as much correct detail about an event as younger adults when both younger and older adults use detailed notes to cue their memory.[41] Thus, a good general recommendation for older adults is to take good notes.

Research also finds that older adults do better on tasks that are more similar to the tasks that they complete in everyday life compared to standardized laboratory tasks.[42,43] This may be due to the fact that many laboratory tasks require older adults to process information quickly and impose time limits, which may reduce older adults' performance. Older adults also perform well on everyday tasks because they are well practiced and the older adult can draw on years of experience.

Many readers of this chapter have probably heard media reports about different techniques for older adults to "train their brain" to lead to better cognitive performance. Many computer programs, training seminars, and Internet-based programs of varying quality are currently on the market. Several studies have found that training participants on specific cognitive abilities can lead to cognitive improvements, such as in inductive reasoning.[44] Reasoning training can also lead to reductions in functional declines, as measured by the IADL, such as preparing a meal or managing money.[45] Further research has found that older adults can train themselves, using materials that researchers provided, just as effectively as when they were trained by researchers.[46] The only downside to the early findings is that training leads to improvements in the area of the training but not necessarily to overall, more general improvements. That is, if a person completes training to improve his or her accuracy on a reasoning task, this does not necessarily translate into improvements on an unrelated memory task. In other words, extensive practice with crossword puzzles will help people retrieve words and particularly the kinds of words used in crossword puzzles, but will not help someone remember the contents of a newspaper article or the name of the president of Afghanistan (unless the name had been a crossword answer). These studies found some evidence that training on processing speed had positive benefits for noncognitive variables, such as improvements in reported health-related quality of life, reduced likelihood of depression, and reduced need for services; however, these results have not been replicated and must be interpreted with caution. More recent research has focused on training that involves coordination of skills, such as using complex video games or tasks that involve dividing one's attention. This type of training has been found to generalize across tasks and suggests that older adults are able to benefit from cognitive training.[47]

Many individuals have heard the phrase "use it or lose it" when it comes to cognition. The idea behind "use it or lose it" is that if you continue to work your brain it will continue to function well. Older adults highly endorse this strategy. In a recent study that asked older adults about their beliefs about how they could control their memory, between 30% and 40% spontaneously reported adopting a "use it or lose it" strategy.[48] So, what does the research say about this phenomenon?

Several longitudinal studies have followed individuals over time and compared activities that people engage in to changes in their cognitive abilities. Participants in these studies are asked whether they engage in activities such as physical activities, hobbies, reading complex material, and social activities. The same participants are tested on measures of fact recall, story recall, working memory, and speed. The research finds that middle-aged and older adults who engage in intellectually stimulating activities show less decline than those who do not engage in such activities, particularly in the areas of reasoning, working memory, and episodic memory.[49,50] Further, several studies have now found that individuals who engage in high levels of intellectual activity were less likely to develop Alzheimer disease.[51,52] Even after controlling for other factors, such as socioeconomic status, social and physical activity, and cognitive activity prior to old age, the association between intellectual engagement and decreased loss in cognitive ability remains.[53]

In summary, there is increasingly strong evidence for a relationship between intellectual engagement and cognitive vitality in the later years. The evidence is clear that older adults should do what they can to engage in intellectual exercise, and our specific recommendation is that they try to mix this with activities that are fun and socially engaging. One of the strongest predictors of happiness in older adulthood is the extent to which individuals feel socially connected.[54] Thus, rather than sitting alone with a crossword puzzle, we recommend getting involved in some of the following types of activities: joining a reading (or film) club, joining a gardening club, taking cooking lessons, taking courses in a lifelong learning program, or volunteering to tutor at a local grade school. In addition, there is a growing body of evidence suggesting that physical changes and cognition are linked and that physical activity can lead to improvements in cognition. This connection will be discussed in the next two sections.

CASE PRESENTATION 5: EFFECTS OF DISTRACTION

Frank is now 74 years old. Cognitively, Frank has remained sharp; however, his health has declined. Frank recently fell down some stairs outside of his home and broke his leg. He now has to work with a physical therapist to learn to use a walker. One afternoon during his therapy session, the therapist asks Frank several questions. Frank is focusing on keeping his balance so his responses come slower. The therapist perceives Frank to be unsure of what the nurse is asking so she repeats herself.

● INTERACTION OF PHYSICAL AND COGNITIVE CHANGES

Thus far, we have discussed the normative changes that occur with age in terms of sensory changes as well as cognitive changes related to memory and cognitive processing. We now turn to the interaction of physical and cognitive changes that occur with age.

As mentioned previously, older adults who experience declines in vision or hearing often compensate in various ways in order to continue functioning in daily life. Vision can be corrected with corrective lenses or surgery and hearing can be corrected through the use of hearing aids. However, if these problems remain uncorrected, they have the potential to impact cognitive ability in negative ways. Researchers who have investigated the relationship between sensory and cognitive decline over time find that there is a moderate relationship between the two.[55,56]

If you ask anyone who has problems with vision, they will likely tell you it can be very frustrating when they misplace their glasses. When information is difficult to see, it takes a person longer to process the information. It becomes more difficult to figure out what the information is in the first place. It also becomes more difficult to find relevant information in a display.[57] These issues mirror the difficulties that older adults have with decreases in processing speed and also difficulties with selective attention. The decrease in processing speed can lead to difficulty storing the information in an effective way for later recall.[58]

With respect to hearing, similar issues arise. Much of what we hear is in the context of an ongoing dialogue with another person. This is a very complex task, because not only does the listener need to parse out what the individual words mean, he or she also has to figure out what those words mean within the context of the knowledge that they have already stored. You need to recall what the conversation partner already knows and what information would be new and informative to share with him or her. When older adults cannot hear properly, they are more likely to misunderstand complex sentences.[59] When sentences are complex and also spoken quickly, the combination exacerbates the effect, and older adults are much more likely to report misunderstandings.[60] Given the deficits in processing resources previously discussed, the more effort that is expended in understanding the information, the fewer resources are available for storing and later remembering that information.[61] Studies that examine loss in both vision and hearing find that individuals with dual impairments, that is, those individuals who need to use the most processing resources, are most likely to report problems in memory, perceptual speed, and reasoning.[62]

In addition to sensory declines, other physical changes also have been found to impact ongoing cognitive processes. For example, as individuals age they tend to notice changes in their balance. Therefore, when older adults walk they need to expend additional cognitive resources and attention to maintain their balance,[63] and this would be expected to affect their memory. To test this, one study asked older adults to walk and also complete a memorization task at the same time. The researchers found that walking was prioritized over the memory task for older adults and therefore performance on the memory task was poor in comparison to young adults.[64] More recent research has replicated this finding.[65]

CASE PRESENTATION 6: PHYSICAL ACTIVITY

When Frank recovers from his broken leg, the first thing that he wants to do is get back out golfing with his friend Dave. He has always thought it was important to keep physically active. His wife, Betty, also tries to keep active by attending low-impact water aerobics at their local senior center. They were pleasantly surprised when they recently read an article in their newspaper saying that physical activity was good for their brains as well as their bodies.

Thus far, the work described in this section has focused on the negative impact of sensory and physical changes on cognitive functioning. Recently, researchers have shifted their attention to examine whether a positive relationship exists between physical health and cognition. This research is finding compelling evidence for the fact that cardiovascular health is strongly related to a healthy brain.

To examine this relationship, initial research examined people completing their typical routines and measured their cognitive performance on a variety of tasks. A study that compared older individuals who vigorously exercised and another group of older adults who did not exercise found that the physically active individuals performed better on tests of working memory, reaction time, and reasoning.[66] Physical activity has also been found to relate to better visual attention,[67] improved performance on tasks that require executive control to block out distracting information,[68] faster reaction times,[69] and enhanced inductive reasoning.[70] In addition to examining the relationship between what older adults do in their daily lives with their cognitive performance, many recent studies have conducted systematic studies to control for additional factors that could influence the relationship between exercise and cognition. In particular, researchers have been interested in whether certain types of exercise are more beneficial than others.

To examine the difference between exercise types, researchers assign older adults to specific exercise groups and then measure the effect on cognitive measures, such as working memory. This body of research on the whole suggests that aerobic exercise has a large impact on working memory, which is particularly impressive given the documented declines in working memory in older adults.[71] Moreover, research shows that modest exercise interventions (eg, a regimen of brisk walking for 45 minutes 3 times per week for 6 months) produce significant changes in cognitive performance.[72] Further, a 6-month randomized clinical trial found significant increases in brain volume in older adults who participated in aerobic fitness training, but not for those in non-aerobic programs.[73] Recently, longitudinal studies that followed the same participants over the span of 5 years found that those with poor cardiovascular health were those who showed largest age-related declines in the structure of their brain and also in cognitive functioning.[74]

Thus far, the evidence suggests that the most beneficial forms of exercise are those that have the largest benefits for cardiovascular health; however, strength training in combination with aerobic exercise can also be beneficial.[75] For individuals who are unable to participate in aerobic exercise, research suggests that tai chi or light exercise are alternative forms of exercise that are also associated with positive cognitive outcomes.[76] Tai chi is a traditional mind-body exercise that involves balance and conscious control of movement. Practitioners of tai chi move through complex sequences of movement that are performed in a particular order. Recent work suggests that tai chi and aerobic activity were equally beneficial for individuals aged 65 to 74 on measures of recall and visual span.[77] Light exercise can be characterized by activities such as walking. Light to moderate walking (eg, twice per week) has been shown to improve memory, vocabulary, and digit span in large representative samples[78] as well as memory in individuals with mild cognitive impairment.[79]

CASE PRESENTATION 7: MORNING PEOPLE VERSUS EVENING PEOPLE

Frank has the sense that he is cognitively sharper in the morning and that he becomes progressively more sluggish throughout the day. As a result, he believes that he has an optimal time of day for cognitive functioning and he reserves his tough mental work for the morning. Is his intuition correct?

It has been known for quite a while that our bodies undergo regular changes or circadian rhythms in their biological functions (including body temperature, hormone secretions, and heart rate) over the course of a day.[80] Recently, research has produced convincing evidence that we have circadian fluctuations in our cognitive capabilities, such that many of us have an optimal time of day for performing demanding mental activities.

To assess one's optimal time of day for cognitive functioning, researchers use a questionnaire that has people indicate their preferred time for waking, for going to bed, their most alert periods, and so forth. It turns out that these self-ratings of optimal and non-optimal times correlate highly with measures of physiologic arousal at those times. Interestingly, large-scale studies reveal that 73% of older adults are morning people (ie, have their optimal time of day in the morning) whereas only 5% of college-age students are morning types.[81]

The research also reveals that performing at your optimal time of day has significant and sometimes very profound benefits on cognitive functioning. Being at one's optimal time of day affects learning, and especially so for effortful tasks (recall that these are the kinds of tasks that are most difficult for older adults). Optimal time of day also affects the ability to concentrate and focus attention. Being at one's optimal time of day, however, has little effect on simple and well-practiced tasks. Thus, Frank's intuition is not only correct, but his strategy for managing his activities across the day is ideal. Older adults *should* consider their optimal time of day when planning their activities. In other words, tasks that require good concentration and that are cognitively complex, such as composing a speech, evaluating one's finances, or comparing various insurance policies, should be done at one's optimal time of day. On the other hand, well-practiced and relatively simple tasks, such as participating in social conversations, working in the garden, and cleaning around the house, can be planned for one's non-optimal time of day.

> ## CASE PRESENTATION 8: EXPERIENCING AGISM
>
> Frank is now 80 years old. He is has remained an avid reader, and volunteers at the local library. Physically, Frank's health continues to deteriorate and he now needs to use a wheelchair to get around. However, he is still functioning cognitively. When Frank visits the doctor, he is discouraged because the doctor speaks directly to his adult child and not to him. The experience makes him second guess his own abilities, and he later is irritated that he didn't speak up to the doctor.

● IMPACT OF SOCIAL FACTORS ON COGNITIVE CHANGE

At the start of this chapter, you were asked to think about your stereotypes of aging. Think back to the list that you generated. Were the traits that came to mind predominately positive, negative, or a mix of both? Research suggests that most people have negative expectations of older adults' abilities, especially in cognitive domains such as memory.[82] When asked about a wide range of memory tasks (eg, memory for remembering names, past events, and facts), individuals report that they expect older adults to do worse.[83] As we have just reviewed, these beliefs are based in some observable facts: older adults do show evidence of slowing with age and difficulty with remembering certain kinds of information. However, the general expectations that we hold for older adults are not always going to match up with the older adult with whom we are currently interacting. You may be able to think of several instances where you have spoken with older adults and they have been much sharper than you would have expected initially based on their age and appearance alone.

Not only do individuals hold different expectations for older adults' abilities, they also attribute different causes to older adults' memory failures than they would give to a young adult's memory failures. For example, you have probably had

the experience where you walk into a room only to forget what you went in there for. An objective observer would likely report that, if you are a young adult, you forgot because you are busy and so you were distracted. This is an example of not putting enough effort into the task. However, if this event happened to an older adult, observers are more likely to report that the older adult forgot because he or she cannot remember as much in his or her old age, that is, that the adult doesn't have the ability. This is an example of providing a "lack of ability" explanation for an older adult's behavior and a "lack of effort" explanation for a young adult's behavior. Research finds consistent evidence for this pattern of attributions of memory failures.[84,85]

It is not only young adults who make these reports; older adults also report feeling lower amounts of control over their abilities.[86,87] Literature examining reports of self-efficacy, or one's beliefs about the ability to perform well on an upcoming task, also shows that older adults report lower self-efficacy on memory tasks than young adults do.[88] Given that individuals hold negative expectations of older adults' performance, researchers have asked the question whether these beliefs have an impact on older adults' cognitive performance.

The answer appears to be yes. Individuals who report higher self-efficacy, or beliefs in their ability, on a memory task are much more likely to set higher goals and invest more effort in the task.[89] Further, it is thought that individuals who believe that they will perform well on a task will also persist at the task for longer periods of time[90,91] and use more effective strategies to complete the task.[92,93] Both cross-sectional and longitudinal research has shown relationships between memory self-efficacy and memory performance.[94]

It may not be surprising that one's personal expectations impact one's performance. My expectations for my golf game are low, and so I don't bother to invest much time into practicing. However, research suggests that it is not only one's personal beliefs that may matter; negative stereotypes in society in general have also been shown to relate to poorer performance in older adults.[95,96] A seminal study[97] on the topic compared the memory performance of young and older Americans with the performance of young and older Chinese adults. In Western cultures, negative aging beliefs are common; however, in Chinese culture elders are stereotyped more positively. This study found that age differences that existed in the American sample were not replicated in the sample of Chinese adults; both young and older adults performed similarly on memory recall tasks. Follow-up research shows that these findings do not hold for all types of memory[98]; however, the evidence that stereotypes impact performance for some forms of memory (eg, recall) has been replicated.[99-101] For example, when negative stereotypes are activated in older adults, their performance suffers, whereas when positive stereotypes are activated, older adults' performance is enhanced.[102]

These effects are impacted by individual differences; older individuals with higher levels of education have been found to show no effects of stereotypes on their performance.[103] Also, one's age identity also has an effect on the impact of stereotypes on performance. Middle-aged adults who identified themselves as having an older age identity were more affected by age stereotypes on their memory performance than individuals who identified as a younger age group.[104] Thus, if a negative stereotype may be perceived as relevant for the individual who is being tested, there is the potential for that stereotype to negatively affect memory performance.

Negative attitudes not only relate to detriments in cognitive performance, but research also suggests that having a negative attitude relates to longevity and poor health outcomes. For example, individuals older than 70 with negative stereotypes had worse hearing performance 3 years later, even after controlling for initial hearing ability and age of participant.[105] Furthermore, individuals under the age of 49 who hold negative age stereotypes early in life have a greater likelihood for cardiovascular health problems (eg, congestive heart failure and stroke) later in life.[106] In addition, the negative age stereotypes held by individuals 50 and older predicted their functional health decreasing over time, based on longitudinal study data collected from 1975 to 1995.[107] Conversely, positive age stereotypes have been linked to longevity, with individuals with positive attitudes toward aging living a median of 7.5 years longer than those with negative attitudes toward aging.[108]

One source of negative stereotypes for older adults is the communication that they receive from those around them. Communication theories suggest that speakers convey their expectations of older adults in the way that they speak to them, often by accommodating their speech to simplify it in various ways.[109] Although some accommodations can be beneficial, such as simplifying the complexity of sentences, many adjustments that individuals think are helpful actually make speech harder to comprehend. Exaggerated prosody is commonly used by young speakers when speaking to older adults; however, exaggerating prosody is detrimental to older adults' language comprehension and results in them making more errors in joint communication tasks.[110] Thus, the ways in which individuals speak to older adults may limit their ability to comprehend the information and/or limit their opportunities to respond, potentially making the older adult appear less competent than he or she actually is.

SUMMARY AND RECOMMENDATIONS

To conclude, we summarize normal age-related changes that health care professionals should keep in mind when working with older adults, as well as some recommendations for how to constructively cope with the physical and cognitive changes that that tend to occur with normal aging.

1. Older adults should be encouraged to see a physician and correct vision and hearing losses. Vision and hearing losses are common in older adulthood, and when left uncorrected they start to limit one's activity level and sense of well-being.

2. Although working memory, processing speed, and the ability to store new information in memory all tend to decline in the course of normal aging, there is a great deal of variability in the rate of decline from individual to individual. In general, given that most individuals show compromised abilities with advancing age, older adults should give themselves more time to learn and should rely more on external cues like notes and lists (see Einstein and McDaniel[38] for a comprehensive presentation of effective techniques that older adults can apply).

3. Older adults should be encouraged to engage in cognitively stimulating behaviors such as playing bridge with friends. Not only will the cognitive activity be beneficial but the social component will also benefit one's well-being.

4. Although physical ailments increase in older adulthood, when possible, engaging in low-impact aerobic exercise can be beneficial to both physical and cognitive health. Any exercise is better than no exercise!

5. Negative attitudes about aging are pervasive in our culture. Keeping a positive attitude has been found to relate to persistence with tasks, increasing one's effort and improvements in performance.

6. Negative attitudes can be conveyed to older adults in many ways. Often, people do not notice that their speech patterns convey negative expectations of older adults. Try to remind yourself when engaging with an older adult that there is a wide range of variability in older adults' abilities. Adjust your speech to the needs of the specific person you are interacting with, rather than using your stereotypes to guide you.

References

1. Hummert ML. Multiple stereotypes of elderly and young adults: A comparison of structure and evaluations. *Psychol Aging*. 1990;5:182.

2. Baltes PB. Theoretical propositions of life-span developmental psychology: On the dynamics between growth and decline. *Dev Psychol*. 1987;23:611.

3. Schiffman SS. Taste and smell losses in normal aging and disease. *JAMA*. 1997;278:1357.

4. Murphy C, Schubert C, Cruickshanks K, et al. Prevalence of olfactory impairment in older adults. *JAMA*. 2002;288:2307.

5. Fozard JL, Gordon-Salant S. Changes in vision and hearing with aging. In: Birren JE, Schaie KW, eds. *Handbook of the Psychology of Aging*. 5th ed. San Diego: Academic Press; 2001:241.

6. Kline D, Schieber F. Vision and aging. In: Birren JE, Schaie KW, eds. *Handbook of the Psychology of Aging*. 2nd ed. New York: Van Nostrand Reinhold; 1985:296.

7. Edwards JD, Ross LA, Wadley VG, et al. The useful field of view test: Normative data for older adults. *Arch Clin Neuropsychol*. 2006;21:275.

8. Lighthouse Research Institute. *The Lighthouse National Survey on Vision Loss: The Experiences, Attitudes and Knowledge of Middle-aged and Older Americans*. New York: Lighthouse; 1995.

9. Katz S, Downs D, Cash HR, Grotz RC. Progress in development of the index of ADL. *Gerontologist*. 1970;10:20.

10. Lawton MP, Brody EM. Assessment of older people: Self-maintaining and instrumental activities of daily living. *Gerontologist*. 1969;9:179.

11. Horowitz A. Vision impairment and functional disability among nursing home residents. *Gerontologist*. 1994;34:316.

12. Heyl V, Wahl HW, Mollenkopf H. Visual capacity, out-of-home activities and emotional well-being in old age: Basic relations and contextual variation. *Soc Indicators Res*. 2005;74:159.

13. Girdler S, Packer T, Boldy D. The impact of age-related vision loss. *OTJR: Occupation Participation Health*. 2008;28:110.

14. Pichora-Fuller MK, Souza PE. Effects of aging on auditory processing of speech. *Int J Audiol*. 2003;42:2S11.

15. Campbell VA, Crews JE, Moriarty DG, et al. Surveillance for sensory impairment, activity limitation, and health-related quality of life among older adults—United States, 1993-1997. *Mor Mortal Wkly Rep CDC Surveill Summ*. 1999;48:131.

16. Gates GA, Cooper JC, Kannel WB, Miller NJ. Hearing in the elderly: the Framingham cohort 1983-1985. *Ear Hear*. 1990; 11:247.

17. Whitbourne SK. *The Aging Individual: Physical and Psychological Perspectives*. New York: Springer; 1996.

18. Fozard JL, Gordon-Salant S. Changes in vision and hearing with aging. In: Birren JE, Schaie KW, eds. *Handbook of the Psychology of Aging*. 5th ed. San Diego: Academic Press; 2001:241.

19. Wingfield A, McCoy S, Peelle J, et al. Effects of adult aging and hearing loss on comprehension of rapid speech varying in syntactic complexity. *J Am Acad Audiol*. 2006;17:487.

20. Erber NP. Use of hearing aids by older people: Influence of non-auditory factors (vision, manual dexterity). *Int J Audiol*. 2003; 42:2S21.

21. Murphy C, Schubert C, Cruickshanks K, et al. Prevalence of olfactory impairment in older adults. *JAMA*. 2002;288:2307.

22. Whitbourne SK. *The Aging Individual: Physical and Psychological Perspectives*. New York: Springer; 1996.

23. Schiffman SS. Taste and smell losses in normal aging and disease. *JAMA*. 1997;278:1357.

24. Murphy C. The chemical senses and nutrition in older adults. *J Nutr Elderly*. 2008;27:247.

25. Stevens JC. Aging and spatial acuity of touch. *J Gerontol*. 1992;47:35.

26. Schiffman SS. Taste and smell losses in normal aging and disease. *JAMA*. 1997;278:1357.

27. Murphy C. The chemical senses and nutrition in older adults. *J Nutr Elderly*. 2008;27:247.

28. Nordin S, Monsch AU, Murphy C. Unawareness of smell loss in normal aging and Alzheimer's disease: Discrepancy between self-reported and diagnosed smell sensitivity. *J Gerontol B Psychol Sci Soc Sci*. 1995;50B:187.

29. Schiffman SS, Graham BG, Sattely-Miller EA, et al. Taste, smell and neuropsychological performance of individuals at familial risk of Alzheimer's disease. *Neurobiol Aging*. 2002;23:397.

30. Suzuki Y, Yamamoto S, Umegaki H, et al. Smell identification test as an indicator for cognitive impairment in Alzheimer's disease. *Int J Geriatr Psychol*. 2004;19:727.

31. Duff K, McCaffrey RJ, Solomon GS. The pocket smell test: Successfully discriminating probable Alzheimer's disease from vascular dementia and major depression. *J Neuropsychiatry Clin Neurosci*. 2002;14:197.

32. Baddeley A. Is working memory still working? *Am Psychol*. 2001;56:849.

33. Zacks RT, Hasher L, Li KZH. Human memory. In: Craik FIM, Salthouse TA, eds. *The Handbook of Aging and Cognition*. 2nd ed. Mahwah, NJ: Erlbaum; 2000:293.

34. Bopp KL, Verhaeghen P. Aging and verbal memory span: A meta-analysis. *J Gerontol B Psychol Sci Soc Sci*. 2005;60B:223.

35. Park DC, Lautenschlager G, Hedden T, et al. Models of visuospatial and verbal memory across the adult life span. *Psychology and Aging*. 2002;17:299-320.

36. Hasher L, Zacks RT. Working memory, comprehension and aging: A review and a new view. In: Bower GH, ed. *The Psychology of Learning and Motivation*. San Diego: Academic Press; 1988:193.

37. Salthouse TA. The processing-speed theory of adult age differences in cognition. *Psychol Rev*. 1996;103:403.

38. Einstein GO, McDaniel MA. *Memory Fitness: A Guide for Successful Aging*. New Haven: Yale University Press; 2004.

39. Einstein GO, McDaniel MA. Prospective memory: Multiple retrieval processes. *Curr Dir Psychol Sci*. 2005;14:286.

40. McDaniel MA, Einstein GO. *Prospective Memory*. Thousand Oaks, CA: Sage; 2007.

41. Cherry KE, Park DC, Frieske DA, Smith AD. Verbal and pictorial elaborations enhance memory in younger and older adults. *Aging Neuropsychol Cognit*. 1996;3:15.

42. Phillips LH, Kliegel M, Martin M. Age and planning tasks: The influence of ecological validity. *Int J Aging Hum Dev*. 2006;62:175.

43. Artistico D, Cervone D, Pezzuti L. Perceived self-efficacy and everyday problem solving among young and older adults. *Psychol Aging*. 2003;18:68.

44. Boron JB, Turiano NA, Willis SL, Schaie KW. Effects of cognitive training on change in accuracy in inductive reasoning ability. *J Gerontol B Psychol Sci Soc Sci*. 2007;62:179.

45. Willis SL, Tennstedt SL, Marsiske M, et al. Long-term effects of cognitive training on everyday functional outcomes in older adults. *JAMA*. 2006;296:2805.

46. Margrett JA, Willis SL. In-home cognitive training with older married couples: Individual versus collaborative learning. *Aging Neuropsychol Cognit*. 2006;13:173.

47. Hertzog C, Kramer AF, Wilson RS, Lindenberger U. Enrichment effects on adult cognitive development: Can the functional capacity of older adults be preserved and enhanced? *Psychol Sci Public Interest*. 2009;9:1.

48. Hertzog C, McGuire CL, Horhota M, Jopp D. Age differences in theories of memory control: Does believing in "use it or lose it" have implications for self-rated memory control, strategy use, and free recall performance? *Int J Aging Hum Dev*, in press.

49. Hultsch DF, Hertzog C, Small BJ, Dixon RA. Use it or lose it: Engaged lifestyle as a buffer of cognitive decline in aging? *Psychol Aging*. 1999;14:245.

50. Schooler C, Mulatu MS. The reciprocal effects of leisure time activities and intellectual functioning in older people: A longitudinal analysis. *Psychol Aging*. 2001;16:466.

51. Wilson RS, Scherr PA, Schneider JA, et al. Relation of cognitive activity to risk of developing Alzheimer disease. *Neurology*. 2007; 69:1911.

52. Verghese J, Lipton RB, Katz MJ, et al. Leisure activities and the risk of dementia in the elderly. *N Engl J Med*. 2003;348:2508.

53. Hertzog C, Kramer AF, Wilson RS, Lindenberger U. Enrichment effects on adult cognitive development: Can the functional capacity of older adults be preserved and enhanced? *Psychol Sci Public Interest*. 2009;9:1.

54. Antonucci TC, Birditt KS, Akiyama H. Convoys of social relations: An interdisciplinary approach. In: Bengston VL, Gans D, Pulney NM, Silverstein M, eds. *Handbook of Theories of Aging*. 2nd ed. New York: Springer; 2009:247.

55. Lindenberger U, Ghisletta P. Cognitive and sensory declines in old age: Gauging the evidence for a common cause. *Psychol Aging.* 2009;24:1.

56. Baltes PB, Lindenberger U. Emergence of a powerful connection between sensory and cognitive functions across the adult life span: A new window to the study of cognitive aging? *Psychol Aging.* 1007;12:12.

57. Gilmore GC, Spinks RA, Thomas CW. Age effects in coding tasks: Componential analysis and test of the sensory deficit hypothesis. *Psychol Aging.* 2006;21:7.

58. Anstey KJ, Butterworth P, Borzycki M, Andrews S. Between and within-individual effects of visual contrast sensitivity on perceptual matching, processing speed, and associative memory in older adults. *Gerontology.* 2006;52:124.

59. Wingfield A, Tun, PA, McCoy SL. Hearing loss in older adulthood: What it is and how it interacts with cognitive performance. *Curr Dir Psychol Sci.* 2005;14:144.

60. Wingfield A, Peele JE, Grossman M. Speech rate and syntactic complexity as multiplicative factors in speech comprehension by young and older adults. *Aging Neuropsychol Cognit.* 2003; 10:310.

61. Pichora-Fuller MK. Cognitive aging and auditory information processing. *Int J Audiol.* 2003;42:2S26.

62. Brennan M, Bally SJ. Psychosocial adaptations to dual sensory loss in middle and late adulthood. *Trends Amplification.* 2007;11:281.

63. Maylor EA, Allison S, Wing AM. Effects of spatial and non-spatial cognitive activity on postural stability. *Br J Psychol.* 2001; 92:319.

64. Li LZH, Lindenberger U, Freund AM, Baltes PB. Walking while memorizing: Age-related differences in compensatory behavior. *Psychol Sci.* 2001;12:230.

65. Siu K, Chou L, Mayr U, et al. Attentional mechanisms contributing to balance constraints during gait: The effects of balance impairments. *Brain Res.* 2009;1248:59.

66. Clarkson-Smith L, Hartley AA. Relationships between physical exercise and cognitive abilities in older adults. *Psychol Aging.* 1989;4:183.

67. Roth DL, Goode KT, Clay OJ, Ball KK. Association of physical activity and visual attention in older adults. *J Aging Health.* 2003; 15:534.

68. Hillman CH, Motl RW, Pontifex MB, et al. Physical activity and cognitive function in a cross-section of younger and older community-dwelling individuals. *Health Psychol.* 2006;25:678.

69. Churchill JD, Galvez R, Colcombe S, et al. Exercise, experience and the aging brain. *Neurobiol Aging.* 2002;23:941.

70. Perrot A, Gagnon C, Bertsch J. Physical activity as a moderator of the relationship between aging and inductive reasoning. *Res Q Exercise Sport.* 2009;80:393.

71. Colcombe SJ, Kramer AF. Fitness effects on the cognitive function of older adults: A meta-analytic study. *Psychol Sci.* 2003;14:125.

72. Kramer AF, Hahn S, Cohen NJ, et al. Aging, fitness and neurocognitive function. *Nature.* 1999;400:418.

73. Colcombe SJ, Erickson KI, Scalf PE, et al. Aerobic exercise training increases brain volume in aging humans. *J Gerontol B Biol Sci Med Sci.* 2006;61.1166.

74. Raz N, Rodrigue KM, Kennedy KM, Acker JD. Vascular health and longitudinal changes in brain and cognition in middle-aged and older adults. *Neuropsychology.* 2007;21:149.

75. Colcombe SJ, Kramer AF. Fitness effects on the cognitive function of older adults: A meta-analytic study. *Psychol Sci.* 2003;14: 125-130.

76. Chan AS, Ho Y, Cheung M, et al. Association between mind-body and cardiovascular exercises and memory in older adults. *J Am Geriatr Soc.* 2005;53:1754.

77. Lam LCW, Tam CWC, Lui VWC, et al. Modality of physical exercise and cognitive function in Hong Kong older Chinese community. *Int J Geriatr Psychiatry.* 2009;24:48.

78. Lindwall M, Rennemark M, Berggren T. Movement in mind: The relationship between exercise with cognitive status for older adults in the Swedish National Study on Aging and Care (SNAC). *Aging Mental Health.* 2008;12:212.

79. van Uffelen JGZ, Chinapaw MJM, van Mechelen W, Hopman-Rock M. Walking or vitamin B for cognition in older adults with mild cognitive impairment? A randomised controlled trial. *Br J Sports Med.* 2008;42:344.

80. Yoon C, May CP, Hasher L. Aging circadian arousal patterns, and cognition. In: Park DC, Schwarz N, eds. *Cognitive Aging: A Primer.* New York: Psychology Press; 2000:151.

81. May CP, Hasher L, Stoltzfus ER. Optimal time of day and the magnitude of age differences in memory. *Psychol Sci.* 1993;4:326.

82. Ryan EB. Beliefs about memory changes across the adult life span. *J Gerontol B Psychol Sci Soc Sci.* 1992;47:41.

83. Lineweaver TT, Hertzog C. Adults' efficacy and control beliefs regarding memory and aging: Separating general from personal beliefs. *Aging Neuropsychol Cognit.* 1998;5:264.

84. Erber JT. Young and older adults' appraisal of memory failure in young and older adult target persons. *J Gerontology B Psychol Sci Soc Sci.* 1989;44:170.

85. Erber JT, Prager IG. Age and memory: Perceptions of forgetful young and older adults. In: Hess TM, Blanchard-Fields F, eds. *Soc Cognition and Aging.* San Diego: Academic Press; 1999:197.

86. Lachman ME. Locus of control in aging research: A case for multidimensional and domain-specific assessment. *Psychol Aging.* 1986;1:34.

87. Devolder PA, Pressley M. Causal attributions and strategy use in relation to memory performance differences in younger and older adults. *Appl Cognit Psychol.* 1992;6:629.

88. Berry JM, West RL. Cognitive self-efficacy in relation to personal mastery and goal setting across the life span. *Int J Behav Dev.* 1993;16:351.

89. West RL, Welch DC, Thorn RM. Effects of goal-setting and feedback on memory performance and beliefs among older and younger adults. *Psychol Aging.* 2001;16:240.

90. Bandura A. Regulation of cognitive processes through perceived self-efficacy. *Dev Psychol.* 1989;25:729.

91. Berry JM. Memory self-efficacy in its social cognitive context. In: Hess T, Blanchard-Fields F, eds. *Soc Cognition and Aging.* San Diego: Academic Press; 1999:69.

92. Devolder PA, Pressley M. Causal attributions and strategy use in relation to memory performance differences in younger and older adults. *Appl Cognit Psychol.* 1992;6:629.

93. Hertzog C, McGuire CL, Lineweaver TT. Aging, attributions, perceived control and strategy use in a free recall task. *Aging Neuropsychol Cognit.* 1998;5:85.

94. Valentijn SA, Hill RD, Van Hooren SAH. Memory self-efficacy predicts memory performance: Results from a 6-year follow-up study. *Psychol Aging.* 2006;21:165.

95. Hess TM, Auman C, Colcombe SJ, Rahhal TA. The impact of stereotype threat on age differences in memory performance. *J Gerontol B Psychol Sci Soc Sci.* 2003;58:3.

96. Yoon C, Hasher L, Feinberg F, et al. Cross-cultural differences in memory: The role of culture-based stereotypes about aging. *Psychol Aging.* 2000;15:694.

97. Levy B, Langer E. Aging free from negative stereotypes: Successful memory in China among the American deaf. *J Pers Soc Psychol.* 1994;66:989.

98. Yoon C, Hasher L, Feinberg F, et al. Cross-cultural differences in memory: The role of culture-based stereotypes about aging. *Psychol Aging.* 2000;15:694.

99. Andreoletti C, Lachman ME. Susceptibility and resilience to memory aging stereotypes: Education matters more than age. *Exp Aging Res.* 2004;30:129.

100. Chasteen AL, Bhattacharyya S, Horhota M, et al. How feelings of stereotype threat influence older adults' memory performance. *Exp Aging Res.* 2005;31:235.

101. Hess TM, Auman C, Colcombe SJ, et al. The impact of stereotype threat on age differences in memory performance. *J Gerontol B Psychol Sci Soc Sci.* 2003;58:3.

102. Levy B. Improving memory in old age through implicit self-stereotyping. *J Pers Soc Psychol.* 1996;71:1092.

103. Andreoletti C, Lachman ME. Susceptibility and resilience to memory aging stereotypes: Education matters more than age. *Exp Aging Res.* 2004;30:129.

104. O'Brien LT, Hummert ML. Memory performance of late middle-aged adults: Contrasting self-stereotyping and stereotype threat accounts of assimilation to age stereotypes. *Soc Cognit.* 2006; 24:338.

105. Levy B, Slade MD, Gill TM. Hearing decline predicted by elders' stereotypes. *J Gerontol B Psychol Sci Soc Sci.* 2006;61:82.

106. Levy B, Zonderman A, Slade M, Ferrucci L. Age stereotypes held earlier in life predict cardiovascular events in later life. *Psychol Sci.* 2009;20:296.

107. Levy B, Slade M, Kasl S. Longitudinal benefit of positive self-perceptions of aging on functional health. *J Gerontol B Psychol Sci Soc Sci.* 2002;57:409.

108. Levy B, Slade M, Kunkel S, Kasl S. Longevity increased by positive self-perceptions of aging. *J Pers Soc Psychol.* 2002;83:261.

109. Nussbaum JF, Hummert ML, Williams A, Harwood J. Communication and older adults. In: Burleson BR, ed. *Communication Yearbook 19.* Thousand Oaks, CA: Sage; 1996:1.

110. Kemper S, Harden T. Experimentally disentangling what's beneficial about elderspeak from what's not. *Psychol Aging.* 1999; 14:656.

POST-TEST

1. **In which type of task do older adults tend not to show a deficit?**
   A. Processing speed
   B. Working memory
   C. Semantic memory
   D. Episodic memory

2. **Aerobic exercise has been shown to have the largest positive effect on:**
   A. Selective attention
   B Working memory
   C. Semantic memory
   D. Episodic memory

3. **The optimal time of day for most older adults, which affects performance on effortful tasks, is:**
   A. Mid-day
   B. Morning
   C. Evening
   D. 2 hours before bedtime

ANSWERS TO PRE-TEST
1. D
2. C
3. A

ANSWERS TO POST-TEST
1. C
2. B
3. B

4

The Global Demography of Aging

Nina Tumosa, PhD
Margo-Lea Hurwicz, PhD

● **LEARNING OBJECTIVES**

1. Describe the historical and ongoing demographic and epidemiologic transitions in human populations.
2. Explain how population aging affects the needs and resources for health and supportive care.
3. Discuss late-life disability from the perspective of social, cultural, and psychological factors.
4. Describe the role of gender in population aging.
5. Discuss the consequences of population aging on use of health care services, the service delivery system, and professional training and workforce development.
6. Explain how migration influences health care delivery.

PRE-TEST

1. **Likely contributors to the epidemiological transition include all of the following EXCEPT:**
   A. Better management of communicable disease
   B. Greater availability of chronic disease treatments
   C. Increases in formal education
   D. More food availability and better nutrition

2. **The greatest proportional change seen in populations will be in those aged:**
   A. ≥ 85 years old
   B. ≥ 65 years old
   C. ≥ 55 but < 65 years old
   D. < 55 years old

3. **The better measure of population fertility is:**
   A. Annual number of births per thousand in a population
   B. Number of children born per woman across a population
   C. Annual number of live births per thousand
   D. Number of infant deaths across a population

INTRODUCTION

The population of most countries of the world is aging. Around the globe, the proportion of the population age ≥ 60 will rise from about 10% (2005) to 22% by mid-century, with the steepest rate of increase in the next 25 years.[1] During this century, the population age ≥ 85 is the fastest growing age-segment, and life spans of 100 years for women will become commonplace in many of the developed countries.[2] Population aging has had—and will have—profound impacts on society, domestic living arrangements, care and support of older family members, the training of health care providers, and the delivery and social and health services. In this chapter, we review historical and ongoing changes in the demographic structure of human populations, as well as some of the epidemiologic and social drivers and concomitants of these changes. Further, we discuss some of the ways in which an aging population affects the needs and resources for health and supportive care.

WHO AND WHAT IS "OLD"—MULTIPLYING DEFINITIONS

Definitions of who is "old" and what comprises aging are profoundly social, and vary across history and cultures (Chapter 5). The conventional, modern *operational* definition of "old age" as beginning at age 65 has a specific social history and rationale related to pension schemes[3] and cultural materials (an individual person's age reckoned in *years*, supported by individual vital statistics records). But there are many ways of assigning or recognizing the status "old," even in medical or scientific contexts (see, for example, definitions of old-age "frailty" in Chapters 2 and 36); these may have more or less to do with phase transitions in the human life span or scientists' evolving understanding of senescence (Chapter 2). It is important to recognize how the terms "old" and "aging" can be used appropriately, as very *contingent* constructs.

POPULATION AGING: DEMOGRAPHIC AND EPIDEMIOLOGIC TRANSITIONS

In most parts of the world, increasing numbers of older people are evident in most aspects of life. Older people are the fastest increasing segment of most the populations of many communities and countries. Countries in Western Europe and Japan have well over 20% of people over age 60; by 2100, more than half of the Japanese population will be aged ≥ 60.[1] The *median age* (dividing the population into two parts of equal size) of the world's population is also increasing, and is projected to be almost 38 years in 2050.[4] In 2000, Japan's median age was 41, followed closely by Germany, Switzerland, and Sweden, which all have median ages of 40 years. Yemen, demographically the world's youngest country, had a median age of 15. However, all countries have aging populations. Projections for median ages in 2050 show 15 African countries with median ages around 25 and 19 European countries with median ages of 50+, led by Spain, Slovenia, Italy, and Austria with median ages of 54+ years.[5] Although it took Sweden

TABLE 4–1 US Census Bureau Projected World Population of People Age 65 and Older		
Year	Age Group	Number
2010	65-69	178,029,550
	70-74	144,127,315
	75-79	101,422,161
	80+	105,799,057
2030	65-69	336,562,186
	70-74	259,395,702
	75-79	194,059,282
	80+	215,507,961
2050	65-69	440,911,150
	70-74	369,611,199
	75-79	311,785,476
	80+	470,254,497

Source: US Census Bureau, 2000.[6]

85 years to double its 65+ population from 7% to 14%, it will take China only 26 years to accomplish the same feat.

In 2010, almost 530 million people are aged 65 and older (7.7% of the world's population; Table 4–1).[6] By 2025, in all regions of the world, the elderly population will grow faster than any other age segment. These elderly populations will rise above 10% of the populations of individual countries in large sections of South America, most of Asia, and all of Europe, North America, and Australia. By 2030, that number will reach 1 billion, making one in eight of the world's inhabitants 65 or older. In 2050, 1.6 billion people (16.7% of the world's population) will be 65 or older. The number of persons ≥ 80 will more than quadruple by 2050. Therefore, not only does the number of elderly persons increase absolutely, with three times more elderly persons in 2050 as there are today, but the relative number increases also, from 7.7% of the world's population today to nearly 17% in 40 years. The greatest proportional change will occur in the oldest-old, those aged ≥ 85, with a 151% increase between 2005 and 2030, as opposed to a 104% increase in those ≥ 65 or older and a 21% increase in the population < 65 during the same period.

Population aging has been and is being achieved historically and in different parts of the globe through a finite number of steps and developmental or transitional stages, with specific socioeconomic and epidemiologic concomitants. The demographic steps have been (1) a reduction of population *mortality* (typically a rate expressed in units of deaths per 1000 individuals per year) accompanied by population *growth*, and (2) more or less complete transitions to lower rates of *fertility*.

Fertility is not equivalent to the *crude birth rate*, which is the annual number of births per thousand in a population. The *total fertility rate* (TFR), which is the number of children born per woman across a population, more directly measures population fertility than the crude birth rate, and is a key to population growth and decline. Two children per woman is considered the *replacement rate*, resulting in relatively stable numbers. TFRs above replacement indicate growing

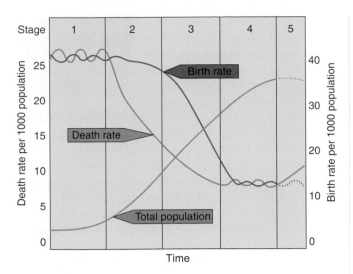

FIGURE 4–1. Five stages of the demographic transition.

The first stage is the condition in pre-industrial (pre-agricultural and agricultural) society in which death rates and birth rates are high relative to subsequent stages; the rates are approximately equal, meaning that population size is in theory roughly stable (Figure 4–1, stage 1) and adapted to traditional modes of subsistence and life conditions. Of course, during this pre-industrial stage and since, pandemic diseases, famine, and natural and human disasters could greatly increase mortality and suppress live births in any given time and place, and life expectancy at birth is generally quite low.[11] High fertility is maintained as a principal survival strategy against such uncertainties. The age structure of the pre-industrial population (Figure 4–2, stage 1) shows a low median age, represented by a broad base of male and female infants and children, with a decelerating decline in population at older age groups. Still, the proportion of population at "advanced" ages (eg, > 65) is almost never greater than 5% of the total. Stage two (Figures 4–1 and 4–2) characterizes earlier states of now developed societies as well as presently developing countries. Mortality begins to drop rapidly (Figure 4–1, stage 2) because of nutritional and sanitation improvements, affecting most directly infant and maternal mortality, but also the general population death rate. The age structure (Figure 4–2, stage 2) begins to reflect an increase in mean age, with improvement in child and maternal survivorship represented by a flattening of the sides of the pyramid. The "age of pandemics" recedes, increasing life expectancy and spurring population growth. Increasing adult survivorship helps reinforce the conditions of declining death rates and improves society's adaptations: technological, agricultural, health, educational, and industrial innovations begin to allow hedging against pre-industrial simple subsistence. Fertility lags, remaining high, as the changes related to increasing population and declining deaths take time to affect individual-level procreative and household economic decisions.

With industrialization, fertility begins to fall in the third stage of demographic transition, and the rate of population growth holds constant or begins to decelerate. Population growth begins to level off (Figure 4–1, stage 3). Two notable results for the population age structure are (1) the "bulging" of the pyramid, as people born during the historical high-fertility

populations with declining median ages. As will be noted later, higher rates indicate challenges for families and communities in raising children, as well as barriers to women obtaining paid work outside the home. The top ten countries in TFR are all sub-Saharan, with rates ranging between 5.8 and 7.8.[7] Rates *below* replacement indicate populations decreasing in size and growing older, as noted above for industrialized and Western European countries. Globally, fertility rates are in general decline (83 countries are below replacement), and this trend is most pronounced in industrialized countries, especially in Western Europe, where populations are projected to decline dramatically over the next 50 years. In 2009, the US TFR was 2.05.[7]

Interest in *demographic transition* theory, which began in the 1920s and has been a central preoccupation in demography since,[8] posits four (and maybe five) stages of population aging. *Birth, death, and population growth rates* associated with these stages are represented in Figure 4–1.[9] *Population age structures* associated with these stages are represented in Figure 4–2.[10]

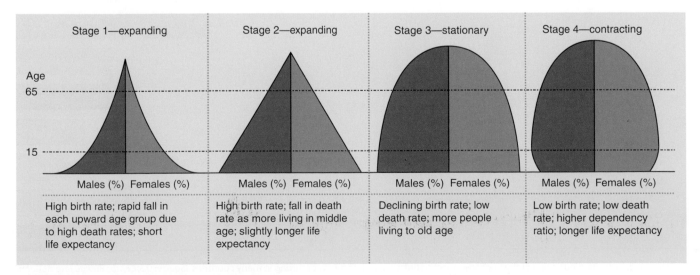

FIGURE 4–2. Population age structure at transitional stages.

stage "age upward" against the smaller number of the more recently born; and (2) the "pushing upward" of persons at the top—at ever greater ages. Instead of < 5% of the population at ages exceeding 65, the proportion climbs, and it becomes reasonable to represent "young-old" versus older-old age groupings. According to Omran's theory of epidemiological transition,[11] this is "the age of degenerative and man-made diseases." Epidemic infectious diseases have widely been suppressed. Further, non-infectious acute illnesses that formerly had high rates of case fatality have—with improvements in wealth, public health, and medical care—become chronic illnesses, increasingly more prevalent among older people, who can live many years with these conditions.

In stage 4 of the demographic transition, crude birth and death rates again come into rough equilibrium, but now at relatively *low* rates, and population growth manifestly slows (Figure 4–1, stage 4). Some posit a stage 5, to characterize the situation in developed countries in which total fertility rates have dropped below replacement levels (population replacement occurs at a rate of two live births per woman— see Figure 4–2, panels 3 and 4), in which population actually declines while life expectancy at birth and at other threshold ages remains high. Over the next 20 years, more than 20 countries are projected to experience population declines (Figure 4–3).[12] In developed countries such as Japan, Germany, and Italy, projected population declines are primarily the result of low fertility and limited immigration of younger, fertile workers. A population that is both aging and shrinking can present challenges to countries whose economies depend on population growth and that need to support through

transfer payments and direct care ever-larger numbers of retired and functionally dependent older people. However, such rising "age-dependency ratios" do not clearly dictate particular social outcomes or solutions. Moreover, they may mask the impact of underlying trends (eg, growing wealth and health in the older population).[13]

Our brief overview of the population transitions risks oversimplifying true processes of historical and contemporary population change. For example, while the four to five stages of transition may adequately describe the histories of Western post-industrial societies that have been through them, there are third world and developing societies that have been at stage 2 for many decades, maintaining high total fertility rates. Also, the impacts of migration are not accounted for (discussed later). Moreover, population declines in some Eastern European countries are attributable not only to declining fertility and immigration but also to rising adult death rates related to unemployment, epidemic alcoholism, and other social and economic problems. Large countries or geographic regions may contain diverse and more or less distinct population groupings whose different dynamics may be concealed at inappropriate levels of aggregation. These are reminders that conceiving population or social dynamics as a series of "stages" risks thinking of observed changes as necessary, predetermined, evolutionary, and universal. Further, as was observed above concerning the interpretation (or misinterpretation) of age-dependency ratios, the transition models—at their level of generality—do not necessarily speak to important demographic and health trends within the aging population segment itself.

Projected Population Decline between 2006 and 2030 (in millions)

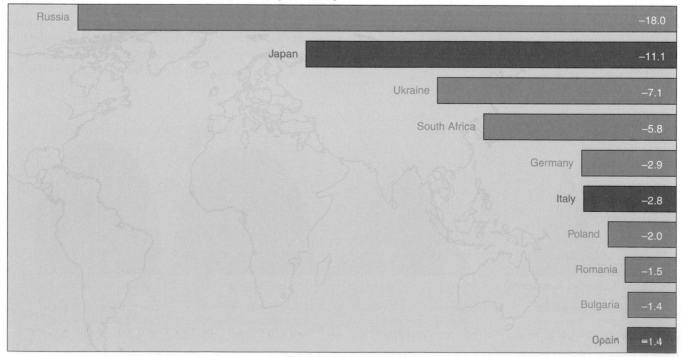

Country	Decline
Russia	−18.0
Japan	−11.1
Ukraine	−7.1
South Africa	−5.8
Germany	−2.9
Italy	−2.8
Poland	−2.0
Romania	−1.5
Bulgaria	−1.4
Spain	−1.4

FIGURE 4–3. Simultaneous aging of the population and population decline is now occurring in many countries. (Source: U.S. Census Bureau International Data Base. http://www.census.gov/ipc/wwwidbnew.html. Accessed January 8, 2007.)

● ARE OLDER PEOPLE LIVING LONGER AND HEALTHIER?

James Fries, writing in 1980, opened three decades of lively debate with his introduction of the "compression" and morbidity and mortality hypothesis.[14] Observing the increases in life expectancy at birth, and the increasing prevalence of age-associated, chronic disease versus burden of acute and infectious diseases at early ages through the improvement in health and medical care, Fries posited that humans would increasingly survive toward an upper age limit, "compressing" the population survival curve (see Figure 2–1, Chapter 2). Compression of survival against an upper age limit would be achieved because morbidity would become similarly compressed, that is, the onset of chronic conditions ultimately resulting in death would occur later in the lives of subsequent birth cohorts. Others, linking incident disability firmly to a medical model, interpolated a notion of the ongoing compression of disability (Figure 4–4) as an eventual outcome of incident chronic disease, occurring prior to death.[15] However, alternative, competing scenarios were also proposed, one of which envisioned "the failure of success," whereby population aging would merely extend years of ill and disabled life, that is, morbidity and disability curves would lag.[16] Kenneth Manton suggested a third theory of population aging, in which incident chronic diseases would lag, but disease severity would be attenuated or progression delayed[17] increases in life expectancy would be paralleled by increases in active (ie, disability-free) life expectancy.[18]

In order to determine whether age-specific disability rates are high, low, changing, or whether disability compression is occurring, (1) disability (a person's capacity to function within social and environmental situations) must be defined fully; and (2) we must be able to measure it on a population level. Disability, even late-life disability, is not a simple end-product of chronic disease but complexly determined, and subject to many different research, social, and even political theories and practical approaches.[19] From the perspective of the geriatrician, disabilities in older patients are usually understood and assessed in terms of difficulties or dependencies in instrumental and basic activities of daily living (Chapters 3 and 7), resulting from trauma or chronic diseases, leading to impairments in organ systems, producing the functional limitations underlying IADL and ADL disabilities.

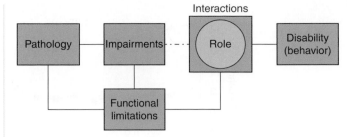

FIGURE 4–5. The Nagi model of late-life disability. (*As adapted by Altman, 2001.*)

This basic model (Nagi[20]) has been criticized as over-medicalized, and subsequently revised or augmented, for example, by the World Health Organization.[21] Altman[22] has pointed out that Nagi's original formulation did in fact incorporate social role and environmental components in the disability pathway (Figure 4–5). First, the model recognizes that functioning, while impacted by the damaged organ, cell, or body part, is an action of the whole person, meaning that functional measurement focuses on the person's capacity rather than the diseases or impairments as such; functioning is thus central in the disability process. Second, both social interaction with friends, family, and community, and the physical environment, provide the situations in which disabilities are manifested. Third, disabilities as "behaviors" in context are social rather than simply biological or medical outcomes. Geriatricians practicing functional assessment accommodate and appreciate this complexity (Chapter 7), but the reason it matters here is that the way disability is understood by society and reported by respondents to surveys affects what can be measured at the population level. "Activity-restricted days," or "difficulty" or "dependence" in using a telephone or dressing, depend not only on the disease-impairment-functional limitation pathway but also on respondent evaluations of the meaning of the terms and question, and on their own social roles, social resources, personal adaptive outlook, ingenuity, and so forth.[23] There are multiple independent social, cultural, and psychological factors bearing on disability rates and trends. So, for example, changes in disability may occur somewhat independently of improvements in management of cardiovascular diseases.

Cross-sectionally, the social aspect of late-life disability is salient in its disparate prevalence. In the 2000 US census, the most prevalent type of limitation/disability among older Americans (≥ 65) was physical (28.6%), followed by limitation in going outside the home (20.4%), sensory limitations (14.2%), cognitive limitations (10.6%), and self-care limitations.[24] The percentage of older adults who reported a limitation or disability was 35% for Asians, 40% for non-Hispanic whites, 49% for white Hispanics, and 53% for African Americans (the overall prevalence was 41.9%, or roughly 14 million Americans). Fifty-six percent of old adults in poverty report a limitation or disability compared with 40% not in poverty. Older Americans who are unmarried (ie, widowed, divorced, or never married) are more likely to report limitations than those who are married. Older Americans with more education or who remain in the workforce are less likely to report limitations than the less educated and unemployed.[24]

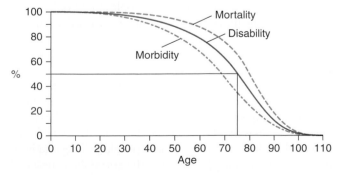

FIGURE 4–4. Hypothetical morbidity, disability, and survival curves for US women born in 1980.

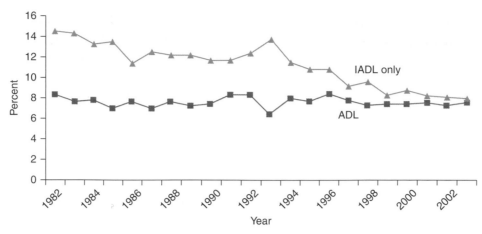

FIGURE 4–6. Percentage of the community-based population age 70 years and older reporting need for help with personal care or only routine care activities, 1982-2004. (Source: *Field MJ, Jette AM, Martin L (eds). Workshop on Disability in America: A New Look—Summary and Background Papers. The National Academies Press.*)

That disability may be undergoing compression is suggested by some evidence that age-specific disability rates are dropping, for example, in the United States. Freedman, using evidence from the National Health Interview Survey (NHIS) between 1982 and 2004,[23] identified a 6 percentage point decline in the population ages 70 years and older needing help only with IADLs such as shopping, preparing meals, and managing money (Figure 4–6). No clear trend was visible for ADLs such as bathing, toileting, and dressing, although she later found consistent declines on the order of 1% to 2.5% per year for two commonly used measures in the disability literature—difficulty with daily activities and help with daily activities—during the middle and late 1990s.[25] An analysis of the National Long Term Care Survey (NLTCS) also found large declines in IADL limitations from 1984 to 1999. However, the author notes that *severity* of disability increased over time for those reporting disabilities.[26] Further, evidence of social disparity in disability trends remains. Researchers using NLTCS data found increasing racial disparities in ADL and IADL prevalence during the 1980s, and diminishing disparities during the 1990s, while studies using NHIS data found no significant changes in the relative difference between whites and minorities.[23] Disparate trends by education level have been found more consistently. Using data from the 1982 to 2002 NHIS, Schoeni and associates[27] found that older people with the least education (0-8 years) showed virtually no improvement in ADL or IADL disability rates, whereas those with 16 or more years of education experienced significant disability declines. The authors found significant increases in ADL disability for the group with the least education and relatively flat trends for those with 16 or more years of education. Consequently, the socioeconomic gap in disability, which favored the more educated group in 1982, became much larger between 1982 and 2002 both in absolute and relative terms.[28]

The question of whether morbidity and disability are undergoing compression is extremely important.[23] If compressions are occurring as hypothesized, then the impact of population aging on future population health care and social security needs is a function of growing numbers of older people, but in absolute terms, and relative to younger people, that is, those of working age. However, the hypothesis depends in part on human mortality reaching an upper limit and the "rectangularization" of the survival curve (again, see Figure 2–1). Biologists estimate this upper limit—the human *maximum life span*—at 122 years,[29] but this estimate is based upon the oldest documented age reached to date (Ms. Jeanne Calment, in France).[30] There is uncertainty whether age 122 in fact represents the maximum potential human life span. What is certain is that life expectancy is being observed to increase in many populations.[2] For example, age at death in Sweden has greatly increased since 1861. However, the compression of mortality as described by Fries occurred only up to 1950 in that country (Figure 4–7). Since then, there has been a parallel shift in the curve due to increased life expectancy,[31] mostly attributable to decreased mortality above age 70.[32] During the same period in Sweden, annual surveys of disability at ages 65 to 84 during the 1980s and 1990s showed disability declines similar to those in the United States overall. However, from 1996 to 2004, successive surveys have shown increasing disability in that age group.[33] In several other national population studies, increases in *life expectancy* (ie, the average number of years to be lived by a group of people born in the same year if mortality at each age remains constant in the future) have occurred along with a growing burden of chronic diseases. The gains in life expectancy may be far greater than for *healthy* life expectancy (again, depending on how the latter is defined and assessed[23]). This suggests that aging is not simply genetically determined, but an interaction between genes and the environment in which there is no biologically fixed upper limit.[34] The social and economic consequences of population aging will be all the more profound where the greater numbers of older people also have longer to live with chronic illnesses and disabilities, that is, decompressing morbidity and disability.[23,33] Meanwhile, the social, health, and economic forces that have driven demographic transition continue to operate toward the extremes of age. For example, pension schemes and universal health insurance coverage in developed countries are clearly related to continuing gains in life expectancy from baseline ages 80 and above.[35-37] The key lesson is that the future burden of co-morbid diseases and disabled life years among older people will depend both on factors influencing health over the entire life course and upon the political will to maintain life and health among older people.

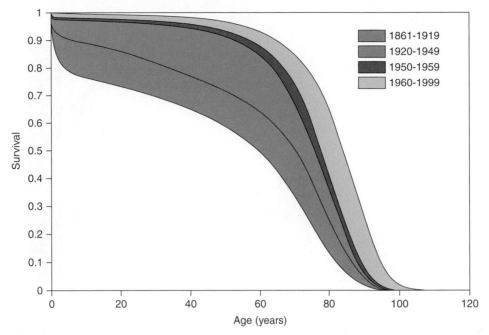

FIGURE 4–7. Historical survival curves in Sweden.

NO COUNTRIES FOR OLD MEN? AGING AND GENDER

To this point, we have not addressed gender differences in population aging. In all populations, girls are outnumbered by boys. However, around the age of 30 or so, women begin to outnumber men due to gender differences in mortality, and the absolute advantage of females increases with age. In the developed countries, the "life expectancy (LE) gap" is about 7 years, while the difference is only around 3 years in developing countries, which may continue to experience high maternal mortality rates and have other impediments to the well-being of women and girls.[38-41] With respect to the developed world, there are two notable trends in LE by gender. First, improvements, especially for males, have been nonlinear (ie, have not been uniform across populations). For example, there was little change in male LE from about 1950 to 1970 for several countries including the United States (and since the 1980s, male LE in much of Eastern Europe and states of the former Soviet Union has declined).[38] Second, while there has been some convergence in LE among the developed nations, the difference between female and male longevity has been widening. Figure 4–8 records the best national performance life expectancies by gender from 1840 to 2000 (countries taking the lead changing during the period). The increase in female LE has been relatively steady, at about 3 months per year.[2]

The causes of the female-male mortality gap and differential morbidity and disability patterns over the life course and in late life are not well understood.[29] These differentials are thought to have both biological and social determinants, although data limitations and research inattention have not helped clarify them. In developed countries, older women have higher rates of chronic conditions associated with later life (eg, osteoporosis, arthritis, chronic bronchitis, and symptoms of depression)[41] as well as higher prevalence of multiple chronic conditions (Figure 4–9).[42] In contrast, men have higher rates of heart disease, cancer, diabetes, and emphysema.[42] Up to age 65 in the United States, men with disabilities outnumber women, but among *older* Americans, women with disabilities (8.3 million, or 43.0% of older women) greatly outnumber disabled men (5.6 million, 40.4% of older men).[24,43] The greater LE of older women combined with higher age-specific disability rates create these vastly disparate numbers, as well as more years of disabled late-life for older women.

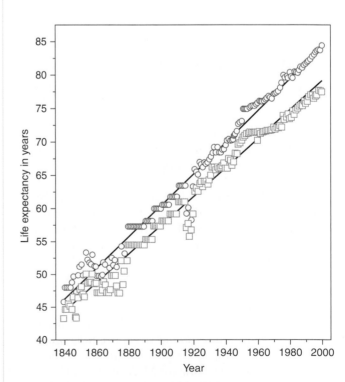

FIGURE 4–8. Female (*red circles*) and male (*blue squares*) life expectancy in the highest ranking country annually, 1840-2000.[2]

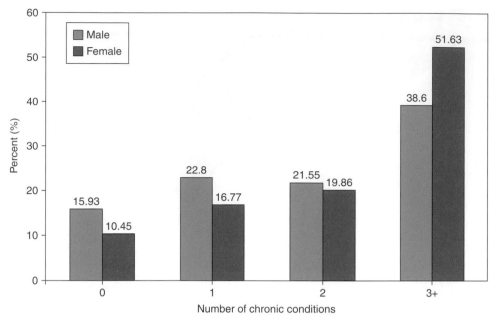

FIGURE 4–9. Distribution of chronic conditions by sex among those 65 years and older, 2001, Canada.

The disparate life expectancies and the different patterns of morbidity, co-morbid illness, and disability of older men and women translate into differences in use of health services. For example, older men tend to have higher rates of acute hospitalization in both the United States and Canada, although more women are hospitalized (given their greater number) and tend to stay longer.[41,42] Further, women are much more likely to use post-discharge rehabilitation and long-term care services,[41] attributable not only to their greater disability burden but to the greater likelihood of being widowed or unmarried, living alone, with lesser access to informal (familial) supportive care.[38]

● HEALTH CARE AND PENSION SYSTEM CONSEQUENCES OF POPULATION AGING

As just suggested, the use of health care services in the United States and in other developed countries is greatly influenced by population aging. Currently, people age 65 or older have the greatest frequency of office visits to doctors, hospital stays, and prescription medicine usage.[44] Average annual expenditures on health care in 2004 for people ages 45 to 54, the age group in the middle of the "baby-boom" generation, was $2695. For those aged 55 to 64, it was $3262; and for those 65 and over, it was $3899.[45] In the United States, from age 50 upward, total health care expenditures will double for every 15 years of life.[46] A casual assessment of public policy debates and public and private planning finds little to suggest how society will adapt to age-related service requirements and expenditure increases as the "boomer" generation retires. Unchecked, expenditures would likely rise from a current level of about 15% to about 29% of GDP in 2040.[46] The sheer number of retirees qualifying for Medicare will place rising demands on a poorly adapted health care system and workforce. Medicare expenditures will outpace economic growth, increasing from 13.5% of federal spending in 2009 to an estimated 18.9% by 2020—an increase that economists characterize as unsustainable.[47]

Service Delivery System

The US health care system is already grappling with the influx of older patients and changing patterns of demand and use. Twenty years ago, most of the growth in Medicare spending was linked to intensive hospital services, for example, for acute heart conditions. Much of the recent growth has been attributable to chronic conditions such as diabetes, arthritis, hypertension, and kidney disease—conditions usually treated by physicians in outpatient settings and by patients at home with prescription drugs.[48] About half of all physician visit time for many specialties is accounted for by patients age ≥ 65—a proportion that is increasing by about 1% every year.[49]

The recent Institute of Medicine report, *Retooling for an Aging America*,[50] puts forward a vision for the future health care of the aging population that must be adopted. This vision is embodied in three principles. First, the health needs of the older population will be addressed comprehensively using a patient-centered, preference-sensitive approach.[51] Preventive services including lifestyle modification will be in greater evidence, as will coordinated treatment of chronic and acute health conditions. Frail and disabled older adults will require integration of health and social services in order to maintain or improve health and function. Patient-centeredness includes taking account for increasing socio-demographic and cultural diversity of older Americans, including language, health beliefs, and living in underserved areas. Second, services will need to be efficient, reducing wasteful and ineffective care. This principle supports training for interdisciplinary teams and delivery systems providing seamless care across various delivery sites, as well as accessible health information systems fitted to emerging care needs and delivery modalities.

Moving from a fee-for-service reimbursement system toward payment mechanisms that promote accountable care and service integration over the long term will be necessary. Third, older persons will be active partners in their own care up until the point that they are too frail or impaired. Such partnerships need to include the adoption of healthy lifestyles, self-management of chronic conditions, and increased participation by the patient in decision making. By becoming participants in their own care, patients can improve their health, reduce unnecessary treatments, and reduce the need for reliance on formal or informal caregivers.

Professional Training and Workforce Development

The current US health care workforce is too small and critically unprepared to meet the health needs for an aging population.[50] Earlier in the chapter, we reviewed the evidence for increased active life among older people in the developed world. If these trends are to continue—and the historical gains in longevity and health are to be maintained—it will depend in part upon matching changes in the health care delivery system with professional training and payment reforms. Certainly, higher salaries and wages are required to attract and retain geriatrics specialists. But much greater numbers of health care providers need to be trained in the basics of geriatric care and should be capable of caring for older patients. The reformed systems of care will need to make use of widened duties and responsibilities of workers at various levels of training.[50]

In addition to training of older patients themselves in the management of their chronic conditions, the system of "informal care"—supportive, usually unpaid care provided by family, friends, and neighbors—will become even more important than in the past. The Institute of Medicine report calls for training programs to be established to help family members, friends, and others acquire the knowledge and skills needed to provide care to their loved ones and to alleviate the stress they may feel from providing this care.[50] Healthy, retired, or semi-retired older people are increasingly being recognized as underutilized human capital. A variety of initiatives are exploring means of activating the healthy, aging population, including offering opportunities for life-long learning, promoting of volunteerism and civic engagement,[52] and training and direct support for familial caregiving.[53]

Migration Policy

In addition to policy inertia, development of a formal and informal geriatric care workforce faces important socio-demographic headwinds. Earlier in the chapter, we described shrinking numbers of children and grandchildren relative to the numbers of aging people in the developed world, affecting the availability of informal caregivers. Moreover, these countries will continue to see the overall workforce shrink.[54] One consequence of this "shortfall" is the service workforce needs of developed countries being filled by immigrants. In 2005, nearly 200 million people (about 1 in 35) lived outside of their country of origin for at least 1 year.[55] About 3 million new people migrate to a different country annually, mainly for financial, religious, political, or safety reasons. Most workforce migration occurs from lower-income to higher-income countries. Europe has the largest number of international migrants (64 million), followed by Asia (53 million), Northern America (44 million), Africa (17 million), Latin America and the Caribbean (close to 7 million), and Oceania (5 million). Individual countries with large numbers of international migrants include the United States (38 million), the Russian Federation (12 million), Germany (10 million), and Ukraine, France, and Saudi Arabia (over 6 million each).[56]

Migration between countries has serious consequences for the delivery of health care to the aging population in both the receiving and the donating countries. Immigration provides a younger workforce in the receiving countries. Many of those workers become employed in the health professions. Some are physicians or nurses but many are in low-paying workforce positions that provide support and services to the elderly population. Emigration leaves a void in the lower-income countries, regions, or rural areas when their older population needs "high-touch" health care and the family members that would normally have provided that care are no longer at home.[57]

Migration tends to occur at the upper and lower ends of the socioeconomic spectrum. At the upper end, international medical graduates (IMGs), the majority of whom are foreign born as well as foreign educated, comprised about 28% of the 2004 US medical residency cohort; furthermore, nearly one-third of practicing US physicians are either immigrants themselves or children of immigrants.[58] In 2005 to 2006, about one-quarter of all visits to office-based MDs were to IMGs.[59] IMGs were more likely than US medical graduates to be practicing internal medicine.[58] With respect to physician care of older patients, the expected source of payment for visits to IMGs was more likely to be Medicare, or Medicare and Medicaid (ie, payers for older and disabled Americans), than for visits to US medical graduates (25.8% versus 23.5%).[59] Focusing on geriatrics, IMGs comprised less than one-third of geriatrics fellows in 1991 to 1992—a proportion that rose to nearly two-thirds in 2008 to 2009.[60] Much of the workforce for long-term care in developed countries is comprised of low-paid, less educated workers. Here too, immigrants are much in evidence. In fact, given the shortfall in workers to meet sharply rising demand in the US, the long-term care industry relies heavily on *undocumented* workers. It is estimated that one in six of all undocumented workers is employed in a long-term care setting.[61] Continuing globalization of labor markets coupled with population aging will further increase the flow of women from source to receiving nations to meet the need for long-term care workers.[62]

Social Security and Income Support

One of the great opportunities for fear-mongering in current political discourse is the status and outlook for the US Social Security system. A frequently cited statistic is that the Social Security Trust Fund is scheduled to run out in 2037, and that after that point if no changes are made, there will only be enough money from tax revenue to pay about 75 cents for each dollar of scheduled benefits. Of course, the imbalance of accounts underlying the crisis is firmly attributable to the demographic changes we have described, coupled to failures to modify the pension system both in accord with the changing demographics and increases in the health and active life of older people. Much of the evidence concerning the health gains of older people in developed countries attributes these gains as much if not more to their growing income security as to their health care. Yet one bulwark of that income security is the public pension systems. At the same time, more healthy years in retirement may deprive national economies of important human capital—capital that they may need to tap to keep these economies vital, as well as to support reformed health care and pension systems on an ongoing basis.

As with reform of the health care system, pension system reforms require great political will, but are ultimately unavoidable. However, a variety of measures can be taken that may help meet the demands of health care and pension system reform as well as take advantage of the improved health, welfare, and capabilities of an aging citizenry. We have already mentioned immigration policy in connection with the services workforce, but it is also much discussed in connection to improvement of pension fund viability.[63] One of the most discussed options is raising the age of retirement, but many adults already work beyond Social Security retirement age not only because they are able and willing, but also due to income security concerns. At the same time, developed countries raise a variety of barriers to continued workforce participation for retired people, which would need to be addressed to facilitate use of this human capital and bolster income support for some proportion of older Americans.

CONCLUSION

The population of the world is aging, and population aging is accelerating in much of the world. Population aging—and its attendant gains in life expectancy—are products of societies undergoing demographic and epidemiologic transitions that have their basis in economic development and public health improvements. Many of the fully developed countries have entered periods in which total population size is stable or even declining, due primarily to very low fertility, while mortality rates continue to drop and life expectancies increase. In these countries, the growth in population age ≥ 85 continues, and questions concerning the future numbers, health, and disability status of the oldest-old are pressing researchers, policymakers, and the public. The implications of population aging for developing and developed counties are huge and affect the social, economic, and political fabric of these societies and cultures. Only by understanding and planning for the future can we anticipate the growing requirements of this aging population and make accommodations to adjust for their unique needs.

References

1. Lutz W, Sanderson W, Scherbov S. The coming acceleration of global population ageing. *Nature.* 2008;451:716-719.

2. Oeppen J, Vaupel JW. Broken limits to life expectancy. *Science.* 2002;296;1029-1031.

3. Clement D. Why 65? Origins of the official retirement age and current trends and policies in other countries. FEDGAZETTE—The Federal Reserve Bank of Minneapolis. March 2004. http://www.minneapolisfed.org/publications_papers/pub_display.cfm?id=1677. Accessed February 10, 2010.

4. United Nations. 2006. http://www.un.org/esa/population/publications/sixbilin/sixbilpart1.pdf. Accessed April 2009.

5. Population Division, DESA, United Nations. World Population Ageing, 1950-2050. 2002. http://www.un.org/esa/population/publications/ worldageing19502050. Accessed June 2009.

6. United Nations. 2006. http://www.un.org/esa/population/publications/sixbillion/sixbilpart1.pdf. Accessed April 2009.

7. CIA World Factbook. https://www.cia.gov/library/publications/the-world-factbook/rankorder/2127rank.html. Accessed February 11, 2010.

8. Caldwell JC, Caldwell BK, Caldwell P, et al. *Demographic Transition Theory.* Dordrecht, The Netherlands: Springer; 2006:418.

9. Wikipedia. Demographic transition. http://en.wikipedia.org/wiki/File:Stage5.svg.

10. Wikipedia. Demographic transition. http://en.wikipedia.org/wiki/File:Dtm_pyramids.png.

11. Omran AR. Epidemiological transition in the United States: The health factor in population change. *Popul Bull.* 1977;32. Washington, DC: Population Reference Bureau; 1977.

12. National Institute on Aging. Why population aging matters: A global perspective. http://www.nia.nih.gov/ResearchInformation/ExtramuralPrograms/BehavioralAndSocialResearch/GlobalAging.htm. Accessed September 2009.

13. Calasanti TM, Bonanno A. The social creation of dependence, dependency ratios, and the elderly in the United States: A critical analysis. *Soc Sci Med.* 1986;23:1229-1236.

14. Fries JF. Aging, natural death and the compression of morbidity. *N Engl J Med.* 1980;303:130-135.

15. Davies AM. Epidemiology and the challenge of aging. In: Brody JA, Maddox G, eds. *Epidemiology and Aging: An International Perspective.* New York: Springer; 1988:17.

16. Gruenberg EM. Failures of success. *Milbank Memorial Fund Q.* 1977;55:3-24.

17. Manton KG. Changing concepts of morbidity and mortality in the elderly population. *Milbank Memorial Fund Q.* 1982;60:183-244.

18. Katz S, Ford A, Moskowitz R, et al. Active life expectancy. *N Engl J Med.* 1983;309:1218-1224.

19. Wikipedia. Disability. http://en.wikipedia.org/wiki/Disability. Accessed February 10, 2010.

20. Nagi S. *Disability and Rehabilitation: Legal, Clinical, and Self-Concepts and Measurement.* Columbus: Ohio University Press; 1969.

21. WHO International Classification of Functioning, Disability and Health (ICF). http://www.who.int/classifications/icf/en/. Accessed February 2010.

22. Altman BM. Disability definitions, models, classification schemes, and applications. In: Albrecht G, Seelman K, Bury M, eds. *Handbook of Disability Studies.* Thousand Oaks, CA: Sage; 2001.

23. Freedman VA. Late-life disability trends: An overview of current evidence. In: Field M, Jette A, Martin L, eds. *Workshop on Disability in America: A New Look.* Washington, DC: National Academies Press; 2006.

24. Freedman VA, Martin LG, Schoeni RF. Disability in America. *Popul Bull.* 2004;59:1-32.

25. Spillman BC. Changes in elderly disability rates and the implications for health care utilization and cost. *Milbank Q.* 2004;82:157-194.

26. Freedman VA, Crimmins E, Schoeni RF, et al. Resolving inconsistencies in trends in old-age disability: Report from a technical working group. *Demography.* 2004; 41:417-441.

27. Schoeni R, Freedman V, Martin L. Socioeconomic and demographic disparities in trends in old-age disability. University of Michigan Center for Demography of Aging Trends Network working paper series 05-01. Ann Arbor: University of Michigan Center for Demography of Aging Trends Network; 2004.

28. Schoeni R, Martin L, Andreski P, Freedman V. Persistent and growing socioeconomic disparities in disability among the elderly: 1982-2002. *Am J Publ Health.* 2005;95:2065-2070.

29. Hazzard WR. The gender differential in longevity. In: Hazzard WR, Blass JP, Ettinger WH, et al., eds. *Principles of Geriatric Medicine and Gerontology.* 4th ed. New York: McGraw-Hill; 1999.

30. Stibich M. Jeanne Calment, world's longest lived person. About.com Guide. Updated November 2, 2008. http:// longevity.about.com/ od/longevitylegends/a/jeanne_calment.htm. Accessed February 24, 2010.

31. Yashin AI, Begun AS, Boiko SI, et al. New age patterns of survival improvement in Sweden: Do they characterize changes in individual aging? *Mech Aging Dev.* 2002;123:637-647.

32. Wilmoth JR, Deegan LJ, Lundstrom H, Horiuchi S. Increase of maximum life span in Sweden, 1861-1999. *Science.* 2000;289:2366-2368.

33. Robine JM, Cheung SLK, Horiuchi S, Thatcher AR. Is the compression of morbidity a universal phenomenon? Paper presented at the Living to 100 and Beyond Symposium, Society of Actuaries, Orlando, January 7-9, 2008.

34. Westendorp RGJ. What is healthy aging in the 21st century? *Am J Clin Nutr.* 2006;83:404S-409S.

35. Manton KG, Vaupel JW. Survival after the age of 80 in the United States, Sweden, France, England, and Japan. *N Engl J Med.* 1995;333:1232-1235.

36. Vaupel JW. The remarkable improvements in survival at older ages. *Phil Trans R Soc Lond B.* 1997;352:1799-1804.

37. Kestenbaum B, Ferguson BR. Number of centenarians in the U.S. 1/1/1990, 1/1/200 and 1/1/2010 based on improved Medicare data. Paper presented at the Living to 100 and Beyond Symposium, Society of Actuaries, Orlando, January 7-9, 2008.

38. Kinsella K, Gist YJ. Gender and aging, mortality and health. International Brief, US Census Bureau, IB/98-2, October 1998.

39. World Health Organization. Maternal mortality ratio falling too slowly to meet goal (press release). http://www.who.int/mediacentre/news/releases/2007/pr56/en/print.html. Accessed February 18, 2010.

40. UC Atlas of Global Inequality. Gender bias and mortality. http://ucatlas.ucsc.edu/gender/gender_mortality.php. Accessed February 18, 2010.

41. Robinson K. *Trends in Health Status and Health Care Use Among Older Women.* Hyattsville, MD: National Center for Health Statistics; 2007.

42. DesMeules M, Turner L, Cho R. Morbidity experiences and disability among Canadian women. *BMC Women's Health.* 2004; 4(suppl 1): S10. doi: 10.1186/1472-6874-4-S1-S10.41.

43. Federal Interagency Forum on Aging Related Statistics. *Older Americans Update 2006: Key Indicators of Well-Being.* Washington, DC: USGPO; 2006.

44. US Census Bureau. Health status, health insurance, and health services utilization, 2001: household economic studies, 2006. http://www.census.gov/prod/2006pubs/p70-106.pdf. Accessed October 2009.

45. Bureau of Labor Statistics. Age of reference person: Average annual expenditures and characteristics. Consumer Expenditure Survey, 2004. http://www.bls.gov/cex/2004/Standard/age.pdf. Accessed October 2009.

46. Fogel RW. Forecasting the cost of U.S. health care in 2040. *J Policy Model.* 2009;31:482-488.

47. Congressional Budget Office. Baseline budget projections, baseline projections of mandatory spending. Table 1-4. http://www.cbo.gov/ftpdocs/105xx/doc10521/budgetprojections.pdf. Accessed February 24, 2010.

48. Thorpe KE, Ogden LL, Galactionova K. Chronic conditions account for rise in medicare spending from 1987 to 2006. *Health Affairs.* 2010;29. doi: 10.1377/hlthaff.2009.0474. Accessed February 24, 2010.

49. US Department of Health and Human Services. Exhibit 2.11. Estimated percentage of physician's time spent providing care to patients, by age of patient. Health Resources and Services Administration, Bureau of Health Professions website. http://bhpr.hrsa.gov/healthworkforce/reports/changedemo/images/2.11.htm. Accessed February 24, 2010.

50. Institute of Medicine, Committee on the Future Health Care Workforce for Older Americans. Retooling for an Aging America: Building the Health Care Workforce. Washington, DC: National Academies Press; 2008.

51. Keirns CC, Goold SD. Patient-centered care and preference-sensitive decision making. *JAMA.* 2009;302:1805-1806.

52. Harvard School of Public Health-MetLife Foundation Initiative on Retirement and Civic Engagement. Reinventing aging: Baby boomers and civic engagement. Center for Health Communication, Harvard School of Public Health. 2004. http://www.hsph.harvard.edu/chc/reinventingaging/Report.pdf. Accessed March 2, 2010.

53. Ministry of Foreign Affairs of Japan. 1997. http://www.mofa.go.jp/POLICY/economy/summit/1997/communique.html. Accessed October 2009.

54. Hayutin A. *Global Aging: The New New Thing: The Big Picture of Population Change.* Issued by SCL, November 2007.

55. Koehn PH, Swick HM. Medical education for a changing world: Moving beyond cultural competence. *Acad Med.* 2006;81:548-555.

56. United Nations. Trends in total migrant stock: The 2005 revision. 2005. http://www.un.org/esa/population/publications/2006_Migration Rep/part_one.pdf. Accessed October 2009.

57. Adams O, Kinnon C. *International Trade in Health Services: A Developmental Perspective.* Geneva: WHO; 1998.

58. Aki EA, Mustafa R, Bdair F, Schunemann HJ. The United States physician workforce and medical graduates: Trends and characteristics. *JGIM.* 2007;22:264-268.

59. Hing E, Lin S. Role of International Medical Graduates Providing Office-Based Medical Care: United States, 2005-2006. NCHS Data Brief no. 13, Hyattsville, MD: National Center for Health Statistics; 2009.

60. American Geriatrics Society Geriatrics Workforce Policy Study Center. Figure 3.2: Distribution of first year geriatric medicine fellows for AY 2001-2002 and 2008-2009. http://www.adgapstudy.uc.edu/figs_fellowship.cfm. Accessed March 2, 2010.

61. Garcia A. Immigration and long-term care. In: AARP International, Immigration: Challenges and Trends in the U.S. Labor Force. 2009. http://www.aarpinternational.org/resourcelibrary/resourcelibrary_show.htm?doc_id=805430. Accessed March 2, 2010.

62. Browne CV, Braune KL. Globalization, women's migration, and the long-term care workforce. *Gerontologist*. 2008;48:16-24.

63. Van de Water PN. Immigration and Social Security. Washington, DC: Center on Budget and Policy Priorities; 2008. http://www.cbpp.org/files/11-20-08socsec.pdf. Accessed March 1, 2010.

POST-TEST

1. **The stage of the *demographic transition* theory associated with decreased mortality but still high birth rate is:**
   A. Stage 1
   B. Stage 2
   C. Stage 3
   D. Stage 4

2. **Which of the following is FALSE regarding aging and gender?**
   A. Around the age of 55 or so, women begin to outnumber men due to gender differences in mortality.
   B. The difference between female and male longevity has been widening.
   C. Among *older* Americans, women with disabilities greatly outnumber disabled men.
   D. Men tend to have higher rates of acute hospitalization in both the United States and Canada.

3. **Migration between countries has serious consequences about the delivery of health care to the aging population. Which of the following is FALSE?**
   A. Immigration provides a younger workforce in the receiving countries.
   B. Most migrating workers into the health care workforce are nurses and physicians.
   C. In the United States, the long-term care industry relies heavily on *undocumented* workers.
   D. Europe has the largest number of international migrants.

ANSWERS TO PRE-TEST

1. B
2. A
3. B

ANSWERS TO POST-TEST

1. B
2. A
3. B

5

Cultural Competence in Geriatric Care

Margo-Lea Hurwicz, PhD

Nina Tumosa, PhD

● LEARNING OBJECTIVES

1. Describe the influence of culture/ethnicity on a person's health.
2. Discuss the impact of the following problem areas on clinical encounter: history, patient identification, and communication.
3. Explain important aspects of explanatory models and how this influences the patient experience.
4. Discuss strategies for culturally sensitive care.

PRE-TEST

1. **All of the following are aspects of explanatory models (EMs) EXCEPT:**
   A. Divine punishment
   B. Weather
   C. Body imbalance
   D. Disease always means illness

2. **Which of the following is FALSE regarding culture?**
   A. Biomedicine is a "culture."
   B. Everyone identifies with just one culture.
   C. Age and social class influence culture.
   D. Compliance is related to culture.

3. **Difficulties in assessing patient cultures include all of the following EXCEPT:**
   A. Inter-group variability in cultures
   B. Tendency to stereotype
   C. Viewing culture as an obstacle
   D. Secretiveness in some cultures

● INTRODUCTION

Patients are becoming empowered as never before, and demanding that health care be delivered in the context of the patient rather than in the context of the provider. Preventive medicine has become more accepted and expected. For older patients with chronic conditions, there are increasing expectations that they be allowed to stay at home and age in place much longer than providers have traditionally thought wise or even possible. Frail patients are asking for more home care, thereby delaying nursing home placement; assisted living options are expanding at a seemingly exponential rate; and nursing home placement is increasingly becoming a series of temporary moves rather than a single, irrevocable move. Indeed, we are entering an age where patient-centered care is becoming a mandate rather than an option.

This chapter will summarize how the cultural characteristics of both patients and providers have added new layers of complication to the already challenging job of providing good geriatric care. It will highlight lessons about cultural context that should be considered and applied when providing health care to the aging population. The ultimate goal of geriatric care providers is to provide good medical care to all older patients. This should be accomplished through collaboration between providers and the patients and their caregivers. We will address some of the barriers to accomplishing that goal that arise from cultural differences. We give examples of culture-related problem areas as well as suggestions on how to deal with them in the clinical encounter. Since there is great variability in the situations encountered in practice, this chapter will serve as a guide for problem-solving rather than as a list of solutions. It will introduce the topic of cultural competence.

● WHAT IS CULTURAL COMPETENCE?

Cultural competence has been defined by a medical anthropologist as the "ability to consider cultural factors in the prevention and treatment of disease; include[ing] the cultural influences on caregivers and patients."[1] *Culture*, according to the same author, is the "shared ideas characteristic of a given social group and the patterns of behavior that result from them."[1] Some of these ideas and behavior patterns are about the maintenance and restoration of health and well-being, and it is important to note that culture constantly changes. The context for these changes in the modern world often is *cultural diversity*, which occurs when many cultural backgrounds are represented in one setting; this term usually refers to members of different *ethnic groups* (individuals who share a sense of race, religion, national origin, or other cultural category[2]) who live in the same country, city, or community. The process by which these changes occur is the *acculturation* of individuals, the degree to which they incorporate the cultural values, beliefs, language, and skills of the mainstream culture[3] or of each other. Ethnic groups are often associated with poor health due to differential access to health care.[3]

Most medical educators have recognized the importance of cultural competence, which is "based on the premise of respect for individuals and cultural differences, and an implementation of a trust-promoting method of inquiry."[4] It is particularly important in geriatrics.

As further evidence that medical education and health care delivery establishments consider these matters important, the American Association of Medical Colleges defines the concept as follows[5]: "Cultural and linguistic competence in health care is a set of congruent behaviors, knowledge, attitudes, and policies that come together in a system, organization, or among professionals that enables effective work in cross-cultural situations." "Culture" refers to integrated patterns of human behavior that include the language, thoughts, actions, customs, beliefs, and institutions of racial, ethnic, social, or religious groups. "Competence" implies having the capacity to function effectively as an individual or an organization within the context of the cultural beliefs, practices, and needs presented by patients and their communities.

Cultural competence in health care combines the tenets of patient/family-centered care with an understanding of the social and cultural influences that affect the quality of medical services and treatment. With the ever-increasing diversity of the population of the United States and strong evidence of racial and ethnic disparities in health care, it is critically important that health care professionals are educated specifically to address issues of culture in an effective manner. Bodies such as the National Academy of Sciences' Institute of Medicine and the American Medical Association have recognized this.

The Liaison Committee on Medical Education (LCME) and the Committee on Accreditation of Canadian Medical Schools (CACMS) believe that aspiring physicians will be best prepared for medical practice in a diverse society if they learn in an environment characterized by, and supportive of, diversity and inclusion. Such an environment will facilitate physician training in:

- Basic principles of culturally competent health care
- Recognition of health care disparities and the development of solutions to such burdens
- The importance of meeting the health care needs of medically underserved populations
- The development of core professional attributes, such as altruism and social accountability, needed to provide effective care in a multidimensionally diverse society[6]

● WHY CULTURAL COMPETENCE IN GERIATRIC PRACTICE?

A laudable goal for all health professionals is to develop increasing awareness of cultural differences and to address them appropriately in the context of providing good health care. This goal is not easily achieved because culture is constantly changing. Thus, the potential for misunderstanding multiplies during interactions between members of different cultural groups. Complicating such interactions even more are cultural differences between generations of people with ostensibly the same cultural background, and differences within those generations based on gender. These differences highlight the fluid nature of culture and remind us that any strategies we create to recognize and address cultural differences in the clinical encounter need to acknowledge the possible existence of these natural changes, even if we do not address them.

Everyone has a culture, and most people have more than one culture. Both providers and patients have their own cultures, which include their ethnic/national/religious culture of origin as well as the results of their exposure (and acculturation) to other ethnic/national cultures over their lifetimes. In addition, providers have the culture of biomedicine in general and of their specific profession (medicine, nursing, therapy, pharmacy, etc.). Finally, both providers and patients have cultural ideas and values that relate to their social class, age cohort, and/or gender.

This chapter will concentrate on cultural differences that exist between older patients and their (usually) younger health care providers (Box 5–1). There are many potential sources of cultural differences between the aging population and their health care providers. The age differential is the most obvious source. The normal challenges of navigating the culture of biomedicine are daunting enough for any adult. They are exacerbated for older adults with physical, mental, and social limitations. The burden that chronic disease puts on older persons when accessing medical support in a timely and appropriate manner is often underappreciated by younger providers. The health care providers have their own challenges when applying their culture of biomedicine to an aging population. They include communicating effectively, providing evidence-based medicine in a timely manner, and developing new health services that target older adults' changing medical needs.

The other large source of cultural differences is the ethnic/national culture of the health care provider (Box 5–2). When cultural differences also exist between older patients and their younger providers, the delivery of optimal health care is even less likely[7] and requires special training. One such Web-based program can be accessed through the Communication and Cultural Competence Program at http://www.img-ccc.ca or through the Canadian Information Centre for International Medical Graduates at http://www.img-canada.ca.

Patients' cultures will influence when they seek treatment, what they expect of care, and whether they will comply with providers' recommendations.[8] Because patient–provider communication is linked to patient satisfaction and the likelihood of compliance with medical instructions,[9,10] poor health outcomes may result if cultural differences are not anticipated,

understood, and addressed. Cultural competence can help providers improve health care delivery in the clinical encounter. It can lead to better provider–patient communication, more accurate diagnosis, more effective treatment, higher patient satisfaction/compliance, and more efficient use of medical resources.

In the past, when dealing with cultural issues it was common to consider the national or ethnic cultures of patients as a source of obstacles to compliance. The impact of the culture of biomedicine on provider–patient communication[1,11] was often ignored. It was thought that medicine had no culture and that students brought no culture to their training (or lost it in school). But providers do bring their cultures with them to the clinical encounter, and current thinking is that they should regularly engage in self-reflection and self-critique. Now cultural competence is becoming a part of general medical competence. Being aware of the potential for culture-related problems in the clinical encounter is the first step in developing strategies to deal with those problems when they arise.

CULTURE-RELATED PROBLEM AREAS THAT MAY AFFECT THE CLINICAL ENCOUNTER

History and Context

Context may be personal or social. The personal context is what each participant—provider or patient—brings to the encounter, based on prior experience. Both may be unaware that their own ethnic or professional culture is influencing the interaction. The social context includes the knowledge and power differential between the patient and the provider.

Patients may distrust their providers based on their own or significant others' previous encounters with biomedicine. The best known example of this in the United States is the distrust engendered in the African American community by the Tuskegee Syphilis Study in which patients identified as

---

● BOX 5–2 How to Assess Your Cultures (Yes, Plural) and the Effect They May Have on Your Practice

The Provider's Guide to Quality and Culture on the Management Sciences for Health website[12] has a "quality and culture quiz" you can take to assess your "start value" for cultural competence. Although the content is not geared exclusively to geriatric practice, this quiz can help you assess what you already know about the potential effect of culture on the clinical encounter.

There are several barriers to developing successful strategies. They include the impossibility of learning about every cultural or ethnic group that might be encountered. Even if it were possible, intra-cultural variation could make it difficult to be sure that what was learned would be relevant to any given patient. There is a real possibility that relying on cultural stereotypes for guidance could result in conflict with patients who might not conform to the conventional wisdom about their group. Also, there remains the danger that culture will be viewed as an obstacle to be overcome, rather than another aspect of the patients' situation (like their history and symptoms), the knowledge of which will help the provider deliver better care.

● BOX 5–1 How to Learn About the Ethnic and National Cultures of Your Patients

There are websites where you can get *a priori* (before working with patients) information about specific cultural, ethnic, and national groups. The culture-specific modules available on the Stanford Ethnogeriatrics website[13] are among the best available. Although these resources are no substitute for asking the patient about his or her unique situation, they are a good place to start to learn about a culture that is completely new to you.

Thus, cultural competence is more a process than an outcome; it is as much about attitude as it is about knowledge. To assist in this process, the following section lists a number of common problems that may arise in clinical encounters between people with different cultural experiences. The next section provides general strategies for addressing these problem areas.

having syphilis were not treated following the discovery of antibiotics that could cure syphilis. It has taken decades for trust in medicine to be restored.[14,15]

Providers may view patients' ethnic cultures as an obstacle based on experience with members of a group. For example, Afghani Muslim women may not be treated by a male doctor. A husband may try to describe his wife's symptoms to his physician in an effort to get advice on how to treat her. If the physician were unaware that the problem was one of gender differences, he might simply refuse to give advice by proxy, when instead he could successfully refer the wife to a female physician.

Providers may also be unaware that members of many ethnic, national origin, or religious groups do not yet feel empowered to express their needs in the clinical encounter. These patients may view the provider as all-powerful and all-knowing, and therefore defer to him or her as a sign of respect. This does not mean that they will follow all the recommendations, however.

Identifying the Patient

Misunderstanding who the patient is may occur because the Western biomedical culture focuses on the individual, and health care is predicated on the idea that the person with the symptoms (the name on the chart) is the patient. In fact, there are many cultures in which the family, or even the entire community, plays a major part in managing illness. This makes it likely that third parties will want to be included in the interview and examination.

Even in Western culture, it is not uncommon for spouses and/or adult children to participate in the clinical encounter, especially when an older patient is involved. Geriatrics has been referred to as a team sport. The central members of that geriatric team are the patient and his or her family. Indeed, providers have found that actively enlisting the family in treatment modalities is often helpful in the acute phase of depression in older men.[16] Therefore, trying to exclude the family could lead to problems. On the other hand, it is important to avoid the "invisible patient" scenario—where the providers and family talk past/around the older patient.

A word of caution must be added here. The health care provider must walk a fine line between respecting the wishes of the patient and those of the family members, especially when there is disagreement. The bottom line is that the family member whose name is on the medical directive must be consulted first and foremost. It is often wise to include all family members in the decision-making process, but the person with power of attorney is the one who has the final word. When there is no power of attorney document, the provider must be careful to take the patient's social support network into account. The child who comes to town to visit annually probably knows less about the patient's physical and mental capacity than the child who lives with the patient. Moreover, the person who takes the patient to medical appointments may not the one who normally cares for the patient. This person may be someone who provides only transportation or caregiver respite time. When in doubt, ask who will be the person most likely to aid the patient with medical compliance issues and how this person may be reached.

Communication

Communication may be verbal or nonverbal, and it is important to use both verbal and nonverbal cues in order to minimize miscommunication. When the patient and the provider do not speak the same language, it is very important to acquire the services of a professional interpreter whenever possible.[4]

Verbal

While the availability of professional interpreters (or lack thereof) falls under the control of the institution, providers should remember that misinterpretations may occur even when the same language is spoken. Providers tend to mix medical jargon and everyday language when they speak to patients, but a word may mean something different to the patient than the provider intended. For example, the provider might ask, "Do you have pain in your stomach?" Some patients refer to their entire abdominal cavity as their "stomach" and so might say "yes" when they have lower abdominal pain. This could lead to misinterpretation of symptoms by the provider, and misunderstanding of treatment by the patient.

Nonverbal

Patients with different cultural backgrounds may have different ways of expressing distress.[17] Some value stoicism while others value the open expression of pain.[2] As a result, a provider from a stoic cultural background could easily mistake culturally appropriate expressiveness for hypochondria. Or, a Japanese or Thai patient might smile or laugh to mask other, more negative emotions, and as a result, the provider might miss underlying fear or pain.

Other potentially problematic areas of nonverbal communication between persons with different cultural backgrounds include the pace of conversation (slow or fast with interruptions); physical proximity (arm's length or closer/farther away); and eye contact (appropriate, disrespectful, or even hostile). The etiquette of touch, hand gestures, and finger pointing also varies across cultures.[2,13] Finally, there is variability in attitudes toward the direct discussion of death and dying (whether discussion is appropriate or not).[2]

For example, a provider may notice that some Hispanic patients keep trying to move closer, and interrupt when the provider tries to speak, while other, Asian patients keep edging farther away and tend to remain silent even when the provider expects a verbal response. A sense of interpersonal discomfort in the clinical encounter might be the result of nonverbal communication that is poorly understood. These uncomfortable situations might be avoided by observing and taking cues from the patients' behavior.

Explanatory Models

While *disease* is defined in biomedicine as "abnormalities in the structure and function of organs and bodily systems," *illness* may be defined as "the patient's subjective experience of physical or mental states, whether based on some underlying disease pathology or not." The term *sickness* is used to refer to both disease and illness.[17]

Explanatory models (EMs) are "the notions about an episode of sickness and its treatment that are employed by all those engaged in the clinical process." EMs typically provide explanations for five aspects of the episode: etiology/cause, timing/onset of symptoms, pathophysiology, natural history/severity, and appropriate treatments.[17]

The way patients and providers understand the nature of illness and/or disease may be different at best and incompatible at worst. Providers and patients may differ greatly in how they interpret/understand and explain a particular episode, with respect to its cause (etiology and onset), diagnosis (pathophysiology and label), appropriate treatment, and prognosis. Providers may not accept patients' supernatural (divine punishment) and interpersonal (hexing) or even alternative physical (imbalance in *qi*, chakras) causes as explanations for etiology or onset. Patients' understanding of the structure and function of the body may differ from what the provider has learned. They may not accept the idea that their suffering is caused by something they cannot see (bacteria or viruses). They may have ideas about the best way to treat the symptoms they perceive, including modalities now recognized by some as complementary and alternative medicine (CAM). Providers may ignore relevant aspects of the situation, especially its meaning to the patient and family, because these are not aspects of the biomedical model of disease. Ultimately, patient compliance with provider recommendations may be compromised because of these incongruities.

For example, some Hispanic immigrants to southern California think breast cancer is a result of spousal abuse or rough sex ("a blow to the breast"). Most providers would disagree. If a woman thinks the diagnosis means she has (or has had in the past) a bad or shameful marriage, she might resist it.[18] A study of veterans in the American Northwest revealed that many of them viewed a diagnosis of hypertension as indicating a combination of being "hyper" and "tense" in the colloquial sense of these words. Their etiologic explanations made it difficult for providers to impress upon them the underlying physiology and the need to continue their medication in the absence of symptoms.[19] The prevalence of weather-related explanations for arthritis flare-ups and folk remedies to deal with them among members of a Medicare HMO in Los Angeles contrasted with the explanations and recommended treatments of their physicians, making communication difficult.[20]

Illness may be present without disease, and disease may be present without illness. Modern technology used during routine screenings may lead to a diagnosis where there are no symptoms. As suggested earlier, if a patient feels fine, it may be difficult to convince the patient to take medications to keep cholesterol or hypertension under control. Or a patient may not feel good, but the provider can find nothing wrong. The diagnosis may be "psychosomatic" or "subclinical," and the danger is that treatable problems may be missed. Subsequent visits may result in the same outcome: the patient may continue to believe that he or she is ill and so leaves the encounter feeling dissatisfied and distrustful. The patient's perception of symptoms is still a symptom that needs to be addressed; an opportunity may be missed to help the patient and gain his or her trust.

Treatment recommendations that do not make sense in terms of the patient's explanatory model may be rejected and ignored. All aspects—purpose, form, speed of action, duration, side effects—must be explained clearly because noncompliance and dissatisfaction are likely to result if the treatment is not well understood. With older adults, conflict may arise if the family feels the proposed treatment is extreme or unnecessary. Patients may not understand the chronic nature of some conditions and therefore resist a recommendation to continue on a medication once the symptoms of a flare-up have resolved (eg, diabetes, heart disease). What is considered successful by the provider may differ from what is considered successful by the patient.

On the other hand, providers sometimes fail to recommend or endorse treatments that are expected or requested by the patient. For example, they may reject culturally familiar CAM treatments that could help, or at least not harm, the patient. They may even recommend discontinuing the annual repetition of screening tests that have yielded negative results in the patient for several consecutive years. They may refuse to prescribe antibiotics requested for colds and the flu.

Stereotyping

Cultural

A provider may have acquired some general background knowledge about a cultural group, and as a result be tempted to think he or she has all the culturally relevant information needed about a specific patient or family. While it is useful to learn about the background, values, and behavioral tendencies of cultural groups in the institution's geographic area, this is not enough. It is important to understand that there is variation within cultural groups. There is no substitute for asking the patient what his or her treatment goals are. For example, a provider may have read about or experienced Asian or Hispanic male dominance. The provider therefore may assume that talking or forming a therapeutic alliance with a wife or adult daughter will not lead to compliance if the husband or father does not understand or agree. This may be true, but some women have achieved autonomy and some men have learned to rely on their female relatives for help in decision-making as a result of acculturation. A provider may have treated very religious African American patients in the past, or may have read that African Americans tend to be religious. The provider therefore may assume that their religious beliefs will be more important than health outcomes, or that prayer will figure prominently in any successful treatment plan. Again, this may be true, but there also are many African Americans who are not religious. Problems may arise when a provider does not ask what does *this* patient really think; what does he or she expect from this encounter; what is the desired outcome?

A patient may also make assumptions about her provider's ethnicity or cultural background, sometimes in surprising ways. For example, an African American patient may request a white male doctor, because the patient feels "they have better training." In one study, it was found that African American primary-care physicians often failed to screen for depression, suggesting that they were culturally predisposed to avoid discussing stigmatized mental health issues.[21] Patients may be aware of cultural barriers to optimal care.

Further, patients often make assumptions about the culture of medicine and its effect on medical decisions: "You are just ordering those tests because you will make more money from them."

Age

The nature of aging may be stereotyped by younger (than the patient) health care providers. This may lead to the decision not to begin treatment (therapeutic nihilism), especially in emergencies such as stroke or traumatic brain injury. However, it is well accepted that nihilism is not an effective treatment strategy.[22] Providers may exaggerate the meaning/impact of functional differences and the sequelae of chronic illnesses and disabilities that increase with age, and therefore neglect to recommend lifestyle changes involving good nutrition and exercise that might help patients continue to live independently for decades. Physicians sometimes decide not to urge patients to quit smoking because they think that if 50 years of smoking has not killed them, then 55 won't either. The evidence for the debilitating effects of smoking has caused the US Veterans Administration to make it a priority to ask every patient at every visit whether he or she smokes and whether he or she wishes to quit.[2,23]

Older patients may disregard the expert advice of health care professionals who are significantly younger than they are (reverse stereotyping) because they feel that the provider does not understand aging due to a lack of personal experience. This may be particularly true when the recommendation is something that restricts the patient's independence, such as stopping driving or beginning to use a cane or a walker.[2]

● SOME SOLUTIONS TO CULTURE-RELATED PROBLEMS IN THE CLINICAL ENCOUNTER

Increase Self-Awareness

Remember that you bring an ethnic and/or national culture with you to the clinical encounter, along with your professional culture. Remember that communication is a two-way street: You too may have ideas that could get in the way of an effective alliance with your patient. Try not to see their culture as merely a problem to be overcome.

CASE PRESENTATION 1: SELF-AWARENESS AND CULTURAL SENSITIVITY

A cancer patient of African descent tells you, "God will decide if I am meant to live." She goes on to tell you that prayer will be the best medicine for her condition and that she will not be making another appointment to see you. You have heard that African Americans are very religious, and that this sometimes gets in the way

of adherence to treatment recommendations. Your training in oncology leads you to believe that a course of aggressive treatment (chemotherapy and/or radiation) would most likely result in a significant increase in life expectancy, and your own religious beliefs do not extend to replacing medical care with prayer. You find yourself feeling annoyed with the patient. You are busy and this appointment is taking longer than scheduled. You know what is best in this case, and you wish the patient would just trust you and follow your advice.

How would you deal with this situation? How could you enlist the patient's family and other members of her religious community to allow each of you to better understand the other's point of view and perhaps allow her to accept your recommendation?

First, you could try to avoid letting the patient see that you are annoyed. You could acknowledge that her beliefs, although not the same as your own, are valid. You could remind yourself that she is scared and that people often turn to religion in times of stress. You could try to point out that her religion might not really suggest that she do nothing beyond prayer, and that she could talk to her minister about what God would want her to do. It could also be helpful to tell her that you would be happy to talk with her minister about topics that she has approved, with her explicit consent, whether they are diagnosis, prognosis, or religious expectations. You could offer to schedule another appointment to meet with her and her family to explain the course of treatment you propose and listen to their concerns. Finally, there are quotations from the Bible that support the idea that medical treatment and prayer are not incompatible, and you could keep a list of these passages on hand if you will be dealing with members of this population on a regular basis.

Would you respond differently if hospice were your recommendation? Members of some conservative Christian groups feel that only God can decide when someone is to die. They take the admonition that "God helps the man who helps himself" literally, and therefore ask that everything possible be done to maintain life, even in the face of overwhelming biomedical evidence that such efforts would be futile and expensive.[24]

In cases such as this, an ethicist should be consulted from the very beginning, as expectations of an easy resolution would be unrealistic. Most hospitals have ethics committees that must be consulted. If not, then a neutral party, acceptable to both the medical staff and the family, should be asked to mediate conversations between the family, family members, and medical staff. Sometimes it is the religious beliefs of medical staff members that are in conflict with the family's religious beliefs and this leads to conflict. In this case, the staff member should not be ignored, but also should be included in the decision making process, as far as the family allows.

Be Culturally Sensitive, and Avoid Stereotyping

Although it helps to familiarize yourself with information about the cultural groups you are most likely to deal with regularly in your institutional setting, superficial knowledge of a culture may lead to stereotyping. Insensitivity can result from making assumptions about older patients' cultures as easily as it can from ignoring their cultures completely.[2] Not all patients identify strongly with their ethnic culture. Educational level, dominant language, religion, gender, year of immigration, and even personality may have more of an effect on interactions with health care providers that cultural identity.[25] The only way to find out what you need to know about the influence of patients' culture on their health is to ask them directly and listen carefully to what they have to say.

In the case example, the patient already made it clear that her religion is influencing her decisions, but it would be a mistake to assume all African American patients are religious. That is, it would not be a good idea to launch into quotations from the Bible before finding out if your patient would be likely to respond positively.

If a patient similar to the one discussed in the case refused to undergo surgery to treat her cancer, you might assume that this decision also is based on religion. In fact, the patient may be afraid of surgery or may have automatically refused the surgery because one of her parents or siblings died during a similar surgery. In order to know the real reason for the rejection of suggested treatments it is necessary to ask the patient about his or her reasons for refusing care and to discuss those reasons until you both understand all options and consequences. It might be possible to suggest chemotherapy or radiation therapy instead.

Improve Communication

Assessment Mnemonics

Over the years, a number of mnemonics for remembering how to conduct an effective patient interview have appeared in the literature.

LEARN suggests that you Listen with sympathy and understanding to the patient's perception of the problem; Explain your perception of the problem; Acknowledge and discuss the differences and similarities; Recommend treatment; and Negotiate (if your recommendation is not accepted).[26] Of concern is that some patients do not tell you that they will not follow your recommendation, so beyond listening carefully, it is important to pay attention to the nonverbal cues.

ETHNIC refers to Explanation (How do you explain your illness?); Treatment (What treatment have you tried?); Healers (Have you sought any advice from folk healers?); Negotiate (mutually acceptable options); Intervention (agreed on); and Collaboration (with patient, family and healers).[27]

The original eight questions for eliciting a patient Explanatory Model (EM), also known as Kleinman's questions,[28] are still used in many contexts, although Kleinman has more recently published an amendment to his recommendations.[25] Other recently published models of effective cross-cultural communication and negotiation and their sources can be found in the Association of American Medical Colleges' Cultural Competence Curriculum,[5] including a Model for Cultural Competency in Health Care,[29] and a "Review of Systems" domains of the Social Context.[30]

What is perhaps more important than any specific mnemonic is to find one that helps you conduct a culturally sensitive patient interview as part of every clinical encounter.

Understand Nonverbal Cues

Communication goes beyond language and medical jargon. Make sure your patient understands what you are saying, especially when you use technical terms, and equally important, make sure that you understand your patient. A "stomach" is not always a stomach; some patients refer to the entire abdominal cavity as their stomach, but if you watch their hands when they talk about it, you may notice where they are pointing while they speak.

Try to be aware of nonverbal signals: Patients may say "yes" while shaking their head "no," or they may use different gestures than you do to mean yes and no. It is important to take nonverbal cues from the patient whenever possible, and ask for clarification if they are doing something you do not understand. Remembering the mnemonic PPPP ("P4") might be useful: Patient Picks Place (to sit) and Pace (of conversation). If you will be dealing with a particular group on a regular basis, you might want to learn more about that group. The Stanford University Ethnogeriatrics[13] Modules are a very good place to start, but keep the dangers of stereotyping in mind.

Use Professional Interpreters When Possible

You may find it advisable to engage a professional interpreter, or to use translated written materials if you do not speak the same language as your patients. Of course, available services will vary depending on your practice/institutional setting. It is a good idea to familiarize yourself with local policies/resources, and if interpretation services are unavailable, to advocate for them. In the absence of a program at your institution, both DiversityRx[4] and Ethnomed[31] provide useful advice.

Although it may be tempting to ask for help from a young relative who accompanies your patient, this is seldom advisable.[4] Children as interpreters are especially problematic, as they often do not have the experience to understand what their older relatives are talking about, even in their own language. However, there will be times when any communication at all is better than none.

Treat Both Illness and Disease If You Can

Understand that illness is distinct from disease, and treat both if you can. Medical interviewing across cultural identities requires taking the time to get a complete illness narrative that includes the patient's explanatory model.[17,25] You will need to collect information about the level of patient/family comprehension and acceptance of the diagnosis, understanding and support of the treatment plan, any concerns about the treatment (including cost and side effects), and alternative suggestions about how to accomplish the treatment (such as CAM practices). Attention to these issues will help you estimate the likelihood of patient compliance and achieve an outcome that all deem successful.

CASE PRESENTATION 2: TREATING BOTH ILLNESS AND DISEASE WHILE BEING CULTURALLY SENSITIVE

A husband tells you about his wife, "She doesn't have Alzheimer's. She's had a stressful life and she's just a bit forgetful like most people her age." You realize, after listening carefully to the husband's story, that the diagnosis of Alzheimer disease is stigmatized in this family's community, considered equivalent to "being crazy," and has implications for how the patient's children and grandchildren will be treated. Their marriage prospects may even be affected. The family caregivers sincerely believe that memory loss is a part of natural aging, perhaps exacerbated by traumatic migration-related events ("a hard life"). You would like to recommend medication, modification of the patient's home to make it safer (to avoid elopement, accidents, elder abuse), and respite/day care (the husband and adult daughter are showing signs of stress).

What would you say to the husband and daughter? How could you make medical treatment and other recommendations more acceptable when the patient and her family are resisting the diagnosis for cultural reasons?

This situation is likely to be found when the patient is of Hispanic or Asian origin. If you are working in a community where the patient's group is concentrated, the local chapter of the Alzheimer's Association most likely sponsors caregiver support groups tailored for members of their ethnic/national origin group. A referral to the Alzheimer's Association is a good first step, because the family members will learn that they are not alone if they participate. Under these circumstances, it might be more effective to suggest this to an adult child, in this case the daughter, because she is likely to have become more acculturated than the father has, and therefore might be more willing to accept the idea that dementia is a disease that can and should be treated. The family also will be able to find out about locally available respite care through the Association. Although acceptance of medication may come more slowly, involvement in a caregiver support group will most likely expose them to other cases where medications have helped.[37] If the family continues to reject a diagnosis of dementia, a referral to a support group for a different disease, such as heart disease or stroke, will still provide both patient and family members with much-needed support.

Promote Health

Good nutrition and exercise, as well as other lifestyle-related changes such as smoking cessation, are the cornerstones of successful aging for all of your patients. Cultural differences in the perception of what is a good diet[33-36] or the proper amount or form of exercise[37,38] may be difficult to address, but it will be worth the effort.

CASE PRESENTATION 3: PROMOTING HEALTH WHILE BEING CULTURALLY SENSITIVE WITHOUT STEREOTYPING

An older woman from Bangladesh presents with a history and symptoms that suggest she has adult-onset diabetes. In addition to medication, you would like to recommend a change in diet (more fresh fruits and vegetables; less saturated fat, salt, and sugar) and exercise or physical activity patterns (taking a walk around the neighborhood every day). But the woman feels she must cook the traditional foods from her homeland for her husband, and as a Muslim woman, she should not be seen sweating or moving quickly in public. Besides, the neighborhood is not safe.

These are very difficult issues to address. First, you will need to distinguish the cultural from the structural barriers to compliance. If you hear "we don't like the taste of the foods you say are healthy," or "we consider baked and grilled meats indigestible," that is cultural. But if there are very few (or no) fresh fruits and vegetables available in the neighborhood, that is structural. If you hear "fast walking and sweating are considered unseemly for an older woman," that is cultural. But if the neighborhood has no sidewalks and/or is unsafe, that is structural. You can't change the living situation.

What would you say to this woman? How could you persuade her to change her cooking habits or ingredients and get some exercise (or engage in some physical activity) that produces sweat?

You could start with not blaming her for her seeming inability to take the initiative in changing her family's diet. She may have very little to say in the matter. You could offer to make another appointment at which you could explain to her husband and sons that she has diabetes and must change what she eats. You could ask her to describe the family's typical menu and look for small changes that might improve her health. If she tells you that women eat separately from (and after) the men, you might suggest that she prepare different food for herself. She could keep elements of the meal, such as sauces, separate. If you will be working with members of her group in future, you could learn what the dietary issues are, and work with allied health professionals to acquire or develop materials with concrete suggestions for dietary change. Or, you could refer diabetes patients to a dietician on staff if there is one available where you work.

Similarly, you could ask the patient to describe her activities on typical day and look for ways to increase her physical activity. She may be able to walk up and down stairs instead of taking an elevator. She may be able to walk with other women. Greenhalgh and colleagues[33] suggest the use of home exercise videos for successfully encouraging increased physical activity among Muslim women, which nicely circumvents the aversion to public perspiration. In particular, the recent availability of the Wii system with its varied exercise software has made home-based exercise programs more fun and, hopefully, more successful for those who can afford it.

● RESOURCES

Cultural competence is a powerful strategy that health care providers can use to help reduce the negative impact of cultural differences on health outcomes. The following is a partial list of Web-based resources that may be useful. A more complete list can be accessed through search engines using key words such as cultural competence, cultural diversity, explanatory model, health promotion programs, and disease self-management.

Cultural Competence in Health Care

http://www.diversityrx.org

The Diversity Rx website promotes language and cultural competence to improve the quality of health care for minority, immigrant, and ethnically diverse communities.[4] It describes how language and culture affect the delivery of quality services to ethnically diverse populations, and provides resources to enable providers to learn about language and cultural competence in health care, design better programs and policies, and network with colleagues and experts.

http://www.hretdisparities.org

The Web-based Health Research and Educational Trust Disparities Toolkit provides guidance on how to collect patient race, ethnicity, and primary language data.[39] The free toolkit provides users with resources on how to collect data from patients, how to do staff training, and how to address legal and privacy concerns. The toolkit identifies the patient's preferred method of communication, any potential language barriers, and the patient's culture. With this information, the provider can enlist any outside assistance needed to ensure proper patient–provider communication.

http://www.Ethnomed.org

EthnoMed focuses on information about cultural beliefs, medical issues, and other related issues pertinent to the health care of recent immigrants to Seattle, Washington or to other parts of the United States, many of whom are refugees fleeing war-torn parts of the world.[31] It offers videos in many languages on basic medical history-taking with interpreters. Hyperlinks on this site may be useful when provider and patient languages differ.

http://www.stanford.edu/group/ethnoger/index.html

The Stanford University Ethnogeriatric Modules website offers a comprehensive curriculum in the health care of elders from diverse ethnic populations for training in all health care disciplines.[13] It contains modules on patterns of health risk, culturally appropriate knowledge, care, and interventions. Ten ethnic-specific modules are also available.

Health Promotion Programs

http://www.move.va.gov/

MOVE! is a national weight management program designed by the Veterans Administration.[40] This program is designed to help veterans lose weight, keep it off, and improve their health. The entire program, from philosophy to handouts, from motivational messages to references, can be found on the Internet and is free. The website has sections for both patients and providers in English and in Spanish. There is a simply stated patient-recruitment message about why this program in important to health and well-being, followed by questionnaires to help patients determine their degree of readiness to participate in the program. Multiple handouts address barriers that patients may face such as depression, lack of time, and boredom. These handouts offer solutions to those barriers.

There are instructions to providers about how to administer the patient questionnaire and how to run successful group sessions. Reference tools are well labeled and accessible and include discipline-specific information on such topics as nutrition, physical activity, medications, and surgery. This program was originally designed to be promoted by providers to the patients and was so successful that the top administrators of the VA promoted it to all of the employees of the VA nationwide. Now one more layer of promotion has been added that would serve as a model for worldwide success. The President of the United States has declared a national President's Challenge to encourage all Americans to be more active and increase their fitness levels.

Chronic Disease Self-Management Program

http://patienteducation.stanford.edu/ programs/cdsmp.html

The Chronic Disease Self-Management Program (CDSMP), developed at Stanford University, is a workshop given for 2½ hours, once a week, for 6 weeks, in community settings such as senior centers, churches, libraries, and hospitals.[41] People with different chronic health problems attend together. Workshops are facilitated by two trained leaders, one or both of whom are non–health-care professionals with a chronic diseases themselves. Subjects covered include (1) techniques to deal with problems such as frustration, fatigue, pain, and isolation; (2) appropriate exercise for maintaining and improving strength, flexibility, and endurance; (3) appropriate use of medications; (4) communicating effectively with family, friends, and health care professionals; (5) nutrition; and (6) how to evaluate new treatments.

It is the process by which the program is taught that makes it effective. Classes are highly participative, where mutual support and success build the participants' confidence in their ability to manage their health and maintain active and fulfilling lives. Each participant in the workshop receives a copy of the companion book, *Living a Healthy Life with Chronic Conditions*, 3rd edition, and an audio relaxation tape, Time for Healing.

The CDSMP Leader's Manual is available in Arabic, Bengali, Chinese, Dutch, German, Hindi, Italian, Japanese, Korean, Norwegian, Somali, Spanish, Turkish, Vietnamese, and Welsh.

References

1. Joralemon D. *Exploring Medical Anthropology*. 2nd ed. Boston: Pearson; 2006.

2. Haber D. *Health Promotion and Aging: Practical Applications for Health Professionals*. 4th ed. New York: Springer; 2007.

3. Institute of Medicine. *Crossing the Quality Chasm: A New Health System for the 21st Century*. Washington, DC: National Academies Press; 2001.

4. Diversity Rx. http://www.diversityrx.org. Accessed July 2009.

5. Cultural Competence Education. http://www.aamc.meded/taact/culturalcomped.pdf. Accessed July 2009.

6. LCME. http://www.lcme.org/functions2008jun.pdf. Accessed March 19, 2010.

7. Lax LL, Russell ML, Nelles LJ, Smith CM. Scaffolding knowledge building in a Web-based communication and cultural competence program for international medical graduates. *Acad Med*. 2009; 84(suppl):S5-S8.

8. Berger JT. Culture and ethnicity in clinical care. *Arch Intern Med*. 1998;159:2085-2090.

9. Ibrahim SA, Whittle J, Bean-Mayberry B, et al. Racial/ethnic variations in physician recommendations for cardiac revascularization. *Am J Public Health*. 2003;93:1689-1693.

10. Rucker-Whitaker C, Feinglass J, Pearce WH. Explaining racial variation in lower extremity amputation. *Arch Surg*. 2003;138:1347-1351.

11. Taylor J. Confronting "culture" in medicine's "culture of no culture." *Acad Med*. 2003;78:555-559.

12. Quality and Culture Quiz. The Providers Guide to Quality and Culture. http://erc.msh.org/mainpage.cfm?file=1.0.htm&module=provider&language=English.

13. Stanford Ethnogeriatrics curriculum. http://www.Stanford.edu/ethnoger/index.hml. Accessed July 2009.

14. Gamble VN. Under the shadow of Tuskegee: African Americans and health care. *Am J Pub Health*. 1997;87:1773-1778.

15. Katz RV, Green BL, Kressin NR, et al. Exploring the "legacy" of the Tuskegee Syphilis Study: A follow-up study from the Tuskegee Legacy Project. *J Natl Med Assoc*. 2009;101:179-183.

16. Apesoa-Varano EC, Hinton L, Barker JC, Unützer J. Clinician approaches and strategies for engaging older men in depression care. *Am J Geriatr Psych*. 2010. doi: 10.1097/JGP.0b013e3181d145ea

17. Helman CG. *Culture, Health and Illness*. 5th ed. London: Hodder Arnold; 2007.

18. Chavez L. Structure and meaning in models of breast and cervical cancer risk factors. *Med Anthropol Q*. 1995;9:40-74.

19. Blumhagen D. The meaning of hyper-tension. In: Chrisman NJ, Maretzki TW, eds. *Clinically Applied Anthropology*. Dordrecht, The Netherlands: D. Reidel; 1982:297-333.

20. Hurwicz M. Lifestyle considerations in physician and patient explanatory models of arthritis. Presented to the Gerontological Society of America, San Diego, 2003.

21. Tai-Seale M, Bramson R, Drukker D, et al. Understanding primary care physicians' propensity to assess elderly patients for depression using interaction and survey data. *Med Care*. 2005;43:1217-1224.

22. Hempill JC III, White DB. Clinical nihilism in neuroemergencies. *Emerg Med Clin North Am*. 2010;27:27-37.

23. Sherman SE, Yano EM, Lanto AB, et al. Smokers' interest in quitting and services received: Using practice information to plan quality improvement and policy for smoking cessation. *Am J Med Qual*. 2005;20:33-39.

24. Hornung C, Eleazer P, Strothers HS, et al. Ethnicity and decision-makers in a group of frail elders. *J Am Geriatr Soc*. 1998;46: 280-286.

25. Kleinman A, Benson P. Anthropology in the clinic: The problem of cultural competency and how to fix it. *PLoS Med*. 2006;3:e294.

26. Berlin EA, Fowkes WC. A teaching framework for cross-cultural health care. *West J Med*. 1983;139:934-938.

27. Levin SJ, Like RC, Gottlieb JE. ETHNIC: A framework for culturally competent ethical practice. *Patient Care*. 2000;34:188-189.

28. Kleinman A, Eisenberg L, Good B. Culture, illness, and care: Clinical lessons from anthropologic and cross-cultural research. *Ann Intern Med*. 1978;88:251-258.

29. Flores G. Culture and the patient-physician relationship: Achieving cultural competency in health care. *J Pediatr*. 2000;136:14-23.

30. Green, AR, Betancourt, JR, Carrillo, JE. Integrating social factors into cross-cultural medical education. *Acad Med*. 2002;77: 193-197.

31. EthnoMed. http://www.Ethnomed.org. 2009. Accessed June 2009.

32. Henderson JN. Dementia in cultural context: development and decline of a caregiver support group in a Latin population. In: Sokolovsky J, ed. *The Cultural Context of Aging, Worldwide Perspectives*. 2nd ed. Santa Barbara, CA: Greenwood Press; 1997.

33. Greenhalgh T, Helman C, Chowdhury AM. Health beliefs and folk models of diabetes in British Bangladeshi: A qualitative study. *BMJ*. 1998;316:978-983.

34. Teufel NI. Development of culturally competent food-frequency questionnaires. *Am J Clin Nutr*. 1997;65(suppl):1173S-1178S.

35. George M. The challenge of culturally competent health care: Applications for asthma. *Heart Lung*. 2001;30:392-400.

36. Wu S, Barker JC. Hot tea and juk: The institutional meaning of food for Chinese elders in an American nursing home. *J Gerontol Nurs*. 2008;34:46-54.

37. Lim K-C, Waters CM, Froelicher ES, et al. Conceptualizing physical activity behavior of older Korean-Americans: An integration of Korean culture and social cognitive theory. *Nurs Outlook*. 2008; 56:322-329.

38. Hovell MF, Mulvihill MM, Buono MJ, et al. Culturally tailored aerobic exercise intervention for low-income Latinas. *Am J Health Promot*. 2008;22:155-163.

39. Hasnain-Wynia R, Pierce D, Haque A, et al. *Health Research and Educational Trust Disparities Toolkit*. 2007. http://www.hretdisparities.org. Accessed June 16, 2009.

40. VA National Center for Health Promotion and Disease Prevention (NCP). MOVE! 2009. http://www.move.va.gov/. Accessed June 2009.

41. CDSMP. 1996. http://patienteducation.stanford.edu/programs/cdsmp.html. Accessed July 2009.

POST-TEST

1. **When considering history and context in cultural assessment it is important to remember that:**
   A. Most patients assume their providers are trustworthy from the start.
   B. If done correctly, a provider can eliminate power differentials.
   C. Context may be personal or social.
   D. Treating all patients alike removes bias.

2. **Which of the following is FALSE regarding cultural sensitivity strategies?**
   A. Improve communication
   B. Watch nonverbal cues
   C. Never use family interpreters
   D. Avoid stereotypes

3. **Which of the following is TRUE?**
   A. Interpersonal discomfort might result from nonverbal communication.
   B. Interpreters eliminate misinterpretations associated with language.
   C. Finger-pointing is universally seen as a sign of disrespect.
   D. Direct discussion of dying and prognosis is always appropriate.

ANSWERS TO PRE-TEST

1. D
2. B
3. D

ANSWERS TO POST-TEST

1. C
2. C
3. A

6

Medical Evaluation of the Older Person

Mark E. Williams, MD

Anna M. Hicks, MD

● **LEARNING OBJECTIVES**

1. Differentiate between a geriatric patient evaluation and the evaluation of a younger individual.
2. Describe specific ways to structure the environment for optimal geriatric interviewing.
3. Discuss barriers to communication with the older patient and approaches to improve information-gathering skills.
4. Describe special features of the physical examination of the older patient.
5. Discuss the influence of atypical presentation of illness and chronic conditions on the medical evaluation of older adults.
6. Explain advanced geriatric physical examination observations and techniques in acute clinical situations.

PRE-TEST

1. **All of the following are specific differences in the approach to physical evaluation of the older patient when compared to younger patients EXCEPT:**

   A. The spectrum of symptoms is broader in younger patients.

   B. The manifestations of distress are more pronounced in younger patients.

   C. Implications for maintaining independence are more compelling in older patients.

   D. Improvement is sometimes less dramatic and slower to appear in older patients.

2. **Which area of inquiry is NOT an essential focus during geriatric evaluation?**

   A. Sensory change

   B. Cognition

   C. Balance, strength, flexibility, and mobility

   D. Nutrition

3. **A part of the geriatric history that should be reviewed at every interval clinical encounter with an older person is:**

   A. Functional review

   B. Immunizations

   C. Previous hospitalizations

   D. Family history

● PRINCIPLES OF GERIATRIC ASSESSMENT

The increasing biologic uniqueness of older persons as they age requires an individualized approach to their medical care. As physicians, we must understand how elderly people behave when they are ill, and know how to interpret a changing constellation of multiple disease possibilities and interrelationships. The physician requires knowledge, skills, and the willingness and discipline to carefully evaluate each situation and to formulate a specifically tailored care plan. The accumulation and constant refinement of these skills reflect the maturity and scientific grounding of the physician.

The elderly person requires an approach and a clinical perspective that differs substantially from the medical evaluation of younger persons. The spectrum of symptoms is broader, the manifestations of distress are more subtle, and the implications for maintaining independence are more compelling. Improvement is sometimes less dramatic and slower to appear. The differential diagnosis is often different in older patients compared to younger patients and chronic illnesses are more common. In addition, the presentation of disease is frequently nonspecific in elderly people. The most common presenting complaints are mental status changes, behavioral changes, urinary incontinence, gait disturbance or falls, and weight loss. As a result of this nonspecific presentation, symptoms are difficult to interpret.

The value of most medical interventions in old age can be measured by their influence on independence and functionality. An older person's ability to manage daily activities cannot be determined confidently from the names of the diseases he or she may have or from the length of the problem list. The crucial issue is the elderly person's ability to function, because the discomfort and disability produced by curable or even incurable conditions often may be substantially modified. The conventional disease-specific perspective may not lend itself to developing strategies that best serve the older patient.

Given the unique feature of geriatric medicine that biological variation increases as we age, assessment of the geriatric patient relies on attentive detail to subtleties of the history and physical examination. "Aging" occurs at different rates across a population with a wide range in the amount and time frame that people age. Due to this increasing biological uniqueness as we age, a "one size fits all" approach simply does not work. Assessment of the geriatric patient is an improvisation of specific strategies to address the realities of the moment and the nature of the patient's predicament. There is no set of stock questions that should occur in the geriatric assessment as each encounter with the older patient should be tailored to his or her individual needs at that particular time.

When assessing the geriatric patient, the primary intention is to appreciate the truth in the light of the moment, the reality behind the appearance, with the goal of maintaining or improving quality of life and functional status. While health promotion, prevention, and screening efforts have a role in geriatric medicine, a balance must be constructed between the benefits of such testing and the patient's preferences, goals of care, and overall life expectancy (Chapter 14). Whether during your first encounter with a patient or a follow-up assessment, evaluation of the geriatric patient should always include evaluation of those things that most threaten the patient's quality of life—loss of mobility, vision, hearing, and cognition. Priority should be given to the specific concerns of the patient and his or her family.

Setting the Proper Environment

Encounters with elderly patients may take place in a variety of settings such as a clinic, hospital, home, or long-term care facility. From the first moment one meets a new patient to every visit thereafter, it is essential to create a healing atmosphere of caring. This is usually accomplished by giving the patient your full undivided attention and by facilitating the communication by putting the person at ease and by minimizing distractions. This improves patient comfort, and also helps the examiner guide the assessment according to the patient's specific concerns.

As sensory impairments occur more frequently in elderly patients, one must ensure that the patient can hear and see you as effectively as possible. Chapter 8 further discusses the nature of sensory impairments in elderly people. Avoid sitting with your back to a window or bright light source because it will put your face in silhouette and will reduce visual clues. Hearing difficulties may be surmounted by sitting close to the patient, talking toward the "good" ear, and avoiding shouting (which increases the pitch). Examiners with higher-pitched voices may try to lower the tone of their voices rather than raising the volume. Aids may be used to augment voice transmission. An example is a "pocket talker," which is a small, portable, battery-powered electronic device consisting of a microphone with amplifier box and earphones for the patient. Similarly, a stethoscope may be placed with the earpieces in the patient's ears while the examiner speaks into the bell. Keeping direct eye contact with patient and speaking calmly may also be helpful.

Optimize the lighting and sit close to patients with visual impairments such as macular degeneration, cataracts, or glaucoma. In the long-term care setting, where rooms tend have lower lighting levels, shades can be opened and patients moved closer to the window. Oftentimes, giving your hand to the patient with visual impairment is reassuring. It is also important to explain to such patients each step of the physical examination prior to proceeding so that they will not be surprised or taken off guard.

In the home, hospital, and long-term care settings, many unique challenges to creating a comfortable environment can exist. Oftentimes, people other than the patient are present in the room or house, which may cause the patient to feel more reserved when discussing personal information. This can be modified by closing the door to the patient's room, using an external examination room within the facility, or asking others to leave the room if possible during examination. Curtains can also create a visual barrier if roommates are unable to leave the room. Televisions and radios should be turned off. In the home setting, one might ask that pets be placed elsewhere during the examination time to reduce distractions.

Case 1 gives an example of how setting the proper environment and putting the patient at ease helps the clinician appreciate the correct diagnosis.

CASE PRESENTATION 1: LOOKING FOR CLUES

A 76-year-old male, Mr. Harris, comes to your office with his daughter for an initial visit. He moved to town in the past week to live with his daughter following the death of his wife 4 months ago. He has a past medical history of hearing loss and hypertension controlled with hydrochlorothiazide and an ACE inhibitor. His daughter states that since moving in with her, the patient has been increasingly confused, easily agitated, and forgetful. He does not have an appetite. She is worried that her father has developed dementia and asks for your help.

On physical examination, blood pressure is 190/88 sitting with a regular pulse of 92 and respiratory rate of 18. You note the patient appears anxious. He does not easily engage with you and is reluctant to answer questions. He appears slightly unkempt with 2 to 3 days of facial hair and a shirt that is not tucked in with food stains on the front. Slight resting tremor is noted in both hands. Skin examination reveals warm, flushed skin. You also note that the patient has wet feet (which raises your suspicion of alcohol abuse).

You feel that the patient may open up more if you can speak with him alone, so you ask his daughter to step outside for a moment. Given his hearing loss, you move your chair close to Mr. Harris, speak slowly, and keep good eye contact with him. Further questioning about the recent loss of your patient's wife triggers a tearful response from Mr. Harris. He states that he deeply misses his wife and has had a difficult time coping with her loss. Mr. Harris admits to a long-time habit of drinking frequently throughout the day, including taking an eye-opener in the morning. This pattern increased since the death of his wife. He also states that he has been treated for depression in the remote past, which he did not previously share with his daughter. Mr. Harris states he has not had access to alcohol in the past 4 days. You determine that he is currently in alcohol withdrawal. He agrees to have his daughter return to the room so that you can reach a plan of treatment for his alcohol withdrawal symptoms.

Prioritizing the Approach

Each encounter with a geriatric patient should begin with the assessment of why the patient seeks your attention that day. Be it an initial evaluation, a follow-up visit, or a consult from another physician, the nature of patient's presentation or "chief complaint" should be acknowledged and addressed. Careful attentive listening may reveal the actual source of distress in a causal "verbal parenthesis" or off-hand remark. The priority of the encounter with that patient will be determined by gathering initial information from the patient and using the examiner's initial impressions of the patient. In order to gain full knowledge of previous health history, disease states, and current concerns of the patient and family, initial visits will be comprehensive evaluations that incorporate all aspects of the history and physical examination. A review of previous medical records, if available, should also be done at initial visits. A thorough initial evaluation will lay a strong foundation for the physician–patient relationship. If there are time constraints that limit a thorough initial assessment, the examination may be divided into two separate visits—the first to focus on the patient's history with a second visit for a complete physical examination. The specific components of the geriatric history and physical are covered in subsequent sections of this chapter.

Consultative visits are also comprehensive in nature. Of utmost importance is the need to identify who referred the patient to you and the reason the consult was placed. If a clear reason for referral is not identified, the referring physician should be contacted prior to visiting with the patient so that goals for the referral may be addressed. Common reasons for referral to a geriatric physician include assessment of mental status and change in functional status. To spare the patient from undergoing duplications in workup, it is also helpful to have the patient's previous records, including any diagnostic studies done in regard to the complaint for which the patient was referred.

Follow-up assessments of patients may be more focused on the specific complaint of the patient on that day or on review of modifications made to treatment at the patient's last visit. During such visits, it is not necessary to revisit all parts of the history or physical. One approach is to focus on what has changed since the patient's last visit and how this has affected health and function. In each contact with a patient, current medications should be reviewed. The review of systems may be tailored to the patient's specific complaint at a return visit, but should generally include review of cognition, vision, hearing, and gait. These elements of the review of systems are important, as disturbances in these systems may lead to change in functional status and, subsequently, loss of independence.

● THE GERIATRIC HISTORY

Structure of History

Given the caveats of increasing biological uniqueness with aging and the limitations of an algorithmic approach to care, the components of a comprehensive geriatric history are listed in Table 6–1. Upon initial visit with the patient, most of these elements should be reviewed. In subsequent contacts with patients, an interval history may be taken by reviewing any changes experienced by the patient and evaluating new symptoms or complaints. Review of functional

● TABLE 6–1 Elements of the Comprehensive Geriatric History

Element of History	Important Components
Chief complaint	• Primary reason for patient's visit
History of present illness	• Timing of symptoms (acute vs. chronic) • Severity and duration of symptoms • Effect of symptoms on function and independence • Relieving/aggravating factors • Interventions previously implemented
Past medical history	• Review of previous acute as well as chronic illnesses • Previous hospitalizations • Previous rehabilitation or long-term care admissions • Review of communicable diseases (hepatitis, tuberculosis) • Surgical history
Review of screening examinations/ immunization history	• Types and dates of immunizations and procedures (mammogram, colonoscopy) • Review of last eye and dental examinations
Social history	• Marital status • Review of children, caregivers • Previous occupation and education level • Hobbies • Cultural/religious affiliations • Code status, living will, power of attorney • Tobacco, alcohol, and illicit drug habits • Sexual history
Family history	• Review of parents', siblings', and children's health
Functional history	• Review of ability to conduct daily activities • Review of who is available to assist patient if needed • Need for assistive devices (cane, walker, wheelchair) • Driving history
Medication review	• Allergies and intolerances to medications • Recently added/discontinued medications • Herbal and over-the-counter supplements
Full review of body systems and symptoms	• Include review of cognition, eyesight, hearing, mobility • May be prioritized to target patient's presenting complaints

status and medications should be considered at each visit. Special attention should be given to herbal and other over-the-counter remedies. These compounds may increase the risk for serious adverse drug interactions depending on the patient's regimen. An abbreviated review of body systems, including the systems affected by current complaints as well as vision, hearing, mobility, and cognition, should be conducted at every geriatric visit.

Special Issues—Collaborating Information

Due to the increased prevalence of cognitive deficits and impaired functional status in elderly patients, care of the geriatric patient often includes an interdisciplinary approach (see Section II, Inter-Professional Geriatrics). Sometimes it is necessary to obtain historical information from persons other than the patient. Caregivers such as family members, long-term care or hospice nurses, or home health aides may be invaluable sources of information regarding the patient's current or past condition. If the individuals are present during the interview, then sometimes the nature of the interaction between the parties can be instructive. For example, significant distance between parties may mirror emotional distance. Key elements of the history from these informants often involve the performance of daily activities. Consider the activities of daily living (ADLs) as a spectrum of handling unpredictable circumstances with the basic ADLs (dressing, bathing, eating, etc.) being the most predictable activities; the instrumental ADLs (shopping, meal planning, handling finances, etc.) being somewhat unpredictable; and the advanced ADLs (independent travel, etc.) as having high unpredictability. By noting where a patient or family member feels most comfortable functioning, you can estimate how much unpredictability the person can handle. Rehabilitation specialists involved in the patient's care such as physical, occupational, or speech therapists may also aid in providing a picture of the patient's function over a given time period. Contact with such rehabilitation specialists, or home health or hospice nurses, may be done directly or in review of documentation provided by that team member. It is important to be aware of patient confidentiality rights when contacting those who may not be directly consulted to provide care for a patient. In such circumstances, the examiner should obtain consent from the patient or the patient's surrogate and be explicit in what will be discussed when contacting outside sources.

● PHYSICAL EXAMINATION

Structure of the Geriatric Physical Examination

Elements of the geriatric physical examination are similar to those of the examination for nongeriatric patients with an increased focus on those body systems that most affect function. The elements of physical examination are listed in Table 6–2.[1] Again, special attention should be given to the systems that play a direct role in functional status such as vision, hearing, mobility, and cognition. As with the geriatric history, the geriatric physical examination must be tailored to include those elements relevant to that day's visit. An initial visit will likely be comprehensive, whereas interval visits may focus on those systems contributing to current distress or health maintenance. Special consideration may be made for patients who are ill and either unable to communicate concerns due to cognitive deficits and communication barriers or in whom the presenting symptoms are vague. In these instances, whether an initial or interval visit, a comprehensive physical examination may be the best way to uncover causative factors.

● **TABLE 6–2** Elements of the Comprehensive Geriatric Physical Examination

Element	Components
Vital signs	• Temperature • Pulse • Blood pressure • Respiratory rate • Oxygen saturation • Pain level
Initial observations	• General appearance • Dress • Language
Head and face	• Observation of complexion and expression • Symmetry of face • Hair texture and distribution • Skull and scalp palpation
Eyes	• Visual acuity and visual field measurement • Evaluation of eyewear • Examination of the eyelid, sclera, cornea, lacrimal duct, pupils, and iris • Assessment of ocular movements • Fundoscopic evaluation
Ears	• External inspection • Examination of the inner ear
Nose and sinuses	• External inspection • Examination of nasal patency and turbinates • Palpation of the sinus cavities
Mouth and throat	• Observation of breath odor • Mandibular and lip examination • Dentition and prosthetic devices • Examination of mucosal membranes • Tongue and palate examination • Uvula position • Posterior pharynx examination
Neck	• Observation of head and tracheal position • Range-of-motion testing • Thyroid and soft-tissue palpation
Lymph nodes	• Palpation for epitrochlear, cervical, supraclavicular, axillary, and inguinal lymph nodes
Back	• Inspection, palpation, and percussion of spine and flanks
Breasts	• Inspection of breasts in sitting and recumbent positions • Palpation of breast tissue including axilla
Respiratory and chest	• Observation of respiratory pattern • Observation of chest shape, posture, and symmetry • Observation of chest and accessory muscle movement and tracheal position • Palpation of chest wall and trachea • Percussion of chest • Auscultation of lungs and trachea
Cardiovascular system	• Palpation of carotid, brachial, radial, femoral, popliteal, and pedal pulses • Inspection of neck veins and carotid pulsations • Palpation of apical pulse and point of maximal impulse • Auscultation of the heart sounds and valves • Auscultation of the carotid, aortic, renal, and femoral pulses • Evaluation and palpation of abdominal and peripheral edema
Abdomen	• Inspection of abdomen • Auscultation of abdomen • Percussion of the abdomen, liver, and spleen • Palpation of abdomen, liver, and spleen • Rectal and prostate examination
Genitourinary system Female	• Inspection of hair, skin, and external genitalia • Palpation of labia • Internal speculum examination • Bimanual examination including rectovaginal examination
Male	• Palpation of scrotum, epididymis, spermatic cord, vas deferens, and testes • Transillumination of any swelling or masses
Extremities	• Observation of positioning of extremities and digits • Observation of symmetry of limbs • Palpation of joints • Assessment of range of motion of joints

Initial Impression—Observations

As mentioned earlier, the fundamental goal of the evaluation is to help the patient by appreciating the nature of the patient's predicament, the truth in the light of the moment. Undivided attention must be paid to all aspects of the physical examination, especially the patient's general appearance, dress, language, and behaviors, which can give many clues to overall well-being and functional status. One must appreciate any incongruities in the patient's presentation (appearance, dress, language, and behaviors) and during the patient's physical examination as these may be critical tools in diagnosis (Table 6–3).

Appearance

The general appearance of a patient can give many clues to underlying disease processes. Does the patient appear his or her stated age? The patient's apparent age may usefully reflect the biological age. While many elderly people may appear much younger than their stated age, chronic illness and impoverishment seem to accelerate biological aging, leading to patients appearing older than their chronological age. Appearance can also provide an indication of how well the patient is able to perform self-care activities. Is the patient well kempt? Does he or she have the fine-motor skills to apply makeup appropriately? Are there stains on the front of the clothing suggesting difficulty with feeding? Are there scars, cuts, bruises, or other signs of trauma on any exposed skin? Bruising on the face or extremities suggests falls or possible abuse. Also important is the patient's body habitus. For example, look for temporal wasting as a sign of significant weight loss, and kyphosis as an indicator of vertebral compression fractures.

Some diseases have specific facial appearances that, in some circumstances, may allow a diagnosis to be made on sight. Examples are the moon face seen in Cushing syndrome and the expressionless mask face that may be present in Parkinson disease. Changes in complexion can be important signs of illness. Patients with anemia often have pallor of the skin. Pernicious anemia can create a "lemon yellow" tint. A generalized increase in pigmentation may suggest Addison disease or hemachromatosis. Acanthuses nigerians or darkening of the skin in the axilla and around the neck may be present in patients with diabetes mellitus or malignancy. Such observations can be combined with other findings of the physical examination and lead to an accurate diagnosis.

Movement abnormalities are also often noted on initial impression. Head bobbing may signify tricuspid (side to side) or aortic insufficiency (front to back). Parkinsonism, thyrotoxicosis, or essential tremors may be appreciated when shaking the patient's hand. Restlessness associated with anxiety may also be apparent. Orofacial chewing or tongue movements may signify tardive dyskinesia from past exposure to medications. Hemiballismus, rapid and violent flailing of one upper extremity, may be seen after a subthalamic stroke. Myoclonus in association with rapidly progressive memory loss can be seen in Creutzfeld-Jakob disease.

● **TABLE 6–3** Observations on Initial Impression and Their Possible Implications

Observations	Examples of Abnormalities or Incongruities	Possible Implications
General Appearance		
Facies: expressiveness, symmetry	A man whose facial expression does not seem to change despite discussing an emotional experience	Degree of interest in interacting, medication effect, illness such as Parkinson disease
Facial grooming: makeup, shaving, skin care	A woman with eye shadow and lipstick applied unevenly and outside of the eye/lip boundaries	Personal tastes, manual dexterity, eyesight, awareness
Hair: coloring, cleanliness, style	A woman whose wig is off-centered and not combed	Personal taste, manual dexterity, joint mobility, eyesight, awareness
Mouth: teeth, cleanliness	A man who with a large, beefy tongue, gum inflammation, and halitosis	Illness, manual dexterity, medication effect, joint mobility, awareness
Nails: polish, cleanliness, trim, number	A woman whose nail polish has grown out to the tips of her long fingernails	Personal taste, awareness, manual dexterity, eyesight
Skin: texture, lesions, cleanliness, tattoos	A man with tanned arms, rough hands, and several tattoos along his forearms	Vocation/hobbies, illness, eyesight, personal taste, manual dexterity, joint mobility
Movement: tremor, gait	A woman who has a pill-rolling tremor and has difficulty getting up out of her chair	Illness, medication effect, joint mobility
Dress		
Style: fabric, color, design, ornamentation	A man who is wearing business attire but has slippers on his feet	Personal taste, cultural influence, awareness, eyesight, degree of interest in appearance, manual dexterity
Fit: tight or loose	A man wearing baggy pants cinched with a belt that has additional holes added	Weight loss/gain, degree of interest in appearance, financial circumstances
Fastenings: open/closed, propriety	A woman whose shirt is mis-buttoned	Manual dexterity, range of joint motion, awareness
Neatness: cleanliness	A man who has dirt on the knees of his pants and under his fingernails	Vocation or hobbies, eyesight, manual dexterity, awareness
Language		
Speech: rate, tone, volume, articulation	A woman who talks very softly and slowly	Personality, general physical or emotional status, illness, medication effect
Content: vocabulary, and topic	A man who speaks in occupational terms regarding his previous employment but uses vague terms when discussing new hobbies	Illness, medication effect, education level, personality, awareness

Dress

Notice the way your patient is dressed when you initially meet him or her. Do clothes fit, or are there signs of weight loss as evidenced by loose clothing or additional holes cut into belts? On average, each belt loop represents about 15 pounds of weight loss or weight gain. Are rings loose or tight? Is the patient dressed inappropriately for the season? Patients with moderate dementia may not consider the weather when they are choosing clothing. The elderly woman wearing a thin cotton dress in the winter may be at increased risk for accidental hypothermia. Those with endocrine disorders affecting the thyroid may also tend to overdress (hypothyroid) or underdress (hyperthyroid) due to the sensation of being cold or flushed. Differences in the type of dress are also important. A patient who comes to the office in a suit may still be active and working. Shoes should also be noted during the general examination. Does the patient wear slippers or slide on shoes suggesting edema of the feet? Is there a pattern of wear on the soles of the shoes suggesting a gait disorder?

Language

Language can give many important clues during physical examination. Does the patient speak rapidly or slowly? Are there signs of difficulty with word finding or comprehension, suggesting a central process such as stroke, Parkinson disease, or dementia? Is the patient able to keep on topic, or are there signs of loss of concentration? In the presence of others, such as family members, it is also important to note who is answering the majority of the questions—the patient or family member. Are the answers each provided congruent with the other? This can give insight into the dynamics of the relationship and the patient's dependence on the family member or can clue the examiner into problems between the patient and family.

Special Features of the Physical Examination of the Older Patient

Visual Examination

Visual disturbances are common in geriatric patients and can lead to decreased function if undiagnosed. Presbyopia, a loss of visual accommodation that makes it difficult to focus on nearby objects, results from a decrease in lens elasticity and atrophy of the ciliary muscle. Presbyopia is one of the common changes in vision that may be seen with aging and can be remedied by corrective lenses. Cataracts, glaucoma, and macular degeneration are other disease processes that may affect vision in the elderly patient. Other visual impairments of the older patient are discussed in Chapter 8. The geriatric physical examination should include examination of the eyes for bulging or prominence. Proptosis, or prominence of the eye, is associated with such things as hyperthyroidism and tumors. Testing of visual acuity by use of vision charts or cards as well as assessment of visual fields should be performed with patients who are able to participate. Eyelids should also be examined for ptosis or asymmetry, which may signify previous stroke, Horner syndrome, myasthenia gravis, cranial nerve III palsy, or other illness. The areas around the eyes should also be observed for periorbital edema, which can be seen with renal failure or myxedema. Discoloration surrounding the eyes may also signify disease. Chronic allergic rhinitis can be associated with black circles underneath the eyes. Sclera examination is also another way an examiner may be clued into underlying disease. Scleral icterus, bright yellow discoloration, is produced by the accumulation of bilirubin to the elastin tissue of the sclera and is a marker for impaired bilirubin metabolism. Conjunctival color should be noted as well, as significant anemia can be associated with pallor. Evaluation of eye movements and pupillary reflexes may reveal abnormalities associated with strokes or cranial nerve disease. Fundoscopic examination should also be done when possible, especially in patients with underlying illnesses such as diabetes and hypertension, which are associated with retinopathies and microvascular eye disease.

Hearing Evaluation

Presbycusis, hearing loss for pure tones, especially those with a higher frequency, increases with age in both men and women. The ability to discriminate pitch also decreases with age. Due to such changes within normal aging, it is important to screen for hearing loss in the elderly person as deficits in hearing can lead to social isolation and inappropriate diagnoses such as dementia or depression. Chapter 8 further discusses hearing loss in the older person.

There are several specific screening examinations that can be done in the office to assess for hearing loss. A good initial screening examination is to stand behind the patient while giving the patient a simple command to follow such as "Raise your hand." This allows you to note if the patient is able to follow the command without visual cues. A finger friction test can also be done by rubbing together your forefinger and thumb by the outside of the ear canals while noting if the patient can hear the sound created. To test for hearing loss due to canal occlusion versus sensorineural hearing loss, a vibrating 512-Hz tuning fork may be placed on the middle of the patient's forehead (Weber test). A 512-Hz tuning fork is used as it creates a frequency in the middle of normal conversational voice range. Hearing the sound of the tuning fork in both ears is normal. Patients who have hearing loss due to occlusion of the canal will localize the tone of the tuning fork in the ear that is occluded. Those who have unilateral sensorineural hearing loss will hear the sound in their good ear, whereas patients who have bilateral sensorineural hearing loss may be unable to hear the sound at all.

In cases of suspected hearing loss, referral can be made for formal audiology testing to determine if assistive devices such as hearing aids would benefit the patient.

Functional Evaluation

The geriatric history and physical examination differ from those of other populations by an intense focus on maintaining the patient's ability to function independently. Initial observations can be used to help the examiner determine the patient's level of independence. The examiner should be able to gain some knowledge of how the patient functions simply by observing the patient in the clinic, home, or long-term care setting. Assessments of gait, muscle strength, joint range of motion, and manual dexterity are all helpful components of functional assessment. Skin assessments are also useful to providing clues regarding the patient's independence as pressure ulcers, skin tears, and bruising may be seen more frequently in patients with functional loss. A more detailed description of functional assessment of the geriatric patient is given in Chapter 7, and frailty/functional decline of aging patients is covered in Chapter 36.

Cognitive Evaluation

Evaluating the elderly person for possible memory impairment is an important medical responsibility. Independent living depends on adequate mental function. The main goal in evaluating the mental function of the geriatric patient is to ascertain whether or not the patient has the ability to identify environmental risks and act on those risks appropriately. The next goal is to identify the underlying cause of cognitive dysfunction and treat any reversible causes.

The geriatric physician is often consulted to assist other physicians in determining the cause of memory impairment. There are numerous causes of memory loss in the elderly including medications, delirium, dementias, depression, and vascular disease. A careful history and physical examination is the cornerstone to appropriate differentiation of these entities.

The physical evaluation of a patient's mental status includes initial observations of the patient (Table 6–3). Further discussion regarding assessment of medical decision-making capacity, delirium, and dementia can be found in Chapters 10, 30, and 31.

Special Considerations
Atypical Disease Presentation

Disease presentation in the elderly population is varied and may not be as obvious as in younger patients. Acute illnesses may be masked by symptoms of chronic disease. Vague complaints like fatigue, anorexia, and confusion may be markers for numerous diseases. Red flags of serious illness or infection such as fever, tachycardia, and chest pain may not be present in elderly persons. Atypical disease presentation in the older person is further discussed in Chapter 9.

Chronic Disease

In the aging population there is an increase in prevalence of chronic illness. Elderly patients are more likely than their younger counterparts to have more than one chronic disease. Chapters 43 through 45 discuss congestive heart failure, stroke (vascular disease), and hypertension in elderly people. Other common chronic diseases in the geriatric population include osteoarthritis, mechanical low back pain, diabetes, chronic kidney disease, chronic obstructive pulmonary disorder, coronary artery disease, and peripheral vascular disease.

Such entities can be assessed during history-taking, by previous medical history, and by current symptoms, and can be monitored by physical examination and laboratory studies.

Special Physical Examination Tests

Geriatric patients can be seen in a variety of settings and the familiar tools for additional diagnostic or radiological testing may not be readily available. Many times, the medical provider must make a choice to treat the presumed illness while waiting on confirmatory tests or to send the patient to another location for testing. This latter option increases the possibility of complications such as falls, pressure ulcers, or confusion, when removing the patient from a familiar location. Physical diagnosis often becomes of greater importance in these instances to aid the provider in making such decisions. Signs and examination findings that may help in potentially emergent situations are outlined next.

Aortic Aneurysm Dissection and Rupture

Typically, patients with a dissecting aortic aneurysm will complain of tearing chest or back pain. If the dissection is leaking, cardiovascular shock may be present. Anterior thoracic aortic dissection can cause aortic regurgitation resulting in a new early diastolic, high-pitched decrescendo murmur heard best at the lower left and upper right sternal borders. Potain sign is dullness to percussion at the right upper sternal border where the underlying aorta can be enlarged during an anterior dissection. One might also note a patient with aortic dissection to have a unilateral pulseless, warm, pale extremity as a result of sympathetic chain ischemia and compromise (similar to harlequin sign, a typically benign finding in newborns). It is very important to measure the blood pressure in all four extremities if aortic dissection is considered.

Coin Test for Pneumothorax

In addition to chest auscultation, the coin test may be a useful bedside diagnostic tool to determine the presence of a pneumothorax. With the patient sitting upright, place a pre-1964 silver dollar flat against the chest 1 inch below the clavicle in the midclavicular line and hold it in place with your ring finger and little finger. While auscultating the chest with your stethoscope, tap this coin with a second coin pinched between your thumb and forefinger. You can also have the patient hold the coin under the clavicle. If a pneumothorax is present, a bell-like ring will be heard rather than the normal metallic tapping.

Long Bone Fracture or Dislocation

Heuter sign is a test to determine the presence of a long-bone fracture or dislocation. If a femur fracture is suspected, place the diaphragm of stethoscope on the pubic symphysis and gently percuss each patella with your forefinger. For a humerus fracture, percuss each olecranon while listening with your stethoscope at the manubrium. Intact bone produces a bright clear tapping sound but the sound is muffled and distant in a fractured or dislocated bone. A tuning fork may also be used.[2]

Pleural Effusion versus Lung Consolidation

Percussion and auscultation techniques can easily differentiate a lung consolidation from a pleural effusion. The areas overlying pleural effusions and lung consolidations will both be dull to percussion. Skodaic hyperresonance is heard as a rim of increased resonance to percussion just above the level of an area of dullness in the lung, suggesting effusion. At the level of a pulmonary consolidation, one will hear an increased intensity of breath sounds, whereas over a pleural effusion, lung sounds will be diminished. Whisper pectoriloquy can differentiate the two conditions. Have the patient whisper "Sixty-six whiskeys, please" while auscultating the area in question. If this sentence is heard clearly at the level of dullness, one is likely listening over consolidated lung. If no sound is heard, a pleural effusion should be suspected. Percussion along the upper border of a pleural effusion may also result in an S-shaped curve (Damoiseau-Ellis sign).

● LABORATORY AND RADIOLOGIC TESTING

The decision to order laboratory and radiologic testing in the geriatric patient should be based on the nature of the patient's presentation and findings of the patient's history and physical examination. Chapter 12 discusses the approach to laboratory and radiologic testing in the aging patient.

● HEALTH PROMOTION AND DISEASE PREVENTION

The approach to screening, health promotion, and disease prevention in the geriatric patient involves knowledge of the patient's preferences, overall life expectancy, and impact that interventions done based on screening and prevention studies would have on the patient's quality of life. These issues are further discussed in Chapters 12 and 14.

Case 2 illustrates how close observation and physical examination skills help to prioritize patient care and lead to appropriate diagnosis.

CASE PRESENTATION 2: IS IT FRACTURED?

You are on your way to the long-term care facility where you make weekly rounds, when you are called by the nurse for your patient, Ms. Jones. Ms. Jones fell this morning while getting out of bed and the nurse was present at the time of the fall. The patient did not hit her head but landed on her left side. Ms. Jones has moderate dementia and normally walks with the assistance of a walker. She falls frequently despite fall precautions and is unable to participate in physical therapy due to her cognitive impairment. Her nurse notes that the patient is complaining of some pain in her left leg and has been in bed since her fall. You decide to see Ms. Jones first when you get to the long-term care facility to decide whether or not she will need a more acute level of care and whether or not she needs an x-ray. If you order a portable x-ray of her left leg and hip it will not be reported until tomorrow.

On your examination of Ms. Jones, she is in bed. Examination of her left leg reveals no foreshortening or abnormal position of the leg and she has full range of motion of her left hip without discomfort. To help determine if a fracture is present, you perform osteophony (Heuter sign). You place the diaphragm of your stethoscope on the pubic symphysis and gently percuss each patella with your forefinger. The intact bone on the right produces a bright clear tapping sound but the sound is muffled and distant on the left. Due to this, the decision is made to transport the patient to the emergency room for expedited evaluation and treatment for presumed left femur fracture.

Diagnostic Testing

Diagnostic testing such as laboratory evaluation or radiologic examinations can be used to support findings of illness found on history and physical examination. Chapter 12 provides information on the approach to laboratory testing and imaging in the aging patient.

• HEALTH PROMOTION AND DISEASE PREVENTION

As briefly discussed within this chapter, health promotion as well as disease screening and prevention remain important parts of medical care throughout life. When discussing screening and routine health maintenance examinations in the geriatric patient, the benefits of such testing should be weighed against the patient's goals of care, life expectancy, and feasibility of testing in regard to functional status. The challenge is that most health promotional efforts have maximizing longevity or avoiding premature death as the goal. For most octogenarians avoiding premature death is problematic. The target of prevention should shift to maintaining function and reducing dependency. With this perspective, many of our traditional preventive measures such as screening for heart disease or malignancy become irrelevant. Chapter 14 discusses these issues in further detail.

CONCLUSION

The medical evaluation of the older person requires knowledge and skills not generally included in the curriculum of most health professional schools. A careful and deliberate approach to assessing the older person—which includes factoring in the impact of disease, disability, co-morbidity, social support systems, mental health, and unique features of the aging body as it relates to disease presentation and function—is imperative to optimizing the treatment of older patients. The medical evaluation should be deliberate and focus on the areas and systems where older adults frequently experience declines in function. Only by evaluating the older adult by using a global approach to evaluating all the important systems can health care and medical care be optimized for that individual.

References

1. Williams ME. *Geriatric Physical Diagnosis: A Guide to Observation and Assessment.* Jefferson, North Carolina: London, McFarland; 2008.

2. Misurya RK, Khare A, Mallick A, et al. Use of tuning fork in diagnostic auscultation of fractures. *Injury.* 1987;18:63-64.

POST-TEST

1. **Heuter sign is a test to determine:**
   A. Lung consolidation
   B. Presence of a fracture
   C. Hearing loss
   D. Hyperthyroidism

2. **An unusual finding in older adults associated with autonomic over-activity during alcohol withdrawal is:**
   A. Damp feet
   B. Bulging eyes
   C. Tachycardia
   D. Unilateral pale extremity

3. **In using a tuning fork to test hearing loss, a patient with an occlusion of one canal will:**
   A. Hear/localize the sound in both ears
   B. Hear/localize the sound in the good ear
   C. Hear/localize the sound in the occluded ear
   D. Not hear/localize the sound

ANSWERS TO PRE-TEST

1. A
2. D
3. A

ANSWERS TO POST-TEST

1. B
2. A
3. C

7

Functional Assessment

Jeffrey De Castro Mariano, MD

David B. Reuben, MD

● LEARNING OBJECTIVES

1. Discuss the process for evaluating functional assessment including BADLs, IADLs, and AADLs, and self-reported and performance-based tools.
2. Explain the importance of knowing baseline function and changes in functional status in the care of the older adult.
3. Identify the impact of functional status on subsequent death and functional decline.
4. Compare and contrast how functional status can be assessed in different settings of care—outpatient, emergency department, hospital, and nursing home.
5. Discuss the impact of functional status on the perioperative period after medical events like hip fracture.
6. Describe the role of functional assessment in the management of cancer patients and frail older demented adults; the management of chronic medical problems such as diabetes, heart failure, and chronic obstructive pulmonary disease; and its impact on discussing advanced care planning.

PRE-TEST

1. **Which impairment in the following activities of daily living is most prevalent?**
   A. Bathing
   B. Dressing
   C. Transferring
   D. Feeding

2. **Which of the following is true concerning the assessment of a decline in functional status?**
   A. It has not been shown to be a risk factor for falls and institutionalization.
   B. Is more common because it accompanies the aging process and affects quality of life.

   C. It is routinely performed in primary care settings.
   D. It is important to assess, as it may reflect a new medical illness and cognitive issues.

3. **In older hip fracture patients, an evaluation of functional status (specifically ADLs and IADLs) is most helpful in anticipating which postoperative outcome?**
   A. Postoperative pain control
   B. Postoperative delirium
   C. Advanced directives
   D. Future ambulatory status

INTRODUCTION: DEFINING PHYSICAL FUNCTION IN OLDER ADULTS

One of the hallmarks of a geriatric approach is the focus on older people's ability to function and the processes that lead to disability. Functional status and disability reflect the interaction between multiple medical conditions, physiologic aging, psychosocial support, cognitive impairment, and the overall health and vitality of the individual.[1] Functional evaluation adds a dimension beyond the usual medical assessment, providing information on well-being and quality of life as well as determining care needs and prognosis.

Function can be conceptualized across a hierarchy of increasing complexity from a focus on specific physical movements, such as lifting and walking, to a focus on more integrated activities such as the ability to maintain occupational and social roles (Figure 7–1).[1] Another way to describe function is by using "building blocks" that are integrated to form a hierarchy of ability (Figure 7–2).[2] The basic building blocks include strength, balance, coordination, flexibility, and endurance. In the first integration level, a specific physical movement is involved, such as an 8-foot walk. In the second integration level, these movements are coordinated into more complex tasks such as dressing, writing, bathing, feeding, and climbing stairs. At the highest level of integration, these tasks are coordinated with cognitive and affective resources to carry out functioning in occupational and social roles.[2]

The maintenance and restoration of functional status is an essential overriding objective of good geriatric care. Health care providers can promote their patients' autonomy and mobilize appropriate medical, social, and environmental supports by conducting careful, comprehensive, and periodic functional assessments. Functional status changes over time. Functional status may also be affected by medical conditions, cognition and mood, hearing and vision, incontinence, nutrition, and the patient's social needs. Therefore, accurate assessments at multiple time points over the course of the patient's life are important.

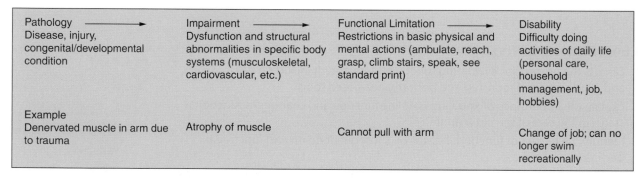

FIGURE 7–1. The theoretical pathway to disability. (*From Guralnik & Ferrucci.*[1])

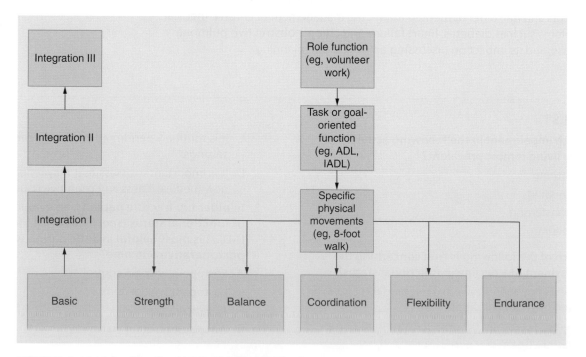

FIGURE 7–2. Hierarchy of functional integration. (*From Reuben.*[2])

● FUNCTIONAL ASSESSMENT TOOLS

Functional impairment cannot be predicted based on the number or severity of medical diagnoses in a specific patient; therefore specific evaluation of function is essential. The choice of functional assessment tools depends upon the characteristics of the population (community dwelling, hospitalized, nursing-home residents) and the level of function being assessed. Function can be assessed by self-report, proxy report, performance-based testing, or a combination of these approaches.[3]

In ambulatory clinical settings, self- or proxy-reported functional status is usually collected by questionnaires or interview with patients or family/caregivers. From a clinical perspective, a functional status assessment that indicates ability to perform specific functional tasks *and* provides information about who provides help, if needed, is more valuable than merely assessing ability. An example is the previsit questionnaire used in the UCLA outpatient geriatric practice (Table 7–1).

A description of the most commonly studied and used assessment tools follows.

Self-Reported Tools

Basic Activities of Daily Living

Basic activities of daily living (BADLs) are the essential elements of self-care (Table 7–2A). The Katz Index is widely used, and includes assessment of:

- Bathing
- Dressing
- Toileting
- Transferring
- Continence
- Feeding

Losses of independence in these skills frequently occur in the order listed, and are regained in the reverse order. Inquiring about difficulty with activities of daily living may provide additional prognostic information.[4] Questions about functional ability are best posed in reference to recent activities; for example, "Did you dress yourself this morning?" rather than "Do you dress yourself?"

Instrumental Activities of Daily Living

Instrumental activities of daily living (IADLs) describe the more complex activities that an individual needs to live independently (Table 7–2B). They provide insight into the functional capacity in older persons whose BADLs are usually intact. These activities include shopping, managing transportation, climbing stairs, managing finances, using the telephone, doing laundry, managing medications, walking outdoors, driving, and preparing meals. Asking "Did you drive here today?" or "When did you last drive?" (rather than "Do you drive?") may elicit a more useful answer. IADLs are less reflective of underlying pathology, impairments, and limitations than BADLs, though, because they include learned skills and assess the impact of the interaction between current patient capabilities and the environment.

Assessment of IADL function must consider gender-related tasks. For example, the ability to do laundry and housekeeping may not be relevant for some male patients who have never performed these tasks, and the assessment of driving may be inappropriate for some female patients.

● TABLE 7–1 Please Tell Us about How Your Health Affects Your Ability to Do Each of the Following Activities			
Task	No Help Needed	Help Needed	Who Helps?
Feeding yourself			
Getting from bed to chair			
Getting to the toilet			
Getting dressed			
Bathing or showering			
Walking across the room (includes using cane or walker)			
Using the telephone			
Taking your medicines			
Preparing meals			
Managing money (eg, keeping track of expenses or paying bills)			
Moderately strenuous housework such as doing the laundry			
Shopping for personal items like toiletries or medicines			
Shopping for groceries			
Driving			
Climbing a flight of stairs			
Getting to places beyond walking distance (eg, by bus, taxi, or car)			

Source: UCLA Previsit Questionnaire 2009.

● TABLE 7–2A Physical Self-Maintenance Scale (Activities of Daily Living, or ADLs)

In each category, circle the item that most closely describes the person's highest level of functioning and record the score assigned to that level (either 1 or 0) in the blank at the beginning of the category.

A. Toilet _____
1. Care for self at toilet completely; no incontinence — 1
2. Needs to be reminded, or needs help in cleaning self, or has rare (weekly at most) accidents — 0
3. Soiling or wetting while asleep more than once a week — 0
4. Soiling or wetting while awake more than once a week — 0
5. No control of bowels or bladder — 0

B. Feeding _____
1. Eats without assistance — 1
2. Eats with minor assistance at meal times and/or with special preparation of food, or help in cleaning up after meals — 0
3. Feeds self with moderate assistance and is untidy — 0
4. Requires extensive assistance for all meals — 0
5. Does not feed self at all and resists efforts of others to feed him or her — 0

C. Dressing _____
1. Dresses, undresses, and selects clothes from own wardrobe — 1
2. Dresses and undresses self with minor assistance — 0
3. Needs moderate assistance in dressing and selection of clothes — 0
4. Needs major assistance in dressing but cooperates with efforts of others to help — 0
5. Completely unable to dress self and resists efforts of others to help — 0

D. Grooming (neatness, hair, nails, hands, face, clothing) _____
1. Always neatly dressed and well groomed without assistance — 1
2. Grooms self adequately with occasional minor assistance, eg, with shaving — 0
3. Needs moderate and regular assistance or supervision with grooming — 0
4. Needs total grooming care but can remain well groomed after help from others — 0
5. Actively negates all efforts of others to maintain grooming — 0

E. Physical Ambulation _____
1. Goes about grounds or city — 1
2. Ambulates within residence on or about one block distant — 0
3. Ambulates with assistance of (check one)
   a ( ) another person, b ( ) railing, c ( ) cane, d ( ) walker, e ( ) wheelchair — 0
   1.___Gets in and out without help. 2.___Needs help getting in and out
4. Sits unsupported in chair or wheelchair but cannot propel self without help — 0
5. Bedridden more than half the time — 0

F. Bathing _____
1. Bathes self (tub, shower, sponge bath) without help — 1
2. Bathes self with help getting in and out of tub — 0
3. Washes face and hands only but cannot bathe rest of body — 0
4. Does not wash self but is cooperative with those who bathe him or her — 0
5. Does not try to wash self and resists efforts to keep him or her clean — 0

For scoring interpretation and source, see note after the next instrument.

In these situations, it is appropriate to ask whether he or she ever performed the task. Acute or subacute changes in functional status are important to elicit, as they may be markers of underlying medical illness, cognitive losses, or other psychosocial issues.

Using the assessment instruments presented, total scores can be calculated for both BADLs and IADLs (Tables 7–2A and 7–2B). BADL total scores range between 0 and 6, and IADL scores between 0 and 8. In some categories, only the highest level of function receives a 1; in others, two or more levels have scores of 1 because each describes competence at some minimal level of function. These screens are useful for indicating specifically how a person is performing at the present time. When they are also used over time,

● TABLE 7–2B Instrumental Activities of Daily Living Scale (IADLs)

In each category, circle the item that most closely describes the person's highest level of functioning and record the score assigned to that level (either 1 or 0) in the blank at the beginning of the category.

A. Ability to Use Telephone _____

1. Operates telephone on own initiative; looks up and dials numbers — 1
2. Dials a few well-known numbers — 1
3. Answers telephone but does not dial — 1
4. Does not use telephone at all — 0

B. Shopping _____

1. Takes care of all shopping needs independently — 1
2. Shops independently for small purchases — 0
3. Needs to be accompanied on any shopping trip — 0
4. Completely unable to shop — 0

C. Food Preparation _____

1. Plans, prepares, and serves adequate meals independently — 1
2. Prepares adequate meals if supplied with ingredients — 0
3. Heats and serves prepared meals or prepares meals but does not maintain adequate diet — 0
4. Needs to have meals prepared and served — 0

D. Housekeeping _____

1. Maintains house alone or with occasional assistance (eg, domestic help for heavy work) — 1
2. Performs light daily tasks such as dishwashing, bed making — 1
3. Performs light daily tasks but cannot maintain acceptable level of cleanliness — 1
4. Needs help with all home maintenance tasks — 1
5. Does not participate in any housekeeping tasks — 0

E. Laundry _____

1. Does personal laundry completely — 1
2. Launders small items; rinses socks, stockings, etc — 1
3. All laundry must be done by others — 0

F. Mode of Transportation _____

1. Travels independently on public transportation or drives own car — 1
2. Arranges own travel via taxi but does not otherwise use public transportation — 1
3. Travels on public transportation when assisted or accompanied by another — 1
4. Travel limited to taxi or automobile with assistance of another — 0
5. Does not travel at all — 0

G. Responsibility for Own Medications _____

1. Is responsible for taking medication in correct dosages at correct time — 1
2. Takes responsibility if medication is prepared in advance in separate dosages — 0
3. Is not capable of dispensing own medication — 0

H. Ability to Handle Finances _____

1. Manages financial matters independently (budgets, writes checks, pays rent and bills, goes to bank); collects and keeps track of income — 1
2. Manages day-to-day purchases but needs help with banking, major purchases, etc. — 1
3. Incapable of handling money — 0

Scoring Interpretation: For ADLs, the total score ranges from 0 to 6, and for IADLs, from 0 to 8. In some categories, only the highest level of function receives a 1; in others, two or more levels have scores of 1 because each describes competence at some minimal level of function. These screens are useful for indicating specifically how a person is performing at the present time. When they are also used over time, they serve as documentation of a person's functional improvement or deterioration.

Source: Lawton MP, Brody EM. Assessment of older people: Self-maintaining and instrumental activities of daily living. Gerontologist. 1969;9:179-186. Copyright by the Gerontological Society of America. Reproduced by permission of the publisher.

they serve as documentation of a person's functional improvement or deterioration. However, it is worth noting that the description of the function is more important than the number total, especially when monitoring function over time.

Advanced Activities of Daily Living

Advanced activities of daily living (AADLs) represent the highest level of function and include vocational, social, or recreational activities that reflect personal choice and add meaning and richness to a person's life. The AADLs are specific to the individual patient and include employment, attending church, volunteering, going out to dinner or the theater, and participating in physical recreational activities. Changes in these activities may reflect a precursor to IADL or ADL dysfunction.[5]

The Vulnerable Elder 13 Survey. The Vulnerable Elder 13 Survey (VES-13) is a 13-item screening tool developed to identify populations of community-dwelling elders at increased risk for functional decline or death over the next 5 years (Table 7–3).[6-8] It can be self-administered or administered by nonmedical personnel over the telephone or in the office in less than 5 minutes. The VES-13 is based upon the ability to perform functional and physical activities, self-rated health, and age, rather than specific medical diagnoses.

Limits of Self-Reported Instruments. Subjective measures that rely on self-report may be inaccurate because a person may overestimate or underestimate his or her capabilities.[9] Studies have shown that race and ethnicity,[10-12] gender,[13] and cognitive impairment[14] may affect how functional impairment is reported. In addition, dependency in the traditionally assessed self-reported items, such as basic and instrumental activities of daily living (ADL), is uncommon among community-dwelling older persons (less than 10% in ADLs and approximately 25% dependent in IADLs).[9,15] As a result, these scales have ceiling effects in which a large proportion receive the top score (ie, are unimpaired).

Although existing self-report measures for basic, instrumental, and advanced activities of daily living are widely used, there is increasing recognition of the need to identify "preclinical disability" that may allow for interventions to modify the disability pathway.[3] As a result, interest in using performance-based measures to assess physical functioning has been increasing.[5]

Performance-Based Instruments

Older adults may not report physical difficulties on self-report measures if they are able to optimize their environment or compensate for their performance deficits by other methods. For example, an older person may answer negatively to the standard self-report on bathing and toileting but may have added grab bars to the bathroom. More objective measures of performance can provide additional information beyond an older adult's self-reported perception of difficulty.[1,9,16] These scales can be used alone or as part of a battery of tests.

Gait Speed and the Get-Up-and-Go Test

Ambulation is an essential prerequisite for completing many of the activities of daily living, and slowing of gait speed is an indicator of future morbidity. For example, gait speeds under 1.0 m/sec, between 0.6 and 1.0 m/sec, and especially below 0.6 m/sec predict hospitalization, cognitive impairment, and mortality.[17-20]

Many performance-based scales were designed for research purposes and are often impractical to use in routine patient care. Of these, the "Get-Up-and-Go" Test is among the few that have been recommended for clinical use.[17,21-23] This assessment procedure does not require specialized equipment but uses an armless chair and has the individual stand up from the chair, walk 3 meters, and sit back down (Table 7–4). It can be performed by the physician, nurse, or other trained health care provider. Not only should the time needed to perform this task be recorded, but observation of poor sitting and standing balance, difficulty rising or sitting down, staggering and discontinuity on turning, short, discontinuous steps,

---

● **TABLE 7–3** The Vulnerable Elders-13 Survey (VES-13)

Age	75-84 years	1 point
	> 85 years	3 points
Self-rated health	Fair or poor	1 point
	Good, very good, or excellent	0 points
Physical disabilities	• Stooping, crouching, or kneeling • Walking ¼ mile • Lifting 10 lbs • Heavy housework • Reaching above shoulder level • Writing or grasping small objects	1 point for each, maximum of 2 points
Functional disabilities (the short 5-item functional screen)	Requiring assistance in any of 5 activities: • Shopping • Light housework • Finances • Walking across room • Bathing	4 points for any activity

---

● **TABLE 7–4** Timed Get-Up-and-Go Test

Examiner asks the patient to:
- Stand up from a chair (without use of armrests, if possible)
- Stand still momentarily
- Walk 10 feet (3 meters)
- Turn around and walk back to chair
- Turn and be seated

Factors to note:
  Sitting balance
  Imbalance with immediate standing
  Pace (undue slowness) and stability of walking
  Excessive truncal sway and path deviation
  Ability to turn without staggering
  Observe and time the patient.

Positive screen: Time of >15 seconds to complete test

excessive truncal sway, and path deviation should be recorded. The patient may use assistive devices (ie, cane and walker) if needed. Severe abnormalities are considered present if the subject appears at risk for a fall at any time during the test. The time needed to complete this task also correlates to some mobility tasks: greater than 15 seconds is considered a positive screen (Table 7–5).

Short Physical Performance Battery

The Short Physical Performance Battery (SPPB) predicts future risk for hospitalization and length of stay, loss of independent living and institutionalization, future risk of mobility-related disability, and mortality (Figure 7–3).[24-27] Developed

● TABLE 7–5	Proportion Able to Complete Mobility Tasks, According to Timed Get-Up-and-Go Test Times			
		Timed Get Up and Go (sec)		
		10-19	20-29	30+
Tub or shower transfers	Self	59%	60%	23%
Climbs stairs	Self	77%	60%	4%
Goes outside alone	Yes	82%	50%	15%
Chair transfer	Self	100%	93%	62%

Source: Adapted from Podsiadlo D, Richardson S. J Am Geriatr Soc. 1991; 39:142-148, and Susan Friedman, MD, MPH, University of Rochester.

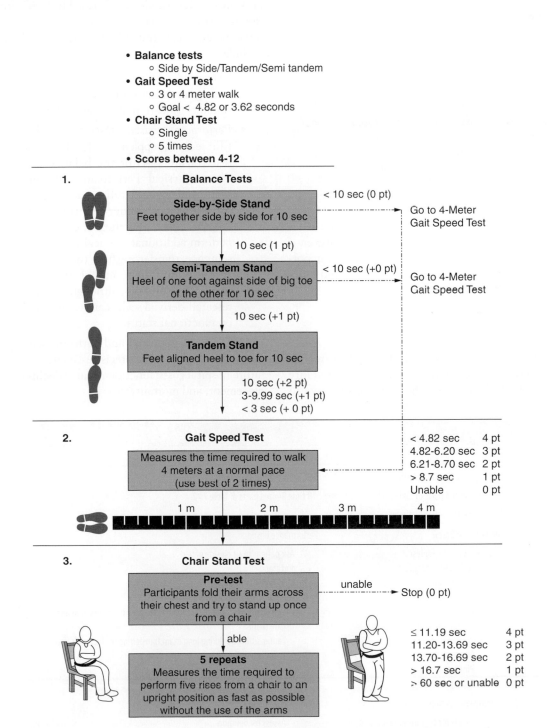

- **Balance tests**
  - Side by Side/Tandem/Semi tandem
- **Gait Speed Test**
  - 3 or 4 meter walk
  - Goal < 4.82 or 3.62 seconds
- **Chair Stand Test**
  - Single
  - 5 times
- **Scores between 4-12**

FIGURE 7–3. Short Physical Performance Battery. (*Accessed: www.niapublications.org/pubs/cdrom/assessingperformance/index.asp. Guralnik et al.*)

● **TABLE 7–6** Physical Performance Test Items

1. Writing a sentence[a]
2. Simulated eating
3. Turning 360 degrees
4. Putting on and removing a jacket[a]
5. Lifting a book and putting it on a shelf
6. Picking up a penny from the floor
7. A 50-foot walk test
8. Climbing stairs one flight
9. Climbing stairs four flights

Mini Physical Performance Test

1. Pick up a penny
2. Walk 50 feet
3. Chair rise 5 times
4. Progressive Romberg Test

Maximum score is 36; 4 points per item.
[a]*Can be used alone during the physician visit.*
Source: Reuben DB, Siu AL. An objective measure of physical function of elderly outpatients. The physical performance test. J Am Geriatr Soc. 1990;38:1105-1112; and Consuelo H. Wilkins CH, Roe CM, Morris JC. A brief clinical tool to assess physical function: The mini-physical performance test. Arch Gerontol Geriatr. 2009.

by the National Institute of Aging, this test may not be as practical for routine use in a busy clinic setting; however, if the clinician has 3 to 5 minutes to perform this test, important information can be gained on gait, balance, and functional lower extremity strength.

Physical Performance Test and Mini-Physical Performance Test

The original Physical Performance Test (PPT)[5] correlates with degree of disability, loss of independence, and mortality (Table 7–6).[28] The PPT has been shown to be sensitive to change as an outcome of interventions (eg, comprehensive geriatric assessment)[29] and detects early physical decline in community-dwelling elderly.[30] Recently, a 4-item scale (the Mini-PPT) based on the Physical Performance Test has been developed.[31] Elements of these tests (sentence writing) may be used to screen patients in a variety of care settings.

Functional Assessment in the Office Setting

Performance-based procedures and tools such as the PPT and SBPP have been widely used in research, but widespread use in clinical practice has been limited by time and resource pressures.[22] Nevertheless, it is feasible to incorporate functional status assessments into busy settings in ways that preserve their clinical utility (Table 7–7). A viable strategy could include:

- *Self-report.* ADLs and IADLs assessed using a questionnaire prior to a visit (Tables 7–2A and 7–2B) with additional clarification, if needed, by the physician.

- *Performance-based tests.* Timed get-up-and-go (Table 7–4), supplemented with the modified Romberg test (Figure 7–4) or the balance component of the Short Physical Performance Battery (side-by-side, semi-tandem, and full-tandem stance), and simple screening in shoulder function and hand function (Figure 7–5).[21] Specifically, one can observe patients perform additional physical tasks, including writing a sentence, transferring from the chair to the exam table, and watching them unhook their bra or unbutton a shirt. These findings, although not specifically put in a research-derived scale, can still give useful information on functional status.

Combining self-reported and performance-based measurements can provide more precise estimates of life expectancy, future hospital costs, functional status decline, nursing-home placement, and mortality[9,32]

● **TABLE 7–7** Functional Status Evaluation

Outpatient	Inpatient
Self-report: BADL/IADL/AADL	Self-report: BADL/IADL/AADL
*If time limited parts of Table 7–2	*If time limited parts of Table 7–2
*Be aware of preclinical disability	
Performance Based	Performance Based
1. Get-Up-and-Go Test	1. Ask patient to sit on side of bed and stand
2. Modified Romberg Test	2. Modified Romberg Test
- Side by side	3. Other physical performance tests
- Semi-tandem	- Personally observed or discussed with other members of health care team
- Full tandem	
3. Shoulder function	- Eating, sitting up during lung exam, transferring to chair, ambulating to bathroom
4. Hand function	
- Grasp or	
- Pinch or	
- Sentence writing	
Cognitive evaluation	Cognitive evaluation
- Assess for cognitive impairment or dementia	- Assess for delirium

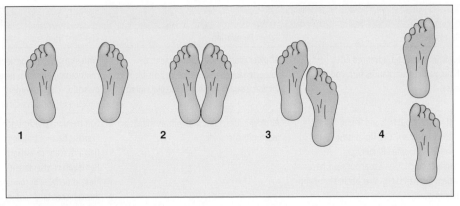

FIGURE 7–4. Modified Romberg Test. **1.** Patient standing, feet comfortably apart (eyes open and then eyes closed); **2.** Feet together (eyes open and eyes closed); **3.** Feet placed heel to instep (eyes open and then closed); **4.** Feet placed heel to toe (eyes open and then closed). Patient is asked, "Do you feel steady?" with successive stress changes. Testing is discontinued when instability is first noticed. (*From Fleming & Evans.*[21])

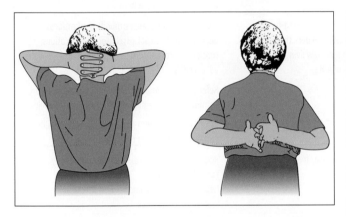

FIGURE 7–5A. Simple screening in shoulder and hand function. *Left.* Patient is asked to put hands together in back at waist level. *Right.* Patient is asked to put both hands together behind neck.

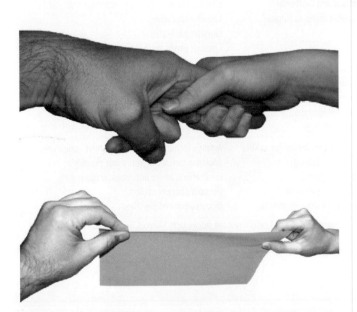

FIGURE 7–5B. Hand Function.[21] 1. Squeeze two of the examiner's fingers with each hand. 2. Pinch strength assessed by having patient firmly hold a piece of paper between the thumb and index finger while the examiner tries to pull the paper out. 3. Observation of patient's ability to write a sentence as part of the Folstein Mini-Mental State Examination (MMSE).

Other Assessment Tools

Since many geriatric syndromes like falls, incontinence, and functional dependence are multi-factorial, researchers and some physicians have advocated additional selected assessment tools to increase the effectiveness of the clinical examination. These assessments overlap with many elements seen in a comprehensive geriatric evaluation, and include evaluations of cognition, special senses (hearing and vision), and psychosocial issues.[21] Several validated short versions of multi-dimensional screens are available,[1,2] but still take considerable staff time to administer. However, in patients who present with physical functional decline or cognitive impairment, these additional assessments should be pursued and applied (Table 7–8).

The following case example highlights the importance of functional status and its evaluation throughout the spectrum of aging.

CASE PRESENTATION: FUNCTIONAL ASSESSMENT IN PRACTICE

Mr. B. is a 78-year-old man with a past medical history of coronary artery disease with coronary artery bypass grafting (CABG), aortic stenosis, atrial fibrillation, diabetes, colon cancer treated by resection, hearing loss requiring hearing aids, and osteoporosis. He recently moved into the state to be near his children after his wife of 60 years died. After his move, he babysat his grandchildren and drove them to and from school. As a retired certified public accountant (CPA), he also volunteered at the local senior center during tax season. He has ambulated with a cane for the past 2 years to increase his stability while walking. He visited his new internist and his functional status revealed intact basic, instrumental, and advanced activities of daily living. His medications were reviewed and he continued to visit his internist with good control of his medical problems.

Two years later, Mr. B. was hospitalized for an episode of decompensated heart failure likely related

● **TABLE 7–8** Summary of Practical Functional Assessment in Elderly Patients

Key Area	Assessment	Target Population	The Next Step
ADL	Basic, instrumental, advanced ADLs Timing and circumstances surrounding losses	All older adults; those with dementia, suspected functional decline, or possible need for home care or nursing-home placement	With impairments, consider underlying or contributing cognitive, neurologic, or musculoskeletal disorders; assistance or adaptive equipment; and physical or occupational therapy
Mobility	Gait—Ask about falls and fear of falling; observe transfers; "Get-Up-and-Go Test" Balance—Modified Romberg Shoulder function—Ask about pain; have patient put hands together behind head and behind waist Hand function—Test grasp strength, pinch strength, dexterity (ie, write a sentence)	All older adults; those with history of falls or indeterminate "spells"	Gait training (physical/occupational therapy) Exercise, balance training (Tai Chi) Gait aids (cane or walker) Home safety assessment Treat underlying or contributory neurologic or musculoskeletal disorders Test hand function and upper extremity strength Consider x-ray study Physical therapy (ROM, pain-relief, and strengthening) Assess ADLs Assess adaptive equipment
Cognitive function (Chapter 33)	Folstein MMSE Mini-cog (clock drawing) ADLs Formal psychometrics	Patients > 80 years old; nursing-home residents, hospitalized elders; those with depression, delirium, new living situations, or impairments of ADLs	Look for reversible causes; modify medications; discuss legal, financial, psychosocial implications; consider depression; discuss placement and advanced directives
Vision (Chapter 7)	Read a newspaper headline and sentence; test vision with Snellen or Jaeger acuity chart	All older adults	Refer to ophthalmology, low-vision aids, adequate lighting, adaptive equipment, test gait and mobility
Hearing (Chapter 7)	Listen for rubbing of fingers or ticking watch; the "whisper test"	All older adults	Refer for audiometry, ENT evaluation, hearing aids, Portable amplifier Test for gait and balance
Continence (Chapter 35)	Ask about incontinence	All older adults (twice as frequent in women)	Request incontinence diary to improve history Formal education Kegel exercises; fluid and voiding schedule, biofeedback, pessaries
Nutrition	Inquire about weight loss and loss of appetite: establish baseline weight to substantiate actual loss	All older adults	Measure weight serially, ENT, abdominal, rectal, neurologic, and CV exam (for cause); add nutritional supplement (nutritional shake) Advise eating with others (avoid isolation) Consider abuse or neglect
Depression (Chapter 39)	Ask about depression: "Do you often feel sad or depressed?" Geriatric Depression Scale PHQ-9	Patients with bereavement, psychosocial losses, dementia, recent functional impairments, severe illness, or surgical procedure	Anticipate depressive symptoms in at-risk elderly patients to increase awareness Consider counseling Consider medication Consider psychiatry if diagnosis difficult, depression severe (psychosis, weight loss)
Alcohol Abuse	ADLs Interview CAGE questionnaire	Hospitalized patients, psychiatric inpatients, new functional impairments, delirium, dementia, new nursing-home admission	Advise abstinence Arrange for formal counseling (AA) Consider abuse or neglect Add multivitamin
Caregiver Needs Assessment (Chapter 17)	Assess ADLs Interview family and caregivers Assess caregiver capacity and burden Nursing or social work interview	For caregivers of patients dependent in ADLs (esp. basic eating and dressing) Bladder/bowel incontinence Dementia/cognitive impairment Prior home health or nursing-home stay	Arrange for home assistance, adaptive equipment, adult day care, social work input, simplify medications, advise firm plans for future care Consider abuse or neglect Discuss advanced directives

Source: Adapted from Fleming KC, Evans JM. Practical functional assessment of elderly persons: A primary care approach. Mayo Clinic Proc. 1995;76: 890-910.

to progression of his aortic stenosis, with new-onset atrial fibrillation and worsening of his hypertension. He was discharged to home and had follow-up with Home Health Care, which provided biweekly nursing and physical therapy visits. His granddaughter agreed to stay with him a few hours a day for about 2 weeks during his summer break.

While staying with him, she noted he was having difficulties taking his pills. Although he used a pill box to help ensure accuracy of administration, pills were found mixed in with pills for other days. Furthermore, he missed paying several bills and was charged late fees. Given these concerns about his ability to live alone, his daughter began arranging for him to live in a local assisted living facility. His daughter called his primary care physician and accompanied him to his next follow-up visit. His physician noticed that his cholesterol level and blood pressure, which had been previously well controlled, were abnormal, and there was suspicion that Mr. B.'s anticoagulation control was becoming erratic. The physician interviewed the patient and his daughter.

By self-report and some clarification with his daughter, the following information was obtained on Mr. B.'s functional status when living at home:

BADLs	IADLs
Bathing—Intact	Medications—Daughter added she has set up a pill box
Dressing—Intact	Grocery shopping—Goes with daughter; however, his wife used to do the grocery shopping
Toileting—Intact	Preparing meals—Making more TV dinners rather than using the stove, although his wife cooked for both of them before her death
Transfers—Intact	Using the telephone—Intact
Grooming—Intact	Handling own finances—Daughter helps
Feeding—Intact	Driving and transportation—Encouraged to abstain by daughter but is still driving near his house
	Housekeeping—Has a housekeeper once a week, which his daughter had requested because his wife did this prior to her death
	Laundry—Housekeeper once a week as, again, his wife used to do this task

BADL score 6/6   IADL score 2/8

The physician also asked about perceived difficulties and how Mr. B. had changed the way he completed tasks. Mr. B. stated that he is doing fine but admits to his daughter helping out more.

Physical Performance-Based Tests

To supplement the self-reported items, the physician administered performance-based testing focusing on gait, and balance with the Timed Get-Up-and-Go and Modified Romberg Tests. The patient was observed to have quadriceps weakness on standing, and impairment in the Modified Romberg Test, with problems with semi-tandem stance without a cane. The Timed Get-Up-and-Go Test was 17 seconds using his cane (normal < 15) (Table 7–4, Figures 7–4, 7–5A, and 7–5B). He was referred to outpatient physical therapy for gait and balance assessment and training on use of adaptive equipment. A handout on home safety was given to his daughter.

Mr. B. returned for follow-up 1 month later. His lab tests, including thyroid function, comprehensive metabolic panel, and complete blood count, were normal. His medications were evaluated and—given his persistent abnormal Mini Mental Status Exam of 22/30 and his decline in functional status—donepezil was started. Based on his IADL impairment, Mr. B. was advised to move to an assisted living facility, and receive medication management service. Furthermore, the physician also clarified his durable power of attorney for health care and began discussing advanced care planning (Chapters 9 and 11).

Assisted Living Facility Setting

Mr. B. moved to a nearby assisted living facility. At the time of admission, his functional status was:

BADLs	IADLs
Bathing—Intact	Administering own medications—Done by facility
Dressing—Intact	Grocery shopping—Done by facility
Toileting—Intact	Preparing meals—Done by facility
Transfers—Intact	Using the telephone—Intact
Grooming—Intact	Handling own finances—Daughter helps
Feeding—Intact	Driving and transportation—Not done
	Housekeeping—Done by facility
	Laundry—Done by facility

BADL score 6/6   IADL score 1/8

The assisted living facility had different care levels including independent apartments with room and board and additional fee-based services including medication management, housekeeping, hourly caregivers, as well as a locked dementia floor.

Four-and-a-half weeks later, Mr. B. began to complain of dizziness and poor appetite. He was unwilling to participate in the group activities or daily exercises as he had just a week ago. He also began to have episodes of fecal incontinence and diarrhea. He had an unwitnessed fall in the dining room after breakfast. Immediately after the fall, he complained of groin pain and was brought to the Emergency Department (ED) for evaluation. X-ray evaluation revealed a right intertrochanteric fracture.

Emergency Room Setting

The ED physician informed the hospitalist and orthopedic consultant that Mr. B. was living in an assisted living facility and ambulated with a cane. Mr. B.'s primary care physician was contacted, who relayed the status of Mr. B.'s ADLs but specifically cited his need for medication management at the assisted living facility, prior ambulatory status with a cane, and known cognitive impairment. Even though Mr. B. had medical co-morbidities including aortic stenosis and coronary artery disease, surgery was appropriate, given his prior ambulatory status and the risks of pain and other adverse outcomes including DVT and pressure ulcers should surgery not be pursued.

Multiple studies not only show functional impairment as being a very common finding in the Emergency Department setting,[33,34] but functional impairments are independent predictors of repeat Emergency Department visits and short-term poor medical outcome in ED patients.[33,35,36] By determining Mr. B.'s functional status and acknowledging his setting of care (assisted living facility), the medical team can anticipate his hospital course (ie, risk for delirium, iatrogenesis, and rehabilitation potential) and clarify the need for surgical or other interventions both during the acute event and in the future.

Inpatient Setting

Mr. B. underwent ORIF (open reduction with internal fixation) with minimal blood loss. On the second postoperative day, he had episodes of confusion and agitation characterized by wanting to pack his bags for an upcoming vacation; he was also pulling at his intravenous lines all night. His postoperative course was further complicated by an episode of atrial fibrillation with rapid ventricular response and a urinary tract infection. After removal of unnecessary intravenous lines and his Foley catheter, and arrangement for a sitter and increased visits by family members, Mr. B. was able to be evaluated by physical therapy. He was able to sit on the side of the bed and stand with moderate assistance, and by his fourth postoperative day, he was able to walk 10 feet with a front-wheeled walker. Mr. B. was discharged to a local SNF (skilled nursing facility) with goals of rehabilitation and return to his previous living situation.

When patients are admitted to the hospital, their functional status should be evaluated and monitored.

Individuals with a poor baseline functional status (ie, impairments in basic activities of daily living, nursing-home residents) usually have underlying combinations of medical, cognitive, or psychosocial co-morbidities that impact many aspects of their hospital care. ADL impairment has been found to be a stronger predictor of hospital outcomes (functional decline, length of stay, institutionalization, hospital cost, 90-day and 1-year mortality, and death) than admitting diagnoses, diagnosis-related group (DRGs), and other physiologic indices of illness burden.[37,38] Functional status is also an important predictor of delirium risk,[39] determinant of discharge planning (ie, hospital to rehabilitation center rather than home), and can help frame goals of care especially in the critically ill.

For Intensive Care Unit patients, baseline functional status, rather than initial abnormal physiologic status, is a major determinant for both early (6 weeks) and late (6 months) recovery.[40] The failure to regain function during hospitalization is associated with higher mortality rate at 3 months, compared with those who regain their baseline functional status.[41]

By knowing Mr. B.'s functional and cognitive status, the health care team can anticipate his hospital course. Measures should be taken to avoid and anticipate his delirium (Chapters 21 and 32), the rehabilitation team (physical therapy, occupational therapy) should use his prior ambulation status to formulate a rehabilitation plan, and finally, members of the multidisciplinary team (ie, discharge planner) should address transitions of care in this case to a rehabilitation facility (Chapters 22 and 19). The following strategy for hospital functional assessment can be employed:

- *Self-report.* Prehospital ADLs and IADLs should be assessed with interview with the patient and/or family members and additional clarification, if needed, by the physician. If time is limited, selected BADLs and IADLs would be helpful to characterize. For example, ambulation, medications, and financial management, with details of how these functional tasks are accomplished. The information can also be obtained by other members of the multidisciplinary team including social work and physical and occupational therapy, and can be mobilized to clarify a baseline functional status.
- *Performance-based.* Although studies have shown the use of the SBPP (Short Physical Performance Battery; Figure 7–3) is correlated with hospital stay,[42] it is not practical because of the time and logistics of applying this test to the inpatient setting. Functional status can be evaluated in other ways—by observing the patient sitting up during the lung exam, sitting to the side of the bed, standing, and possibly doing the Modified Romberg Test. Findings including proximal weakness, imbalance, and symptoms of dizziness should be elicited. These evaluations should be done at admission and regularly throughout the hospital course. Furthermore, input from nursing staff and other members of the health care team about the patient's ability to transfer, to go to the bathroom with assistance, and feeding difficulty should be obtained. Any difficulties noted would merit evaluation by physical and or occupational therapists early in the hospital course.

When functional impairment is noted, other members of the health care team including social work and the discharge planner should be involved (Chapter 19). In addition, bedrest orders should be avoided whenever possible. Restraints, intravenous lines, Foley catheters, or other devices should be evaluated routinely for their use and removed as soon as possible. Patients should be ordered to be out of bed and into a chair during meals and during other times of day.

Skilled Nursing Facility/Short-Term Rehabilitation Setting

Mr. B. was admitted to the local skilled nursing facility, or nursing home, for rehabilitation. On day 7 of his stay, the nursing staff completed the Minimum Data Set (MDS), which documented his need for ADL assistance, mobility prior to admission, balance, and range of motion. Physical therapy was initiated with long-term goals of ambulation with a cane given his prior level of function. Occupational Therapy spent time on his BADLs, specifically focusing on therapy for his lower body to enable independence in dressing. The MDS also corroborated his deficits in vision, cognition, hearing, gait, and cognitive impairment. These functional deficits were supported by members of the rehabilitation team (ie, occupational therapy, certified nurses' aides, activity coordinator). Care plan meetings were held and ongoing discussions confirmed his daughter being his durable power of attorney and that full resuscitation be pursued including hospitalization. He stayed at the SNF for 6 weeks. At the time of discharge from the SNF, Mr. B. was able to walk 200 feet out-and-back with a front-wheeled walker with larger than standard-sized wheels. Physical therapy added a heel lift to address a leg length discrepancy. He had follow-up with the orthopedic surgeon, who maintained the order for weight-bearing as tolerated.

Older persons in nursing homes and receiving home health care are at increased risk of further health deterioration. As a result, the CMS (Center for Medicare and Medicaid Services) in the United States and multiple health care entities around the world have developed comprehensive assessment instruments including the Minimum Data Set (MDS) in the Skilled Nursing Facility and nursing home, and the OASIS (Outcome and Assessment Data Set) for home health. Studies have not clearly shown improved outcomes from the use of these assessment tools, but quality-of-care studies are ongoing.[43-47]

Back in Assisted Living after Short-Term Rehabilitation

Mr. B. was discharged to his assisted living facility with Home Health Care, which included a multidisciplinary team of nursing, physical, and occupational therapy. At his facility, he continued to rely on using a walker. The occupational therapist performed a home safety evaluation and added extra grab bars to the bathroom and a raised toilet seat. He continued to participate in daily exercises and other activities at the assisted living facility. Although he initially had a fear of falling, this improved with physical therapy.

Follow-up with his primary care physician revealed:

BADLs	IADLs
Bathing—Intact	Administering own medications—Done by facility
Dressing—Intact but using reacher and sock aid	Grocery shopping—Done by facility
Toileting—Intact	Preparing meals—Done by facility
Transfers—Intact but using front-wheeled walker	Using the telephone—Increasing difficulty, but using speed dial
Grooming—Intact	Handling own finances—Daughter helps
Feeding—Intact	Driving and transportation—Not done
	Housekeeping—Done by facility
	Laundry—Done by facility

BADL score 5/6   IADL score 1/8

- Timed Get-Up-and-Go (Table 7-4)—25 seconds (prior, 16 seconds).
- Tub transfer and climb stairs—60%, goes outside alone—50%.
- Modified Romberg Test (Figure 7-4)—Impaired side-by-side stance without walker (prior, impaired semi-tandem). He was noted to have a limp (antalgia) when he walked. His primary care provider therefore requested a home health agency to give him weekly updates about his progress and to continue physical therapy with an occupational therapy follow-up to assess for environmental modifications (raised toilet seats, grab bars). He was continued on his regular medications.

Future Issues in Mr. B.'s Care and the Role of Functional Assessment (Dementia, Cancer, Advanced Directives, and Chronic Disease Management)

Since Mr. B.'s pre–hip fracture history pointed to progressive cognitive impairment, his physician anticipated this further decline. Over the next 7 years, he was continued on his donepezil, and started on memantine. A Reisberg Functional Assessment Scale (FAST) was used to document this decline.[48] Prior to this more substantial decline, his physician addressed the issue of feeding and the role of gastrostomy tube placement. Additional discussions were held with his daughter and framed by prior discussions with the patient. Mr. B. made it clear that feeding himself was a very important functional outcome.

Using functional status to frame an intervention can be helpful in advanced care planning. For example, asking "What is something you do on a daily basis that is so important that if you were unable to do it, you would not say you were 'living'?" would be one way to introduce advanced care planning (Chapters 9 and 11). In addition, resuscitation preferences could be explored by adding, "If the doctors could do these life-sustaining procedures to prolong your life but you were still unable to do that special activity you mentioned, would you want that procedure to be done?" Feeding himself was an important functional goal for Mr. B. Therefore, his advanced care goals placed limitations, and focused on not escalating his care given the unlikelihood that interventions like cardiopulmonary resuscitation and intubation would improve his already compromised functional state.

CASE PRESENTATION (continued)

At the age of 88, Mr. B. was noted to have new-onset iron deficiency anemia and weight loss. Concern was for recurrence of his colon cancer. His Karnovsky Scale (Table 7-9)[49] was scored at 50 (moderately disabled). The Reisberg FAST Scale was scored at stage 5 (requires assistance in choosing proper clothing) but with some elements of stage 6 (unable to bathe properly). The VES-13 score was 8 (Table 7-3). His

● TABLE 7–9 Karnofsky Scale

This 10-point scale is a quick and easy way to indicate how a person is feeling on a given day, without going through several multiple-choice questions or symptom surveys.

Score	Description
100	Able to work; normal, no complaints, no evidence of disease
90	Able to work; able to carry on normal activity, minor symptoms
80	Able to work; normal activity with effort, some symptoms
70	Unable to work or carry on normal activity, cares for self independently
60	Mildly disabled, dependent; requires occasional assistance, cares for most needs
50	Moderately disabled, dependent; requires considerable assistance and frequent care
40	Severely disabled, dependent; requires special care and assistance
30	Severely disabled; hospitalized, death not imminent
20	Very sick; active supportive treatment needed
10	Moribund; fatal processes rapidly progressing

Source: Karnofsky DA, Burchenal JH. The clinical evaluation of chemotherapeutic agents in cancer. In: MacLeon CM, ed. Evaluation of Chemotherapeutic Agents. Columbia University Press; 1949:196.

daughter had already been assigned Durable Power of Attorney (DPOA) for health care, as Mr. B. was no longer capable of decision-making. With the help of the above assessment findings, and his family's impression of his increasing functional reliance, a decision was made not to evaluate the cause of his anemia.

In addition, his functional status was helpful in addressing some of his chronic illnesses, including diabetes. His hemoglobin A_{1c} was stable at 7.6%, and given the higher risk of hypoglycemia and the lack of clinical evidence of benefits from aggressive sugar management, additional hypoglycemic agents were not added.

Mr. B.'s functional status took on even more importance in helping stage his dementia, and assisting in the management of a probable colon cancer recurrence. Dementia is defined by both cognitive and functional impairment,[50] and clinical tools used in geriatric oncology involve some type of functional assessment. The ECOG and Karnovsky Scales (Table 7–10) are used to help determine feasibility of surgery, chemotherapy, radiation, or palliation options in geriatric cancer patients.[51-54] Functional status has an impact on prognosis in acute illness such as pneumonia[55] and decompensated heart failure,[56] and has a role in the evaluation and outcomes of chronic conditions such as osteoarthritis,[57] Parkinson disease,[58] diabetes,[59] and end-stage renal disease.[60] The poorer the prior functional status, the worse the outcomes.

In a 10-year longitudinal study of older adults characterizing common medical conditions leading to death and trajectories of functional disability during the last year of life (none, catastrophic, accelerated, progressive, and persistently severe), heterogeneity was found among patients with frailty (weight loss, exhaustion, low physical activity, muscle weakness, and slow gait speed), cancer, organ failure (congestive heart failure, end-stage lung disease, end-stage kidney disease, and cirrhosis), advanced dementia, and sudden death.[61] Personal care needs at the end of life were not easily predicted, which may raise questions about policies whose benefits are solely based on disease-specific criteria in the last year of life.

CONCLUSION

An older person's ability to function can be viewed as a summary measure of the overall effect of medical conditions, lifestyle, and age-related physiologic changes in the context of his or her environment and social support system.[9] Characterizing and appreciating functional status is critical in the evaluation of all older adults. Functional status has been called the sixth vital sign (with pain being the fifth).[62] Unfortunately, physicians often fail to recognize and document functional disability in patients in both the ambulatory and inpatient settings.[62,63] There has been an increasing acknowledgment by governmental agencies (Medicare in the United States) and other groups like the American Geriatrics Society that functional status be evaluated in all levels of care (outpatient, inpatient, nursing homes, and other sites of care).[64]

Changes in Mr. B.'s functional status were associated with loss of independence, increased caregiver burden, and greater financial expenditures. At several time points, changes in functional status were an important presenting symptom of other acute illness. Oftentimes, the appearance of traditional symptoms of medical illness will be preceded by a decline in function, for example, a "failure to go shopping" or "spending more time in bed."

When patients are in the hospital, their functional status becomes an important element in determining further transitions of care (eg, hospital to home). In the care of older adults, establishing a "safe" environment that supplements their functional status is critical. This can be achieved by additional caregivers or other supported care settings (assisted living, nursing home, rehabilitation center). Knowing Mr. B.'s functional baseline was important in his placement in an assisted living facility and transition to a nursing home for rehabilitation after his hip fracture.

Baseline functional information is also important to manage acute illness and determine treatment options. If the prior functional status is not known, how can recovery be framed after a major catastrophic event like Mr. B.'s hip fracture or other events like a stroke? The primary care provider or other members of the health care team (eg, physical therapy, nursing) must be able to convey specific knowledge of the person's previous level of function to assist in setting reasonable targets for recovery. For example, since Mr. B.'s prior functional baseline was ambulating with a walker, surgery to repair his hip was appropriate, as this

● **TABLE 7–10** The KPS and ECOG Scales

(%)	Karnofsky Performance Scale (KPS)	Score	ECOG Performance Scale
100	Normal, no complaints, no evidence of disease	0	Normal activity; asymptomatic
90	Able to carry on normal activity; minor signs or symptoms of disease	1	Symptomatic; fully ambulatory
80	Normal activity with effort; some signs or symptoms of disease		
70	Cares for self, unable to carry on normal activity or to do active work	2	Symptomatic; in bed <50% of time
60	Requires occasional assistance, but is able to care for most of his/her needs		
50	Requires considerable assistance and frequent medical care	3	Symptomatic; in bed 50% of time; not bedridden
40	Disabled, requires special care and assistance		
30	Severely disabled, hospitalization indicated; death not imminent		
20	Very sick, hospitalization indicated; death not imminent	4	100% bedridden
10	Moribund, fatal processes, progressing rapidly		
0	Dead	5	Dead

would be the most reasonable option to restore his mobility. If the patient had impairments in basic ADLs, then perhaps assistance from nurses or nurses' aides would be needed in the hospital or nursing home.

Functional status information also helps in prioritizing individual patient problems and deciding on the intensity and effectiveness of treatment. When multiple medical, psychosocial, and cognitive co-morbidities are present, the problem that most affects the person's daily life may be more important than the severity of any individual condition. For example, Mr. B.'s hip fracture must be understood to assess the risk-benefit ratio of each intervention. Earlier in his long course of care with his primary care physician, repair of his hip fracture was more clearly indicated given Mr. B.'s initial functional status, but—given his functional status and dementia later in his life—the evaluation and treatment of recurrent colon cancer and tight control of his diabetes were not.

Functional assessment findings should be accurately recorded so that the degree of change over time and the speed of functional change can be monitored. In this manner, the potential functional impairment due to chronic conditions like congestive heart failure, depression, or changes in care setting (eg, to an assisted living facility) can be accurately measured and monitored.

For the busy outpatient practice, BADL, IADL, and AADL assessment by questionnaire and appropriate follow-up questioning, the Timed Get-Up-and-Go Test, Modified Romberg Test or Short Physical Performance Battery balance test, shoulder and hand function, as well as a cognitive assessment screen are useful. This should be done routinely on the first visit, on a yearly basis, and at the time of any changes in functional status or cognition.

Conducting careful, comprehensive, and periodic functional assessments, health care providers can promote their patients' autonomy and mobilize appropriate medical, social, and environmental supports on their behalf (Tables 7–11 and 7–7).

● **TABLE 7–11** Some Reasons to Screen for and Describe Functional Status

1. Changes in functional status can be **a symptom of acute or worsening chronic illness** (congestive heart failure, urinary tract infection, malignancy)

2. Critical in **determining appropriate level of care and transitions of care**
   a. Can the patient stay home safely or does he or she need a caregiver or more family help?
   b. Can the patient safely return home after his or her hospitalization?
   c. Should the patient be in an assisted living facility or nursing home?

3. Important in **managing acute illness and determining prognosis and treatment options** (cerebrovascular accident, cancer, myocardial infarction)
   a. Should this patient undergo cardiac catheterization with findings of a non–Q wave myocardial infarction?
   b. Should a surgical procedure be offered for management of this patient's breast cancer?

4. Prioritizing individual patient problems and **deciding on the intensity and effectiveness of treatment**
   a. What benefit would a functionally frail patient get from management of his or her diabetes?
   b. How much does the patient's incontinence impact his or her daily functional status?
   c. In a patient with cognitive impairment and chronic constipation, would starting an anticholinergic be helpful?

References

1. Guralnik JM, Ferrucci L. Assessing the building blocks of function: Utilizing measures of functional limitation. *Am J Prev Med.* 2003; 25(suppl):112-121.

2. Reuben DB. Performance-based measures of physical function: Concepts and roles. Presented at NIA Behavioral and Social Research Physical Performance Protocols meeting, December 12, 2003.

3. Fried L. Relationships between performance measures and self-report: Examples from the Women's Health and Aging Studies. Presented at the National Institute on Aging Behavioral and Social Research Physical Performance Protocols meeting, December 12, 2003.

4. Gill TM, Robison JT, Tinetti ME. Difficulty and dependence: Two components of the disability continuum among community-living older persons. *Ann Intern Med.* 1998;128:96-101.

5. Reuben DB, Siu AL. An objective measure of physical function of elderly outpatients. The Physical Performance Test. *J Am Geriatr Soc.* 1990;38:1105-1112.

6. Saliba D, Elliott M, Rubenstein LZ, et al. The Vulnerable Elders Survey: A tool for identifying vulnerable older people in the community. *J Am Geriatr Soc.* 2001;49:1691-1699.

7. Min L, Yoon W, Mariano J, et al. The Vulnerable Elders-13 Survey predicts 5-year functional decline and mortality outcomes among older ambulatory care patients. *J Am Geriatr Soc.* 2009;57:2070-2076.

8. Min LC, Elliott MN, Wenger NS, Saliba D. Higher vulnerable elders survey scores predict death and functional decline in vulnerable older people. *J Am Geriatr Soc.* 2006;54:507-511.

9. Reuben DB, Seeman TE, Keeler E, et al. Refining the categorization of physical functional status: The added value of combining self-reported and performance-based measures. *J Gerontol A Biol Sci Med Sci.* 2004;59:1056-1061.

10. Spencer SM, Albert SM, Bear-Lehman J, Burkhardt A. Relevance of race and ethnicity for self-reported functional limitation. *J Am Geriatr Soc.* 2008;56:553-557.

11. Shih VC, Song J, Chang RW, Dunlop DD. Racial differences in activities of daily living limitation onset in older adults with arthritis: A national cohort study. *Arch Phys Med Rehabil.* 2005;86:1521-1526.

12. Sims T, Holmes TH, Bravata DM, et al. Simple counts of ADL dependencies do not adequately reflect older adults' preferences toward states of functional impairment. *J Clin Epidemiol.* 2008;61:1261-1270.

13. Merrill SS, Seeman TE, Kasl SV, et al. Gender differences in the comparison of self-reported disability and performance measures. *J Gerontol A Biol Sci Med Sci.* 1997;52A:M19-M26.9.

14. Jefferson AL, Byerly LK, Vanderhill S, Characterization of activities of daily living in individuals with mild cognitive impairment. *Am J Geriatr Psychiatry.* 2008;16:375-383.

15. Lawton MP, Brody EM. Assessment of older people: Self-maintaining and instrumental activities of daily living. *Gerontologist.* 1969;9:179-186.

16. Cesari M, Kritchevsky SB. Added value of physical performance measures in predicting adverse health-related events: Results from the Health, Aging And Body Composition Study. *J Am Geriatr Soc.* 2009;57:251-259.

17. Studenski S, Perera S. Physical performance measures in the clinical setting. *J Am Geriatr Soc.* 2003;51:314-322.

18. Hardy SE, Perera S. Improvement in usual gait speed predicts better survival in older adults. *J Am Geriatr Soc.* 2007;55:1727-1734.

19. Ostir GV, Kuo YF. Measures of lower body function and risk of mortality over 7 years of follow-up. *Am J Epidemiol.* 2007;166:599-605.

20. Fitzpatrick AL, Buchanan CK, Ginkgo Evaluation of Memory (GEM) Study Investigators. Associations of gait speed and other measures of physical function with cognition in a healthy cohort of elderly persons. *J Gerontol A Biol Sci Med Sci.* 2007;62:1244-1251.

21. Fleming KC, Evans JM. Practical functional assessment of elderly persons: A primary-care approach. *Mayo Clinical Proc.* 1995;70:890-910.

22. Moore AA, Siu AL. Screening for common problems in ambulatory elderly: Clinical confirmation of a screening instrument. *Am J Med.* 1996;100:438.

23. Hurria A, Lichtman SM, Kelly E. Identifying vulnerable older adults with cancer: Integrating geriatric assessment into oncology practice. *J Am Geriatr Soc.* 2007;55:1604-1608.

24. Guralnik JM, Ferrucci L, Pieper CF, et al. Lower extremity function and subsequent disability: consistency across studies, predictive models, and value of gait speed alone compared with the short physical performance battery. *J Gerontol A Biol Sci Med Sci.* 2000;55:221-231.

25. Vasunilashorn S, Guralnik JM. Use of the Short Physical Performance Battery score to predict loss of ability to walk 400 meters: Analysis from the InCHIANTI study. *J Gerontol A Biol Sci Med Sci.* 2009;64:223-229.

26. Volpato S, Guralnik JM. Performance-based functional assessment in older hospitalized patients: Feasibility and clinical correlates. *J Gerontol A Biol Sci Med Sci.* 2008;63:1393-1398.

27. Miller DK, Miller JP. Adverse outcomes and correlates of change in the Short Physical Performance Battery over 36 months in the African American health project. *J Gerontol A Biol Sci Med Sci.* 2008;63:487-494.

28. Reuben DB, Siu AL. The predictive validity of self-report and performance-based measures of function and health. *J Gerontol.* 1992;47:M106-M110.

29. Reuben DB, Frank JC. A randomized clinical trial of outpatient comprehensive geriatric assessment coupled with an intervention to increase adherence to recommendations. *J Am Geriatr Soc.* 1999;47:269-276.

30. Brach JS, Krista AM. Identifying early decline of physical function in community-dwelling older women: Performance-based and self-report measures. *Phys Ther.* 2002;82:320-328.

31. Wilkins CH, Roe CM, Morris JC l. A brief clinical tool to assess physical function: The mini-physical performance test. *Arch Gerontol Geriatr.* 2009;50:96-100.

32. Reuben DB, Seeman TE, Keeler, Guralnik JM. The effect of self-reported and performance-based functional impairment on future hospital costs of community-dwelling older persons. *Gerontologist.* 2004;44:401-407.

33. Miller DK, Morley JE. Controlled trial of a geriatric case-finding and liaison service in an emergency department. *J Am Geriatr Soc.* 1996;44:513-520.

34. Denman SJ, Ettinger WH, Zarkin BA, et al. Short-term outcomes of elderly patients discharged from an emergency department. *J Am Geriatr Soc.* 1989;37:937-943.

35. McCusker J, Healey E, Bellavance F, et al. Predictors of repeat emergency department visits by elders. *Acad Emerg Med.* 1997;4:581-588.

36. Chin MH, Jin L, Karrison TG, et al. Older patients' health-related quality of life around an episode of emergency illness. *Ann Emerg Med.* 1999;34:595-603. *J Gerontol A Biol Sci Med Sci.* 2006;61:53-62.

37. Inouye SK, Peduzzi PN, Robison JT, et al. Importance of functional measures in predicting mortality among older hospitalized patients. *JAMA.* 1998;279:1187-1193.

38. Covinsky KE, Justice AC, Rosenthal GE, et al. Measuring prognosis and case mix in hospitalized elders. The importance of functional status. *J Gen Intern Med.* 1997;12:203-208.

39. Robinson TN, Moss M. Postoperative delirium in the elderly: Risk factors and outcomes. *Ann Surg.* 2009;249:173-178.

40. Roche SML, Kramer A, Hester E, et al. Long-term functional outcome after intensive care. *J Am Geriatr Soc*. 1999;47:18-24.

41. Sleiman I, Trabucchi M. Functional trajectories during hospitalization: A prognostic sign for elderly patients. *J Gerontol A Biol Sci Med Sci*. 2009;64:659-663.

42. Volpato S, Cavalieri M, Guerra G, et al. Performance-based functional assessment in older hospitalized patients: Feasibility and clinical correlates. *J Gerontol A Biol Sci Med Sci*. 2008;63:1393-1398.

43. Zingmond DS, Wenger NS. Measuring the quality of care provided to dually enrolled Medicare and Medicaid beneficiaries living in nursing homes. *Med Care*. 2009;47:536-544.

44. Sangl J, Hittle DF. Challenges in measuring nursing home and home health quality: Lessons from the First National Healthcare Quality Report. *Med Care*. 2005;43(suppl):I24-I32.

45. Achterberg WP, Ribbe MW. Effects of the Resident Assessment Instrument on the care process and health outcomes in nursing homes. A review of the literature. *Scand J Rehabil Med*. 1999;31:131-137.

46. Mor V. A comprehensive clinical assessment tool to inform policy and practice: Applications of the minimum data set. *Med Care*. 2004;42(suppl):III50-III59.

47. Gindin J, Walter-Ginzburg A, Geitzen M, et al. Predictors of rehabilitation outcomes: A comparison of Israeli and Italian geriatric post-acute care (PAC) facilities using the minimum data set (MDS). *J Am Med Dir Assoc*. 2007;8:233-242.

48. Reisberg B. Functional assessment staging (FAST). *Psychopharmacol Bull*. 1988;24:653-659.

49. Karnofsky DA, Burchenal JH. The clinical evaluation of chemotherapeutic agents in cancer. In: MacLeon CM, ed. *Evaluation of Chemotherapeutic Agents*. New York: Columbia University Press; 1949:196.

50. Naeim A, Reuben D. Geriatric syndromes and assessment in older cancer patients. *Oncology (Williston Park)*. 2001;15:1567-1577.

51. Mayo AM. Measuring functional status in older adults with dementia. *Clin Nurse Spec*. 2008;22:212-213.

52. Cohen-Mansfield J, Frank J. Relationship between perceived needs and assessed needs for services in community-dwelling older persons. *Gerontologist*. 2008;48:505-516.

53. Schubert CC, Gross C, Hurried A. Functional assessment of the older patient with cancer. *Oncology (Williston Park)*. 2008;22:916-922; discussion 925, 928.

54. Pal SK, Kahteria V, Hurria A. Evaluating the older patient with cancer: Understanding frailty and the geriatric assessment. *CA Cancer J Clin*. 2010;60:120-132.

55. Pilotto A, Franceschi M. The multidimensional prognostic index predicts short- and long-term mortality in hospitalized geriatric patients with pneumonia. *J Gerontol A Biol Sci Med Sci*. 2009;64:880-887.

56. Formiga F, Pujol R. Admission characteristics predicting longer length of stay among elderly patients hospitalized for decompensated heart failure. *Eur J Intern Med*. 2008;19:198-202.

57. Burns R, Martindale-Adams J. Differences of self-reported osteoarthritis disability and race. *J Natl Med Assoc*. 2007;99:1046-1051.

58. Schneider MG, Shardell M. Parkinson's disease and functional decline in older Mexican Americans. *Parkinson Rel Disord*. 2008;14:397-406.

59. Sinclair AJ, Conroy SP, Bayer AJ. Impact of diabetes on physical function in older people. *Diabetes Care*. 2008;31:233-235.

60. Cook WL, Jassal SV. Functional dependencies among the elderly on hemodialysis. *Kidney Int*. 2008;73:1289-1295.

61. Gill TM, Gahbauer EA, Han L, Allore HG. Trajectories of disability in the last year of life. *N Engl J Med*. 2010;362:1173-1180.

62. Bogardus ST Jr, Inouye SK. What does the medical record reveal about functional status? A comparison of medical record and interview data. *J Gen Intern Med*. 2001;16:728-736.

63. Calkins DR, Rubenstein LV, Delbanco TL. Functional disability screening of ambulatory patients: A randomized controlled trial in a hospital-based group practice. *J Gen Intern Med*. 1994;9:590-592.

64. Haffer SC, Bowen SE. Measuring and improving health outcomes in Medicare: the Medicare HOS program. *Health Care Finance Rev*. 2004;25:1-3.

POST-TEST

1. **Which of the following combinations of functional assessment tools would be practical in the busy outpatient clinic setting?**
   A. Physical Performance Test
   B. Short Physical Performance Battery, BADL, IADL
   C. Get-Up-and-Go Test, BADL, IADL, Modified Romberg Test
   D. VES-13, Physical Performance Test, BADL, IADL

2. **Which of the following is FALSE regarding functional status?**
   A. Return to baseline functional status is unrealistic in frail elders.
   B. Change in functional status can be a presenting symptom of illness.
   C. Functional status is an important element in determining transitions of care.
   D. Functional status should be considered when prioritizing patient problems.

3. **Pain is considered the fifth vital sign. What have some health care providers called the sixth vital sign?**
   A. Gait and ambulation
   B. Cognitive impairment
   C. Functional status
   D. Chronologic age

ANSWERS TO PRE-TEST

1. A
2. D
3. B

ANSWERS TO POST-TEST

1. C
2. A
3. C

8

Aging and Sensory Loss: Vision, Hearing, Somatosensory, and Vestibular

Anne L. Harrison, PT, PhD

Anne Olson, MA, CCC-A

Scott Shaffer, PT, PhD, ECS, OCS

● **LEARNING OBJECTIVES**

1. Describe age-associated changes in function with age-associated changes in the somatosensory, vestibular, auditory, and visual sensory systems.
2. Discuss examination strategies for identifying sensory and functional loss related to each of these systems.
3. Compare and contrast interventions that modify or compensate for age-associated-sensory loss and the associated functional loss.

PRE-TEST

1. **Which of the following is a typical age related change in sensation of older adults?**

   A. Increased sensation in feet

   B. Increased response of the stretch reflex

   C. Hyperactive vestibular function

   D. Reduced proprioception of joints

2. **How does vertigo differ from dysequilibrium in older adults?**

   A. Vertigo implies a problem with the somatosensory system.

   B. Vertigo involves the sensation of the room spinning or moving.

   C. Dysequilibrium involves the sensation of the room spinning or moving.

   D. Dysequilibrium is generally much more problematic for older adults than vertigo.

3. **What are the functional implications for older adults experiencing dual sensory loss of hearing and vision?**

   A. Symptoms may include clumsiness, disorientation, and depression.

   B. They can easily compensate with other senses as they interact with the environment.

   C. There are no easily accessible interventions to address this problem.

   D. It is difficult for primary care physicians to assess this problem.

INTRODUCTION

Older adults often face challenges related to changes in physical and cognitive function that result in increased risk of injury, reduced independence, and altered quality of life. Sensory losses associated with both typical aging and age-associated pathologies contribute substantially to these challenges by impeding the ability of the older adult to navigate and interact within his or her world. Motor and cognitive functions are regulated in part by sensory inputs. Sensory information gained through the auditory, visual, tactile, proprioceptive, and vestibular senses provides essential information that is integrated at the central nervous system level in the performance of both motor and cognitive functions.

Proper execution of a motor task requires dynamic sensory processing of the changing environment, providing information that allows comparison of the actual outcome with the intended outcome to ensure functional accuracy. This is accomplished through feedback and feed-forward circuits initiated and monitored by the sensory systems.[1] Cutaneous and proprioceptive sensory inputs provide essential feedback for the execution of meaningful motor functions, but healthy adults over the age of 65 have been found to have over 70% loss of cutaneous sensation in the fingertips and feet compared to healthy younger adults.[2] It is established that older people with limited abilities in physical function, such as gait instability, are likely to have sensory impairments across increased numbers of domains compared to those with higher functional abilities.[3]

Moreover, multisensory impairments are associated with increased falls. Older adults fall more often than younger adults, and sustain more life-threatening or disabling injuries as a result. Falls are a major public health problem, injuring one in ten older US adults annually.[4,5] Individuals with vestibular pathology and subsequent dizziness are also eight times more likely to fall. In fact, 31% of patients who sustained a hip fracture had evidence of vestibulopathy.[6]

Competent cognitive processing depends in part on sensory input from the visual and auditory systems to interpret environmental information and create new thought processes. Hearing loss may be present in approximately 15% of adults under age 65,[7] and up to half of adults over the age of 75,[8] resulting in difficulty understanding speech and engaging in social activities. An estimated 17% of adults between the ages of 65 and 75 present with vision loss, increasing to almost 25% of adults over 75 years of age,[9] creating serious obstacles to completing daily activities. Furthermore, many older adults present with both vision and hearing losses, known as dual sensory impairments (DSI). Dual sensory impairments related to hearing and vision are associated with cognitive decline.[10] While the prevalence of DSI ranges anywhere from 8% to 20% of adults over the age of 70,[10,11] the clinical reality is that health care practitioners rarely encounter older adults with a single sensory issue. These numbers and the resulting vulnerabilities highlight the importance of identification of the impairment(s) associated with sensory loss and interventions to facilitate recovery or compensation.[12]

Biological variability, distinct from recognizable pathology, is characteristic of the aging population. Variations in sensory function contribute to the fact that some individuals thrive physically and cognitively until late in life while others experience declines unrelated to diagnosed pathologies. An understanding of the complexity of variables that converge to influence function is foundational to the design of interventions to modify the disablement process. In order to adequately characterize the complexity of multisensory decline, it is useful to examine the changes at the cellular and subcellular levels and link these with changes at the organism level. To do this, we present two case studies of individuals seeking support from their primary care provider for functional problems related to multisensory deficits. By focusing on the salient aspects of sensory loss, we will provide a lens through which practitioners can consider increased options for targeted interventions to improve function of older adults. Primary care practitioners are well positioned to identify early signs of loss when equipped with the appropriate screening mechanisms.

CASE PRESENTATION 1: FALLS AND LOSS OF BALANCE EVENTS

Mr. George is a 64-year-old African American male with a 14-year diagnosis of type 2 diabetes mellitus. He comes to the physician's office today with complaints of leg pain ("pins and needles stabbing my feet") and report of frequent stumbles, with three falls in the last year. He reports, "It was like the ground suddenly came up to meet me." He was a high school athletics referee for 20 years, and has been calling various younger children's sports events for the last 6 years. He was an army officer for 10 years prior to his work in high school athletics. He reports pain and stiffness in both of his knees and in his neck and low back with "too little or too much" physical activity. He is married to a supportive spouse, although she has medical issues as well. He wears glasses and his last eye exam was approximately 5 years ago. His medications are glipizide (Glucotrol) for diabetes and acetaminophen (Tylenol) for pain. His wife complains that he either "can't hear" or "is not listening." Mr. George asks you, "Can you help me with this pain and stumbling so I can keep up with my work?"

CASE PRESENTATION 2: HOW MANY CONTRIBUTORS TO UNSTEADY GAIT?

Ms. Muir is an 80-year-old woman who arrives at the physician's office with her daughter. Her chief complaint, according to her daughter, is that she feels unsteady on her feet. Her daughter thinks she has fallen recently due to substantial bruising of her lateral thigh area. Ms. Muir denies this, and indicates that she has "just a little stumble now and then which causes me to bump into my tables and chairs." Ms. Muir lives alone and does not drive. She does acknowledge that she is occasionally dizzy. "When I turn to look over my shoulder or try to stand up from lying down, I feel funny in my head." She has hearing aids, but does not wear them. "Darn things are so much trouble to get in my ears." Medications include sertraline (Zoloft), propoxyphene (Darvocett) prn for pain, alendronate (Fosamax), lisinopril (Zestril), and omeprazole (Prilosec). Her last glasses update was "several years ago." She rarely goes out anymore ("Just don't want to"). Her daughter thinks she is afraid of falling.

● HEARING AND VISION

Both hearing and vision loss are commonly observed in older adults, and these sensory losses occur across a continuum from mild to severe deficits. Interestingly, the prevalence of hearing loss appears to vary along gender/racial/ethnic lines. Men consistently report hearing loss more often than women regardless of ethnicity or race.[13] In fact, the odds of having a hearing loss were reported 5.5 times more often by men compared to women. Asian and black males report hearing loss up to 70% less frequently than white or Hispanic males.[11,13] Furthermore, researchers have identified additional risks for hearing loss which include diabetes,[14] noise exposure, smoking, and cardiovascular disease.[13]

While up to one quarter of older adults are estimated to have substantial vision loss, the severity of impairments varies along racial ethnic lines. The Eye Disease Prevalence Research group reported that blindness was 2.77 more prevalent in black persons compared to white and 3.13 times more prevalent compared to Hispanic persons. Low vision was more common in Hispanic persons (OR = 1.39) or black persons (OR = 1.9) compared to white persons.

Impact: Hearing Loss

The primary effect of hearing loss is difficulty in recognizing speech, particularly in the presence of other noise.[15-17] One reason for this is that most hearing loss caused by aging results in threshold reductions for higher frequencies,[18] and higher frequencies contribute the most to our ability to understand speech.[19,20] Left untreated, and in combination with other age-associated changes, there are likely to be fewer opportunities for social interaction, reductions in emotional well-being, feelings of being excluded, increased risk of depression, and overall reductions in quality of life.[11,21]

Impact: Vision Loss

Research suggests that the loss of vision appears to have its greatest impact through the ability to execute daily living activities.[22] Visual deficits in older adults may result in increased difficulties with driving, recognizing a friend across the room, reading a newspaper, or watching television. Reductions in visual acuity are primarily due to age-related changes in the eye involving the ciliary muscle and crystalline lens.[23] Specifically, as the crystalline lens loses elasticity and becomes stiffer, less light reaches the retina. Additional illumination or corrective lenses are needed for older adults to read as well as discriminate contrasts between surfaces when walking. The useful field of view (UFOV), which is the area that one can quickly scan, is also reduced. This reduction may affect an older person's ability to drive as well as maintain balance when walking. Finally, adaptation to darkness takes longer, so that older adults may be at higher risk for falling at night or in low-illumination conditions.[24] Since changes in visual skills often occur gradually, many people may be unaware if their condition is due to natural aging or is actually a treatable visual condition.

Dual Sensory Impairment

Helen Keller once explained that the difference between vision and hearing loss is that visual loss affects your ability to interact with things, while hearing loss affects your ability to interact with people.[25] This distinction is consistent with research demonstrating that visual loss predominantly affects activities of daily living whereas hearing loss affects our communication ability, compromising our psychosocial well-being.[26] People with sensory loss in one area will compensate through increased reliance upon another. For example, individuals with visual impairment will use hearing to enhance their awareness of their environment during mobility.[27] However, older adults with dual sensory impairment (DSI) will not have the full benefit of sensory compensation. Symptoms of undiagnosed DSI may include clumsiness in daily activities (eating, walking, using the telephone), disorientation, and depression.[10] Figure 8–1 illustrates the impact of dual sensory loss as Ms. Muir has trouble seeing and hearing the telephone when it rings in her home.

In order to reduce the impact of hearing and vision loss, primary care practitioners must intervene in a timely manner through routine screening. The American Speech and Hearing Association has published guidelines for screening hearing in

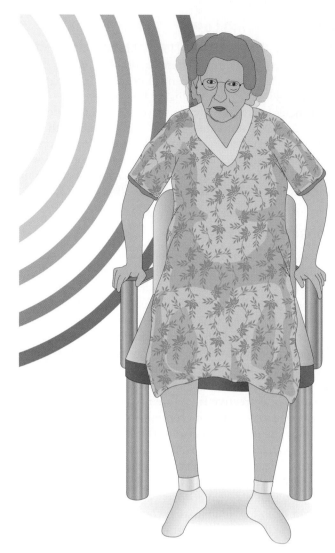

FIGURE 8–1. Ms. Muir hears a noise, thinks it might be the phone and is unsteady getting up because of DSI.

● **TABLE 8–1** Strategies to Improve Communication[32]
Improving Verbal Communication
· Introduce yourself by name.
· Let the patient know when you enter or leave the room.
· Speak before touching the person.
· Approach the patient on the side of his or her better eye.
· Allow the person with visual loss to speak for himself or herself; talk directly to the person with the visual impairment.
· Let the person with visual loss do as much as possible; this builds confidence.
Making Text More Legible for Persons with Visual Impairment and Low Vision
· Keep in mind that text should be printed with the highest possible contrast light against dark.
· Keep in mind that printed material is most readable in black and white.
· Use wide spacing between letters.
· Use extra-wide margins, especially for bound material; makes it easier to use on a flat surface.
· Use large fonts, 16-18 point.
· Use ordinary typeface, upper and lower case, and/or boldface print.
· Do not use paper with glossy finish.
Telephone Features for Patients with Visual Impairments
· Telephones with large buttons
· Telephones with good color contrasts
· A paging feature
· Memory and redial features
Improving Communication with Hearing-Impaired Elderly Persons
· Obtain the person's attention before beginning a communication exchange.
· Speak face to face.
· Paraphrase if you have to repeat what has been said.
· Speak at a normal level or slightly louder.
· Speak slowly, but not exaggerated.
· Stand within 2-3 feet of the listener.
· Reduce background noise.
· Pause at the end of a sentence.
· Avoid appearing frustrated.
· If the person can read, write down key words.
· Have the person with the hearing loss repeat what you have said to verify that the message was understood.
Data from reference 32.

adults[28] and provides additional resources at its website www.asha.org. Similarly, the US Preventive Services Task Force recommends vision screening for older adults,[29] which may help reduce falls and associated fractures.[30] Although such screenings are covered by Medicare Part B as part of the Initial Preventative Physical Examination (IPPE), they are currently underutilized in primary care settings.[31] Compounding the problem of screening is the challenge in communication faced by people with hearing and/or vision loss. Weinstein discusses a wide range of communication strategies for health care practitioners to adopt to insure optimal interactions during examination and education (Table 8–1).[32] Both vision and hearing screens would be appropriate for Mr. George, particularly since he is at higher risk for loss because he is male, diabetic, and has a history of noise exposure.

Auditory System: Structure and Function

The ear is divided into four components: the outer ear, middle ear, inner ear (cochlea), and auditory nerve (Figure 8–2).[33] In most situations, the outer ear funnels sound down the ear canal to the tympanic membrane. Here the acoustic energy is transformed into mechanical energy, which is then transmitted along the ossicular chain of the middle ear. The ossicular chain is comprised of the malleus, incus, and stapes. The footplate of the stapes articulates with the oval window and connects to the cochlea. Within this fluid-filled cochlea is a membranous labyrinth that houses the end-organ of hearing called the organ of Corti along with the vestibular sensory organs within the semicircular canals (Figure 8–2). Thousands of inner and outer hair cells reside within the organ of Corti and are deflected when the cochlear fluids are displaced. Mechanical deformation of the hair cells allows cellular changes to occur, which results in either a depolarization or hyperpolarization of the hair cell. This triggers a cascade of electrochemical activity that transmits the auditory signal from the hair cell to the auditory cortex, both ipsilaterally and contralaterally.[33] Damage or dysfunction to any structure along this pathway may result in hearing difficulties. The ipsilateral auditory pathway is shown in Figure 8–2.

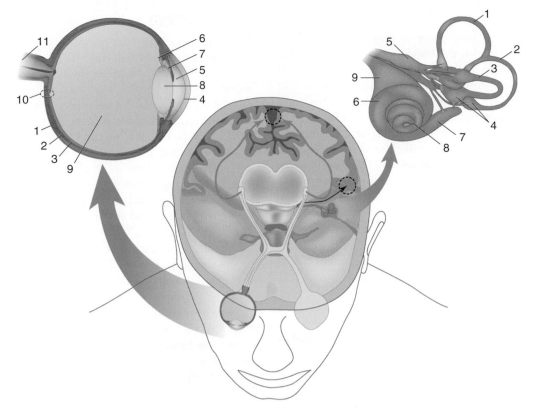

FIGURE 8–2. Vision, auditory, and vestibular anatomy. Ear/vestibular landmarks: **1.** Superior SC canal, **2.** Posterior SC canal, **3.** Horizontal SC canal, **4.** Ampulla, **5.** Vestibular nerve, **6.** Cochlea, **7.** Basal end of cochlea, **8.** Apical end of cochlea, **9.** Auditory nerve. Eye landmarks: **1.** Fibrous tunic, **2.** Vascular tunic, **3.** Retina, **4.** Cornea, **5.** Anterior chamber, **6.** Ciliary muscle, **7.** Iris, **8.** Lens, **9.** Vitreous chamber, **10.** Fovea/macula, **11.** Optic nerve. *Permission for use granted by University of Kentucky Department of Arts and Graphics, Tom Dolan, Medical Illustrator.*

Hearing loss associated with middle or outer ear problems is called *conductive hearing loss*, while hearing loss associated with cochlear pathologies is called *sensorineural hearing loss*. Central hearing losses are caused by damage to key structures important in the processing of auditory information.

Auditory System: Age-Related Change

Presbycusis

An often reported observation from older adults is "I can hear, but I just can't understand." This complaint is symptomatic of age-related, bilateral, high-frequency hearing loss called presbycusis. The hearing loss is typically symmetrical and sensorineural in nature.[32] The onset of presbycusis may begin around the sixth decade and decreases more rapidly in the high frequencies.[34] Those who have been exposed to excessive noise (such as Mr. George, because of his military background) may present with additional hearing loss. Speech recognition ability is also reduced.[16,35] The inability to hear high-frequency sounds such as *f* or *s* negatively affects speech understanding.

The loss of outer hair cell function in the basal turn of the cochlea appears to be responsible for the typical declines in hearing observed with age,[36] yet deterioration of other structures including structures in the central auditory nervous system have also been identified.[37] These findings may explain why central processing factors also contribute to speech understanding ability by older adults.[35] The hearing loss

observed in older adults may either be a result of damage to one structure, or more likely, a combination of changes in inner ear structures[32] and associated neural pathways.

Tinnitus

While there are several ways to describe tinnitus (ringing, buzzing, whistling, humming, clicking, etc.), it can be defined as any sound that is perceived in the absence of an external stimulus.[38] Most tinnitus is subjective, ranging in severity from slight to severe,[39] and can be disabling enough to warrant medical consultation. There is a strong correlation between tinnitus and hearing loss,[40] and it is not surprising that tinnitus also occurs more often in older adults[41] and in those with noise exposure.[38] Persons with vascular disease, diabetes, high blood pressure, and autoimmune disorder may be at risk for tinnitus without concomitant hearing loss as well.[38]

The mechanisms underlying tinnitus are not well understood but may relate to abnormal signal processing in the central auditory pathways.[12] To date, interventions for tinnitus include a variety of strategies such as education, reassurance, biofeedback, masking, counseling, and hypnosis. While these may offer relief for some patients, there is no clear evidence that these interventions can improve the actual condition of tinnitus.[12] Clinical trials using tinnitus retraining therapy are under way in hopes that such therapies may alleviate symptoms of tinnitus and improve quality of life.[42-44] Persons needing assessment and intervention for tinnitus should be referred to an audiologist and otolaryngologist.

Cerumen Impaction

Cerumen impactions may occur in one-third of geriatric patients.[45] In older adults, this build-up may result in a *mixed* hearing loss caused by both a conductive component (wax) and a sensorineural component (presbycusis). Removal of wax can improve hearing as well as communication function[46] and improve function of hearing aids. This may be an additional reason that Ms. Muir is not using her hearing aids. Impacted wax may increase the likelihood of feedback or squealing from the hearing aid because amplified sound essentially bounces off the wax, leaks out of the ear canal, and becomes re-amplified. Treatment options include irrigation, curettes, self-administration with bulb syringe, and cerumenolytics (ear drops to soften cerumen).[47] It should be noted that while ear candling has gained some popularity in recent years, it is not considered to be an effective treatment option for wax removal and may in fact be dangerous.[48]

Pathologic Conditions of the Aging Ear

Several pathological conditions of the ear are summarized in Table 8–2.[49] Two of these conditions may be of particular relevance for primary health care practitioners. Sudden sensorineural hearing loss (SSHL) is defined as a recent onset of unilateral hearing loss that occurs within 72 hours and should be considered a medical emergency.[50] Additional symptoms may also include fullness in the ear, tinnitus, and dizziness. While some patients recover spontaneously, others may experience improved hearing following timely treatment with corticosteroids[51] and referral to an otolaryngologist.

Several medications and environmental toxins can result in ototoxicity, unleashing a variety of auditory symptoms including hearing loss, balance disorders, and tinnitus. Some of these medications will require routine monitoring of hearing such as cisplatinum or carboplatin (commonly used in chemotherapy)[52] or aminoglycoside antibiotics particularly associated with loop diuretics.[53] Both of these drugs result in high-frequency hearing loss, which may be permanent or reversible. For patients on these medications, routine monitoring of hearing with high-frequency pure tone testing is recommended.

Hearing Screen

A multiple-component screening may be necessary in order to (1) identify the medical disorder, (2) determine future risk of loss, and (3) describe activity limitations and participation restrictions (Table 8–3).[32] The first screening step is to examine the patient's ears. Visual otoscopy will provide insight about the medical condition of the outer and middle ear and particularly the extent of wax problem that may be contributing to the hearing loss. To identify who is most likely to present with hearing loss, most clinical settings today have adopted electronic tests over tuning forks because of their superior sensitivity and specificity.[28] A portable (calibrated) audiometer is used and screening for adults occurs at 1000, 2000, or 4000 Hz at 25 dB HL. If a person fails to detect a tone at any of these frequencies at 25 dB HL, in either ear, he or she should be referred for audiologic evaluation. While many facilities use separate equipment to perform these two tests, the audioscope combines both otoscopic and audiometric screening functions. Research with this instrument has suggested that results are in agreement with conventional pure tone hearing screening procedures.[54] To more fully understand how a person's hearing loss impacts daily life, health care practitioners may use a self-assessment questionnaire such as the Hearing Handicap Inventory for the Elderly-Screening (HHIE-S).[55] It includes 10 questions across both social and emotional domains, is considered a reliable and valid clinical tool, and is available in several languages. In general, persons who perceive their hearing loss as more problematic have higher HHIE-S scores. A copy of this questionnaire can be found at http://audiologyawareness.com/hearingtest.asp.

For patients who fail the pure tone hearing screening, or score above 10 on the HHIE-S, audiologic or otologic referral is necessary. If a patient is referred to an audiologist for an in-depth assessment of hearing, a basic battery of tests (pure tone air and bone conduction testing, speech recognition ability, and thresholds for speech) will be conducted to determine the type and degree of hearing loss. These tests help quantify and describe the hearing loss so that appropriate interventions are identified. Typically, *conductive* hearing losses require additional medical (otologic) consultation for possible treatment.[49] In contrast, *sensorineural* hearing losses are more permanent in nature and often slowly progressive

● **TABLE 8–2** Selected Pathologic Conditions of the Ear[49]

Condition	Site of Pathology	Symptoms
Noise-induced hearing loss	Inner ear	Difficulty hearing in noise, hears male voices better than female, tinnitus
Ménière disease	Inner ear	Ear fullness, hearing loss, vertigo, nausea, tinnitus
Otosclerois	Conductive	Gradual hearing loss, hears better in noisy environments
Acoustic neuroma	Inner ear and or auditory nerve	Unilateral hearing loss, dizziness, fullness, tinnitus
Ototoxicity	Inner ear	High-frequency hearing loss, tinnitus, balance
Sudden sensorineural hearing loss (SSHL)	Inner ear	Unilateral hearing loss, tinnitus, fullness, dizziness

Data from reference 49.

● **TABLE 8–3** Hearing Screens

Type of Screening	Purpose	Outcomes
Otoscopy	Medical condition of the outer and middle ear	Wax, redness, discharge, foreign body
Questionnaire Hearing Handicap Inventory for the Elderly (HHIE-S)[55]	Functional impact of hearing loss as perceived by patient	< 10 Pass > 10 Refer (> 14, usually benefit from amplification)
Pure tone test[54] 1000, 2000, 4000 Hz at 25 dB HL in each ear	Determine who is at risk for hearing impairment	Pass if detect all tones in each ear Refer if fail to detect any tone in either ear at 25 dB HL

in older adults. A *mixed* hearing loss is a combination of both a sensorineural and a conductive hearing loss. The magnitude of the hearing loss is expressed by the degree of hearing loss in each ear and can range from mild to severe. Speech recognition scores are also performed to document how well patients understand speech. Abnormally poor scores may suggest neural involvement.[49]

Hearing Loss: Interventions

Amplification

Hearing Aids. The best and most common rehabilitative tool for hearing loss is amplification. Extensive research on the benefit of hearing aids documents improved speech understanding,[56] reductions in perception of disability,[57-59] and improved communication function and quality of life.[60,61] However, overall hearing aid use in the United States is considered low.[62] For example, in the Epidemiology of Hearing Loss study, only 14% of adults with hearing deficits actually reported using a hearing aid.[62] Several factors such as cost, stigma, cosmetics, lack of perceived benefit, and concern about handling technology have all been identified as factors related to the low compliance of hearing aid use in adults.[63-65] Prior to hearing aid fitting, patients should be examined by a physician, preferably an otolaryngologist, to rule out any contraindications to hearing aid use. Some examples of conditions that require medical management before hearing aid use, as outlined by the Food and Drug Administration,[66] are listed in Table 8–4.

There are several different styles of hearing aids, which vary in size and how they are coupled to the ear (in the ear, behind the ear, in the canal, and completely in the canal). Manual dexterity is essential for proper insertion and removal of hearing aids. Ms. Muir is a perfect example of a typical hearing aid user who suffers from decreased manual dexterity, due in part to an age-related reduction in somatosensation in the fingers. To address this, she should be referred back to her hearing aid dispenser for additional education and practice. Additionally, hearing aids are available in different types of circuits, which can be broadly described as analog or digital.[67] Because there are so many types and features of hearing aids, selection for older adults should be individualized based on their communication needs. Hearing aids are not currently covered by Medicare; however, the diagnostic evaluation,

if ordered by a physician, is covered. One option for accessing funding for amplification is Hear Now—the Starkey Hearing Foundation, www.sotheworldmayhear.org. Another useful organization for education on hearing loss is the Hearing Loss Association of America, www.hearingloss.org.

Assistive Listening Devices. Sometimes additional devices are needed to improve an individual's ability to understand in specific settings. For example, frequency modulation (FM) units typically consist of a microphone that is used by the primary speaker and a receiver that is directly coupled to a listener's hearing aid. This allows amplification of the primary speaker and eliminates unwanted background noise.[67] Television listening systems that are either hard wired or wireless can provide amplification for the television only. A variety of personal amplifiers are also helpful for persons without hearing aids, to improve communication in a one-on-one setting and may be particularly useful in primary care.

Cochlear Implants. Individuals with severe to profound hearing loss may receive only modest, if any, benefit from conventional hearing aids. For such individuals, a cochlear implant (CI) is increasingly being considered as a treatment option. A cochlear implant is an electronic, class III medical device that requires surgical placement of an electrode within the cochlea.[68] This technology essentially bypasses the damaged hair cells and directly stimulates the auditory nerve. Individuals continue to wear an external microphone to pick up sound, which is then coded, processed, and sent across the skin via FM waves to the underlying receiver unit and ultimately sent to the implanted electrode.

The number of adults who are eligible for cochlear implants has expanded in the past decade.[69] The vast majority of them obtain substantial benefit for recognition of everyday speech and environmental or warning sounds.[70-73] Furthermore, outcomes for older adults with implants offer similar improvements as in younger adults.[74] Many factors, such as duration of deafness, age at implantation, degree of hearing loss, expectations, and surviving neural populations have been identified as influencing an individual's ability to utilize electrical stimulation.[71,75,76]

Auditory Training

Specific training may be necessary to re-teach an individual to make perceptual distinctions about sounds to enhance understanding of speech.[67] Recently, several researchers have examined the effects of computerized auditory training programs in adults with hearing aids and cochlear implants.[77-82] Overall these studies show promise for the benefits of home auditory training programs.

Counseling

Finally, group or individual counseling may be needed to address psychosocial issues related to the hearing loss or identify communication strategies to enhance speech understanding. A systematic review conducted by Hawkins[83] examined the effectiveness of support groups for adults with hearing loss. Support groups may empower older adults in ways in which a clinician simply cannot because most clinicians have not experienced the impact of sensory loss with aging.

● **TABLE 8–4** Conditions Requiring Medical Management Prior to Hearing Aid Use[66]
Visible congenital or traumatic deformity of the ear
History of or active drainage from the ear within the previous 90 days
History of sudden or rapidly progressive hearing loss within the previous 90 days
Acute or chronic dizziness
Unilateral hearing loss of sudden onset within the previous 90 days
Significant air-bone-gap (from pure tone air and bone conduction testing)
Foreign body or cerumen in ear canal
Ear pain or discomfort
Data from reference 66.

Visual System: Structure and Function

The eye globe is composed of three major layers; the retina, vascular tunic, and fibrous tunic (Figure 8–2).[84] The outer layer of connective tissue is the fibrous tunic, which functions in a protective manner and consists of the cornea, the outermost optical structure, and the sclera, the opaque white of the eye. Most of the refractive power of the eye is performed by the cornea.[84] The pupil is located directly behind the cornea, and regulates the amount of light that reaches the inner layer or the retina.[85] The inner layer, located at the posterior wall of the eye, houses the retina's photoreceptors, and converts electromagnetic information into neural impulses. Near the center of the retina is the macula, a small oval yellowish spot that is critical for central vision.[85] In between the fibrous tunic and the retina is the vascular tunic, a highly metabolic area that serves as the blood supply.

The three major chambers of the eye are the anterior, posterior, and vitreous chambers.[85] The anterior chamber is enclosed in front by the cornea and posteriorly by the iris. The posterior chamber lies behind the iris and encircles the lens. Aqueous humor fluids fill both the posterior and anterior chambers. The larger vitreous chamber is enclosed in front by the lens and posteriorly by the inner retinal layer and is filled with a semigelatinous substance. The crystalline lens lies in the posterior chamber. When the ciliary muscles contract, the curvature of the lens changes and projects an inverted image on the retina. Specifically, the lens is flattened when focused on more distant objects and more curved for nearer objects.

Two major types of receptor cells are found in the retina. The rods are distributed along the periphery of the retina and are maximally responsive in darkness or dim light. In contrast, cones are densely distributed near the fovea and are maximally responsive to light and color, making them responsible for much of our near vision. No receptors are observed where the ganglion cells exit the retina, resulting in a "blind spot." Optic nerve fibers travel to the optic chiasm, where nasal fibers cross to the contralateral pathway, and temporal fibers course ipsilaterally. Visual information travels from here to the lateral geniculate nucleus and ultimately to the striate cortex. Damage or dysfunction to any structure along these pathways may result in visual field difficulties.[33]

Visual System: Age-Related Change

Age-associated reduction in visual function is primarily related to changes in the physical structure of the eye.[23] Senile miosis is a reduction in pupil size and is commonly seen in both older men and women.[86] As the dilator muscle fibers atrophy, the pupil diameter becomes smaller when illuminated. This change in structure results in a reduction in retinal illumination and ultimately leads to reduced vision.

As the crystalline lens enlarges and hardens with age, less light reaches the retina and results in presbyopia, which makes focusing on near objects more difficult. The yellowing of the lens also affects the absorption rate of different wavelengths, which causes older adults to have greater difficulty detecting violet hues (at the higher end of the spectrum).[23] These physiologic changes may affect a variety of visual skills such as visual acuity (both near and distance), contrast discrimination, depth perception, useful field of view (UFOV), color discrimination, and dark adaptation.[22] Refractive errors due to presbyopia are typically corrected with glasses or contact lenses. Interestingly, cone density (in the fovea) remains stable throughout the lifespan, whereas rod density does not.[87] Therefore, the loss of acuity with age does not appear to be related to the loss of photoreceptors.

Pathologic Conditions of the Aging Eye

Cataracts

Several ocular diseases are associated with increased age and account for almost all of the visual loss in persons over 70 years of age. The Eye Diseases Prevalence Research Group[88] summarized findings from several population studies conducted after 1990. According to this report, cataracts are the leading cause of vision loss among adults, regardless of race, and are reported in up to half of adults over the age of 65.[88] They typically develop in the translucent area of the lens, which becomes cloudy or opaque and decreases acuity (especially at night), and increases sensitivity to glare.[23] Risk factors such as smoking or exposure to toxic substances can hasten the development of a cataract.[89,90] Fortunately, cataract surgery with lens implantation is highly successful and correlated with improved subjective and objective measures of vision.[91]

Age-Related Macular Degeneration

Age-related macular degeneration (AMD) is the leading cause of blindness among Americans, affecting more than 3.5 million persons.[88] Degeneration of the macula can occur in two forms: dry (early-stage AMD) and wet (later-stage AMD). AMD is more common in women (over the age of 70) and among Caucasians compared to African American or Hispanic adults. Increased incidence may be observed in persons who smoke[92] or are obese.[93] Patients may initially report that images are wavy or distorted, but vision is later compromised by dense blind spots (scotomas).[94] Often persons lose their central vision and thus have difficulty performing near vision tasks. Currently there is no treatment to reverse the visual loss associated with AMD, but clinical trial results with Lucentis and Macugen along with high-dose antioxidants and zinc regimens may slow the disease process.[95]

Diabetic Retinopathy

Diabetic retinopathy is a complication of Diabetes Mellitus (DM). In the early stages of the disease, it results in low vision, but if left untreated, it can result in blindness.[96] The prevalence is higher in black adults with DM; more research is needed to ascertain the influence of mediating factors such as co-morbidities and health care access.[88] As mentioned earlier, vigilant treatment of DM may slow the progression of additional visual loss in most patients. Therefore, best practice suggests that persons with DM (such as Mr. George) receive annual dilated eye (fundoscopic) examinations.

Glaucoma

Glaucoma occurs when there is an increase in intraocular pressure resulting from inadequate drainage of fluids from the anterior chamber. This increased pressure can cause damage to the optic nerve. Open-angle glaucoma is twice as common in black older adults compared to white older adults.[88] If left untreated, this can result in irreversible loss of peripheral vision and possibly blindness. This gradual loss can affect orientation and mobility such that individuals have difficulty navigating safely through environments. Also, since peripheral vision is reduced, appearance of persons and objects that exist outside the field of view can appear suddenly. In contrast, angle-closure glaucoma is rare, but occurs more often in Caucasians, Eskimos, and Asians due to the shallower anterior chamber depth.[97] Patients usually present with a rapid onset of blurred vision, eye pain, headache, or nausea.[98] Since early diagnosis and treatment of both forms of glaucoma gives patients the best chance of improved visual function, health care practitioners can educate patients at risk for glaucoma, make timely referrals (for anyone over the age of 40), and discuss proper medical management to improve vision outcomes.[99]

Vision Screening

Since the onset of symptoms related to visual loss may be gradual and go undetected, screenings for vision can be a crucial first step in the treatment process. Current best practice endorsed by the American Optometric Association suggests that persons over the age of 61 have annual vision screening,[100] although a recent systematic review questions this.[101] Primary care physicians are in an ideal position to provide simple in-office examinations to differentiate age-related changes from possible underlying disease process.[101]

Guidelines for screening vision are available through the American Optometric Association.[100] An ophthalmologic exam is used to determine the extent of any identifiable visual medical conditions that warrant immediate attention such as glaucoma, diabetic retinopathy, or cataracts. While these exams are within the scope of practice for primary care physicians, specific training and practice in the use of ophthalmoscope and dilation of eyes are recommended to gain competency.[102]

A Snellen Eye Chart is typically used to screen visual acuity for distance vision (at 20 feet) and for near vision (at 16 inches).[100] Patients are to use their best corrected glasses for both near and far conditions. Each eye is examined separately, beginning at the top line on the chart and working down until the person falters. Acuity is recorded as fraction with normal vision described as 20/20 and legal blindness as 20/200.[102] Patients should be referred for in-depth ophthalmologic assessment if they measure 20/60 or worse. Near vision is assessed using the Snellen Near Card, in a well-lit environment. Persons failing these screenings should be referred to an eye care professional for full evaluation of visual loss.

There can be additional problems, beyond acuity, experienced by persons with visual problems, such as sensitivity to glare, limited depth perception, and color contrast difficulties. Any of these problems may negatively affect function.

● TABLE 8–5 Visual Screens[100]

Type of Screening	Purpose	Outcomes
Ophthalmological exam	Evaluate external and internal health of eye	Opacity of lens Scattered spots at macula Cupping of optic disc Microaneurysm or hard exudates
Visual Functioning Questionnaire[103]	Functional impact of vision loss as perceived by patient	No specific threshold criteria Use to guide intervention plan
Visual Acuity[102] Distance (20"), Near (16") Performed in each eye and with best available glasses for each condition	Determine who is at risk for visual impairment	Threshold: 20/40 or better Refer: 20/60 or worse

Data from reference 100.

The National Eye Institute's Visual Function Questionnaire-25 (NEI-VFQ 25) can be used to describe the extent of disability related to the visual impairment. This 25-item questionnaire measures the effect of vision on emotional well-being, social functioning, and daily visual functioning and is considered to be a valid and reliable screening tool.[103] In general, the higher scores represent better functioning. This questionnaire is readily accesible via the Internet. See Table 8–5 for an overview of vision screening.

Interventions: Vision Loss

A variety of low-vision rehabilitative services may provide older adults with additional resources needed to regain their independence. These resources include devices, skills, and strategies that can be implemented to optimize performance of daily activities. Referrals to optometrists and ophthalmologists are ideal for obtaining prescription or magnification devices. For persons needing additional resources, vision rehabilitation professionals are uniquely qualified to develop an intervention plan to address needs related to reading, mobility, and daily activities.[22] These professionals can provide training in use of residual vision, determine appropriate environmental modifications, and provide counseling or training for safe mobility. Community-based service aging organizations or the state agency for visual impairment may be good entry points to locate vision rehabilitation specialists. Lighthouse International (www.lighthouse.org) and Vision Aware (www.visionaware.org) are self-help vision resource centers for additional information about vision therapy, services, and research on low-vision devices.

A broad range of optical devices are available to enhance vision. Use of simple strategies such as large print, lamps, reading stands, and high-contrast colors should be reinforced when appropriate. Magnification devices, however, may require a prescription.[22] Magnifiers can be hand held, stand alone, or mounted on glasses depending on the application. Mounted telescopes can even be provided for some older drivers. Electronic magnification is possible through use of a closed circuit television system (CCTV). A camera is focused on the desired visual task (reading, picture) and projects an image onto a monitor or wall.

Environmental Modifications

Since mobility is a key determinant of independent living among older adults, skills that enhance safe movement in the home and travel outside of home are important to include in rehabilitation plans. Some skills may include use of a cane, electronic devices, or even public transportation. Additionally, improved lighting, increased contrast between objects and backgrounds, and use of bright clear colors can be used in homes to improve visual function.[22]

● THE VESTIBULAR SYSTEM

Vestibular disorders with subsequent dizziness and postural instability are common reasons that older adults seek medical care.[104] In fact, it is estimated that 12.5 million Americans over 65 years of age are affected by dizziness, with reported prevalence of 28% to 34% in adults over age 60,[105] and 47% and 61%, respectively, in males and females over 70 years.[106] Although dizziness can result from various medical conditions, approximately half of the reported cases are due to vestibular disorders with subsequent vertigo and postural instability.[107] A recent study by Agrawal and colleagues examined 5084 adults and identified vestibulopathy as measured by postural testing in 49%, 69%, and 85% of adults between the ages of 60 and 69, 70 and 79, and 80 and 89 years, respectively.[108] Investigators also discovered that those with vestibulopathy were significantly more likely to have a past history of falls (OR = 6.9) or diabetes (OR = 1.7).[108] Pothula and associates have also reported that 80% of their older patients with a history of falls had symptoms of vestibular dysfunction.[109] Additionally, research by Aktas and Celik and Herdman and associates found that 31% of older adults who sustained hip fractures had vestibular disease.[110,111] Collectively, these findings stress the importance of understanding the age-related and pathologic conditions that impact optimal vestibular function, and the need for assessment and treatment techniques that can assist older adults who exhibit vestibular dysfunction and postural instability. Ms. Muir and Mr. George have a past history of falls, and Ms. Muir also has episodes of dizziness associated with head movement, suggestive of vestibular dysfunction. Mr. George also has diabetes, a risk factor for postural instability related to both the vestibular and somatosensory systems.

Vestibular System: Structure and Function

The vestibular system allows for precise three-dimensional orientation, accurate visual acuity, and postural stability. This is accomplished by peripheral vestibular receptors located within the inner ear that detect tilt and angular and translational motion of the head. This sensory information is then sent to the CNS, specifically the vestibular nuclear complex and the cerebellum, and used to control the vestibulo-ocular, vestibulocollic, and vestibulospinal reflexes that are integral to visual acuity and postural stability. The vestibulo-ocular reflex (VOR) allows visual images to remain tightly focused on the fovea of the retina during high-velocity head and body movements, allowing for rapid responses for the maintenance of visual acuity during rapid movements.[112,113] The vestibulocollic reflex stabilizes the head by facilitating a contraction of the neck musculature, and the vestibulospinal reflex provides rapid compensatory body movements to assist with postural stability and prevent falls. The contributions and speed that the vestibular system contributes to postural stability cannot be overstated, and it has been suggested that older adults who cannot recover from a trip within 145 ms are likely to fall.[114] Typical and pathologic age-related disturbances in optimal vestibular structure and function contribute to reduced visual acuity, vertigo, nausea, and postural instability.[113]

Peripheral Vestibular Anatomy and Physiology

The peripheral part of the vestibular system, or membranous vestibular labyrinth, is located in the inner ear and lies within the petrous portion of the temporal bone. Each vestibular labyrinth has three semicircular canals (superior or anterior, horizontal or lateral, and posterior) and two otolith organs (utricle and saccule) (Figure 8–2). The three semicircular canals (SCC) respond to rotation of the head (angular acceleration) via specialized neuroepithelial hair cells (sterociliium and kinocilia) that are located in a gelatinous barrier or cupula, which is found in the ampulla at the end of each SCC. It is important to point out that the SCCs work as functional pairs. For example, when the head is rotated to the right, the hair cells within the cupula of the right SCC are excited, and the hair cells within the left lateral SCC inhibited.[115-117]

The utricle and saccule are also key components of the membranous labyrinth and provide information regarding linear acceleration.[117] The utricle and saccule also utilize sensory hair cells, but the sterocilium and kinocilium are in contact with a gelatinous membrane that is embedded with calcium carbonate crystals (otoconia). The function of the otoconia is to provide the gelatinous membrane with mass that is extremely sensitive to linear head movement and tilt. The utricle's orientation allows it to respond to horizontal linear acceleration (eg, running or driving in a car) or static head tilt, whereas the saccule detects vertical linear acceleration (eg, going from sit to stand or going up an escalator).[116]

Peripheral vestibular information from the SCCs, saccule, and utricle are transported along peripheral afferent pathways towards the cell bodies located in the vestibular or Scarpa ganglion. The central processes for the cell bodies of the vestibular ganglion then form the vestibular nerve and travel within the internal auditory meatus as the vestibulocochlear nerve (Figure 8–2). The majority of vestibular nerve fibers terminate within the vestibular nuclei, while the remaining fibers actually terminate directly within the flocculo-nodular lobe of the cerebellum.[116]

Central Vestibular Anatomy and Physiology

The vestibular nuclei project information along secondary vestibular fibers to various structures within the central nervous system. All of the vestibular nuclei contribute secondary vestibular fibers that travel within the medial longitudinal fasciculus to terminate on the extraocular motor nuclei (oculomotor, trochlear, and abducens) and axial motor neurons of the neck. Collectively these connections contribute to the vestibular ocular reflex (VOR) and contribute to the control of head and eye movement. The lateral vestibular nucleus sends secondary fibers forming the lateral vestibulospinal tract that travels to all spinal levels to regulate extensor muscle tone.[116] The medial and inferior nuclei send fibers to the flocculo-nodular lobe and uvula of the cerebellum. The cerebellum connections assist in maintenance of postural control, coordination of the limbs, and calibration of the VOR. Vestibular neurons connect with other central nervous system structures to play a role in arousal, body awareness, and movement of self versus the environment.[117]

Vestibular System: Age-Related Change

Aging impacts the structural and functional integrity of the vestibular system.[118] Specifically, research reveals that the volume and number of otoconia in the utricle and saccule are significantly reduced in older individuals.[118,119] The fragmentation and migration of otoconia to the semicircular ducts have also been well documented and result in benign paroxysmal positional vertigo (BPPV), which is more common with advanced aging.[118,120]

Age-related degeneration of vestibular neuroepithelial hair cells, peripheral vestibular neurons, and the vestibular nuclear complex have also been reported.[121-124] The age-related anatomic changes that occur in the vestibular system also correlate with physiologic and functional changes. For example, a longitudinal study investigating the vestibulo-ocular reflex in 57 older adults (mean age 82 years) revealed increased latencies and reduced gain of the VOR during the 5-year follow-up.[125] This is cause for concern, as reduced function of the VOR results in impaired gaze stability, retinal slip, and reduced visual acuity.[111,126-128] Dynamic visual acuity testing performance, which measures the ability to maintain gaze stability during fast head perturbations, has also shown a significant relationship with age.[129,130]

It is suggested that age-related vestibular changes result in progressive bilateral vestibular dysfunction that potentially contributes to dysequilibrium commonly reported in older community dwelling adults.[131] Slow and progressive degradation of the multiple components of the vestibular system leads to a mismatch between vestibular and visual mechanisms, resulting in dysequilibrium. Dysequilibrium, unlike vertigo, is categorized by a feeling of unsteadiness or postural imbalance that occurs only when the patient is erect.[132] In addition, unilateral degeneration, dislodgement of otoconia (eg, BPPV), or a shift in fluid pressure within the canal (eg, Ménière disease) can lead to unilateral dysfunction in older adults with an acute onset of vertigo and postural instability.[131]

Vertigo: Screening and Interventions

Although dizziness occurs in approximately one-third of older adults, it is not appropriate to attribute it to the normal aging process.[133] Primary care providers need to be familiar with the diagnosis and management of dizziness, and in particular vertigo, as it comprises approximately half of those who present with dizziness.[107] *Vertigo* is typically defined as a sensation in which a patient feels that his or her environment is moving or that he or she is spinning or falling.[133] Vertigo often begins abruptly, is episodic, and can involve nausea and vomiting. Although Ms. Muir is not experiencing nausea or vomiting, she does report vertigo, or the sensation that the environment is spinning with certain positions. Damage to the vestibular membranous labyrinth, vestibulocochlear nerve, or vestibular connections in the central nervous system can result in vertigo.

Central Vertigo

One of the immediate challenges for primary care providers is to determine if the cause of vertigo is the result of a peripheral or central disorder. Epidemiologic studies estimate that 25% of dizziness cases are the result of dysfunction within or influencing (eg, presyncope) the central nervous system.[134] Typically central vertigo results in severe postural instability, inability to ambulate, less prominent movement illusion and nausea than peripheral vestibular disorders, and spontaneous nystagmus that does not suppress with optic fixation. Nystagmus is involuntary rhythmic oscillations of the eyes; the direction of the fast phase defines nystagmus direction.[134] Bidirectional gaze-evoked nystagmus (right-beating nystagmus with gaze to the right, and left-beating nystagmus with gaze to the left), spontaneous vertical nystagmus (usually downbeating), and pure torsional nystagmus are also identified with central nervous system dysfunction.[132] Additional neurologic signs such as Horner syndrome, dysarthria, dysphagia, facial weakness or numbness, severe gait ataxia, pathologic reflexes, and limb incoordination or weakness also indicate a possible central lesion and need for enhanced MRI and neurology consultation.

Potential *central vestibular* causes of vertigo include migraines, cerebrovascular disorders (eg, brainstem ischemia, lateral medullary infarction, cerebellar infraction), tumors (cerebellopontine angle, brain), infection or central nervous system disease (multiple sclerosis), presyncopal dizziness, and panic attacks.[135] Fortunately, serious causes of central vertigo (nonvestibular) are limited and include cerebrovascular disease (6-7%), cardiac/circulatory problems (1.5-3.6%), and posterior fossa tumors (less than 1%).[134,136] In general, it is recommended that older adults who have an unclear diagnosis of vertigo, remain symptomatic following treatment, or have multiple concurrent vestibular disorders receive a referral for vestibular function testing and a consult to an otolaryngologist or vestibular specialty clinic.[132] For further details regarding the causes and differential diagnosis of central vertigo and dizziness the reader is referred to a recent review by Karatas.[134]

Peripheral Vestibular Vertigo

In contrast to central nervous system causes of vertigo, peripheral vestibular dysfunction typically involves more pronounced nausea, vomiting, and the potential for hearing loss. Although postural instability and ataxia occur in both central and peripheral vestibular dysfunction, patients with peripheral disorders usually are able to walk and have less severe postural instability. Peripherally induced nystagmus also has a delayed onset and is inhibited with optic fixation.[134,137]

The most common peripheral vestibular conditions associated with vertigo include: (1) benign paroxysmal positional vertigo, (2) acute labyrinthitis (vestibular neuritis), and (3) Ménière disease.[134]

Benign Paroxysmal Positional Vertigo. Benign paroxysmal positional vertigo (BPPV) is the most commonly identified cause of vertigo across the lifespan,[138] and the incidence of idiopathic BPPV peaks at 60 to 70 years of age.[131,137] As previously mentioned, the primary pathology associated with BPPV involves otoconia inadvertently breaking away from the otolithic gelatinous membrane and moving into the semicircular canals. Once the otoconia are in the SCC they can either adhere to the cupula (cupulolithiasis) or enter the canal (canalithiasis), thus influencing endolymph flow and subsequent afferent firing rates. Although it is estimated that 85% to 95% of BPPV cases are the result of posterior canal dysfunction,[139] particles can enter the lateral and superior canals.[131] Similar to Ms. Muir, individuals with BPPV often report brief episodes of vertigo that are associated with a change in head position. Common reports of activities that result in brief (20-60 seconds) vertigo include turning from supine to side lying in bed, getting out of bed, and extending the neck to look up.[133] Key diagnostic features of BPPV are that vertigo is induced with head or positional maneuvers, lasts less than 1 minute, and patients are normal in between episodes and provocative maneuvers.[132] The diagnosis of posterior canal BPPV also requires positional testing (Figure 8–3A and B, Dix-Hallpike maneuver) aimed at provoking vertigo and upbeating and torsional nystagmus toward the side tested. The onset of nystagmus following the Dix-Hallpike maneuver is typically 5 to 20 seconds, but has been reported as long as a minute.[139] This maneuver should also reproduce the patient's presenting symptoms of vertigo and both vertigo and nystagmus should subside within 1 minute from the start of nystagmus. Although clinical practice guidelines published in 2008 recognize the Dix-Hallpike

maneuver as the gold standard for the diagnosis of BPPV,[139] false negatives have been reported, and use of Frenzel lenses and repeat testing or referral to a specialist is recommended.[139-141] The guidelines also point out that the test should be avoided in individuals with spinal pathology (eg, cervical stenosis/radiculopathy), disease processes resulting in cervical instability (rheumatoid arthritis, Paget disease, Down syndrome), spinal cord injuries, retinal detachment, and morbid obesity. Care should also be exercised in patients with severe vascular disease and those at risk for vertebrobasilar insufficiency.[139] The Dix-Hallpike test was positive for Ms. Muir on the right side.

Individuals with a positive Dix-Hallpike test can also be treated from the final testing position with a continuation known as the Epley or canalith repositioning maneuver (Figure 8–3). The purpose of this positional maneuver is to attempt to reposition otolithic debris from the posterior SCC.[132] Five separate meta-analyses, including a 2007 Cochrane review, have summarized that the canalith repositioning maneuver (CRP) was superior to placebo for the treatments of posterior canal BPPV.[142-145] Additionally, six separate randomized control trials have exhibited significant vertigo resolution within 1 to 4 weeks with small numbers needed to treat (NNT) statistics (NNT = 1.3-3.4). The majority of these trials were conducted in specialty clinics, potentially limiting the generalizability of the findings to primary care clinics.[139] Mild complications (eg, nausea, vomiting, fainting, conversation to horizontal canalithiasis) with the CRP for posterior canal BPPV were reported in 12% of patients, and no serious complications were reported in these trials.[139] Current clinical practice guidelines suggest there is a preponderance of evidence for the benefit of using the CRP technique in patients with posterior canal BPPV.[139] Ms. Muir is a good candidate for this technique. For additional information and details regarding the assessment and treatment of BPPV, to include horizontal canalithiasis, the reader is referred to the American Academy of Otolaryngology—Head and Neck Surgery Clinical Practice Guidelines.[139]

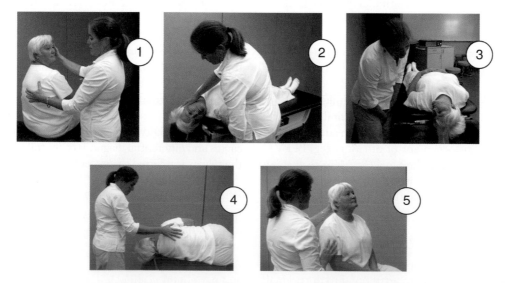

FIGURE 8–3. Dix-Hallpike maneuver; **1.** Sitting on exam table, physician turns the patient's head 30-45 degrees to one side; **2.** While maintaining this head position the physician rapidly lowers the patient to the supine position such that the head hangs over the edge of the table; observe 30-60 seconds for nystagmus; **3.** Repeat steps 1 and 2 with head turned in the opposite direction; **4.** For canalith repositioning, physician holds position 2 and/or 3 until cessation of nystagmus, or up to one minute, and then turns head to a face down position; **5.** Patient is then brought back up to the sitting position and the eyes are observed again.

Acute Labyrinthitis (Vestibular Neuritis). Acute labyrinthitis or vestibular neuritis is the second most common cause of vertigo.[131] A viral infection is also suspected as the primary cause as 50% of patients have a history or current bout of an upper respiratory infection.[146] This condition is characterized by rapid onset of intense rotational vertigo resulting in visceral symptoms including nausea, vomiting, and diaphoresis.[146] During acute symptoms postural stability and gait are also impaired. Hearing loss is not typically associated with vestibular neuritis and alerts physicians to other possible diagnoses (eg, Ménière disease, acoustic neuroma, herpes zoster). Intense symptoms usually last from 1 to 5 days with gradual resolution over weeks to months.[132] Patients evaluated in the first few hours of symptom onset present with spontaneous unilateral horizontal-rotary nystagmus with the fast or beating phase moving toward the good ear. After this initial period, visualization of nystagmus requires gaze testing (having the patient look to one side) or blocking of optical fixation (put a blank piece of white paper a few inches in front of patient).[132] The head thrust test is a noninvasive means of testing the VOR. To conduct this test, the examiner holds the head with both hands, passively flexes the cervical spine 30 degrees, instructs the patient to fixate on the examiner's nose, and randomly provides quick passive rotations to the head of 5 to 10 degrees. A lesion, such as damage to the labyrinth or peripheral vestibular nerve, results in a delayed VOR and corrective eye movement known as a saccade. In a normal VOR the patient can stay focused on the nose and no corrective eye movement is noticed. The reported sensitivity and specificity of the head thrust test for the diagnosis of unilateral vestibular hypofunction are 71% and 82%, respectively.[147]

Initial treatment is directed at control of symptoms and involves vestibular suppressants such as Meclizine. Bed rest can also be helpful for the initial 24 to 72 hours, but patients are encouraged to resume activities as tolerated and vestibular suppressants are diminished after intense symptoms have subsided. Strupp and colleagues also found some later benefit with corticosteroids used in the initial stages of the diagnosis.[148] Increased physical activity and specifically formal vestibular rehabilitation programs have also demonstrated short-term (1-month) improvements in symptoms, disability, balance, and postural stability.[149,150] For a detailed review of vestibular rehabilitation the reader is referred to the 2007 Cochrane review.[142]

Ménière Disease. Ménière disease is a disorder of the inner ear resulting in episodic vertigo lasting from a few minutes to a few hours. The condition occurs equally in males and females and onset is typically between 40 and 60 years of age. Vertigo caused by Ménière disease is often severe and can result in nausea, vomiting, and postural instability. Patients also experience fluctuating low-frequency hearing loss that is often described as "roaring" tinnitus and fullness of the ear.[135] The pathophysiology is related to excessive endolymphatic fluid pressure and endolymphatic hydrops causing displacement and inflammation on inner structures (eg, cochlea and labyrinth). The head thrust test is usually negative due to an intact vestibular nerve, but patients can exhibit peripheral patterns of nystagmus.[132] Audiograms and electronystagmography (ENG) are useful tests for the diagnosis of Ménière disease, and typically demonstrate low-frequency sensorineural hearing loss and unilateral vestibular weakness with caloric testing. Brainstem-evoked potentials are also helpful if retrocochlear disease is found on routine audiometry, and abnormal findings warrant an MRI to assess for CNS pathology and cranial nerve VIII schwannoma.[131] Due to the episodic nature of symptoms it also important to consider transient ischemia attacks in the differential diagnosis, especially if attacks are becoming more frequent.[132]

The goal of treatment during the acute phase is similar to vestibular neuritis and includes treatment of symptoms with vestibular suppressants. Dietary restrictions of salt, water, alcohol, caffeine, nicotine, and the use of diuretics are also utilized in the remission phase with the hopes of reducing the frequency and intensity of attacks. Surgery is required in only 1% to 3% of patients with chronic Ménière disease.[131] Vestibular exercises are not recommended for patients with Ménière disease unless patients exhibit long-standing vestibular damage between attacks or are postsurgical with the need for accommodation exercises.[146]

● THE SOMATOSENSORY SYSTEM

Postural instability and slowing of motion are hallmarks of the aging process. Motor control in its broadest sense implies the development and performance of a physical function that solves a movement problem such as walking across the street, dressing, and putting on hearing aids. Besdine noted in his introduction to *The Merck Manual for Geriatrics* that decreased independence in functional ability is often the only identifiable complaint from the older patient receiving a medical exam.[151] It is no surprise that functional independence is an independent predictor of quality of life[152] and nursing home placement.[153]

Both Mr. George and Ms. Muir have problems with postural control. Postural control requires the development of a precise motor outcome based on the integration of complex sensory inputs received through environmental interactions. This integration occurs through both direct environmental interaction and also through anticipatory interactions that occur through the senses of vision and hearing. The somatosensory system is comprised of the sensory information provided from the cutaneous and musculoskeletal systems. Somatosensory information converges at the level of the spinal cord and is processed reflexively and/or travels along spinal pathways for processing at higher centers. In order to accurately place her hearing aid, Ms. Muir must process and integrate joint motion in the hands with tactile sensation in both the hands and the ears. Mr. George is integrating somatosensory, visual, and vestibular sensory information to stay upright as he runs down the sports field as a referee.

Proprioception

Proprioception is the sensory domain that provides information about joint position (joint position sense) and joint motion (kinesthesia). It results from the complex integration of converging sensory inputs from the muscle, tendon, and joint structures, forming the awareness of body parts in relation to one another. This awareness is essential to balance, motor control, and coordination.[1]

Proprioception: Structure and Function

Accurate proprioception relies upon the viability of sensory end-organs (receptors), the sensory neurons that are activated by the end-organs, and central nervous system (CNS) integration. Proprioceptive sensory receptors are the joint mechanoreceptors, free nerve endings (FNEs), the muscle spindle, and the Golgi tendon organ. The joint mechanoreceptors are located in the joint capsule and ligaments, and include Pacinian, Ruffini, and Meissner corpuscles. During mechanical deformation, these receptors activate sensory neurons that have large myelinated fast-conducting axons that converge at the CNS to provide information about joint end range of motion, dynamic movement, and tension (Figure 8–4).[154] Muscle spindles lie in parallel to muscle fibers, are deformed by muscle stretch, register changes in muscle length and velocity, and remain dynamically sensitive during varying lengths and force outputs of a muscle contraction. Muscle spindles are considered the dominant influence in proprioceptive awareness, particularly those of the distal lower extremities during weight-bearing activities.[155] The Golgi tendon organ is located near the muscle tendon transitional zone and activates sensory neurons during tendon stretch, as occurs during muscle contraction (Figure 8–4). The joint receptors, muscle spindle, and Golgi tendon organ collectively provide overlapping and redundant information about joint position and movement and are key regulators of balance and postural control.[154,156] Proprioceptive information converges in the spinal cord on internerons and alpha motor neurons that facilitate reflexes such as the stretch reflex (examined clinically through the deep tendon reflex) and/or activate secondary neurons that deliver information to higher centers.[156]

Somatosensation: Age-Related Change

Typical age-associated changes occur to both muscle and joint proprioceptive sensory organs, and to the sensory nerves that transmit the information.[157] It has been documented in human and animal studies that age-related changes in the muscle spindle result in a reduction in muscle spindle sensitivity.[158] There is an age-associated decline in the number of joint proprioceptors, particularly in joints with arthritic changes,[159] and many studies have demonstrated an age-associated reduction in joint position and motion sense.[157] A relationship between reduced lower extremity proprioceptive abilities (eg, toe, knee, ankle position and motion sense) and reduced balance in older adults has been repeatedly demonstrated.[155,160] Reduced proprioceptive ability in the lower extremities is associated with a history of falls[155] and difficulties completing activities of daily living (ADLs).[161]

It should be noted that people with knee arthritis have an exaggerated loss of knee proprioception,[162,163] reduced postural stability,[164,165] and increased fall risk.[166] This is an impressive finding given that at least 30% of people over 60 are estimated to have knee arthritis,[167] and many more are likely to have subclinical or early-stage joint changes. Mr. George relies upon the integration of cutaneous receptors on the soles

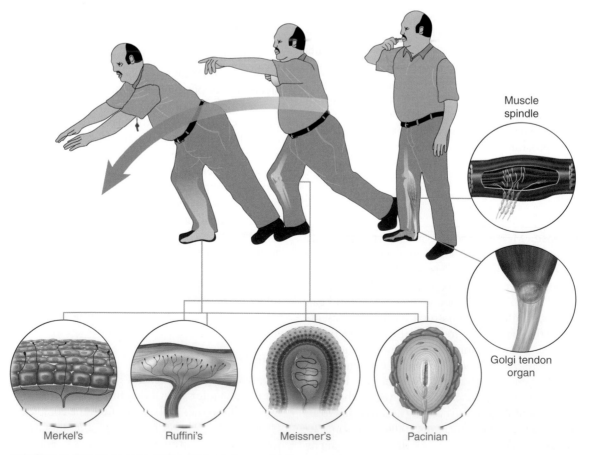

FIGURE 8–4. Cutaneous and proprioceptive sensory receptors.

of his feet and proprioceptors in his lower extremity joints and muscles to provide information about weight-bearing pressure changes and joint movements in order to maintain balance while calling athletic events. His history is suggestive of peripheral neuropathy and knee osteoarthritis, both of which add to the reduction in proprioception that is already associated with the normal aging process (Figure 8–4).

Proprioceptive Screening

Examination of joint position sense and kinesthesia is performed for research purposes with more sophisticated equipment than is typical in most clinical settings. An efficient and commonly cited clinical approach involves manual movement of the great toe up or down, with the patient (vision occluded) indicating the direction of the movement. Table 8–6 describes this method. The research findings of reduced lower extremity proprioception in people with conditions affecting lower extremity joint function (eg, knee osteoarthritis) and lower extremity sensation (eg, peripheral neuropathy) suggest that proprioception in areas key to balance and stability is reduced in people with these conditions in addition to the typical age-associated reductions.[160,162,168] The medical history itself may be suggestive of problems with proprioception.

Proprioception: Interventions

There is evidence of a positive plastic adaptation in the proprioceptive systems of younger and older adults with appropriate interventions. Improved proprioceptive abilities have been demonstrated in younger adults in response to proprioceptive training.[169,170] Several cross-sectional studies have demonstrated improved proprioceptive abilities in the lower extremities in physically active older people.[171] In particular, tai chi interventions have demonstrated an improvement in joint proprioceptive abilities, and older adults who played golf were found to have increased proprioceptive abilities compared to those who did not.[172] Waddington and Adams trained older people on a wobble board and found an improved ankle joint proprioception as a result.[173] Westlake

and associates found improved lower extremity proprioception (motion sense) and balance in older adults who participated in balance training that challenged specific sensory domains by altering sensory specific conditions.[174] These studies demonstrate the importance of challenging the system through physical activity and therapeutic exercise, and underscore the importance of targeted interventions to achieve the desired effect. Primary care providers can refer older adults to a physical therapist for individually prescribed therapeutic exercise, and/or to a community exercise program designed with a focus on balance activities.

Cutaneous Sensation

The integration within the CNS of a broad array of cutaneous information is required for complex sensory experiences such as stereognosis (discriminating familiar objects through touch) and texture recognition. Cutaneous sensation is also integrated with proprioceptive, vestibular, and visual information to play an important role in postural stability and coordination.

Cutaneous Sensation: Structure and Function

Cutaneous sensation occurs as a result of (1) mechanical deformation of end-organs (Meissner, Ruffini, and Pacinian corpuscles, Merkel receptors, and hair cells) in response to deep and light pressure, vibration, tension, and movement across skin (Figure 8–4); (2) activation of thermal receptors (heat and cold); and (3) stimulation of free nerve endings by noxious stimuli. As with proprioceptors, stimulation of cutaneous receptors results in activation of sensory axons that deliver information to the CNS for reflexive or higher-center processing.[154,156] The fingertips, lips, and plantar surface of the feet have a much higher density of cutaneous end-organs than do other areas of the body. These broad and densely populated sensory fields result ultimately in central projections to relatively enlarged representations on the somatosensory cortex. Figure 8–6 depicts the sensory homunculous.[154] Cutaneous sensation from the receptors in the fingertips plays a very

● TABLE 8–6 Somatosensory Screens for the Feet[134]

Mode	Light Touch Monfilament 5.07/10 gram	Sharp/Pain Neurological Pin	Vibration Tuning Fork	Vibration Biothesio-Meter	Proprioception
Site	Dorsum of great toe, proximal to nail bed, noncalloused	Dorsum of great toe, proximal to nail bed, noncalloused site	Bony prominence on dorsum of great toe, proximal to nail bed	Dorsum of great toe	Great toe[147]
Method	Apply monofilament perpendicularly 4 trials each toe. Patient reports "now" upon feeling touch.	Apply gentle pressure with sharp end 4 trials each toe. Patient reports "now" when felt	1. Place vibrating fork, then dampen, twice each site. Patient identifies vibration on and then vibration off. 2. Patient indicates when vibration stops, and time to lose vibratory sense is noted.[61]	Place tip perpendicular to site, turn up voltage slowly. Patient indicates when vibration felt. Perform 3 trials, and record the mean volts.	Move great toe up or down in 1-cm increments. Patient (vision occluded) identifies when movement occurs and in what direction. 10 trials each toe.
Threshold norms	≤ 1 insensate	≤ 1 insensate	1. ≤ 1 insensate (foot) 2. < 8 seconds: reduced vibration sense[61]	≥25 volts: reduced vibration sense	<8/10 correct[147]: reduced sensation

Data from reference 134.

important role in object manipulation and protective sensation, and the sensation from the soles of the feet is critical for postural stability in the upright position.

Cutaneous Sensation: Age-Related Change

Human cross-sectional studies examining healthy people of all ages have demonstrated an age-associated decrease in number and density of cutaneous receptors. Several studies have demonstrated that healthy older adults have reduced tactile and vibration sense bilaterally in the hands and the feet,[157] which has implications not only for motor control but also for protection of the skin in response to damaging stimuli. In one study, older subjects (> 65 years) had a decline of cutaneous sensation of 91% in the foot, 70% in the fingertips, and 22% in the forearm.[2] Vibration perception thresholds in the feet doubled in people at around the age of 72 to 73,[175] supporting other evidence that the rate of loss has a much steeper incline with advanced age.

Animal studies also demonstrated an age-associated reduction in axonal transport speed along peripheral nerves,[176] a reduction in number of peripheral nerve fibers, and a reduction in myelin thickness.[177] These physiologic findings are paralleled by behavioral human research demonstrating an age-associated reduction in sensory nerve conduction velocity.[178,179] The distal to proximal cutaneous and proprioceptive sensory declines associated with aging are consistent with the evidence of slowed sensory axonal transport and the reduced number and viability of sensory end-organs.

Ms. Muir has difficulty manipulating her hearing aids, and she may also be at risk of burning her hands if she does not perceive thermal stimuli adequately. Mr. George's age and long-standing diagnosis of diabetes with burning, numbness, and tingling are highly suggestive of peripheral neuropathy, which potentially has resulted in a loss of tactile acuity and proprioception in his feet and ankles. He must compensate with vision, although it has been several years since his last eye exam. The sensory loss in his feet is a major contributor to his history of falls and places him at serious risk for future falls as well as injury to the joints and dermis of his feet. Further examination of the sensation in his fingertips would likely reveal a reduction also.

Cutaneous Sensation: Screening

Common approaches to examining the integrity of cutaneous sensation include the use of light touch, vibration, sharp-dull, two-point, and warm and cold temperature stimuli. One conventional approach to sensory screening is light touch with cotton or tissue with vision occluded ("Tell me when you feel me touching you?" or "Does this side feel the same as the other?"). This approach has limited utility if sensation has declined bilaterally in age-associated sensory loss or peripheral neuropathy. One efficient and valid approach is to test sharp-dull sensation using a neurologic pin with a dull and sharp surface, with the patient's vision occluded, taking care not to puncture the skin (the tip can be filed down slightly as needed). Disposable neurologic pins are inexpensive, but this approach is not optimal for people with peripheral neuropathy.

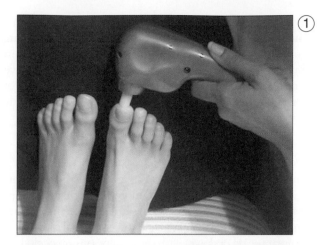

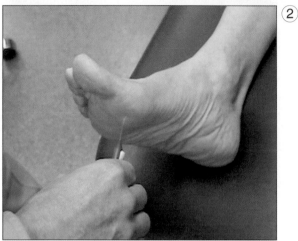

FIGURE 8–5. 1. Vibration perception threshold testing; 2. Monofilament touch sensation testing.

A more precise approach involves use of monofilaments calibrated to bend with specific amounts of pressure. Using a few key monofilaments to test sensation will provide useful information. The 5.07 monofilament bends with 10 g of pressure and discerns the presence of protective sensation in both the hands and the feet (Table 8–6, Figure 8–5).[180,181] Two-point discrimination testing of the fingers using an aesthesiometer caliper designed to measure varying distances provides valid information about this specific aspect of sensation. Six millimeters of separation accurately perceived ≥ 8/10 trials is considered the threshold for normal two-point discrimination in the fingertips. In lieu of a caliper or more sophisticated equipment, a paperclip with distance between ends accurately measured will suffice for a screen. If only one point is perceived at the fingertips, the individual is considered to have a loss of protective sensation.[182,183]

Vibration perception threshold testing (VPT) is also a valid approach for detecting early sensory loss in subclinical neuropathy.[180,184] Vibration sensation involves the fast-adapting mechanoreceptors and the large sensory neurons, both of which are affected by diabetes. Consistent with the increased density of receptors in the hands and feet and the increased representation of the hands and feet on the somatosensory cortex (Figure 8–6), VPT is typically lower (ie, more sensitive) in the distal aspect of the extremities and becomes progressively greater (less sensitive) proximally. This proximal-to-distal

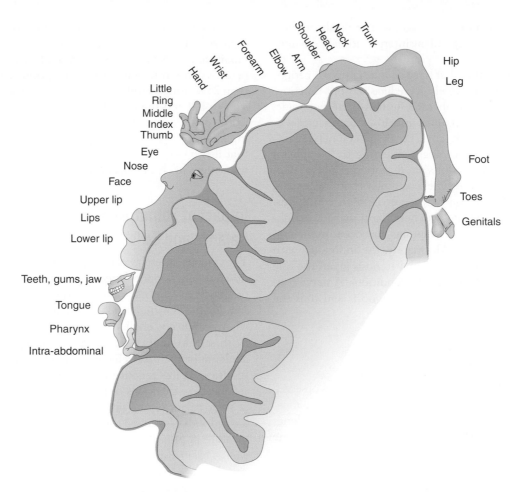

Little
Ring
Middle
Index
Thumb
Eye
Nose
Face
Upper lip
Lips
Lower lip

Teeth, gums, jaw
Tongue
Pharynx
Intra-abdominal

Hand
Wrist
Forearm
Elbow
Arm
Shoulder
Head
Neck
Trunk

Hip
Leg

Foot
Toes
Genitals

FIGURE 8–6. The sensory homunculous.

increase in sensitivity is reversed in people with PN as a result of the distance required for vessels and nerves to reach the distal extremities.[184]

Vibration perception threshold testing can be performed with either a 128-Hz tuning fork or the electronic vibrometer (often called an "electronic" tuning fork) (Figure 8–5). The manual tuning fork method is commonly used, although approaches and norms are not consistently applied.[181] The biothesiometer is a vibrometer that provides stimulation from 0 volts (no vibration) to 50 volts (most vibration), with 25 volts as the threshold for indicating sensory loss and the likely development of foot ulceration in people with diabetic PN.[185] This method correlates significantly with the outcomes from the lesser expensive tuning fork, but the application and norms are more objectively applied.[186]

Cutaneous Sensation: Interventions

Richerson and Rosendale found improved vibratory sense (using a vibrometer) in people with diabetic sensory loss and also in those without diabetes and little to no sensory loss with a 6-month intervention of tai chi training.[187] Individuals in this study (mean age 73.1 yrs) who did not have diabetes had an improvement in hemoglobin A_{1C} levels, which is likely the mediating factor for the sensory improvement. The authors speculated that increased blood flow to the feet might also be a mediating factor for improved vibratory sense in both groups. Balance measures also improved in both groups.

Vitamin B is commonly used to address peripheral neuropathy because it plays an important role in energy metabolism. A recent Cochrane review concluded that more research is needed to establish causality, but at least one controlled study found short-term improvement in vibration sensation in a group of older adults taking a vitamin B compound.[188] Anodyne monochromatic infrared photo energy has been shown in one study to enhance sensation and reduce pain in people with peripheral neuropathy,[189] but recent research questions the validity of these findings.[190] While additional research concerning these and other interventions is necessary, they provide preliminary foundations for further investigation of interventions that will prevent or modify cutaneous sensory loss in older adults.

Pathologic Conditions Affecting Somatosensory Function

The vestibular nucleus, cerebellum, somatosensory cortex, and cortical associative areas play key roles in processing, sorting, prioritizing, facilitating, and inhibiting a multitude of incoming sensory information. Pathologies and injuries to the central nervous system such as stroke, cerebral aneurysm, traumatic brain injury, tumors, and spinal cord injury will have a negative impact on sensory function. The PNS and CNS are interactive in terms of delivering and receiving sensory information; when one is affected, the other must also be in terms of losing interactive access. The result can be a devastating loss of stability and misinterpretation of environmental cues.[191]

Pathologies or injuries that have an impact on the peripheral nervous system are likely to reduce sensory function, including lymphedema, diabetes, Guillian-Barré syndrome, spinal stenosis, respiratory failure, arthritis, atherosclerosis, or trauma (laceration, stretch, crush) to peripheral nerves. Two of the more common pathologies affecting the peripheral nervous system in older adults are diabetic peripheral neuropathy and spinal stenosis. The symptoms of burning leg pain and hyper- or hypoalgesia may occur in both conditions. While a diagnosis of diabetes will help clarify diabetic peripheral neuropathy, neurologic symptoms may occur in the preclinical stage of diabetes. Alternately, the individual with diabetes may well suffer with spinal stenosis given the role that body mass index plays in both conditions. A nerve conduction study can help clarify the diagnosis and thus the intervention.

Diabetic Peripheral Neuropathy

A distal to proximal sensory loss in the extremities is observed in the increasingly prevalent pathology of peripheral neuropathy (PN). Neuropathy affects over 50% of people with long-term diabetes, and represents a general degeneration of the peripheral nerves, affecting both the autonomic as well as the somatic nerves. This is manifested in Mr. George's complaint of "stabbing pins and needles" in his feet. The individual's length of time of exposure to hyperglycemia and the severity of the condition have a direct impact on the extent of PN present as glycation products collect in the vascular structures. There is a gradual decline in nerve conduction as measured in longitudinal studies of people with diabetic PN, and this decline is significantly related to current and past history of glycemic control.[192,193] The UK Prospective Diabetes Study Group demonstrated through longitudinal research that improving glucose control in people with diabetes types 1 or 2, even in the early stages (impaired glucose tolerance), can improve sensory signs and symptoms.[193]

Boulton and associates[185] provide a thorough overview of the types of diabetic neuropathy, clinical manifestations, physiologic basis, and evidence for interventions. The authors provide multiple sources of evidence that fluctuating glucose contributes substantially to PN, and that stabilizing glucose levels over time reduces the signs and symptoms of PN, highlighting the importance of glucose "flux" to the health of the peripheral nervous system. In fact, one condition known as acute peripheral neuropathy is considered to result from large glucose flux and is reversible with tighter and consistent glucose control. It has been shown that once reduced sensation (as measured through quantitative sensory testing such as vibration or monofilament testing) is clinically evident, the rate of progression of DPN increases. Moreover, the greatest risk factor for foot ulceration among people with diabetes is peripheral neuropathy.[180] The risk of foot ulceration requires educational interventions to teach individuals to use visual inspection of feet and hands to compensate for the loss of cutaneous sensation.

These facts highlight the importance of recognition of early sensory loss to initiate appropriate interventions and modify as possible the progression of PN. In people with diabetes, vibration thresholds of perception requiring greater than 25 V using a biothesiometer were predictive of progression to PN and the risk of foot ulceration.[180] Richardson's work examining the Achilles reflex, vibration sensation (tuning fork), and position sense of the great toe demonstrates that if two out of three of these clinical signs are impaired, the patient likely has electrodiagnostic signs of PN.[194]

Impact of Somatosensory Loss: Balance and Falls

The complex interplay of multiple sensory domains is foundational to functional balance. Individuals rely primarily upon proprioceptive and cutaneous information during undisturbed standing.[155] The visual and vestibular systems are called upon when stability is challenged and sensory conflicts arise.[195] With sensory inputs declining in multiple domains, older adults must increase reliance on higher center processing, resulting in less reliance on the more efficient automatic reflexive contributions to motor control. A simple measure of static balance is the single-leg stance measure. When performed with eyes closed this test provides a salient functional measure of proprioceptive and/or cutaneous integration as well as balance abilities. Objective application and norms by decade of age have been established for single-leg stance eyes open and single-leg stance eyes closed.[196] When Mr. George performed single-leg stance eyes open, he was slightly below the threshold considered normal for his age. However, he was unable to perform single-leg stance with his eyes closed, suggestive of his inability to rely on his proprioceptive and cutaneous senses in the distal aspect of his lower extremities.

Reduced balance is a predictor of falls and both Mr. George and Ms. Muir are seeking help for balance problems and fall prevention. Research has demonstrated conclusively that the risk for falling increases substantially with increased numbers of risk factors identified.[197,198] Nevertheless, in one study only 34% of older patients seeking medical care received any fall risk evaluation,[199] and referrals were typically made only after a serious fall had already occurred.[200] The optimal approach to a comprehensive fall risk examination involves a team: physicians to assess medical conditions and pharmacologic issues; physical therapists for a focused examination of sensation, strength, balance, gait, function, and home hazards; and vision specialists for eye examination.[4,5] The American Geriatric Society Panel on Falls Prevention uses the findings from two Cochrane reviews[4,5] to support these approaches.[197] The reader is referred to Chapter 34 for more specifics regarding interventions.

● CASE CONCLUSIONS

The heterogeneity that is characteristic of aging results in the need for individual examination. Indeed, Ms. Muir and Mr. George are quite different when examining their sensory domains individually, and this necessitates interventions

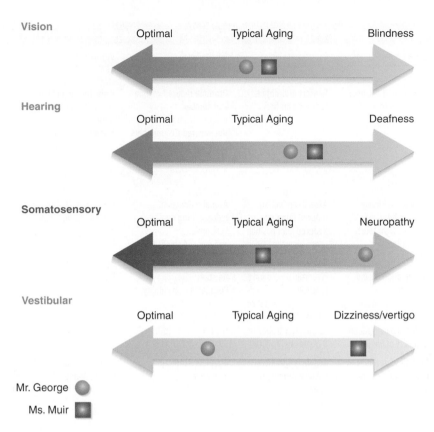

FIGURE 8–7. Where patients Mr. George and Ms. Muir lie on the spectrum of sensory function.

specific to each (Figure 8–7). Ms. Muir's function improved substantially with medication adjustments, glasses update, and increased education from the hearing aid specialist. She was referred to a vestibular rehabilitation specialist who performed the canalith repositioning maneuver and reduced her dizziness immediately ("I just couldn't believe it!"). A home health PT initiated a therapeutic exercise program that improved her balance and strength, and provided her with appropriate options for assistive device use when outside the home, making her feel more secure in varied environments. She started going out again with the help of friends and family. Mr. George received enhanced medical management for his diabetes, cerumen impaction removal which improved his hearing, and glasses update. He received outpatient PT targeted toward improving his balance, and this was followed by participation in a falls prevention community program. Mr. George's balance and function improved, although he also reduced the component of his work that required running activities. Both he and his wife found an improvement in their quality of life from these interventions and modifications.

● CONCLUSION

It is abundantly clear that typical and pathologic age-related sensory deficits have profound impacts on function and quality of life. Table 8–7 provides a summary of those deficits covered in this chapter using the World Health Organization International Classification of Function Model as a framework.[201] Age-associated changes in the body's anatomy and physiology result in functional impairments that often lead to less participation and engagement and can contribute to a reduced quality of life. Approaches to measurement of the impact of each sensory domain on participation and engagement are provided in Table 8–7.[55,103,202,203] The sensory domains examined in this chapter—visual, auditory, somatosensory, and vestibular—are critical for function, but other debilitating age-associated dysfunctions such as dysphagia, urinary stress incontinence, and loss of appetite are often directly related to sensory declines.[204] Furthermore, pathologies such as HIV, cancer, and cardiorespiratory disease are known to aggravate loss in multiple sensory domains.[205]

The primary care practitioner is well positioned to identify early or progressed signs of sensory decline and link patients with the appropriate resources to support therapies that facilitate compensation and/or recovery. Strategies and resources presented in this chapter provide an overview of and rationale for these processes. The convergence of expertise represented in a transdisciplinary team provides the best hope for promoting optimal function for older adults who are experiencing typical or pathological sensory loss resulting in functional decline.

ACKNOWLEDGMENTS

Special thanks to Tom Dolan, MS, medical illustrator and multimedia developer, University of Kentucky Department of Arts and Graphics, for providing his creativity, substantial talents, and copyright permission. We also thank Linda Allen for modeling the Dix-Hallpike maneuver.

● **TABLE 8–7** Summary: Age-Related Sensory Change Translated Across International Classification of Function Domains[201]

Sensory System	Cutaneous	Proprioceptive	Vestibular	Vision	Auditory
Functional Domain					
Body Structure	Sensory end-organs: reduced numbers	Sensory end-organs: reduced numbers	Otoconia: reduced volume and number Fragmented hair cells Neurons: reduced numbers	Reduction in pupil diameter Yellowing of lens Atrophy of iris Thinning of retinal nerve fiber	Sensory end organs: reduced numbers Stiffening of tympanic membrane Calcification of middle ear joints, atrophy of middle ear muscles Neurons: reduced numbers
Body Function Impairments	Axonal conduction: reduced firing rate Reduced light touch & vibration	Axonal conduction: reduced firing rate Reduced joint position sense, kinesthesia	Axonal conduction: reduced firing rate VOR: prolonged latency and reduced amplitude	Reduced light absorption and retinal illumination Reduced adaptation, field of view	Reduced conduction of sounds Reduced function sensorineural pathways
Activity Limitations, Participation Restrictions	Reduced balance & coordination during function Postural gait instability Slowed function Reduced participation & quality of life (QOL)	Reduced balance & coordination during function Postural gait instability Slowed function Reduced participation & quality of life (QOL)	Dizziness or vertigo during function Postural gait instability Slowed function Reduced participation & quality of life (QOL)	Reduced vision Difficulty scanning while driving Postural gait instability Slowed function Reduced participation & quality of life (QOL)	Reduced hearing Difficulty understanding conversation Withdrawal social interaction Reduced participation & quality of life (QOL)
Participation/Disability Measure	Activities Specific Balance Confidence Scale[203]	Activities Specific Balance Confidence Scale[203]	Dizziness Handicap Inventory[202]	Visual Function Questionnaire-25[103]	Hearing Handicap Inventory for the Elderly[55]

Data from reference 201.

References

1. Ghez C, Krakauer J. The organization of movement. In: Eric Kandel JS, Thomas Jessell, eds. *Principles of Neural Science*. 4th ed. Columbus, OH: McGraw-Hill; 2000:653-673.

2. Stevens JC, Alvarez-Reeves M, Dipietro L, et al. Decline of tactile acuity in aging: A study of body site, blood flow, and lifetime habits of smoking and physical activity. *Somatosens Mot Res*. 2003; 20:271-279.

3. Duncan PW, Chandler J, Studenski S, et al. How do physiological components of balance affect mobility in elderly men? *Arch Phys Med Rehabil*. 1993;74:1343-1349.

4. Gillespie LD, Gillespie WJ, Robertson MC, et al. Interventions for preventing falls in elderly people. *Cochrane Database Syst Rev*. 2003;4:CD000340.

5. Gillespie LD, Robertson MC, Gillespie WJ, et al. Interventions for preventing falls in older people living in the community. *Cochrane Database Syst Rev*. 2009;2:CD007146.

6. Colledge N, Lewis S. Magnetic resonance brain imaging in people with dizziness: A comparison with non-dizzy people. *J Neurol Neurosurg Psychiatry*. 2002;72:587-589.

7. Lethbridge-Cejku M, Schiller JS, Bernadel L. Summary health statistics for U.S. adults: National Health Interview Survey, 2002. Vital and Health Statistics. Series 10: Data from the National Health Survey. Jul 2004:1-151.

8. Adams PF, Marano MA. Current estimates from the National Health Interview Survey, 1994. Vital and Health Statistics. Series 10: Data from the National Health Survey. Dec 1995:1-260.

9. Lee DJ, Arheart KL, Lam BL, et al. Trends in reported visual impairment in United States adults. *Ophthal Epidemiol*. 2009;16: 42-49.

10. Brennan M, Horowitz A, Su YP. Dual sensory loss and its impact on everyday competence. *Gerontologist*. 2005;45:337-346.

11. Campbell VA, Crews JE, Moriarty DG, et al. Surveillance for sensory impairment, activity limitation, and health-related quality of life among older adults—United States, 1993-1997. *MMWR CDC Surveill Sum*. 1999;48:131-156.

12. Ahmad N, Seidman M. Tinnitus in the older adult: Epidemiology, pathophysiology and treatment options. *Drugs Aging*. 2004;21:297-305.

13. Agrawal Y, Platz EA, Niparko JK. Prevalence of hearing loss and differences by demographic characteristics among US adults: Data from the National Health and Nutrition Examination Survey, 1999-2004. *Arch Inter Med*. 2008;168:1522-1530.

14. Vaughan N, James K, McDermott D, et al. A 5-year prospective study of diabetes and hearing loss in a veteran population. *Otol Neurotol*. 2006;27:37-43.

15. Dreschler WA, Plomp R. Relations between psychophysical data and speech perception for hearing-impaired subjects. II. *J Acoust Soc Am*. 1985;78:1261-1270.

16. Humes LE. Speech understanding in the elderly. *J Am Acad Audiol*. 1996;7:161-167.

17. Pichora-Fuller MK, Schneider BA, Daneman M. How young and old adults listen to and remember speech in noise. *J Acoust Soc Am*. 1995;97:593-608.

18. Gates GA, Cooper JC. Incidence of hearing decline in the elderly. *Acta Otolaryngol*. 1991;111:240-248.

19. French NR, Steinberg JC. Factors governing the intelligibility of speech sounds. *J Acoust Soc Am*. 1947;19:90-119.

20. Rankovic CM. Factors governing speech reception benefits of adaptive linear filtering for listeners with sensorineural hearing loss. *J Acoust Soc Am*. 1998;103:1043-1057.

21. Arlinger S. Negative consequences of uncorrected hearing loss—a review. *Int J Audiol*. 2003;42 (Suppl 2):2S17-2S20.

22. Watson G. Low vision in the geriatric population: Rehabilitation and management. *J Am Geriatr Soc*. 2001;49:317-330.

23. Haegerstrom-Portnoy G, Morgan M. Normal age-related vision changes In: Rosenbloom A, ed. *Vision and Aging*. St. Louis: Butterworth-Heinemann; 2007.

24. Ivers RQ, Cumming RG, Mitchell P, Attebo K. Visual impairment and falls in older adults: The Blue Mountains Eye Study. *J Am Geriatr Soc.* 1998;46:58-64.

25. Keller H. *The Story of My Life*. New York: Doubleday, Page and Company; 1905.

26. Karlsson-Espmark A, Scherman M. Hearing confirms existence and identity—Experiences from persons with presbyacusis. *Intern J Audiol.* 2003;42:106-115.

27. Wahl HW, Oswald F, Zimprich D. Everyday competence in visually impaired older adults: A case for person-environment perspectives. *Gerontologist.* 1999;39:140-149.

28. American Speech-Language-Hearing Association Panel on Audiologic Assessment. *Guidelines for Audiologic Screening*. Rockville, MD: American Speech-Language-Hearing Association; 1997.

29. Coffield AB, Maciosek MV, McGinnis JM, et al. Priorities among recommended clinical preventive services. *Am J Prev Med.* 2001;21:1-9.

30. Day L, Fildes B, Gordon I, et al. Randomised factorial trial of falls prevention among older people living in their own homes. *BMJ.* 2002;325:128.

31. Wallhagen MI, Pettengill E. Hearing impairment: Significant but underassessed in primary care settings. *J Gerontol Nurs.* 2008;34: 36-42.

32. Weinstein BE. *Geriatric Audiology*. New York: Thieme; 2000.

33. Moller A. *Sensory Systems*. San Diego: Elsevier; 2003.

34. Wiley TL, Chappell R, Carmichael L, et al. Changes in hearing thresholds over 10 years in older adults. *J Am Acad Audiol.* 2008;19:281-292; quiz, 371.

35. Jerger J. Can age-related decline in speech understanding be explained by peripheral hearing loss? *J Am Acad Audiol.* 1992;3:33-38.

36. Willott JF, Parham K, Hunter KP. Comparison of the auditory sensitivity of neurons in the cochlear nucleus and inferior colliculus of young and aging C57BL/6J and CBA/J mice. *Hear Res.* 1991;53:78-94.

37. Schuknecht HF, Gacek MR. Cochlear pathology in presbycusis. *Ann Otol Rhinol Laryngol.* 1993;102:1-16.

38. Henry JA, Dennis KC, Schechter MA. General review of tinnitus: Prevalence, mechanisms, effects, and management. *J Speech Lang Hear Res.* 2005;48:1204-1235.

39. Nondahl DM, Cruickshanks KJ, Dalton DS, et al. The impact of tinnitus on quality of life in older adults. *J Am Acad Audiol.* 2007;18:257-266.

40. Rosenhall U. The influence of ageing on noise-induced hearing loss. *Noise Health.* 2003;5:47-53.

41. Sindhusake D, Golding M, Wigney D, et al. Factors predicting severity of tinnitus: A population-based assessment. *J Am Acad Audiol.* 2004;15:269-280.

42. Henry JA, Loovis C, Montero M, et al. Randomized clinical trial: Group counseling based on tinnitus retraining therapy. *J Rehab Res Dev.* 2007;44:21-32.

43. Herraiz C, Hernandez FJ, Plaza G, de los Santos G. Long-term clinical trial of tinnitus retraining therapy. *Otolaryngol Head Neck Surg.* 2005;133:774-779.

44. Herraiz C, Hernandez FJ, Toledano A, Aparicio JM. Tinnitus retraining therapy: prognosis factors. *Am J Otolaryngol.* 2007;28: 225-229.

45. Yueh B, Shapiro N, MacLean CH, Shekelle PG. Screening and management of adult hearing loss in primary care: Scientific review. JAMA. 2003;289:1976-1985.

46. Lewis-Cullinan C, Janken JK. Effect of cerumen removal on the hearing ability of geriatric patients. *J Adv Nurs.* 1990;15:594-600.

47. Meador JA. Cerumen impaction in the elderly. *J Gerontol Nurs.* 1995;21:43-45.

48. Ernst E. Ear candles: A triumph of ignorance over science. *J Laryngol Otol.* Jan 2004;118(1):1-2.

49. Martin F, Clark J. *Introduction to Audiology*. 9th ed. Boston: Pearson; 2006.

50. Wei BP, Mubiru S, O'Leary S. Steroids for idiopathic sudden sensorineural hearing loss. *Cochrane Database Syst Rev.* 2006: CD003998.

51. Chen CY, Halpin C, Rauch SD. Oral steroid treatment of sudden sensorineural hearing loss: A ten year retrospective analysis. *Otol Neurotol.* 2003;24:728-733.

52. Rybak LP, Whitworth CA, Mukherjea D, Ramkumar V. Mechanisms of cisplatin-induced ototoxicity and prevention. *Hear Res.* 2007;226:157-167.

53. Arslan E, Orzan E, Santarelli R. Global problem of drug-induced hearing loss. *Ann NY Acad Sci.* 1999;884:1-14.

54. Bienvenue GR, Michael PL, Chaffinch JC, Zeigler J. The Audio-Scope: A clinical tool for otoscopic and audiometric examination. *Ear Hear.* 1985;6:251-254.

55. Ventry IM, Weinstein BE. The hearing handicap inventory for the elderly: A new tool. *Ear Hear.* 1982;3:128-134.

56. Shanks JE, Wilson RH, Larson V, Williams D. Speech recognition performance of patients with sensorineural hearing loss under unaided and aided conditions using linear and compression hearing AIDS. *Ear Hear.* 2002;23:280-290.

57. Marttila TI, Jauhiainen T. Hearing disability assessment in evaluating hearing aid benefit. *Scand Audiol.* 1996;25:121-125.

58. Newman CW, Weinstein BE, Jacobson GP, Hug GA. The Hearing Handicap Inventory for Adults: Psychometric adequacy and audiometric correlates. *Ear Hear.* 1990;11:430-433.

59. Saunders GH, Forsline A. The Performance-Perceptual Test (PPT) and its relationship to aided reported handicap and hearing aid satisfaction. *Ear Hear.* 2006;27:229-242.

60. Chisolm TH, Johnson CE, Danhauer JL, et al. A systematic review of health-related quality of life and hearing aids: Final report of the American Academy of Audiology Task Force on the Health-Related Quality of Life Benefits of Amplification in Adults. *J Am Acad Audiol.* 2007;18:151-183.

61. Takahashi G, Martinez CD, Beamer S, et al. Subjective measures of hearing aid benefit and satisfaction in the NIDCD/VA follow-up study. *J Am Acad Audiol.* 2007;18:323-349.

62. Popelka MM, Cruickshanks KJ, Wiley TL, et al. Low prevalence of hearing aid use among older adults with hearing loss: The Epidemiology of Hearing Loss Study. *J Am Geriatr Soc.* 1998;46: 1075-1078.

63. Franks JR, Beckmann NJ. Rejection of hearing aids: Attitudes of a geriatric sample. *Ear Hear.* 1985;6:161-166.

64. Garstecki DC, Erler SF. Hearing loss, control, and demographic factors influencing hearing aid use among older adults. *J Speech Lang Hear Res.* 1998;41:527-537.

65. Kochkin S. MarkeTrak VI: 10 year customer satisfaction trends in the US hearing instrument market. *Hear Rev.* 2002;9:14-46.

66. Food and Drug Administration Code of Federal Regulations. *Hearing Aids*. 2008. https://www.accessdata.fda.gov/scripts/cdrh/cfdocs/ cfCFR/CFRSearch.cfm?fr=801.420. Accessed August 18, 2009.

67. Schow R, Nerbonne M. *Introduction to Audiologic Rehabilitation*. Vol 5. Boston: Pearson Education; 2007.

68. Fabry D. Creating the evidence: Lessons from cochlear implants. *J Am Acad Audiol*. 2005;16:515-522.

69. Waltzman SB. Cochlear implants: Current status. *Exp Rev Med Dev*. 2006;3:647-655.

70. Dorman MF, Ketten D. Adaptation by a cochlear-implant patient to upward shifts in the frequency representation of speech. *Ear Hear*. 2003;24:457-460.

71. Hamzavi J, Baumgartner WD, Pok SM, et al. Variables affecting speech perception in postlingually deaf adults following cochlear implantation. *Acta Otolaryngol*. 2003;123:493-498.

72. Valimaa TT, Maatta TK, Lopponen HJ, Sorri MJ. Phoneme recognition and confusions with multichannel cochlear implants: consonants. *J Speech Lang Hear Res*. 2002;45:1055-1069.

73. Valimaa TT, Maatta TK, Lopponen HJ, Sorri MJ. Phoneme recognition and confusions with multichannel cochlear implants: vowels. *J Speech Lang Hear Res*. 2002;45:1039-1054.

74. Sterkers O, Mosnier I, Ambert-Dahan E, et al. Cochlear implants in elderly people: Preliminary results. *Acta Otolaryngol Suppl*. 2004;552:64-67.

75. Khan AM, Handzel O, Burgess BJ, et al. Is word recognition correlated with the number of surviving spiral ganglion cells and electrode insertion depth in human subjects with cochlear implants? *Laryngoscope*. 2005;115:672-677.

76. Ruffin CV, Tyler RS, Witt SA, et al. Long-term performance of Clarion 1.0 cochlear implant users. *Laryngoscope*. 2007;117:1183-1190.

77. Burk MH, Humes LE. Effects of training on speech recognition performance in noise using lexically hard words. *J Speech Lang Hear Res*. 2007;50:25-40.

78. Burk MH, Humes LE, Amos NE, Strauser LE. Effect of training on word-recognition performance in noise for young normal-hearing and older hearing-impaired listeners. *Ear Hear*. 2006; 27:263-278.

79. Miller JD, Watson CS, Kistler DJ, et al. Preliminary evaluation of the speech perception assessment and training system (SPATS) with hearing-aid and cochlear-implant users. *J Acoust Soc Am*. 2007;122:3063.

80. Stecker GC, Bowman GA, Yund EW, et al. Perceptual training improves syllable identification in new and experienced hearing aid users. *J Rehab Res Dev*. 2006;43:537-552.

81. Sweetow R, Sabes J. The need for and development of an adaptive Listening and Communication Enhancement (LACE) program. *J Amer Acad Audiol*. 2006;17:538-558.

82. Sweetow R, Sabes J. Listening and communication enhancement (LACE). *Semin Hear*. 2007;28:133-141.

83. Hawkins DB. Effectiveness of counseling-based adult group aural rehabilitation programs: A systematic review of the evidence. *J Am Acad Audiol*. 2005;16:485-493.

84. Snell R, Lemp MA. *Clinical Anatomy of the Eye*. Malden, MA: Blackwell Science; 1998.

85. Remington L. *Clinical Anatomy of the Visual System*. St. Louis: Elsevier; 2005.

86. Winn B, Whitaker D, Elliott DB, Phillips NJ. Factors affecting light-adapted pupil size in normal human subjects. *Invest Ophthalmol Vis Sci*. 1994;35:1132-1137.

87. Curcio CA, Owsley C, Jackson GR. Spare the rods, save the cones in aging and age-related maculopathy. *Invest Ophthalmol Vis Sci*. 2000;41:2015-2018.

88. Eye Diseases Prevalence Research Group. Causes and prevalence of visual impairment among adults in the United States. *Arch Ophthalmol*. 2004;122:477-485.

89. Christen WG, Glynn RJ, Ajani UA, et al. Smoking cessation and risk of age-related cataract in men. *JAMA*. 2000;284:713-716.

90. Rowe S, MacLean CH, Shekelle PG. Preventing visual loss from chronic eye disease in primary care: scientific review. *JAMA*. 2004;291:1487-1495.

91. Applegate WB, Miller ST, Elam JT, et al. Impact of cataract surgery with lens implantation on vision and physical function in elderly patients. *JAMA*.1987;257:1064-1066.

92. Smith W, Assink J, Klein R, et al. Risk factors for age-related macular degeneration: Pooled findings from three continents. *Ophthalmology*. 2001;108:697-704.

93. Peeters A, Magliano DJ, Stevens J, et al. Changes in abdominal obesity and age-related macular degeneration: The Atherosclerosis Risk in Communities Study. *Arch Ophthalmol*. 2008;126:1554-1560.

94. Bressler NM, Bressler SB, Fine SL. Age-related macular degeneration. *Surv Ophthalmol*. 1988;32:375-413.

95. Hazin R, Freeman PD, Kahook MY. Age-related macular degeneration: A guide for the primary care physician. *J Natl Med Assoc*. 2009;101:134-138.

96. Elner SG. Gradual painless visual loss: Retinal causes. *Clin Geriatr Med*. 1999;15:25-46, v-vi.

97. Wang N, Wu H, Fan Z. Primary angle closure glaucoma in Chinese and Western populations. *Chinese Med J*. 2002;115:1706-1715.

98. Shindler KS, Sankar PS, Volpe NJ, Piltz-Seymour JR. Intermittent headaches as the presenting sign of subacute angle-closure glaucoma. *Neurology*. 2005;65:757-758.

99. Lin AP, Orengo-Nania S, Braun UK. The PCP's role in chronic open-angle glaucoma. *Geriatrics*. 2009;64:20-28.

100. American Optometric Association. American Optometric Association Older Adult Vision Screening Guidelines. http://www.aoa.org/documents/OlderAdultVisionScreeningGuide.pdf. Accessed August 4, 2009.

101. Smeeth L, Iliffe S. Community screening for visual impairment in the elderly. *Cochrane Database Syst Rev*. 2006;3:CD001054.

102. Frith P, Gray R, MacLennan S, Ambler P. *The Eye in Clinical Practice*. 2nd ed. Malden, MA: Blackwell Science; 2001.

103. Mangione CM, Lee PP, Gutierrez PR, et al. Development of the 25-item National Eye Institute Visual Function Questionnaire. *Arch Ophthalmol*. 2001;119:1050-1058.

104. Kroenke K, Mangelsdorff AD. Common symptoms in ambulatory care: Incidence, evaluation, therapy, and outcome. *Am J Med*. 1989;86:262-266.

105. Sloane PD, Coeytaux RR, Beck RS, Dallara J. Dizziness: State of the science. *Ann Intern Med*. 2001;134:823-832.

106. Luxon LM. Disturbances of balance in the elderly. *Br J Hosp Med*. 1991;45:22-26.

107. Kroenke K, Lucas CA, Rosenberg ML, et al. Causes of persistent dizziness. A prospective study of 100 patients in ambulatory care. *Ann Intern Med.* 1992;117:898-904.

108. Agrawal Y, Carey JP, Della Santina CC, et al. Disorders of balance and vestibular function in US adults: Data from the National Health and Nutrition Examination Survey, 2001-2004. *Arch Intern Med.* 2009;169:938-944.

109. Pothula VB, Chew F, Lesser TH, Sharma AK. Falls and vestibular impairment. *Clin Otolaryngol Allied Sci.* 2004;29:179-182.

110. Aktas S, Celik Y. An evaluation of the underlying causes of fall-induced hip fractures in elderly persons. *Ulus Travma Acil Cerrahi Derg.* 2004;10:250-252.

111. Herdman SJ, Schubert MC, Tusa RJ. Role of central preprogramming in dynamic visual acuity with vestibular loss. *Arch Otolaryngol Head Neck Surg.* 2001;127:1205-1210.

112. Huterer M, Cullen KE. Vestibuloocular reflex dynamics during high-frequency and high-acceleration rotations of the head on body in rhesus monkey. *J Neurophysiol.* 2002;88:13-28.

113. Minor LB, Lasker DM, Backous DD, Hullar TE. Horizontal vestibuloocular reflex evoked by high-acceleration rotations in the squirrel monkey. I. Normal responses. *J Neurophysiol.* 1999;82:1254-1270.

114. Pavol MJ, Owings TM, Foley KT, Grabiner MD. Mechanisms leading to a fall from an induced trip in healthy older adults. *J Gerontol A Biol Sci Med Sci.* 2001;56:M428-M437.

115. Goldberg JM, Fernandez C. Physiology of peripheral neurons innervating semicircular canals of the squirrel monkey. I. Resting discharge and response to constant angular accelerations. *J Neurophysiol.* 1971;34:635-660.

116. Tascioglu AB. Brief review of vestibular system anatomy and its higher order projections. *Neuroanatomy.* 2005;4:24-27.

117. Schubert MC, Minor LB. Vestibulo-ocular physiology underlying vestibular hypofunction. *Phys Ther.* 2004;84:373-385.

118. Walther LE, Westhofen M. Presbyvertigo-aging of otoconia and vestibular sensory cells. *J Vestib Res.* 2007;17:89-92.

119. Igarashi M, Saito R, Mizukoshi K, Alford BR. Otoconia in young and elderly persons: A temporal bone study. *Acta Otolaryngol Suppl.* 1993;504:26-29.

120. Baloh RW, Sloane PD, Honrubia V. Quantitative vestibular function testing in elderly patients with dizziness. *Ear Nose Throat J.* 1989;68:935-939.

121. Lopez I, Ishiyama G, Tang Y, et al. Regional estimates of hair cells and supporting cells in the human crista ampullaris. *J Neurosci Res.* 2005;82:421-431.

122. Rauch SD, Velazquez-Villasenor L, Dimitri PS, Merchant SN. Decreasing hair cell counts in aging humans. *Ann NY Acad Sci.* 2001;942:220-227.

123. Rosenhall U. Degenerative patterns in the aging human vestibular neuro-epithelia. *Acta Otolaryngol.* 1973;76:208-220.

124. Fernandez JA, Suarez C, Navarro A, et al. Aging in the vestibular nuclear complex of the male golden hamster (*Mesocricetus auratus*): Anatomic and morphometric study. *Histol Histopathol.* 2007;22:855-868.

125. Enrietto JA, Jacobson KM, Baloh RW. Aging effects on auditory and vestibular responses: A longitudinal study. *Am J Otolaryngol.* 1999;20:371-378.

126. Demer JL, Honrubia V, Baloh RW. Dynamic visual acuity: A test for oscillopsia and vestibulo-ocular reflex function. *Am J Otol.* 1994;15:340-347.

127. Grossman GE, Leigh RJ. Instability of gaze during locomotion in patients with deficient vestibular function. *Ann Neurol.* 1990; 27:528-532.

128. Pritcher MR, Whitney SL, Marchetti GF, Furman JM. The influence of age and vestibular disorders on gaze stabilization: A pilot study. *Otol Neurotol.* 2008;29:982-988.

129. Herdman SJ. Role of vestibular adaptation in vestibular rehabilitation. *Otolaryngol Head Neck Surg.* 1998;119:49-54.

130. Schubert MC, Herdman SJ, Tusa RJ. Vertical dynamic visual acuity in normal subjects and patients with vestibular hypofunction. *Otol Neurotol.* 2002;23:372-377.

131. Herdman SJ. *Vestibular Rehabilitation.* Philadelphia: Davis; 2007.

132. Kerber KA. Vertigo and dizziness in the emergency department. *Emerg Med Clin North Am.* 2009;27:39-50, viii.

133. Eaton DA, Roland PS. Dizziness in the older adult, part 1. Evaluation and general treatment strategies. *Geriatrics.* 2003;58:28-30, 33-26.

134. Karatas M. Central vertigo and dizziness: epidemiology, differential diagnosis, and common causes. *Neurologist.* 2008;14:355-364.

135. Chan Y. Differential diagnosis of dizziness. *Curr Opin Otolaryngol Head Neck Surg.* 2009;17:200-203.

136. Sekine K, Sato G, Takeda N. [Incidence of vertigo and dizziness disorders at a university hospital]. *Nippon Jibiinkoka Gakkai Kaiho.* 2005;108:842-849.

137. Baloh RW. Vertigo. *Lancet.* 1998;352:1841-1846.

138. Neuhauser HK. Epidemiology of vertigo. *Curr Opin Neurol.* 2007; 20:40-46.

139. Bhattacharyya N, Baugh RF, Orvidas L, et al. Clinical practice guideline: Benign paroxysmal positional vertigo. *Otolaryngol Head Neck Surg.* 2008;139:S47-S81.

140. Nunez RA, Cass SP, Furman JM. Short- and long-term outcomes of canalith repositioning for benign paroxysmal positional vertigo. *Otolaryngol Head Neck Surg.* 2000;122:647-652.

141. Viirre E, Purcell I, Baloh RW. The Dix-Hallpike test and the canalith repositioning maneuver. *Laryngoscope.* 2005;115:184-187.

142. Hillier SL, Hollohan V. Vestibular rehabilitation for unilateral peripheral vestibular dysfunction. *Cochrane Database Syst Rev.* 2007;4:CD005397.

143. Lopez-Escamez J, Gonzalez-Sanchez M, Salinero J. [Meta-analysis of the treatment of benign paroxysmal positional vertigo by Epley and Semont maneuvers]. *Acta Otorrinolaringol Esp.* 1999;50: 366-370.

144. Teixeira LJ, Machado JN. Maneuvers for the treatment of benign positional paroxysmal vertigo: A systematic review. *Braz J Otorhinolaryngol.* 2006;72:130-139.

145. Woodworth BA, Gillespie MB, Lambert PR. The canalith repositioning procedure for benign positional vertigo: A meta-analysis. *Laryngoscope.* 2004;114:1143-1146.

146. Eaton DA, Roland PS. Dizziness in the older adult, part 2. Treatments for causes of the four most common symptoms. *Geriatrics.* 2003;58:46, 49-52.

147. Schubert MC, Tusa RJ, Grine LE, Herdman SJ. Optimizing the sensitivity of the head thrust test for identifying vestibular hypofunction. *Phys Ther.* 2004;84:151-158.

148. Strupp M, Zingler VC, Arbusow V, et al. Methylprednisolone, valacyclovir, or the combination for vestibular neuritis. *N Engl J Med.* 2004;351:354-361.

149. Giray M, Kirazli Y, Karapolat H, et al. Short-term effects of vestibular rehabilitation in patients with chronic unilateral vestibular dysfunction: A randomized controlled study. *Arch Phys Med Rehabil.* 2009;90:1325-1331.

150. Strupp M, Arbusow V, Maag KP, et al. Vestibular exercises improve central vestibulospinal compensation after vestibular neuritis. *Neurology.* 1998;51:838-844.

151. Besdine R. *The Merck Manual of Geriatrics.* Whitehouse Station, NJ: Merck; 1990.

152. Atchley R. Adaptive capacity. In: *Continuity and Adaptation in Aging: Creating Positive Experiences.* Baltimore: Johns Hopkins Press; 1999:76-132.

153. Gaugler J, Duval S, Anderson K, Kane RL. Predicting nursing home admission in the US: A metaanalysis. *Biomed Central Geriatr.* http://www.biomedcentral.com/1471-2318/7/13. Accessed June 19, 2007.

154. Gardner EP, Martin J. Coding of sensory information. In: Kandel ER, Schwartz JH, Jessell TM, eds. *Principles of Neural Science.* Norwalk, CT: Appleton & Lange; 2000:411-428.

155. Lord SR, Sturnieks DL. The physiology of falling: Assessment and prevention strategies for older people. *J Sci Med Sport.* 2005;8:35-42.

156. Lundy-Eckman L. *Neuroscience: Fundamentals of Rehabilitation.* 2nd ed. Philadelphia: Saunders; 2002.

157. Shaffer SW, Harrison AL. Aging of the somatosensory system: A translational perspective. *Phys Ther.* 2007;87:193-207.

158. Liu JX, Eriksson PO, Thornell LE, Pedrosa-Domellof F. Fiber content and myosin heavy chain composition of muscle spindles in aged human biceps brachii. *J Histochem Cytochem.* 2005;53:445-454.

159. Swash M, Fox KP. The effect of age on human skeletal muscle. Studies of the morphology and innervation of muscle spindles. *J Neurol Sci.* 1972;16:417-432.

160. Lord SR, Rogers MW, Howland A, Fitzpatrick R. Lateral stability, sensorimotor function and falls in older people. *J Am Geriatr Soc.* 1999;47:1077-1081.

161. Hurley MV, Rees J, Newham DJ. Quadriceps function, proprioceptive acuity and functional performance in healthy young, middle-aged and elderly subjects. *Age Ageing.* 1998;27:55-62.

162. Hewitt BA, Refshauge KM, Kilbreath SL. Kinesthesia at the knee: The effect of osteoarthritis and bandage application. *Arthritis Rheum.* 2002;47:479-483.

163. Marks R. Further evidence of impaired position sense in knee osteoarthritis. *Physiother Res Int.* 1996;1:127-136.

164. Harrison AL. The influence of pathology, pain, balance, and self-efficacy on function in women with osteoarthritis of the knee. *Phys Ther.* 2004;84:822-831.

165. Hinman RS, Bennell KL, Metcalf BR, Crossley KM. Balance impairments in individuals with symptomatic knee osteoarthritis: A comparison with matched controls using clinical tests. *Rheumatology (Oxford).* 2002;41:1388-1394.

166. Sturnieks DL, St George R, Lord SR. Balance disorders in the elderly. *Neurophysiol Clin.* 2008;38:467-478.

167. Felson DT, Naimark A, Anderson J, et al. The prevalence of knee osteoarthritis in the elderly. The Framingham Osteoarthritis Study. *Arthritis Rheum.* 1987;30:914-918.

168. Armstrong B, McNair P, Taylor D. Head and neck position sense. *Sports Med.* 2008;38:101-117.

169. Benjuya N, Melzer I, Kaplanski J. Aging-induced shifts from a reliance on sensory input to muscle cocontraction during balanced standing. *J Gerontol A Biol Sci Med Sci.* 2004;59:166-171.

170. Hutton RS, Atwater SW. Acute and chronic adaptations of muscle proprioceptors in response to increased use. *Sports Med.* 1992; 14:406-421.

171. Petrella RJ, Lattanzio PJ, Nelson MG. Effect of age and activity on knee joint proprioception. *Am J Phys Med Rehabil.* 1997;76: 235-241.

172. Tsang WW, Hui-Chan CW. Effects of exercise on joint sense and balance in elderly men: Tai Chi versus golf. *Med Sci Sports Exerc.* 2004;36:658-667.

173. Waddington GS, Adams RD. The effect of a 5-week wobble-board exercise intervention on ability to discriminate different degrees of ankle inversion, barefoot and wearing shoes: A study in healthy elderly. *J Am Geriatr Soc.* 2004;52:573-576.

174. Westlake KP, Wu Y, Culham EG. Sensory-specific balance training in older adults: Effect on position, movement, and velocity sense at the ankle. *Phys Ther.* 2007;87:560-568.

175. Perry SD. Evaluation of age-related plantar-surface insensitivity and onset age of advanced insensitivity in older adults using vibratory and touch sensation tests. *Neurosci Lett.* 2005;21.

176. Stromska DP, Ochs S. Axoplasmic transport in aged rats. *Exp Neurol.* 1982;77:215-224.

177. Verdu E, Ceballos D, Vilches JJ, Navarro X. Influence of aging on peripheral nerve function and regeneration. *J Periph Nerv Syst.* 2000;5:191-208.

178. Bouche P, Cattelin F, Saint-Jean O, et al. Clinical and electrophysiological study of the peripheral nervous system in the elderly. *J Neurol.* 1993;240:263-268.

179. Taylor PK. Non-linear effects of age on nerve conduction in adults. *J Neurol Sci.* 1984;66:223-234.

180. Boulton AJM, Armstrong DG, Albert SF, et al. Comprehensive foot examination and risk assessment: A report of the Task Force of the Foot Care Interest Group of the American Diabetes Association, with endorsement by the American Association of Clinical Endocrinologists. *Diabetes Care.* 2008;31:1679-1685.

181. Perkins BA, Olaleye D, Zinman B, Bril V. Simple screening tests for peripheral neuropathy in the diabetes clinic. *Diabetes Care.* 2001;24:250-256.

182. Callahan AD. Sensibility assessment for nerve lesions in continuity and nerve lacerations. In: EJ M, ed. *Hunter-Mackin-Callahan Rehabilitation of the Hand and Upper Extremity.* St. Louis: Mosby; 2002:233.

183. Magee DJ. Forearm, wrist, and hand. In: Magee DJ, ed. *Orthopedic Physical Assessment.* 5th ed. St. Louis: Saunders Elsevier; 2006.

184. Manivannan M, Periyasamy R, Narayanamurthy VB. Vibration perception threshold testing and the law of mobility in diabetes mellitus patients. *Primary Care Diabetes.* 2009;3:17-21.

185. Boulton AJM, Armstrong DG, Albert SF, et al. Comprehensive foot examination and risk assessment. *J Am Podiatr Med Assoc.* 2009;99:74-80.

186. Tochman-Gawda A, Paprzycki P, Dziemidok P. A tuning fork or a biothesiometer: Which one to choose in the outpatient diabetes care? *Diabetologia.* 2007;7:13-19.

187. Richerson S, Rosendale K. Does Tai Chi improve plantar sensory ability? A pilot study. *Diabetes Technol Ther.* 2007;9: 276-286.

188. Ang OD, Mhha MJ, Dario AD, et al. Vitamin D for treating peripheral neuropathy. Cochrane Database Syst Rev. 2009;CD004573.

189. Leonard DR, Farooqi MH, Myers S. Restoration of sensation, reduced pain, and improved balance in subjects with diabetic

peripheral neuropathy: A double-blind, randomized, placebo-controlled study with monochromatic near-infrared treatment. *Diabetes Care.* 2004;27:168-172.

190. Lavery LA, Murdoch DP, Williams J, Lavery DC. Does anodyne light therapy improve peripheral neuropathy in diabetes? *Diabetes Care.* 2008;31:316-321.

191. Fredricks CM. *Pathophysiology of Motor Systems.* Philadelphia: Davis; 1996.

192. Vinik AL, Park VS, Stansbury KB, Pittinger GL. Diabetic neuropathies. *Diabetologia.* 2000;43:957-973.

193. Group UPDS. Intensive blood-glucose control with sulphonylureas or insulin compared with conventional treatment and risk of complications in patients with type 2 diabetes (UKPDS 33). *Lancet.* 1998;352:837-853.

194. Richardson JK. The clinical identification of peripheral neuropathy among older persons. *Arch Phys Med Rehabil.* 2002;83:1553-1558.

195. Shumway-Cooke A, Woollacott M. *Motor Control: Theory and Practical Applications.* Baltimore: Williams & Wilkins; 1995.

196. Springer BA, Marin R, Cyhan T, et al. Normative values for the unipedal stance test with eyes open and closed. *J Geriatr Phys Ther.* 2007;30:9-15.

197. Prevention AGSPoF. Guideline for the prevention of falls in older persons. *J Am Geriatr Soc.* 2001;49:664-672.

198. Tinetti ME. Clinical practice. Preventing falls in elderly persons. *N Engl J Med.* 2003;348:42-49.

199. Wenger NS, Solomon DH, Roth C. The quality of medical care provided to vulnerable community dwelling older patients. *Ann Inter Med.* 2003;139:740-747.

200. Baker DI, King MB, Fortinsky RH. Dissemination of an evidence-based multicomponent fall risk assessment and management strategy throughout a geographic area. *J Am Geriatr Soc.* 2005;53: 675-680.

201. World Health Organization. *Classification of Functioning, Disability and Health.* WHO; 2009.

202. Jacobson GP, Newman CW. The development of the Dizziness Handicap Inventory. *Arch Otolaryngol Head Neck Surg.* 1990;116: 424-427.

203. Myers AM, Fletcher PC, Myers AH, Sherk W. Discriminative and evaluative properties of the activities specific balance confidence (ABC) scale. *J Gerontol A Biol Med Sci.* 1998;53: M287-M294.

204. Schiffman SS. Critical illness and changes in sensory perception. *The Proceedings of the Nutrition Society.* 2007;66:331-345.

205. Watters MR, Poff PW, Shiramizu BT, et al. Symptomatic distal sensory polyneuropathy in HIV after age 50. *Neurology.* 2004;62: 1378-1383.

POST-TEST

1. **What type of hearing loss would be observed if a patient has both presbycusis and cerumen impaction?**
   A. Conductive
   B. Sensory
   C. Neural
   D. Mixed

2. **Which of the following distinguishes vertigo from disequilibrium?**
   A. Vertigo is more likely to begin as a mild problem and grow progressively.
   B. Dysequilibrium is a feeling of unsteadiness only when in the upright position.
   C. Dysequilibrium typically causes nausea and occasionally vomiting.
   D. Vertigo is more common than dysequilibrium with aging.

3. **Which of the following is true in regard to somatosensory loss and aging?**
   A. Reduced numbers of somatosensory receptors contribute to age-related somatosensory decline.
   B. There are no known interventions for age-associated proprioceptive decline.
   C. Arthritis does not impact the proprioception of joints.
   D. Measurement of cutaneous sensation is more precise with the tuning fork than the electronic vibrometer.

4. **Which of the following is true in regard to people with peripheral neuropathy?**
   A. No interventions have been identified to address the signs and symptoms.
   B. Vibration detection requiring greater than 10 volts (electronic vibrometer) is predictive of a progression to PN.
   C. Sensory loss occurs in a distal to proximal direction.
   D. PN affects only the sensory nerves.

ANSWERS TO PRE-TEST

1. D
2. B
3. A
4. B

ANSWERS TO POST-TEST

1. D
2. B
3. A
4. C

9

Atypical Presentation of Diseases in the Older Adult

Keerti Sharma, MB, BS

● LEARNING OBJECTIVES

1. Describe physiologic changes in the aging adult that contribute to atypical disease presentation.
2. Discuss the role of functional and cognitive decline in atypical disease presentation.
3. Explain the optimal approach to diagnosis and treatment of atypical diseases in older adults, including urinary tract infection, pneumonia, and myocardial infarction.

PRE-TEST

1. **Elderly patients with sepsis are LEAST likely to present with:**
   - A. Altered mental status
   - B. High fever
   - C. No fever
   - D. Loss of appetite

2. **Elderly patients with pneumonia are MOST likely to present with:**
   - A. Pleuritic chest pain
   - B. Fever of 102-102.5°F
   - C. Altered mental status
   - D. Copius sputum production

3. **Which of the following is TRUE regarding UTI in older adults?**
   - A. It is usually a diagnosis of exclusion.
   - B. It is associated with dysuria and fever.
   - C. Dipstick testing is useful in predicting UTI.
   - D. Pyuria is an accurate predictor of bacteriuria among the elderly.

INTRODUCTION

The physiologic changes and accumulation of co-morbidities accompanying chronological aging predispose older adults to having unusual presentations of common ailments. Older patients are subject to physiologic and pathologic processes changing the normal, predictable physiologic states, and resulting in atypical signs and symptoms when common illnesses develop.

For decades, training in medicine has taught clinicians to base the diagnostic workup on conclusions drawn from a detailed history, followed by focused or complete physical examinations. Clinicians are taught to identify patterns and reach a diagnosis when the clinical scenario meets most of the diagnostic criteria. The usual prerequisite to this diagnostic model is a cognitively and physically intact patient who is not only aware of his or her symptoms, but also is able to communicate a reliable account of symptoms to the clinician. However, multiple barriers often arise for older adults that limit their ability to develop, perceive, and/or communicate their symptoms. Limitations in ability to communicate secondary to impaired cognition may occur in various clinical syndromes affecting memory and language skills. These can be compounded with an inability to effectively vocalize symptoms (secondary to aphasia, dry mouth, lack of teeth, etc.) and a decreased perception of symptoms (due to decreased sensory input, lack of typical symptoms, or other causes), thereby complicating the presentation. Blunting or absence of typical or classic signs and symptoms are also well described in many conditions in older adults, including myocardial infarction and pneumonia.[1-3]

In addition to the physical and cognitive barriers, diminished physiologic reserves in older adults produce weakened compensatory mechanisms, which may allow a disease to present at an earlier, less severe stage, or at a later stage with the absence of severe symptoms.[1] In this patient population, it may be difficult to reach a diagnosis based on a history and physical examination alone. Instead, we often must employ a multi-pronged approach that targets multiple possible etiologies and anticipates the possibility of other systems declining while the presenting illness is being treated.

APPROACH TO HISTORY-TAKING IN THE OLDER ADULT

CASE PRESENTATION 1: "SHE'S NOT EATING"

Mrs. Smith is an 89-year-old African American nursing home resident who presents to the emergency room with a transfer sheet that reads, "She's not eating." The nurse conducting the assessment reports to the ER physician, "She doesn't talk or really respond at all. It looks like she probably doesn't even walk because she has contractures in both her arms and legs." In a call to the nursing home to determine her baseline function, the ER physician finds that Mrs. Smith is nonverbal and dependent in all ADLs. She eats with assistance, but for the past day has not been willing to be fed.

The approach to obtaining a history must be modified in the assessment of very old or frail patients. Not infrequently, the account obtained from family members and formal (paid) caregivers concerning current changes in status is the only clue to the possible diagnosis. Here, it is imperative to determine what Mrs. Smith's baseline function was prior to the change, and then inquire specifically what change has occurred. The busy, noisy emergency room environment may limit the clinician's ability to get a reliable history from older patients with hearing or cognitive impairments. The clinician may need to return when feasible and reassess the patient or make accommodations such as moving the patient to a quieter area in order to obtain a reliable history. Patient's medical records brought in by the patient or family members or records sent in from the nursing home may be the sole source of written information available to guide the clinician concerning the patient's baseline functional status, cognitive status, current medications, and co-morbidities.

A fair number of older adults will present with symptoms consistent with or typical for common diseases or conditions. However, clinicians must pursue a careful workup for any acute illness or acute exacerbation of a chronic illness when encountering a sudden worsening in a person's functional status; changes in intake of solids or liquids; changes in mental status, mood, sensorium, or alertness; or change in bladder and bowel habits.

Circumstances of the recent changes should also include a search for any recent change in medications, the external environment (a move to new surroundings), social stressors, and roles.

APPROACH TO THE PHYSICAL EXAMINATION

CASE PRESENTATION 2: "I HAVE NO ENERGY"

Mrs. Simpson is a 76-year-old woman who lives independently in her own home. She presents to her regular physician for a 3-day history of increasing fatigue, poor energy, and lack of appetite. Her history is notable only for hypertension well controlled on a hydrochlorothiazide, and degenerative arthritis of her knees, for which she takes acetaminophen. Her vital signs include temperature of 98.0°F (36.7°C), heart rate of 76, respirations of 22, blood pressure of 106/70, and room air oximetry of 88%.

An assessment of vital signs marks the initial step toward the likely etiology for the change in the patient's condition. Fever may indicate the possibility of an underlying infection; tachycardia should make the clinician search for infection (especially if associated with fever), blood loss, or change in volume status or possible cardiac condition; and tachypnea may be the only indicator of an underlying pulmonary or cardiopulmonary pathology.

Physiologic changes in the older adult in combination with co-morbidities and medications may make standard interpretations of vital signs less than reliable indicators of which organ systems are involved or what problems are occurring. However, vital signs give important clues to possible etiologies or clinical conditions. In Mrs. Simpson's case, the history of symptoms is nonspecific, but the vital signs—which initially look unremarkable—show an elevated respiratory rate. A perceptive nurse technician obtained a low room-air oximetry reading, indicating that Mrs. Simpson may be suffering from a community-acquired pneumonia or early congestive heart failure.

Heart Rate and Blood Pressure

Maximal heart rate and maximal aerobic capacity decline progressively with age, but may be modified by habitual physical activity, owing in part to decreased catecholamine responsiveness due to fewer beta-receptors on the aging heart.[2]

Absence of compensatory tachycardia in an older adult is suggestive of autonomic insufficiency, sinus node dysfunction, or a medication side effect. The cardiovascular response to sympathetic stimulation has been seen to slow with aging: chronotropic response (heart rate), inotropic response (myocardial contractility), and vasodilatation of blood vessels all reduce with age. The clinical implication of these predictable changes is an age-related reduction in maximal cardiac output during stress, and an increased risk of congestive heart failure and dysrhythmias.

The number of pacemaker cells in the sinoatrial (SA) node and number of bundle branch fibers decrease with age, with loss of SA pacemaker cells being more pronounced.[4] Loss of sinus node pacemaker cells and fatty infiltration around the sinoatrial node with aging can lead to sick sinus syndrome. Atrioventricular block, intraventricular conduction delay, and bundle branch blocks may be caused by fibrosis and calcium deposition in the cardiac skeleton. These problems can be accentuated by drugs used to treat hypertension and coronary disease, such as beta-blockers and calcium antagonists.

Blood Pressure

Blood vessel changes with age include increased intimal thickness, increased wall thickness, and hypertrophy of smooth muscle. The clinical implications of these changes are an increase in systolic blood pressure, a drop in diastolic blood pressure, and an increase pulse pressure (SBP-DBP). Arterial blood pressure and pulse in older adults should be measured in both arms, and in the lying, sitting, and standing positions, in order to exclude significant stenosis distal to the origin of the subclavian artery as well as evaluate for orthostatic hypotension.

In about 20% of persons ≥ 65 years, standing causes systolic blood pressure to decrease by > 20 mm Hg. This is orthostatic hypotension. Orthostatic hypotension occurs in 15% to 20% of community-dwelling and in about 50% of institutionalized elderly persons.[5] Its prevalence increases with age and with basal blood pressure elevation, and is higher among patients with cardiovascular disease. Many elderly persons have wide variations in postural blood pressure, which is closely associated with basal supine systolic blood pressure; that is, when basal supine blood pressure is highest, the decline in postural systolic blood pressure is greatest. Among elderly nursing home residents, orthostatic hypotension is most prevalent in the morning when residents first arise, after basal supine systolic blood pressure has been highest. Orthostatic hypotension in the elderly may be due to age-related physiologic changes in blood pressure regulation, to certain disorders such as Parkinson disease, or the use of certain drugs such as diuretics, vasodilators, or ACE inhibitors.[5]

Temperature

Fever is a warning sign for potentially life-threatening diseases. The rise of body temperature in response to pyrogens such as IL-6 is blunted or absent with increasing age, hence the febrile response may be absent in the older person with infection. Consequently, the absence of fever in an older patient with a high suspicion for infection based on physical findings or laboratory data does not exclude infection. Of note, a change in temperature of 2.4°F (1.3°C), even if the temperature is still "normal" (< 97.6°F [36.4°C]), identifies a significant number of persons with infection in the nursing home.[6] Older patients are also more likely to present with hypothermia when septic. This may be missed if the thermometer does not measure low temperatures, or the clinician is unaware of this fact. Thermoregulatory defenses in humans are dependent on autonomic and behavioral responses to temperature changes. In cognitively or functionally compromised older adults, the ability to protect oneself from extreme temperature changes may be limited, thus increasing the risk of hypothermia in extreme cold or heat stroke–related injuries in hot weather.

Clinical encounters with geriatric patients, as previously discussed, whether acute or chronic, are often marked by ambiguous historical detail, equivocal physical findings, variable laboratory values, and atypical responses to therapeutic treatments. In addition, geriatric patients presenting with disorders of thermoregulation have a greater morbidity and mortality than others.[7] Table 9–1 lists the sensitivity and specificity of different temperature cut-points in determining the presence of infection in long-term care patients. A high fever usually indicates the presence of infection. However, it missed a large number of cases that were infected but with lower temperatures.

● TABLE 9–1 **Sensitivity and Specificity of Oral Temperature in the Presence of Documented Infection in Nursing Home Residents**

Definition	Sensitivity (%)	Specificity (%)
T > 101°F (38.3°C)	40.0	99.7
T > 100°F (37.7°F)	70.0	98.3
T > 99°F (37.3°C)	82.4	89.9

Data from Castle SC, Yeh M, Toledo S, et al. Lowering the temperature criterion improves detection of infections in nursing home residents. Aging Immunol Infect Dis. 1993;4:67-76.

Respiratory Rate

A rate of > 25 breaths/minute may signal a lower respiratory tract infection, congestive heart failure, or other disorder before the signs and symptoms appear.[8] Careful monitoring of the respiratory rate or a change in patient's breathing pattern may be the only clue to an underlying pneumonia or congestive heart failure in a non-communicative, physically limited patient.

CASE PRESENTATION 3: THE COGNITIVELY AND FUNCTIONALLY IMPAIRED OLDER PATIENT

Mrs. Reiger, an 89-year-old resident of a long-term care facility, is sent to the emergency department for "confusion and decreased oral intake." The transfer sheet reports that she has Alzheimer disease, hypertension, degenerative arthritis, stroke, gastroesophogeal reflux (GERD), and a greater-than-50 pack/year history of smoking. Her medications include treatment for diabetes, hypertension, GERD, and hypercholesterolemia. She recently moved to the Memory Care Unit of the facility, as her function has been gradually worsening. She is currently wheelchair bound and dependent in most ADLs. The patient's physical examination is remarkable for temperature of 97.5°F (37.4°C), heart rate of 108/minute, blood pressure of 94/50 mm Hg, and a respiratory rate of 28 breaths/min. The patient appears confused; her lung exam reveals bilateral expiratory wheezing. Cardiac examination reveals tachycardia with a hyperdynamic precordium, and a systolic murmur grade II/V along the right upper sternal border. No pedal edema is noted. Neurologic examination is limited because of patient's baseline cognitive status and lower extremity contractures, although she is moving her upper extremities.

The physician calls the facility to obtain further information. The nurse for the Memory Care Unit reported that patient had seemed listless since the day prior and had refused both lunch and dinner. In addition, physical therapy reported that she would not participate in restorative therapy. This morning the nurse's aide had noticed the patient appeared confused and short of breath while being turned in bed. The nurse denied having noticed any cough and mentions that patient may have been wheezing. The ED physician is concerned that this constellation of symptoms could represent MI, pneumonia, urinary tract infection, or congestive heart failure and requests the following tests: troponin, CPK, UA, CBC, electrolyte panel with BUN and creatinine, chest x-ray, and an EKG.

The physician often needs to obtain the details of a patient's decline from a number of individuals involved in providing care, particularly for patients transferred from nursing homes. Often changes are noticed not only by the nurse but by nurses' aides, who provide direct care; physical therapists, who direct daily exercise; kitchen staff, noticing whether meals have been consumed; or activity therapists, recognizing lack of interest in activities usually enjoyed. The relatively acute change in Mrs. Reiger's oral intake noticed by all involved in her care serves as a red flag that there is a likely acute change in her medical condition. Given the patient's age, co-morbidities, and dependence on others for her activities of daily living, the nursing home staff and physician must be vigilant to evaluate the cause of her decline.

CASE PRESENTATION 3 (continued)

Additional Data

Leucocyte count: 7000/µL (7×10^9/L)

Serum blood urea nitrogen: 56 mg/dL (20 mmol/L)

Serum creatinine: 2.6 mg/dL (230 µmol/L)

Sputum Gram stain is requested

Blood cultures are drawn

UA: Gravity is 1.020, leukocyte esterase negative, WBC 0-5, RBC 0-5, nitrate negative

EKG: Normal sinus rhythm, Q-waves in II, III, and aVF, unchanged from previous

Chest x-ray: New right lower lobe infiltrate suspicious for pneumonia

The characteristic clinical features of pneumonia—fever, cough, and sputum production—are often subtle or absent in elderly patients. As few as 33% of elderly patients present with a high fever in the presence of pneumonia.[9] Clinical characteristics of community-acquired pneumonia in the elderly have traditionally been described by a lack of respiratory symptoms and an absence of fever in 40% to 60% of cases, but an increase in altered mental status in 20% to 50%.[9] Few large studies quantify the clinical symptoms and their frequency.

Fernandez-Sabé and associates examined a cohort of 1,474 patients hospitalized with community-acquired pneumonia, including a subgroup over 80 years of age.[10] The clinical presentation of older and younger groups was similar with regard to the presence of an acute onset (60% in younger patients vs. 63% in the very elderly), shock (3% vs. 2%), chills (51% vs. 45%), and purulent sputum production (55% vs. 53%). However, very elderly patients complained less frequently of pleuritic chest pain (45% in younger vs. 37% in the elderly; $p = 0.007$), headache (21% vs. 7%; $p < 0.001$), and myalgias (23% vs. 8%; $p < 0.001$). Confirming other studies, very elderly patients were more likely to have an absence of fever (22% in younger patients vs. 32% in the very elderly; $p < 0.001$), to have an altered mental status (11% vs. 21%, $p < 0.001$), and to have examination findings of rales (77% vs. 84%; $p < 0.005$).[11]

Nursing home residents tend to present with more atypical and less characteristic symptoms. There are fewer studies of elderly patients in nursing homes compared to the community. Muder[12] reviewed pneumonia in long-term care facilities and found that patients presented with a higher frequency of nonspecific symptoms, such as altered mental state, incontinence, generalized weakness, and decreased appetite. Prevalent dementia may account for nonspecific symptoms.[9]

A decline in mental status may be the only presenting feature, and this is found in 21-73% of patients. It is therefore important to consider pneumonia in patients who present with nonspecific symptoms, and to look for tachypnea—a common sign in elderly patients, occurring in 70% of cases.[8] Tachypnea is also a sensitive indicator of the presence of lower respiratory infections in the elderly.

Physiologic Changes in the "Aging Lung" That Increase Risk for Pulmonary Infections

Lung function gradually declines after age 20. In the absence of respiratory insults (eg, smoking, exposure to environmental toxins, prior respiratory infections), most elderly people have sufficient respiratory reserve to avoid symptoms. The reduction of respiratory reserve, which tends to cause no symptoms in healthy people, often increases the risk and severity of pulmonary disorders, particularly in those with underlying impairment.[13] Aging is associated with a decline in lung performance, with the most important physiologic changes being a decrease in elastic recoil of the lung, chest wall compliance, and respiratory muscle strength. Changes also occur in the lung parenchyma with enlargement of the alveoli, a condition that is also called "senile emphysema."[13] This combination leads to an increase in functional residual capacity, causing older patients to breathe at higher lung volumes, increasing the workload on respiratory muscles. Where there is an added stress such as pneumonia, elderly patients are at risk for respiratory failure. More than 70% of elderly patients with community-acquired pneumonia develop a blunted cough reflex (compared with only 10% of age-matched controls), probably due to accompanying hypoxia, drug-induced sedation, and neurologic disorders.[14]

Elderly patients often have co-morbidities, such as heart failure and cerebrovascular disease, also affecting respiratory function. Because mucociliary clearance and the cough reflex are also impaired, elderly patients frequently have difficulties expelling sputum, or may have an ineffective cough. Older patients also have a lower sensitivity to hypoxia and hypercapnia and a diminished ventilatory response to acute conditions, because peripheral and central chemoreceptor responses diminish, as do their integration of CNS pathways. Effects are greater in people who are deconditioned. These factors may delay the clinical manifestations of pneumonia, namely tachypnea and dyspnea.[15,16]

Approach to Diagnostic Workup

The chest x-ray is usually diagnostic, but may be falsely negative when profound volume depletion is also present. Progression and multilobe involvement are seen more often in elderly patients. Leukocytosis with immature white blood cells develops less often in elderly patients.[17] Blood cultures should be performed routinely, particularly in hospitalized patients. The diagnosis should not be based on expectorated sputum, because expectorated sputum is unlikely to distinguish colonization from true pulmonary infection. However, expectorated sputum is useful for culturing M. tuberculosis, pathogenic fungi (Histoplasma, Blastomyces, and Coccidioides), and Legionella spp. A Gram stain of expectorated specimens may be useful if a predominance of one organism is seen along with a large number of neutrophils (Chapter 42).

Pneumonia in the Older Adult

Pneumonia is one of the most common and significant health problems in older people. It is the fourth leading cause of death and the leading infectious cause of death in this age group. The major risk factor for developing pneumonia is the presence of other serious illness. The likelihood of a serious outcome with pneumonia, including death, is directly related to the number of co-morbid conditions.[12] Elderly patients are likely to experience more complications from pneumonia, such as bacteremia, empyema, and meningitis.[12]

The annual incidence of pneumonia in the elderly is between 25 and 44/1000 for noninstitutionalized patients—four times that of patients younger than 65.[18] For the elderly in residential care, the incidence increases to 33 to 114 cases/1000 per year.[18] Other studies have reported that the rate of pneumonia for those who are in residential care facilities is six to ten times higher than for community-dwelling elderly.[15-17] The mortality rate from nursing home-acquired pneumonia is as high as 44% to 57%, whereas mortality for community-acquired pneumonia in hospital-based studies is reported to be as high as 30%.[11,12,15]

CASE PRESENTATION 3 (continued)
Early Hospital Course

Mrs. Reiger is found to have right lower lobe pneumonia, and is started on an intravenous third-generation cephalosporin. She is admitted, and transferred to a medical floor with telemetry. She remains afebrile and her respiratory status begins to improve. She appears to be more alert on day 2 and eats 60% of her meals with assistance. Physical therapy advises that the patient may be transferred out of bed into a chair. Range-of-motion exercises are assisted by the nurses during her routine care. The results of blood culture are pending, and the plan is to discharge Mrs. Reiger back to the long-term care facility if she continues to improve and remains afebrile. The nursing home is contacted in anticipation of the transfer with an update on her condition as well as anticipated therapy, medications, and dietary needs.

CASE PRESENTATION 4: THE COGNITIVELY INTACT, FUNCTIONALLY IMPAIRED OLDER ADULT

Ms. Allen, a 93-year-old woman, is brought to the Emergency Department by her daughter, following a witnessed episode of loss of consciousness. The patient was in the bathroom, and was being helped off the toilet when she suddenly slumped over and lost consciousness for approximately 30 seconds. She was initially groggy but quickly returned to her previous level of alertness. An hour earlier, she had taken all her medications with a small breakfast. She takes metoprolol 50 mg, lisinopril 10 mg, atorvastatin 10 mg, aspirin 81 mg, furosemide 40 mg, and senna 2 tablets daily for the last 2 years, and there has been no recent change in her medication regimen. Her medical history includes hypertension, stable two-vessel coronary artery disease, chronic congestive heart failure with a left ventricular ejection fraction of 35%, and osteoporosis. The patient has been living with her daughter for the last few months since a fall, during which she sustained an undisplaced right lesser trochanter fracture managed without surgery. Since then, Ms. Allen has significantly limited her activities, using a wheelchair outside the house and ambulating with a walker inside. Since the fracture, she has needed help getting up from a seated position.

On evaluation in the emergency department, the patient is alert and says she feels tired. She denies any dizziness or light-headedness prior to the episode. The physical examination is remarkable for a pulse of 100/min and blood pressure of 110/72 mm Hg lying, and upon two minutes of standing a pulse of 105 with a blood pressure of 105/70. Her mental status is at baseline according to the daughter. Coarse bibasilar crackles are noted, and a grade 2/6 systolic murmur is audible at the left sternal border, with an S3 gallop. Electrocardiogram shows sinus tachycardia; Q-waves in leads II, III, and aVF, unchanged from previous. Chest x-ray shows cardiomegaly but no infiltrates.

Laboratory Studies

Hemoglobin: 10.6 g/dL (106 g/L)
Blood urea nitrogen: 40 mg/dL (14.3 mmol/L)
Serum creatinine: 1.2 mg/dL (106 μmol/L)
Serum troponin: 2.0 ng/mL (2.0 μg/L) (normal range < 0.4 ng/mL)
Creatinine kinase: 637 U/L with 12% MB fraction
Serum ProBNP: 8000 ng/L (normal range 180-254 ng/L)

APPROACH TO THE HISTORY IN A FUNCTIONALLY IMPAIRED OLDER ADULT

Age-related changes in a person's daily routine may mask classic symptoms. For example, exertional angina pectoris and dyspnea may not occur if a patient no longer walks far or fast enough to experience them. Other symptoms may be atypical; for example, the age-related decrease in left ventricular compliance may produce exertional dyspnea rather than angina in patients with myocardial ischemia. Memory or attention deficits may prevent a patient from accurately recalling or describing a cardiac symptom. A syncopal event can affect the patient's ability to recall what happened before and sometimes shortly after the event.

Elderly patients should be asked about cardiovascular risk factors, including smoking, hypertension, hyperlipidemia, family history for heart disease, and diabetes mellitus. Chest pain as the presenting manifestation of acute MI is less frequent in elderly individuals.[19] Classic chest pain is reported by only one-third of patients older than 85 years. Elderly patients have an increased prevalence of co-morbid illness associated with painless infarction, such as diabetes and hypertension. There may be lesser or altered sensitivity to pain with aging. Although the myocardial infarction may be painless, the clinical presentation is often not asymptomatic, and may include acute dyspnea, exacerbation of heart failure, or pulmonary edema; syncope, vertigo, palpitations, nausea and vomiting, or more subtle changes involving altered mentation, including acute confusion or agitation, profound weakness or fatigue, and changes in eating pattern or in other usual behaviors. The onset of symptoms of MI is more likely to occur at rest or during sleep in elderly patients.[19] Drugs commonly used by older patients may affect cardiac function. For example, a nonsteroidal anti-inflammatory drug may cause sodium retention, exacerbating heart failure. Looking for classic symptoms of chest pain and exertional dyspnea as indicators of coronary symptomatology may delay the diagnosis.

Unrecognized MI is more common in elderly women than in elderly men. In the Gothenburg Study, 60% of patients with ECG evidence of MI gave no history of an acute episode.[20] Mrs. Allen's case is an example of atypical presentation of myocardial ischemia and consequent congestive heart failure in an elderly woman with functional limitations. The patient did not describe any chest pain or typical symptoms that might be described by a functionally intact younger individual.

DIAGNOSTIC WORKUP FOR MYOCARDIAL ISCHEMIA

Asymptomatic or atypical presentations of MI frequently result in elderly patients not experiencing the potential benefits of acute coronary interventions. Acute MI in elderly patients is often non–Q-wave and, as is the case with angina pectoris, more often precipitated by an intercurrent medical or surgical problem associated with hypovolemia, blood loss, infection, and hypotension. Atypical symptoms may partly explain the delayed hospital presentation in older patients.[21] Acute myocardial infarction—because of its atypical presentation—is often unrecognized in aged patients, despite the fact that infarction in elderly persons is characteristically of increased severity, has a greater occurrence of complications, entails a longer hospital stay, and results in a higher mortality than in a younger age group.[21]

The diagnosis of MI may be further obscured in that the electrocardiographic diagnosis is limited by the higher prevalence of non–Q-wave infarction,[8] as well as normal total creatine kinase (CK) levels in the presence of elevated myocardial band (MB) fractions (indicating MI) as a result of decreased lean body mass.[22]

IMPACT OF PHYSIOLOGIC CHANGES IN THE CARDIOVASCULAR SYSTEM ON THE PHYSICAL EXAMINATION

Heart sounds are usually softer in older patients, probably because the distance between the heart and the chest wall increases with age. Splitting of the second heart sound (S_2) can be heard in only about 30% to 40%. Wide splitting that increases with inspiration suggests right bundle branch block.

In the elderly, the heart relies on atrial contraction to compensate for diminished early left ventricular filling. Consequently, a fourth heart sound (S_4) is normal, but a third heart sound (S_3) is always abnormal. Kyphoscoliosis and other deformities of the chest wall complicate interpretation of the apical impulse and other precordial movements. Systolic ejection murmurs (most often aortic) are present in about half of elderly patients.[23] These benign murmurs are distinguished from murmurs due to significant aortic valve stenosis or hypertrophic obstructive cardiomyopathy by their short duration, low intensity (usually grade 1 or 2), and failure to radiate.

Pulmonary rales are more likely to represent atelectasis, pulmonary edema, pulmonary fibrosis, or an acute inflammatory process in elderly patients than in younger ones. Chronic obstructive lung disease (COPD) may mask or attenuate abnormal lung sounds that otherwise would be evident upon careful auscultation.

Peripheral edema may be secondary to right-sided heart failure or to venous varicosities, lymphatic obstruction, or low serum albumin.[23]

MYOCARDIAL INFARCTION IN THE ELDERLY

Elderly patients have a significantly different presentation, clinical course, and prognosis of MI compared to younger persons.[24] Unrecognized MI portends a serious prognosis.[22] There is a marked increase in morbidity and mortality,[25] with 80% of all MI deaths occurring after age 65. Mortality from acute MI increases 6-fold at ages 75 to 84 years and 15-fold after 85 years, compared with persons aged 55 to 64 years.[25]

Functional disability before MI importantly predicts MI severity and post-infarction survival.[26] Although age adversely affects MI survival in part because prior MI, hypertension, and heart failure all increase with increasing age, the contribution of less aggressive therapies requires study.[27] In the Myocardial Infarction Triage and Intervention (MITI)

project, MI mortality was increased 10-fold in elderly patients (17.8% at 75 years or more vs. 2% at less than 55 years).[28] The prognosis was worse for elderly women than elderly men,[28] although data from the U.S. National Registry of Myocardial Infarction-1 suggest that younger women and not older women have higher rates of death during hospitalization than men of the same age.[29]

CASE PRESENTATION 4 (continued)
Hospital Course
Mrs. Allen is admitted to the hospital, and is placed on cardiac telemetry. She is started on oxygen, deep venous thrombosis prophylaxis, given aspirin, and continued on most of her outpatient medications except furosemide, which is changed to 40 mg twice a day intravenously. Senna is stopped. The patient, after discussion with her daughter, refuses a cardiac catheterization. Strict input and output is maintained, and physical therapy is asked to evaluate her gait and mobility. Over the next 3 days, her troponin peaks at 6 ng/mL (6 µg/L) and her CK MB fraction at 15%. She improves and is back to her baseline and ready for cardiac rehabilitation 4 days later.

CASE PRESENTATION 5: THE COGNITIVELY AND FUNCTIONALLY INTACT OLDER ADULT

An 80-year-old woman, Mrs. Johns, is brought by her daughter to her primary care physician's office, as she has been "feeling tired." Mrs. Johns lives in her own home and is able to manage her affairs including light housework and cooking. She continues to be active at her local church and usually meets her daughter for brunch after church every Sunday. She enjoys these weekly outings and usually spends the entire week preparing for them. The daughter reports that she became concerned that something may be wrong with her mother this morning when a friend came by to pick her up for a church outing. Mrs. Johns refused to go, saying she was "feeling tired." On further questioning, the patient thinks she may be tired because she has not slept well for the last 2 nights. She was awake most of last night because she had to use the bathroom multiple times. She requests that a sleeping pill be prescribed to help her sleep. Mrs. Johns has osteoporosis, and is taking calcium and vitamin D supplements and a weekly bisphosphonate. Her physician advises the patient that he is concerned that her difficulty sleeping may not be the primary problem and that he recommends that additional tests be performed.

On physical examination, the patient is noted to appear tired and is noted to have a blood pressure of 100/60 mm Hg, pulse 90/min, and temperature of 98.8°F (37.1°C). The rest of her examination is unremarkable. Laboratory data reveal:

Leucocyte count: 11,000/μL (11 × 10⁹/L)
Plasma glucose: 150 mg/dL (8.3 mmol/L)
Blood urea nitrogen: 34 mg/dL (12.1 mmol/L)
Urinalysis: 2+ bacteria, nitrates positive, WBC 40-50/hpf
Urine culture results are pending

The diagnosis of UTI among geriatric patients is more difficult than in younger persons because many elderly patients have a greater prevalence of baseline urinary symptoms. The high prevalence of co-morbidities, asymptomatic pyuria, and asymptomatic bacteriuria in this population increases the ambiguity of diagnostic testing and interpretation. As such, the majority of presumably "uncomplicated" UTIs among the elderly would be characterized as "complicated" UTI in all other age groups, because older patients have a higher prevalence of co-morbidities and an increased risk of drug–drug and disease–disease interactions.[30] In comparison to the relative homogeneity of UTI in younger populations, there is significant demographic and clinical diversity in the geriatric population with UTI. Most research on UTI in older patients has focused on the 5% who are institutionalized, overlooking the 95% who live in the community.[31] Because of the prevalence of asymptomatic bacteriuria (ASB) among the elderly, diagnosis of frank UTI may be more difficult to distinguish than in younger adults.

The diagnosis of UTI in older patients is often a diagnosis of exclusion. Older patients frequently present with atypical nonurinary symptoms, and many common urinary symptoms, such as frequent urination and incontinence, are already present in the older patient. Nonurinary symptoms, including delirium, are most likely among patients with other medical problems (dehydration or multiple chronic diseases). As a result, clinicians often rule out other serious illnesses, such as pneumonia, acute myocardial infarction, and dehydration, before they can confidently attribute the presenting symptomatology to a UTI. Conventional diagnosis relies on identifying a potential urinary pathogen from culture of a midstream specimen of urine (MSU) in a symptomatic patient with a urinalysis suggestive of UTI. In elderly patients, obtaining a midstream urine specimen may be impossible given the presence of incontinence or impairment of manual dexterity. In fact, almost one in three specimens taken from the elderly is "contaminated."[32] In and out catheterization is usually indicated for a definitive evaluation in patients in whom a midstream catch urinalysis is not possible.

In a study of chronically incontinent nursing home residents, 45% had pyuria and 43% had (presumably) asymptomatic bacteriuria; 34% of the residents had pyuria without bacteriuria.[33] An earlier study of elderly ambulatory women found pyuria without bacteriuria present in 52%.[34] High-titer bacteriuria, however, was almost always (94%) associated with pyuria. There are differences in the sensitivity and specificity of leukocyte esterase tests between nursing home residents and office patients. In both cases, dipstick testing is far more useful in ruling out than in confirming UTI.[32]

● URINARY TRACT INFECTIONS IN THE OLDER ADULT

Urinary tract infection is the second most common cause of infectious disease hospitalization in adults 65 years or older, after lower respiratory tract infections.[35] The diagnosis of UTI in community dwelling older adults follows a similar paradigm to the diagnosis in younger adults, requiring significant bacteriuria (≥ 10⁵ cfu/mL), pyuria, and other suggestive markers such as leucocyte esterase as well as genitourinary symptoms. In most older adults who are cognitively intact and can report symptoms, the diagnosis of UTI can be made relatively easily. Among institutionalized older adults, however, particularly when they are cognitively impaired, distinguishing ASB from UTI is often challenging.[36]

Studies in younger adults have shown that the presence of urinary tract symptoms increases the likelihood that the person has a UTI. This relationship is less clear in the older adults, in whom disease may present atypically.[37-39] Guidelines often rely on the presence of urinary tract symptoms to distinguish asymptomatic bacteriuria from symptomatic UTI, but it is a common experience among clinicians treating elderly patients with cognitive impairment that some may present without any urinary tract symptoms.

CASE PRESENTATION 5 (continued)
Outpatient Course

Mrs. Johns is started on treatment for UTI with a sulfa drug and is sent home with a follow-up appointment scheduled in one week. Her urinary frequency begins to improve by day 2 and she begins to sleep better.

CASE PRESENTATION 6: THE COGNITIVELY IMPAIRED, FUNCTIONALLY INTACT OLDER ADULT

Mrs. Willard, a 90-year-old resident of an assisted living facility, is transferred to the emergency room after being found to be extremely confused at the breakfast table. She usually enjoys sitting at the corner table during meals and talking to dining room staff. She has been residing at this facility for the last 5 years, after a hospitalization for a left middle cerebral artery embolic stroke that left her with some weakness on her right side. Atrial fibrillation was detected at the time of the stroke, and warfarin was started.

At baseline, she is pleasant and communicative; she speaks in short clear sentences and can follow simple commands. She has very poor short-term memory and ambulates with a walker. The staff attempt to get her up from the dining room chair but she stares at them and is unable to stand up. A staff member calls the ambulance. She is brought to the emergency department. There, she is noted to be confused, and her neurologic examination is essentially unremarkable except for right-sided weakness, which seems unchanged from her baseline. Her vital signs at initial presentation are: heart rate 68/min, blood pressure 140/90, respiratory rate 22/min, and temperature 98°F (36.7°C). An initial set of labs are drawn, an EKG is performed, and the patient is sent for a CT scan.

This case is a typical presentation of cognitively impaired older patients brought to the emergency department following changes in mentation. Cases such as this present an interesting diagnostic dilemma since the evaluation for "acute-onset confusion," and hence the approach to initiating or assessing the need to initiate a diagnostic workup, is based on the knowledge of the patient's baseline mental status and the duration of the noted change. This information should be obtained from the patient's family or others involved in the care of the individual for a significant period. Frequently, for institutionalized patients, the changes are noticed not only by nurses, but also by nurses' aides who provide direct care.

Relying on information obtained from persons too recently or too remotely involved in care may not only be misleading but also expose the patient to the risk of unnecessary diagnostic evaluation and subsequent treatment. Circumstances around the recent change should also include a search into changes in medications, changes in the external environment (move to new surroundings), loss of loved ones, and role changes.

● APPROACH TO PHYSICAL EXAMINATION

The mental status examination remains the first step of neurologic examination. In normal aging, not all cognitive functions decline in parallel, and some may not decline at all. However, speed of processing, attentional capacity, or visuospatial perception may be impaired with age, as well as certain aspects of memory (mainly episodic memory). Moreover, dementia, delirium, and depression all alter the mental status.[40]

In Mrs. Willard's case, the account we get from caregivers unfortunately does not provide much information, except that there is a new noted change in this patient's level of mentation. Co-morbidities make it essential to

have a multi-pronged approach to the possible causes for the change in mental status. It is not unusual to have more than one explanation for the change in the patient's condition. Given our patient's history of a prior stroke, arrhythmia, and her age, it becomes essential to look for neurologic, cardiac, and infectious etiologies to explain the sudden change in her condition.

CASE PRESENTATION 6 (continued)
Additional Data
Results of laboratory tests are as follows:

Serum glucose: 90 mg/dL (5.0 mmol/L)

Blood urea nitrogen: 56 mg/dL (20 mmol/L)

Serum creatinine: 2.6 mg/dL (230 µmol/L) (baseline creatinine 2.0-2.3 mg/dL)

INR: 1.5

Serum troponin: < 0.5 ng/mL (0.5 µg/L)

Electrocardiogram: Atrial fibrillation with ventricular rate 74/min.

Patient has been unable to provide a urine specimen and the results of CXR and CT of the head are still pending. A Foley catheter is inserted and a concentrated-appearing urine specimen is obtained and sent to the laboratory.

While awaiting the results of the imaging studies and laboratory data, the initial set of laboratory data has provided us with some lead about our patient's status. Her BUN and creatinine suggest that she may be in a negative fluid balance. At this time, it is unclear if this is contributing to the change in her overall condition. Her INR being subtherapeutic raises concern that she may have had a recurrent embolic event causing the change in her mental status. With her rate under control, and no other changes on her EKG as well as a negative troponin, the likelihood of a coronary event contributing to her clinical presentation is effectively ruled out.

CASE PRESENTATION 6 (continued)
Additional Data
Urinalysis: Specific gravity 1.028, leucocyte esterase and nitrate negative

CT scan: Lacunar infarct in right internal capsule, new compared to previous scans

Delirium, also referred to as acute confusional state, is the most common reason for acute cognitive dysfunction in hospitalized elderly patients.[41] The syndrome occurs in about 10% to 25% of all acute admissions to a general hospital and in 20% to 40% of elderly patients.[40] The incidence of delirium after ischemic or hemorrhagic stroke is between 13% and

48%.[42-45] Delirium is more common in acute stroke than in acute coronary patients, suggesting a causal relationship between brain damage and the occurrence of delirium after stroke.[44] Several specific locations of cerebral infarcts have been associated with delirium, such as the territory of one or both posterior cerebral arteries, especially thalamic infarction,[46-48] the territory of the anterior cerebral artery,[44] and the capsular genu.[49] Delirium as the isolated sign of stroke has been reported more often in right-sided[43,45] than after left-sided lesions,[42] probably related to the superiority of the right hemisphere in attentional processes[50] (for more on delirium please see Chapter 30). Obtaining an accurate history for the diagnosis of TIA or stroke in older adults can be compromised by problems of obtaining a reliable history because of the absence of a witness, dysphasia, dementia or confusion, unusual symptoms or signs due to pre-existing cerebrovascular disease, as well as the nonspecificity of symptoms (especially if they involve the vertebrobasilar territory).[51] The examiner must be aware of unique clinical difficulties associated with motor examination of elderly people. First, certain muscle groups, like the iliopsoas and glutei, are particularly difficult to test compared to younger adults. Thus, functional testing (eg, rising from a chair with arms folded) may be more appropriate. Second, dexterity is a complex motor function related to pyramidal, extra-pyramidal, proprioceptive, and cerebellar functions influenced by other medical conditions (eg, rheumatoid arthritis).[52] Some have found that strength of both upper and lower extremities gradually decreased with increasing age,[53] while others reported that these changes were infrequent.[54]

PHYSIOLOGIC AND PATHOLOGIC CHANGES IN THE HUMAN BRAIN

With normal aging, cerebral blood flow decreases by about 20% on average; decreases are even greater in persons with small-vessel cerebrovascular disease due to diabetes and hypertension. Although blood flow in women is usually greater than in men until age 60, the subsequent rate of decrease is slightly more rapid. Decreases are greater in certain areas of the brain (eg, the prefrontal region) and are greater in gray matter than in white matter.[55]

Atherosclerosis of the extracranial internal carotid and vertebral arteries is twice as common among white men as among white women; it correlates highly with coronary and peripheral vascular occlusive disease and hyperlipidemia. Lacunar infarcts are small, deep infarcts caused by occlusion of penetrating brain arteries. The small arteries that penetrate deeper brain structures (basal gray nuclei, internal capsule, thalamus, pons) are especially susceptible to degenerative changes caused by hypertension. Plaques within arteries and microatheromas are more common among patients with diabetes. Lacunes are more common in the posterior circulation and prevalence increases with age. Cerebral embolization can result from valvular heart disease, atrial fibrillation, and myocardial ischemia, prevalent in this age group.

CEREBROVASCULAR EVENTS IN THE ELDERLY

Each year, about 750,000 Americans have a stroke, and about 150,000 die. Stroke is the third leading cause of death in the United States and in most other industrialized countries. At any time, there are about 2 million stroke survivors in the United States. Stroke incidence and mortality rate increase with age, especially after age 65. About 72% of persons who have a stroke in a given year are ≥ 65, and > 88% of persons who die of stroke are ≥ 65. Prevalence in the United States is generally higher among men and African Americans. More impressive than the mortality rates are the ways in which stroke changes the survivor's quality of life. Daily functioning in the workplace, home, and community is often reduced, and many stroke patients are impaired in their ability to walk, see, and feel. Some cannot read, recall, think, speak, or otherwise communicate as well as they could before the stroke.[56] Dementia may be the end result, especially if multiple lacunar infarcts occur.

CASE PRESENTATION 6 (continued)
Hospital Course

Mrs. Willard is admitted for observation, started on intravenous fluids, and placed on cardiac monitoring. Her outpatient medications are restarted. An echocardiogram is done and carotid Doppler is planned. Her coumadin dose is increased to maintain the INR between 2 and 2.5. On day 2, the family requests avoidance of excessive testing, and a focus on keeping Mrs. Willard comfortable, and asks that she be discharged to the nursing home once stable. They feel she is most comfortable in her familiar surroundings.

SUMMARY

Elderly patients are likely to have an atypical presentation of common diseases. Multisystem approaches to diagnosis during workup serve the best interests of the patient. Further workup is warranted for "red flags," such as recent functional decline, limitation of already limited functional ability, change in oral intake, change in bowel or bladder habits, change in mental status, or significant changes in mood or sensorium. Infection without fever is more common in elderly patients.

Atypical presentation of disease in older adults should be viewed as the norm, particularly for common conditions in impaired older patients. With increasing frailty and co-morbidities, disease presentations will frequently vary from what is described as typical in medical texts, such that nonspecific symptoms including fatigue, loss of appetite, poor energy, and changes in mental status are often the only symptoms. The astute clinician obtains information from various sources including caregivers, aides, friends, and others when the patient is unable to provide a cogent history or is felt to be unreliable. In addition, the clinician should be vigilant for medication changes and other minor stresses that can upset the delicate balance of homeostasis of many older adults. With proper training, patience, and diligent workup, older adults will be more likely to have an accurate diagnosis made and appropriate treatment provided in a timely manner.

References

1. Brieger D, Eagle KA, Goodman SG, et al.; GRACE Investigators. Acute coronary syndromes without chest pain, an underdiagnosed and undertreated high-risk group: Insights from the Global Registry of Acute Coronary Events. *Chest*. 2004;126:461-469.

2. Canto JG, Shlipak MG, Rogers WJ, et al. Prevalence, clinical characteristics, and mortality among patients with myocardial infarction presenting without chest pain. *JAMA*. 2000;283:3223-3229.

3. Halm EA, Teirstein AS. Clinical practice. Management of community-acquired pneumonia. *N Engl J Med*. 2002;347:2039-2045.

4. I Shiraishi, T Takamatsu, T Minamikawa, et al. Quantitative histological analysis of the human sinoatrial node during growth and aging. *Circulation*. 1992;85:2176-2184.

5. Gupta V, Lipsitz L. Orthostatic Hypotension in the elderly: Diagnosis and Treatment. *Am J Med*. 2007;120:841-847.

6. Castle SC, Yeh M, Toledo S, et al. Lowering the temperature criterion improves detection of infections in nursing home residents. *Aging Immunol Infect Dis*. 1993;4:67-76.

7. Harchelroad F. Acute thermoregulatory disorders. *Clin Geriatr Med*. 1993;9:621-639.

8. McFadden JP, Price RC, Eastwood HD, et al. Raised respiratory rate in elderly patients: A valuable physical sign. *Br Med J (Clin Res Ed)*. 1982;284:626-627.

9. Johnson JC Jr., Baccash PD, et al. Nonspecific presentation of pneumonia in hospitalized older people: Age effect or dementia? *J Am Geriatr Soc*. 2000;48:1316-1320.

10. Fernandez-Sabé NCJ, Rodon B, et al. Community acquired pneumonia in very elderly patients:ccausative organisms, clinical characteristics and outcome. *Medicine*. 2003;82:159-169.

11. Metlay JP, Li YH, et al. Influence of age on symptoms at presentation in patients with community-acquired pneumonia. *Arch Intern Med*. 1997;157:1453-1459.

12. Muder RR. Pneumonia in residents of long-term care facilities: Epidemiology, etiology, management, and prevention. *Am J Med*. 1998;105:319-330.

13. Aging and the lungs. Section 10, Chapter 75. In: *Merck Manual of Geriatrics*. 3rd ed. NJ: Merck; 2000.

14. El-Solh AA, Ramadan F, et al. Etiology of severe pneumonia in the very elderly. *Am J Respir Crit Care Med*. 2001;163:645-651.

15. Janssens JP. Pneumonia in the very old. *Lancet Infect Dis*. 2004; 4:112-124.

16. Medina-Walpole AM. Nursing home-acquired pneumonia. *J Am Geriatr Soc*. 1999;47:1005-1015.

17. Marrie TJ. Pneumonia in the long-term-care facility. *Infect Control Hosp Epidemiol*. 2002;23:159-164.

18. Beers MH, Berkow R. Section 10. Pulmonary disorders—Chapter 76: Pulmonary infections. In: *Merck Manual of Geriatrics*. 3rd ed. Whitehouse Station, NJ: Merck; 2000.

19. Solomon CG, Cook EF, et al., for the Chest Pain Study Group. Comparison of clinical presentation of acute myocardial infarction in patients older than 65 years of age to younger patients: The Multicenter Chest Pain Study experience. *Am J Cardiol*. 1989;63: 772-776.

20. Lapidus L, Bengsston C, Larsson B, et al. Distribution of adipose tissue and risk of cardiovascular disease and death: A 12 year follow up of participants in the population study of women in Gothenburg, Sweden. *Br Med J*. 1984;289:1257-1260.

21. Gurwitz JH, Willison DJ, et al. Delayed hospital presentation in patients who have had acute myocardial infarction. *Ann Intern Med*. 1997;126:593-599.

22. Hong RA, Wei JY, et al. Elevated CK-MB with normal total creatine kinase in suspected myocardial infarction: Associated clinical findings and early prognosis. *Am Heart J*. 1986;111:1041-1047.

23. Beers MH, Berkow R. Section 1: Basics of geriatric care—Chapter 3: History and physical examination. In: *Merck Manual of Geriatrics*. 3rd ed. Whitehouse Station, NJ: Merck; 2000.

24. Devlin W, Jacks M, et al. Comparison of outcome in patients with acute myocardial infarction aged >75 years with that in younger patients. *Am J Cardiol*. 1995;75:573-576.

25. Marcus FI, McCans J, et al. Age-related prognosis after acute myocardial infarction (the Multicenter Diltiazem Postinfarction trial). *Am J Cardiol*. 1990;65:559-566.

26. Vaccarino V, Mendes de Leon CF, et al. Functional disability before myocardial infarction in the elderly as a determinant of infarction severity and postinfarction mortality. *Arch Intern Med*. 1997; 157:2196-2204.

27. Paul SD, Mahjoub ZA, et al. Geriatric patients with acute myocardial infarction: Cardiac risk factor profiles, presentation, thrombolysis, coronary interventions, and prognosis. *Am Heart J*. 1996;131:710-715.

28. Kudenchuk PJ, Maynard C, Martin JS, et al. Comparison of presentation, treatment, and outcome of acute myocardial infarction in men versus women (the Myocardial Infarction Triage and Intervention Registry). *Am J Cardiol*. 1996;78:9-14.

29. Chandra N, Ziegelstein R, Rogers W, et al. Observations of the treatment of women with myocardial infarction: A report from the National Registry of Myocardial Infarction-1. *Arch Intern Med*. 1998;158:981-988.

30. Dairiki Shortliffe LM. Urinary tract infection at the age extremes: pediatrics and geriatrics. *Am J Med*. 2002;113:55s-66s.

31. Ruben FL, Norden CW. Clinical infections in the noninstitutionalized geriatric age group: Methods utilized and the incidence of infections. *Am J Epidemiol*. 1995;141:145-157.

32. Hamilton-Miller, JMT. Issues in urinary tract infections in the elderly. *World J Urol*. 1999;17:396-401.

33. Ouslander JG, Schnelle JF, Fingold S. Pyuria among chronically incontinent but otherwise asymptomatic nursing home residents. *J Am Geriatr Soc*. 1996;44:420-423.

34. Boscia JA, Levison ME, Pitsakis MG, Kaye D. Pyuria and asymptomatic bacteriuria in elderly ambulatory women. *Ann Intern Med*. 1989;110:404-405.

35. Curns AT, Sejvar JJ, et al. Infectious disease hospitalizations among older adults in the United States from 1990 through 2002. *Arch Intern Med*. 2005;165:2514-2520.

36. Juthani-Mehta M, T.M., Perrelli E, et al. Diagnostic accuracy of criteria for urinary tract infection in a cohort of nursing home residents. *J Am Geriatr Soc*. 2007;55:1072-1077.

37. Jarrett PG, Carver D, et al. Ilness presentation in elderly patients. *Arch Intern Med.* 1995;155:1060-1064.

38. Berman P, Fox RA. The atypical presentation of infection in old age. *Age Ageing.* 1987;16:201-207.

39. Boscia JA, Abrutyn E, et al. Lack of association between bacteriuria and symptoms in the elderly. *Am J Med.* 1986;81:979-982.

40. Fick DM, Inouye SK. Delirium superimposed on dementia: A systematic review. *J Am Geriatr Soc.* 2002;50:1723-1732.

41. Meagher DJ, O'Mahony E, Casey PR, Trzepacz PT. Relationship between etiology and phenomenologic profile in delirium. *J Geriatr Psychiatr Neurol.* 1998;11:146-149; discussion 157-178.

42. Gustafson Y, Erikkson S, Bucht G. Acute confusional state (delirium) in stroke patients. *Cerebrovasc Dis.* 1991;1:257-264.

43. Henon H, Durieu J, et al. Confusional state in stroke: Relation to preexisting dementia, patient characteristics, and outcome. *Stroke.* 1999;30:773-779.

44. Caeiro L, Albuquerque R, Figueira MI. Delirium in the first days of acute stroke. *J Neurol.* 2004;251:171-178.

45. Dunne JW, Edis RH. Inobvious stroke: a cause of delirium and dementia. *Aust NZ J Med.* 1986;16:771-778.

46. Vatsavayi V, Franco K. Agitated delirium with posterior artery infarction. *J Emerg Med.* 2003;24:263-266.

47. Verselegers W, Saerens J, et al. Slow progressive bilateral posterior artery infarction presenting as agitated, complicated with Anton's syndrome. *Eur Neurol.* 1991;31:216-219.

48. Bogousslavsky J, Regli F, Assal G, et al. Manic delirium and frontal-like syndrome with paramedian infarction of the right thalamus. *J Neurol Neurosurg Psychiatry.* 1988;51:116-119.

49. Tatemichi TK, Probhovnik I, et al. Confusion and memory loss from capsular genu infarction: A thalamocortical disconnection syndrome? *Neurology.* 1992;42:1966-1979.

50. MM. Large scale neurocognitive networks and distributed processing for attention, language, and memory. *Ann Neurol.* 1990;28:597-613.

51. Hankey G. Recent advances in cerebrovascular disease. *Rev Clin Gerontol.* 1992;2:187-206.

52. Assal F. Neurological signs in old age. In: *Brockelhurst's Textbook of Geriatric Medicine and Gerontology.* 6th ed. New York: Churchill Livingstone; 2003:541-548.

53. Potvin AR, Tourtellotte WW, et al. Human neurologic function and the aging process. *J Am Geriatr Soc.* 1984;28:1-9.

54. Kokemen E, Barney J, et al. Neurological manifestations of aging. *J Gerontol.* 1977;32:411-419.

55. Beers MH, Berkow R. Chapter 42: Aging and the nervous system. In: *Merck Manual of Geriatrics.* 3rd ed. NJ: Merck; 2000.

56. Beers MH, Berkow R. Section 6: Neurologic disorders—Chapter 44: Cerebrovascular disease. In: *Merck Manual of Geriatrics.* 3rd ed. NJ: Merck; 2000.

POST-TEST

1. **A 92-year-old woman is brought to your office for evaluation of new-onset urinary incontinence. Her attendant reports that in spite of her poor memory she has usually been able to self-toilet. The attendant is concerned that for the last 2 days the patient has not been able to get to the bathroom in time and has been having accidents. The only change in her medications has been a low-dose diuretic that was started by her cardiologist as he noted her to have some leg edema about 10 days back. The possible etiology for this patient's recent change in ability to self-toilet could include all the following EXCEPT:**

   A. Urinary tract infection

   B. Fecal impaction

   C. Diuretic use

   D. Worsening dementia

2. **Which of the following is FALSE regarding MI in older adults?**

   A. Asymptomatic or atypical presentations of MI commonly exclude elderly patients from the potential benefits of thrombolytic therapy or acute coronary angioplasty.

   B. Acute MI in elderly patients is often a non–Q-wave MI.

   C. Elderly patients with MI are more likely to be male; to have associated hypertension, diabetes mellitus, and cerebrovascular accident; and to have a history of prior infarction and heart failure.

   D. Elevated myocardial band (MB) fractions of creatine kinase (CK) are common in the presence of a normal total CK level because of decreased lean body mass with aging.

3. **An 87-year-old nursing home resident with advanced dementia is noted to be spending increasingly more time in her bed for the past 3 days. Her usual routine is to pace the hallways or spend time around the nurses' station after breakfast. This acute change in functional status (spending more time in her room) is likely to be of:**

   A. No concern; it's probably personal choice

   B. Concern, as it may be fatigue from anemia

   C. Concern, as it may be acute infection

   D. No concern; it's probably normal aging

4. An 89-year-old man is brought to the emergency room by his daughter. She is concerned he may have suffered a stroke. The family reports that he had a stroke 15 years previously, following which he developed left-sided weakness but recovered completely with physical therapy. Since then he has been on treatment for hypertension and hypercholesterolemia and takes an aspirin on a daily basis. He was diagnosed with benign prostatic hyperplasia about 2 years ago and his symptoms are currently well controlled. He lives with his daughter and per the daughter his blood pressure and laboratory tests during a recent visit to his primary care physician were described as "excellent." Today's visit to the emergency room is a result of the daughter noting that her father seemed extremely listless this morning and had refused to get out of bed. As the emergency department physician evaluating this patient, your FIRST step after ruling out stroke will be to:

A. Reassure the patient's daughter that he has not had another stroke, it's just normal aging.
B. Perform an EKG, and if negative, discharge the patient to rest.
C. Perform an EKG and do workup for a possible source of infection.
D. Get a baseline account of patient's usual routine, and explore the possible recent use of any new drugs including over-the-counter medications.

ANSWERS TO PRE-TEST

1. B
2. C
3. A

ANSWERS TO POST-TEST

1. D
2. C
3. C
4. D

10

Assessing Decisional Capacity in Older Adults

Diane Chau, MD, FACP

Patricia Lanoie Blanchette, MD, MPH

Sreekanth Donepudi, MD, MPH

Reed Dopf, MD

● **LEARNING OBJECTIVES**

1. Define decision-making capacity and describe the basic elements of decision-making capacity.
2. Compare and contrast competency and capacity.
3. Describe key components of the diagnostic interview.
4. Discuss medical conditions (including mental health) that can alter a person's capacity.
5. Describe the surrogacy process in decision-making.

PRE-TEST

1. **The most appropriate statement with the initiation of a new medication is:**

   A. "I think you should consider medication X. It works very well with few side effects. I'll write the prescription and you can fill it."

   B. "What is your understanding of why I am recommending this medication, and what concerns do you have about this medication treatment plan?"

   C. "You have essential hypertension and I am starting this drug based on a study I just read about. It is cutting-edge science and you will like it."

   D. "This medication will work well for your blood pressure problem."

2. **In its broadest definition, autonomy is best explained as:**

   A. The right to make decisions free from undue influence or coercion

   B. The obligation to restore health and relieve suffering

   C. The intention to do no harm

   D. The goal of doing "good" as part of actions

3. **Which of the following may MOST limit a person's capacity?**

   A. Congestive heart failure

   B. Delirium

   C. Mild depression

   D. Age over 90

CASE PRESENTATION 1: DEPRESSED PATIENT

Mr. G. is a 75-year-old male with underlying hypertension, well controlled, and type 2 diabetes with no known complications. His wife died over 6 months ago, but he still has depressed mood most of the day. He started treatment for depression 1 week ago. He still describes himself as very sad and is adjusting to life without his wife. You are evaluating him in the emergency room after he presented with a ground-level fall and resultant right ankle fracture. The emergency room doctor had consulted orthopedics; however, when the orthopedic doctor attempted to get consent, Mr. G. replied, "What is the point?" Mr. G. has difficulty understanding the benefits of surgical repair and expresses his hopelessness in living without his wife.

Does this patient with uncontrolled depression possess capacity to refuse surgery?

● BACKGROUND

The concept of decisional capacity relies upon a patient's understanding of the specific question being asked, the ability to weigh alternatives to the decision, and the ability to communicate a reasoned decision. Traditionally, medical practices within paternalistic models have allowed physicians to decide what is in the best interest of patient care. As society moves toward a model of care where the patient has a right to make a better-informed decision, patient autonomy and personal choice has become a priority in many cultures. The role of the physician in this case is to provide the patient with the education needed for the patient to make such an informed decision. When a patient is unable to make a decision, he or she may elect a surrogate or have a surrogate assigned. Physicians often assume patients have decisional capacity if they are in agreement with the treatment recommendations. It is commonly only the patients who refuse treatment recommendations whose capacity is questioned. However, patients may communicate an agreement to a treatment without possessing any understanding of the treatment, the alternatives, or consequences. Thus, it is important for physicians to understand concepts of decisional capacity, how to access capacity, and conditions where capacity might be limited.

CASE PRESENTATION 1 (continued)

You proceed with an evaluation of Mr. G.'s depression using a geriatric depression assessment tool; he tests positive, but he expresses no suicidal ideations or suicidal attempts. During the assessment, he reports his hopelessness and that he sees no point in improving his health. In this case, the patient has undertreated depression which could impair his decisional capacity. Did the patient possess adequate capacity despite his depression to give informed consent?

How would you approach the assessment of this patient's capacity?

The next sections describe the foundations of decisional capacity and provide the fundamentals of determining capacity. This will include the types of capacity and introduce the concept of surrogacy in decision-making. Example cases will demonstrate how limits in decisional capacity can occur in older adult populations, either transiently or permanently.

● THE CHANGING ROLE OF PHYSICIANS

Historical Considerations

Historically, decisions about health care have predominantly relied upon application of bioethical principles and deductive reasoning. Medical decisions were primarily made by a beneficent physician, acquiesced to by the patient, in a traditional authoritarian model. With society's greater emphasis on autonomy, medicine has transformed to include the incorporation of personal cultural values and the right of the competent adult to make uncoerced informed decisions to accept or refuse treatment.

There have been many cases where failure to understand autonomy as core to decisional capacity has led to human injustices. In the United Kingdom, it has been reported to cause egregious errors that have led to mass institutionalization, loss of individual choice, loss of personal finances, and loss of voting rights.[1] It would not be impossible to imagine similar events occurring commonly in other countries; thus it is important to understand decisional capacity within the context of bioethical principles.

Modern Expectations

Today, personal values of quality of life, cultural values, and personal experience have moved into the forefront of medical decision-making. As medical decision-making has evolved in complexity, the paternalistic model of medicine has evolved to a more informative model that includes input from a team of caregivers and the patient's personal preferences. The interdisciplinary team may consist of a mental health provider, social workers, nurses, pharmacists, and other allied health workers. The physician works collaboratively and leads this interdisciplinary team of educators to make treatment plan recommendations. To be effective in this role, physicians should consider not only the additional data generated by team members, but also the patient's personal and cultural values that factor into informed medical decision-making. The individual should be involved to the furthest extent he or she is capable within the decision-making process.

Role of Ethics and the Law

Whereas ethics define and establish for a society what is good and how individuals should act, the law establishes the rules that must be followed. There are many ethical dilemmas wherein the relationship between the law and ethics leaves a clinician without clear guidance. For example, an older person with mild dementia may want to continue driving short distances despite failing an annual cognitive screening exam threshold set by your state's laws. Respecting the patient's autonomy and wishes to continue driving may conflict with the law in the state that requires practicing physicians to report the patient to an appropriate regulating agency. The physician's professional opinion regarding the patient's ability to drive might differ from the laws that may limit the patient's driving. In the United States, laws governing informed consent and capacity for decision-making are under the jurisdiction of each state. Physicians should become familiar with the laws under which they are practicing. In the United States, each state's statutes are generally available through their legislative offices and websites. In the United Kingdom, these are published through the UK Office of Public Sector Information (OPSI). The United Kingdom has published statutes—the Mental Capacity Act 2005 (MCA), with amendments in 2006, 2008, and 2009—that provide guidance on mental capacity, the MCA Code of Practice, the Independent Mental Capacity Advocates (IMCA) service, and the new crimes associated with violating rights of those who have impaired capacity.[1] In the United States, the American Bar Association has published summaries and reviews of each state's elder law available on its website through http://www.abanet.org. Often, these medical reporting statutes are also incorporated into the State Medical Board Regulations. However, as state statutes and revisions are different and subject to changes, practicing providers must maintain their updated information through their local published laws. An opinion regarding capacity is what clinicians render. However, legally competency judgments are only made by the courts according to state laws.

● BIOETHICS AS THE BASIS OF CAPACITY

In bioethics and in the law, the most common principles are beneficence, nonmaleficence, justice, and autonomy. The concept of beneficence guides the physician to do good by restoring health and relieving suffering. The natural companion of beneficence is nonmaleficence, requiring physicians to do no harm whether intentional or unintentional, and to carefully consider the possible negative ramifications of medical decisions. The concept of justice in medicine concerns the overall distribution of medical resources. The principle of autonomy allows that competent adult patients may accept or refuse any medical treatment providing they have been appropriately informed and free from coercion or undue influence.[2]

In the United States, patients are allowed, within the extent allowed by law, to dictate the course of many aspects of their medical care, including choices with regard to end-of-life care. This right requires that patients are well informed and understand their medical condition, the potential risks and benefits of treatment, and the potential outcomes from accepting or refusing treatment. This means that they must be able to process and use information. Dictated by both law and medical ethics, it is the responsibility of the clinician to determine whether patients have capacity for medical decision-making

and when a responsible surrogate should be authorized to act as an agent for the patient.

In the United Kingdom, the government has published five principles as part of the MCA Code of Practice[3]:

1. A person must be assumed to have capacity unless it is established that he or she lacks capacity.
2. A person is not to be treated as unable to make a decision unless all practicable steps to help the person to do so have been taken without success.
3. A person is not to be treated as unable to make a decision merely because he or she makes an unwise decision.
4. An act done, or a decision made, under this Act for or on behalf of a person who lacks capacity must be done, or made, in his or her best interests.
5. Before the act is done, or the decision is made, regard must be taken to whether the purpose for which it is needed can be as effectively achieved in a way that is less restrictive of the person's rights and freedom of action.

This Code of Practice was created to support the national legislation, MCA 2005, and provide day-to-day guidance for caregivers and practitioners, lawyers, and others appointed by the courts who affect the lives of those with decreased capacity. The purpose for having clearly written principles is twofold: to protect those who lack capacity and to allow them to take part in the decisions that affect them.[3] A key element in this pioneering legislation is the respect for autonomy.

Autonomy's Role in Capacity

Medicine relies on the concept of autonomy and that, by law, adults are considered to have capacity unless determined by a court to be lacking competence. Physicians may be requested by the court to render an opinion with regard to a patient's capacity, but only the court has authority to legally determine a person's competency. Autonomy allows that rational people have the capacity to render an educated, uncoerced decision representing the expression of their choices. Morally speaking, it is the patients who will carry the responsibility for the outcome of those decisions, provided they have been well informed about the potential outcomes of treatment decisions. In clinical treatment, questions about capacity occur when patients refuse treatment without logical rationale, when a provider questions a patient's cognitive abilities to understand treatment, when patients are inconsistent about their choices, or when family members or other loved ones question the patient's choices. Unfortunately, a formal capacity assessment is often only undertaken when the interaction between the physician and the patient leads the physician to question the patient's capacity. In ideal practice scenarios, capacity assessment should be part of any informed consent process and not limited to occasions of disagreements.

Concepts of Agency and Liberty in Capacity

The concept of agency with regard to medical decision-making refers to the concept of carrying out one's decisions or will to have something done.[4] An agent is by definition one who acts. In other words, we are the agents over our own decision-making and can initiate our own actions, unless we designate our agency to another person. However, external influences can move an individual to act in ways that undermine his or her autonomy, that is, through coercion or undue influence. The concept of liberty overlaps with the concepts of autonomy and agency. Liberty refers to freedom, and it is the extent to which actions are possible and free of obstacles. Liberty or freedom may have numerous definitions, but their applicability in capacity and medical decision-making are based upon the idea that actions are consistent with a person's beliefs, desires, and values and free from undue influence or coercion.[5]

Consider undue influence to be present when all of the factors of "SODR"—susceptibility, opportunity, disposition, and resulting suspicious transaction—are present. Examples of SODR:

Susceptible—Mental illness, severe dementia, or delirium.
Opportunity—A trusting confidential relationship, such as patient and religious advisor, physician, spouse, or other family member.
Disposition—The patient is prevented from obtaining independent advice and is heavily encouraged in the direction desired by another.
Resulting suspicious transaction—The decision is inconsistent with previous decisions or with long-held beliefs.

The clinician should also be observant of factors suggesting undue influence; besides SODR, there are more subtle findings such as the patient simply repeatedly expressing one decision without being able or willing to discuss options. Patients unduly influenced will rarely provide evidence of reasoning in arriving at a particular decision. In some instances there will be overt pressure brought by individuals to manipulate the course of decision-making.

In clinical practice, clinicians should be aware of patients who may be vulnerable to someone who is exerting undue influence through threats of psychological, physical, or financial harm to make a choice. Coercion may even occur at the level of the medical practice itself. Extreme examples of this can be found through physician influence on a pregnant patient's agreement to a cesarean section procedure by using the threat of harm to an unborn fetus if she refuses to consent.[6] Coercion factors can be very subtle and difficult to detect, even by most skilled clinicians, and many may not recognize their repeated efforts to educate patients and to persuade them to certain actions as coercive. They may justify their excessive persuasion as advocating for the vulnerable. These subtle cases may take higher legal court action to resolve. If a clinician finds that the care of an older adult involved obvious coercive practices, the clinician should take appropriate action, even to the extent of reporting the case to his or her local authorities. Although undue influence is not a defined form of abuse, it is a method wherein exploitation of the victim is committed. Obvious coercive tactics might include the threat of physical or psychological abuse to gain or maintain power over an older adult patient by the abuser. The abuser may be a caregiver, family member, partner, or even court-appointed guardian. In the United States, the proper agencies for reporting reside within the Elder Protective Services (EPS) or the State Attorney General's office. Each state has a separate threshold for EPS eligibility, reporting guidelines, and sanctions for failing to report. Many informative resources about elder abuse can be found on the Internet through the National Center on Elder Abuse (NCEA).[7] Each state has its own interpretation within its laws regarding undue influence, and these can be found through the NCEA "Undue Influence: Context, Provisions, and Citations in Adult Protective Services Laws, by State" Chart[7] or the American Bar Association Commission on Law and Aging.[8] Again, physicians should be aware of their individual state laws.

● ESTABLISHING CAPACITY

A capacity assessment should be considered on all clinical cases wherein consent from a patient must be documented. It is common law that a patient has presumed decisional capacity until proven otherwise.

CASE PRESENTATION 1 (continued)

In going through the review of systems with our depressed patient, Mr. G., he reveals dry skin, fatigue, constipation, wanting to sleep most of his day, and having poor energy. His social history reveals a daughter living out of state in California, but he lives alone. He drinks 1 gin cocktail daily and has smoked 1 pack of cigarettes per day for 40 years. His physical exam reveals an otherwise normal-appearing heavyset man with a heart rate of 52, respiratory rate of 20, pulse oxygenation on room air at 88%, dry skin, barrel chest, mild clubbing, and a right ankle fracture as found in the emergency room. Labs are pertinent for a markedly elevated thyroid-stimulating hormone value of 89 mIU/L and mildly low serum sodium of 130 mEq/L (130 mmol/L).

There are many reversible factors that may render a person unable to act as his or her own agent due to a lack of judgment. A first step in assessing capacity is to determine if there are potential conditions that may be affecting the patient's capacity, such as delirium, dementia, depression, substance abuse, recent head injury, or other illnesses. In Mr. G.'s case, there are elements of hypothyroid-related depression. Other potentially reversible conditions in this situation could include electrolyte or metabolic derangements, hypoxia, and chronic intoxication. The second step is to determine if these conditions are affecting the patient's ability to make a decision. In the United Kingdom, these basic first steps are exemplified in the Code of Practice.[3] Given the high potential for this patient not to have capacity due to the cognitive impact from his medical conditions, the physician proceeds to perform and document the decisional capacity of this patient through a meaningful interview.

CASE PRESENTATION 1 (continued)

The physician clarifies, "Mr. G., I have some questions that can help me better understand your decision." The patient is alert, responds slowly, but is oriented to time, date, place, and person. "Mr. G., what is your understanding of your condition?" The patient replies, "I have a broken ankle." The physician proceeds, "I am asking for your permission to fix your broken ankle. What is your understanding of what I am asking of you?" The patient slowly responds, "You don't understand."

Mr. G.'s physician incorporates his assessment of capacity within the history and physical exam. He notes the patient's level of alertness, function, mood, and mental status. If there is a decision being asked of the patient, the assessment of capacity should be integrated into the clinician's interview, as was done in the case. During the interview, the patient's personal statements should be noted with regard to their ability to:

- Understand what is the decision being asked
- Weigh the options and alternatives of the decision
- Communicate the actual decision in question

Does the Patient Understand the Decision Being Asked?

In understanding the decision being asked of the patient, the clinician must provide enough relevant information to help the patient make a decision. The information must be provided on a level and in a language patients can understand. Poor health literacy can contribute to many patient-physician failures in communication (Chapter 11). Often patients may fail to make a decision because they are either overwhelmed with too much information, or were not given enough information. They may lack the understanding of the health care terminology. The communication style of the clinician may be ineffective. In order to understand information, patients must be able to retain information long enough to mentally process it. This does not mean that patients have to retain the information indefinitely, but rather just long enough to make the decision. People with memory impairment may still be able to process enough relevant information to make a decision. Mild memory impairment by itself should not exclude a person from having decisional capacity. Decisional capacity really depends on the level of complexity of the question asked in people with cognitive disorders. People with memory impairment may require repetition of the information, visual support, or other memory cues to help them come to the decision. When possible, patients should be given the opportunity to gather more support and have more time to help them come to a decision. To understand the decision being asked of them, patients should understand why they need to make a decision. Often cultural factors or life patterns of not being a decision-maker may contribute a patient not

wanting to make a decision. In this case, the patient understands that he has a fracture, but does not understand the surgical options and alternatives required to make a reasoned decision.

CASE PRESENTATION 1 (continued)

The doctor proceeds, "I want to better understand your reasoning. I would like to fix your broken ankle, which would help you walk again. The alternative is that we leave it broken, which will likely impair your ability to walk and you may suffer from prolonged pain. What are your thoughts on this?"

Can the Patient Weigh the Options and Alternatives of His or Her Decision?

Although in this case, the physician presented in simple language the options for the patient, the patient has not demonstrated his understanding of the treatment options. The patient understands he has a fracture, but his medical conditions (ie, hypoxia, hypothyroidism, and depression) are impairing his ability to process the information presented to come to a decision. Patients must be able to use the information provided to them in way that allows them to consider their options and make a reasoned decision using the information. Patients who are unable to use such information have impaired decisional capacity.

CASE PRESENTATION 1 (continued)

The patient replies, "It won't help me."

Are There Barriers in Patient Communication?

In this case, the patient is verbally communicating without any obvious barriers. Some challenging cases might be clouded by communication barriers, and clinicians should be aware of factors such as hearing loss, sign language, or foreign language barriers wherein patients may require additional support. Verbal and nonverbal support should be provided, such as translators, writing tablets, or picture blocks.

CASE PRESENTATION 1 (continued)

Since the patient has not affirmed that he understood the relevancy of the decision being asked, the physician persists with further questions: "Mr. G., I need you to tell me in your words what you mean by 'it' and what is your understanding of what might help your broken ankle." The patient replies sadly, "I've tried to tell you, it doesn't matter."

Are there additional tools for assessment that could help in this case? Would performing a mini-mental status exam help the capacity assessment?

Are There Additional Tools to Aid in the Assessment?

The gold standard for assessing capacity is a diagnostic examination and interview by a clinician skilled in such assessments, including a discussion of the pertinent topics, such as the diagnoses and options being presented. In the United Kingdom, clinicians can utilize the five sets of comprehensive training materials that support the MCA 2005 to improve their knowledge of capacity assessment; the information is available through their Department of Health[1] and on the Internet (http://www.dh.gov.uk/en/link Social Care then Delivering Adult Social care/MentalCapacity). To gain skills in capacity assessment requires clinical experience in applying this knowledge. In the United States, increasing capacity assessment skills are available through additional years of fellowship training in subspecialties such as geriatric medicine, geriatric psychiatry, geriatric psychology, and geriatric social work, wherein high volumes of capacity cases and experienced trainers are available.

In the general practice of capacity assessment, the clinician should note the patient's level of alertness, and review the medication history, physical examination, laboratory tests, and any neuroimaging studies to determine whether there may be a reversible component to a current diminished capacity. The patient's mood and mental status should be observed. To ascertain whether the patient is putting forth his or her best effort, the clinician should be attuned to the level of engagement of the patient in the interview. Since there are many potential causes of reversible or irreversible losses of decisional capacity, the clinician performing the assessment should have enough medical background to consider a diagnosis of delirium and all of its potential causes. There are many medical conditions that require knowledge and experience to recognize, conditions that could contribute to reversible cognitive changes. Some of these conditions include fecal impaction, urinary retention, hypo/hyperthyroidism, drug effects and interactions, hypoxia, hypercarbia, electrolyte disorders, renal failure, liver dysfunction, and a host of other medical illnesses. The clinician should also understand that it may take as many as 6 weeks for the patient's baseline mental status to be regained following appropriate treatment for delirium. If a decision is not urgent, patients should be allowed the time to resolve their delirium to participate in their decision-making process.

Possibly because of varying experience and skill in decisional capacity assessment or the lack of a longitudinal patient-physician relationship, single-point clinical assessments of decisional capacity have shown low inter-rater reliability.[9] Attempts have been made to develop structured tools to evaluate capacity to consent to treatment and to participate as a subject in research trials.[10] Structured tools are available and used in research, but rarely used or indicated in clinical practice, especially when the clinician knows the patient and can ascertain a patient's decisional consistency.

Formal tests of mental status may be used to supplement the clinician's diagnostic interview. However, caution should be used in their interpretation, since they lack face validity with regard to specific capacity. A certain score on a mental status test, unless the score is extremely low, does not correlate well with specific capacity tasks, such as testamentary capacity or the designation of a surrogate decision-maker. A patient may have an MMSE score that is abnormal such as 23 out of 30 on the commonly used Folstein exam, but an abnormal score does not by itself denote that a person with dementia has no decisional capacity. Decisional capacity would be based on the complexity of any decision being asked and the ability of the patient to exhibit components of capacity for question asked. In other words, an advanced dementia patient may be able to decide if he or she wants to join a group in a recreational activity or have a skin biopsy, but lack decisional ability for a laparotomy to remove a necrotic gall bladder.

In documenting the diagnostic interview, clinicians should include the patient's verbatim responses, using the patient's own words, as part of the clinical note. If ever questioned, this portion of the documentation within the medical record will serve as the voice of the patient as part of the capacity assessment.

CASE PRESENTATION 1 (continued)

Despite repeated questioning and attempts at further education, Mr. G. has only communicated an understanding of his diagnosis. The missing element of decisional capacity rests on the patient's inability to use the information of the surgery, weigh the options of the interventions or no intervention, and then communicate that decision to the physician.

The general components of evaluating decisional capacity include the ability of the patient to understand the relevant information, to appreciate the consequences of the situation, to reason about choices, and to communicate a choice.[11] Patients do not need to show complex levels of understanding, such as understanding of percentages or statistics. If this patient had simply stated he understood that fixing his ankle meant taking him to surgery so he could walk or have less pain, and that the alternative was natural healing with the possibility of impaired function or pain, this would have been sufficient to have decisional capacity. However, in this case the patient's mild hypoxia, depression, and hypothyroidism may all contribute to impair his level of alertness and his decision-making abilities.

It is important to remember that, while the patient may lack capacity at this time due to the combined effects of medical illness, he will likely regain decisional capacity when his thyroid, depression, and hypoxia are corrected. Several factors, including many medications—such as pain medications, sedative hypnotics, antipsychotics, antianxiety agents, and antidepressants—can diminish a patient's level of alertness and ability to attend to mental status tasks. They may diminish the patient's ability to process information. Polypharmacy, which is common in various settings, can compound this problem. Other factors that may temporarily affect any patient's decisional capacity include delirium, untreated depression, anxiety-provoking aspects of being in a hospital or a clinic, pain associated with diagnostic and treatment procedures, difficulties with language, and being in an unfamiliar culture.[12]

CASE PRESENTATION 1 (continued)

The physician comes to the opinion that Mr. G. does not have capacity to render a decision regarding a surgical repair of his right ankle. Since the patient is unable to provide informed consent for the surgery, the physician consults with the Emergency Room social worker on call, who replies, "I can't get a court competency hearing or guardianship for him anytime soon. However, I think we can probably obtain consent from his daughter under our surrogate decision-maker law. Let me check with the hospital attorney to make sure we would be acting within the state law." When the physician asks Mr. G. if it would be okay for his daughter to help with the decision regarding surgery or not, he replies, "I think that would be okay, she has helped me with medical appointments and other things."

It is not uncommon in clinical practice for professionals to confuse the terms "capacity" and "competency." In this case, the patient has diminished decisional capacity regarding surgery needed to repair his ankle. However, the patient may well have retained the capacity to designate a surrogate decision-maker. In this case, the patient designates his daughter as a decision-maker. He states that his daughter has always helped him with medical appointments and medical decisions, and that he trusts her. His daughter was then contacted for consent.

Differences between Capacity and Competence

The terms "capacity" and "competence" are often used interchangeably. The determination of competence is a legal decision rendered by a judge, albeit generally relying on the opinion of one or more physicians in this regard.[13] Capacity determination does not require a lawyer, judge, or court hearing. Clinicians who are trained in examining patients for decisional capacity can render a valid opinion without extensive formal psychiatric or psychological testing. Decisional capacity assessments do not require advanced cognitive status testing or any mini-mental status examination scores, although these may be helpful to support an opinion and to follow a patient's progress over time. Later in the chapter, we will discuss decision-making when patients lack capacity and why this patient's daughter was chosen as the person to contact.

CASE PRESENTATION 2: ACUTE DELIRIUM

An 88-year-old man, who lives with his daughter, is brought to the hospital emergency department for an acute abdomen. He is found to have a bowel perforation, by CT scan, and it is recommended that he be admitted to the hospital for an urgent surgical repair. His baseline functioning is that he is ambulatory, and has required progressive assistance with his personal care and financial affairs. After being informed of the urgent need for surgery, the patient states that he wishes to decline surgery and to return home with pain medication so that he can continue to take care of his cat. The hospital physician consults the geriatrics team for further evaluation. On examination the patient is pleasant but disoriented. His history and exam are supportive of long-standing dementia with a baseline mini-mental state examination (MMSE) score of 23 out of 30. Due to his pain and decompensated medical state, an MMSE could not be obtained accurately, but based on his answers to the medical student on the surgery service, she reports the patient's score as 10 out of 30. The geriatrician notes the patient's level of alertness, baseline function, mood, and mental status. The geriatrician performs a detailed physical exam and reviews all of the patient's medications to see if any could be contributing to the patient's cognitive decline in addition to his acute abdomen. Despite further discussion, he is convinced that his perforated abdomen will heal by itself without surgery and he mentions nothing regarding the risks of death. During his exam, it is clear the patient is inattentive with acute delirium. The geriatrics team recommends that a surrogate decision-maker be contacted for consent.

When Patients Lack Capacity

Patients who are considered to have capacity to make informed medical decisions can understand the decision, weigh the options and alternatives of the decision, and communicate their decision. A patient who does not have capacity to make an informed medical decision may have the capacity to designate a surrogate decision-maker who will act as the patient's agent. In both cases discussed, since the patient could not demonstrate an understanding of the risks and outcomes of refusing surgery, the physician needs to seek out the patient's surrogate decision-maker. This surrogate could be appointed by the patient when he possessed capacity at an earlier point in time, but in emergency situations many states or countries have lists, in order of priority, for acceptable surrogates. If the patient has a written document declaring a durable power of attorney (DPOA) for health care decisions, then the physician should contact that DPOA. In situations where there are no surrogate decision-maker(s) appointed, the physicians must rely upon the state laws. Each state has a legal order for surrogacy that can be found through the Office on Aging or the State Attorney General's office/website. In the United Kingdom, the MCA 2005 added in 2007 statutory use of Independent Mental Capacity Advocate services.[14] Their services are particularly useful in cases where there are no family or friends to support a patient's decision-making abilities. Some states in the United States, such as Nevada, offer similar independent capacity advocates for seniors. The availability is not uniform, and information about these advocates (if they are available) can be found through your local Office on Aging. Although each state has its own list order for whom to contact for decision-making, many are based on family order.

A typical hierarchy for decision-making when a patient lacks capacity is the following:

1. The legal guardian of the patient
2. The spouse
3. The adult children
4. The living parents
5. Other relatives

However, some states have recognized that long-time partners who have no marital or family relationship may be the best surrogate decision-makers, and list long-time friends as potential decision-makers as well. Some states do not have a list order, allowing for interested parties to agree on the most appropriate decision-maker. Where there is disagreement about which person should act as the surrogate, a court order may be necessary.

Advance Directives

Patients who lack decisional capacity may have previously voiced their wishes for care in oral statements to their physicians, family, or friends, or expressed their wishes in written documents. The patient's advance directives (ADs) reflect personal values and represents their autonomy. The AD may contain a living will, or may designate a health care proxy or surrogate who would interpret the patient's health care wishes and represent the patient when the patient lacks capacity. As each state has different statutory laws governing ADs, physicians again need be aware of the AD rules in their state. In some states, oral advance directives made to physicians and recorded in the physician's medical record are recognized by the courts. Oral ADs such as comments to relatives about their health care or the health care of others may have limited utility depending on the context in which they were spoken. Oral ADs are limited by inaccurate recall, disagreements, or specificity. Written directives are more formal and considered more accurate than oral ADs. Written ADs also have limitations in being too vague, outdated, and not representative of the patient's wishes for care are when he or she is not terminally ill. Patients with written ADs should update their AD with changes in their life status and yearly to prevent them from becoming outdated. In clinical practice, if there is a written AD, it may have been written years before the current event and not reflect all of the changes in that person's life that may have impacted his or her decision-making process, such as the birth of a new grandchild. In these cases, it is best to discuss the best course of care with the surrogate who would help interpret the patient's wishes.

Surrogate Decision-Makers, DPOA

When patients demonstrate a lack of capacity in medical decision-making, the next step would be to determine whether the patient has a durable power-of-attorney (DPOA) or alternative agent who can make the decision on the patient's behalf who could reflect his or her beliefs and actions prior to the illness.

In preparing for the possibility of future medical conditions that could impair decision-making, patients should routinely be counseled to execute a DPOA. To be valid, the DPOA must have been executed at a time when the person understood the DPOA. DPOAs should be read carefully, as they differ with regard to when they come into play, which powers are conveyed to another person (medical and/or financial affairs), whether there are successor persons who may act if the primary named decision-maker cannot or refuses to serve, and whether one or more persons must both decide on a course of action for the decision to be valid. DPOAs also may contain specific instructions with regard to medical interventions, such as tube feeding, in the event of certain conditions being present. The most common reason for a DPOA to be challenged successfully in US court is by demonstrating that the affected person did not or could not have understood what he or she was signing at the time the DPOA was executed.

At the time of signing the DPOA, did the patient possess capacity to understand it? Again, a diagnostic interview with an accompanying medical note is the gold standard in helping validate the DPOA.

Other Types of Capacity

Although this chapter deals with decisional capacity for health care decisions, there are other terms relating to capacity with which clinicians should be aware. These differ somewhat in assessment style and documentation requirements.

Capacity to Provide Informed Consent for Research

In research studies, issues of capacity often involve informed consent and vulnerable subjects such as those with dementia, depression, or other clinical situations where impaired decisional capacity may be present. Obtaining informed consent for such research studies is guided by differing government/state law, research ethics, and by Institutional Review Boards. In the United States and United Kingdom, people with limited capacity for informed decision-making must assent to the study and must have informed consent provided by another person entitled to be their agent.[15,16] In keeping with ethics in research, they can also only participate in research studies where the condition studied relates to the illness that impairs their capacity. That is, a patient with dementia may only participate in studies of dementia.[15,16]

Testamentary Capacity

A person's mental ability to make or break a will defines testamentary capacity. Wills are often challenged in court for various reasons, such as when a significant change from a previous will has been made, when there is a lack of consistency with the will and the verbally expressed wishes of the person, when more than one will is uncovered, and when wills surface that are unknown to exist by some of the beneficiaries. A charge of undue influence, as described above, is another common reason to challenge a will. In the course of these challenges, physicians' medical records may be subpoenaed and physicians may be asked to testify with regard to the health and mental status of the patient during the time the will was made.[10] Unless the physician has specific knowledge of the patient's testamentary capacity at the time the will was made, he or she should not do more than offer objective information. Testamentary capacity is often retained even though other capacities have declined.

Financial Capacity

It is not uncommon in the practice of medicine for the physician to be asked for a formal opinion as to whether the patient has capacity for making financial decisions, such as transferring title to property, or making or breaking a will. These issues are outside of the usual practice of medicine, and may or may not be related to the specific issue of medical decision-making. Unless skilled in the assessment of these issues, and willing to appear in court to defend one's assessments and opinion, often years after the assessment has occurred, the clinician is advised to refer the patient to a clinician who by training and experience is skilled in handling these topics. Some patients require the assistance of representative payees for the management of their retirement or financial benefits. In this case, if the clinician is comfortable in this area, the clinician may offer an opinion limited to the management of funds from federal benefits. Any misuse of the patient's funds will be under the jurisdiction of the respective government agency. A representative payee is often necessary for the patient's medical or nursing home bills to be paid. In these cases, to prevent misuse of the clinician's opinion about a patient's ability to manage his or her retirement benefits, the clinician would be well advised to limit his or her opinion to this issue and to define the cause of the lack of ability as due to the patient's "medical condition."

CONCLUSION

Assessing and understanding the components of decision-making capacity is a critical skill for providers of care to older adults. All older patients should have their decision-making capacity assessed prior to any procedure or surgery. Providers should also recognize that consent to a procedure, consistent with the expectations of the medical provider, does not automatically imply that the older patient has adequate decision-making capacity. Usually disagreements in approaches to care between the provider and the patient are what generate a discussion and assessment of capacity. A thoughtful and sequential approach to assessing decision-making capacity is necessary to provide the optimal care consistent with the preferences of the patient and when decision capacity is impaired an understanding of laws regarding surrogate decision-makers and the assistance of social workers and others skilled in these areas are essential.

References

1. University of Central Lancashire; Social Care Workforce Research Unit (King's College, London); and various authors. Mental Capacity Act 2005. May 8, 2007. Accessed Feb. 2-7, 2010. Available through the UK Department of Health in .pdf training documents and websites:
http://www.dh.gov.uk/dr_consum_dh/groups/dh_digitalassets/@dh/@en/documents/digitalasset/dh_074624.pdf
http://www.dh.gov.uk/en/publicationsandstatistics/publications/publicationspolicyandguidance/DH_074491

2. Wallace KA. Common morality and moral reform. *Theory Med Bioethics*. 2009;30:55-68.

3. Mental Capacity Act 2005. Code of Practice. Issued by the Lord Chancellor on April 23, 2007 in accordance with sections 42 and 43 of the Act by the Department of Constitutional Affairs in London. http://www.opsi.gov.uk/acts/acts2005/related/ukpgacop_ 20050009 _en.pdf. Accessed Feb. 7, 2010.

4. Agency. *Merriam-Webster Online Dictionary*. 2009. Retrieved from http://www.merriam-webster.com/dictionary/agency.

5. Positive and negative liberty. *Stanford Encyclopedia of Philosophy*. http://plato.stanford.edu/entries/liberty-positive-negative/#TwoConLib. Accessed Oct. 8, 2007.

6. American Civil Liberties Union. 1997. *Coercive and Punitive Governmental Responses to Women's Conduct During Pregnancy*. http://www.aclu.org/reproductive-freedom/coercive-and-punitive-governmental-responses-womens-conduct-during-pregnancy.

7. National Center on Elder Abuse through the Administration on Aging. http://www.ncea.aoa.gov/ncearoot/Main_Site/index.aspx. Accessed Feb. 7, 2010.

8. American Bar Association Commission on Law and Aging. http://www.abanet.org/aging/about/elderabuse.shtml. Accessed Feb. 7, 2010.

9. Marson DC. Consistency of physician judgments of capacity to consent in mild Alzheimer's disease. *J Am Geriatr Soc*. 1997;45: 453-457.

10. Sturman ED. The capacity to consent to treatment and research: a review of standardized assessment tools. *Clin Psychol Rev*. 2005; 25:954-974.

11. Appelbaum PS. Clinical practice. Assessment of patients' competence to consent to treatment. *N Engl J Med*. 2007;357:1834-1840.

12. Grisso T, Appelbaum PS. *Assessing Competence to Consent to Medical Treatment*. Oxford: Oxford University Press; 1998.

13. Snyder L, Leffler C; Ethics and Human Rights Committee, American College of Physicians. Ethics manual, 5th ed. *Ann Intern Med*. 2005;142:560-582.

14. Mental Capacity Act 2005. Independent Mental Capacity Advocate Service. http://www.dh.gov.uk/en/SocialCare/Deliveringadultsocialcare/MentalCapacity/IMCA/DH_4134876. Accessed Feb. 7, 2010.

15. Mental Capacity Act 2005. Fact Sheet for Social Scientists. http://www.dh.gov.uk/dr_consum_dh/groups/dh_digitalassets/@dh/@en/@pg/documents/digitalasset/dh_106217.pdf. Accessed Feb. 7, 2010.

16. Research Involving Individuals with Questionable Capacity to Consent. US Department of Health and Human Services, National Institute of Health, November 2009. http://grants.nih.gov/grants/policy/questionablecapacity.htm. Accessed Feb. 7, 2010.

POST-TEST

1. **Which of the following is required to determine a person's decisional capacity?**

   A. The person must be able to communicate a reasoned choice.

   B. The person must have a caregiver, parent, or guardian.

   C. The person must have been evaluated by psychology or psychiatry.

   D. The person must have a normal mini-mental examination.

2. **Which of the following is the most CORRECT statement regarding durable power-of-attorney (DPOA)?**

   A. Once signed, a DPOA can make all decisions for a patient at any time.

   B. A lawyer is needed to make a DPOA.

   C. A complete mental health exam is required as part of the DPOA draft document.

   D. The DPOA may have specific instructions pertaining to medical interventions.

3. **Which of the following is TRUE regarding decisional capacity?**

   A. A person with mild memory loss does not meet the requirements for patient understanding.

   B. Formal tests of mental status are required in assessment of decisional capacity.

   C. Patients do not need to show complex levels of understanding.

   D. A person must verbally provide his or her understanding.

ANSWERS TO PRE-TEST

1. B
2. A
3. B

ANSWERS TO POST-TEST

1. A
2. D
3. C

11

Health Literacy Assessment and Practice

Carolyn Crane Cutilli, MSN, RN, ONC, CCRN

Cynthia T. Schaefer, RN, MSN

● LEARNING OBJECTIVES

1. Define health literacy and describe its impact in the geriatric population.
2. Explain aspects of literacy including prose, document, and quantitative literacy.
3. Discuss the risk of geriatric populations for low health literacy.
4. Identify and describe patient behaviors and characteristics that may indicate low health literacy.
5. Describe strategies that can minimize the effect of low health literacy in the geriatric population.

PRE-TEST

1. In the 2003 National Assessment of Adult Literacy (NAAL), the majority of people were found to be in what category of health literacy?

   A. Proficient
   B. Intermediate
   C. Basic
   D. Below basic

2. A task in health literacy where a person has the ability to comprehend and use information from a food label is:

   A. Readability
   B. Document
   C. Suitability Assessment of Materials (SAM)
   D. Proficient

3. A factor that is NOT considered by research to be well linked to lower literacy levels is:

   A. Race
   B. Age
   C. Education
   D. Gender

CASE PRESENTATION 1: "WHAT DOES THIS MEAN?"

Mr. John Taylor, age 69, is a widower who lives by himself. He retired last year from an accounting firm where he was a certified public accountant. He was recently given a new diagnosis of type 2 diabetes mellitus. He was given a new medication to start, by his doctor, as well as an instruction sheet to read about diabetes. When he gets home he reviews the materials and notes that he does not eat any "concentrated sweets," in fact he does not even know what those are. When he gets to the section on "starches," he gets completely lost and puts the papers away.

INTRODUCTION

Health literacy has come to the forefront of health care literature in the last decade. The emphasis on this concept stems from the impact it has on our country's health and fiscal management. Individuals with adequate health literacy are able to make appropriate health care decisions and achieve desired health goals. However, individuals with inadequate health literacy, representing approximately one-third of our population, struggle with making appropriate decisions and are at risk for poor health outcomes.[1] The older adult population (age 65 or older) has the lowest health literacy of all age groups and represents approximately 30% of the population with low health literacy.[2] Coupled with the extensive use of the health care system by older adults, the impact of low health literacy in the older adult population can have a large impact on health expenditures and outcomes.[3] Meeting the health literacy demands of the older adult population is key to achieving individual well-being, societal health, and financial goals.

DEFINITION OF LOW HEALTH LITERACY

Like the term "literacy", "health literacy" is often viewed as simply the ability to read printed health care material. However, this simple definition does not describe the full meaning and scope of health literacy. The concept and definition of health literacy has evolved over time. The Institute of Medicine's report "Health Literacy: A Prescription to End Confusion" defines health literacy as "The degree to which individuals have the capacity to obtain, process and understand basic health information and services needed to make appropriate health decisions."[4] From this definition, it is evident that health literacy refers to a broader skill set than simply reading written health information but rather is essential for appropriate decision-making. This definition has been utilized in numerous publications including the government initiative, *Healthy People 2010*.[5]

To highlight the areas of knowledge and skill that are needed to be health literate, Zarcadoolas and associates describe four domains in their health literacy model: fundamental literacy (reading, writing, speaking, and numeracy),

science literacy (human biology), civic literacy (government programs), and cultural literacy (cultural health values/perspectives).[6] This implies that for individuals to be health literate, they need skills and knowledge in these four domains. The National Assessment of Adult Literacy (NAAL) 2003 focused the concept of health literacy on the functional aspects of using printed material. The NAAL defines health literacy "as the ability of US adults to use printed and written health-related information to function in society, to achieve one's goals and to develop one's knowledge and potential."

From these definitions, it is evident that health literacy is not simply the ability to read health information. Rather, it is ability to use knowledge and skills to comprehend health information in various formats to make appropriate health care choices and ultimately achieve one's goals.

PREVALENCE

The National Assessment of Adult Literacy (NAAL) was a large-scale 2003 federal study examining literacy in the US population with an embedded health literacy section.[7] The NAAL examined several different aspects of literacy including prose, document, and quantitative literacy. **Prose tasks** require the ability to search, comprehend, and use information from continuous texts such as articles and instructional materials. An example of this type of health literacy is using instructional materials to prepare for a diagnostic test. **Document tasks** require the ability to search, comprehend, and use information from non-continuous texts such as forms and food labels. An example of this would be to complete a health history form when beginning care with a new provider. **Quantitative tasks** require the ability to identify and perform computations using numbers embedded in printed materials.[1] Examples include determining the amount not covered by insurance and then paying the provider of service.

Based on the participants' responses, the literacy/health literacy was categorized as below basic, basic, intermediate, and proficient.[1] At the proficient levels, one can perform complex and challenging literacy activities; at intermediate levels, one can perform moderately challenging literacy activities; at basic levels people can perform simple everyday literacy activities; and at "below basic" one can perform no more than the most simple and concrete literacy activities.

The NAAL noted that 5% of the United States population (approximately 11 million individuals) was not literate in English. In looking at health literacy specifically, 22% of adults (approximately 47 million) had a score in the basic level, and another 14% (approximately 30 million) had a score in the below basic range.[2] A total of 36% of the adult population has basic/below basic health literacy—more than one-third of the population. The majority of people were in the intermediate level. The characteristics that place individuals most at risk for below basic and basic health literacy include low oral reading fluency, not a high school graduate, non-English speaking prior to starting school, poor health, Hispanic, below poverty threshold, age ≥ 65, no medical insurance, no use of Internet for health information, African American, one or more disabilities, and prison inmate. In the NAAL, adults age 65 and older comprised 31% of the population with the lowest health literacy, and had the lowest health literacy of all age groups. Twenty-nine percent of those age 65 or older had below basic, while 30% had basic health literacy.[2] The older individual with one or more of the characteristics associated with health literacy has an even greater probability of having low health literacy.

● CONTRIBUTING FACTORS

Research focused on geriatric health literacy began in the 1990s. Several studies used data collected on 3,000 geriatric patients enrolled in a managed care program.[8-12] The majority of studies focused on individuals who could read or speak English or Spanish to determine health literacy in either language. The studies collected various demographic information such as socioeconomic status, language, gender, age, education, and race. In addition, most studies obtained health status information: visual acuity, specific diseases, and cognitive function.[13]

Age

Age is a critical demographic marker in many of the geriatric health literacy studies. An inverse relationship with age and health literacy was noted in several studies. In studies that examined various groups over age 65, older individuals usually had lower health literacy.[1,13] However, in one study with all older patients, age was not consistently the most significant variable impacting health literacy; adjusting for age showed that education was the most significant variable.[14] Thus, age impacts health literacy, but may not be the only variable that has a strong relationship with health literacy.

Gender

Gender-based differences in health literacy are not clearly delineated by research.[13] Data from the NAAL 2003 show that the average health literacy score for women is 6 points higher than men, more men had below basic health literacy, and more women had intermediate literacy. This information suggests that males have lower health literacy; however, the difference between men and women with basic or proficient health literacy was not significant.[1] Wilson and associates demonstrated that women have higher health literacy scores than men when using the Rapid Estimate of Adult Literacy in Medicine (REALM).[15] No significant link between health literacy and gender was demonstrated in two other studies.[10,16]

Race

The research on race and health literacy is very dependent upon the races included in the research studies.[13] The NAAL noted that Asian/Pacific Islanders and whites had higher average health literacy than Hispanic, Black, American Indian/Alaska Natives, and multiracial adults.[1] Other studies had mostly Caucasian and African American participants and report that those of African American background had higher rates of inadequate or marginal health literacy.[9,10,17] Of the studies with Hispanic participants, the Hispanic population had higher rates of inadequate or marginal health literacy.[9,18]

Education

Most studies indicate that there is a relationship between education and health literacy; however, educational attainment and health literacy level are not identical.[13] Two studies demonstrated that the grade level completed in formal education does not match the health literacy grade level.[19,20] Most health literacy grade levels were at least 2 years below the highest level of formal education. In the majority of studies the relationship between education and health literacy is positive; for most adults, the higher the level of education, the higher the health literacy grade level.[8,16,18] The NAAL results support this trend by demonstrating that those with below basic health literacy had the following education level: 3% with 4-year college/graduate degree, 4% with a 2-year college degree, and 12% to 15% with education equal or less than trade/business school post high school.[2]

Socioeconomic Variables

No relationship between marital status and health literacy was identified in multiple studies focused on geriatric health literacy.[13] Socioeconomic variables include income, use of public assistance, marital status, and car ownership. Multiple studies indicate a relationship between low income and health literacy.[1,9,21] However, some researchers felt that income was not the best indicator of economic status, and focused instead on the participant's type of work (blue or white collar), car ownership, and use of public assistance.[13] Blue collar occupations, lack of car ownership, and use of public assistance for food were negatively correlated with medication adherence.[10,22] Williams and associates found that socioeconomic status markers were not consistently correlated with functional health literacy in the elderly group.[18]

Overall Health

Multiple studies have examined the relationship between health and health literacy.[13] The NAAL notes that adults who had good, very good, or excellent health (by self-report) had increasingly higher health literacy when compared to those with fair or poor reported health.[2] Some studies demonstrated an association between low health literacy and poor health/specific diseases, such as worse physical functioning, mental health, and diabetes.[8,9,12,17]

Elderly Cognition

The ability to understand health care information is impacted by the cognitive function of older individuals. The cognitive changes with aging result from alteration in function, structure, and behavior.[13] Older individuals are viewed as having cognitive resources that are divided into sensory functioning, working memory, processing speed, and inhibition. The consequences of sensory impairment such as significant visual or hearing impairments are obvious; however, research has noted that when sensory impairments are corrected, older individuals may still have problems with accurate perception.[23]

Working memory involves the ability to use new information to complete tasks, which mandates cognitive processes to retain, work with, and transform the information.[24] Older individuals often have a decrease in their working memory. Processing speed is the blending of various cognitive functions to complete tasks in a timed situation.[23] The older individual's processing speed is slowed. Older individuals also struggle with ignoring irrelevant information, which leads to distraction when completing a task.[24] These changes are general observations for the older population; they vary from individual to individual and are impacted by disease processes.

Culture

The need for health care professionals to provide culturally competent care has evolved over the last 50 years, especially as the diversity of the US population has continued to grow. Models have been developed to guide health care professionals in understanding various cultures or developing cultural competence skills.[25-28] To maximize the health literacy of an individual, health care and information should be provided in a manner that is congruent with the cultural values of the patient whenever possible.[29] The only way to determine congruency is for the health care professional to become familiar with the patient's culture, including health care values and language. When assessing a patient, the health care provider needs to understand the patient's perception of the problem including the cause, how the illness impacts the patient, the illness severity, and treatment.[27]

Although English is the predominant and official language of the United States, the number of individuals who do not have English as their first language is increasing.[30] Key to adequate health literacy is being able to communicate in a language that is understood by both the patient and the health care provider. The NAAL 2003 clearly demonstrates that components of culture such as language are associated with health literacy. Individuals who spoke another language (not English) prior to their formal education years have lower health literacy than those who spoke English only or English and another language.[1]

● OUTCOMES ASSOCIATED WITH HEALTH ILLITERACY

Low health literacy in the older population has been associated with significant deficits in health knowledge, specifically concerning anticoagulation, chronic diseases, and medications.[10,11,21] Examples of these outcomes noted in the literature include patients with asthma unable to correctly use their inhaler, patients with diabetes unable to detect signs and symptoms of hypoglycemia, and individuals less likely to understand health care information advertised on the television.[31,32] In addition,

geriatric individuals with low health literacy are more likely to be hospitalized and utilize fewer preventive health care services.[9,12] Besides health outcomes, the cost of low health literacy impacts society. Older individuals with low health literacy had higher emergency room and inpatient care costs when compared to those with adequate health literacy.[33] The geriatric patients are at risk for low health literacy due to cognitive changes that occur with age and disease, and multiple demographic and socioeconomic factors that impact health literacy. The difficulties faced by these individuals are understandable and a challenge for the patient and health care provider. Health care providers are obligated to recognize individuals at risk for low health literacy and utilize approaches/interventions that will help increase the knowledge of these individuals, and in the end, increase health literacy.

● ASSESSMENT OF HEALTH LITERACY

Identifying who has low health literacy can be difficult.[34] The NAAL shows that individuals who graduate from high school and college can still have low health literacy.[2] There are several approaches used to identify whether a patient has adequate health literacy. Tools to measure health literacy have been developed over the past 15 years; however, no universally accepted tool to use in the clinical setting has emerged.[35] Due to numerous factors, the current sentiment among health literacy experts does not support formal testing of patients.[36] However, knowledge about health literacy assessment/testing is critical to a full understanding the current knowledge about health literacy.

Educational Attainment

One of the most common approaches to assessing health literacy (although not the most accurate) is to ask for the patient's education level. This approach assumes that a patient's highest level of education correlates with his or her ability to read material written at a certain grade level. Unfortunately, this correlation does not exist, and research has shown that patients' health literacy level is usually two grades less than the stated grade completed.[19] Educational attainment should only be used in conjunction with other health literacy assessment processes.

Assessment Tools

In an effort to formally identify the health literacy level of patients, health care practitioners and researchers attempted to develop tools that are efficient and effective in determining those patients with low health literacy in the clinical setting. The first tools developed had the ability to accurately identify those with low health literacy and worked well in the research setting, but were found to be cumbersome to implement in the everyday clinical setting. The health literacy tools most often found in the literature include the Rapid Estimate of Adult Literacy in Medicine (REALM), the Test for Functional Health Literacy in Adults (TOFHLA), and the Newest Vital Sign (NVS).[37-39] These tools have been used in research studies and rarely for clinical purposes. REALM and TOFHLA have been extensively evaluated. TOFHLA is the tool most often used now in the research setting. This tool even in its shortened form takes 7 to 8 minutes on average to administer. REALM has undergone revision and in its shortened form takes an average of 3 to 5 minutes to administer. NVS takes the least amount of time to administer, with an average of 2 to 3 minutes for completion.[39,40] Providers continued to look for efficient ways to identify patients with low health literacy. Several health care providers have developed tools that have a single-item screener. The screener asks one question and takes less than 1 minute to administer.[21,41,42] This tool offers another perspective on the skills needed to have adequate health literacy and a way to identify patients who lack skills to achieve adequate health literacy.

Rapid Estimate of Adult Literacy in Medicine

Rapid Estimate of Adult Literacy in Medicine (REALM) is a 66-word recognition test that begins with one-syllable health-related words and progresses to multi-syllable words. The words are arranged in three columns beginning with one-syllable words like *fat*, *pill*, and *eye*, and progressing to multi-syllable words like *osteoporosis*, *impetigo*, and *gonorrhea*. The patient is asked to read the word aloud starting with the first column. The patient reads down the list until the patient can read no further. The patient is then asked to review the remaining words and pronounce any other words. The words that are pronounced correctly become the raw score. The raw scores are converted into a reading grade range. A raw score of 0 to 18 correlates with a reading level of third grade or below, a score of 19 to 44 correlates with a fourth- to sixth-grade reading level, a score of 45 to 60 correlates with a seventh- to eighth-grade reading level, and 61 to 66 indicates a reading level of ninth grade and above.[37] Although REALM, which reports the grade level, correlates well with other standardized reading tests, it does not examine all skills needed for adequate health literacy. Some critics question whether it measures the comprehension and numeracy skills needed to function in today's health care environment.[43] Additionally, researchers have shown that the results of REALM are not consistent across racial groups.[44] The benefit of a tool that can be used quickly in the clinical setting must be weighed against the potential that it does not adequately evaluate all the health literacy skills required to function in the health care environment.

The Newest Vital Sign

Newest Vital Sign (NVS) is the most recently developed health literacy tool to provide a quick way for health care professionals to assess health literacy. It is available in English and Spanish. NVS uses a nutritional label from an ice cream container and six questions that focus on literacy and numeracy. The NVS score ranges from 0 to 6, with a score greater than 4 indicating adequate health literacy and a score less than 2 indicating inadequate health literacy skills. The average time to complete this tool is 3 minutes.[39] NVS was more likely to misclassify adequate health literacy as inadequate health literacy when compared with REALM and the short

TOFHLA,[45] though it has been seen by patients as a relevant link to a health-related skill of reading nutrition labels.

Test for Functional Health Literacy in Adults

Test for Functional Health Literacy in Adults (TOFHLA) was developed to assess functional health literacy using health-related material that a patient would encounter when interacting in a health care setting. For research purposes, this tool has become the instrument of choice. The items used include prescription vials, appointment slips, informed consents, information regarding an upper GI x-ray, or Medicare forms. The reading section uses a modified Cloze method in which a blank is inserted every 5 to 7 words. The patient then has to choose from a list of words to fill in the blank. The numeracy section involves reading instructions that involve numbers, such as a prescription label, and answering questions about the readings. The recommended scoring of this tool is on a scale of 0 to 100. A score of 0 to 59 is considered inadequate functional health literacy, a score from 60 to 74 is considered marginal functional health literacy, and a score from 75 to 100 is considered adequate functional health literacy. TOFHLA is the only health literacy tool that has been translated into Spanish. The short TOFHLA takes about 7 minutes to complete and the full TOFHLA takes about 22 minutes to complete.[38] Disadvantages of TOFHLA are the length of time to complete and the fact that it is not public domain and is only available for a fee.

Single-Item Question Screens

Health care providers have recently developed and tested a single-question screener to identify patients who may be at risk for inadequate health literacy. Several single-item questions have been evaluated. Questions include: How happy are you with the way you read? How often do you have someone help you read hospital materials? How often do you need to have someone help you when you read instructions, pamphlets, or other written material from your doctor or pharmacy? How confident are you filling out medical forms by yourself?

The questions focus on asking the patients if they need help reading written health care information or do they feel confident in completing medical forms by themselves.[21,34,41,42,46] If a patient indicates that he or she needs help with reading materials or does not feel confident in completing medical forms, then the health care profession should suspect that that this patient may have inadequate health literacy.

Learning Styles

The Institute of Medicine encourages providers to use more informal approaches to determine their patients' health literacy levels and learning styles. This can be done by asking questions related to the patients learning style. Examples of questions: How do you learn best? What kinds of learning material are you most comfortable with: visual, oral, or printed material? The answers to these questions can help providers identify health literacy deficits and design education that matches the health literacy demands of the patient.[4]

UNIVERSAL APPROACH FOR HEALTH LITERACY

During the same time period when tools were being developed, the health care industry was being increasing pressured to be more productive, resulting in health care practitioners assessing more patients in a shorter amount of time. When the time of an average health care visit is 18 minutes, taking time to administer a formal health literacy test is not an effective use of time.[47] Practitioners also began to realize that all patients, regardless of their health literacy levels, struggle to understand health information when dealing with an illness. In addition, it was noted that patients may feel shame when being tested and turn the health care encounter into a negative experience. A study that looked at patient's shame related to health literacy found that almost half (47.6%) of the patients with low health literacy admitted feeling embarrassed and ashamed about their inability to read.[48]

Based on these factors, most practitioners and health care facilities are not pursuing formal health literacy testing. Instead, providers are attempting to meet the health literacy demands of older adults by understanding the meaning of health literacy, the prevalence of low health literacy in the practice setting (especially with the elderly population), subtle patient behaviors that suggest low health literacy, and teaching methods to use with patients of all different health literacy levels. At this point in time there is no known benefit to using health literacy screening tools in clinical practice.[36] Instead, the suggestion is to use the Universal Precautions approach related to health literacy.[49] This approach assumes a uniform procedure in patient care and interactions. By using this approach to address every patient's health literacy needs, without regard to socioeconomic, ethnic, age, or educational background, the end result is that information is provided in simple, everyday language (Table 11–1).[49]

Suitability Assessment of Materials

When evaluating the appropriateness of health education material, the Suitability Assessment of Materials (SAM) provides the health care provider with a scoring guideline to assist in determining the suitability of written information.[50] SAM was developed by Doak, Doak, and Root as a validated tool to assess the suitability of health care information. SAM focuses on several areas: content criteria, literacy demand, graphics, layout and typography, learning stimulation and motivation, and cultural appropriateness.

Teach-Back Technique

One of the best methods to determine if the patient understands health care information and/or instructions is to have the patient teach the information back to the health care provider. This is known as the "teach-back" technique.[34] This approach is commonly used in the hospital environment when teaching a complicated task such as a dressing change or exercises, to confirm that the patient understands the task. However, this technique can be used in any health care setting.

Teaching Terminology

The words that are used by health care providers can be a communication barrier to patients. Banja stressed that medical jargon affects all patients and that physicians are infamous for using vocabulary that far surpasses many patients' understanding.[51] Verbal instruction is the most common way health care providers teach patients. Patients report that it would be helpful if health care providers were aware that patients do not understand many medical terms.[48] Providing education in simple everyday language rather than complex medical terms promotes understanding of health information.

● TABLE 11–1 Health Literacy Intervention Strategies

Intervention Strategy	Description
Suitability Assessment of Materials (SAM)	A tool to determine the suitability of written health information and provide information on how to write appropriate health material.
Written document readability	Written information needs to be in simple language, at the lowest reading level possible, in at least 14-point font.
Audiovisual aids	Audiovisual aids provide another way to learn. Common examples of audiovisual aids include videos/DVDs, pictures, computer programs, and models. Audiovisual aids support learning through multiple senses.
Teaching terminology	When teaching, the terminology should be clear and understood by the patient avoiding the use of medical jargon.
Utilization of past experiences	Learning is enhanced in older individuals when new information is connected to past experiences.
Use of support person(s)	The support person assists the individual in remembering and understanding health care instructions during and after the interaction with the health care provider.
Interpreter	Key to adequate health literacy is being able to communicate in a language that is understood by both the patient and the health care provider.
Cultural broker	A member of the community, such as a health care professional, leader, or respected elder, who aids the patient and the health care provider in reaching mutual understanding of the health care issues.
System nonclinical intervention	Interventions that occur outside of the clinical interaction and aid in meeting the health literacy demands of the older adult population. Intervention examples include assistance with document completion, appropriate signage, and user-friendly phone systems.

Audiovisual Aids

While providing written health care material is a common educational approach, several other approaches using various sensory organs are available.[52] Examples of audiovisual aids include videos, computer assisted programs, pictures, audiovisual aids, multimedia, and bullet lists.

• SUPPORT PERSON(S)

For patients who exhibit signs of low health literacy, the health care practitioner may recommend that the individual utilize a support person. The support person accompanies the patient during interactions with health care providers; especially when critical health care information or decisions are being discussed. New technology offers creative ways to have a support person engaged even if he or she cannot be physically present.

Interpreters/Cultural Brokers

Recent mandates by the federal government through the Office of Minority Health clearly describe the language services required to support patients in the health care setting. The availability of a trained and certified interpreter is essential for the full understanding of health care information in patients who speak languages other than English.[53]

Often there are cultural barriers besides language that impact an older individual's ability to comprehend health information. To overcome these barriers, a cultural broker is utilized. A cultural broker is an individual who works between the patient and Western medicine when the services of an interpreter are not sufficient.[54] The cultural broker is a member of the community, such as a health care professional, leader, or respected elder, who aids the patient and the health care provider in reaching mutual understanding of the health care issues.

To understand Mr. Taylor's situation better, the health care provider will need to determine what the barriers are and what can be done to eliminate the barriers. By understanding Mr. Taylor's health literacy level, the provider will effectively treat Mr. Taylor by individualizing the education and communication.

Clinical assessment of health literacy is usually an informal process. One of the ways to identify patients with low health literacy is to look for certain behaviors and responses that are often subtle. Subtle patient behaviors that may indicate low health literacy include repeatedly not having reading glasses, exhibiting unusually angry behavior when asked to complete forms, lack of adherence with medical regimen, and asking to review information with significant other before making health care decisions. The patient with low health literacy may fail to complete, or give inaccurate information on, registration forms, frequently miss appointments, and not follow up with referrals for lab work, x-rays, and specialists. Further behaviors related to medical regimens may be noted such as patients stating that they are following recommendations and taking medication but the laboratory tests or other parameters show no improvement. Other indicators are the inability of the patient to name the medications, explain the purpose of medications, or explain the routine timing of the medications. Refer to the list of subtle behaviors in Table 11–2. Knowledge of these behaviors as well as the risk factors for low health literacy will guide health care professionals in providing education at the appropriate health literacy level.[34]

CASE PRESENTATION 1 (continued)

Mr. John Taylor has come to the office for a follow-up visit after being diagnosed with type 2 diabetes 3 months ago. Mr. Taylor has voiced his surprise at the diagnosis since he states that no one in his family has diabetes. He was placed on medication and a no-concentrated-sweet diet but neglects to mention that he does not know what "concentrated sweets" are. There is a concern because his diabetic lab work shows no improvement. His hemoglobin A_{1c} was 9.4%, up from the time of diagnosis of 8.7%. Mr. Taylor insists he is taking his medication at supper each day, has 3 days' worth left, and is hoping to get a new prescription today. When questioned about his diet, he says that he has stopped eating snacks and only eats three times a day. He states he never learned to cook and since the death of his wife last year has been eating frozen meals. He says that he has switched to the meals that say "healthy" on them. He understands that he needs to keep the amount of sugar down and he feels he has done this.

• TABLE 11–2 Low Health Literacy Behaviors

Behaviors
Incomplete and/or inaccurate registration forms
Missed appointments or comes on incorrect date or at incorrect time
Does not adhere to medication regimen
Does not complete tests or referrals to consultants
Lab tests and physiologic responses indicate that patient is not following treatment plan
Becomes unusually angry when asked about the completion of a particular form
Simply nods "yes" to all questions
Fills out forms incorrectly or inconsistently

Responses to Written Materials
Forgot glasses and wants to read material at home or wants health care team to read
Does not even accept or glance at any written material offered
Wants to discuss all care decisions with family at home or simply passes materials to family
Demonstrates undue anger when presented with forms
Focuses attention on something else when talking about written material

Responses to Questions about Treatment Plan
Unable to state medication names, purposes, or administration
Unable to describe tests and purpose

CASE PRESENTATION 1 (continued)

During the visit with Mr. Taylor his lab values are discussed. His diet becomes the focus of the discussion once he acknowledges that he has been very religious about taking his medications daily. He does not like fruits or vegetables. You explain to him that while these "healthy" dinners might be better choices, he will need to look at the nutritional label to see what the number of calories is and the amount of carbohydrates in the dinner. He states, "I have been doing everything I can. I do not know what else you expect me to change." He becomes more anxious, looking at the floor and avoiding any type of eye contact. While it is known that Mr. Taylor is educated, he is having trouble understanding the dietary restrictions that have been imposed because of his diabetes. Here is an opportunity to assess Mr. Taylor's health literacy level by asking "Mr. Taylor, how do you learn best? Is it by looking at diagrams that explain the information, or by talking with someone about the information, or reading a booklet?" Mr. Taylor states, "I do best if I can see an example of what I need to understand. Sometimes I do not understand what is being told to me, and if the directions are just a bunch of words I seem to get lost."

By understanding that Mr. Taylor's low health literacy is a barrier to his success in following the prescribed treatment regimen, you as the health care provider can help by providing information in a manner that is understandable to him. For Mr. Taylor it appears that having visual aids with brief written educational material would be most helpful. One suggestion would be to give Mr. Taylor information on the appropriate amount of carbohydrates for a meal. If possible, it would be helpful to have a nutritional label to review with him. Encourage him to take the time in the grocery store to read the labels of the prepared foods he plans on purchasing. Since he has told you that he does best with words and pictures you can pre-select the diabetic information that will be best for him.

● EVALUATION OF WRITTEN MATERIAL: SUITABILITY ASSESSMENT OF MATERIALS (SAM)

When evaluating the appropriateness of health education material, Suitability Assessment of Materials (SAM) provides the health care provider with a scoring guideline to assist in determining the suitability of written information.[50] SAM focuses on several areas: content criteria, literacy demand, graphics, layout and typography, learning stimulation and motivation, and cultural appropriateness. To view the specific SAM criteria and scoring system, please refer to http://www.beginningsguides.net/pdfs/SAM-for-Beginnings.pdf. The best

time to evaluate the educational material you use in your practice is when it is first presented to you. Having an understanding of the suitability of the educational material will help in providing the best educational information for each of your patients.

For content criteria, SAM evaluates purpose, content topics, scope, and summary/review. Excellent written patient education has a clear purpose, focuses on essential information for the patient, and has a concise summary.[50] It would be helpful for Mr. Taylor if the purpose of the information provided focused on making good food choices and provided him with examples of what those choices might be. It would be helpful if the information summarized the most important points at the end of the document in a simple, easy-to-read manner.

CASE PRESENTATION 1 (continued)

To help Mr. Taylor understand the dietary information, you look for material that has diagrams, written information, and examples that will help him understand his diet. At the end of the information sheet you then summarize the most important information for him to understand. You also discuss that it might be a good time to meet with a dietitian who will be able to go over the information in more depth.

The next consideration is assessing the literacy demands of the material. This includes the need to review the reading level, writing style, vocabulary, context, and learning aids. Superior patient education material contains common everyday words, explanation of medical terminology, organizers (ie, subheadings), and context information to prepare the patient for the next information in the text.[50] Although all criteria in SAM are important, making sure that the readability level is appropriate is a major priority. Readability refers to how difficult a written passage is to read.[50]

The most frequently used formulas to measure the readability of health care information noted in the literature include the Flesch-Kincaid and McLaughlin's Simple Measure of Gobbledygook (SMOG).[55] The Flesch-Kincaid is very accessible, since it is part of the Microsoft Word program located with the spell-check function. However, care must be taken when using this formula because it tends to place the reading level lower than it actually is when compared to SMOG.[56,57] SMOG has been found to be the most accurate and overall best to use.[55] SMOG can be calculated either manually or by a computer-based program. The computer-based program requires that a minimum of 30 sentences or a maximum of 2000 words be placed in software to calculate an accurate grade level. The website is easy to use and is located at http://www.harrymclaughlin.com/SMOG.htm.

Doak, Doak and Root recommend a sixth-grade reading level for health-related text. The sixth grade was chosen because approximately 75 percent of all Americans can read at this level without difficulty.[50] Several research studies have examined the best way to educate older adult patients with written health care information. One study took place in three rural hospital emergency rooms where an individualized discharge sheet (a geragogy-based medication instruction) was given to elderly patients versus the usual discharge information. Geragogy focuses on how geriatric adults learn and considers their special needs. The results of this study showed that older individuals who received the individualized discharge sheets geared toward older individuals showed an increased knowledge about the prescribed medications when compared to older individuals who received the usual standard discharge information.[58]

CASE PRESENTATION 1 (continued)

Mr. Taylor confides in you that there is a lot of information that he does not understand. You ask him to bring in a copy of this information on his next visit so that you can see what he has been using. You think about the information available from the Centers for Disease Control and Prevention, and especially the book "Take Charge of Your Diabetes," which you have used in the past. You find that the font size is large, the use of illustrations is good, and there seems to be a lot of white space on each page. Taking 10 sentences from the beginning, middle, and end of the book and placing them into the SMOG calculator, you find that the book is written at an 8.86 grade level.

The next section of SAM evaluates learning stimulation and motivation, which includes interaction, behavioral modeling, and motivation in the written information. Excellent educational material promotes interaction with the reader through problems or questions, and models specific behavior for the patient. Also complex topics are divided into small parts so the learner can accomplish small successes before moving on to the next part of the information.[50] The following nutritional information and questions about a frozen dinner appear in a diabetic information pamphlet and demonstrate how to engage the patient in the learning activity.

A healthy frozen pasta and fish dinner has the following nutritional information:

Calories 290
Total fat 8 g
Cholesterol 30 mg
Sodium 590 mg
Potassium 510 mg
Total carbohydrate 40 g
Protein 15 g

What is the total carbohydrate and protein in this dinner?

a. 30 mg, 510 mg
b. 290, 8 g
c. 40 g, 15 g
d. 9 g, 2 g

The correct answer can be found on the next page.

The final set of criteria involves cultural appropriateness, which examines cultural match (logic, language, experiences) and cultural image and examples. Superior written information has key concepts and ideas that match the target culture, and images and examples present the culture in a positive manner.[50]

CASE PRESENTATION 1 (continued)

To provide nutritional information that is a cultural match, you inquire about Mr. Taylor's favorite foods, including those that he has enjoyed since his childhood. Mr. Taylor states that he really enjoys Italian foods such as pasta and Italian bread (both his wife and mother were great Italian cooks). He also enjoys sweets such as cookies and ice cream, but has stopped eating them due to the diabetes. He states that he is eating his usual amount of pasta and bread. Because Italian food is culturally important to Mr. Taylor, you recognize that you need to make recommendations about his diet that continue to include Italian foods, but find substitutes for the pasta and bread, which contain large amounts of carbohydrates. You discuss the carbohydrate content of pasta and bread and the need for him eat less pasta and bread and more proteins such as chicken and beef, which are part of Italian dishes. You encourage him to talk about foods that are important to him with the dietician so that they can find ways to keep these foods in his diet, but decrease the overall carbohydrate content.

Mr. Taylor is engaged in the information you provided as he is able to answer the questions that are at the end of each section. He is starting to ask more questions about what should be included in his diet and comments that he might need to bring his friend Harry with him to see the dietitian since the two of them have started to eat more meals together. He comments that "two heads are always better than one." You encourage Mr. Taylor to bring his friend and any family members who might help him. He tells you that his daughter lives in another state and he and Harry try to help each other out. As you walk out of the exam room Mr. Taylor thanks you for spending the time with him and tells you that he feels better about what he needs to do. "I will start checking labels on my food and will set up the appointment with the dietitian as soon as I can."

Although SAM was designed to evaluate written patient education materials, it is an excellent tool to use when developing new patient education. The criterion guides the author in developing appropriate written information. The website with specific SAM criteria is located in the Health Literacy Resource (Table 11–3).

● **TABLE 11–3** Health Literacy Resources

Resource	Web Address
American Medical Association Foundation *The Health Literacy and Patient Safety: Help Patients Understand Educational Kit*	http://www.ama-assn.org/ama/pub/about-ama/our-people/affiliated-groups/ama-foundation/our-programs/public-health/health-literacy-program/health-literacy-kit.shtml
Partnership for Clear Communication *Clear Communication Askme3*	http://www.npsf.org/askme3
US Department of Health and Human Services Health Resources and Services Administration *Unified Health Communication 101: Addressing Health Literacy, Cultural Competency, and Limited English Proficiency is a free online learning resource*	http://www.hrsa.gov/healthliteracy/training.htm
Suitability Assessment of Materials (SAM) *Systematic method to objectively assess the suitability of health-related material*	http://www.beginningsguides.net/pdfs/SAM-for-Beginnings.pdf
Simple Measure of Gobbledygook *Measures readability of health-related material*	http://www.harrymclaughlin.com/SMOG.htm
Information on various cultural groups *Websites provide information on cultural groups*	http://erc.msh.org/mainpage.cfm?file=1.0htm&module=provider&language=English www.tcns.org

CASE PRESENTATION 2: LOW HEALTH LITERACY AND CULTURE

Mary Lopez is a 76-year-old female who presented to the hospital with a hip fracture sustained after a fall at home. Mary has been healthy with a past medical history limited to bunion surgery and childbirth. The orthopedist determines that Mary will need to have her hip surgically repaired. She is admitted to the orthopedic unit where her preparation for surgery begins. The staff reviews her outpatient office records, which state that Mary has low health literacy. Mary is a retired housekeeper who completed elementary education in Mexico before moving to the United States as a teenager. She speaks and understands English, but is it her second language after Spanish. Mary tells the staff that she is nervous about the surgery and would like to know what to expect before, during, and after the procedure.

● INFORMED CONSENT: THE TEACH-BACK METHOD AND UTILIZATION OF PAST EXPERIENCES

The goal of the consent process is to confirm and verify that the patient is informed before agreeing to have the surgery. The process of becoming informed involves the education of the patient. The providers chose to use the teach-back technique with Mary because it is an effective means of confirming whether a patient understands health care information. The teach-back method has been employed by health care providers for decades. However, its importance as a teaching strategy has been re-emphasized as our health care system places more demands on individuals to learn how to manage their health. In addition, the teach-back method has been associated with better health outcomes, lower health care costs, and increased patient safety.[59]

During the educational process, patients should not be asked if they understand, because they usually state "yes" whether or not they do understand. Instead, patients should ask to teach the information back to the provider to determine comprehension.[34] The teach-back technique is only effective if questions are framed in a manner that puts the responsibility for the patient's understanding on the provider and avoids the patient feeling embarrassment and shame. For example, the provider can ask the patient, "Can you tell me how you will be using this medication at home? I want to make sure that I have correctly explained how to use it," or "Could you please show me how to use the ointment so I can make sure that I have given you clear instructions."[34] Two important keys to successfully using this method are to not appear rushed, annoyed, or bored while using teach-back; and to assume that the teaching was faulty if a patient is unable to explain/demonstrate the information adequately.[34] If the patient fails to comprehend the information, the provider must teach in another manner or make other arrangements so that the patient receives appropriate support for optimal health.

CASE PRESENTATION 2 (continued)

In Mary's situation, the health care provider describes the surgical procedure, risks, and alternative treatments. The provider informs Mary that hip fracture surgery has the following risks: infection, blood clot formation, nerve and/or muscle damage, and non-healing of the bone. After this information is given to Mary, the provider states, "I want to make sure that I have been clear in describing the risks involved in having your hip fracture repaired. Could you please tell me in your own words the risks of having the surgery?" Mary responds, "If I have this surgery, I may get a blood disease and my bone will not heal." From Mary's response the provider knows that she does not totally comprehend the risks and cannot provide informed consent. The provider explains the risks in greater detail using simple language. "From this surgery you may get an infection. Germs can get into the place where the surgery is done and cause the area to get red, tender, swollen, and have pus. This will need to be treated with medication. Mary, can you describe this first risk so I can make sure that I have told you the information clearly?" Mary responds, "This is like the time I cut my finger. It got all red, sore, swollen, and had pus. So with this surgery there is a chance I could get the same problem." The provider continues, "Yes, that is right. You could also have a clot (thick clump of blood cells) form in your leg and possibly move into your heart, lungs, or brain, which could lead to a heart attack, breathing problems, or a stroke. Once again, I need to make sure that I am clear, so could you please tell me about this risk?" Mary states, "I had an aunt that had a stroke. So with this surgery, my blood could get clogged and it could cause problems with my heart, lungs, or brain." The provider goes on, "Yes, that's correct. With this surgery you can also have problems with the nerves and/or muscles in your leg, but this is rare. Please explain the last risks to make sure that I have explained the risks of surgery fully." Mary responds, "With this surgery I could have nerve, muscle, or bone problems in my leg, but it doesn't happen often." The provider states, "From your description of the risks, I feel that you understand the risks. Before we move on to the alternative treatments, do you have any questions?" Mary responds, "I do not have any questions about the risks."

By using the teach-back technique, the provider was able to determine Mary's comprehension and adjust teaching to increase her comprehension. The teach-back technique will also support the therapeutic provider–patient relationship. By the end of the consent process, the provider felt that the patient understood the information and signed the consent indicating that she was informed and agreed to the surgery.

● BUILDING ON PAST EXPERIENCES

During the teaching, Mary responded to the provider by using past experiences to give herself a foundation for new learning. Older adults naturally relate new learning to past experiences to assist them in comprehension.[60] A skilled provider utilizes this attribute of older individuals to teach new health information. If Mary did not comprehend the information, the provider could utilize her past experiences to link the new information to her previous knowledge. Using individuals' past experiences with the teach-back method provides an effective approach to teaching and verifying comprehension.

CASE PRESENTATION 2 (continued)

When Mary is having trouble understanding the risks, the provider utilizes her past knowledge. The provider says to Mary, "One of the risks of surgery is infection. Have you ever had an infection?" Mary replies, "Yes I had an infection on my finger last year." The provider asks, "How did your finger look and feel with the infection?" Mary states, "It was red, big, hurt, and some yellow liquid came out." The provider states, "With hip surgery, you can get an infection on the skin which would make the skin look and feel like your finger. You can also get an infection in the bone. Both of these risks are very small, less than three surgeries in one hundred. To make sure that I have clearly explained, can you tell me about the risk of infection with hip surgery?" Mary says, "I have a very small chance of getting an infection with this surgery. It may look and feel like my finger when it was infected. My bone could also get infected."

● AUDIOVISUAL AIDS: WHAT TO EXPECT BEFORE, DURING, AND AFTER SURGERY

Many audiovisual aids are available for health education. Examples include videos, pictures, computer programs, and models. For patients with low health literacy, using audiovisual strategies offers a way for patients to receive health information that does not tax their reading skills. However, many audiovisual strategies are not produced by the providers working with the patient and need to be evaluated for appropriateness. SAM, described in the previous case study, can also be used to evaluate the appropriateness of audiovisual materials.[50]

There are several other considerations when using audiovisual aids with older individuals. For changes in the older adult's vision, the teaching environment should be well lit, but not have a glare. Primary colors are the best to use and fine shades of colors such as blue, blue-green, or violet should be avoided because older individuals have difficulty discriminating shades of colors. Avoid describing pills by their colors because blue, green, and yellow pills may all appear gray to an older individual. When providing auditory education, the environment should be free of distracting noises. The health care professional needs to face the learner directly and keep his or her mouth uncovered. The pitch and rate of speaking are key; speaking in a low tone and slowly (not more than 140 words per minute) will promote appropriate auditory stimulation. The older individual will also need time to process the audiovisual information, so information should not be presented in a rushed manner and time should be available to ask questions and verify what the patient has learned.[60] Refer to Chapter 8 for further information on sensory changes associated with aging.

While interacting with the health care team, Mary indicated that she likes learning about health information from the local cable TV shows. The staff suggests that Mary view a DVD on hip surgery, which includes information on preparing for the surgery, what happens during surgery, and how to take care of herself after surgery. The DVD received an overall superior SAM criteria rating because the content was clear and focused, the literacy demand was low, detailed graphics depicted the teaching, learner involvement was present with each key point, and information about cultural differences was presented. The staff gave Mary a headset for the DVD and limited distracting noises. Mary was also offered the opportunity to view the DVD as often as she felt necessary, and then the provider asked Mary to describe what she had seen. Mary accurately described the key points of the surgery and recovery. At multiple points in this interaction, Mary was asked if she had any questions or needed further clarification.

• CULTURAL CONSIDERATIONS: RECOVERY PHASE

During her hospital admission the health care team asks Mary if she has any cultural or religious practices that would impact her surgery and recovery that she would like to tell the staff. Mary shares that it is important for her family members to be with her. The staff makes arrangements for at least one family member to stay with her at all times, and Mary's daughter stayed with her mother most of the time. The staff began to notice that Mary does little for herself and that her daughter often did things for Mary that she was capable of doing. Mary described herself as independent prior to her hip fracture and she desires to return to that level of independence once her hip is repaired. The staff became concerned.

The family is one of the most important social structures in Mexican-American culture. It is common for extended family members to live together or in close proximity (with frequent interaction). Family members often care for one another, and children feel that they need to care for parents who need help because their parents cared for them when they were young.[61] The Mexican-American culture also values having an interpersonal relationship with health care providers. With each interaction, the Mexican-American patient prefers to have a social exchange that personalizes the interaction.[61] The staff used this knowledge to approach Mary's daughter about her mother's recovery from hip surgery.

The health care provider enters Mary's room and asks about Mary's grandchildren and praises Mary's daughter for her concern about her mother and the support she has given her. The provider goes on to explain that he is concerned that Mary is not recovering as quickly as she could be because she is not doing as much as she is capable of doing for herself. The provider emphasizes that Mary will need to be mobile and take care of herself as much as possible to recover quickly from the surgery and avoid complications. The provider acknowledges the daughter's desire to help her mother, but states that the best way to help her mother is to encourage her to be independent. The daughter is encouraged to talk to the staff if her mother is having difficulty with a task, rather than just doing the task for her, so the staff can problem-solve with Mary and her daughter. Mary and her daughter state that they want Mary to be independent and want to avoid complications. Mary will try to complete as much as she can on her own and her daughter will communicate with the staff if Mary is having difficulty with a certain task.

In Mary's situation her culture clashed with health information about mobility and activities of daily living after surgery. The health care providers utilized knowledge about Mexican-American culture to help increase their understanding of Mary and her daughter's interactions, and to help them effectively discuss health concerns.

Although Mary did not need an interpreter because she spoke and understood English, she could not communicate via writing in Spanish or English, so providers need to consider a language barrier when addressing health literacy. If a language barrier exists, the health care provider needs to utilize an interpreter to overcome this barrier. The US Department of Health and Human Services, Office of Minority Health, developed the National Standards for Culturally and Linguistically Appropriate Services (CLAS).[53] The standards require language assistance services in a timely manner at all points of contact free of charge, provision of information in the preferred language, assurance of competent interpreters, and provision of information in the language used by the community served by the health care provider/facility.[53] One of the most challenging aspects of these standards is the non-use of family members and friends as interpreters unless requested by the patient. Most family members and friends do not have training to effectively interpret medical information. In most health care facilities, interpreter services are provided in person and via a phone service.

When working with a patient or patient population with cultural barriers that impede the restoration of health, a provider can consult a cultural broker. A cultural broker is an individual who works between the patient and Western medicine when the services of an interpreter are not sufficient.[54] The cultural broker is a member of the community, such as a health care professional, leader, or respected elder, who aids the patient/community and the health care provider in reaching mutual understanding of the health care issues.

● SUPPORT PERSON: PREPARING FOR DISCHARGE

CASE PRESENTATION 2 (continued)

Mary had surgery 2 days ago, and the staff started her discharge teaching. Despite using low health literacy strategies the staff realized that Mary was struggling with comprehending how to care for herself when she returned home. The staff identified that Mary needed a support person to aid her in remembering and organizing her care at home. As noted in the prior situation, Mary's daughter is very involved in the care of her mother. Upon discharge, Mary will be living with her daughter until she is able to return to her own home.

For patients who exhibit signs of low health literacy and are struggling with managing their health, the health care provider should recommend that the individual utilize a support person. The support person accompanies the patient during interactions with health care providers, especially when critical health care information or decisions are being discussed. New technology offers creative ways to have a support person engaged even if that person cannot be physically present. The use of the speaker phone option on current cell phones allows the support person to hear the information being shared with the patient and ask questions for clarification.

Although the use of a support person appears to be a simple intervention, it may be complicated to implement. An important element of this intervention is for the older individual to agree to a support person's presence during interactions with the health care system. If the health care professional is concerned that the patient will not be receptive to a support person, the provider needs to use expert interpersonal and communication skills to discuss the benefits of this intervention in a manner that does not cause the patient to feel unable to care for himself.

Another potential obstacle to this intervention is the availability of the support person. For the older individual, the most likely support person is a spouse, sibling, or child; however, it can be any individual chosen by the patient. Due to societal demands, the availability of this individual cannot be assured, and thus the intervention may not be available. One final consideration when implementing this intervention is the health literacy level of the support person. Inadequate health literacy of the support person cancels the benefit of this intervention.

CASE PRESENTATION 2 (continued)

Mary told the team that her daughter recently resigned her job as a secretary for an engineering company to spend more time with her children. During a social exchange with the provider, Mary's daughter states that in her secretarial position she developed written agendas for meetings and proofed material being sent out from the engineers. This information told the health care team that Mary's daughter was able to read and write, although it did not provide information on her level of understanding about health concepts. Mary's daughter commented that she prefers to learn through demonstration and have handouts available to use at home. Through the teach-back method the health care team was able to verify that Mary's daughter had adequate health literacy, comprehended the information, and was able to act as an advocate for her mother's health concerns.

The use of a support person can enhance the health literacy of older individuals, especially those with known inadequate literacy. An effective support person needs to have adequate health literacy, availability to participate in interactions with the health care team, and a strong desire to help individuals optimize their health.

● SYSTEM-LEVEL INTERVENTION

There are system-level, nonclinical interventions that assist in meeting patients' health literacy demands that need to be considered. Most of these interventions focus on patient interactions with support staff (non–health care providers) and facility systems such as phone systems and signage. A patient's encounter with the health care system usually begins with the administration staff interactions (secretaries, administrative assistants, and medical assistants).[62]

To meet the health literacy demands of patients, all staff need to approach patients with an attitude of helpfulness and utilize simple everyday language. This approach is beneficial when scheduling appointments/tests and assisting with forms. In addition, the staff should notify the health care provider when a patient needs assistance with completing forms or scheduling appointments/tests because this may be an indicator of inadequate health literacy. The phone system works well with those who have low health literacy when instructions are provided in plain and simple terms and an obvious opportunity to talk to a receptionist/operator is offered on the phone menu. Signage throughout a health care facility provides another opportunity to help patients with various health literacy levels. Signs throughout a facility should be clearly displayed; use consistent, plain, everyday terms; and have a consistent color scheme. Large facilities (hospitals and multiple specialty complexes) should have a welcome/information desk and clearly written maps displayed in various locations.[62]

CASE PRESENTATION 2 (continued)

Unfortunately, Mary's daughter needs to take care of her sick child on the day of her mother's follow-up appointment with the orthopedic surgeon. The only person available to take Mary to the appointment was her younger sister, who like Mary has Spanish as her first language, understands and speaks English fairly well, but cannot read either Spanish or English well. When Mary and her sister enter the facility, a staff member greets them at the welcome desk, asking them if they need assistance finding their doctor's office. The staff member gives them a simple map with hand-drawn arrows to show them exactly where to go. Mary has no difficulty finding the office because there are large color-coded signs throughout the facility. Mary and her sister arrive at the office, where the staff greet them with papers to be completed and offer to help Mary complete the paperwork. Mary provides the health information while the staff member completes the form. The staff member tells the orthopedic surgeon that Mary cannot read English well and needed help completing her forms. During the office visit, the surgeon provides information appropriate to Mary's health literacy level and speaks to her daughter via cell phone about the next stage of her recovery. When leaving, the staff offers to set up outpatient physical therapy and gives Mary instructions on how to get to the front door of the facility. Mary tells her daughter that her visit to the surgeon went smoothly and she understands the next step in her recovery process.

The staff and facility provided the necessary interventions for an older adult with inadequate health literacy like Mary to successfully complete an interaction with the health care system. Mary has a greater chance of having a positive health outcome from her hip fracture because she had a follow-up with her surgeon, understands what she needs to do, and has resources available to assist her in the recovery.

● SUMMARY

Large national studies have shown that older adults suffer more often from inadequate or low health literacy than any other age group in our population. Approximately 30% of those with low health literacy were older adults.[1] The cause of low health literacy in this population is associated with age-related changes in cognition and disease processes. Low health literacy has been linked to poor health outcomes and increased health care costs in the older adult population.[10,11,21] To meet the health literacy demands of this population, several interventions need to be used by health care providers and respective support staff.

Although identifying individuals with low health literacy would appear to be a logical first step, the assessment tools currently developed are too time consuming or inaccurate to be beneficial in the clinical setting. An understanding of health literacy assessment tools adds to the overall understanding of the issues with inadequate health literacy and interventions, but is not essential for working with low health literacy patients. However, there are subtle behaviors that can indicate that a patient suffers from low health literacy such as always forgetting reading glasses, needing help with forms, becoming unusually angry when being asked to complete forms, and missing appointments and tests.[34]

The second step in meeting the health literacy demands of a patient is for health care providers to approach the teaching of health care information using the concept of Universal Precautions. The health care provider assumes that all patients have low health literacy, and thus is prepared to provide information in a very simple clear manner and verifies that the patient understands or makes arrangements for the patient who does not understand.[49]

To provide information at the appropriate level, the provider can use SAM to evaluate written and audiovisual information or as a guide when developing information. SAM provides criteria to rate education material as superior, adequate, or unsuitable based on several factors (content criteria, literacy demand, graphics, layout and typography, learning stimulation and motivation, and cultural appropriateness).[51]

For the older adult, verbal and written health care information should be presented in simple, clear everyday language, and the reading level should be approximately sixth grade. Print should be at least 14-point size, illustrations or pictures should clearly show the information meant to convey, and there should be adequate white space. The information should highlight key points, and should be presented with subheadings (or in chunks) so the patient is not overwhelmed. In addition, the material should motivate the learner by having interaction sections and have appropriate material that reflects the culture of the learner. The SAM tool and related resources can be located at http://www.beginningsguides.net/pdfs/SAM-for-Beginnings.pdf.

Often health care providers verify that a patient understands health information by asking the patient if he or she understands. In most cases, patients state that they understand even if they do not. Thus other methods for verifying the comprehension of health information are needed. The teach-back technique is a method where the provider verifies understanding by asking the patient to teach what has been learned. When using the technique, the provider asks the patient to provide information in order to verify that the provider has been clear in giving instructions, thus taking away the shame associated with the patient not being able to understand. The provider must keep trying different educational methods or seek support of others if the patient is not able to understand how to care for himself or herself.

The older adult population benefits from a number of interventions during the educational process, including the following:

- Ask patients how they best learn, and provide information in that format.

- Consider cultural values and background that may impact understanding and use of health information.
- Relate new teaching to the learner's past experiences.
- Provide a well-lit teaching environment.
- Use primary colors and avoid fine shades of colors or colors such as blue, blue-green, or violet.
- Do not describe pills by their colors. Blue, green, and yellow pills may all appear gray to an older individual.
- Auditory education should be provided in a distraction-free environment with the health care professional facing the learner and the mouth uncovered. Speaking should be done in a low tone and slowly.
- Give the older individual time to process the audiovisual information and ask questions.[59]

RESOURCES

The number of resource regarding health literacy continues to grow. The AMA has developed a program that includes several different aspects of health literacy. The primary purpose of this is to raise the health care provider's awareness of health literacy. There are CEUs available with the content. Another good resource is the Partnership for Clear Communication sponsored by Pfizer. The program, called "Ask Me 3," provides information on health literacy for a variety of audiences including health care providers, patients, employers, and the media. The website provides brochures in English and Spanish. The patient brochures include information regarding the three most important questions to ask a doctor, nurse, or pharmacist. There is an entire program to assist health care providers in understanding and assisting their patients with low health literacy.

The US Department of Health Resources and Services Administration offers a free online training program—Unified Health Communication 101: Addressing Health Literacy, Cultural Competency and Limiter English Proficiency. The program and can be taken for credit (CEU/CE, CHES, CME, or CNE) or not for credit. The purpose of the program is to improve the health care provider's ability to communicate with patients and improve health outcomes. This program addresses skills regarding health literacy, cultural competency, and patient communication. A summary of resources with corresponding websites is contained in Table 11–3. You will also find a website with information on various cultural groups to help health care provides deliver quality care to multi-ethnic populations.

The older adult population experiences low health literacy at a higher rate than any other age group. To meet the literacy demands of this population, providers must recognize the prevalence of this issue in the older adult population, realize the impact on health outcomes and costs, and develop the skills necessary to provide and verify learning of health information in an effective manner. The interventions for low health literacy require specialized knowledge and persistence of the health care provider. The health care provider's goal of educating the patient to manage his or her health is not accomplished until the patient is able to describe how to care for himself or herself or, if that is not possible, an advocate with adequate health literacy is identified to support the older adult. Health outcomes depend on meeting the health literacy needs of the older population.

References

1. Kutner M, Greenberg E, Paulsen C. *The Health Literacy of America's Adults: Results from the 2003 National Assessment of Adult Literacy.* (NCES 2006-483). U.S.Department of Education.Washington, DC: National Center for Education Statistics.

2. White S. *Assessing the Nation's Health Literacy: Key Concepts and Findings of the National Assessment of Adult Literacy (NAAL).* American Medical Association Foundation; 2008. http://www.ama-assn.org/ama/pub/about-ama/ama-foundation/our-programs/health-literacy-program/assessing-nations-health.shtml

3. Tabloski P. *Gerontological Nursing.* Upper Saddle River, NJ: Pearson; 2006.

4. Nielsen-Bohlman L, Panzer AM, Kindig DA. *Health Literacy: A Prescription to End Confusion.* Washington, DC: National Academies Press; 2004.

5. US Department of Health and Human Services (HHS). *Healthy People 2010.* 2000. http://www.healthypeople.gov/document/html/uih/uih_2.htm.

6. Zarcadoolas C, Pleasant A, Greer DS. Understanding health literacy: An expanded model. *Health Promotion Int.* 2005;20:195-203.

7. National Center for Education Statistics, US Department of Education, Institute of Education Sciences. *National Assessment of Adult Literacy (NAAL): A First Look at the Literacy of America's Adults in the 21st Century.* NCES 2006-470:1; 2006.

8. Baker D, Gazmararian JA, Sudano J, Patterson M. The association between age and health literacy among elderly persons. *J Gerontol B Psychol SciSoc Sci.* 2000;55:S368-S374.

9. Baker D, Gazmararian JA, Williams MV, et al. Functional health literacy and the risk of hospital admission among Medicare managed care enrollees. *Am J Public Health.* 2002;92:1278-1283.

10. Gazmararian J, Baker D, Williams M, et al. Health literacy among Medicare enrollees in a managed care organization. *JAMA.* 1999; 281:545-551.

11. Scott TL, Gazmararian JA, Williams MV, Baker DW. Health literacy and preventive health care use among Medicare enrollees in a managed care organization. *Med Care.* 2002;40:395-404.

12. Wolf MS, Gazmararian JA, Baker DW. Health literacy and functional health status among older adults. *Arch Intern Med.* 2005; 165:1946-1952.

13. Cutilli CC. Health literacy in geriatric patients: An integrative review of the literature. *Orthop Nurs.* 2007;26:43-48. http://proxy.library.upenn.edu:2054/login.aspx?direct=true&db=cin20&AN=2009507554&site=ehost-live.

14. Buchbinder R, Hall S, Youd J. Functional health literacy of patients with rheumatoid arthritis attending a community-based rheumatology practice. *J Rheumatol.* 2006;33:879-886.

15. Wilson FL, Racine E, Tekieli V, Williams B. Literacy, readability and cultural barriers: Critical factors to consider when educating older African Americans about anticoagulation therapy. *J Clin Nurs.* 2003;12:275-282.

16. Benson JG, Forman WB. Comprehension of written health care information in an affluent geriatric retirement community: use of the Test of Functional Health Literacy. *Gerontology.* 2002;48:93-97.

17. Sudore R, Mehta K, Simonsick E, et al. Limited literacy in older people and disparities in health and healthcare access. *J Am Geriatr Soc.* 2006;54:770-776.

18. Williams MV, Parker RM, Baker DW, et al. Inadequate functional health literacy among patients at two public hospitals. *JAMA.* 1995;274:1677-1682.

19. Wilson FL, McLemore R. Patient literacy levels: A consideration when designing patient education programs. *Rehabil Nurs.* 1997;22:311-317.

20. DeWalt DA, Pignone M, Malone R, et al. Development and pilot testing of a disease management program for low literacy patients with heart failure. *Patient Educ Couns.* 2004;55:78-86.

21. Chew L, Bradley K, Boyko EJ. Brief questions to identify patients with inadequate health literacy. *Fam Med.* 2004;36:588-594.

22. Raehl CL, Bond CA, Woods TJ, et al. Screening tests for intended medication adherence among the elderly. *Ann Pharmacother.* 2006; 40:888-893.

23. Craik F, Salthouse T. *The Handbook of Aging and Cognition.* 2nd ed. Mahwah, NJ: Erlbaum; 2000.

24. Park D, Schwarz N. *Cognitive Aging: A Primer.* New York: Psychology Press Taylor & Francis Group; 2000.

25. Leininger M. Culture care theory: A major contribution to advance transcultural nursing and practices. *J Transcult Nurs.* 2002;13:189-192.

26. Giger JN. The Giger and Davidhizar Transcultural Model. *J Transcult Nurs.* 2002;13:185-188.

27. Kleinman A. *The Illness Narratives: Suffering, Healing, and the Human Condition.* New York: Basic Books; 1988.

28. Campinha-Bacote J. The process of cultural competence in the delivery of healthcare services: A model of care. *J Transcult Nurs.* 2002;13:181-184.

29. Cutilli CC. Do your patients understand? Providing culturally congruent patient education. *Orthop Nurs.* 2006;25:218-226. http://proxy.library.upenn.edu:2054/login.aspx?direct=true&db=cin20&AN=2009206870&site=ehost-live.

30. Grieco E. English Abilities of the US Foreign-Born Population. Updated 2003. http://wwww.migrationinformation.org/USfocus/display.cfm?id=84. Accessed July 9, 2009.

31. Williams MV, Baker DW, Parker RM, Nurss JR. Relationship of functional health literacy to patients' knowledge of their chronic disease. A study of patients with hypertension and diabetes. *Arch Intern Med.* 1998;158:166-172. http://proxy.library.upenn.edu:2054/login.aspx?direct=true&db=cin20&AN=2009795105&site=ehost-live.

32. Kaphingst KA, Rudd RE, DeJong W, et al. Literacy demands of product information intended to supplement television direct-to-customer prescription drug advertisement. *Patient Ed Counsel.* 2004;55:293-300.

33. Howard DH, Gazmararian J, Parker RM. The impact of low health literacy on the medical costs of Medicare managed care enrollees. *Am J Med.* 2005;118:371-377.

34. Weiss B. *Health Literacy and Patient Safety: Help Patients Understand.* Chicago: American Medical Association Foundation; 2007.

35. Johnson K, Weiss BD. How long does it take to assess literacy skills in clinical practice? *J Am Board Fam Med.* 2008;21:211-214.

36. Paasche-Orlow M, Wolf M. Evidence does not support clinical screening of literacy. *JGIM: J Gen Int Med.* 2008;23:100-102. http://proxy.library.upenn.edu:2054/login.aspx?direct=true&db=keh&AN=32486412&site=ehost-live.

37. Davis TC, Long SW, Jackson RH, et al. Rapid estimate of adult literacy in medicine: A shortened screening instrument. *Fam Med.* 1993;25:391-395.

38. Parker R, Baker D, Williams M, Nurss J. The test of functional health literacy in adults: A new instrument for measuring patients' literacy skills. *J Gen Intern Med.* 1995;10:537-541.

39. Weiss BD, Mays MZ, Martz W, et al. Quick assessment of literacy in primary care: The newest vital sign. *Ann Fam Med.* 2005;3:514-522.

40. Paasche-Orlow MK, Parker RM, Gazmararian JA, et al. The prevalence of limited health literacy. *J Gen Intern Med.* 2005;20:175-184.

41. Morris NS, MacLean CD, Chew LD, Littenberg B. The Single Item Literacy Screener: Evaluation of a brief instrument to identify limited reading ability. *BMC Fam Pract.* 2006;7:21.

42. Wallace LS, Rogers ES, Roskos SE, et al. Brief report: Screening items to identify patients with limited health literacy skills. *J Gen Intern Med.* 2006;21:874-877.

43. Mika VS, Kelly PJ, Price MA, et al. The ABCs of health literacy. *Fam Commun Health.* 2005;28:351-357.

44. Shea JA, Beers BB, McDonald VJ, et al. Assessing health literacy in African American and Caucasian adults: Disparities in rapid estimate of adult literacy in medicine (REALM) scores. [see comment.] *Fam Med.* 2004;36:575-581.

45. Osborn CY, Weiss BD, Davis TC, et al. Measuring adult literacy in health care: Performance of the newest vital sign. *Am J Health Behav.* 2007;31:S36-S46.

46. Cornett S. Assessing and addressing health literacy. *OJIN: Online J Issues Nurs.* 2009;14.

47. Grey L. Rx for time crunched physicians: Communication skills that increase physician efficiency and patient satisfaction. *University of Washington News.* July 14, 2008.

48. Wolf MS, Williams MV, Parker RM, et al. Patients' shame and attitudes toward discussing the results of literacy screening. *J Health Communication.* 2007;12:721-732.

49. Brown DR, Ludwig R, Buck GA, et al. Health literacy: Universal precautions needed. *J Allied Health.* 2004;33:150-155.

50. Doak C, Doak L, Root J. *Teaching Patients with Low Literacy Skills.* 2nd ed. Philadelphia: Lippincott; 1996.

51. Banja J. My what? *Am J Bioethics.* 2007;7:13-14.

52. Schwartzberg JG, Cowett A, VanGeest J, Wolf MS. Communication techniques for patients with low health literacy: A survey of physicians, nurses, and pharmacists. *Am J Health Behav.* 2007;31:S96-S104. http://proxy.library.upenn.edu:2054/login.aspx?direct=true&db=cin20&AN=2009658222&site=ehost-live.

53. US Department of Health and Human Services, Office of Minority Health. National Standards for Culturally and Linguistically Appropriate Services in Health Care, Executive Summary. 2001.

54. Rankin SH, Stallings KD. *Patient Education: Principles & Practice.* 4th ed. Philadelphia: Lippincott Williams & Wilkins; 2001.

55. Daly JM, Jogerst GJ. Readability and content of elder abuse instruments. *J Elder Abuse Neglect.* 2005;17:31-52.

56. Ledbetter C, Hall S, Swanson JM. Readability of commercial versus generic health instructions for condoms. *Health Care Women Int.* 1990;11:295-304.

57. DuBay WH. The principles of readability. *Online Submission.* 2004;76.

58. Hayes KS. Randomized trial of geragogy-based medication instruction in the emergency department. *Nurs Res.* 1998;47:211-218.

59. Flowers L. Teach-back improves informed consent. *OR Manager.* 2006;22:25-26.

60. Bastable S. *Nurse as Educator: Principles of Teaching and Learning for Nursing Practice.* Sudbury, MA: Jones & Bartlett; 2003.

61. Leininger M, McFarland MR. *Transcultural Nursing: Concepts, Theories, Research & Practice.* 3rd ed. New York: McGraw-Hill; 2002.

62. Rudd RE, Anderson JE. The Health Literacy Environments of Hospitals and Health Centers, Partners for Action: Making Your Healthcare Facility Literacy-Friendly. Updated 2007. http://www.hsph.harvard.edu/healthliteracy/HealthLiteracyEnvironment.pdf?id=1163. Accessed February 6, 2010.

POST-TEST

1. **An important key to successful use of teach-back technique is that the:**
   A. Patient describes care in a detailed manner using correct medical terminology
   B. Provider must schedule at least 30 minutes of time for the education
   C. Patient is responsible for all education and must get help if not understanding
   D. Provider appears interested and assumes fault if teaching is not understood

2. **Along with number of syllables in a word, which factor impacts the readability of educational materials?**
   A. Length of sentence
   B. Number of pages
   C. Number of vowels and consonants
   D. Passive voice

3. **The best way to explain health care information to patients is to:**
   A. Use proper medical terminology to describe all aspects of information
   B. Instruct the patient to read the health care information in a brochure
   C. Use simple everyday language and explain medical terms
   D. Instruct the patient to review an educational video at the end of the office visit

ANSWERS TO PRE-TEST

1. B
2. B
3. D

ANSWERS TO POST-TEST

1. D
2. A
3. C

12

Approach to Laboratory Testing and Imaging in Aging

Allan S. Brett, MD

Caroline Powell, MD

● **LEARNING OBJECTIVES**

1. Discuss questions that clinicians should consider before ordering a clinical or imaging test.
2. Describe two tests where "normal" values in older adults often indicate clinical or subclinical disease states.
3. Define and list at least one type of "incidentaloma."
4. Describe two circumstances where the "spectrum effect" may alter the diagnostic accuracy of a test when utilized on older adults.

PRE-TEST

1. **Which of the following is the KEY requirement to justify screening for a particular disease in asymptomatic persons?**

   A. A test is available that can detect the disease.

   B. A test is available that can detect the disease before it becomes symptomatic.

   C. A treatment exists for the disease that will add significant years to the life span.

   D. A test is available that can detect the disease when asymptomatic and so can reduce long-term morbidity or mortality.

2. **In deciding whether the benefits of a diagnostic test outweigh the harm in an elderly person, which of the following is the LEAST important consideration?**

   A. The patient's preferences

   B. The patient's co-morbidities

   C. The patient's specific age

   D. The discomfort or burdens associated with testing

3. **In general, the range of "normal" is unrelated to age for which of the following tests?**

   A. Glomerular filtration rate

   B. Hemoglobin and hematocrit

   C. Forced vital capacity on pulmonary function testing

   D. Bone mineral density

● GENERAL OVERVIEW

Basic Concepts

CASE PRESENTATION 1

A 75-year-old man presents with a several-week history of persistent upper abdominal discomfort and poor appetite; he thinks he might have lost 5 or 10 pounds during this interval, and his daughter has noted yellowish discoloration in his eyes. A physical exam clearly reveals scleral icterus; his mid-abdomen and right upper quadrant are mildly tender, without any definite mass or organomegaly.

CASE PRESENTATION 2

A 75-year-old man presents with a several-week history of intermittent upper abdominal discomfort, usually relieved with antacids. He has had similar episodes over many years that resolve spontaneously; this episode has lasted a bit longer, prompting a visit to the physician. The patient is not sure whether symptoms are consistently related to eating. There is no weight loss, and appetite and bowel movements are normal. He takes one aspirin daily for cardiovascular prophylaxis. Physical examination is entirely normal.

The primary purpose of diagnostic testing is to inform clinical reasoning and decision-making in order to benefit patients. When tests are chosen rationally and performed appropriately, they reduce clinical uncertainty by increasing or decreasing the likelihood of various diagnostic considerations. In some cases, the main goal is to "rule in" one of several plausible conditions suggested by the patient's clinical presentation. For example, the patient in Case 1 clearly has a hepatobiliary disorder that is likely obstructive (eg, pancreatic cancer or a common bile duct stone), but could conceivably represent a hepatocellular process (eg, viral or drug-induced hepatitis). Blood testing and imaging will almost certainly confirm one of these disorders. In contrast, in other cases the main goal is to "rule out" an unlikely but lethal diagnosis, and not necessarily to arrive at a specific medical explanation for the patient's symptoms. For example, the clinician in Case 2 will consider ordering an upper endoscopy to rule out gastric cancer or peptic ulcer in an older person with vague dyspepsia. Although the absence of "alarm" symptoms and the suggestion that these symptoms are chronic and recurrent suggest a low probability of cancer, the clinical impression (based on the history and physical examination) may not be sufficiently accurate in this case.[1,2] In both Cases 1 and 2, the clinician starts—overtly or subliminally—with some idea about the likelihood of certain clinical entities (so-called "pre-test probabilities"), and assumes that testing will provide additional information that reduces uncertainty.

Concepts that convey the accuracy of diagnostic testing—sensitivity, specificity, and predictive value—are discussed thoroughly in numerous textbooks, review articles, and websites, and are summarized in Table 12–1. In brief, the intrinsic relationship between a diagnostic test and a clinical disorder is captured by sensitivity and specificity. Sensitivity is the probability of having a positive test if one has the disease; as the sensitivity increases, the false-negative rate decreases. Specificity is the probability of having a negative test if one does not have the disease. As the specificity increases, the false-positive rate decreases. Typically, there is a tradeoff between sensitivity and specificity: The higher the sensitivity of a test, the lower the specificity (and vice versa).

When a clinician orders a test and the result is positive for the disease under consideration, the clinician wants to know if the result is likely to be a true positive, suggesting that the patient really has the disease, and not a false positive. Conversely, the clinician wants to know the probability that a negative test result is truly or falsely negative for the disease in question. In these instances, the clinician is thinking about the concept of positive and negative predictive value.

● **TABLE 12–1** Sensitivity, Specificity, and Predictive Value. The letters A, B, C, and D represent numbers of people with and without a disease in a hypothetical population.

	Disease Present	Disease Absent	Total
Test positive	A (True positive)	B (False positive)	A + B (All positives)
Test negative	C (False negative)	D (True negative)	C + D (All negatives)
Total	A + C (All those with disease)	B + D (All those without the disease)	A + B + C + D (All people being tested)

Sensitivity = the proportion of diseased people who test positive = A/(A + C).

Specificity = the proportion of non-diseased people who test negative = D/(B + D).

Pre-test probability = background prevalence of the disease = (A + C)/(A + B + C + D).

Positive predictive value = the proportion of test-positive people who actually have the disease = A/(A + B).

Negative predictive value = the proportion of test-negative people who don't have the disease = D/(C + D).

Positive predictive value is the chance that the patient has the disease when the test result is positive. Negative predictive value is the chance that the patient does not have the disease when the test result is negative.

Predictive value depends not only on the intrinsic characteristics of the test (sensitivity and specificity), but also on the known or estimated background prevalence of the disease in the population that is being tested—the so-called "pre-test probability." The closer the positive predictive value is to 100%, the greater the clinician's confidence that a patient who tests positive actually has the disease. However, in some instances (eg, when a disease is rare, and when false-positive test results are relatively common), the positive predictive value may not be high enough to guide the clinician confidently; in such cases, false-positive results from non-diseased people may "drown out" true positives.

Diagnostic test accuracy can also be expressed through likelihood ratios. Discussion of likelihood ratios is beyond the scope of this chapter, but several references provide good overviews of this topic.[3,4]

The Fundamental Question: Will Testing Change Management?

Those who teach clinical decision-making often propose that we ask the following question each time we think about ordering a test: Will testing change our management of this patient's problem? This question is more complex than it seems at first glance: The question is stated in a "yes-no" format, when in fact it should be stated in probabilistic terms because we do not really know whether testing will change management before we know the outcome of the test. Thus, a more appropriate question is the following: *What is the probability* that testing will change our management of this patient's problem? To answer this question, we need to break it down into a series of component questions that, taken together, can inform decisions to order tests:

- What are plausible test results in this patient, and what are their probabilities?
- What clinical diagnoses would be suggested by each plausible test result, and what are the probabilities of these diagnoses?
- What treatments (if any) exist for these diagnoses?
- For each diagnosis, would the benefits of treatment likely outweigh the harm in this patient?
- Would this patient be willing to undergo any of these treatments?

At first glance, the task of addressing these questions routinely in clinical practice seems daunting, if not impossible. After all, the first two bullets require substantial quantitative knowledge about a test's intrinsic characteristics and predictive value in the relevant patient population; the third and fourth bullets require familiarity with treatment options and their effectiveness; and the fifth bullet requires anticipation of the patient's preferences. Nevertheless, expert clinicians consider these items routinely—perhaps subliminally in some instances—drawing on their fund of knowledge and clinical experience. When the cases are complex and the stakes are high (for example, when invasive tests with potential adverse effects are contemplated), such clinicians may review the relevant medical literature or involve trustworthy consultants.

In addition, expert clinicians take short-cuts that obviate the need to dwell on each item. For example, suppose that only one treatable diagnosis is a plausible outcome of testing, and that we know in advance (by asking the patient) that the patient would reject that treatment because he or she considers it too burdensome. In such a case, testing immediately becomes unnecessary: If we know confidently that testing will not change management of the problem, we do not need to worry about exact probabilities. The next case exemplifies this sequence.

CASE PRESENTATION 3

A 65-year-old man presents with a 1-week history of right-sided low back pain that radiates down the leg; it began after a day of heavy lifting, bending, and twisting while doing yard work. Physical examination reveals a positive straight leg-raising maneuver on the right, decreased sensation to pinprick in the right great toe webspace, and slight weakness of great toe dorsiflexion. The probability of L5 radiculopathy, caused by a herniated disc, seems high. The clinician wonders whether to order an MRI.

A herniated disc is likely, and MRI is a reasonably accurate way to document the diagnosis. However, we know that initially conservative (nonsurgical) management of herniated discs is appropriate,[5] that most nonsurgical interventions do not require MRI corroboration of the diagnosis, and that the main role of MRI is to depict the anatomic problem before surgery. If this patient tells us during the initial clinical encounter that "I would do anything to avoid surgery unless it's absolutely necessary," an MRI becomes unnecessary, and we do not need to dwell excessively on the sensitivity, specificity, and predictive value of MRI for diagnosing herniated discs that cause radiculopathy.

In the discussion so far, the primary role of testing has been to confirm or refute new clinical diagnoses. However, laboratory and imaging tests are used commonly to monitor the progress of certain diseases, to follow a patient's response to certain types of treatment, or to screen for drug side effects. These uses of testing are discussed in the sidebar on page 163.

Time and Therapeutic Response as "Diagnostic Tests"

Laboratory testing and imaging should be situated in the larger context of the clinical encounter (and in many cases, a series of encounters over time). When a patient presents with a new problem, the encounter begins as a "blank slate"; history-taking and physical examination maneuvers suggest various diagnoses and their probabilities, and thus can be considered diagnostic tests themselves. Sometimes the degree of certainty resulting from the history and physical examination is so high that no further diagnostic testing is necessary. For some clinical presentations, researchers have developed and validated clinical scores or rules—based exclusively on the history and physical examination—that safely eliminate or reduce the need for additional diagnostic testing.[6,7]

Even when substantial uncertainty remains after careful history-taking and physical examination, immediate testing is not always necessary: Observing the progression (or resolution) of a patient's symptoms over time is a valid "diagnostic test" in some instances, as long as it does not compromise the ability to intervene effectively later on. Similarly, observing a patient's response (or lack of response) to empiric therapy can provide valuable diagnostic information. For example, in Case 2, one might offer the patient a choice between a time-limited therapeutic trial (eg, acid-suppressive therapy) and immediate diagnostic testing (eg, endoscopy or blood testing for *Helicobacter pylori*). The point here is that laboratory testing and imaging are tools that complement, but do not replace, other sources of information that help clinicians refine diagnostic probabilities. When observation or a therapeutic trial is being used diagnostically, close follow-up of the patient is essential, particularly when serious disorders are among the diagnostic possibilities.

Problematic Influences on Test-Ordering

CASE PRESENTATION 4

An 80-year-old man who is taking several antihypertensive medications (but is otherwise well) briefly passes out on his way to the bathroom in the middle of the night. He regains consciousness and feels fine; however, his son drives him to the emergency department and the patient is admitted to the hospital. Physical examination is normal except for orthostatic hypotension; a 12-lead electrocardiogram is normal. The admitting physician orders a head CT scan, carotid Doppler ultrasound, a transthoracic echocardiogram, and a Holter monitor.

CASE PRESENTATION 5

A healthy 68-year-old man with no medical problems comes for a "routine" physical examination. Just as the physician is leaving the room at the end of the visit, the patient asks, "Oh Doc, could you order that new heart test, you know, the CRP test? I heard about it on TV."

CASE PRESENTATION 6

For many years, a 72-year-old woman has had intermittent low back pain that responds to a heating pad and brief courses of acetaminophen or ibuprofen. Last year, plain films of the lumbar spine revealed mild osteoarthritis. Because her last few exacerbations have lasted a bit longer than previous ones, she makes an appointment and asks, "Isn't it time to get an MRI so we can really see what's going on in my back?" She has no radicular symptoms, no alarm symptoms, a normal lower-extremity neurologic examination, and no functional impairment.

In daily practice, the problem-solving rationale for diagnostic testing is influenced or distorted by other motivations for testing. Clinicians sometimes order tests out of sheer habit, or because the tests are mistakenly perceived as indicated in every evaluation of a specific medical problem. For example, the clinician in Case 4 is likely pursuing his standard "syncope work-up," even though studies have shown repeatedly that a one-size-fits-all approach to diagnostic testing for syncope is illogical and wasteful.[8] In other instances—Cases 5 and 6, for example—tests might be ordered simply because a patient asks for them. In such cases, granting the patient's request will likely be less time-consuming than explaining the pros and cons of a controversial test (Case 5) or talking to the patient about a difficult-to-treat chronic problem such as back pain (Case 6); however, ordering tests simply to avoid discussion or save time is not acceptable practice. In addition, clinicians frequently perceive tests as providing protection against malpractice litigation. And unfortunately, financial conflicts of interest (eg, ownership of imaging equipment) can drive unnecessary testing.[9] These various influences on testing are powerful, or even dominant, in some situations, and they detract from the primary goal of using diagnostic testing to benefit patients.

● TEST PERFORMANCE IN GERIATRICS: SPECIAL CONSIDERATIONS

The general principles discussed so far in this chapter are broadly applicable to all age groups. But are there specific issues in diagnostic testing with special relevance to geriatric populations? At least four such issues are worth considering: (1) normal limits of test results, (2) incidental findings on diagnostic testing, (3) test accuracy in different age groups, and (4) age limits for screening tests.

Normal Limits of Test Results

Normal limits for laboratory tests in adults, as specified on lab reports, usually do not vary by age. Determining whether normal limits should differ for elderly persons is conceptually problematic, because we know that for some internal organs, physiologic function and anatomic structure change "normally" with age. For example, age-related declines in renal function as indicated by glomerular filtration rate,[10] lung volumes as measured by spirometry,[11] and bone mineral density as measured by dual energy x-ray absorptiometry (DEXA) are well documented. Thus, measurements of renal function, lung volumes, and bone density that are "normal" for an 80-year old person (in the sense of being near the average for apparently healthy octogenarians) would be subnormal for healthy 40-year-olds. For each of these three examples, the influence of aging on the interpretation of test results is handled somewhat differently:

- Most clinicians use the serum creatinine as the marker for renal function. But the situation is complicated in older adults: A tendency for serum creatinine to rise with age (because of declining glomerular filtration rate [GFR]) is opposed by a tendency for serum creatinine to decrease with age (reflecting age-related decrease in muscle mass). Thus, formulas that incorporate age (eg, the Cockcroft-Gault and the Modification of Diet in Renal Disease formulas) have been developed to convert the patient's serum creatinine into an age-adjusted estimate of creatinine clearance or GFR.[10]

- For spirometry, the laboratory provides a "predicted" normal value for forced vital capacity (FVC) that incorporates the specific patient's age, sex, and height; the patient's FVC is reported as a percentage of that predicted normal value. Thus, a patient's lung volumes are declared to be normal or abnormal in relation to similarly aged people.

- For bone mineral density (as measured by DEXA), the laboratory generally provides so-called "T-scores" and "Z-scores." The T-score is the number of standard deviations by which the patient's bone density departs from the average value for a healthy person around 30 years old; the Z-score is the number of standard deviations by which the patient's bone density departs from the average value for people whose age is the same as the patient's. Somewhat arbitrarily, osteoporosis has been defined as a T-score ≤ -2.5. Thus, older patients are usually labeled as normal or abnormal in relation to young adults, and not to their similarly aged peers.

For some blood tests, the distribution of test results may change slightly among healthy aging adults. These observations tend to be controversial because "normal ranges" are usually established by sampling apparently healthy populations, but apparently healthy 80-year-old people are more likely to have subclinical co-morbidities than apparently healthy 40-year-old people. Thus, it may be unclear whether a slightly high or low laboratory value reflects normal aging or a pathologic process. Consider the next case.

CASE PRESENTATION 7

A previously healthy 80-year-old woman presents with mild fatigue and vague myalgia. She relates her symptoms to several recent stressful events in her family, but seeks reassurance that her symptoms do not reflect an insidious organic condition. Physical examination is normal. The clinician orders a chemistry panel, thyroid tests, complete blood count (CBC), and sedimentation rate. Everything is normal except for a thyroid-stimulating hormone (TSH) level of 5.5 mIU/L (labeled as "high"; the laboratory's upper limit of normal is 4.5), a hematocrit of 34.5% (labeled as "low"; the laboratory's lower limit of normal for a woman is 35), and a sedimentation rate of 30 mm/hr (labeled as "high"; the laboratory's upper limit is 20). Notably, the patient's free thyroxine level is in the middle of the normal range, and the rest of her CBC, including the mean cell volume (MCV), is normal.

The medical literature addresses the laboratory abnormalities in Case 7 as follows:

- In a recent population-based survey, researchers measured thyroid-stimulating hormone (TSH) levels in about 15,000 people who reported no history of thyroid disease and who had normal levels of serum thyroxine (T4) and no antithyroid antibodies. In this population, TSH levels were > 4.5 mIU/L in 11% of people aged ≥ 70, but in only about 3% of younger people.[12] Whether this age-related shift in the frequency distribution of TSH should be considered normal or pathologic remains controversial.

- The upper limit of normal for the erythrocyte sedimentation rate (ESR) appears to rise modestly with normal aging, according to several survey studies.[13] In fact, some authors have proposed simple rules to calculate age-adjusted upper limits of normal (eg, for men, age in years ÷ 2; for women, [age in years + 10] ÷ 2).[14] However, the clinical relevance of these observations is limited, given that the ESR is subject to so many influences and is nonspecific. In addition, ESR values just above the upper limits of normal tend to be of limited value for clinical decision-making in any age group.

- Bone marrow cellularity decreases with aging, and some studies show slight decreases in mean blood hemoglobin levels in otherwise healthy older adults.[13] However, because this effect appears to be modest at best, experts generally recommend not attributing slightly low hemoglobin levels to age alone. The extent of the workup in an elderly patient with mild anemia will obviously depend on the clinical context, extent of change from previous values, and the presence or absence of other abnormalities in the complete blood count.

A comprehensive review of subtle abnormalities in thyroid and hematologic testing is beyond the scope of this discussion. The take-home point, however, is that no universally applicable principles exist for determining what should count as "normal" when clinicians interpret test results for elderly patients. Intelligent clinical decision-making requires reasonable knowledge of the physiology of aging, understanding of how test results are reported, and familiarity with published literature on the natural history of borderline test results.

Incidental Findings on Imaging and Laboratory Testing

CASE PRESENTATION 8

A 78-year-old man presents to the emergency department with left lower quadrant abdominal pain and tenderness. Abdominal CT scan shows mild diverticulitis, which clearly explains the patient's symptoms. In addition, the radiologist reports a 7-cm abdominal aortic aneurysm and a smooth 2-cm right adrenal mass. He recommends that "an adrenal MRI or CT protocol could be considered to further characterize the lesion."

Radiologic imaging has advanced remarkably during the past few decades. One consequence is the identification of incidental findings that are unrelated to the reason the test was ordered. In some cases, the fortuitous identification of a potentially lethal condition at a curable stage (eg, the asymptomatic abdominal aortic aneurysm discovered in Case 8) might benefit the patient. But in other cases, clinicians and patients must decide whether further evaluation of an incidental finding—such as the adrenal lesion in Case 8—is worthwhile at all.

The term "incidentaloma" has been coined to describe incidentally discovered mass lesions. While this term has been used particularly for adrenal and pituitary lesions, the literature also refers to incidentalomas in other locations, including the thyroid, liver, kidneys, and pancreas. In general, incidentalomas are more common in older than in younger populations. For example, the prevalence of adrenal incidentalomas on abdominal CT scanning rises from less than 1% among people aged 20 to 29 to about 7% in people over 70 years of age.[15]

Sometimes, imaging characteristics of incidentalomas suggest either benignity or malignancy with a high degree of accuracy. But in other cases, imaging characteristics are ambiguous, and additional radiologic studies or biopsies will be necessary if one chooses to pursue the diagnosis further. To facilitate sensible decision-making in such cases, clinicians should enlist the help of patient-oriented radiologists who are capable of discussing the pros and cons of further diagnostic assessment in relation to the patient's particular clinical circumstances and preferences. For example, in Case 8, if the density of the adrenal mass is less than 10 Hounsfield units on noncontrast CT, the probability of malignancy is so low that additional evaluation to rule out malignancy may be unnecessary.[15]

Clinicians must also remain up to date with published literature on the natural history of incidentally found mass lesions. For example, several recent studies suggest that small, incidentally discovered, solid renal masses—most of which are renal cell carcinomas histologically—can be observed safely without intervention in elderly patients; in most cases, these tumors are slow growing and do not result in morbidity or mortality.[16,17]

Not all age-related incidental findings on imaging are mass lesions or tumors; some findings appear to reflect "normal" aging. For example, in a large community-based cross-sectional study of magnetic resonance imaging (MRI) of the brain, researchers documented that ventricular and sulcal size increased with age in apparently healthy older adults with no history of neurological disease and no obvious cognitive impairment.[18] Because these findings suggest brain atrophy, clinicians may be tempted to use such findings to explain clinical signs and symptoms; however, that temptation should be resisted.

Outcomes analogous to radiologic "incidentalomas" also occur frequently with laboratory testing in elderly populations. For example, clinicians frequently encounter incidental mild hypercalcemia in asymptomatic older patients when automated chemistry panels are ordered for other reasons. Not infrequently, this finding represents primary hyperparathyroidism, the prevalence of which increases with age.[19] Another example is illustrated in the next case.

CASE PRESENTATION 9

A comprehensive metabolic panel is obtained in a 75-year-old woman to monitor renal and hepatic function because she is taking several antihypertensive drugs and a statin. Because the total protein and globulin are mildly elevated, the clinician orders a serum protein electrophoresis, which shows a monoclonal IgG protein measuring 0.8 g. The patient is asymptomatic; a complete blood count and the rest of her chemistry panel are normal.

Monoclonal gammopathy of unknown significance (MGUS) is usually discovered incidentally, as in Case 9. MGUS occurs almost exclusively in older patients: In one recent study, the prevalence of MGUS ranged from 1.7% in people aged 50 to 59 to 6.6% in those aged ≥ 80. Published data—which should be shared with patients—provide probabilities of the transition from MGUS to multiple myeloma over time.[20,21]

Test Accuracy in Older Patients: The "Spectrum Effect"

Spectrum effect, also known as spectrum bias, is another issue in diagnostic testing that may have particular relevance to older patients.[22,23] The sensitivity and specificity of a diagnostic test is initially derived when researchers apply the test to people known to have the disease in question (to calculate sensitivity) and to people who do not have the disease (to calculate specificity). Clinicians often view published values for sensitivity and specificity as immutable attributes of a test. However, when the test is actually applied by practicing clinicians, its sensitivity and specificity in the "real world" may not necessarily approximate the published values. For sensitivity, this problem occurs if the spectrum of disease severity among patients typically seen by clinicians differs from the spectrum of disease severity among research subjects in whom the test was initially evaluated. For specificity, the analogous problem occurs if the spectrum of conditions that cause false-positive test results was not properly represented in study populations. The use of carcinoembryonic antigen (CEA) as a test for colorectal cancer provides one of the first examples in which spectrum effect was described.[22] The test was initially evaluated in patients with advanced colorectal cancer, among whom the test sensitivity was very high. But later on, when the test was applied to early, localized cases of colorectal cancer, sensitivity was much lower.

Although published discussions of spectrum effects tend to involve disease severity, patient age is another characteristic that can cause spectrum effects. Tests performance may differ in older and younger populations if anatomic and physiologic effects of aging change the threshold at which the test becomes positive. For example, the sensitivity of mammography for breast cancer is higher in postmenopausal than in premenopausal women, because breast density generally declines after menopause, and mammography is better able to detect cancers in less dense breasts. In a study of first screening mammograms, the sensitivity of mammography for breast cancer was 77% in women in their 30s, 87% in women in their 40s, and more than 90% in all decades thereafter; in contrast, specificity was similar (range, 92-95%) in all decades.[24]

CASE PRESENTATION 10

On the same day, a clinician sees two patients who come to the office worried about prostate cancer. Both patients had prostate-specific antigen (PSA) tests at a local community center that advertised free prostate cancer screenings; both got letters stating that their tests were abnormal. The first patient is a 50-year-old man with a PSA of 6 ng/mL; the second patient is an 80-year-old man with the exact same result, 6 ng/mL. Neither patient has a nodule or induration on prostate examination.

Prostate-specific antigen (PSA) testing to detect prostate cancer provides another example of spectrum effect. Although PSA levels increase in most patients with clinically important prostate cancer, an anatomic and physiologic effect of aging—benign prostatic hyperplasia (BPH)—also causes PSA levels to rise. For example, in a study of healthy volunteers with no clinical evidence or history of prostate disorders, the cutoff value of PSA that defined 97.5% of men as "normal" ranged from 2.5 ng/mL among men in their 40s to 6.5 among men in their 70s[25]; BPH was almost certainly responsible for most of this age-related shift in the distribution of PSA levels. Analyses show that in the presence of BPH, the ability of a PSA test to distinguish between presence and absence of prostate cancer is substantially diminished.[26] Thus, if one uses the typical cutoff of 4 ng/mL as the upper limit of normal regardless of age, the implications of a mildly elevated PSA test will differ in younger and older men. The implications

for the two patients in Case 9 are apparent: An 80-year-old man without prostate cancer is more likely to have a mildly elevated PSA level (eg, 6 ng/mL) than is a 50-year-old man without the disease.

When spectrum effects are responsible for age-related differences in test performance among diseased people, sensitivity is affected. When spectrum effects are responsible for age-related differences in test performance among non-diseased people, specificity is affected. When the prevalence of a disease (ie, pre-test probability) changes with age, positive and negative predictive values are affected (Table 12–1). When *both* spectrum effects *and* increased disease prevalence occur in older populations, as is the case with breast cancer and prostate cancer, the overall interpretation of test results may differ considerably from that in younger populations. Unfortunately, published age-specific sensitivities and specificities are not available for many tests. Thus, clinicians must develop at least a qualitative understanding of how aging may distort the performance of common diagnostic tests.

Screening Tests in Older Populations

CASE PRESENTATION 11

An 86-year-old woman with hypertension and osteoarthritis is seeing her primary care clinician for a yearly problem review. She asks, "Do I still need to have mammograms?"

CASE PRESENTATION 12

During an office visit, an 82-year-old man with no history of cardiovascular disease reminds the clinician that he hasn't had his lipids measured during the past several years. "Shouldn't we recheck my cholesterol?" he asks. On previous lipid profiles, LDL and HDL cholesterol levels have been in the range of 130 mg/dL (3.37 mmol/L) and 50 mg/dL (1.30 mmol/L), respectively.

Screening tests are performed to detect medical conditions before they become clinically evident. The target of screening can be a disease itself (eg, cancer) or a risk factor for disease (eg, serum cholesterol). In either case, the underlying premise is that early detection through screening will improve clinical outcomes that are meaningful to patients.

An important and often controversial issue is the timing of screening during a person's life span. Ideally, screening tests should be performed only during periods in the life span when benefits clearly exceed harm. Mammographic screening for breast cancer is a good example. Too-early screening—for example, performing routine mammograms in average-risk women in their 30s—exposes large numbers of women to harm (eg, radiation, unnecessary biopsies, and cost) at a time when few cancers are detected. Too-late screening is equally problematic: At some point near the end of a person's life span, screening will neither extend life nor improve quality of life, but might result in interventions that are both harmful and costly.

Several other issues are particularly relevant regarding screening tests in older persons. First, even when randomized screening trials exist, they are unlikely to have involved elderly persons. Thus, robust evidence to support the efficacy of screening is often absent for geriatric populations. For example, the large clinical trials of screening mammography generally enrolled women in the age range of 40 to 70 years.[27]

Second, the benefit of screening generally does not accrue until some time in the future, when the disease in question would have become clinically evident if early detection by screening had not occurred. For some screening tests, this "lead time" (ie, the interval between the date of screening and the date when symptomatic disease would have developed) can be considerable. For the woman in Case 11, a small mammographically detected breast cancer might not become clinically evident during her lifetime. The probability that some other source of morbidity or mortality would arise after age 86 is substantial enough to diminish the potential value of mammography.[28]

Third, risk factors may not have the same relevance in older populations as in younger and middle-aged populations. For example, the association between total or LDL cholesterol levels and subsequent coronary events or mortality becomes tenuous in the very old.[29] For the patient in Case 12, repeated cholesterol screening has no proven value.

Clinicians and elderly patients would benefit by authoritative and unbiased clinical guidelines that address upper age limits for screening. Unfortunately, such guidance has been largely absent until recently. In 2008, the US Preventive Services Task Force (USPSTF) recommended against screening for prostate cancer in men aged 75 or older.[30] That same year, the USPSTF recommended against colorectal cancer screening after age 85; for ages 75 to 85, the Task Force recommended against "routine" screening, but allowed for individualized decisions to screen in selected cases.[31] These recommendations are not made arbitrarily; rather, they reflect a careful balancing of benefits and harm that are discussed thoroughly in supporting documents. As of this writing, the USPSTF has specified no formal upper age limit for lipid screening, although the discussion accompanying its guideline does address the potential benefits and harms of lipid screening in older populations.[32] In 2009, the USPSTF published an updated guideline on breast cancer screening. Biennial screening mammography was recommended between ages 50 and 74; for older women, the Task Force made no specific recommendation because it concluded that evidence is insufficient to assess the benefits and harm of mammography in that age group.[33]

● ADDITIONAL PATIENT-CENTERED CONSIDERATIONS

Three additional factors can influence decisions to order laboratory tests and imaging studies in geriatric populations.

First, some frail elderly patients with chronic pain or limited mobility may find certain procedures (eg, a prolonged MRI study that requires uncomfortable positioning) to be unacceptable, particularly when the anticipated test results are unlikely to contribute importantly to the patient's clinical care. Similarly, some debilitated elderly patients may reject interventions that require frequent monitoring by diagnostic tests; for example, when the indications for warfarin are marginal, the inconvenience and complexity of INR monitoring may be a factor in the patient's decision whether to initiate warfarin therapy.

A second issue is the frequent existence of multiple co-morbidities in geriatric populations. When the potential benefits of diagnostic testing outweigh the burdens or harms, the patient's preferences—and not the mere presence of background co-morbidities—should dictate whether the test is performed. However, co-morbidities can complicate every step of the sequence from choice of diagnostic tests, to interpretation of test results, to treatment. Clinicians should not order tests when co-morbidities will predictably render the results uninterpretable, or when co-morbidities will preclude meaningful changes in treatment after testing. In addition, tests with intrinsic adverse effects (eg, CT scanning or arteriography with iodinated contrast agents that may cause renal failure) should be used especially judiciously in frail patients with multiple co-morbidities.

Third, we have observed that some older patients—both those with multiple chronic illnesses and those who are robust and healthy—reach a point at which they simply do not wish to "medicalize" their lives further, preferring to forgo diagnostic tests or screening tests that younger but otherwise similar patients might choose to have. If the potential benefits of testing appear clearly to outweigh the burdens in such situations, the clinician should offer persuasive arguments in favor of testing—as long as the clinician avoids manipulation or coercion. But ultimately, the patient's preferences should be accepted and supported. Finally, a patient's decision to forgo a potentially beneficial diagnostic test is not irreversible; an initial period of watchful waiting followed by testing later on may be a strategy that is favored by some patients.

CONCLUSION

The responsible conduct of laboratory testing and imaging in older patients follows the same general principle as testing in any age group: Tests should be ordered only if they are likely to inform clinical judgment in a way that benefits patients. Testing that does not adhere to this primary objective wastes resources, exposes patients to potential harms without redeeming value, and breeds illogical or sloppy clinical reasoning. In geriatric populations, however, additional considerations arise: The performance characteristics of tests may change with patient age, the value of screening tests may diminish, and personal preferences of patients may evolve predictably or unpredictably as they grow older. Clinicians cannot be expected to have detailed encyclopedic knowledge about every available diagnostic test. But they can be expected to cultivate a style of judicious test ordering that reflects both evidence-based medicine and attention to individual patient characteristics.

A CLINICAL EXAMPLE OF LABORATORY TESTING AND MONITIORING IN THE OUTPATIENT SETTING

In outpatient settings, laboratory tests and imaging studies are ordered frequently to follow chronic conditions or to screen for adverse effects of medications. An approach to outpatient laboratory monitoring is illustrated by the case of Mr. Benson, a 79-year-old man whom I have followed for 13 years. Mr. Benson has five longstanding, stable medical problems. *Primary hypothyroidism* was diagnosed 15 years ago, when his TSH was elevated and free T4 was low. That same year, *pernicious anemia* was documented by a low serum B_{12} level and an abnormal Schilling test. About 12 years ago, soon after I met Mr. Benson, I initiated drug therapies for *hypertension* and *hyperlipidemia*. And finally, the patient has *aortic stenosis*. An echocardiogram 15 years ago showed aortic sclerosis but not stenosis; 5 years ago, when his murmur had grown louder and harsher, I repeated the study and it revealed moderate aortic stenosis by valve area and gradient.

I see Mr. Benson every 6 months. At his most recent visit, he reports that he's feeling well. He works part-time at a local hardware store, and takes his dog for a daily 1-mile walk that includes a small hill. He denies chest pain, dyspnea, syncope, near-syncope, claudication, edema, abdominal symptoms, or weight loss. His medications are lisinopril, hydrochlorothiazide, pravastatin, L-thyroxine, and vitamin B_{12}. On physical examination, his blood pressure is normal and his cardiac examination reveals his usual harsh systolic outflow murmur of aortic stenosis; he has no physical findings of heart failure. How do I decide what tests to order?

- Hydrochlorothiazide and lisinopril can cause asymptomatic electrolyte abnormalities and renal dysfunction—sometimes unexpectedly. A periodic basic metabolic profile (electrolytes, BUN, creatinine, and glucose), which might detect these abnormalities before they cause adverse clinical outcomes, seems reasonable. However, we lack evidence-based data supporting a specific laboratory screening interval for drug-treated hypertensive patients.
- Dosing requirements for hypothyroidism sometimes change with age; thus periodic measurement of TSH is reasonable. Measurement of free T4 is unnecessary if TSH is normal and the patient is asymptomatic.

- Is it necessary to measure yearly lipid levels in a 79-year-old man whose LDL and HDL cholesterol levels have consistently averaged about 120 mg/dL (3.11 mmol/L) and 40 mg/dL (1.04 mmol/L), respectively, during a decade of pravastatin therapy? The patient has neither diabetes nor known coronary disease, conditions that might mandate adjustment of drug therapy to achieve more stringent targets. Thus, one could argue that annual lipid testing is unnecessary, because results that would change management are highly unlikely. However, if one does decide to check Mr. Benson's lipids periodically, one could consider ordering only a total and HDL cholesterol. Recent data indicate that non-HDL cholesterol (total minus HDL cholesterol) predicts cardiovascular outcomes as well as LDL cholesterol does.[1] Because total and HDL cholesterol can be measured in nonfasting specimens, they can be drawn conveniently during the afternoon, when Mr. Benson prefers to schedule office visits.
- Must we check liver enzymes indefinitely in patients on long-term statin therapy? Several manufacturers advise measuring liver enzymes 3 months after starting these drugs and "periodically" thereafter (including after a dose increase). However, studies have shown that hepatotoxicity virtually never occurs in patients who have tolerated statins for years.[2] Thus, I would argue that liver tests are unnecessary in this patient.
- The patient's macrocytic anemia resolved with B_{12} replacement 15 years ago; several subsequent determinations of hemoglobin and serum B_{12} were normal. Because the patient complies with supplemental B_{12} therapy and is asymptomatic, there is no reason to check a blood count or B_{12} level.
- What about echocardiography, which was last performed about 5 years ago? In general, guidelines recommend against aortic valve replacement in asymptomatic patients, because surgical morbidity and mortality (plus subsequent risks associated with having a prosthetic valve) outweigh the benefits for asymptomatic patients.[3] Some cardiologists believe that surgery should be considered for asymptomatic patients who develop symptoms or hypotension on exercise stress testing. However, Mr. Benson is active and has no symptoms on exertion; in addition, his general philosophy is to avoid invasive interventions unless compelling evidence exists to support them. Hence, repeated echocardiography is unnecessary in this case, because there is no plausible result that will change management.

Although clinicians will vary in their approaches to laboratory monitoring for patients like Mr. Benson, test-ordering decisions should reflect careful deliberation and not rote behavior. According to the reasoning just outlined, I completed Mr. Benson's latest visit by ordering only a basic metabolic profile (BUN, creatinine, electrolytes, glucose) and a TSH level. I check these tests annually, recognizing that a 1-year interval is somewhat arbitrary. I have been checking nonfasting total and HDL cholesterol every 2 years. Finally, in my view, a blood count, B_{12} level, liver tests, and echocardiography are not necessary in this case.

—Allan S. Brett, MD

References

1. The Emerging Risk Factors Collaboration. Major lipids, apolipoproteins, and risk of vascular disease. *JAMA.* 2009;302:1993-2000.

2. Charles EC, Olson KL, Sandhoff BG, et al. Evaluation of cases of severe statin-related transaminitis within a large health maintenance organization. *Am J Med.* 2005;118:618-624.

3. Otto CM. Valvular aortic stenosis: Disease severity and timing of intervention. *J Am Coll Cardiol.* 2006; 47:2141-2151.

References

1. Vakil N, Moayyedi P, Fennerty MB, et al. Limited value of alarm features in the diagnosis of upper gastrointestinal malignancy: Systematic review and meta-analysis. *Gastroenterology.* 2006; 131:390.

2. Moayyedi P, Talley NJ, Fennerty MB, et al. Can the clinical history distinguish between organic and functional dyspepsia? JAMA. 2006;295:1566.

3. McGee S. Simplifying likelihood ratios. *J Gen Intern Med.* 2002;17:646.

4. Richardson WS, Wilson MC, Keitz SA, et al. Tips for teachers of evidence-based medicine: Making sense of diagnostic test results using likelihood ratios. *J Gen Intern Med.* 2008;23:87.

5. Peul WC, van Houwelingen HC, van den Hout WB, et al. Surgery versus prolonged conservative treatment for sciatica. *N Engl J Med.* 2007;346:2245.

6. LeGal G, Righini M, Roy PM, et al. Prediction of pulmonary embolism in the emergency department: The revised Geneva score. *Ann Intern Med.* 2006;144:165.

7. Bachmann LM, Kolb E, Koller MT, et al. Accuracy of Ottawa ankle rules to exclude fractures of the ankle and mid-foot: Systematic review. *BMJ.* 326:417, 2003.

8. Mendu ML, McAvay G, Lampert R, et al. Yield of diagnostic tests in evaluating syncopal episodes in older patients. *Arch Intern Med.* 2009;169:1299.

9. Hillman BJ, Joseph CA, Mabry MR, et al. Frequency and costs of diagnostic imaging in office practice—A comparison of self-referring and radiologist-referring physicians. *N Engl J Med.* 1990;323:1604.

10. Choudhury D, Raj DSC, Levi M. Effect of aging on renal function and disease. In: Brenner BM, ed. *The Kidney.* 7th ed. Philadelphia: Saunders; 2004:2305.

11. Kohansal R, Martinez-Camblor P, Agusti A, et al. The natural history of chronic airflow obstruction revisted: An analysis of the Framingham Offspring Cohort. *Am J Respir Crit Care Med.* 2009;180:3.

12. Surks MI, Hollowell JG. Age-specific distribution of serum thyrotropin and antithyroid antibodies in the U.S. population: Implications for the prevalence of subclinical hypothyroidism. *J Clin Endocrinol Metab.* 2007;92:4575.

13. Shayne M, Lichtman MA. Hematology in older persons. In: Lichtman MA, Kipps TJ, Kaushansky K, et al., eds. *Williams Hematology.* 7th ed. New York: McGraw-Hill; 2006:111.

14. Miller A, Green M, Robinson D. Simple rule for calculating normal erythrocyte sedimentation rate. *BMJ.* 1983;286:266.

15. Young WF. The incidentally discovered adrenal mass. *N Engl J Med.* 2007;356:601.

16. Volpe A, Panzarella T, Rendon RA, et al. The natural history of incidentally detected small renal masses. *Cancer.* 2004;100:738.

17. Wehle MJ, Thiel DD, Petrou SP, et al. Conservative management of incidental contrast-enhancing renal masses as safe alternative to invasive therapy. *Urology.* 2004;64:49.

18. Yue NC, Arnold AM, Longstreth WT, et al. Sulcal, ventricular, and white matter changes at MR imaging in the aging brain: Data from the Cardiovascular Health Study. *Radiology.* 1997;202:33.

19. Fraser WD. Hyperparathyroidism. *Lancet.* 2009;374:145.

20. Kyle RA, Therneau TM, Rajkumar SV, et al. Prevalence of monoclonal gammopathy of undetermined significance. *N Engl J Med.* 2006;354:1362.

21. Kyle RA, Therneau TM, Rajkumar SV, et al. A long-term study of prognosis in monoclonal gammopathy of undetermined significance. *N Engl J Med.* 2002;346:564.

22. Ransohoff DF, Feinstein AR. Problems of spectrum and bias in evaluating the efficacy of diagnostic tests. *N Engl J Med.* 1978;299:926.

23. Mulherin SA, Miller WC. Spectrum bias or spectrum effect? Subgroup variation in diagnostic test evaluation. *Ann Intern Med.* 2002;137:598.

24. Kerlikowske K, Grady D, Barclay J, et al. Effect of age, breast density, and family history on the sensitivity of first screening mammography. *JAMA.* 1996;276:33.

25. Oesterling JE, Jacobsen SJ, Chute CG, et al. Serum prostate-specific antigen in a community-based population: Establishment of age-specific reference ranges. *JAMA.* 1993;270:860.

26. Meigs JB, Barry MJ, Oesterling JE, et al. Interpreting results of prostate-specific antigen testing for early detection of prostate cancer. *J Gen Intern Med.* 1996;11:505.

27. Humphrey LL, Helfand M, Chan BKS, et al. Breast cancer screening: A summary of the evidence for the U.S. Preventive Services Task Force. *Ann Intern Med.* 2002;137:347.

28. Schonberg MA, Silliman RA, Marcantonio ER. Weighing the benefits and burdens of mammography screening among women age 80 years or older. *J Clin Oncol.* 2009;27:1744.

29. Psaty BM, Anderson M, Kronmal RA, et al. The association between lipid levels and the risks of incident myocardial infarction, stroke, and total mortality: The Cardiovascular Health Study. *J Am Geriatr Soc.* 2004;52:1639.

30. U.S. Preventive Services Task Force. Screening for prostate cancer: U.S. Preventive Services Task Force recommendation statement. *Ann Intern Med.* 2008;149:185.

31. U.S. Preventive Services Task Force. Screening for colorectal cancer: U.S. Preventive Services Task Force recommendation statement. *Ann Intern Med.* 2008;149:627.

32. U.S. Preventive Services Task Force. Screening for lipid disorders in adults: Recommendation statement. http://www.ahrq.gov/clinic/uspstf08/lipid/lipidrs.htm. June 2008. Accessed Sept 20, 2009.

33. U.S. Preventive Services Task Force. Screening for breast cancer: U.S. Preventive Services Task Force recommendation statement. *Ann Intern Med.* 2009;151:716.

POST-TEST

1. **Which of the following questions is MOST important when a clinician is deciding whether to obtain a diagnostic test for a symptomatic patient?**
   A. What is the test's sensitivity for the most likely diagnosis?
   B. Is there a reasonable chance that the test results will change management of this patient's problem?
   C. Does a validated treatment exist for each of the diagnoses under consideration?
   D. Is the cost of the test worth the benefit to the patient?

2. **"Incidentalomas" (incidental mass lesions on imaging) commonly create diagnostic dilemmas for elderly patients in all of the following organs EXCEPT:**
   A. Kidney
   B. Adrenal
   C. Spleen
   D. Thyroid

3. **"Spectrum effect" or "spectrum bias" in diagnostic testing occurs when:**
   A. The sensitivity or specificity of a test, as applied to real clinical populations, differs from the sensitivity or specificity originally described in research populations.
   B. The positive or negative predictive values of a test, as applied to real clinical populations, differ from the predictive values originally described in research populations.
   C. A new test methodology is created, resulting in different normal limits for test results.
   D. The clinician uses a test that is inappropriate for the patient's condition.

ANSWERS TO PRE-TEST

1. D
2. C
3. B

ANSWERS TO POST-TEST

1. B
2. C
3. A

13

Considerations Prior to Drug Prescribing in the Elderly

Edmund H. Duthie, Jr., MD

Kathryn M. Denson, MD

Elizabeth Cogbill, MD

● **LEARNING OBJECTIVES**

1. Discuss the pharmacokinetic and pharmacodynamic changes that occur with aging.
2. Describe important considerations to use when prescribing medications to older adults.
3. Identify barriers to patient medication adherence.
4. Describe physician and patient solutions for better adherence.
5. Explain medication classes to avoid or prescribe with caution in older adults.

PRE-TEST

1. **The best indicator of the concept of polypharmacy in older adults is to look at the:**
   A. Number of drugs
   B. Appropriateness of use of drugs
   C. Presence of drug interactions
   D. Presence of side effects

2. **Decreased pharmacodynamic sensitivity requires higher dosing of:**
   A. Beta blockers
   B. Opioids
   C. Anesthetics
   D. Benzodiazepines

3. **Ms. Martin developed hypertension and was prescribed amlodipine. She was seen a month later and had developed lower extremity edema, for which furosemide was prescribed to treat a new diagnosis of congestive heart failure. Several weeks later, your clinic nurse tells you that Ms. Martin has been hospitalized with dehydration and acute renal insufficiency.**

   This adverse drug reaction is an example of which prescribing pitfall to avoid?
   A. Abrupt addition of medications
   B. Increasing medication dose too quickly
   C. Polypharmacy
   D. Prescribing cascade

PHARMACEUTICAL USE IN OLDER ADULTS

Elderly people, while a minority of the population, consume a disproportionate amount of health care resources. Drug therapy is an important part of this consumption. As much as 30% of prescription use and 40% of over-the-counter (OTC) use can be attributed to this group of patients.[1] Adverse drug reactions (ADRs) account for a substantial amount of emergency department (ED) use, hospital admissions, and health care expenditures. One US study reported an estimated 177,504 ED visits annually in response to adverse drug events.[2] The most common conditions and classes of drugs that geriatric patients receive during ambulatory visits are noted in Table 13–1. Not surprisingly, many of these drugs relate to the common chronic illnesses of old age (eg, arthritis, hypertension, and heart disease). Clinicians must give high priority to the agents contained in these classes since use in elderly patients is frequent. Given this high use of drugs, adverse reactions, and cost, it is critical that physicians and all health care providers use drugs properly. The American Association of Medical Colleges has promulgated competencies that all graduating medical students should be able to demonstrate in regard to geriatric pharmacology (Table 13–2). The concept of polypharmacy has been utilized to measure the quality of geriatric care. Polypharmacy has several definitions. Many studies define polypharmacy as the taking of more than 5 or 6 medications, which may lead to adverse drug events, drug-drug interactions, decreased medication compliance, poor quality of life, and unnecessary drug expense. The number of agents is related to drug interactions and adverse outcomes; however, simply enumerating the number of agents may not result in the best understanding of the quality of care being rendered to a geriatric patient. Appropriateness of use may be a more valid construct. This should assess crucial prescribing errors and drug overuse as well as errors of omission where indicated agents were not utilized to positively impact outcomes.

● **TABLE 13–1** Most Commonly Prescribed Drugs by Class (Office-Based and Hospital Outpatient Departments) 2004-2005 for Ages 65 and Over

Hypertension control drugs

Hyperlipidemia control drugs

Non-narcotic analgesics

Diuretics

Beta blockers

Blood glucose/sugar regulators

Acid peptic disorders control drugs

ACE inhibitors

Vitamins, minerals, dietary supplements

Calcium channel blockers

Source: CDC/NCHS, National Ambulatory Medical Care Survey and National Hospital Ambulatory Medical Care Survey. http://www.cdc .gov/nchs/data/hus/hus08.pdf#097. Accessed June 28, 2009.

● **TABLE 13–2** Minimum Geriatric Competencies for Medical Students

The graduating medical student, in the context of a specific older adult patient scenario (real or simulated), must be able to:

1. Explain the impact of age-related changes on drug selection and dose based on knowledge of age-related changes in renal and hepatic function, body composition, and central nervous system sensitivity.

2. Identify medications, including anticholinergic, psychoactive, anticoagulant, analgesic, hypoglycemic, and cardiovascular drugs, that should be avoided or used with caution in older adults and explain the potential problems associated with each.

3. Document a patient's complete medication list, including prescribed, herbal, and over-the-counter medications, and for each medication provide the dose, frequency, indication, benefit, side effects, and an assessment of adherence.

Source: Leipzig RM, Granville L, Simpson D, et al. Keeping granny safe on July 1: A consensus on minimum geriatrics competencies for graduating medical students. Acad Med. 2009;84:604-610.

CASE PRESENTATION: HE'S "JUST NOT HIMSELF"

You are providing care in the geriatric psychiatry clinic. You have received consultation to "please see Mr. Brown and make suggestions regarding his anxiety." You want to address this issue in a comprehensive manner to maximize his health. The patient and his wife come to the clinic, and you obtain more pertinent history from both of them. His wife is concerned that her husband is just "not himself" lately and has been showing little interest in activities. She wonders if he is "losing his memory." On reviewing the chart, you find that Mr. Edward Brown is an 80-year-old man who has been generally very healthy. He has been married 54 years. He and his wife have two children. Mr. Brown has a number of new complaints.

Chief Complaints

- He is having *difficulty eating*. His dentures are creating sores in his mouth and he has a hard time swallowing because he feels that his mouth is so dry. He went to see his dentist and was given artificial saliva.

- He is *constipated*. He went to the drugstore and is self-medicating with laxatives.

- He is having *difficulty urinating*. He tells you that his urine stream is slow. While at the drugstore, he also bought saw palmetto and is self-medicating. He asks if you could prescribe that medication he saw on television for men with urinary problems.

- At the end of the visit he mentions that he is having *trouble focusing*, that his "head seems like it is just in a fog."

HPI: Recently a number of Mr. Brown's friends and family members have died and he is very worried about his retirement funds and whether he will have enough money to pay his bills. These worries have resulted in his inability to get a good night's sleep. Typically he has had no trouble sleeping and has been very active. Now he is waking up in the middle of the night, often thinking about all these concerns and being unable to get back to sleep. He was seen in the urgent care clinic and the clinician suggested that he "try some medication that would help (him) sleep."

PMH: Mr. Brown has been extraordinarily healthy and active all his life with only one surgery, an appendectomy (ruptured) when he was 16 years old.

Medications: Mr. Brown reports using a "sleep medication" which is listed in the electronic medical record as amitriptyline 50 mg at bedtime. His only other medication listed is a multivitamin.

● PHARMACOLOGIC CHANGES WITH AGING

Pharmacokinetics

Pharmacokinetics is the relationship between the administered dose of a drug and the concentration of the drug in the systemic circulation. The typical classification scheme is absorption, distribution, and elimination. Age-related changes in physiology can affect pharmacokinetics. The influence of age on pharmacokinetics is addressed in Table 13–3. Although some intestinal atrophy occurs with aging, there is much intestinal surface area reserve to permit effective drug absorption into late life. Some drugs that are actively absorbed (eg, calcium) do require greater doses to overcome the less efficient absorption. Decreased absorption due to gastroparesis, drug–drug interactions, or gut passive congestion from heart failure is the result of diseases or concomitant drug use in elderly people and not normal aging.

Drug distribution is affected by a loss of lean mass and body water as a result of aging. Water-soluble agents may result in a higher drug concentration for a given dose of drug (eg, digoxin, alcohol). There is also a concurrent increase in the percentage of body fat with age, resulting in agents that distribute according to body fat having a higher volume of distribution (Vd). Vd is proportional to a drug's clearance (Cl), assuming a constant half life. The practical result is that a geriatric patient administered a highly fat-soluble agent may have more drug deposited in the lipid compartment, resulting in prolonged drug clearance from the body and a prolonged drug effect.

Drug elimination can involve the hepatic and renal systems. There are declines in liver size and hepatic blood flow with aging. Thus, agents that rely on first-pass metabolism in the liver (eg, morphine, propranolol, verapamil) may not be initially metabolized to the same extent in geriatric patients. Phase 1 hepatic metabolism involves the endoplasmic reticulum, and microsomal reactions of oxidations and reductions. The cytochrome P450 system is involved with these metabolic processes and may be influenced by aging. Some agents shown to be affected by aging are listed in Table 13–4. Interestingly, phase 2 hepatic metabolism (glucuronidations, sulfations, acetylations, methylations) does not seem to be influenced by aging. Therefore, to make patient management easier and safer, drugs metabolized through the phase 2 hepatic process are preferable in the geriatric patient. For example, while diazepam does undergo phase 1 metabolism influenced by aging, lorazepam does not undergo this metabolic step and its metabolism is unaffected by age. Liver disease can occur in geriatric patients and drug modification may be required. Genetics, environment, other drugs, and habits can also influence hepatic function and drug metabolism in any age group, including the elderly.

Renal physiology has important changes with aging. Kidney size declines, and there is a physiologic loss of glomerular filtration rate with aging. Drugs that rely on renal excretion require some measure of glomerular filtration to assist with drug management. This is critical for agents with serious toxicity potential

● TABLE 13–4 Drugs Influenced by Hepatic Metabolism	
Age-Related Decrease in Hepatic Clearance Found	No Age-Related Difference Found
Alprazolam	Ethanol
Amlodipine	Isoniazid
Barbiturates	Lidocaine
Chlordiazepoxide	Lorazepam
Desmethyldiazepam	Oxazepam
Diazepam	Prazosin
Flurazepam	Salicylate
Imipramine	Warfarin
Meperidine	
Nortriptyline	
Propranolol	
Quinidine, quinine	
Theophylline	

Source: Modified from Katzung BG. Special aspects of geriatric pharmacology. In: Katzung BG, ed. Basic & Clinical Pharmacology. 11th ed. New York: McGraw-Hill; 2009.

● TABLE 13–3 The Influence of Age on Pharmacokinetics	
Pharmacokinetic Process	Age-Related Influence
Absorption	Little or no change
Distribution	Increased body fat and decreased body water
Elimination Hepatic	Phase 1 enzyme activity reduction, phase 2 unchanged
Renal	Decline in glomerular filtration rate

(eg, aminoglycosides, vancomycin, methotrexate, chemotherapeutic agents). Serum creatinine alone is not a reliable indicator of renal function as the loss of lean body mass with age results in decreased creatinine production. A "normal" serum creatinine can be seen when there is actually significant reduction in renal elimination capacity. The Cockcroft-Gault equation is utilized in many electronic medical records to aid in the calculation of glomerular filtration rate (GFR). The equation is:

$$GFR = [(140 - age) \times Wt] \div (72 \times S\,Cr)$$

The age is measured in years, Wt is body weight in kilograms (kg), and S Cr is the serum creatinine in mg/dL. This value is multiplied by 0.85 in women, due to the smaller muscle mass. In the case where S Cr is reported in International Units (μmol/L), the conversion to mg/dL requires dividing the S Cr (μmol/L) by 88 and then inserting the value into the above equation. The Cockcroft-Gault equation generates an average GFR value for the population and individual patients may vary from this average, potentially requiring further drug monitoring and management. Pharmacokinetic profiling is available in many facilities when precise dosing is needed for use of agents with significant toxicity in geriatric patients. This is typically done through consultation with a pharmacist who guides the initial drug dose and arranges for serum drug level testing in order to ensure the precise subsequent dosing. Pharmacokinetic profiling is often utilized when dosing aminoglycosides or vancomycin. Renal disease is common in geriatric patients and requires further adjustments of drug therapy when it occurs.

Pharmacodynamics

Pharmacodynamics is the relationship between the concentration of the drug in the systemic circulation and the observed pharmacologic response. Unbound drug concentrations are a critical determination in pharmacodynamic evaluations. Drug receptors, drug–receptor interactions (eg, receptor numbers, receptor affinity, second messenger, and cellular responses) are also important in these analyses. In essence, pharmacodynamics is the measure of whether a geriatric patient is truly more or less sensitive to an agent. A large body of work on this topic is summarized in Table 13–5.[3] Clinical implications include enhanced responses of certain benzodiazepines when used for conscious sedation or anxiety,

and potential blunted responses to beta agonists used in elderly patients in an ICU setting or cardiac tilt lab. The endogenous insulin receptor becomes less sensitive with aging, with increased insulin resistance resulting in the relatively easy induction of hyperglycemia with stress and the administration of glucocorticoids. A number of medications have not been shown to have any pharmacodynamic changes with aging, including alpha-receptor blockers, angiotensin-converting enzyme inhibitors, and sulfonylureas. Diuretics show decreased diuretic and natriuretic responses in elderly subjects, but these appear to be more pharmacokinetic related.

● FACTORS AFFECTING MEDICATION ADHERENCE

Adherence to a complex medication regimen is challenging. About 40% of older patients do not take their medications as prescribed.[4] Rates of adherence to medication regimens in an older population are similar to those in other age groups, however, and this adherence correlates primarily with the number of medications that are being taken.[5] Non-adherence to medication regimen is a prevalent problem among older adults that affects health care costs, clinical outcomes, and quality of life.[6] Factors associated with medication non-adherence in older adults include greater number of prescribed medications or doses, multiple health care providers prescribing medications, higher medication costs, medication side effects, limited family support, depression, and cognitive impairment.[6] Medication non-adherence may be unintentional or intentional. Intentional non-adherence may occur because patients either need or want to save money by extending the medication or by not filling the prescription. Denial of the illness, or belief that the medications are unhelpful, as well as dissatisfaction with the clinician or pharmacist may also result in non-adherence.[5] In the case of Mr. Brown, he might not adhere to the sleeping medication if he felt it was causing his new symptoms. Unintentional non-adherence is common and is often caused by complex regimens; a lack of understanding of the illness, drug, or regimen; or poor instructions.[7]

Barriers to Adherence

Physical illness or disability may contribute to difficulty with medication adherence. Poor vision may prevent patients from reading the medication list or the pill bottle labels, while arthritis, neuropathy, and weakness may contribute to difficulty in opening pill containers. Physical side effects of some medications may be substantial, leading patients to discontinue their medications. This can be desirable non-adherence and, in Mr. Brown's case, might actually have been advantageous to him.

Cognitive loss and psychological conditions may also lead to medication non-adherence. Dementia and delirium can lead to patients either over- or under-dosing their medications, or to stopping medications completely. This can occur in more mild cognitive loss, where the patient may not initially comprehend the instructions of the clinician and pharmacist, or may occur with unrecognized dementia as the patient is unable

---

● TABLE 13–5 Pharmacodynamic Changes with Aging

Increased pharmacodynamic sensitivity to:

- Benzodiazepines
- Anesthetics
- Opioids
- Dihydropyridines (transient in naïve patients)

Decreased pharmacodynamic sensitivity:

- Beta adrenergic receptor

Source: Modified from Bowie MW, Slattum PW. Pharmacodynamics in older adults: A review. Am J Geriatr Pharmacother. 2007;5:263-303.

to remember the medications or dosing schedule. Mood and other psychiatric disorders may also affect medication adherence. Depression may lead to apathy in caring for oneself, anxiety may lead to increased self-medication, and paranoid schizophrenia may result in a wariness and reluctance to take prescribed medication.

Functional and social factors influence adherence. Once the prescription is written, the patient must be able to access the pharmacy and afford the medications. Low literacy and lack of social support decrease the ability of elderly patients to take medications as prescribed. Health beliefs and cultural backgrounds may influence adherence to medications and care. Patient perception that the medication does not improve the disease or condition may lead to treatment of the health problem with solely non-medication therapies (eg, nutrition, social contacts, exercise, herbal remedies). These barriers are summarized in Table 13–6.

Solutions to Non-Adherence

Consider each patient as an individual. Carefully evaluate the need for various treatments by weighing the risks and benefits for the particular patient. Consideration of the patient's overall physical and cognitive health, as well as functional status in the context of the patient's goals and quality of life, will help bring necessary balance to the treatment decision process. Including patients and families in medication decisions is crucial as they may have information regarding past medication use, intolerances, and allergies. This approach enables the clinician to thoughtfully recommend appropriate medication treatment, and to recommend against other medication treatment, as these factors are evaluated (eg, certain medication therapy in a healthy 90-year-old may be more advantageous than that same therapy in a 70-year-old patient with end-stage dementia). Reassess patients carefully over time, as changes in cognition, mood, vision, hearing, driving, and finances may all influence medication adherence.

Take a careful "medication history." Do not assume that simply because the medications are listed on the medication record that the patient is taking these medications as prescribed (Table 13–2). Inquire about medications in a nonjudgmental manner. Ask the patient if it is difficult to take the medications as prescribed, and if so, which medications are being missed. Discussing and identifying barriers to adherence will help the physician, patient, and family to either (1) discontinue or reduce the medication or (2) identify strategies to overcome barriers.

Components of a medication history may include current and previous prescription and over-the-counter (OTC) medications, home remedies (may include alcohol or other drugs), medication allergies or adverse drug events, and drug interactions (Table 13–2). In the case of Mr. Brown, the OTC complementary drug use of saw palmetto and laxatives was detected. An adherence assessment including eyesight, dexterity, cognition, literacy, and ability to obtain medications is essential. Multiple clinicians and pharmacies may lead to incomplete knowledge of the patient's entire medication list. Encouraging patronage of only one pharmacy is helpful for simplicity, while the "brown bag" approach is advocated to help obtain a more complete medication list by encouraging the patient and family to bring all of the current medications to the clinic visit.

Employ geriatric prescribing principles. Be alert to medications that are considered inappropriate in older persons, and try to minimize or avoid them (see "Drugs of Concern in Older Adults" later in this chapter). In Mr. Brown's case, many of his problems were the result of the use of amitriptyline, an agent not preferred in a geriatric patient. Minimize the number of medications as much as possible and then simplify the medication-dosing regimen. Evaluate each medication to determine whether it is the safest option available, with the most appropriate dose and administration. Discuss with the patient and family whether the medication is effective, acceptable, and affordable. If not, consider discontinuation or other possible medication options. Watch for the "prescribing cascade" (discussed later), as careful recognition of drug side effects may minimize other unnecessary prescribing. Mr. Brown has begun the cascade by using the OTC saw palmetto to treat

● **TABLE 13–6** Barriers and Possible Solutions in Medication Non-Adherence

Barrier	Solution
Physical Illness/Disability	Consider patient as an individual. Weigh risk and benefit of medications. Determine patient goals and quality of life.
Arthritis/neuropathy	Easy-to-open pill bottles/pill box.
Visual loss	Work with low-vision center to provide visual aids.
Weakness	Easy-to-open pill bottles/pill box.
Medication Side Effects	Avoid the prescribing cascade. Educate patient/caregiver about possible side effects. Minimize medications and lower dosing frequency. Nursing/pharmacy to educate and assess adherence.
Cognitive Loss	Evaluate and treat potential underlying causes.
Delirium	Increase family/caregiver/social support.
Dementia	Use of reminders, calendars, pill box.
Psychological Conditions	
Mood disorders	Assess and treat underlying disorder. Consider counseling for patient. Encourage increased family/caregiver support.
Culture/belief systems	Attempt to understand patient's perspective. Respectful dialogue with medication education.
Functional Loss	
Access to medications	Encourage patient use of one pharmacy. Enlist the help of family members/caregiver. Consult social work to suggest transportation assistance. Easy-to-open bottles/pill box.
Financial loss	Consult social work to determine financial assistance.
Social Loss	
Low literacy	Patient/caregiver medication education.
Decreased family/social support	Consult social work to **assess** community services. Encourage patient to consider other people who may be willing to assist.

● **TABLE 13–7** Interdisciplinary Contributions to Medication Adherence

Nursing/Case Management

- Assessment of the patient's response to medications
- Compile an accurate, complete medication list (gather all medications/OTC/herbals/vitamins in the home)
- Education of patient/caregivers regarding correct medication use
- Gather medication history information at patient appointments

Pharmacy

- Alerting clinicians to medication interactions, allergies, and side effects
- Anticoagulation dosing and monitoring
- Dosing simplification
- Education of patients, caregivers, and clinicians in regard to new or existing medications
- Education regarding the most economic medication regimen for the patient
- Ensuring pill packaging is appropriate/accessible for the patient's condition
- Medication dosing adjustment for renal or hepatic dysfunction
- Medication reconciliation
- Recommending reminder devices to improve adherence

Social Work

- Assist patient/caregiver with accessing available community services (transportation, home care)
- Assist patient/caregiver understand possible financial resources available

an effect of the amitriptyline on his ability to urinate effectively, as well as laxatives for his drug-induced constipation and a mouth moisturizer for his drug-induced dry mouth with denture irritation.

Emphasize patient medication education, as an informed patient and family are more likely to take medications as prescribed. Education may occur in a variety of ways, through discussions with the clinician, nurse, and pharmacist, or through a trusted website or patient education handout. Instruct patients and families on what to do if doses are missed. Suggest that the patient tie the medications to the daily routine or identify someone to offer reminders. Try to schedule medications to be given at the same time each day, but be aware that many medications taken at mealtime with water may decrease the appetite. Enlist the help of other care providers. Nursing, pharmacy, and social work play a crucial role in the patient's care in regard to medication adherence (Table 13–7).

● GENERAL PRESCRIBING CONSIDERATIONS IN OLDER ADULTS

Adverse reactions to medications is one of the most frequent causes of admission to the hospital in elderly patients, and side effects of many medications are associated with a high level of morbidity and, in some cases, mortality. Though the list of medications that are potentially harmful in the elderly is long, practitioners have little guidance on how to avoid adverse reactions to necessary medications. Many medications, particularly older medications, do not have geriatric dosing guidelines, creating prescribing challenges.

Multiple co-morbidities in geriatric patients can result in the need for many medications to prevent and treat these conditions. As a result, patients may be prescribed a large number of medications, all with valid indications. While this would constitute appropriate prescribing, it does raise concerns of the number of drugs, potential for drug–drug interactions, and a higher probability of adverse drug reactions. Further complicating matters is the absence of any financial incentives for dose reduction or medication removal. As a result, frail elders, such as nursing home residents, can accumulate large medication profiles.

General Principles in Prescribing

Careful attention to preventing adverse reactions to medications, identifying adverse reactions to medications when they do occur, and modifying the medication or regimen in the case of an adverse reaction will help minimize potential adverse reactions and their associated morbidity in the elderly patient. Prevention of adverse drug reactions includes identifying and avoiding initiation of potentially troublesome medications, and dosing medications properly in the context of geriatric physiology. Consideration must be given to the patient's co-morbidities as well as baseline renal and liver function, which may alter a medication's metabolism. The Beers list, as detailed in the next section of this chapter, is an excellent resource that identifies potentially inappropriate medications in the elderly patient. Medication lists should be reviewed at every appointment, and any new medications must be considered in light of medications the patient is already taking, to minimize metabolic interactions. Therapeutic alternatives to troublesome medications should be considered (eg, alternative antibiotics to avoid quinolones or trimethoprim/sulfamethoxazole in patients currently prescribed warfarin, as these antibiotics may increase the prothrombin time). Additionally, family members should be educated on possible adverse reactions and encouraged to seek medical attention if they are concerned about the patient's response to a medication.

Prescribing high-risk medications often cannot be avoided, so clinicians should diligently seek to identify adverse reactions or morbidity that may be medication related. Assessing the temporal relationship between medication initiation and the onset of symptoms helps determine the presence of a medication-induced adverse reaction. This is critical in Mr. Brown's case. Careful history does show the relationship of his mouth, bowel, urinary, and concentrating problems to his new sleeping agent. This careful assessment assists the practitioner in avoiding the "prescribing cascade," in which mis-attribution of symptoms to a new disease rather than to the side effect of a medication can result in the prescription of further unnecessary and potentially harmful medications (Table 13–8). For example, Mr. Brown was prescribed amitriptyline. This produced the anticholinergic effects of dry mouth, constipation, and decreased urinary stream. He is now taking an oral lubricant, laxatives, and saw palmetto to treat these drug-induced symptoms. He has the increased expense of these agents as well as the cost of the dental and medical visits.

● **TABLE 13–8** Prescribing Cascade

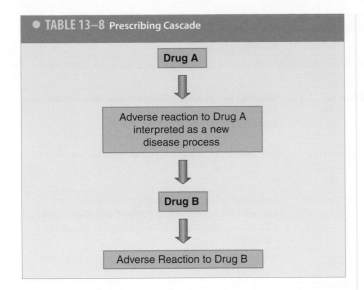

A prescribing principle that can be useful in avoiding the prescribing cascade is the concept of "start low, go slow" in which one medication is added or changed at a time, and doses are increased or changed slowly. This minimizes potential adverse reactions, enabling the practitioner to identify likely adverse reactions to a medication change prior to initiating another drug.

When medication-induced adverse reaction is suspected, discontinuing or modifying the culprit medication can decrease the potential for the adverse reaction to result in hospital admission or a life-threatening event due to associated morbidity. Stopping Mr. Brown's amitriptyline may result in resolution of many of his symptoms. Clinicians should avoid abrupt withdrawal of medications and instead consider switching to a therapeutically comparable medication that is less likely to cause an adverse reaction. Documenting the adverse reaction clearly and informing the patient's family members of the suspected offender is important to prevent similar events in the future.

● DRUGS OF CONCERN IN OLDER ADULTS

Adverse Drug Reactions

Adverse reactions to medications are far-reaching and range from minor disruptions to life-threatening events. Cognitive impairment such as delirium or confusion is a very common adverse reaction with a very high level of associated morbidity, such as falls. Mr. Brown is having problems with his cognition as the result of the amitriptyline. While some medications are notoriously implicated as causing increased morbidity due to adverse reactions in the elderly, no medication is entirely without risk. Adverse drug events may occur even when appropriately indicated medications are used carefully and correctly. Many medications carry high adverse-risk profiles and must be prescribed with caution, such as insulin, warfarin, digoxin, and NSAIDs. Medications such as these should be monitored closely by the physician, and alternative therapies if equally as efficacious should be considered. There are certain medications that as a rule should not be used in elderly

patients. The antihistamine diphenhydramine (Benadryl) should be avoided due to the side effect of sedation, placing patients at risk for falls. In addition, its anticholinergic properties can worsen or exacerbate chronic medical conditions such as cognitive impairment and urinary retention.

A list of medications to be avoided in the elderly was created by a group of clinicians led by geriatrician Dr. Mark Beers. This list has been periodically updated since its inception, and the 2003 revision is currently in use. The list is divided into medications to be avoided in all elderly patients if possible, and medications to be avoided in elderly patients with certain diseases.[8] The risk of an adverse reaction to a medication increases with prescription of the highest-risk medications such as those on the Beers list, including those with anticholinergic and sedative effects.[9] Amitriptyline has both these effects and was provided to Mr. Brown. An amalgamation of the Beers list as well as two other sources is shown in Table 13–9, including concerning medications and suggested medication alternatives.

Drug–Drug Interactions

Polypharmacy increases the risk that a patient will develop a medication adverse reaction. Interactions between medications pose as much concern as the development of an adverse reaction to one medication. This underscores the importance of a complete medication history and list review at each patient visit, and maintaining a high level of suspicion for an adverse reaction to a medication when a patient presents with a new complaint. All new medications must be considered in light of the patient's current medications, to minimize potential interactions and adverse reactions.

● CASE SUMMARY: LESSONS LEARNED FROM MR. BROWN

Mr. Brown is a healthy octogenarian. His initial sleep problems are significant and require exploration. Nonpharmacologic approaches should always be considered as the first line of therapy in any geriatric patient. Clinicians must also recall that geriatric prescribing requires different approaches than what might be commonly done in younger patients. Amitriptyline may be the clinician's favorite soporific for younger people, but should be reconsidered in geriatric practice. Amitriptyline is a tricyclic antidepressant (TCA). Prior to prescribing, recall that it will be well absorbed and has a long half-life (31-46 h) with active metabolites. TCAs are dependent on phase 1 hepatic metabolism, so Mr. Brown may experience an even more prolonged course with this agent compared to published literature from younger individuals. Interestingly, patients may sometimes detect the connection between a drug and onset of symptoms. Nonadherence in this instance may benefit the patient and would be a desirable outcome. Mr. Brown did not make the connection between his prescription and constellation of symptoms. Since his drug regimen was simple, he was adherent to the amitriptyline and experienced the typical side effects of an anticholinergic agent: dry mouth, constipation,

● TABLE 13–9 Froedtert Acute Care for the Elderly (FACE) Medication List

Medication/Class	Potential Adverse Effect	Notes & Alternative(s)[a]
The Froedtert ACE List is a reference list of medications to avoid in elderly patients based on a compilation of the Beer's Criteria,[1] The Medical Letter,[2] Chutka et al[3] and Froedtert geriatric specialists' expert opinions.		
Class: Benzodiazepines, anxiolytics: Alprazolam (*Xanax*), Diazepam (*Valium*), Flurazepam (*Dalmane*), Chlordiazepoxide (*Librium*), Meprobamate (*Equanil*)	Prolonged sedation, cognitive impairment, dependence, increased fall risk, addiction risk	Lorazepam, oxazepam (*lowest dose, shortest duration of therapy, possible*) Lorazepam doses > 3 mg = excessive sedation
Class: Antidepressants: Amitriptyline (*Elavil*), Chlordiazepoxide/amitriptyline (*Limbitrol*), Doxepin (*Sinequan*)	Anticholinergic effects, orthostatic hypotension, sedation, cardiac arrhythmias	SSRIs (other than fluoxetine), eg, **sertraline, paroxetine**
Class: Non-steroidal anti-inflammatory (NSAIDs): Ibuprofen (*Motrin*) Indomethacin (*Indocin*), Naproxen (*Aleve, Avaprox, Naprosyn*), Piroxicam (*Feldene*), Oxaprozin (*Daypro*)	Serious GI toxicity; *if used, titrate to lowest effective dose and monitor for GI toxicity* Possible renal toxicity	Acetaminophen (< 4 g/day), tramadol, non-acetylated salicylates (*Trilisate*), morphine[3] (Ketorolac: *If used, titrate to lowest effective dose and monitor for GI toxicity [15mg QID × 5 days maximum]*)
Class: Analgesics (misc.): 1. Propoxyphene, including combos (*Darvon, Darvocet*) 2. Pentazocine (*Talwin*) 3. Merperidine (*Demerol*)	1. Propoxyphene: Convulsions, CNS toxicity, limited effectiveness 2. Pentazocine: Psychotropic effects, hallucinations, seizure risk 3. Meperidine: Confusion, convulsions, tremors, myoclonus	Acetaminophen (< 4 g/day), tramadol, non-acetylated salicylates (eg, *Trilisate*), morphine[3]
Class: Antihistamines: Diphenhydramine (*Benadryl*), Chlorpheniramine (*Chlor-Trimeton*), Hydroxyzine (*Vistaril, Atarax*)	Anticholinergic, highly sedating, delirium, cognitive decrease	Loratadine (*Claritin*) Cetirizine (*Zyrtec*)
Class: Muscle Relaxants: Carisprodol (*Soma*), Cyclobenzaprine (*Flexeril*), Methocarbamol (*Robaxin*), Metaxalone (*Skelaxin*)	Anticholinergic symptoms, limited effect	
Class : Barbiturates (eg, Phenobarbital *[Luminal]*, secobarbital *[Seconal]*, pentobarbital *[Nembutal]*)	Sedation, decreased attention (risk of falls), respiratory depression, addiction risk, hallucinations	Benzodiazepines (lorazepam, oxazepam) May be appropriate as an anticonvulsant[3]
Class: Antiemetics Trimethobenzamide (*Tigan*), Promethazine (*Phenergan*)	Extrapyramidal effects, lower potency, sedating	Prochlorperazine (*Compazine*) 5HT3-antagonists: ondansetron (*Zofran*)
Class: Gastrointestinal Agents 1. Cimetidine (*Tagamet*) 2. Dicyclomine (*Bentyl*) 3. Hyoscyamine (*Levsin, Levsinex*) 4. Propantheline (*Pro-Banthine*) 5. Belladonna alkaloids (*Donnatal*)	1. Confusion, potential for drug interactions 2. Anticholinergic sx, uncertain effectiveness 3. Anticholinergic effects 4. Potent anticholinergic, effectiveness uncertain Potent anticholinergic, uncertain effectiveness	1. Other H_2 antagonists preferred: famotidine 20 mg daily
Miscellaneous Agents: 1. Chlorpropamide (*Diabinese*)	Long half-life, hypoglycemia	Shorter acting sulfonylureas, thiazolidinediones (rosiglitazone [*Avandia*], pioglitazone [*Actos*]) and alpha-glucosidase inhibitors (acarbose [*Precose*])
2. Digoxin (*Lanoxin*)	Decreased renal function, potential toxicity	**Dose "125 mcg/day**[3] unless clinically indicated. Monitor serum concentrations.
3. Ferrous Sulfate (*Iron*)	Constipation	Dose "325 mg/day
4. Nitrofurantoin (*Microdantin*)	Limited efficacy in renal impairment	
5. Zolpidem (*Ambien*)	Risk of impaired motor and/or cognitive performance with 10-mg dose	**Avoid zoipiden doses > 5mg** Trazodone 25-150mg every evening

[a]Alternative agents represent only suggestions, not appropriate substitutions for all patients. Patient-specific factors and response to therapy should be included in choosing alternatives.

Anticholinergic side effects include: drowsiness, fatigue, disorientation, delirium, increased thirst, pupillary dilation, blurred vision, constipation, tachycardia, decreased nasal, throat and bronchi secretions, dry mucous membranes, decreased gastric/small intestine and colon motility, urinary retention, inhibited sweat gland activity.[3]

References for Table 13–9:

1. Fick DM, Cooper JW, Wade WE, et al. Updating the Beers criteria for potentially inappropriate medication use in older adults. *Arch Intern Med.* 2003;63:2716-2724.

2. Drugs in the elderly. *Med Lett.* 2006;48:6-7.

3. Chutka DS, Takahashi PY, Hoel RW. Inappropriate medications for elderly patients. *Mayo Clinic Proc.* 2004; 79:122-139.

Updated: April 23, 2008

and urinary difficulties as well as central effects of prolonged sedation and trouble concentrating. The treating physician in this case was well served by obtaining a complete history and recognizing the OTC drug use that was occurring to treat the drug-induced symptoms. Mr. Brown did begin the prescribing cascade by medicating himself for the symptoms induced by the prescribed drug. An astute clinician should always look for drugs as a source of symptoms and avoid needless testing and prescribing in geriatric patients. Health care systems should take measures to alert clinicians about agents that are not preferred in geriatric patients. In this case, it would have been helpful if the original clinician had an algorithm to follow for geriatric patients experiencing sleep complaints. This certainly would have avoided the use of the TCA. Another safeguard could be a compiled listing, readily available to prescribers, that indicates agents that are not preferred in geriatric patients and suggests safer alternatives. Finally, synergy between the prescriber and the pharmacy might also help avoid the use of agents that are not preferred. In Mr. Brown's case, a sedating, long-acting anticholinergic agent, known to be associated with falls, is clearly not what Mr. Brown needed.

CONCLUSIONS

Drug use, both prescription and over-the-counter, is a common occurrence in clinical care of elderly adults. Health care providers must inventory medications on a regular basis and insure proper reconciliation at transitions of care. When prescribing for a geriatric patient, the clinician must recall the age-related changes in physiology that impact pharmacokinetics and pharmacodynamics. Knowing the properties of a drug and then applying these properties to the elderly patient should result in more predictable outcomes. To reiterate one example, an agent that is primarily renally excreted will require dose adjustment to account for the age-related decline in renal function.

Medication adherence is a challenge under the best of circumstances. As the number of agents and frequency of doses increases, there is a greater likelihood of non-adherence. Clinicians should anticipate adherence challenges and take measures to minimize these. When non-adherence is encountered, then an organized strategy should be employed to identify the issues leading to this problem so that specific solutions can be offered to improve adherence. Interdisciplinary team approaches to patient education can be helpful.

Clinicians must be aware that certain agents are not appropriate for elderly patients. If possible, these agents should be avoided and alternatives selected. To also further better outcomes when prescribing for elderly patients, the clinician should avoid the prescribing cascade. New symptoms should be considered for their relationship to existing agents patients are taking. When possible, consider stopping an agent to see if a symptom abates. Reflexively adding another agent should be avoided. Adverse drug events can result in significant morbidity, and some agents (eg, anticoagulants and hypoglycemics) need close monitoring to minimize problems. Once again, geriatrics care teams and systems of long-term care may aid the clinician in providing excellent pharmacologic care to the elderly patients.

References

1. Berardi RR, Kroon LA, McDermott JH, et al. *Handbook of Nonprescription Drugs: An Interactive Approach to Self-Care.* 15th ed. Washington, DC; American Pharmacists Association; 2006.

2. Budnitz DS, Shehab N, Kegler SR, et al. Medication use leading to emergency department visits for adverse drug events in older adults. *Ann Intern Med.* 2007;147:755-765.

3. Bowie MW, Slattum PW: Pharmacodynamics in older adults: A review. *Am J Geriatr Pharmacother.* 2007;5:263-303.

4. Ives TJ. Pharmacotherapeutics. In: Ham RJ, Sloane PD, Warshaw GA, eds. *Primary Care Geriatrics: A Case-Based Approach.* 4th ed. St. Louis: Mosby; 2002:146-147.

5. Gurwitz J, Monane M, Monane S, Avorn J. Polypharmacy. In Morris JN, ed. *Quality Care in the Nursing Home.* St. Louis: Mosby; 1997.

6. Schlenk EA, Dunbar-Jacob J, Engberg S. Medication non-adherence among older adults: A review of strategies and interventions for improvement. *J Gerontol Nurs.* 2004;30:33-43.

7. Ives TJ. Pharmacotherapeutics. In: Ham RJ, Sloane PD, Warshaw GA, eds. *Primary Care Geriatrics: A Case-Based Approach.* 4th ed. St. Louis: Mosby; 2002:142.

8. Fick DM, Cooper JW, Wade WE, et al. Updating the Beers criteria for potentially inappropriate medication use in older adults: Results of a US consensus panel of experts. *Arch Intern Med.* 2003;163:2716-2724.

9. Hilmer SN, Mager DE, Simonsick EM et al. A drug burden index to define the functional burden of medications in older people. *Arch Intern Med.* 2007;167:781-787.

POST-TEST

1. Mr. Anderson is a 78-year-old man with depression. He is felt to have bipolar illness and lithium is going to be needed to manage his depression. In considering geriatric prescribing principles, which of the following is most important to keep in mind when reviewing his medications?

   A. Drug absorption
   B. Drug protein binding
   C. Drug hepatic metabolism
   D. Drug renal excretion

2. Mr. Smith, a 76-year-old man, is scheduled for a surveillance colonoscopy. A benzodiazepine, midazolam, is employed for conscious sedation. The typical dose that is utilized in a younger patient is employed. He has an exaggerated response and is over-sedated. What might explain this reaction?

   A. Drug absorption (pharmacokinetic effect)
   B. Drug disease interaction
   C. Drug sensitivity (pharmacodynamic effect)
   D. Drug renal excretion (pharmacokinetic effect)

3. Ms. Andrews, an 85-year-old woman, visited her physician with an initial complaint of insomnia. She was prescribed a medication to help her sleep. Over the next 2 weeks she developed further physical symptoms and returned to her physician. During this visit she complained of dry mouth, constipation, urinary hesitancy, and some changes in her thinking. What is the unifying diagnosis that could explain these complaints?

   A. Depression
   B. Medication effect
   C. Prescribing trend
   D. Urinary outlet obstructions

ANSWERS TO PRE-TEST

1. B
2. A
3. D

ANSWERS TO POST-TEST

1. D
2. D
3. B

14

Health Promotion and Disease Prevention

David Haber, PhD

William Logan, MD

Sarah Schumacher, DO

● **LEARNING OBJECTIVES**

1. Describe the challenge of health promotion for older adults.
2. Discuss a "typical" geriatric patient.
3. Explain common disease screening recommendations associated with older adults.
4. Discuss healthy lifestyle recommendations for older adults.
5. Describe the process of follow-up for disease screening and health promotion activities, including the use of health contracts.

PRE-TEST

1. **Which of the following is FALSE regarding the challenges of health promotion counseling for older adults?**

   A. No two older adults experience the same chronic disease through the same set of symptoms.

   B. As individuals age, they become more similar in attitude and willingness to change.

   C. Older adults have usually established and experienced lifestyle patterns based on prior decisions.

   D. Health care providers need to be willing to take the time to establish rapport.

2. **Which of the following is NOT a typical concern with US geriatric patients?**

   A. Use of dietary supplements

   B. Access to health insurance

   C. Medication mismanagement

   D. Financial vulnerability

3. **A US Preventive Services Task Force recommendation of "I" indicates:**

   A. Data are present to allow strong recommendation for performance.

   B. Data are present to recommend against performing screening.

   C. There are not enough data to make a recommendation.

   D. A recommendation is under review.

INTRODUCTION TO GERIATRIC HEALTH PROMOTION

There are many contributors to a person's sense of health and personal well-being, including family, friends, institutions, educational attainment, environment, and medical care.[1] Health promotion is the provision of any education, health services (including procedures), or lifestyle support that leads to ongoing health and well-being for patients. Medical providers can contribute to health promotion by teaching patients about health and wellness, health services (including procedures), and lifestyle support that lead to ongoing health and well-being. It is important to note that in this discussion "health" means more than being free of disease and disability, especially for the many older persons who live with disease and are vulnerable to disability. Being able to manage the symptoms and complications of disease, and being open to lifestyle change and medical screenings, are fundamental goals of health promotion and disease prevention. As Americans live longer, quality of life supersedes quantity of life as the primary concern of older adults.[2]

All too often medical providers remain narrow in their thinking about health promotion, tending to think in terms of disease screening and prevention rather than healthy lifestyle promotion.[3] Complicating the picture is that the applicability of disease screening and prevention recommendations is complex for many of the oldest people in the context of variable patient preferences, co-morbidities and life expectancy, as well as a small evidence base concerning the effectiveness of much screening and preventive care in late life. Even in the area of healthy lifestyle promotion, a review of the literature reveals a high volume of information, but information that may often be summarized by "eat right, get enough sleep, exercise, and deal effectively with the stresses of life."[3] Despite the simplicity and seeming intuitiveness of this, many individuals, both young and old, remain ignorant or misinformed about how to best improve their own health. Therefore, there is still tremendous opportunity for health professionals to provide advice, health services, and education.

Health promotion for older adults presents unique challenges for both the patient and the provider. Unlike working with young or even middle-aged individuals, assessing an older adult's current health needs and building a set of personal health goals initially involves determining a number of other things. As individuals age, they do not become more similar, they become more unique and differentiated. For example, by age 70, a person has usually established and experienced lifestyle patterns based on prior decisions, whether conscious or unconscious. Understanding a person's preferences for exercise, diet, and daily time management requires getting to know them a bit as a person—their background, experiences, family composition, prior work experience, and activities in retirement. If someone is retired on a small pension, he or she will likely not wish to join an expensive health club or participate in extensive dietary counseling and education. On the other hand, an individual who has chosen daily exercise and pursued education on diet and healthy lifestyles might be a great candidate for further classes or supervised exercise toward a training goal.

Another way in which patients can differ vastly is belief in the medical system as a source for healthy goals. Because of some patients' backgrounds, experiences, and choices, they may be very negatively biased against information that comes from established medical research while being very open to alternative therapies. Unless health care providers are willing to take the time to establish rapport and ask about these things, attempts to counsel older patients about any health promotion ideas may be met with smiling and polite "noncompliance."

Each aging patient has her own complement of health challenges, including diseases resulting from prior lifestyle choices or family genetic tendencies. The average 70-year-old, for instance, may have three or more chronic diseases. To make things more complex, no two older adults experience the same chronic disease through the same set of symptoms or with the same severity. One older adult may control high blood pressure with exercise and limited salt intake, and another older patient's blood pressure may be unresponsive to lifestyle modifications and taking multiple medications. Thus, with older patients especially, approaches to care planning need to be very patient specific.

CASE PRESENTATION 1: WHAT DOES SHE NEED?

Doris Doe is a 78-year-old white woman who comes to a new-patient appointment in your office. As you introduce yourself to her and begin to chat, you find that her primary reason for the visit is seeking relief from her knee pain. She currently takes Aleve twice a day with partial relief. After seeing a TV commercial, she added glucosamine and chondroitin. She currently lives alone and handles all of her own affairs including finances. She still drives. She reports difficulty recently with these tasks and is afraid of falling. Her BMI is 28. Her blood pressure in the clinic today was 148/88. She last saw a physician about a year ago and has been taking hypertension medication on a regular basis.

When you ask about her daily physical activity, she admits to doing very little outside of walking to the street to get the newspaper. Alone in the home, she has low motivation for cooking her own meals and relies mostly on frozen foods that she puts in the microwave. She has not had any influenza vaccine during any flu season or any prior pneumococcal vaccinations. While her previous physician asked her about breast cancer screening with mammograms and osteoporosis screenings with bone densitometry, she has refused in the past, because she felt the testing was inconvenient and she did not understand the potential benefit.

Her church is a very important outlet for her socially and she attends faithfully. She has Medicare coverage for physician office visits, but she has to pay for her medications out of pocket (she could not understand any of the Medicare part D plans and chose not to sign up).

In terms of health promotion and disease prevention, what will you do in the future for Ms. Doe?

SNAPSHOT OF HEALTH IN OLDER ADULTS

Ms. Doe is a typical geriatric patient in several ways. Clinicians are more likely to encounter geriatric female than male patients. Women represent 56% of the population aged 65 to 74, but 72% of those over age 85.[4] In addition, older females are more likely to have an acute or chronic condition, more likely to visit a provider, and more likely to seek immediate medical care if they are sick or in pain.[5] Older adults with chronic impairments have a high likelihood of turning toward complementary or alternative medicine (CAM). One study reported that up to 88% of older adults used CAM techniques.[6] Dietary supplements are widely used by older adults in the United States, the most popular being ginkgo biloba (advocated for forgetfulness), St. John's wort (depressive symptoms), and glucosamine/chondroitin (arthritic pain and discomfort). In one study, 58% of Medicare recipients did not discuss dietary supplement usage with their physician,[7] and 65% of the supplements were not documented in a medical chart.[8] These supplement omissions are significant due to the risk of side effects or interactions with prescribed or over-the-counter medications, food, and drink.

Adults in their late 70s and beyond may decline in their ability to conduct Activities of Daily Living (ADLs)—eating, bathing, dressing, toileting, transfer, and walking (with walking the most common ADL limitation); and Instrumental Activities of Daily Living (IADLs)—home management, money management, meal preparation, making a phone call, and grocery shopping (with grocery shopping the most common IADL limitation). These vulnerabilities increase dramatically from age 65 to 74 to age 75+: fourfold for ADLs and threefold for IADLs.[9] Adults aged 75 and older account for 59% of fall-related deaths, even though make up only 5% of the population.[4] Another well-known geriatric syndrome, fear of falling, can lead to a cycle of inactivity, functional decline, and greater likelihood of falling. Two interventions that have been shown effective for fall prevention are exercise programs and reduction of environmental hazards in the home.

Medication mismanagement is a major concern with older adults, with about 50% of prescriptions not being taken properly according to the National Council on Patient Information and Education. About 5% of Medicare patients are made ill by their medications during the course of a year, leading to as many as 1.9 million drug-related injuries.[10] Among those with high blood pressure, a symptomless medical condition, only 25% remain in treatment and consistently take their medication in sufficient amounts to achieve adequate blood pressure control.[11]

By age 75, an average of 50% of women engage in no discretionary physical activity.[12] Sedentary behavior leaves older adults vulnerable to a wide array of conditions including cardiovascular disease, cancer, diabetes, depression, cognitive decline, osteoporosis, osteoarthritis, falls, and insomnia.[4] While many older adults report being conscientious about managing their diets, they may not be educated as to which dietary components need to be managed. For instance, a substantial percentage of hypertensive older persons are sodium sensitive and need to focus on reducing sodium intake. Those who are obese need to focus on reducing caloric intake (versus fat intake, which can distract from overall caloric consumption). Those with osteoporosis or osteopenia need to focus on calcium intake and vitamin D supplementation.

Almost half of older adults remain unvaccinated for pneumonia, with more vulnerability among older blacks and Hispanics.[13] Almost one-third did not receive an annual influenza vaccination, with African Americans at greatest risk.[14] Many more older adults have passed on the opportunity to take advantage of Medicare-covered medical screenings such as mammography, colonoscopy, densitometry, PSA and digital rectal exam, Pap smear and pelvic exam, cardiovascular screening, and diabetes screening.[4]

Both obesity (particularly up to age 75) and malnutrition (especially after age 75) increase with age. About one-third of older adults in their 70s are obese. Obesity exacerbates arthritis, and increases the probability of heart disease, diabetes, cancers of the breast, colon, and prostate, as well as premature mortality.[4] Between 16% and 30% of older Americans are malnourished or at high risk, with even higher percentages among older hospital patients and nursing home residents.[15] Malnourished older adults take 40% longer to recover from illness, have two to three times as many complications, and have hospital stays that are 90% longer.[4]

About 43% of women age 65 and older are widowed, in contrast to 14% of men in this age group,[9] which raises issues around whether older women have adequate financial, social, and emergency support. More than 80% of Americans past age 65 claim that their religious faith is the most important influence in their lives.[16] Recognizing the importance of religion in the health of older adults, about 70 medical schools offer instruction on how to address patients' religious beliefs.[17] Among older minorities, religious institutions may be the only community organization deemed trustworthy for providing health information.[18] Health programs implemented at religious institutions have improved mammography adherence,[19] reduced hypertension,[20] increased fruit and vegetable intake,[21] decreased weight,[22] and improved other physical and mental health measures.[23]

Financial vulnerability increases with age, particularly among older women. Social Security provides more than 50% of the total income level for 75% of single older women.[9] In 2004, the average monthly Social Security check was $826 for women, compared to $1076 for men. This can affect how older adults allocate for out-of-pocket expenses and medications as well as transportation to medical facilities. Choosing between medical care and food, utilities, and other essential expenses is a dilemma for low-income elders.

SCREENING

When assessing an older adult for health promotion or disease screening, the process can seem overwhelming for the novice and seasoned provider alike. There are multiple sources of expert opinions, guidelines, and recommendations including the US Preventive Services Task Force (USPSTF), American Geriatrics Society, American Cancer Society, National Osteoporosis Foundation, Centers for Disease Control and Prevention, ACOVE project (Assessing Care of Vulnerable Elders), American Heart Association, American College of Cardiology, Prevention Advisory Committee on Immunization Practices (ACIP), World Health Organization (WHO), and the Cochrane Reviews. As more data accumulate, recommendations often change and sometimes contradict what was previously recommended. Usually, individualized patient health promotion recommendations cannot be addressed in a single office visit and will evolve over several encounters.

The USPSTF provides recommendations on preventive services for patients at various stages of life. Formed in 1984, the goal of the task force was to reduce confusion among clinicians regarding effectiveness of preventive medicine interventions. Many recommendations are applicable to all age groups. Others are unique, specific guidelines for health promotion as it pertains to older adult patients. The USPSTF issues updated medical screening guidelines (http://www.ahrq .gov/clinic/pocketgd.htm). These guidelines are based on a rating system that gives the most weight to randomized controlled trials, followed by well-designed research trials without randomization. The rating system gives the least weight to other types of research as well as to the opinions of respected authorities or representatives of professional societies. Guidelines are rated from A (good evidence that intervention is *effective*) to D (good evidence that intervention should be *excluded*). An "I" recommendation means that the evidence is *insufficient* to recommend for or against the service—the service may or may not be useful, but has not been studied in sufficient detail for the task force to make a recommendation. Medicare coverage of health promotion adheres closely to the recommendations of USPSTF.[24]

MEDICARE

While it is true that many of Medicare's disease-prevention coverage decisions have been influenced by medical lobbyists rather than derived solely from evidence-based medicine,[25,26] a review of Medicare prevention coverage is a good initial exercise in understanding what needs to be discussed with an older patient.

It should be noted, though, that Medicare reimbursement policy has not only favored medical screenings over lifestyle changes, but that reimbursement decisions for medical screenings have exceeded evidence-based medical recommendations. For instance, Medicare provides coverage for an *annual* mammography for women, though based on evidence-based medicine, biannual mammograms would be sufficient. Also, routine annual coverage past age 65+ for prostate cancer screening and the baseline EKG past age 65+ have not been substantiated, but they are still covered by Medicare. Additionally, the efficacy of continuing medical screening coverage after age 75 or 80 is still being hotly debated in the research community (Table 14–1).[27-31]

TABLE 14–1

Screening[a]
Cardiovascular Health
Blood Pressure: Begin early adulthood, annually, ending around age 80.
Cholesterol: Begin early adulthood, every 2-3 years, ending around age 80.
Diabetes:
Cancer
Colorectal Cancer: Begin age 50, every 5-10 years for colonoscopy, ending around age 80.
Breast Cancer/Mammogram: Begin age 40, every year or two; begin age 50 annually; begin age 65 every 2 years; ending around age 80.
Cervical Cancer/Pap Smear: Begin with female sexual activity, two normal consecutive annual screenings, followed by every 3 years; two normal consecutive annual screenings around age 65, then discontinue.
Prostate Cancer: Do not do routinely, except if there is a family history or African-American heritage.
Bone Health
Osteoporosis/Bone Density: Begin early adulthood for women (no frequency recommended); every 2-3 years after age 65 for women, less frequently for men.
Immunizations
Tetanus: Routine Td vaccination of persons aged ≥ 65 years every 10 years.
Influenza: Annual influenza vaccination for all adults age 50 years and older.
Pneumococcal Polysaccharide (PPSV): Vaccination of persons aged ≥ 65 years with one dose; one revaccination for those who were initially vaccinated before age 65, provided that at least 5 years have elapsed since the initial vaccination.
Zoster: Single vaccination of persons aged ≥ 60 years with one dose.

[a]*These are estimates of what researchers recommend, relying most heavily on the US Preventive Services Task Force recommendations, but not exclusively on them.*

CASE PRESENTATION 1 (continued)

Based on your assessment of Ms. Doe, you create a problem list of health promotion issues that you will address with her over the next few visits. These include:

- Breast cancer screening
- Colon cancer screening
- Physical activity counseling
- Osteoporosis screening
- Immunizations
- Cervical cancer screening
- Nonmedical approaches to hypertension and degenerative arthritis management
- Overweight
- Lipids and cardiovascular health screening
- Screening for diabetes

GUIDELINES FOR DISEASE SCREENING IN OLDER ADULTS

This section includes evidence-based guidelines based primarily, but not exclusively, on USPSTF guidelines.

Cardiovascular Health

Cardiovascular disease is a major cause of death worldwide and the number one killer of Americans. A number of factors influence the development of cardiac disease and the course of illness. Three areas of particular importance for cardiovascular health include blood pressure screening and control, lipid screening and management, and diabetes screening and management.

Blood Pressure

Blood pressure screenings are not specifically covered by Medicare as they are considered standard practice for a patient visit. Even without a patient visit to a provider over the course of a year, blood pressure screenings are recommended annually throughout adulthood. The screening should be conducted in a physician's office where it is likely to be done more accurately than in the community and accompanied by counseling when needed.

In 2003, a panel of experts from the NIH issued updated federal guidelines stating that readings between 120 and 139 mm Hg systolic and 80 and 89 mm Hg diastolic should be considered pre-hypertensive. The NIH panel believed there was solid evidence that damage to blood vessels begins at pressure levels lower than the standard 140/90.[4]

Sixty-five percent of Americans aged 60 and over have high blood pressure; those who do not face a 90% chance of developing hypertension over the remainder of their lives.[32] Complicating the problem is the undertreatment of hypertension by providers, affecting perhaps as many as 75% of older patients.[33,34]

Overtreatment, however, also becomes a concern after the age of 80. There has been disagreement over whether blood pressure screenings should be discontinued at age 80 due to their uncertain impact on morbidity and mortality.[35-38] One study suggested that we should think twice before initiating drug therapy and attempting to lower mild-to-moderate systolic hypertension among persons aged 85 and over because of *increased* mortality when treated with blood pressure medication.[32] For more on hypertension, see Chapter 45.

Hyperlipidemia

In 2004, the National Cholesterol Education Program (NCEP) updated its Adult Treatment Panel III guidelines for management of lipidemia. Guidelines recommend high-risk patients should aim for a low-density lipoprotein (LDL) goal of below 100 mg/dL (2.59 mmol/L), with an optional goal of below 70 mg/dL (1.81 mmol/L) for patients at very high risk. Moderate-risk patients should aim for an LDL below 130 mg/dL (3.37 mmol/L) and lower-risk patients below 160 mg/dL (4.14 mmol/L). High risk is defined as the presence of coronary heart disease or its risk equivalent (such as diabetes with end-organ effect such as microalbuminuria), moderate risk is 2+ risk factors, and lower risk is zero to one risk factor. The major risk factors are cigarette smoking, hypertension, high-density lipoprotein below 40 mg/dL (1.04 mmol/L), family history of premature coronary heart disease, and age (men over 45 and women over 55). A high-density lipoprotein score above 60 mg/dL (1.55 mmol/L), however, removes one risk factor from the total count.

Additional counseling recommendations include a multifaceted lifestyle approach to reduce the risk for coronary heart disease including the reduction of saturated fat (below 7% of total calories) and cholesterol (below 200 mg per day), increased fiber (10-25 g/day), weight reduction, and increased physical activity. A review of the NCEP report, however, reveals limited attention to this lifestyle approach, and provides unrealistic lifestyle recommendations, such as a daily limit on dietary cholesterol to less than the amount in the yolk of a single large egg. There appears to be a clear bias toward statins and other drugs as the best way to reduce the cholesterol level.

The medication recommendations for hyperlipidemia raise several questions. Following the recommendations, the number of Americans taking cholesterol-lowering drugs would be 43 million. Can the health system afford the expenditures for medication costs? What are the long-term clinical effects of treating persons at earlier ages and more aggressively over longer periods? Finally, do screening and treatment of patients over the age of 80 lower mortality?[39] Cholesterol screening is covered every 5 years by Medicare without a deductible or a copayment.

CASE PRESENTATION 1 (continued)

You ask about Ms. Doe's family history and find out that her mother lived to be 92 and died in her sleep. She had hypertension but no other problems. Her father fell off a ladder and broke his hip at age 67. He later developed Alzheimer disease. There is no history of stroke or heart attack in her family, and no history of cancer. Based on your review of the literature, you believe that it is worthwhile to treat Ms. Doe's hypertension. However, given her age and lack of family history for stroke or heart disease, you discuss with her that it would be reasonable not to test her lipids.

Diabetes

Diabetes is a major co-morbid condition associated with cardiovascular disease. The USPSTF recommends screening for type 2 diabetes in asymptomatic adults with sustained blood pressure (either treated or untreated) greater than 135/80 mm Hg. The American Diabetes Association (ADA) recommends that the fasting plasma glucose test for screening patients with levels of 126 mg/dL (6.99 mmol/L) or greater needs confirmation with repeat testing. The optimal screening interval is unknown. Based on expert opinion, the ADA recommends screening every 3 years.

Annual diabetes screenings are covered by Medicare, and patients with pre-diabetes (fasting glucose 100-125 mg/dL, 5.55-6.94 mmol/L) may be screened every 6 months, with no deductible or copayment. While not covered routinely, the diabetes screening recommendations include most older persons on Medicare, because eligibility includes persons who are overweight, have a family history of diabetes, or who have pre-diabetes, hypertension, or dyslipidemia. The USPSTF had concluded that there was insufficient evidence to recommend for or against routine screening for diabetes in asymptomatic adults.

Pre-diabetes, or what was previously referred to as "glucose intolerance," has become more of a target of health professionals because diet, exercise, and weight loss are more effective during this stage, with an estimated 60% risk reduction for those who would otherwise develop diabetes with its associated complications.[4]

Cancer

Cervical Cancer

Cervical cancer screening is covered by Medicare every 2 years, with no deductible (but a copayment applies). Pap smear and pelvic examination are included in the screening. Until the 1940s, more American women died of cervical cancer than any other type of malignancy. However, the Pap test, named for its creator, George Papanicolaou, has reduced the death rate by 70%. Screenings are recommended to begin at the age at which women first engage in sexual intercourse, and should be repeated every 3 years after women have had at least two normal annual screenings.

For women aged 65 and older, routine screening for cervical cancer is NOT recommended in those who have had adequate recent screening with normal Pap smears and are otherwise at low risk for cervical cancer. The USPSTF

concluded that the harms of continued routine screening, such as false-positive tests and invasive procedures, outweigh the benefits. About 75% of older women, however, have not had adequate screening; and nearly half have never received a Pap test. The American Cancer Society suggests stopping cervical cancer screening at age 70.

Colorectal Cancer

Colorectal cancer screening is covered annually for fecal occult tests with no deductible or copayment, every 4 years for sigmoidoscopy or barium enema with deductible and copayment, and every 10 years for colonoscopies with deductible and copayment. USPSTF recommends screening all adults beginning at age 50 and continuing until age 75. USPSTF recommends against routine screening for colorectal cancer in adults 76 to 85 years old, but recognizes that individual patient factors may support screening. Screening for colorectal cancer in adults over 85 years old is NOT recommended.

The US Preventive Services Task Force reports that digital rectal examinations are of limited value (10% detection rate), fecal occult blood tests produce a high percentage of false-positives (5-10%), and a sigmoidoscopy accesses just 40% of the colon. Colonoscopies, therefore, are the colorectal screening option of choice. While there is no upper age limit with Medicare coverage, researchers have argued that this screening test may be discontinued at age 80 with minimal loss in life expectancy.[29,31] Limited life expectancy, in contrast to the likelihood of slow-growing tumors, and the risk of perforation of the older intestinal lining during colonoscopy, become factors to consider after age 70.[40]

Breast Cancer

Mammography is covered annually by Medicare with no deductible, but a copayment applies. The effectiveness of mammograms has been hotly debated since 2001, though at the time this chapter is being written this medical screening is being widely endorsed again. The latest USPSTF recommendations have been updated and are a change from previous recommendations. They state that women without risk factors should start screening at age 50 instead of the previous recommendation of 40. Women between the ages of 50 and 74 without symptoms or risk factors should undergo mammography every other year rather than annually. There is insufficient evidence either for or against a screening recommendation for women ages 75 and over. Physicians can stop teaching patients to perform breast self-examinations, because there is no evidence they are effective.

In addition to the challenge regarding the effectiveness of mammograms,[41] Medicare does not cover the full cost of mammograms. This inadequate reimbursement rate combined with the risk of legal liability has increased the waiting time for this screening test. Legal liability is a concern because between 15% and 40% of cancers are not detected by mammography clinics[42]—that is, they are false-negative tests; while 50% of women who have had 10 mammograms will have had one result that led to unnecessary further testing that is, false-positive tests, with 20% of these women undergoing a breast biopsy.[43]

The real challenge when investigating screening for breast cancer lies in making recommendations for older women. The precise age at which to discontinue screening mammography is not certain. There are very few randomized, controlled studies in older women. It is well known that as women advance in age there is a higher probability of developing and dying from breast cancer. Unfortunately, so is the chance of dying from other causes. Decision-making must include potential mammography benefits (earlier detection of breast cancer, reducing chance of dying from breast cancer) versus potential harm (false-positive results, unnecessary biopsies, etc.). Older women with multiple co-morbid conditions that limit their life expectancy are unlikely to benefit from screening. Clinical breast exams alone and routine self-breast exams have insufficient data regarding effectiveness as breast cancer screening tools, although most providers continue to teach and recommend these procedures. Although men are not screened for breast cancer, it is imperative for providers to recognize that men can also be affected by this disease. Any breast signs or symptoms in patients of either gender warrant further discussion, examination, and evaluation in accordance to the patient's health care wishes.

CASE PRESENTATION 1 (continued)

Over the next few visits, you discuss with Ms. Doe diabetes screening, breast cancer, colon cancer, and cervical cancer screening. She reports that she had regular Pap screening in the past with no history of abnormal tests before stopping screening at age 60. She is interested in being tested for diabetes since this just involves drawing some blood. She is a bit more reluctant to consider mammography and colon cancer screening. She has had two mammograms in the past but did not want to continue because they were very uncomfortable. She feels her risk is low since no one in her family has had breast cancer, and she had two friends who had biopsies for abnormal mammograms that turned out not to be cancer. Her preference would be no further mammograms. She says she will consider colon cancer screening with a colonoscopy but she needs to "think about it," as she has never had the test and thinks that perhaps having it at least once might be a good idea. You agree and decide to bring this up at her next follow-up visit.

CASE PRESENTATION 2: UP MORE AT NIGHT

Mr. Schafer is a 68-year-old male who lives with his wife of 45 years in their single-level home with two small dogs. He has underlying hypertension treated with lisinopril and hydrochlorothiazide, degenerative arthritis for which he takes acetaminophen when the pain is severe, and osteoporosis for which he takes calcium, vitamin D, and a once-weekly oral bisphosphonate. The osteoporosis was diagnosed after he slipped and fell in his bathroom shower, fracturing his right wrist, 3 years ago. He comes to you today stating that his urinary stream is getting slower and that he has to get up two or three times per night to urinate. Two years ago, he was just getting up once a night as he had for the past 20 years.

Prostate Cancer

Annual prostate cancer screenings are covered by Medicare through digital rectal examinations and prostate-specific antigen screening tests (PSA tests), with no deductible or copayment. Over the past few years, the controversy over the effectiveness of prostate cancer screening tests has grown. Most men who undergo a biopsy for an abnormal PSA test do not turn out to have prostate cancer, because high PSA readings often signal a benign enlarged prostate. Of those who do have cancer, some are fast growing and have already spread before treatment can be implemented and others are slow growing and will have no effect on life expectancy or symptoms. Moreover, finding an early tumor forces men to choose between watchful waiting and several non-benign treatment modalities—surgery, radiation, and hormone therapy—that can cause incontinence, impotence, painful defecation, or chronic diarrhea. Men whose tumors would not have resulted in symptoms or limited life expectancy can suffer serious side effects for no net gain.

The prior national health guideline, which recommended that men over age 75 NOT undergo a routine PSA screening, has not affected Medicare policy regarding coverage of an annual screening without discontinuation. It remains to be seen how two new rigorous studies—one involving 182,000 men in several European countries[44] and the other 77,000 men at 10 medical centers in the United States[45]—will affect practice. Both studies reported that prostate cancer screening saved few lives. Prostate cancer screening has been highly promoted in the United States despite past controversies, in contrast to Europe, where it is not widely recommended on a routine basis.

Bone Health

Bone Density

Biannual densitometry screenings are covered by Medicare, with a deductible and copayment applicable. Osteoporosis (bone density that is 2.5 or more standard deviations below the young adult peak bone density) was found in 7% of more than 200,000 reportedly healthy women aged 50 and older, and osteopenia (T-Score 1-2.5 standard deviations) in an additional 40% of women.[46]

While the USPSTF recommends that routine screening begins at age 65 for all women, it is still not known how often women should undergo screenings (typically every 2 or 3 years is recommended) and at what age if at all that screenings should be discontinued. Routine screening should begin earlier (age 60) for women at increased risk for osteoporotic fractures. Because only one of five cases of osteoporosis affect men, screenings for men are thought to be needed less frequently; specific screening intervals for men are not given.

Interventions for reducing or reversing bone loss are effective and include an increase in dietary calcium, calcium and vitamin D supplementation, weight-bearing exercise, hormone replacement therapy, and medications such as the bisphosphonates. (For more on bone health and osteoporosis, see Chapter 41.)

CASE PRESENTATION 2 (continued)

You examine Mr. Schafer and find that he has a moderately enlarged prostate which is smooth, rubbery, and without nodules. You discuss with him that this likely represents benign prostatic hyperplasia, which you explain to him, and that there may be some medications that could help his urinary symptoms. He asks about whether he should have PSA testing. You discuss with him that his symptoms would generally not be suggestive of prostate cancer, though at his age and given the unclear data, whether he has a PSA test or not is really his choice. He reports that his neighbor had to have a prostate biopsy after finding an elevated PSA, and he told him that the biopsy felt like someone "shooting a nail gun up my rear end." He decides to defer on PSA testing. Before leaving Mr. Schafer asks if he should have another bone density DEXA scan, since the last one was 3 years ago and he was told that it should be rechecked regularly by his orthopedist. You tell him it would be reasonable, but again there are no specific recommendations as to frequency of bone density retesting, but since it is noninvasive, you and he agree to schedule a retesting of his bone density before the next visit.

● GUIDELINES FOR HEALTHY LIFESTYLE PRACTICES IN OLDER ADULTS

What is covered by Medicare and secondary insurance is variable, but it is worth understanding what may be covered and what is not. Regarding lifestyle changes covered by Medicare, clinicians need to do a better job of recommending that older adults take advantage of an increasing amount of prevention and health promotion coverage that is being provided for older adults by Medicare. For instance, after 2 years of a "Welcome to Medicare" physical examination provided at no charge, only 2% of eligible seniors have taken advantage. Many clinicians are unaware that Medicare now covers smoking cessation, as well as health promotion programs for persons with cardiovascular disease.

The average patient in a family practice waiting room needs 25 preventive services.[47] Using a base of 2500 patients, researchers conservatively estimated that 7.4 hours a day would be needed to provide the recommended preventive care in a typical practice. Disease prevention and health promotion, therefore, require prioritizing among the many available medical screenings, immunizations, and risk reduction counseling areas.

CASE PRESENTATION 3: ARE YOU INTERESTED IN GETTING HELP?

Mrs. Lee is a 74-year-old Japanese-American who is moderately overweight and knows she is much too sedentary. When she comes to the office, she is approached by one of the medical staff. "Mrs. Lee, are you interested in getting help with improving your health? We have two options in our medical clinic. You can pick up a self-help brochure from our receptionist who will review how to use the document, and then we will briefly check on your progress each time you come for a medical visit. This option is a free service.

"Or, we have affiliated with a health educator who will provide one-to-one guidance at our clinic. This option is $60 an hour, and we estimate the total cost will be $180 for two visits and five phone calls. Also, we will follow up with you during your medical visits at the clinic. Are you interested in either option?"

"Yes, I am. My daughter has been encouraging me to do something like this for years and has promised to pay for health counseling if I would follow through on it. I really appreciate this opportunity."

The above conversation needs to be embedded within a host of practices that converts a medical clinic into a health clinic. In addition to telling all patients that the health care team values health and provides options for them to improve health, office staff need to be educated about health values and how they can each contribute to the achievement of patient health goals. The health-promoting protocol can start with the receptionist, who informs patients that the health clinic offers a variety of health information and services. Other staff, however, also need to know what is expected of them and how they will be held accountable.

The front office waiting area needs to contain up-to-date health promotion and disease prevention materials, along with charts and pictures pertaining to health hanging on the walls. One health priority area can be prioritized by a medical practice, with specific health education material on this topic personally given to all suitable patients who visit the clinic, or mailed to the appropriate segment of the patient population.

One strategy for selecting which health goal to prioritize is to find out if there is a high percentage of the older patient population in your individual or group practice with a specific problem, such as skipping flu shots, underutilization of mammograms, obesity, or sedentary behavior. Another strategy is to check whether the city, county, or state has a particularly urgent gerontologic health issue that needs to be addressed. These data can be obtained by contacting your local public health department. It is important that a baseline percentage is obtained among your patient population and then compared 6 months later to assess whether progress has been made.

Two good sources of information for the conversion of a medical clinic into a health clinic are the Put Prevention Into Practice initiative, developed by the US Public Health Service's Office of Disease Prevention and Health Promotion[48] and the Community-Oriented Primary Care model.[49]

Exercise/Physical Activity

Physical activity has long been linked with optimal health. Clearly, multiple benefits of regular exercise in older adults include reduced risk of cardiovascular disease, stroke, hypertension, breast and colon cancer, diabetes, and falls.[50] Exercise can also benefit older adults as a therapeutic option for several chronic diseases, including congestive heart failure, mood disorders, dementia, chronic pain syndromes, and stroke. Exercise is beneficial at any age, and reduces mortality while maintaining independence.

Exercise prescriptions for older adult patients should build up over time to include a minimum of 30 minutes of aerobic activity 5 days each week. In addition to aerobic exercise, training focus should include weight training, resistance, flexibility, and balance work. The American Heart Association emphasizes a step-wise introduction of physical activity for adults beginning an exercise program. This improves patient safety and adherence to the exercise plan.

Unhealthy Habits

Smoking

The current older generation has a long history of high rates of tobacco use and smoking-related mortality from lung cancer, cardiovascular disease, and COPD. Clinicians should screen all adults for tobacco use and provide tobacco cessation interventions for those who use tobacco products. Smoking cessation can reduce mortality risks. One study reports that at 5 years post smoking cessation, older adults have reduction in mortality rates when compared to peers who continue to smoke.[51] Several smoking cessation approaches are effective for patients, including provider recommendation, smoking cessation counseling programs, and pharmacotherapy.

Alcohol

Approximately 15% of adults over age 65 experience health problems due to the complications of alcohol consumption with medications or chronic diseases. Alcoholism is identified in 2% to 4% of all older adults.[52] Alcohol use in older adults can negatively impact function and cognition. Providers are encouraged to screen all older adults for alcohol misuse by inquiring about specific frequency and quantity of alcohol consumption. Providers may have a positive impact through recommendations and advice for patients to reduce and cease alcohol ingestion.

UNIQUE GERIATRIC ISSUES

Injury Prevention and Falls

Fall prevention is an assessment category important to patients 65 and older. The annual incidence of falls in older adults who live independently is quite significant at 25% for 65-year-olds and 50% for patients older than 80. Falls are not benign and are responsible for considerable morbidity and mortality. Several factors can contribute to falling. Intrinsic factors include age-related changes in vision and hearing, gait, and musculoskeletal strength. Chronic and acute disease can contribute to a person falling. For assessment and screening guidelines for falls, refer to Chapter 34.

Driving

Driving is a key part of independence for older adults. As the population ages, more and more of the drivers on the road will be older. The rate of crashes involving older adults, adjusted for miles driven, is higher than the rate for all other age groups; older adults are also more susceptible to physical and cognitive debility that might interfere with driving fitness. Noticing sensory impairment (vision especially), cognitive impairment, and/or significant declines in reaction time, strength, and flexibility that could impact driving fitness should lead to further evaluation. Discussing driving fitness assessments and decisions when patients are doing well can establish a baseline for further discussion if driving fitness problems develop in the future. In cases where future physical or cognitive difficulties are anticipated, it is helpful to have the patient and family agree to allow the provider or a key family member to make the decision about when driving capabilities are no longer sufficient for safe driving. Currently, while there are guidelines for driving fitness evaluation in the elderly from the AMA, AARP, and other groups, there is no gold standard for driving fitness assessment. (See Chapter 15 for additional information on evaluating the older driver.)

Vaccinations

Influenza

Influenza is a serious viral infection in the elderly with significant morbidity and mortality. In fact, older adults comprise the majority of influenza-related deaths (more than 90%). Data from several studies confirm that influenza vaccination is associated with reduced hospitalization, death, and overall incidence of influenza in older adults.[53] Annual influenza immunization for individuals 50 and older is recommended through the Advisory Committee on Immunization Practices (ACIP). Note that older adults should NOT receive the live attenuated intranasal preparation of the influenza vaccine, as this vaccine is only approved for "healthy" adults up to the age of 49 with no co-morbid conditions.

Tetanus

Tetanus is a rare condition in most developed countries, with the majority of cases occurring in unvaccinated or underimmunized older adults. In the United States, 60% of all reported tetanus cases are in adults over the age of 60.[54] Tetanus is preventable by immunization. Current ACIP recommendations include a single Td booster after age 50 in patients who have completed the primary series and have not had a booster within the last 10 years. Booster doses of adult-type tetanus and diphtheria toxoid should otherwise be administered every 10 years.

Pneumococcal Vaccine (PPV)

Community-acquired pneumonia in older populations is associated with hospital mortality and 30-day mortality rates of 11% to 20%.[55] In 2008, rates of pneumococcal invasive disease in these groups were 40.8 per 100,000 population.[56] *Streptococcus pneumoniae* is the most common cause of community-acquired bacterial pneumonia, occurring most frequently among the elderly.

The ACIP recommends pneumococcal vaccine for all persons age 65 years and older. The ACIP does NOT recommend routine revaccination with the vaccine every 5 years. The ACIP recommends that persons age 65 years and older who were initially vaccinated before age 65 should receive only one revaccination, provided that at least 5 years have elapsed since the initial vaccination.

Zoster Vaccine

Herpes zoster, also known as shingles, is associated with significant morbidity in older adults. One million cases of herpes zoster occur annually in the United States, and individuals age 60 and older comprise nearly half of all cases.[57] In addition to the pain of the acute phase of this disease, older adult patients are at markedly increased risk for long-term complications including debilitating post-herpetic neuralgia, vision loss, and depression. In the late 1990s, Oxman and colleagues initiated the Shingles Prevention Study, evaluating the Oka/Merck VZV vaccine and vaccination outcomes affecting incidence, severity, and complications of herpes zoster.[58] This randomized, double-blind, placebo-controlled, multicenter trial has confirmed the hypothesis that the zoster vaccine is beneficial in older adults who had previous varicella infection but never had primary zoster. Patients receiving the vaccine had a nearly 52% reduction of the incidence of zoster disease. Those people who developed zoster disease despite vaccination had less severe disease than the placebo group and a nearly 50% reduction in the incidence of post-herpetic neuralgia. The vaccine was generally safe and well tolerated, with the most common adverse effect being a mild injection site reaction.

Zoster vaccine is recommended for all persons aged ≥ 60 years who have no contraindications, including persons who report a previous episode of zoster or who have chronic medical conditions. It is not appropriate for treatment in patients with acute zoster or postherpetic neuralgia. Currently, Medicare does not cover the cost of zoster vaccinations in the outpatient office setting. Many prescription plans will pay for part or all of the vaccine if prescribed as a medication.

● MISCELLANEOUS CONSIDERATIONS

Ethnic Diversity

The diversity of the older adult population is increasing. Between 1990 and 2030, the increase in the population age 65+ will be 131% among African Americans, 147% among Native Americans, 285% among Asians and Pacific Islanders, and 328% among Hispanic Americans.[59]

Much progress has been made in recent years in the area of cross-cultural health promotion. Realizing that every culture potentially has different beliefs and priorities that shape its view of the concept of health and what constitutes a healthy lifestyle will prepare any health care provider to be sensitive to these cultural and ethnic differences when he or she is providing health promotion. The older a patient is, often the more deeply held his or her beliefs will be. Communicating respect for these beliefs to the elder may open the provider–patient dialogue even further for health promotion counsel and education.

Health professionals need to learn new knowledge and skills to improve the adherence of older ethnic clients to their health goals. Additional knowledge and improved communication skills may lead to better adherence to health recommendations and to enhanced health outcomes.[60,61] Most fundamental to this endeavor is to establish trust and sensitivity toward effective communication. Different ethnic groups, for instance, relate better to extended silence as a natural part of conversation, to eye contact, to spatial proximity, to the expression of emotion, or to touching or hand gestures.[62]

Other relevant questions include: Are there cultural traditions that influence your diet? Do you believe regular exercise is a desirable goal in late life? What type of help or assistance do you expect from family or friends? What prevention or health promotion practices are different in your heritage from mainstream health care in the United States?

Additional information on cultural and ethnic issues is available in Chapter 5. For a list of health-promoting questions of relevance to ethnic elders, see Haber.[62]

Health Information on the Internet

Information (whether evidence based or not) is more available now than ever. With the growth of Internet technology, even previously non–computer-literate older adults are now able to access and indeed are often bombarded with huge amounts of information through Web searches and e-mail. Due to time constraints, face-to-face communication with health professionals has become increasingly limited and more patients are using the Internet for health information. According to a 2005 national survey conducted by the Pew Internet and American Life Project, 80% of American Internet users have sought information on health topics.

The fastest growing segment using the Internet is the age 50+ category. Much of this growth in computer usage is taking place among the boomers, the next generation of older adults. A national Kaiser Family Foundation survey in 2005 reported that 31% of persons age 65+ have gone online, but over 70% of the boomers have done so.

It is not uncommon for older patients to download and print information to bring to their provider's visit for review and discussion. Often how a provider responds to this will also determine whether that patient will continue to be receptive to counsel or simply write off the provider as biased and uninformed. It is worth careful consideration of anything that the patient brings in or wishes to discuss. Such respect will go a long way toward promoting ongoing health promotion dialogue. Internet users need to be cautioned about the credentials of the contributors to websites, whether the contributor has a financial stake in the products or information (particularly among ".com" sites), and if there are other sources of information with competing points of view.

Health Counseling

When considering the topic of health promotion and disease prevention with older patients, providers communicate to older patients considerably less cardiac risk reduction advice on diet, exercise, weight control, smoking, and stress management than they give their younger clients.[63] Using audiotapes and other research tools, investigators have found that physicians seem more reluctant to discuss prevention and psychosocial issues with older patients than with younger ones.[64]

Communication between clinician and patient can be impeded by differences in age, educational attainment, ethnic beliefs, socioeconomic status, religion, and gender. Clinicians who are most similar to their patients are viewed as better communicators and more participatory. For example, physicians receive highest ratings on participatory decision-making style when they and their patients are of the same gender and race.[65]

Clinics, however, are not blessed with the resources to match patients with clinicians who are similar to them. Moreover, communication and trust take time, which is not a luxury afforded to anyone in most health care settings. Access to a health educator, therefore, can be a major asset in a medical practice that wants to promote health and prevent disease. Time spent with a health educator is less expensive than time with a clinician, and health educators are specialized in the important skill of health behavior change. According to the US Preventive Services Task Force,[66] patient education and counseling may be more important to client health than conventional clinical activities such as diagnostic testing.

● FOLLOW-UP OF HEALTH PROMOTION/ DISEASE PREVENTION

Follow-up can be performed on a facility-wide or individual basis. *Facility-wise*, let us say that the baseline percentage of mammograms for one clinical practice is particularly low, about 48% for female patients age 50 and over during the past 2 years. A 6-month follow-up allows for enough time to reach the stated goal of 70% for this practice, which is approximately equal to the national average. Six months is not too long a period in which the focus of the goal may be diluted over time among clinic staff, and it is not too short a period of time to make time itself the issue rather than the effectiveness of the facility-wide intervention.

It is also important to give feedback to staff on the success or failure of a facility-wide health goal, and to meet as a team at the end of 6 months to discuss the prospect of another health goal or the continuation of the previous one. Success should be celebrated through individual praise of staff members and a social gathering of the entire health care team. Failures need to be analyzed as a group and future modifications discussed.

With *individual patients*, follow-up contact can be performed in a variety of ways: through a patient visit or telephone contact with a health educator, through written or telephone contact by a receptionist or another staff person, or incorporated into a routine medical visit.

Using the health contract technique with a health educator, the patient can receive a second scheduled visit with the health educator at the end of the 1-month health contract period (Figure 14–1). The purpose of this follow-up visit is to assess the month-long success ratio of the patient in achieving his or her health goal, and to help determine a potential future

My health goal is:_____

My motivation for my health goal is:	Problems that may interfere with reaching my health goal and solutions:
1._____	_____
2._____	_____
3._____	_____
My Plan of Action	_____
For social or emotional support I will...	_____
	_____
To remind me of new behaviors I will...	_____
My signature/date Support person's signature/date	

FIGURE 14–1. Health contract.

goal. It should be noted that prior to this follow-up interview, a phone call from the health educator to the patient takes place at the end of each of the first 3 weeks to offer encouragement, assess progress, and suggest modifications if needed.

After these phone calls and the follow-up monthly meeting, another two telephone calls are conducted. One occurs at the end of 2 weeks to assess whether there is continued progress on the health goal, if that option is selected, or whether there is progress on the next health goal selected and whether modifications are needed. The other phone call takes place at the end of the second month to determine if the continued or new health goal was accomplished. If longer-term success is to be evaluated, additional phone calls or in-person visits can be scheduled.

If patients opt for receiving a self-help guide by the receptionist, the ideal follow-up is a phone call by the receptionist in about 2 weeks. If the patients are having some success with their health goal, praise is given to them and reinforced during their next regularly scheduled medical visit. If patients have not been successful with their health goals, the health educator option can be offered once again.

If the entire population pool receives a mail-out from the practice for any reason, this opportunity can be seized for recommending the health-promoting priority of the practice to individual patients who have failed to take advantage of this initiative previously. For those who have demonstrated some degree of success with a previous health priority, a follow-up congratulatory letter signed by the nurse or physician can be highly motivating to patients.

CONCLUSION

Medical care is not synonymous with health care. To be concerned about health promotion and disease prevention among older patients, a systematic plan must be designed, implemented, and evaluated. In addition to the health benefits received by patients, a health perspective can provide tremendous professional satisfaction to the provider as well as an effective strategy for growing a practice. When potential patients hear about the unusual emphasis of a medical clinic or medical professional in caring for the health promotion and disease prevention of geriatric patients, there is a strong interest among older adults in being a part of this endeavor.

References

1. Glanz K, Bishop DM. The role of behavioral science theory in the development and implementation of public health interventions. *Ann Rev Public Health ePub*, January 2010.

2. Resnick B. *Topics in Advanced Practice Nursing eJournal*. 2001;1.

3. Goldberg TH, Chavin SI. Preventive medicine and screening in older adults. *J Am Geriatr Soc*. 1997;45:344-354.

4. Haber D. *Health Promotion and Aging: Practical Applications for Health Professional*. 5th ed. New York: Springer; 2010.

5. Shelton D. Men avoid physician visits, often don't know whom to see. *Am Med News*. 2000;1-33.

6. Ness J, Cirillo DJ, Weir D, et al. Use of complementary medicine in older Americans: Results from the Health and Retirement Study. *Gerontologist*. 2005;45:516-524.

7. Astin J, Pelletier KR, Marie A, Haskell WL. Complementary and alternative medicine use among elderly persons: One-year analysis of a Blue Shield Medicare supplement. *J Gerontol Series A: Biol Sci Med Sci*. 2000;55:M4-M9.

8. Cohen R, Ek K, Pan CX, et al. Complementary and alternative medicine (CAM) use by older adults: A comparison of self-report and physician chart documentation. *J Gerontol Series A: Biol Sci Med Sci*. 2002; 57:M223-M227.

9. Hooyman N, Kiyak H. *Social Gerontology: A Multidisciplinary Perspective*, Boston: Allyn & Bacon; 2008.

10. Gurwitz J, Field TS, Avorn J, et al. Incidence and preventability of adverse drug events among older persons in the ambulatory setting. *JAMA*. 2003;289:1107-1116.

11. National Heart, Lung, and Blood Institute. *Report of the Joint National Committee on Treatment of High Blood Pressure*. Washington, DC: US Department of Health and Human Services; 1997.

12. *Surgeon General's Report on Physical Activity and Health*. Washington, DC: US Government Printing Office; 1996.

13. Mieczkowski T, Wilson S. Adult pneumococcal vaccination: A review of physician and patient barriers. *Vaccine*. 2002;20:1383-1392.

14. Medicare screenings, vaccines underused. *Am Med News*. June 17, 2002:7.

15. Beers M, Berkow R. *The Merck Manual of Geriatrics*. 3rd ed. Whitehouse Station, NJ: Merck; 2000.

16. Moberg D. The ecological fallacy: Concerns for program planners. *Generations*. 1983;8:12-14.

17. Duenwald M. Religion and health: New research revives an old debate. *New York Times*, May 7, 2002:D1-D4.

18. Williams M. Increasing participation in health promotion among older African-Americans. *Am J Health Behav*. 1996;20:389-399.

19. Duan N, Fox S, Derose KP, Carson S. Maintaining mammography adherence through telephone counseling in a church-based trial. *Am J Public Health*. 2000;90:1468-1471.

20. Smith E, Merritt S, Patel M. Church-based education: An outreach program for African Americans with hypertension. *Ethnicity Health*. 1997;2:243-253.

21. Resnicow K, Jackson A, Wang T, et al. A motivational interviewing intervention to increase fruit and vegetable intake through black churches: Results of the Eat for Life Trial. *Am J Public Health*. 2001;91:1686-1693.

22. Kumanyika D, Charleston J. Lose weight and win: A church-based weight loss program for blood pressure control among black women. *Patient Ed Counsel*. 1992;19:19-32.

23. Randsdell L. Church-based health promotion: An untapped resource for women 65 and older. *Am J Health Promotion*. 1995;9:333-336.

24. US Preventive Services Task Force. *The Guide to Clinical Preventive Services*. Rockville, MD: Agency for Healthcare Research and Quality; 2005.

25. Haber D. Medicare prevention: Movement toward research-based policy. *J Aging Social Policy*. 2001;13:1-14.

26. Haber D. Medicare prevention update. *J Aging Social Policy*. 2005; 17:1-6.

27. US Preventive Services Task Force. Screening for prostate cancer. *Ann Intern Med*. 2008;149:185-189.

28. US Preventive Services Task Force. Screening for colorectal cancer. *Ann Intern Med*. 2008;149:627-637.

29. Lin O, Kozarek RA, Schembre DB, et al. Screening colonoscopy in very elderly patients: Prevalence of neoplasia and estimated impact on life expectancy. JAMA. 2006;295:2357-2365.

30. Rastas E, Pirttila T, Viramo P, et al. Association between blood pressure and survival over 9 years in a general population aged 85 and older. J Am Geriatr Soc. 2006;54:912-918.

31. Rich J, Black W. When should we stop screening? Effective Clin Pract. 2000;3:78-84.

32. Vasan R, Beiser A, Seshadri S, et al. Residual lifetime risk for developing hypertension in middle-aged women and men. JAMA. 2002;287:1003-1010.

33. Hyman D, Pavlik V. Characteristics of patients with uncontrolled hypertension in the United States. N Engl J Med. 2001;345:479-486.

34. Oliveria S, Lapuerta P, McCarthy B, et al. Physician-related barriers to the effective management of uncontrolled hypertension. Arch Inter Med. 2002;162:413-420.

35. Amery A, Birkenhäger W, Brixko R, et al. Efficacy of antihypertensive drug treatment according to age, sex, blood pressure and previous cardiovascular disease in patients over the age of 60. Lancet. 1986;2:589-592.

36. Gueyffier F, Bulpitt C, Boissel J, et al. Antihypertensive drugs in very old people: A subgroup meta-analysis of randomized controlled trials. Lancet. 1999;353:793-796.

37. Rigaud A, Forette B. Hypertension in older adults. J Gerontol Series A Biol Sci Med Sci. 2001;56:M217-M225.

38. Staessen J, Fagard J, Thijs L, et al. Subgroup and per-protocol analysis of the randomized European trial on isolated systolic hypertension in the elderly. Arch Inter Med. 1998;158:1681-1691.

39. Foody J, Rathore S, Galusha D, et al. Hydroxymethylglutaryl-CoA reductase inhibitors in older persons with acute myocardial infarction. J Am Geriatr Soc. 2006;54:421-430.

40. Ko C, Sonnenberg A. Comparing risks and benefits of colorectal cancer screening in elderly patients. Gastroenterology. 2005;129:1163-1178.

41. Gotzsche P, Nielsen M. Screening for breast cancer with mammography. Cochrane Database Syst Rev. 2006;art. no. CD001877. DOI.10.1002/14651858.CD001877.pub2.

42. Moss M. Senator says it's time to upgrade standards. New York Times, October 24, 2002:12.

43. Elmore J, Barton M, Moceri V, et al. Ten-year risk of false positive screening mammograms and clinical breast examinations. N Engl J Med. 1998;338:1089-1096.

44. Kolata G. Prostate cancer screening found to save few, if any, lives. New York Times, March 19, 2009:27.

45. Andriole G, Crawford D, Grub R, et al. Mortality results from a randomized prostate cancer screening trial. N Engl J Med. 2009;360:1310-1319.

46. Siris E, Miller P, Barrett-Connor E, et al. Identification and fracture outcomes of undiagnosed low bone mineral density in postmenopausal women: Results from the National Osteoporosis Risk Assessment. JAMA. 2001;286:2815-2822.

47. Yarnall K, Pollak K, Østbye T, et al. Primary care: Is there enough time for prevention? Am J Public Health. 2003;93:635-641.

48. Melnikow J, Kohatsu ND, Chan BK. Put prevention into practice: A controlled evaluation. Am J Public Health. 2000;90:1622-1625.

49. Nutting P. Community-oriented primary care: From principle to practice. In: Nutting P, ed. Community-Oriented Primary Care. Albuquerque: University of New Mexico Press; 1987:xv-xxv.

50. Vogel T, Brechat PH, Lepretre PM, et al. Health benefits of physical activity in older patients: A review. Int J Clin Pract. 2009;63:303-320.

51. Russell MA, Wilson C, Taylor C, Baker D. Effect of general practitioners advice against smoking. BMJ. 1979;2:231.

52. American Geriatrics Society. Clinical Guidelines for Alcohol Use Disorders in Older Adults. Position Statement. 2003.

53. Nichol K, Nordin J, Nelson D, et al. Effectiveness of influenza vaccine in the community-dwelling elderly. N Engl J Med. 1994;357:1373-1381.

54. Pascual F, McGinley E, Zanardi L, et al. Tetanus surveillance— United States, 1998—2000. MMWR Surveil Sum. 2003;52:1-8.

55. Fernandez-Sabé N, Carratalà J, Rosón B, et al. (2003). Community-acquired pneumonia in very elderly patients: Causative organism, clinical characteristics, and outcomes. Medicine (Baltimore). 2003;82:159-169.

56. National Center for Immunization and Respiratory Diseases/Division of Bacterial Diseases. ABCs Report: Streptococcus pneumoniae, PROVISIONAL 2008 Active Bacterial Core Surveillance (ABCs): Emerging Infections Program Network. CDC; September 1, 2009. CDC.gov.

57. Insigna R, Itzler R, Pellissier J, et al. The incidence of herpes zoster in a United States administrative database. J Gen Inter Med. 2005;20:748-753.

58. Oxman MN, Levin MJ, Johnson GR, et al. A vaccine to prevent herpes zoster and postherpetic neuralgia in older adults. N Engl J Med. 2005;352:2271.

59. Administration on Aging. Cultural Competency Guidebook. 2001. Available at: http://www.aoa.gov/prof/addiv/cultural/addiv. cult.asp.

60. Betancourt J. Cultural competence: Marginal or mainstream movement? N Engl J Med. 2004;351:953-955.

61. Smedley B, Stith A, Nelson A. Unequal Treatment Confronting Racial and Ethnic Disparities in Health Care. Washington, DC: National Academies Press; 2003.

62. Haber D. Cultural diversity among older adults. Educational Gerontol. 2005;31:683-697.

63. Young R, Kahana E. Age, medical advice about cardiac risk reduction, and patient compliance. J Aging Health. 1989;1:121-134.

64. Callahan E, Bertakis KD, Azari R, et al. The influence of patient age on primary care resident physician-patient interaction. J Am Geriatr Soc. 2000;48:30-35.

65. Cooper-Patrick L. Race, gender, and partnership in the patient-physician relationship. JAMA. 1999;282:583-589.

66. Lehtinen M, Paavonen J. Vaccination against human papillomaviruses shows great promise. Lancet. 2004;364:1731-1732.

POST-TEST

1. **A screening that should be performed every 5 years is:**
   A. Blood pressure
   B. Diabetes/glucose
   C. Bone density
   D. Cholesterol

2. **Which of the following is FALSE regarding physical activity?**
   A. Exercise should be limited in frail patients with chronic illness.
   B. Training focus should include weight training, resistance, flexibility, and balance work.
   C. Exercise promotes independence in older adults.
   D. Older adults should have a minimum of 30 minutes of aerobic activity 5 days each week.

3. **A vaccine that should be given annually to older adults is:**
   A. Zoster
   B. Influenza
   C. Pneumococcal
   D. Tetanus

● DISCUSSION QUESTIONS

Health Contract Discussion: An Example with Mrs. Doe

For those who want to individualize their health promotion and disease prevention priorities with older patients, the health contract approach (which would be used by the health educator in Case Presentation 1) provides a systematic technique for reviewing a wide variety of health goals, and a step-by-step procedure for achieving a priority goal with each willing older patient.

Starting the Conversation

"Mrs. Doe, there are a number of health goals that are relevant for you, including your use of dietary supplements, blood pressure medication adherence, inactivity, inadequate diet, lack of recommended vaccinations and medical screenings, and need for additional social support. Let's go over these briefly one by one before you make up your mind. My strategy is to encourage *you* to make the choice of a health goal and then to decide whether you will accomplish this on your own with my assistance, or perhaps visit with an appropriate community health service or join a community health program or group. For these latter two options I have compiled a list of local community health resources that I am giving to you, which includes type of health activity or service, contact person, address, telephone number, and cost."

Discussion between clinician and geriatric patient ensues.

"You have decided to choose an exercise routine that consists of walking in your neighborhood. There are surveys that report that exercise is the number one option chosen by older adults when offered a range of options by a health educator. Perhaps it is because the value of exercise is so well known, and the benefits are so numerous. Let me briefly review the benefits from exercise that apply to you. This will be helpful to you later when you identify the most meaningful motivations for choosing your health goal and recording them on your health contract."

Selecting a Health Goal (Exercise)

"It is important to make your health goal modest and measurable. Modesty increases your chances of success with your current monthly goal and your subsequent confidence level for continued progress in the future. Measurability allows you to assess progress on your current health goal and, when completed, to set an appropriate future goal.

"Modesty means that you do *not* choose an overly ambitious *daily* exercise routine as your goal, but perhaps exercise four times a week. If you exceed this goal—great, but this allows you not to exercise on occasion and still have success. You are also going to limit yourself to one goal, and postpone your desire to select an additional nutrition goal (the second most likely chosen health goal with a health educator). If you want to work on additional goals on your own, that's fine, but we will focus on a single goal. You have chosen the modest, measurable, and safe goal of walking four times a week.

"Four times a week, or frequency, is one aspect of measurability, but so is duration and intensity level. We have chosen to gradate your duration, starting at 10 minutes per session during week one and eventually reaching 45 minutes each session. We want a safe intensity level, so we have chosen brisk walking, which is about twice as fast as normal walking speed. You will warm up with slower walking for a few minutes—and *not* with stretching muscles that are cold—and cool down with slower walking as well."

Motivation

"Among the many potential benefits of exercise we discussed and that I have also listed for you to examine, which ones are the most motivating for you? You note that increasing your energy level is the most important motivation. You have also identified two other motivations: ability to do your daily activity routines more easily, and to prevent gaining more weight, or even lose a little if possible. I want to encourage you to think about your motivations on a daily basis, perhaps leaving little written reminders of your motivations in key places that you are likely to see every day."

Social Support

"While it is not essential that you identify a support person or two, it tends to be a helpful technique for most clients. Please review this list of possible support persons—ranging from family and friends to pastor and neighbors—and decide on who you want to receive support from, the way you want it to be provided, and how often you want this support.

"Social support options range from someone who accompanies you on your walks, to someone who reminds you, encourages you, brainstorms with you, or shares in your success. Frequency of support can range from every day, to exercise days only, to weekly, to spontaneously, to only when asked."

Remembering a New Habit

"There are many tips for remembering a new habit. Attach the health calendar with a magnet to your refrigerator. Associate the new behavior with an established habit, such as walking just before breakfast or dinner. Place a cue card on the dinner table to remind you to exercise, or place your walking sneakers next to the door in a visible place. Exercise at the same time each day. Hang a picture on the wall that shows you exercising."

Health Contract Discussion: An Example with Mrs. Doe (Continued)

Problem-Solving

"Consider previous problems that arose when similar goals were set in the past and brainstorm around them. Anticipate new problems that might arise in the coming month, such as the week-long visit to your daughter's home that you noted and that could upset your exercise routine. Are you a negative thinker? Deliberately verbalize positive thoughts about being able to exercise four times a week. Are your knees sore in the morning? Are you fatigued later in the day? Consider changing your exercise time to minimize the barriers of aches and fatigue."

Signing the Health Contract

"Unlike a legal contract, no one sues you for being unable to fulfill a health contract. However, the structure of a contract can be useful. Choose someone to co-sign it with you whom you are not willing to disappoint. This may or may not be your support person. This may or may not be your nurse or physician. If no one comes to mind, I will co-sign it with you as your health educator."

Keeping Records with a Calendar

"A month may be an ideal length of time for you to set a health goal. It is short enough so that you are not as likely to drop out. It is long enough to provide a test for whether this is a worthwhile goal for you to achieve. The blank calendar allows you to fill in today's or tomorrow's date on the appropriate day of the week and begin to checkmark the days that you exercise over a 1-month period on a single sheet of paper. You can also use your regular calendar or an appointment book.

"At the end of each week you add up your checkmarks and place that number next to the number of days you had contracted to exercise. At the end of the month add the numbers and come up with a success ratio. To further encourage success, set 75% as your success ratio. Anything above that is gravy, with some achieving more than a 100% success ratio by exercising on average more than four times a week."

CASE PRESENTATION 4: GETTING HEALTH EDUCATION

John Doe (no relation to the Doris Doe cited in the beginning of this chapter) is a 75-year-old African American male. For educational purposes, let us say that—coincidentally in terms of similarity to Doris Doe—John Doe also takes analgesics as well as glucosamine and chondroitin. While still able to perform Activities of Daily Living independently, he too reports increasing difficulty with these tasks and a concern with falling. His BMI is also 28. He is also concerned about rising blood pressure (148/88) even though he reports taking hypertension medication on a regular basis.

The patient also reports sedentary behavior, low motivation for preparing healthy foods, no influenza or pneumococcal vaccinations, and no recent cancer, cardiovascular, or osteoporosis screenings.

The patient is also widowed and lives alone, but manages to attend church regularly. Although covered by Medicare, he too relies on Social Security for most of his income, which creates a financial hardship.

Five questions and answers concerning this case will be given.

Question 1

Can you complete a 1-month health contract for Mr. Doe that identifies an exercise health goal? You may use material from this chapter with Mrs. Doe, but also share some of your own original ideas. Be specific with the exercise goal in terms of type of activity, frequency, duration, and intensity level.

- Identify three likely motivations for his wanting to accomplish this health goal.
- Identify two hypothetical persons who might provide social support to him in the accomplishment of this goal, what type of support each will provide, and how often this support will be offered.
- Describe two techniques to remember this health goal. Identify two potential problems likely to arise in the next month, and describe how they can be avoided with prior planning.
- Identify someone to sign this health contract and explain why you chose this person.

Answer 1

The health contract can include some of the content listed next.

Health Goal (Exercise)

- *List of likely exercise goals can include:* join a community exercise class, brisk walking, counting steps with a pedometer, bicycling, dancing, an aerobic routine at home, swimming, strength-building, flexibility, balance, etc.
- *In terms of frequency and duration, include:* number of days per week, and minutes per day (either continuous single session or accumulating shorter segments over the course of a day).
- *In terms of intensity level include:* very light (no physical signs of exertion), fairly light (breathing rate increased), somewhat hard (warmth, slight sweat, breathing rate increased), or hard (sweat); exclude very hard intensity level (heavy sweat, difficult to talk).

Motivation

- *List of likely motivations in terms of function can include:* more energy, better sleep, mental acuity, ADL/IADL improvement, reduction in constipation, less stiffness, weight maintenance or loss, fall prevention, and additional strength.
- *In terms of disease prevention or control can include:* heart disease, diabetes, stroke, cancer (some research support for lowering the probability of breast cancer or colon cancer), cognitive decline, depression, arthritis, osteoporosis, stress, hypertension.

Social or Emotional Support

- *List of potentially social supportive people can include:* spouse, child, grandchild, parent, sibling, extended family member, friend, neighbor, physician, nurse, pastor, co-worker, or announcement of intent to acquaintances in general. If the spouse is selected, make sure he or she is a socially supportive person to your client, and not just selected because of marriage and expectations of duty.
- *In terms of ways you want support, this may include:* participation in activity, reminders to do the activity, discussion of progress, encouragement to continue, help with celebrating success, brainstorming around barriers, seeking and obtaining additional involvement of clinical staff, or reduction of contact with an unsupportive person.
- *In terms of how often to receive support, this may include:* every day, on exercise days, weekly, spontaneously, or when asked.

Memory

- *List of memory techniques:* Attach health contract to refrigerator with magnet, use own calendar/appointment book/computer reminder (Figure 14–2), associate new habit with established one, keep visible signs of exercise paraphernalia around the home, exercise the same time each day, ask the support person to remind you over the first couple of weeks.

Problems/Solutions

- *List of problem areas may include:* fatigue, aches and pain, lack of time, negativity, unsupportive housemate, unsupportive environment, too much stress.

- *List of solutions may include:* change the time of day one exercises, time the taking of pain medication to when the exercise will begin, use ice or heat as appropriate, state or write affirmations, spend more time with supportive persons or in a more supportive environment, learn and use stress management techniques.

Signature

- *Signing the health contract may include:* the support person in your health contract, or see the list of socially supportive people for suggestions of another person to sign the contract. The support person in the health contract may be the wisest choice, or selecting another person adds yet another individual to be accountable to. One rule of thumb to consider: Select the person to sign the health contract who will make you feel the worst if you do not succeed.

Question 2

How many safety tips can you identify for older patients who are beginning an exercise routine, with a particular emphasis on older adults who have multiple functional or disease limitations?

Answer 2

Your answer may include: Limit range of motion, find an alternative exercise movement, avoid or limit strength movements above the heart level, support one's back in a chair, use gentle or slower movements, implement fewer sets or repetitions or build in longer rest periods in between sets or repetitions,

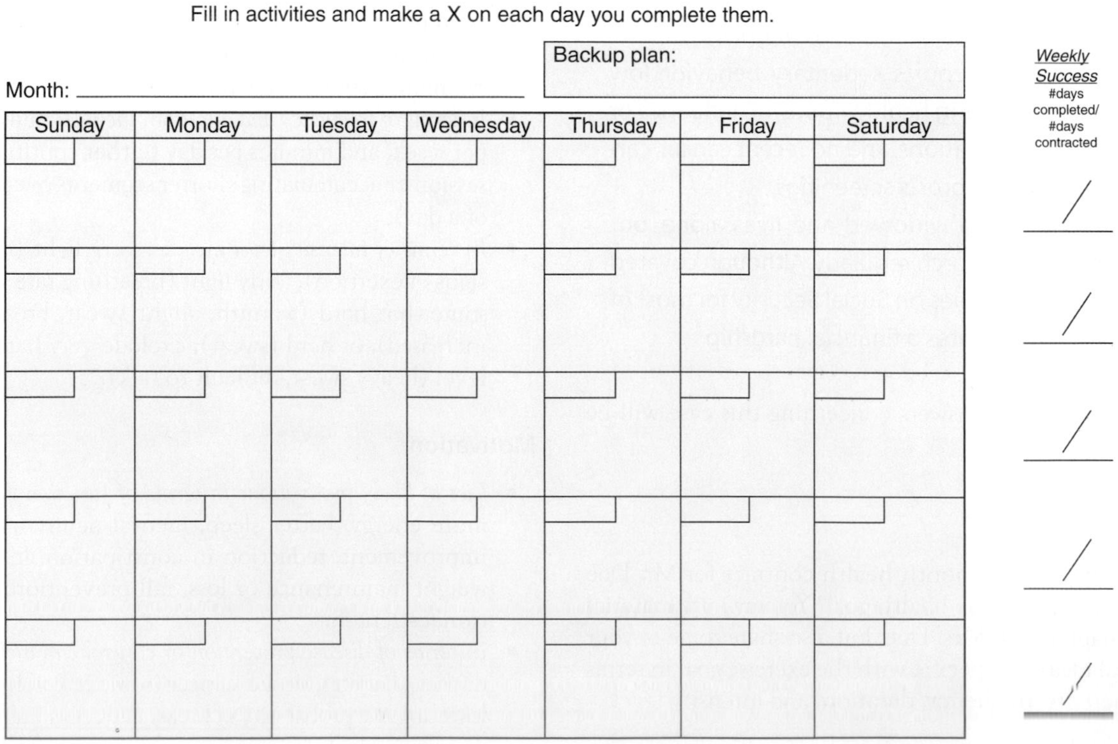

Fill in activities and make a X on each day you complete them.

FIGURE 14–2. Health calendar.

avoid jarring impact exercises (perhaps consider water aerobics), lower intensity level, use warm-up and cool-down periods, be conscious of breathing during strength-building exercises rather than holding one's breath, use the pursed-lip breathing technique if needed, employ proper posture, apply heat or ice as appropriate, and avoid or limit the following: unusual fatigue, excessive sweating, dizziness, shortness of breath, nausea, headache, chest pain, leg cramping, as well as uneven surfaces to exercise on, prolonged sitting or standing, and all or some bending and twisting movements.

Question 3

Suppose you conduct a health contract with two older patients—Doris Doe and John Doe—who are equivalent in all aspects described previously, except for two: sex and ethnicity. For this question, can you select *three* components of the health contract, and identify *one way* in which you would make the contract different for *a female older adult versus a male older adult*, in order to better serve each patient?

Answer 3

Health Goal. Older females are more likely to join a community exercise group for fun and sociability. This option should definitely be presented to older women and, if possible, provide information on a few community exercise choices to enhance accessibility. Older males should be given this opportunity as well but they are more likely to value individual convenience versus sociability.

Motivation. Older females are more interested in weight maintenance or loss and physical appearance. Older males may be more motivated to improve their fitness level. Older males may be more interested in achieving strength gains, but this goal is even more important for older females as they have less lean muscle tissue and more body fat.

Social Support. Older females may be likely to select a spouse or another support person because they think they ought to include them, and do not want to hurt their feelings. They should be cautioned against doing this. Older males are more likely to decline the social support option altogether and may need more encouragement to try this component of the health contract, perhaps in the spirit of experimentation.

Memory. Older females are more likely to join a community health class that will help them to remember a new habit. Older males may enjoy the prospect of a record-keeping technique for establishing a new habit.

Barriers/Solutions. Older females are more likely to have ADL/IADL limitations and will need to devise a way to work around these limitations. Older males may be more likely to set a health goal that is too ambitious and may need help in adjusting their goal to offset a high, perhaps too high, initial confidence level.

Signing the Contract. The same general principle applies to both older males and older females. Select the person you would least likely want to disappoint.

Please note: The "are" statements above are backed by evidence, while the "may" statements are based on commonly recognized differences between the sexes. Commonly recognized differences are more likely to be inaccurate than evidence-based statements. Nonetheless, thinking about sexual differences may be sensitizing to the options that are available.

Question 4

Select *three* components of the health contract. Can you identify *one* way in which you would make the contract different for *a white older adult* versus *a black older adult*, in order to better serve each patient?

Answer 4

Health goal. Older blacks are more likely to think of exercise as harmful in later life after having completed a work career that is more likely to involve heavy physical labor. The benefits of exercise will need to be reinforced more for older blacks than for older whites, and the implementation of an exercise goal will have to work around the greater number of ADL/IADL limitations, chronic diseases, and acute diseases that afflict older blacks more than older whites.

Motivation. Black elders are more motivated by religion. In motivating older blacks it may be useful to quote scripture such as "to take care of God's temple [the body]" and "above all else, guard your heart for it provides health to a man's whole body." The higher educational level and the slightly lower involvement and intensity level in church activities of white elders may lead to the greater influence of scientific evidence on the benefits of exercise.

Social Support. The black congregation is a major source of support for black elders, and the investigation of whether there is a health program associated with a neighborhood church is important. This issue, however, may be more sex-sensitive than race-sensitive, with older females more trusting and involved in church activities than older males.

Memory. No differences identified between ethnicities.

Barriers/Solutions. Older blacks are more likely to have the aches and pains associated with greater ADL and IADL limitations and will need to work around these barriers. The strategies for increasing safety in question 2 are relevant here. Extra time will be needed to build and maintain motivation levels for older blacks than older whites.

Signing the Contract. The black pastor or an influential church elder may be the most important person to sign the health contract for the black elder. This option may be easily overlooked as black churches have not been associated with health promoting practices. Churches with a parish nurse program can be helpful for either ethnicity.

Some black elders are trusting of physicians and other health professionals and take the authority of the role very seriously. Others, however, are somewhat suspicious of white health professionals who dominate the health care industry. This potential difference should be recognized when contemplating the suggestion of a white health professional to sign the health contract of a black elder.

Please note: The danger of positing about racial or ethnic differences is that stereotypes may get reinforced. Nonetheless, being aware of evidence-based differences and, to a lesser extent, commonly believed differences that have not been subjected to research, can still be sensitizing and motivating for searching for more options that may be available.

Question 5

When it comes to recommending medical screenings for Mr. John Doe and Mrs. Doris Doe, can you identify one important difference to consider (other than the obvious difference that you recommend some screenings exclusively for men—prostate cancer screening, and others exclusively for women—breast cancer and cervical cancer)?

Answer 5

Among medical conditions that pertain to both genders, African American older men are at much greater risk than Caucasian older women for glaucoma, hypertension, dyslipidemia, diabetes, stroke, and heart disease. Thus, medical screenings may be even more urgent for African American older men. However, physicians who treat African American patients may be less well trained clinically and refer fewer African American patients for medical screenings and other important clinical resources.[56]

Caucasian older women are at much greater risk than African American older men for osteoporosis and for sarcopenia (muscle weakness). Caucasian women, however, may be more amenable to seeking medical screenings and lifestyle changes than African American men. On the negative side, older women are more likely to be involved with intense caregiving responsibilities that can affect both their health as well as their ability to follow up on medical screening referrals.

Medical screening controversies rise up from time to time, and currently older black men and older women each have a different controversial medical screening to consider. PSA testing is under greater scrutiny than ever before for men regarding its effectiveness. However, African American heritage is a risk factor for prostate cancer that was not isolated by the two large studies published in 2009 that suggested routine PSA screenings were suspect.

For older women, mammographies are under less scrutiny than they were between 2001 and 2007, but new research published in 2009 may revive this controversy. It has been difficult to compare the costs (effectiveness of mammography, additional unnecessary procedures, and anxiety) and the benefits (reduced breast cancer death rates).

ANSWERS TO PRE-TEST

1. B
2. B
3. C

ANSWERS TO POST-TEST

1. D
2. A
3. B

15

Older Drivers: Safe Mobility in the Later Years

Karlene Ball, PhD

Rachel Benz, RN, BSN

● **LEARNING OBJECTIVES**

1. Describe the process by which older patients may be properly assessed for mobility impairment.
2. Discuss common risk factors for unsafe driving.
3. Explain the elements and approach to communicating with patients who may be at risk for unsafe driving.
4. Describe specific disease states and medications that may place a patient at risk for unsafe driving.

PRE-TEST

1. **Which of the following statements is TRUE?**
   A. Older drivers are less likely to wear their seatbelts.
   B. The hazard posed by an impaired older driver is primarily to himself or herself.
   C. Older drivers are usually unaware of their declining function.
   D. Impairments in visual, cognitive, and physical activities are not better predictors of driving competence than age alone.

2. **Primary care physicians should evaluate patients for warning signs associated with increased driving risk. Which of the following is LEAST relevant?**
   A. Slow gait
   B. Reduced visual acuity
   C. Difficulty with memory, attention, and understanding
   D. Poor hygiene

3. **Motor abilities important for safe driving do NOT include:**
   A. Ability to perceive movement
   B. Lower limb strength
   C. Ability to turn one's head
   D. Strength

4. **Which of the following statements is FALSE?**
   A. Vision impairments associated with unsafe driving can frequently be managed or corrected.
   B. There are no licensing standards with respect to glaucoma and macular degeneration.
   C. Following cataract extraction, patients should be advised not to drive at night.
   D. Licensing requirements related to visual function are inconsistent across states.

● OLDER DRIVERS

Driving is such an important aspect of everyday life that most people take it for granted, assuming they will always be able to drive to meet their mobility needs. In most areas of the United States driving is the only means of transportation for shopping, getting to work, and attending social events. Thus losing one's driving privileges for many can be equivalent to losing one's freedom and independence.

CASE PRESENTATION 1: A WARNING SIGN

John is discussing an accident with his friend. "The way Sarah was carrying on last night you would have thought I had really hurt myself. That minor accident I had …it was nothing …just a few dents and scratches. I really need my car to be able to get around. If I didn't have it I don't know what we'd do …have to live somewhere else, I guess. We've lived in this house all of our married life, and I think I'm still fine to drive. I can still see pretty well. I didn't notice that other driver right away because these young kids drive so darn fast. They need to slow down! I just had a few bumps and bruises and I'm going to cover the cost of fixing the cars myself rather than let my insurance company know. It's a small price to pay. Everything will be fine." (Figure 15-1.)

The Older Driver Dilemma

What people think about older drivers is frequently portrayed in cartoons and jokes depicting impaired individuals (Figure 15–1). The truth is that most older drivers are very safe and careful drivers.[1,2] They are more likely to wear their seatbelts and to avoid tailgating, drinking and driving, and driving at night.[3,4] However, the behavior of a few impaired individuals can easily become a stereotype for an entire group. Age is frequently cited in the media, for example, when an older driver is at fault. It is not commonly mentioned for other age groups. Therefore it is important to be able to identify warning signs when they occur, and to identify any impairments that may be more common with increasing age.

From a driver's perspective, the loss of a driver's license is an emotional if not a traumatic event. Losing the ability to drive, especially if forced to give up the keys, has been associated with depression, social isolation, and poorer quality of life.[5-10] Therefore balancing risks associated with continued driving against the negative impact of driving cessation can be a very difficult decision for older adults themselves, concerned family members, and even health care providers and personnel in Departments of Motor Vehicles.

Compounding this is the fact that the hazard posed by an impaired older driver is primarily to himself or herself; this may not be the public perception since there have been some highly publicized instances where innocent bystanders were hurt and/or killed by an older driver. Due to increased frailty in older age, older individuals are much more likely to be injured in a car accident than younger persons.[2] In fact, motor vehicle crashes are the number one cause of injury-related fatalities in the 65- to 74-year-old age group.[11] These facts understandably leave family members afraid for their loved one, and there is also frequently fear for the safety of grandchildren or others who may ride with the older adult. In addition, family members commonly believe that the older person may be unaware of his or her declining function. These discussions, however, can be very difficult to initiate among family members. Consider the next case.

CASE PRESENTATION 2: WHEN THE FAMILY IS CONCERNED

Daughter: "Mom, the family has been talking and we are all concerned about your ability to drive."
Mother: "What do you mean you have been talking? I drive myself where I need to go, and I have been just fine."
Daughter: "No, Mom, you are not just fine. We will all pitch in and drive you wherever you need to go, but we don't want you driving. The kids are scared to death when you drive them anywhere."
Mother: "I can't be dependent on you or your sisters to take me everywhere. I need my car to go to church, to the doctor, or just over to visit with a friend."
Daughter: "I know, Mom, but we all love you and don't want you to get hurt. You don't seem to realize that you are not seeing very well. You keep scraping the sides of your car when you try to park it in the garage. Haven't you noticed the scratches on the car, or the damage you did to the garage door?"
Mother: "I don't know what you are talking about."
Daughter: "That is exactly what I mean. You aren't even aware that you are having a problem."
Mother: "My doctor hasn't said anything about it."
Daughter: "Well, will you at least let us go with you and speak to your doctor about driving, we are all worried to death."

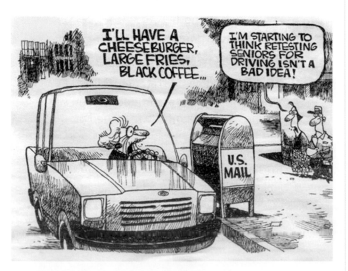

FIGURE 15–1. The older driver stereotype.

At times family members may become so frustrated and concerned that they have avoided further discussion and resorted to disabling the vehicle, or moving it to another location. These approaches, however, may or may not be successful, and the driver, in some instances, may have been able to continue driving with evaluation and successful intervention.

Older adults today are living longer and healthier lives than ever before, and many older adults continue to drive well into their 80s and 90s. The number of older drivers on the road will be at all-time highs with the aging of the baby boomers, in addition to the increased numbers of women who drive in that age cohort. These changing demographics have led to increased study into the health-related factors that place some older drivers at increased risk for crash involvement. The findings of this research are also important for physicians and other health care providers who will need to become even more involved with the issues of driving safety with their patients.

With respect to issues of driving safety, studies have found that those older drivers who self-impose limits to their driving (for example, avoiding highways, night driving, and unfamiliar roads) may incorrectly assume they have compensated for any impairments they might have.[12,13] These behaviors can actually increase risk, because highway driving is usually safer with fewer signs, less traffic, and fewer other hazards to negotiate. Thus, even though some drivers may limit their driving, they may not actually be at reduced risk. In fact, it is frequently the drivers who do limit their driving, those who are concerned or aware of some functional impairments, who are the most at risk.[13]

Most studies investigating functional impairments as risk factors have focused on the visual, cognitive, and physical capabilities of older drivers. While changes in these abilities are frequently associated with age, these abilities themselves are better predictors of driving competence than age per se.[14-17] It is important not to assume that a given individual is at increased risk based on the appearance of advanced age or frailty. Health care providers, however, may be unsure of how to assess whether or not a given patient should continue driving, and may also have concerns about reporting a patient to a licensing authority and potentially losing that patient's trust. Some physicians are uncomfortable talking to patients about driving because they know it can lead to emotions such as anger, denial, resistance, or rejection. They also may not be aware of other mobility options that might work for their patient. The issue of safe driving, however, is so important that health care providers should learn about the various ways of handling the problem if safe driving is no longer an option.

● COUNSELING OLDER DRIVERS

CASE PRESENTATION 3: LOSING THEIR WAY

Mr. Bellville comes to your office for a regular follow-up appointment. You notice that he is 15 minutes late and he told the nurse that he forgot to take his medications this morning. When you enter the room you notice that he is unshaven and his shirt is tucked out on one side. this is unusual for him, as he is generally very neat. He recognizes that he is late and apologizes and says, "I'm sorry, Doc, but I got turned around on my way here and had to backtrack a couple of blocks to find your office." When you ask him if he has gotten lost driving before, he shrugs and says, "I've gotten lost a couple times in the past few weeks." You ask him if he has gotten any tickets lately, and he says he was stopped by a police officer for running a red light but was just given a warning. He also reports that his wife has been complaining more about his driving as well.

Primary care physicians and other health care providers are in a unique position to detect potential risk factors for unsafe driving. The American Medical Association (AMA) recommends that physicians evaluate their patients for functional impairments, such as slow gait, falls, frailty, and poor vision, that could have an impact on driving competence. In speaking with patients, physicians should pay close attention to issues with hygiene (clothing soiled, wrinkled, or worn), any visual problems (cataracts, glaucoma, or macular degeneration), disorientation, difficulty walking or rising from a sitting position, or difficulty with memory, attention, or understanding. If concerned, health care providers should ask the patient if he or she or another family member is concerned about the patient's driving. In taking the patient's history, physicians should look for warning signs such as diseases that can impact visual function, acute events such as a stroke, psychiatric or neurologic issues, any history of certain events such as syncope or seizure, and any medications known to have an impact on cognitive function.

If concerns persist, health care providers are encouraged to have a conversation to include the following types of questions (Figure 15–2):

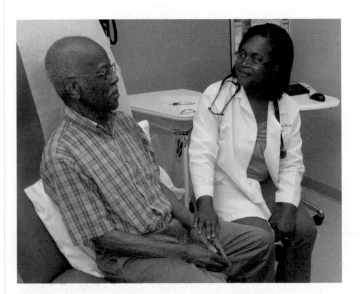

FIGURE 15–2. Having a conversation with the older patient.

- Did you drive here today?
- Did you drive here alone?
- Have you ever had any problems when you were driving? What kind?
- Have you ever gotten lost?
- Have you had any accidents or fender benders in the past 2 years—even if it wasn't your fault?
- Have you had any traffic tickets or warnings?
- Have your family members or friends ever insisted on driving when you were with them?
  - If you couldn't drive for any reason, what other options do you have for getting around?"

According to the AMA, the rate of fatality for drivers in vehicle collisions over the age of 85 is 9 times that of drivers aged 25 to 69.[18] For this reason the AMA has guidelines in place to address not only the physician's responsibilities for recognizing those individuals who may pose a danger on the road, but also help assess and refer patients for further screening. It is the physician's responsibility to assess any physical or cognitive impairment that may make driving a matter of public safety. Physicians are first encouraged to tactfully discuss with their patient the issues of driving to see if an agreement can be reached, including a more formal driving assessment, seeing an occupational therapist for possible intervention, or complete driving cessation.

Screening for these types of impairments may be left up to the physician if no policies are in place at the physician's practice. Mental status with an Mini-Mental State Exam (MMSE) or Mini-Cog, vision examinations with a Snellen eye chart or referral to an optometrist or ophthalmologist, impulsivity as evidenced by large purchases or rash decision-making, and executive function are all things that may be assessed at this time. The physician may also choose to review the patient's medical history as well as current medications for interactions or impairment that may be caused by these. It is the responsibility of the physician to warn the patient about any side effects from medications, especially new medications or new dosages of any medication, or conditions that may have an effect on the ability to drive. Specific tools for screening of patients are discussed later in this chapter.

A physician, if uncertain about a patient's driving ability, may choose to refer the patient to the state licensing agency for arrangement of a driving test. If the physician chooses this option, the person's ability to drive will only be tested in the manner that it is tested for all drivers, which may include a driving test, written exam, or vision test. Another option is referral to a driving assessment clinic for evaluation by a driver rehabilitation specialist, if one is available. Unfortunately, these clinics are very limited in their availability and are frequently only located in larger metropolitan areas. These clinics assess not only the ability to drive safely, but also mental status, cognitive function, executive function, and vision.

If, after the assessment by the physician, and the driving evaluation if needed, it is found that the person should not be driving, a candid discussion with the patient is necessary. The physician should include the patient's family, if the patient consents. It is important to address the emotional components of driving, and the feelings the patient may have about his or loss of independence when discussing driving cessation.

Every effort should be made to include different options that are available to the patient to ensure adequate mobility in the person's community. However, it should be made very clear that the physician feels that there is a strong threat to the patient's and public safety if the person continues to drive. The physician must also inform the patient that if he or she does not agree to stop driving, the physician has the ethical responsibility to report the patient to the Department of Motor Vehicles because the patient creates a risk to public safety. Policies and procedures for this vary from state to state, and each physician must be familiar with his or her own state's laws and policies regarding the reporting of unsafe drivers.

If a health care provider has any concerns regarding a patient's ability to drive safely, he or she can administer some assessments to provide help in the decision-making process (eg, mental status examination, visual examination). While these assessments, described in more detail later in this chapter, may not fully indicate a person's ability to drive safely, they do provide an indication that further evaluation may be needed. Some patients may refuse to be tested and/or become defensive due to their fear of being told not to drive.

CASE PRESENTATION 4: ASSESSING THE OLDER DRIVER

James Park is a 75-year-old white male who has been living alone for 6 years since his wife passed away. He has 4 children who are concerned about his safety, not only because he lives alone, but also because of his driving. Mr. Park has a history of hypertension and type 2 diabetes mellitus, neither of which are very well controlled with medication, myocardial infarction with CABG 10 years ago, and prostate cancer status post radiation. He does not always remember to take his medications as directed, and his children want to make sure that he is safe to live as well as drive alone. Mr. Park and his children received a referral from his primary care physician to a driving assessment clinic because they are worried about "Dad's driving safety." Mr. Park has been driving for 60 years and has had 3 at fault and 2 not at fault accidents in the past 3 years.

Mr. Park comes to the Driving Assessment Clinic for evaluation. He states that he is "fine to live alone" and "a very good driver." Mr. Park appears to be physically robust and is able to rise from a chair and walk 20 feet and sit down again (Timed Get Up and Go) in less than 10 seconds, which is a normal result. Mr. Park was then given several cognitive tests to determine his mental abilities. Mr. Park was given the Trails A (use a pen to connect pre-printed dots numbered 1, 2, 3, etc.) and B (connect dots with numbers and letters; 1-A, 2-B, 3-C, etc.) tests. He was able to complete Trails A in 100 seconds but he was unable to complete Trails B within

5 minutes. He was also given the UFOV test (Task 1 and Task 2, described in next section). He was unable to complete Task 2 on the UFOV test and received the lowest possible score. His Dementia Rating Scale score was 94/144 (with a score greater than 135 as normal and scores less than 125 usually indicating an inability to pass an on-road driving test), indicating a high level of impairment. Mr. Park was not taken on the road test with the occupational therapist due to the findings of cognitive impairment and his inability to pass a visual acuity test at the legal limit for driving in that state.

When interviewed, Mr. Park reported the need to drive himself and live alone. He does not want to live with any of his children and feels that he would be a burden to them. The assessment of the driving evaluation concluded that he was unable to recognize his impairments and is probably not safe to live alone. His history of crash involvement plus his cognitive impairment increased the risk that he would be involved in another crash. His inability to recognize his own limitations increases the risk that he will not be able to take care of himself. The driving assessment clinic recommended that, based on his testing and recent history, he no longer drive and that arrangements for some sort of supervised living be made.

The report from the Driving Assessment Clinic was sent to the patient, his family (with his permission), and the referring physician. It was determined that he was unfit to drive based on his performance on the UFOV and the Dementia Rating Scale and his history of frequent accidents. The patient was then referred for development of an Activities of Daily Living plan, which is a plan developed with the patient and family in mind that will assist the patient to complete everyday tasks such as bathing, dressing, and eating, as well as safe mobility within his or her environment. His family plans to allow him to live with one of them as he chooses.

● ASSESSMENT TOOLS

As illustrated in this case study, safe driving relies primarily on three key functions:

- Vision
- Cognition
- Motor function

There are obviously a number of potential assessments that can be used to evaluate these functions. Several assessments, most commonly used to evaluate driving competence, will now be described in more detail.

Adequate visual function is obviously very important for safe driving. Two aspects of visual function commonly assessed in health care settings include visual acuity and visual fields,

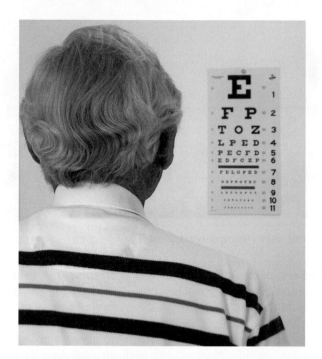

FIGURE 15–3. Testing visual acuity.

both of which have some predictive ability for safe driving. Far visual acuity is needed for driving (reading street signs and seeing potential hazards), but near visual acuity is also needed to see dashboard instruments. Acuity is typically measured using an eye chart such as the one depicted here. If a patient has adequate visual acuity (better than 20/40), then he or she is not restricted from driving due to central visual impairment. If acuity is poorer than 20/40 (eg, 20/40 to 20/70), patients should be referred to an ophthalmologist for evaluation for eye disease and consideration of corrective lenses followed by an on-road assessment by a driver rehabilitation specialist. Patients may be allowed to continue driving based on the results of this assessment in some states (Figure 15–3).

While logically it is recognized that an adequate visual field is important for safe driving, there is not sufficient evidence to define what is "adequate" for safe driving. As a result, visual field requirements are inconsistent across states, varying from 100 degrees or more along the horizontal meridian to no requirements at all. If a visual field deficit is suspected based on medical history, patient history, or confrontation testing, the patient should be referred to an ophthalmologist for more specialized testing, as this may be a sign of early glaucoma, occipital stroke, or other problem.

If concerns persist relative to the size of the visual field, a driver evaluation (including on-road assessment) performed by a driver rehabilitation specialist is recommended. This specialist is trained to teach patients to compensate for decreased visual fields while driving, and may also prescribe specialized side and rear view mirrors as aids for safe driving.

A more sophisticated test of visual processing speed throughout the visual field is called the Useful Field of View. The UFOV test uses a commercially available software program to assess the speed with which individuals perform increasingly difficult attentional tasks. Unlike conventional measures of visual field, which assess visual sensitivity, this test relies on

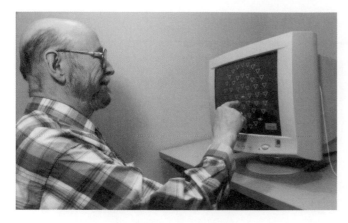

FIGURE 15–4. Testing the Useful Field of View.

higher-order processing skills such as selective and divided attention and rapid visual processing speed. Multiple studies from different laboratories have shown this test to have excellent ability to identify elevated crash risk in older adults.[19] These studies imply that visual attention and visual processing speed are important indices when evaluating safe driving skills. The strength of the association between the visual/cognitive measures and driving competence is consistently much stronger than with visual sensory function alone (Figure 15–4).

In addition to the Useful Field of View, other measures of executive function that have shown promise in identifying drivers at risk are the Trail-Making Test and the Clock Drawing Test.[15,19-21] The Trail-Making Test A entails connecting the dots, numbered 1 through 12, as quickly as possible. Recall that Mr. Park was able to complete Trails A in 199 seconds. This time is considerably slower than would normally be expected. In Trails B (depicted here), the patient must connect the dots, alternating between numbers and letters that have been randomly placed on the page (eg, 1 to A to 2 to B to 3 to C, etc.). Any mistakes made are pointed out by the examiner and must be corrected by the examinee, thus increasing the time required to finish the test. If the patient completes Trails B in fewer than 3 minutes, the results are considered to fall within normal limits. Mr. Park was unable to complete Trials B within 5 minutes. Therefore the test was discontinued. His performance clearly demonstrated impairment in this area (Figure 15–5).

Performance on the Clock Drawing Test reflects a patient's memory, visuospatial ability, and executive function. To administer the test, a patient is given a pencil and a blank sheet of paper. The patient is asked to draw the face of the clock, including all the numbers, and to draw the time at 10 minutes past 11. Patients must include all 12 hours, in correct order and placement, with no duplicates or omissions. The numbers must be inside the clock circle, spaced nearly equally, with correct placement of only two hands. Several examples from impaired individuals are depicted in Figure 15–6. In some cases patients may be experiencing visual field defects in addition to cognitive ones. For example, the upper left clock shows numbers only on the right side of the clock face. All criteria must be met to be considered within normal limits.

Driving also requires motor abilities such as the capability to turn the head, the ability to perceive movement, and the capacity to move the foot quickly from the accelerator to the brake pedal. These abilities can be affected by arthritis and

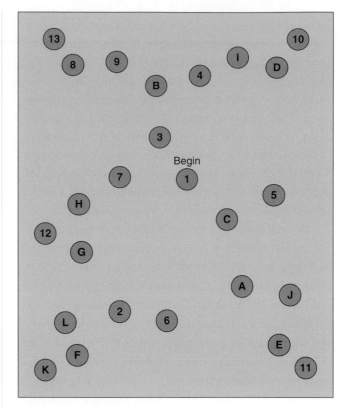

FIGURE 15–5. Trail-Making Test.

musculoskeletal problems, which are more common among older adults. Motor function is most usually evaluated through a rapid-pace walking assessment that measures lower limb strength, range of motion, balance, and proprioception. Patients are asked to walk 10 feet (3.05 m), turn around, and walk back as quickly as possible. The time in seconds for the patient to walk the 20 feet (6.1 m) is recorded. Patients who complete this test in 9 seconds or less are considered to be performing within normal limits. Slower times may require intervention or additional evaluation.

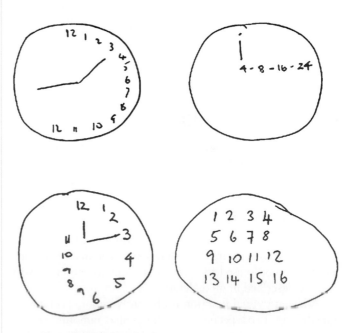

FIGURE 15–6. Clock Drawing Test.

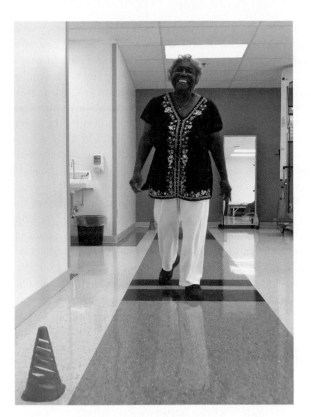

FIGURE 15–7. Rapid-pace walking assessment.

Recall from the case study that Mr. Park was able to walk 20 feet in less than 10 seconds. Thus his lower limb mobility was sufficient to safely operate a motor vehicle. His visual function, however, was poor (falling outside of the range allowed by the state Department of Motor Vehicles), and most significantly Mr. Parks performed poorly on two measures of cognitive function, as well as the Dementia Rating Scale, indicating an elevated risk of crash involvement (Figure 15–7).

● PATIENT REFUSAL

Despite the concerns of family members and the recommendation of one or more health care providers, some patients will refuse to participate in further evaluation. Under such circumstances the patient's refusal, and the basis for concerns related to driving, should be documented in the patient chart. A follow-up on driving issues should be conducted during any subsequent appointments to evaluate any changes in either underlying conditions or amenability to further evaluation.

● MEDICAL CONDITIONS AND SAFE DRIVING

Certain medical conditions are associated with potential changes in visual, cognitive, and motor function. If a patient presents with a diagnosed condition known to be associated with these functional deficits, and therefore driving competence, further evaluation of function should be explored as described earlier. Under such circumstances, the medical condition should first be treated, if possible, to correct any functional problems and prevent further decline. If any decline in function cannot be medically corrected, the patient should be referred to a driver rehabilitation specialist for further evaluation. This specialist may be able to prescribe adaptive equipment or techniques, train the patient in how to use them, and potentially compensate for functional declines. If in the opinion of the specialist compensation is not possible, the patient should be advised about the risks associated with his or her condition, and a recommendation of driving cessation may be warranted. If a patient is hospitalized, discharge should not occur without a discussion about driving and a recommendation that the patient not resume driving until cleared by the physician.

● VISION IMPAIRMENTS

Certain medical conditions, such as cataracts, glaucoma, macular degeneration, and diabetic retinopathy, are associated with declines in visual function, and may affect visual acuity, night vision, the size of the visual field, and other aspects of visual function. Quite frequently, visual deficits can be managed and/or corrected. For example, cataracts can be removed, restoring visual function after a relatively brief recovery period. Prior to extraction, however, patients should be advised to avoid night driving and any driving situations involving glare. Glaucoma and macular degeneration are also eye diseases more common with advancing age. No restrictions for these diagnoses are needed provided licensing standards for visual acuity and visual fields are met within that state. Patients with hemianopia or quadrantanopia resulting from a stroke should in most instances be referred to a driver rehabilitation specialist for assessment and possible rehabilitation. Licensing requirements for these conditions vary by state, and road tests should be administered prior to licensing.

● COGNITIVE IMPAIRMENTS

There are several diseases that can affect cognitive functioning in drivers. Often the person may continue to drive in the earliest stages of some of these conditions, such as Alzheimer disease and other forms of dementia. Regular screening of these patients for changes in function by physicians, and monitoring of the person by his or her family, should take place until the person's deficits increase to a point at which driving may be unsafe. Unfortunately, determining when this point has been reached can be difficult. Some drivers with Alzheimer disease can be safe to more advanced stages when they travel with a spouse (as a copilot), and others, who may have mild disease but more impaired judgment, might need to stop driving sooner. Diseases that cause dementia—such as Alzheimer disease, Parkinson disease, Lewy body dementia, multiple strokes, and less commonly HIV in the older population—are the most frequent causes of dementia and each probably has a different impact on driving function both among individuals with the same disease and between different diseases. Epilepsy is another disease affecting the brain that may cause cognitive and motor impairment of the person in the form of seizures. People with epilepsy that is uncontrolled despite medications or surgical intervention are generally prohibited from driving in most states and should be told by their providers that they cannot drive. However, people who have been without seizures for a period of time may be allowed to drive based upon the physician's assessment and the state's regulations.

● MOTOR IMPAIRMENTS

Adequate motor functioning is crucial for safe mobility in every part of one's environment. There are many diseases that may produce peripheral neuropathy (such as diabetes mellitus, vitamin B_{12} deficiency, and shingles) as well as certain treatments for diseases (such as chemotherapeutic agents for cancer). This may lead to problems with proprioception as well as sensation and motor function. Health care providers should pay attention to complaints of numbness or tingling in persons who have been diagnosed with these diseases or administered these treatments, and their abilities should be assessed in a case-by-case manner. Certain types of degenerative musculoskeletal diseases, such as multiple sclerosis and Parkinson disease, should be routinely monitored for their impact on function, as should some other treatable or transient musculoskeletal diseases that may not lead to permanent weakness or loss. People with these diagnoses may have a range of functional abilities, and should be further assessed for their capability to maintain control of a motor vehicle through assessment by a driving rehabilitation specialist. In certain cases of motor impairment, affected persons may be able to drive a modified vehicle that is equipped to accommodate their needs.

● MEDICATIONS THAT MAY CAUSE IMPAIRMENTS

Any new medication prescribed has the potential to create deficits that could impair driving ability. The level of impairment varies from patient to patient, between different medications within the same therapeutic class, and in combination with other medications or alcohol.

Medication side effects that can affect driving performance include drowsiness, dizziness, blurred vision, unsteadiness, fainting, and slowed reaction time. In many cases, medication side effects are dose related and are often reduced over time. Often medications that cause this have sedative effects: medications for pain (especially opioid analgesics), allergies (primarily first-generation antihistamines, but others may as well), antidepressants, anxiolytics, chemotherapeutic agents, sedatives including medications for insomnia, or cough and cold medicines. People may be taking these medications by prescription or over the counter, so it is important to assess patients for every medication or supplement they take, as there may be interactions or the potential for over-medicating. Older adults are particularly prone to polypharmacy, and may be susceptible to delirium as a result of medication interactions or medications that are unable to be metabolized as effectively as they are in younger persons.

Physicians need to teach their patients that their driving ability may be impaired without them realizing it. Medications that cause drowsiness, euphoria, and/or anterograde amnesia can diminish insight and self-awareness. In the case of these medications, the concerned physician and patient may wish to consider formal psychomotor testing (up to and including driving simulation) or driver evaluation (including on-road assessment) performed by a driver rehabilitation specialist, while off and on the medication to determine the extent of impairment. Often the patient may be told to avoid driving until the patient knows how the medication will affect him or her, and may resume driving when either deemed capable of driving or no longer take the medication.

When prescribing new medications, the physician should always consider the patient's existing regimen or prescription and nonprescription medications, including medications taken seasonally (Chapter 13). Physicians should add new medications at the lowest dosage possible, counsel the patient to be alert to any impairing side effects, and adjust the dosages of individual medications as needed to achieve therapeutic effects with a minimum of impairment. Patients should temporarily cease driving and for at least 3 months thereafter when an anticonvulsant is initiated or during withdrawal, or dosage change due to the risk of recurrent seizure and potential medication side effects that may impair driving performance.

Benzodiazepines can impair vision, attention, motor coordination, and driving performance. Evening doses of long-acting benzodiazepines have been shown to markedly impair psychomotor function the following day, while comparable doses of short-acting compounds produce a lesser impairment.[22] Patients should be prescribed evening doses of the shortest-acting hypnotics whenever possible. Patients who take longer-acting compounds or daytime doses of any hypnotic should be advised of the potential for impairment, even in the absence of subjective symptoms. These patients should also be advised to avoid driving, particularly during initiation and the initial phase of dosage adjustment(s). Most skeletal muscle relaxants (eg, carisoprodol, cyclobenzaprine) have significant central nervous system effects. Patients should be advised not to drive during the initial phase of dosage adjustment(s) if they experience side effects severe enough to affect safe driving performance. All narcotic analgesics (opioids) can impair driving even in the absence of subjective symptoms. Patients should not drive while these medications are being started or dose adjusted; however, patients with chronic pain on stable doses are generally safe to drive on these medications.

Alcohol use should also be assessed in older drivers since alcohol may be contraindicated for use with many medications. In addition, alcohol abuse is generally under-recognized in older persons and may manifest as frequent falling, incoordination, and variable cognition. Assessment for alcohol use with the CAGE questions or other tool should be performed if there is any suspicion of alcohol abuse.

● LEGAL CONSIDERATIONS

As noted earlier, physicians and other health care professionals may have conflicting issues with respect to the driving privileges of their patients. These touch on ethical considerations and practical ones, as well as potential legal ramifications.

The legal requirements for reporting patients with diagnoses or impairments that may impact driving competence vary from state to state. However, lawsuits against physicians by their patients, or by another person who was injured as a result of his or her patient driving a car, are a concern for all physicians. Obviously physicians are bound ethically to protect the confidentiality of their patients. Furthermore, no physician can state with certainty that a particular patient will cause a vehicular crash, and it is not the physician's responsibility to determine whether or not someone is competent to drive. However, physicians also have a responsibility to protect their patients and the public health, and they should report serious concerns to the licensing agency and advise their patients about those concerns.

The primary responsibility of the health care provider is to care for a patient's health through the treatment and/or prevention of illness, as well as provide advice relative to a patient's safety. This involves counseling patients about both medical conditions and medications that could potentially impair their ability to drive safely. Failure to provide such warning can be considered negligent, and physicians should document in patient files when such counsel has been provided.

There has been considerable debate concerning state requirements to report certain medical conditions to licensing authorities. Many physicians feel that these reporting requirements have a negative impact on their relationships with their patients, and that they may result in older individuals not seeking medical help when they need it. However, court cases have found physicians liable for third-party injuries caused by their patients when it becomes clear that the physicians did not advise their patients not to drive.[23] Furthermore, as in cases of child abuse, patient confidentiality is not absolute, and preserving confidentiality is not the primary concern when it may lead to the harm of others.

Some physicians are reluctant to report impaired drivers to the DMV out of fear of violating the Health Insurance Portability and Accountability Act of 1996. The HIPAA privacy rules, however, *permit* health care providers to disclose protected health information without individual authorization *as required by law*. The rules also permit disclosure of protected information to public health authorities authorized by law to collect or receive such information for preventing or controlling disease, injury, or disability.

The first step in reducing exposure to a lawsuit related to an impaired driver is thoroughly and repeatedly advising *all* patients of medical conditions, procedures, and medications that may impair their driving performance. This is, of course, simply good medical practice, but it is also essential from a legal standpoint because failure to advise and counsel will leave physicians and their employing entities vulnerable in the event of a lawsuit.

If a health care provider believes that a patient's driving is unsafe and cannot be made safe by any available medical treatment, adaptive device, or adaptive techniques it should be recommended that the patient retire from driving. This is much easier said than done. The key point here is that, from a legal standpoint, physicians and other health care providers need to protect themselves by taking this step. As always, clinical judgment should be based on the patient's *function* rather than age, number of medical conditions, medications, or gender.

Because being denied the right to drive can evoke such powerful emotions, patients may sometimes react inappropriately or irrationally despite the best efforts of a physician. A patient who threatens legal action is one of the most difficult quandaries a physician will face. Occasionally, a patient refuses to stop driving despite a physician's best efforts to encourage driving retirement. In fact, sometimes people continue to drive even after their license has been revoked. If either of these situations exists, health care providers may have a legal obligation to report the patient (or re-report the patient) to the appropriate state agency. Even in the case that there is no legal requirement in a state, health care providers may still need to report the situation both to uphold responsibility for protecting public safety and to minimize exposure to legal liability. In any situation, legal counsel should be sought from the employing entity before proceeding, since responsibility to report may conflict with legal obligation to protect patient confidentiality.

This can be a very difficult thing for both physician and patient, but as always honesty and candor are very important in this situation. Techniques of "how to break bad news" can be helpful in these situations. Many times it can be useful to include family members if the patient allows it, and understanding that this is a difficult time for the patient and his or her family must be expressed. Assessment of options available to the patient should take place and referral to a social worker for medical transportation needs can be arranged, depending on the facility.

CASE PRESENTATION 5: TELLING THE OLDER ADULT TO STOP DRIVING

Doctor: "Jim, I received your driving clinic evaluation back and the results are not favorable for your continued driving."

James Park: "What do you mean, I feel fine."

Doctor: "I understand you feel fine, which is great, but I'm talking about the tests they did to evaluate your ability to drive. The clinic sent me a report, and their conclusion is that you should stop driving because you are not safe."

James Park: "I can't stop driving. How will I get anywhere? Those tests didn't say anything about my driving. I didn't even get in the car."

Doctor: "I know we are asking you to make a big change, but look at this as a transition. You are no longer safe to drive, if you keep driving you place yourself and others at risk for harm. I know you don't want that. Let me have our social worker come in and talk to you about a number of alternatives you have to driving and we'll see about making this work for you and your family. I'm sorry but I think this is really in your best interest and though it's hard to take now, I think you'll get used to it as many of my other patients have. Let me have you speak to Kelly, our social worker, and she will give you some ideas about alternative transportation options."

This conversation, though difficult, should be handled firmly and directly. It is important to point out the choices that patients have in terms of transportation alternatives and give them support throughout this process.

It is important, as a health care provider, to know your state's reporting laws when talking to patients who have demonstrated impairments. Obtaining permission to bring in family members for discussion may be helpful. It is also important in discussions to reiterate an obligation to report medical conditions that increase the risk of an accident and to document the discussion in the patient's chart. It is also imperative to follow up and assess people who stop driving for signs or symptoms of depression, isolation, and neglect. Often these people rely on others to take them to doctor's appointments, the grocery store, and to run other errands, and this can be quite distressing, particularly if they have fewer social networks or family relationships.

CASE PRESENTATION 5 (continued)

"Hi, Mr. Park, my name is Kelly and I've been asked to talk to you about driving alternatives. Did you get a chance to fill out the form that the doctor gave you while you were waiting for me?" Mr. Park turns over a sheet that lists what he spends on maintaining his car. The list has the following items.

1. Car loan or lease payment	"None, the car is paid for."
2. Yearly insurance costs	$675
3. Yearly licensing fees	$225
4. Average spent on maintenance (oil, tires, repairs)	$525
5. Average miles per year driven	4000
6. Average gas mileage you get	22 miles per gallon

"When I total up your yearly expenses for operating your car it looks like you spend about $1970 per year just to run your car. This is less than many of our other patients, but I think you'll find that we can develop a very nice budget for alternative transportation that will get you where you need to go and maybe even leave some money over for a longer trip if you like, how does that sound?" Mr. Park replies, "I had no idea that I was spending that much money on my own car, and it's not even a very new one. I am encouraged that if I get rid of my car I will have plenty of money to still get around and maybe even save some money. You didn't even include the money I will get when I sell my car. Thank you, this gives me hope that I won't be stuck in the house and will still be able to get around."

SUMMARY AND CONCLUSION

It is important to recognize that driving is probably the single most important aspect of older adults' independence, and the loss of driving privileges is often accompanied by a significant sense of loss; however, there are a few things to emphasize. First, most older persons do not have problems with driving. It is important to assess each person based upon his or her clinical presentation, diagnoses, functional impairments, and history. These are much stronger indicators of driving competence than age alone. All patients should be counseled on safe driving behaviors, and any restrictions they may need to place on themselves, such as the avoidance of night driving prior to cataract surgery or driving in unfamiliar areas. Regular follow-ups should be scheduled for any person for whom driving may be or may become a problem (for example signs of cognitive impairment). Treatment for the cause of any impairment should begin, and follow-up on the efficacy of that treatment should take place.

If a person presents with any risk factors for unsafe driving, referral to a driving assessment clinic, if available, should be made. In some cases older drivers may be able to complete a driving rehabilitation program that would allow them to continue driving safely, or would identify any particular restrictions that should be made on their driving.

Health care providers should be alert to things that may impair driving, or may make driving unsafe. Discussions with the patient and their family (if agreed to) should be initiated and revisited as necessary. Patients should be encouraged to assess their own driving, and report any problems they may see or anything brought up by a family member. If possible, review past driving history with the patient. Documentation of any counseling or follow-up should be made, and any concerns of the health care provider, patient, or family should be noted. This will make follow-up easier, and may serve as a reminder, while allowing the health care provider to track any changes or decline in function. If driving cessation is indicated, documentation of refusal should also be kept. As always, the effects of any intervention made by the health care team should be documented and the effects noted.

References

1. Ball KK, Owsley C. Driving competence: It's not a matter of age. *J Am Geriatr Soc.* 2003;51:1499-1501.

2. Evans L. Risks older drivers face themselves and threats they pose to other road users. *Int J Epidemiol.* 2000;29:315-322.

3. Cook LJ, Knight S, Olson LM, et al. Motor vehicle crash characteristics and medical outcome among older drivers in Utah, 1992-1995. *Ann Emerg Med.* 2000;35:585-591.

4. Ball K, Owsley C, Stalvey B, et al. Driving avoidance and functional impairment in older drivers. *Accident Analysis Prev.* 1998;30: 313-322.

5. Anstey KJ, Windsor TD, Luszcz MA, Andrews GR. Predicting driving cessation over 5 years in older adults: Psychological well-being and cognitive competence are stronger predictors than physical health. *J Am Geriatr Soc.* 2006;54:121-126.

6. Fonda SJ, Wallace RB, Herzog AR. Changes in driving patterns and worsening depressive symptoms among older adults. *J Gerontol Series B Psychol Sci Social Sci.* 2001;56:S343-S351.

7. Freeman EE, Gange SJ, Muñoz B, West SK. Driving status and risk of entry into long-term care in older adults. *Am J Public Health*. 2006;96:1254-1259.

8. Mann WC, McCarthy DP, Wu SS, Tomita M. Relationship of health status, functional status, and psychosocial status to driving among elderly with disabilities. *J Phys Occup Ther Geriatr*. 2005;23:1-24.

9. Marottoli RA, Mendes de Leon CF, Glass TA, et al. Consequences of driving cessation: Decreased out-of-home activity levels. *J Gerontol Series B Psychol Sci Social Sci*. 2000;55:S334-S340.

10. Marottoli RA, Mendes de Leon CF, Glass TA, et al. Driving cessation and increased depressive symptoms: Prospective evidence from the New Haven EPESE. *J Am Geriatr Soc*. 1997;45:202-206.

11. Dellinger A, Kresnow M, White D, Sehgal M. Risk to self versus risk to others: How do older drivers compare to others on the road? *Am J Prev Med*. 2004;26:217-222.

12. Freund B, Colgrove LA, Burke BL, McLeod R. Self-rated driving performance among elderly drivers referred for driving evaluations. *Accident Analysis Prev*. 2005;37:613-618.

13. Ross LA, Clay OJ, Edwards JD, et al. Do older drivers at-risk for crashes modify their driving over time? *J Gerontol Series B Psychol Sci Social Sci*. 2009;64:163-170.

14. Anstey KJ, Wood J, Lord S, Walker JG. Cognitive, sensory and physical factors enabling driving safety in older adults. *Clin Psychol Rev*. 2005;25:45-65.

15. Ball KK, Roenker DL, Wadley VG, et al. Can high-risk older drivers be identified through performance-based measures in a Department of Motor Vehicles setting? *J Am Geriatr Soc*. 2006;54:77-84.

16. Bieliauskas LA. Neuropsychological assessment of geriatric driving competence. *Brain Injury*. 2005;19:221-226.

17. Wood JM, Anstey KJ, Kerr GK, et al. A multidomain approach for predicting older driver safety under in-traffic road conditions. *J Am Geriatr Soc*. 2008;56:986-993.

18. American Medical Association. *How to Help the Older Driver*. 2009. Retrieved from http://www.ama-assn.org on May 9, 2009.

19. Clay OJ, Wadley VG, Edwards JD, et al. Cumulative meta-analysis of the relationship between useful field of view and driving performance in older adults: Current and future implications. *Optom Vis Sci*. 2005;82:724-731.

20. Freund B, Gracenstein S, Ferris R, et al. Drawing clocks and driving cars: Use of brief tests of cognition to screen driving competency in older adults. *J Gen Inter Med*. 2005;20:240-244.

21. Goode KT, Ball K, Sloane M, et al. Useful field of view and other neurocognitive indicators of crash risk in older adults. *J Clin Psychol Med Settings*. 1998;5:425-440.

22. Dubois S, Bedard M, Weaver B. The impact of benzodiazepines on safe driving. *Traffic Injury Prev*. 2008;9:404-413.

23. Henry TA. Court: Physician liability limited in third-party cases. 2009. www.ama-assn.org/amendnews/2009/07/20/prsco720.htm.

POST-TEST

1. **Which of the following statements is FALSE?**

   A. Losing the ability to drive is associated with a reduced quality of life for older persons.

   B. Motor vehicle crashes are the number one cause of injury-related fatalities in the 65- to 74-year-old age group.

   C. Increased numbers of older women drivers are on the road.

   D. Older drivers can eliminate any increased crash risk due to functional impairments by self-imposing limits to their driving.

2. **The Useful Field of View:**

   A. Measures higher-order visual processing skills

   B. Is an automated perimetry test

   C. Has not been found useful in identifying elevated crash risk in older adults

   D. Is a vision test evaluating contrast sensitivity

3. **Measures of executive function used to evaluate older drivers do NOT include:**

   A. The Trail-Making Test

   B. The Clock Drawing Test

   C. The Useful Field of View

   D. The Mini Mental Status Test

4. **If a physician determines that a patient should not be driving, he or she should FIRST:**

   A. Call family members to discuss the physician's conclusions.

   B. Have a discussion with the patient about driving cessation, and note the discussion in the patient's file.

   C. Inform the DMV of his or her concerns.

   D. Run further tests.

ANSWERS TO PRE-TEST

1. B
2. D
3. D
4. C

ANSWERS TO POST-TEST

1. B
2. A
3. C
4. B

16

Changing Living Environments for Older Adults: Environmental Supports for Aging in Place

J.L. Warren, PhD

S. Rodiek, PhD, NCARB

● **LEARNING OBJECTIVES**

1. Identify the multiple dimensions that must be considered by the health care team in recommending environmental support for aging in place.
2. Describe the role of allied health professionals in determining environmental modification to enhance aging in place.
3. Identify the eight domains of daily activity important in determining needed environmental modifications.
4. Explain how the Personal Living Profile (PLP) and Personal Environmental Summary (PES) can be used to identify significant gaps in environmental support for aging in place.
5. Describe simple, economical modifications that can enhance ease and safety of mobility for functionally impaired elders.

PRE-TEST

1. **Which health professional is LESS LIKELY to be called on to help assess the home environment for possible modifications?**

   A. Family physician
   B. Physical therapist
   C. Occupational therapist
   D. Nursing staff

2. **One of the most important reasons for including the family and other caregivers in determining environmental modifications is:**

   A. To provide continuity of care
   B. To give multiple perspectives on the home environment
   C. To help settle disputes between caregivers and family members
   D. To help older adults realize they are valued by everyone.

3. Which environmental support DOES NOT enhance feelings of independence and control for older adults with impaired mobility?
    A. Ramps
    B. Grab bars
    C. Brighter lighting
    D. Portable toilets

4. What percentage of older adults living in the community requires considerable support and assistance from others?
    A. 5-8%
    B. 10-15%
    C. 20-25%
    D. Over 30%

• INTRODUCTION

What features of the living environment are needed for a person to "age in place," to continue living in one's own home, despite changing functional abilities? This chapter will review important factors to consider in modifying existing home environments to help older adults, with and without functional impairments, achieve the goal of staying at home (aging in place) as long as possible. Most of the features described in this chapter can be feasibly incorporated in the design and construction of new homes, and builders are increasingly taking advantage of the opportunity of "universal design" to appeal to a broader market.[1,2] However, for a majority of older adults, buying a new house is not an option, and their goal is to remain in the home they are living in now. A case study approach will be used to illustrate how modifications in the home and near-home environment can provide support for aging in place, and how health care providers can contribute to older adults remaining in the personal and familiar surroundings of their own home and community.[3] This chapter introduces a *Personal Living Profile (PLP)* for completion by the older adult patient. This profile incorporates questions that focus on identifying the needs and assets of each older adult living environment, as well as the meaning of home, history of home modifications, and attitude toward modifications. The process of evaluating the level of support afforded by the current environment, and introducing modifications to improve functioning by older adults, and their families and caregivers, will be demonstrated through the case study. Finally, a *Personal Environment Summary (PES)* is presented for use in the office visit to fill in any gaps identified in the Personal Living Profile and prescribe environmental changes to help the older adult age in place.

• DEFINITIONS

Some of the important terms used in this chapter are defined here.

ADL/IADL: Activities of Daily Living and Instrumental Activities of Daily Living are routine activities that people typically complete on a daily basis. ADL are self-care tasks such as eating, dressing, or bathing, while IADL activities such as shopping, paying bills, or housework can be delegated to others. See Chapter 7 for further detail.

Aging in place: Being able to remain in one's present residence despite changing functional abilities, usually requires securing necessary supportive services and home modifications in response to changing needs.

Caregiver: A person who provides direct physical and emotional care for a dependent adult, whether paid or unpaid, a health professional, friend, neighbor, or family member.

Care network: The health and allied health organizations and professionals, as well as nonprofessional caregivers, that provide a full complement of health and mental health services.

Environmental affordances: Refers to the ways in which an environment can provide (or afford) support for specific behaviors, and the ways in which those behaviors take place in that environment.

Environmental hazards: Features of the home, community, or built environment that increase risks to human health and safety.

Health care provider: An organization or person who delivers health care in a systematic way professionally to an individual in need of health care services.

Home modification: Alterations made to the interior or exterior of a home or to the near environment that improve safety, accessibility, and the potential for independent living.

Self-care behaviors: Decisions and actions by an individual to improve his or her health, reduce health risks, and/or cope with a health problem.

Social support: Physical and emotional comfort and resources given by family, friends, neighbors, and the other people encountered in daily life.

Universal design: The design of products and environments to be usable by all people, with or without disabilities, without the need for further adaptation by those with special needs.

• THE CASE FOR "GOING HOME"

CASE PRESENTATION 1: ADAPTING TO NEW DISABILITIES

Mr. W., age 69, had a severe left hemisphere stroke with resulting Broca aphasia 3 months ago. He has nearly completed 3 months of intensive inpatient rehabilitation at a geriatric care facility and is ambulatory with the use of a quad cane for balance. He still favors his left side and has some difficulty with fine motor function in his right hand. He is able to complete most of his daily activities effectively at the rehabilitation facility, which is a well-designed, supportive environment, with highly trained health professionals.

He is a highly motivated, outgoing, cognitively intact individual with many friends in the community. His spouse is still in reasonable health though she has had heart bypass surgery, is being treated for high blood pressure and arthritis, and cannot be depended on to assist with any weight-bearing tasks. The couple lives in a 1960s split-level home in a rural community where Mr. W. operated a successful small business. He has three married daughters—two living several states away and one living next door with her husband and two daughters. Mr. W. wants to go home. But home is not equipped like the rehabilitation center.

This health crisis in Mr. W.'s life represents a host of challenges that could potentially lead to quite different outcomes. Initially, after the stroke, his family physician indicated that placement in a nursing home was likely, since most people with such extensive damage have not recovered the ability to walk, talk, or feed themselves. The speech therapist agreed with the family physician and indicated that the aphasia was so severe that only limited language use could be expected. Fortunately, the attending physician at the hospital had been through a geriatric rehabilitation rotation in medical school and had seen a physiatrist-led (physician specializing in physical medicine, rehabilitation, and restoring optimal function) team of allied health professionals in an adapted environment "work miracles" with highly impaired but motivated individuals—so she wrote the orders for rehabilitation. That Mr. W. made such a significant recovery in rehab—regaining the ability to walk, perform daily routines, and communicate (even though hesitantly), with the hope of returning to his home and community—indicates that there is still much to learn about maintaining independence and health in the face of apparently clear medical conditions but with differing medical opinions about potential functional improvements. While the family physician saw Mr. W. as a disabled person with nursing care needs whose wife could not be expected to take care of him, the attending physician sought to return Mr. W.'s capacity to the highest level possible.

This case sets the stage for a perspective that sees the crucial role of physicians and other health care providers in understanding the complex components affecting health, aging, and independent living. Medical practitioners who are able to effectively draw upon the latest research to improve health outcomes will be the leaders of the future. Twenty-five percent of our population, known as the "baby boomers," will soon reach retirement age—the period of life where the majority of health crises typically occur. With health costs continuing to rise (currently consuming 16.5% of the US GDP), it is imperative to assist individuals and families, especially in this large cohort, with preventive and rehabilitative practices that maintain people in the community as long as possible, regardless of perceived physical limitations.[4]

In the following section, the research on maintaining functioning in older adults and improving or stabilizing functioning in older impaired adults will be reviewed in terms of both the risks and the resources of the living environment. Research on people with functional limitations who remain in home and community settings has shown the importance of considering the whole person—physical, social and personal aspects—in the context of his or her physical environment. The case of Mr. W. will be used to illustrate the complexity of managing "aging in place."

● REVIEW OF RELEVANT LITERATURE

The Effects of Environment on Living Independently in Later Life

The home environment becomes increasingly important as people age. While only 5% of those over 65 live in institutions such as nursing homes and 95% live in the community, it is estimated that between 10% and 15% of community-dwelling elders require considerable support and assistance from others.[5] Today, there are also many more older adults who are single and live alone. In the last 20 years, alternative housing options such as assisted living and congregate senior apartments have increased, as well as the availability of home care, giving older adults a range of options beyond depending on adult children, spouses, or having to go into a nursing home. In spite of attractive new options, however, the goal of staying at home and avoiding institutionalization, at almost any cost, is important for many older adults. Studies show that 90% of older adults strongly prefer to continue living in the same home or county where they live now.[6] Home remains a "symbol of self," the center of the physical world, and the center of social activities.[7] To the elder, home means comfort and security, in spite of the fact that it is sometimes a burden and may potentially be unsafe.[8]

Functional Abilities of the Person

Early work in gerontology pointed to stressors that the environment presented to older adults experiencing physical and health-related changes. Activities of Daily Living (ADL) and Instrumental Activities of Daily Living (IADL) were developed as scales measuring a person's physical and cognitive mastery of tasks necessary for independent living (Chapter 7 provides greater detail about these measures). They were used by health care providers and social workers to assess the level of task functioning of older adults and to determine needed assistance and accompanying reimbursement level. ADLs include bathing, grooming, dressing, eating, toileting/continence, and transferring in and out of a chair or bed.[9] IADLs include tasks such as telephone use, driving, shopping, laundry, housekeeping, medication management, food preparation, and handling finances.[10] Assessment of individual functioning through ADL and IADL evaluation provides an initial source of information useful in identifying potential environmental modifications that could compensate for deficits in functioning. It is also a first-level predictor of risk for further decline.

The role of the environment, however, should not be understated. A review of studies on environmental factors identified several design features associated with active behaviors and fall prevention, including flooring, lighting, grab bars, and room layout.[11] For example, in a person with incontinence, a bathroom located far away or on another level may render that person "toileting dependent." Providing a bedside commode or urinal can support toileting independence and allow a person to remain at home with minimal expense. A talking microwave may provide a person with vision impairment with adequate support for meal preparation. While single impairments may occur and be managed with a simple modification or intervention, multiple impairments may indicate broader and more complex environmental supports including intermittent or around-the-clock personal care.

The outdoor environment also presents opportunities for modification to improve safety, so the older adult can maintain outdoor activity, social contacts with neighbors, and gain psychological benefits from the natural environment.[12] Accessible views of the outside encouraged older adults to sit by windows for enjoyment of nature. Other features noted that encouraged outdoor engagement included walkable areas, continuous paths, and areas for gardening. A built-up garden or a table for potting plants can work well for a person with balance problems who can sit on a walker or in a chair and tend the roses.

A meta-analysis of peer-reviewed research and reviews published between 1997 and 2006 found evidence based on randomized controlled trials showing that improved home environments can enhance functional ability outcomes, aside from falls that may involve medication issues.[13] Some specific findings cited were that environmental support reduced the need for assistance by wheelchair users; independence in bathing was linked to modified bathroom environments[14]; improved lighting was linked with higher independent function; and overall, barriers in the home resulted in increased hours of assistance being required.

The issue with fall-accident related outcomes seems to be that falls particularly have multiple influences aside from the environment, including muscle weakness and medication. Studies that included environmental modifications with exercise and balance training and medication review have found a reduction in falls.[15] With an aging population, even stabilizing a condition would be a positive effect.

Hazards in the Home Environment

Home safety checklists have been developed to identify particular features of the environment that increase risk for specific injuries such as falls.[16,17] These environmental assessment tools are used by health care providers, family members, and social workers to identify high-risk features whose removal would improve safety, and to identify environmental features that could be added or modified to increase safety. Permanent upgrades to the environment can continue to support the functioning and independence of older adults as they age; however, further changes in their health status and functioning may require additional modifications in the future. Specific checklists for home modification to improve functioning and safety for persons with dementia have also been developed.[18,19] Again, these tools provide another source of information to target specific home modifications. Where adoption of specific home modifications has been studied, there have been documented improvements in functional outcomes, such as fewer falls and slower rates of decline in functional ability.[20,21]

An analysis of potential environmental hazards in the homes of community-dwelling adults over age 72 identified known hazards in each room. Over 90% of the homes had two or more hazards present, with many hazards found in more than one room (Table 16–1).[22]

When present, stairs were often hazardous. Staircase-related hazards were identified separately and are shown in Table 16–2. Two or more hazards were present in 44.1% of homes with stairs.

When hazards were classified by the person's level of ADL disability, this study showed that hazards were equally present at all levels of functional ability. One difference found between age-restricted housing and community housing was the presence of tub/shower grab bars in 90.7% of bathrooms

● TABLE 16–1 Home Environment Hazards (Excluding Stairs)	
Home Hazards	Percent of Homes
Loose throw rugs, runners, mats, slip or trip hazards	77.9
Light switches not clearly visible in dark	67
Grab bars not present in tub/shower	61
Obstructed pathways with small objects, cords, or tripping hazards	46.7
Dim lighting, shadows, or glare	44.1
Bathtub/shower surface slippery, nonskid mat or abrasive strips not present	41.2
Carpet edges curling or tripping hazards	35.7
Low chair that is difficult to get out of	18.1
Toilet seat too low or wobbly	17.2
Stepstool not sturdy	13
Chair not sturdy, moves easily or needs repair	12.2
Frequently used items stored too low or too high to easily reach	7.8
Area slippery, if not carpeted	7.5
Table not sturdy or moves easily	5.1

Source: Gill TM, Williams CS, Robison JT, Tinetti ME. A population-based study of environmental hazards in the homes of older persons. Am J Public Health. 1999;89:553-556.

● TABLE 16–2 Staircase-Related Hazards	
Stair Hazards	Percent of Homes
Night light not present or not near stairway	67.6
Dim lighting, shadows, or glare	26.9
Light switches not at both top and bottom of stairway	21
Some steps narrower, higher, lower than others	15.1
Handrail not present, sturdy, or full length of stairway	14.5
Steps in need of repair, loose treads or carpeting	14

Source: Gill TM, Williams CS, Robison JT, Tinetti ME. A population-based study of environmental hazards in the homes of older persons. Am J Public Health. 1999;89:553-556.

in age-restricted housing. Bathrooms were found to be the most hazardous room in community dwellings, some having multiple hazards. Although it is clearly important to address the environmental hazards described, many older adults and their families have not made modifications that would improve their ability to continue living in the community. Health care providers are often influential with their patients, and are in a better position to prescribe environmental modifications when using tools for assessing a person's capabilities (ADL-IADL) in combination with safety checklists of environmental risks.

Care Network

Allied professionals such as occupational and physical therapists, social workers, and nurses are important members of the health care team. These team members provide a bridge between the acute care or rehabilitation environment and the older adult's home. They start with the medical status of the person and then apply data from a person's ADL assessment and home environment safety analysis to determine a care plan. These professionals are trained to use a multidimensional framework of care that includes elements beyond the physical environment, such as coping strategies and expressed needs and preferences of the older adult, as well as the level of social support from family and friends. They can also focus on proper implementation of home modification with the user. This is a critical factor, since adherence to recommended home modifications has been reported to occur in fewer than 15% of cases without support; even intermittent follow-up increased adherence rates to only 50%.[23] Other factors that may influence adherence include financial constraints, personal reluctance, lack of knowledge and family support, and the specific type of residential situation. Home assessments by an appropriate allied health professional can help identify such factors, and determine potential funding sources as well as educational and training programs that may be available within the community.

One component of "aging in place" is the person's social support system. Older adults living alone with a network of friends who are willing and able to assist with such tasks as grocery shopping, picking up medications, and other intermittent tasks may be able to continue living at home, even

with some decline in IADLs. The presence of a spouse is the highest predictor of remaining in the community during ADL decline, when environmental modifications and assistive devices may not be sufficient to aid a person to remain at home. While a spouse caregiver, or an adult child—typically a daughter—is found to be a critical component of support, paid caregivers can also perform this role to some extent. For example, a weekly housekeeper or yard worker may take on additional roles such as grocery shopping or driving an older person to a doctor's appointment.

It is essential to involve any significant caregivers in health care conferences, and in situations where cognitive deficits are present in the patient, the caregiver can contribute valuable information about behavioral issues. Studies have shown that it is also important to understand and address the level of environmental support needed by the caregiver.[24,25] For example, if a person with Alzheimer-type dementia attempts to leave the house while unattended, the environment can help alleviate this problem through modifications such as positioning door locks at floor level, where they will not be noticed by the patient, or disguising the door with wallpaper having a bookcase motif. Caregivers can also benefit from training on the proper use of assistive devices, safe moving and lifting techniques, and techniques such as the use of music to calm an agitated person.

Self-Care Behaviors of the Patient

People who have had a tendency to emphasize prevention throughout life may be more willing to adopt and use environmental supports in later years. In addition, having a proactive approach and valuing personal control over the environment have been shown to improve functional outcomes when home modifications are introduced. Beliefs about the environmental deficits present and the effectiveness or applicability of home modifications seem to influence this self-care attitude.[26-28] Determining a person's willingness to make and use interventions can be one predictor for improving adoption and ultimately outcomes. Similarly, when quite old people live in accessible homes and believe their situation to be supportive, meaningful, and not entirely dependent on others, they have been found to exhibit better well-being, less depression, and be more independent in their daily activities.[29,30] People who resist environmental changes may have an idea that "asking for help" is a sign of personal weakness. Psychologists have successfully employed the use of cognitive reframing to adjust this perspective. Speaking about environmental changes as representing a sign of strength and the use of devices as "smart" and promoting independence can help break down barriers to acceptance and promote behavior change.

Personal Aspects of Home

By including the meaning of home in patient discussions, the health care provider will have greater success in recommending environmental modifications that support the person who wishes to remain at home. Understanding how an older adult views self, what supports his or her feelings of "being intact," and where the older person is in the process of "environmental centralization" can aid the health care provider in recommending environmental changes. Environmental centralization refers to an age-related tendency to spend time in certain favored places within the home. This seems to occur in both healthy and functionally impaired older adults. It is important to identify such favored places, as they represent comfort, ease of access, and a sense of control.[31,32] The health care provider can help develop a more accurate understanding of the patient's specific preferences and goals, and can partner with the patient and care network in achieving these goals.

ASSESSMENT TOOLS

Personal Living Profile (PLP)

The Personal Living Profile (Appendix 16–1) was developed to incorporate personal traits and meaning, history of modifications, and environmental affordance opportunities in a very brief profile that can be used with ADL/IADL evaluations to identify the most critical and potentially successful areas for modification in the living environment. It would be completed by the older adult and family member prior to the office visit.

The concept of "environmental affordances" is an effective way to visualize the capacity of the home and nearby environment to support multiple dimensions of a person's life. These dimensions include the medical, physical, cognitive, psychological, and functional capabilities of the person, as well as his or her preferences, social support, and care network—all in the context of the person's physical environment.[33] The term "affordance" refers to the ways in which an environment can provide (or afford) support for specific behaviors and the ways in which those behaviors take place in that environment.[34] Other researchers use terms such as an "enabling environment" to acknowledge the interactive nature of the person operating at a specific functional level within a physical environment to which the person attaches meaning.[35]

Personal Environment Summary

The Personal Environment Summary (PES) (Appendix 16–2) was developed as an additional tool for the health care provider to use after reviewing the PLP that was completed by the older adult or family member. This simple matrix gives the health care provider a framework for making notes on each of the major dimensions of the person's life as it relates to his or her home environment, and provides added assurance that important issues will not be overlooked. Each cell in the PES would be used to note additional relevant data on which the health care team could act.

APPLYING THE TOOLS

CASE PRESENTATION 2: THE PERSONAL LIVING PROFILE APPLIED

Mrs. Smith completed the Personal Living Profile (PLP) for her recently widowed mother Angela, who lives alone.

A. *Sleeping and waking.* "Mom seems to be sleeping later and later each day I stop by to check on her. She complains about having a hard time getting to sleep."

B. *Bathing, grooming, dressing.* "She is not bathing every day and sometimes doesn't take care of her personal appearance. The arthritis in her hip and back make it hard for her to move."

C. *Cooking, eating, vitamins, and medications.* "She seems to have lost interest in food, but her medication organizer is helping me track that she is taking her meds every day."

D. *Utilitarian chores and tasks.* "Mowing the yard is the only thing she does every week—it takes her longer and longer to get it done. The house is a mess—I think we need to hire a cleaning service."

E. *Leisure activities.* "She is very focused on keeping her favorite roses alive. This is a worry because she always got compliments on them and now she can't bend down to work on the soil like she used to."

F. *Interaction at or near home.* "Her two favorite neighbors moved—to be near their children or in a retirement community. One woman had helped her with gardening tips, and had joined the community Master Gardener Group when she lost her garden."

G. and H. Nothing was filled in/blank.

Upon reviewing Angela's PLP, Dr. Jones noted possible symptoms of depression in items A, B, C, and D. He used the Personal Environment Summary (PES) to remind him of additional questions related to items G and H. He asked Angela about her husband, who had also been a patient for many years. Angela seemed relieved to be able to talk about him. A referral was made to a clinical social worker in the community who specialized in grief counseling. Dr. Jones also noted the possible impact of arthritis on Angela's activities of daily living such as bathing, dressing, preparing food, and caring for her yard from items B, C, D, and E. The PES reminded him to ask Angela about her preferences in these areas. Dr. Jones suggested that Angela increase her frequency of anti-inflammatory medication and referred her to a physical therapist. The therapist reviewed the PLP and

APPENDIX 16–1: PERSONAL LIVINGI PROFILE (PLP)

Date: _____

PERSONAL LIVING PROFILE (PLP) for _____(Name)

Completed by _____ (Relationship to person above) _____
This should be completed before the office visit, preferably by the older adult patient. If necessary, a family member or friend familiar with their living situation can complete the form for them.
(Circle) your answers.

1. Being able to live at home during the later part of life is important to some older adults.
   How important is it to **you** to continue living in your own home?

   Very important   Somewhat important   Not important

2. Which of the following ideas might be easier to achieve if you could **continue living in your own home**? Please circle any that apply.

Freedom	Privacy	Daily variety	Enjoy life
Security	Have choices	See nature	See neighbors
Safety	Care for home	Do hobbies	Prepare meals
Comfort	Stay active	Have pets	Contact with friends

3. What changes have you made in your home to make life **easier, safer, or more comfortable**?

Tub mat	Clear pathways	Sturdy or higher chair	Shower wand
Night light(s)	Brighter lighting	Raised toilet seat	Ramp
Electric cord safety	Secure loose rugs	Grab bars	Door handles
Stair safety	Use lower cabinets	Bath seat	Add light switches

   Other changes: _____
   _____
   _____
   _____

4. How do you feel about **making changes** to help you continue living at home?

   Things are OK as is   Not sure   Willing to make changes

DAILY BEHAVIOR: CONCERNS AND PREFERENCES
A day in YOUR life: Please respond in terms of your typical activities.
Look at the Daily Behavior list below. Under each category note any <u>concerns</u> you have about comfort, safety, or ease in completing the activity. Also note any <u>preferences</u> you have related to each activity.

A. Sleeping and waking. Includes going to bed, getting up at night, waking and getting up in the morning
_____
_____
_____
_____

B. Bathing, grooming, dressing. Includes brushing teeth and hair, shower or bath, drying, putting on lotions, dressing and undressing
_____
_____
_____
_____

C. **Cooking, eating, vitamins, and medications.** Includes food preparation, eating meals and snacks, taking vitamins, supplements, and medications

_____
_____
_____
_____

D. **Utilitarian chores and tasks.** Includes housekeeping, laundry, making the bed, paying bills, sweeping the porch, mowing the lawn, weeding and watering the garden

_____
_____
_____
_____

E. **Leisure activities and hobbies.** Includes watching TV, knitting, arts and handicrafts, using the computer, gardening for pleasure

_____
_____
_____
_____

F. **Interaction at or near home.** Includes interaction with pets, having friends or family over, talking on the phone, visiting with neighbors outdoors

_____
_____
_____
_____

G. **Activities away from home.** Includes shopping, medical/ dental appointments, visiting

_____
_____
_____
_____

H. **Physical activity, exercise.** Includes indoor and outdoor exercise, stretching, walks in nearby neighborhood or in the yard

_____
_____
_____
_____

APPENDIX 16–2: PERSONAL ENVIRONMENT SUMMARY

Personal Environment Summary for _____

Completed by _____ Date _____

(To be completed by the healthcare professional during the client/patient visit)

	RISKS/HAZARDS What causes problems with…	PREFERENCES What would you like to have…	NEEDS/EQUIPMENT What would make it easier…	SOCIAL SUPPORT Can people help with…	HEALTH/FUNCTION What makes it harder to…
SLEEPING In and out of bed Up at night Sleeping comfort					
BATHING Grooming Dressing Shower/bath					
EATING Food preparation Taking vitamins Medications					
CHORES Household Paying bills Yard work					
HOBBIES TV/computer Arts & crafts Golf/sports					
SOCIAL Friends/family Neighbors Interact with pets					
OUTINGS Appointments Visiting Shopping					
EXERCISE Walking Being outdoors Stretching					

the PES with Dr. Jones' notes before making a home visit, noting the areas of the home that presented hazards (item B) and opportunities (items D, E, and F). She suggested to Angela and her daughter, Mrs. Smith, that a bath chair, a hand grip attached to the tub, and a hand-held shower wand be installed to provide a safer bathing and dressing environment. She also suggested placing a patio chair near the rose bed for easier access and possibly building the flower bed higher so Angela would not have to bend over. She encouraged Angela to join the community Master Gardener Program run by the local Cooperative Extension Service, where she could learn about rose care, become more physically active, and maintain contact with her former neighbor.

In Angela's case, the PLP and PES brought both environmental and social-emotional issues to light that if addressed, could improve her opportunities for aging in place. Her daughter would then be able to return to a social support role rather than taking on a full-time caregiver role.

CASE PRESENTATION 1 (continued)

Once Mr. and Mrs. W. completed the Personal Living Profile, important behavioral patterns, attitudinal assets or barriers, and specific aspects of the living environment needing attention could more easily be identified. The data from this profile showed that some safety measures were already present, but no specific accessibility-oriented home modifications had been made. There was a high willingness to do whatever it took to return Mr. W. to his home. A physical therapist from the rehabilitation center was assigned to do an on-site home assessment with Mrs. W. and the adult daughter.

This assessment of Mr. W.'s home environment was an important step, preferably before his release from the rehabilitation facility. For example, adding an extra railing along the staircase wall would allow Mr. W. to climb the stairs independently when he arrived home. Next, it was important for the therapist to observe Mr. W. functioning in his own environment, in order to accurately determine his use of environmental modifications and identify additional modifications that would improve his functioning. Modifications can be made in ways that retain a home-like character, which is important to Mr. W. and to others (spouse, family, guests) who also use areas in the home.

In each of the PLP sections below, Mr. W.'s daily behavior patterns are considered in light of his recent functional changes and challenges. Environmental modifications that are both acceptable and improve safety are discussed in terms of the Personal Living Profile for each behavior pattern typically experienced in a 24-hour period.

Sleeping

Comfort

Because sleep is an important daily behavior that extends for several hours, it is important that environmental conditions support healthy sleeping patterns. Mr. W. no longer has as much muscle and fat tissue as when he was younger, so he needs a mattress with a softer surface layer, such as a pillow top or memory foam. At the same time, he needs a firm under layer to support his back, in part because his back muscles are no longer as strong as they were. Mr. W. likes to have his toes free to move around in bed. Their housekeeper used to tuck the sheets in tightly, but he noticed that it cut off circulation and sometimes made his feet cramp or go numb, so he asked her to leave the sheets untucked. They compromised when she tucked the sheets in more loosely, leaving an intentional loose fold at the foot of the bed in which he could move his toes freely. This small change made a big difference in how his feet and legs felt the next morning. Other products such as special elasticized top sheets with toe room or an interior rail providing space for foot movement are available.

Safe Movement at Night

Mr. W. does wake during the night to go to the toilet. In reviewing the Daily Behavior section of the Personal Living Profile, Mr. W.'s spouse noted that one bathroom is easily accessed from the bedroom and that a nightlight has been used for years, since they both have to get up at least once during the night. They purchased a small portable bed cane, secured between the mattress and box spring to the bed frame, to make it safer and easier to get in and out of bed (Figure 16–1).

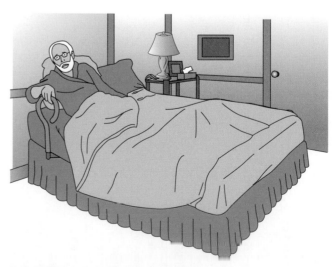

FIGURE 16–1. Bed cane.

Mrs. W. indicates that a higher toilet seat without bars was added to the existing toilet because of her arthritis pain. Side grab bars were added to the wall by the toilet to provide stability while standing, as well as support to stand up from a sitting position. The bathroom doorknob was replaced by a lever-style handle to improve ease of access by Mr. W.; this also benefited Mrs. W., who has arthritis in her hands.

Bathing, Grooming, Dressing

Mr. W. is still able to bathe and dress himself, but he would prefer to be able to sit in the shower and use a spray wand to bathe, rather than standing. He also finds it easier to sit for some aspects of dressing. He stands for other grooming activities such as shaving and brushing hair and teeth. He leans against the cabinet, though, because of some weakness in his right leg.

There are many easy and inexpensive modifications that can improve the ease and safety of reaching the bathroom and performing tasks there, including the following:

Shower seating: A portable seat, a chair with back and arms, or a fold-down seat installed in the shower. These devices, obtained from a medical supply company or ordered online, are useful for maintaining independent bathing when balance, weakness, low energy, pain from arthritis, and limited mobility due to surgery are concerns. Chair legs should be adjustable to obtain the preferred seating height. The least-intrusive device would be a wall-mounted fold-down seat, but this requires installation skills and awareness of exactly where to attach the seat to the studs in a location that optimizes the user's access to shower controls. Such a seat can be folded up for standing and while others use the shower/bath. Mr. W. elected to use a portable seat that could be removed from the shower by his wife. A shower wand was installed, giving the option of a hand-held shower or the fixed shower head (Figure 16–2).

Nonslip mat: For tub/shower, low-pile carpet or nonslip rug for floor outside bath/shower. These were already present in Mr. W.'s bathroom.

Grab rails/bars: In strategic places, grab rails or bars enable Mr. W. to move securely into and to stand in the bathtub or shower; to move from the bath/shower to the dressing area and back into the adjacent room; and to move onto and off the toilet. Grab bars also improve his stability if standing. Grab rails/bars may assist functioning in a small space where a full-size walker would not be functional. These also require skilled installation, so they are securely attached to the studs in the wall and will bear the user's weight as needed (Figure 16–2).

Seating for dressing: A seat for dressing can be managed by adding a straight-back chair or a shower chair with arms and back, if space permits, to the bathroom or dressing area. Mr. W. decided to use the commode with the lid down. A fabric lid cover increased comfort. Having a nearby surface or wall hooks on which clean clothing can be assembled is another feature that can aid independent dressing.

Appliance safety: Mr. W. stands by the sink and uses an electric razor to shave each day. The outlet was updated

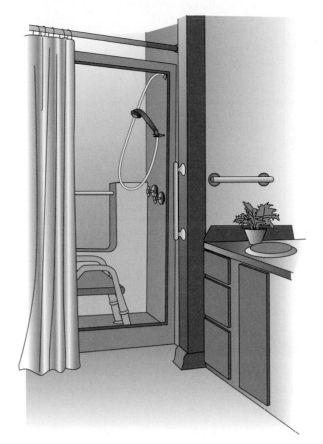

FIGURE 16–2. Shower seating, shower wand, and grab rail.

by an electrician to meet safety standards with a ground fault circuit interrupter (GFCI).

Adequate lighting: The bathroom has full ceiling lighting and accent lighting over the sink, which provides sufficient light, although this feature has been found to be deficient in many older adult's homes.

Negotiating doorways: There is currently adequate space for Mr. W to easily pass through the doorway with his cane. The future likelihood of needs for a walker or a wheelchair should be considered before beginning any remodeling requiring a larger financial investment such as widening the doorway. Removing a door, and the inner molding, and installing an attractive curtain on a tension rod easily secured with Velcro to the door frame is a cost-effective solution for assuring privacy and visual warmth, while widening the doorway to allow access with assistive devices (Figure 16–3).

Cooking, Eating, Supplements, and Medications

Maintaining Nutrition

Mr. W. has always been involved in some aspects of food preparation, including preparing the holiday turkey, preparing fish and seafood, and grilling meats. Accomplishing such tasks contributes greatly to his self-esteem. He enjoys eating

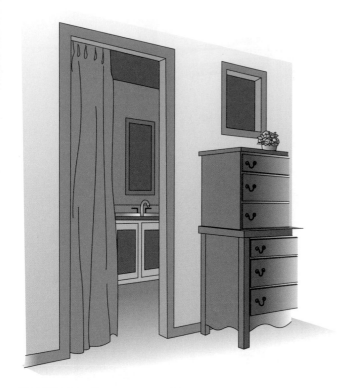

FIGURE 16–3. Doorway removed for access with assistive devices.

favorite and familiar foods prepared by Mrs. W., and he has a sweet tooth. Mr. W. is able to eat independently and does not require a plate with a built up rim/guard. He does have difficulty cutting meat with a knife and fork using both hands, so Mrs. W. cuts his meat prior to serving up the evening meal, or else serves easily cut chicken, fish, or shrimp.

Mr. W. fixes his own lunch in the kitchen. This is usually a sandwich, fruit chunks, a glass of milk, and a cookie. A grab bar was mounted with hardware to base cabinets giving a raised bar at the front edge of the kitchen counters (Figure 16–4) to enhance his stability.

Moving Safely and Easily

One aspect of helping Mr. W. maintain his role in food preparation is assuring that his transition from house to patio to use the BBQ grill, and then returning to house, is as safe as possible. This means that the pathway should be unobstructed, and the door threshold should be level with interior and exterior floors (Figure 16–5). Evaluation of the pathway from the kitchen through the family room and sliding glass doors to the patio identified one barrier and one "naturally-occurring aid." A large area rug under the dining table and chairs was the hazard, but at least it was highly visible because its color contrasts with the floor. Securing the rug's edges with two-sided tape reduced the tendency of the edge to turn up

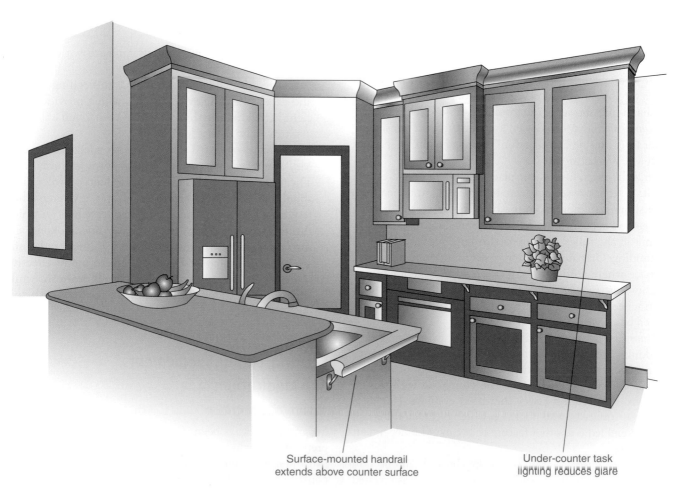

Surface-mounted handrail
extends above counter surface

Under-counter task
lighting reduces glare

FIGURE 16–4. Handrail and lighting in a modified kitchen.

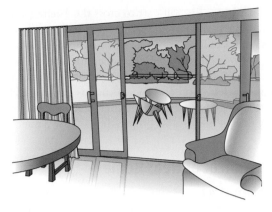

FIGURE 16–5. Unobstructed pathway to patio.

and create a fall hazard. With reduced grasp function in his right hand, Mr. W. needs to put down the tray with meat he is carrying to the grill to open the sliding door. The dining table is a naturally occurring aid, close enough to the door to serve as a place to put things, or for him to grip and rest on his way through.

Conserving Energy, Being Safe in Household Tasks

A second aspect of Mr. W. maintaining his role in food preparation is the need for a sitting area for accomplishing tedious tasks like shrimp deveining. The dining table, near a pass-through to the kitchen, has a view to the outside through the glass doors. The table has a polyurethane finish so "kitchen tasks" may be done without damaging the wood. A large plastic cutting mat can be used for food preparation work while sitting down. The wooden chairs are sturdy and have a secured seat cushion. Their old refrigerator with overhead freezer has been replaced with a side-by-side model, which allows both Mr. and Mrs. W. easier access to the food items they use most often, both fresh and frozen. This environment enables Mr. W.'s continued involvement in meal preparation. Increasing socialization, sensory satisfaction, and continuity of involvement and activity around mealtime is especially important to enhancing health outcomes in older adults.

Safe and Convenient Medication Access

Managing medications for compliance is very important to an older adult's health. Mr. W. takes three medications— Betoptic (betaxolol) for glaucoma, Flomax (tamsulosin) for urinary urgency at night, and Lopurin (allopurinol) for gout— and a multivitamin. The Betoptic drops are kept by his bed for nighttime dosage; the Flomax in the bathroom to take when he brushes his teeth after dinner; and the Lopurin and multivitamin in the kitchen to take with meals. Mrs. W. administers the Betoptic but Mr. W. takes the other medications independently. After the stroke, he did get two daily pill managers, simple plastic boxes in different colors with seven sections (one for each day) in which he keeps the Flomax, Lopurin, and multivitamins.

Utilitarian Chores and Tasks

Stair Safety

In the past, Mr. W. was responsible for making trips to the basement to the large chest freezer to obtain food items Mrs. W. used in preparing meals. This entailed walking down and up one long flight of stairs with handrails on both sides, and one short flight with a handrail on only one side. As he appears to still be capable of this activity, which contributes strength training to his daily behavior, it was important to add a handrail to the opposite side for safe continuance of this task (Figure 16–6). The existing light switches at the top and bottom of the stairs were replaced with wide rocker switches that can easily be engaged by the heel of the hand. The new switches have a built-in backlight to help Mr. W. find them at night, in case he needs to check the water, furnace, or power located in the basement.

Mobility and Connectedness

Mr. W. raises cattle as well as growing the needed food for his small Angus herd. One everyday task was driving his SUV over the farm to "check the cows." After the stroke, he could not drive for a year until he completed the driver retraining course designed for brain-impaired people. His son-in-law looked after the cows for that year. Mr. W. stayed engaged by riding along or by sitting on the patio or by the large sliding glass doors and watching the cattle in the field near the home. He could also drive his golf cart to certain parts of the farm to see the crops. His son-in-law would regularly report in on the status of crops and ask Mr. W. what work he wanted completed that day.

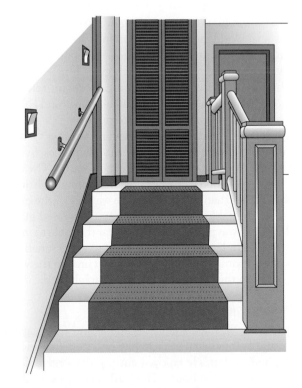

FIGURE 16–6. Stairway with handrail and rocker light switches added.

Involvement in Important Life Roles

Mr. W. had managed the household and farm accounts prior to his stroke. He requested his adult daughter to work with him on this task because his signature with his left hand is not clearly legible. He is able to review accounts and checks, but this function now takes place at the dining table rather than at his office desk so the two can work together. The ability to continue this responsibility in full partnership with his adult daughter has provided a feeling of control over the assets that Mr. W. had worked hard to create for his family.

Task Continuity Through Assistive Tools

In earlier years, Mr. W. also helped with routine household and yard maintenance, such as minor repairs, pruning, and hedge trimming. Hoping to continue these activities, he purchased specially designed ergonomic hand tools, which made some of these activities much easier. He can still use the riding mower to maintain the lawn. However, some tasks still require more strength than he has, so he has hired a local handyman to do repairs, reduced the high-maintenance ornamental plantings in their yard, and asked his grandson to help with some of the heavier yard work. He puts proceeds from the sale of a calf each year into a bank account for his grandson.

Leisure Activities and Hobbies

Managing Losses

Mr. W. was an avid golfer. His stroke affected his ability to drive long shots, but his putting has remained quite good. Golf was an important physical and social activity with friends. With the partial aphasia, Mr. W. often hesitates in finding the right word, and then gets frustrated. He is acutely aware of becoming a burden to his friends, and because he was never the most patient golfer when the group ahead was slow, he now refuses to play the game. This represents a loss in his social world, as many of his friends are unsure how to communicate with him. He will, however, putt balls in the yard with his granddaughters, which gives him satisfaction. And he has always enjoyed watching sports on television. One good friend comes to watch football games and golf tournaments with him every Sunday afternoon.

This same friend comes by on Tuesday evenings for a game of dominoes. They now use the oversize dominoes, available through the Web, to handle and see more easily. The dining table serves as a good game table, but additional lighting was needed. Rather than just boosting the wattage of the existing light over the table—which could have increased glare—a standing lamp was placed in a corner near the table to increase the overall light levels. It was important to make sure that the cords of additional lighting were firmly secured to the walls or baseboards, so they did not create a tripping hazard.

Continuing Roles with Adaptive Tools

Mr. and Mrs. W. have a large vegetable and flower garden. Mr. W. has always taken pride in having a pest-free and well-maintained garden. He enjoyed cutting the vegetables and bringing them to the house. The yard is fairly even, but the branches and debris that often fall from trees can be a hazard.

Now Mr. W. uses his golf cart to cross the 1-acre yard to the garden, brings several small containers to gather different vegetables, and is able to continue this task using scissors rather than a knife to cut through cucumber and squash stems. He has adapted to the diminished strength in his right hand by engaging his left hand and increasing his dexterity. He continues to take pride in the vegetable garden and the harvesting activity that helps Mrs. W. prepare home-grown meals.

Interaction at or Near Home

Importance of Pets

Mr. and Mrs. W. have always been quite social. They have had friends into their home for dinner, hosted family reunions and local gatherings. They are also both fond of animals, though they do not have a pet currently. They are able to "take advantage" of their daughter's pets that she brings over for companionship during her workday. There is sufficient outdoor seating out of the sun and rain, to sit and entertain the "pups." Each dog has its own water and food bowl for those extra treats from Mr. W.

Maintaining Engagement

Because they live in the country—over 2 miles from town—their visitors have to drive out to see them rather than merely walking next door. However, friends and neighbors still drop by, and they visit with people by phone nearly every day. Their out-of-state daughters phone frequently to visit with their parents, so having a portable telephone nearby at all times is important. Mr. W. keeps the portable phone by his chair, so he can easily respond to these calls, as well as the calls from friends and neighbors.

A nearby neighbor, who is also a cousin of Mrs. W. and has an adjoining farm, is a frequent visitor. He brings news of current happenings in town, on the farm, and meetings of local civic groups. He is a good person to reminisce with because their families have been lifelong friends. He often stays for dinner since he was recently widowed and would otherwise be eating alone.

Should Mr. W. lose mobility in the future, it would be important to arrange seating in a comfortable area near a window or glass door with visible outdoor activity so he can continue his "engagement" with the world beyond his household. Watching the seasons change—the crops grown through harvest, the newborn calves, the animals grazing, the loading of livestock for market—helps maintain interest in life. Creating or revitalizing a "living center" within the existing home environment can change a person's interest in life and emotional state, as well as influencing health outcomes. Having a table with necessary items within reach such as a portable phone, TV remote, phonebook, drink, and tin of favorite snacks can return "control" to a chair-bound person.[30]

Activities Away From Home

Access to Friends and Community

During the first year following his stroke Mr. W. was dependent upon his spouse, daughter, and friends for transportation. Because of their rural location, there were no services, such as a store, library, or post office he could walk to. Once he regained the ability to drive safely, he initially drove short distances on the quiet roads near their home, and then eventually was able to drive to visit his two out-of-state daughters. Because there is no local public transportation where they live, he might have been confined to the immediate area around his home during the year following the stroke, had he not had a transportation support system. Several of his close friends offered to pick him up for civic functions in the community, such as Lions Club. Mr. W. was able to engage his personal support system of friends and family by asking for a ride—a crucial step to maintain engagement. Mr. and Mrs. W. attended weekly church services, including their adult Sunday school class. This offered continuing social contact with long-term acquaintances.

Travel

They also took trips south to visit their two out-of-state children, driving 2 days to the first daughter's home, and staying several weeks, before driving another day to reach the second daughter's home. Each adult child had grab rails installed in bathrooms to provide a safe environment for their father while away from his home.

By checking with motels, the W.'s were able to have a fully accessible room available for overnight stays. This assured a ground-floor room and safe bathing environment for Mr. W. Their travels south during the winter also helped them escape the harsh cold and snowy conditions of their more northerly region that were a hazard to their mobility.

Physical Activity and Exercise

While many daily activities, such as chores, gardening, and shopping, help to maintain physical mobility and strength, it is important to assess physical activity as a separate domain, and work toward an optimal level for each individual. When considered separately, this domain can provide insight about a person's commitment to and capacity for remaining physically active.

Adaptive Equipment

Mr. W. was an active person with a lot of energy. He never stayed still unless he was watching TV, taking an afternoon nap, or enjoying his meal—however, he was not an avid exerciser. Following the stroke, he had some weakness in his lower right leg but was still able to walk with his quad cane. He tried "exercising" on a stationary bike, but his right foot kept slipping off, and he felt unstable. His daughter found a recumbent exercise bike that worked well for Mr. W. There was a strap for securing his feet, and he could easily get on and off. Positioning the bicycle so it had the full view of the pasture where his cattle grazed improved the motivation and pleasure for Mr. W. This exercise also strengthened his right leg, improved coordination, and he was again able to walk without the cane (Figure 16–7).

Accessible Environment

The external environment is an important setting for physical activity by many older adults, who may associate the outdoors with exercise. There is great variation in the type and extent

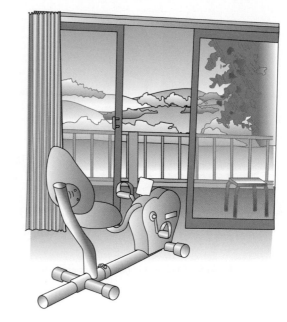

FIGURE 16–7. Recumbent exercise bike.

of outdoor space available; it may include the area around the home, the nearby walkable neighborhood, and workout stations or other amenities in the community. The quality, extent, and location of these environmental features have been found to substantially influence levels of outdoor activity. To fully support outdoor activities and avoid falls, these areas should ideally be reachable by smooth and level walking surfaces, and should provide comfortable, safe seating at frequent intervals.[12,36-38] However, Mr. W. lives on a farm. There are no sidewalks, and the walking trails are just the ones made by the cattle, very unsuitable for an older person with any mobility problems to navigate safely. So Mr. W. relies on a golf cart to check areas of the yard, drive to get the mail down the mile-long paved driveway, and to go to his daughter's home which is about a quarter of a mile through the woods, via a paved driveway. The home patio area is one step down from a large carport, used in the summer as a living area with a carpet and furniture. This step was not clearly visible and did not have a handrail. A small wooden ramp was added, with a handrail along one side, to make this transition safer (Figure 16–8). Good external lighting is available as an additional safety measure.

The Personal Living Profile provided adequate information about Mr. W. and his daily patterns for the health care provider to recommend changes that would contribute to improved functioning and provide a safe and supportive environment. For patients who provide minimal information on the Profile, or for patients who may not have identified all areas of concern, an additional tool may be useful as a summary for health care providers to fill in during the office visit to help ensure that the main dimensions of environmental support are taken into account for each daily behavior pattern. The Personal Environment Summary (Appendix 16–2) was developed as an additional tool for the health care provider to use after reviewing the PLP completed by the older adult or family member. Each cell in the PES would be used to note additional relevant data on which the health care team could act.

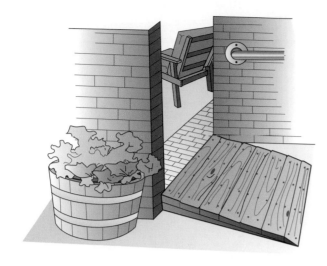

FIGURE 16–8. Addition of a ramp and handrail for easier transition.

CONCLUSION

The description of Mr. W.'s case illustrates the level of consideration needed for each dimension of an impaired person's daily living environment. Some modifications required merely adjusting tools like switching from a knife to scissors to gather vegetables. Some modifications were simple and required minimal resources such as the simple ramp, grab bars in the bath, and adding a shower wand and bath seat. Other modifications such as installing light switches or an attractive handrail at the stairs required a greater investment. Mr. W. represents those older adults who have sufficient resources to make the environmental changes that can allow him to continue living at home as long as possible. He also represents the group of older adults who are highly motivated, and have a spouse and strong ties with family and friends; these social resources help support important needs such as self-esteem, and his continued role of in the family as a provider, rather than being merely a receiver.

With the 65+ population having 44% of women widowed and living alone,[39] there are clearly issues that have not been addressed through this case study. Women living alone are more likely to have fewer resources than a woman whose spouse is still living in the later years. However, remaining in the community is often so important that even older adults with limited financial and social resources choose to stay in less-supportive environments, even when risks are clear. Particular attention is needed to link this population group with community resources.

Most communities have multiple resources that can offer information, and possibly support, to older adults in need. These include the local area agency on aging, state agencies such the Commission for the Blind or Disability Council, city home repair programs, AARP, Retired Senior Volunteer Program, state cooperative extension programs, civic and non-profit groups, and churches. Some of these agencies and organizations may have specific programs to assist in home modification or provide volunteer handyman services. In many regions, for example, the United Way produces a resource directory of available services and programs that can be useful to older adults. However, many older adults may not

even know that these resources are available, and because of decreased mobility are unlikely to find out about them. Thus, for an older person to remain living in his or her own home, it is important for the person's support and health care provider networks to find out what services are available, and help introduce the older person to these resources.[40,41] Helping older adults remain at home should make it possible to save significant amounts of money. For example, with a one-time investment of between $5000 and $50,000, one state projected annual cost savings of $44,896 per functionally impaired person that would otherwise have been spent on expenses related to nursing home care.[42]

Implementing many solutions for environmental support and safety does not need to be expensive. For example, one older single woman with type 2 diabetes was able to return to her ground-level apartment after a below-the-knee amputation required the use of a walker and sometimes a wheelchair. The apartment manager removed the carpet pad and put in low-pile carpeting to ease her mobility; she also added an inexpensive plug-in, motion-sensing night light in the hallway to improve safety. Because her family lived far away and because she met the economic and health guidelines for a community-based alternative program, a caseworker became involved in assisting her with the type of environmental supports needed to reduce her risk of moving to a more costly nursing home setting. Many states have implemented such programs to save state dollars by simple environmental modifications that allow people to stay at home.

As health care providers work with the rapidly increasing population of aging baby boomers, it is clearly important to open the conversation about supportive environments in later life as part of the routine annual checkup. Older adults can be resistant to environmental modifications, seeing these as a sign of infirmity. Addressing environmental concerns early, while an aging person's functionality is still relatively intact, may allow an older adult to make appropriate modifications in a timely manner, to avoid the potential tragedies caused by hazards in the home while allowing the person to continue living in his or her own home as long as possible. Introducing risk-reduction strategies related to the home environment will help boomers "age in place," whether in a long-term family home or a downsized home built to accommodate older adults in all phases of functionality.

References

1. Null RL, Cherry KE. *Universal Design: Creative Solutions for ADA Compliance.* Belmont, CA: Professional Publications; 1998.

2. 55+ Housing. Builders, Buyers, and Beyond. MetLife Mature Market Institute. September 2009. 42-page report available at MatureMarketInstitute@MetLife.com.

3. Clark PG. Values and voices in teaching gerontology and geriatrics—Case studies as stories. *Gerontologist.* 2002;42:297-303.

4. Centers for Disease Control and Prevention and the Merck Company Foundation. *The State of Aging and Health in America 2007.* Whitehouse Station, NJ: Merck Company Foundation; 2007.

5. He W, Sengupta M, Velkoff VA, DeBarrow KA. *65+ in the United States: U.S. Census Bureau Current Population Reports.* Washington, DC: US Government Printing Office; 2005, 23-209.

6. Prisuta R, Barrett L, Evans, E. Aging, Migration, and Local Communities: The Views of 60+ Residents and Community Leaders: An executive summary. *AARP*, 2006.

7. Brummett W. *The Essence of Home*. New York: Von Nostrand Reinhold; 1997:25-29.

8. Oswald F, Wahl H, Schilling O, et al. Relationships between housing and healthy aging in very old age. *Gerontologist*. 2007; 47:96-107.

9. Katz SJ, Ford AB, Moskowitz RW, et al. Studies of illness in the aged. The index of ADL: A standardized measure of biological and psychosocial function. *JAMA*. 1963;185:914-919.

10. Lawton MP, Brody EM. Assessment of older people: Self-maintaining and instrumental activities of daily living. *Gerontologist*. 1969;9: 179-186.

11. Wang Z, Shepley M. Site-level environmental support of active behavior and fall prevention for seniors. *Seniors Housing Care J*. 2008;16:97-121.

12. Wang Z, Rodiek S, Shepley M. Residential site environments and yard activities of older adults. *AIA 2006 Report on University Research*. American Institute of Architects; 2007:1-15.

13. Wahl H, Fange A, Oswald F, et al. The home environment and disability-related outcomes in aging individuals: What is the empirical evidence? *Gerontologist*. 2009;49:355-367.

14. Allen S, Resnick L, Roy J. Promoting independence for wheelchair users: The role of home accommodations. *Gerontologist*. 2006;45: 115-123.

15. Tinetti ME, Baker DI, Gottschalk M, et al. Effect of dissemination of evidence in reducing injuries from falls. *N Engl J Med*. 2008;359:252.

16. Kirby SD. A Housing Safety Checklist for Older People. http://www.ces.ncsu.edu/depts/fcs/pdfs/FCS-461.pdf.

17. Check for Safety: A Home Fall Prevention Checklist for Older Adults. http://www.cdc.gov/ncipc/pub-res/toolkit/Falls_ToolKit/DesktopPDF/English/booklet_Eng_desktop.pdf.

18. Home Safety for People with Alzheimer's Disease. http://www.nia.nih.gov/Alzheimers/Publications/homesafety.htm.

19. Safety at Home. Adapting the Home to Support the Person with Dementia. http://www.alz.org/national/documents/brochure_homesafety.pdf.

20. Cummings RG, Thomas M, Szonyi G, et al. Home visits by an occupational therapist for assessment and modification of environmental hazards: A randomized trial of falls prevention. *J Am Geriatr Soc*. 1999;47:1397-1402.

21. Liu S, Lapane K. Residential modifications and decline in physical function among community dwelling older adults. *Gerontologist*. 2009;49:344-354.

22. Gill TM, Williams CS, Robison JT, Tinetti ME. A population-based study of environmental hazards in the homes of older persons. *Am J Public Health*. 1999;89:553-556.

23. Yuen HK, Carter RE. A predictive model for the intention to implement home modifications: A pilot study. *J Appl Gerontol*. 2006;25: 3-16.

24. Gitlin LN, Winter L, Corcoran M, et al. Effects of the home environment skill-building program on the caregiver-care recipient dyad: 6-month outcomes from the Philadelphia REACH Initiative. *Gerontologist*. 2006;43:532-546.

25. Allen S, Resnik L, Roy J. Promoting independence for wheelchair users: The role of home accommodations, *Gerontologist*. 2006;46: 115-123.

26. Lawton MP. Environmental proactivity in older people. In: Bengtson VL, Schaie KW, eds. *The Course of Later Life*. New York: Springer; 1989:15-23.

27. Stearns S, Bernard SL, Fasick SB, et al. The economic implications of self-care: The effect of lifestyle, functional adaptations, and medical self-care among a national sample of Medicare beneficiaries. *Am J Public Health*. 2000;90:1608-1612.

28. Stineman MG, Ross RN, Maislin G, Gray D. Population-based study of home accessibility features and the activities of daily living: Clinical and policy implications. *Disabil Rehabil*. 2007;29: 1165-1175.

29. Oswald F, Wahl HW, Schiling O, et al. Relationships between housing and healthy aging in very old age. *Gerontologist*. 2007;47: 96-107.

30. Nygren C, Oswald F, Iwarsson S, et al. Relationships between objective and perceived housing in the very old age. *Gerontologist*. 2007;47:85-95.

31. Rowles GD, Chaudhury H, eds. *Home and Identity in Late Life*. New York: Springer; 2005.

32. Rowles GD. The surveillance zone as meaningful space for the aged. *Gerontologist*. 1981;21:304-311.

33. Rodiek S. A new tool for evaluating senior living environments. *Seniors Housing Care J*. 2008;16:3-9.

34. Gibson JJ. *The Ecological Approach to Visual Perception*. Boston: Houghton Mifflin; 1979.

35. Oswald F, Schilling O, Wahl HW, et al. Homeward bound: Introducing a four domain model of perceived housing in very old age. *J Environ Psychol*. 2006;26:187-201.

36. Rodiek S. *Access to Nature for Older Adults*. Three-part DVD series, 90-minute running time. College Station, TX: Center for Health Systems & Design; 2009. www.accesstonature.org.

37. Takano T, Nakamura K, Watanabe M. Urban residential environments and senior citizens' longevity in megacity areas: The importance of walkable green spaces. *J Epidemiol Community Health*. 2002;56:913-918.

38. Li W, Keegan THM, Sternfeld B, et al. Outdoor falls among middle-aged and older adults: A neglected public health problem. *Am J Public Health*. 2006;96:1192-1200.

39. US Census Bureau. http://www.census.gov/Press-Release/www/releases/archives/facts_for_features_special_editions/004210.html.

40. Pynoos J, Nishita CM. The cost and financing of home modifications in the United States. *J Disabil Policy Stud*. 2003;14: 68-73.

41. Andrus Gerontology Center. *The National Directory of Home Modification and Repair Resources*. Los Angeles: University of Southern California Andrus Gerontology Center. http://www.homemods.org/directory/index.shtml.

42. Naughton E. Fact Sheet—Home Modifications Revolving Fund for People with Disabilities and the Elderly. Rhode Island House Bill-H7629, 2008.

ACKNOWLEDGEMENTS

We would like to thank Dillon J. Phillips for the illustrations; Kristen Unteidt for original photography, and Drs. E. Berigan, W. Birdwell, and J. Shafer for their review of the chapter.

POST-TEST

1. **Which of the following statement does NOT correctly describe how the Personal Living Profile (PLP) should be used?**
   A. By surveying the home using the PFP when the owner is present
   B. By asking the owner and/or family members to fill out the PLP in advance of the office visit
   C. By mailing the PLP to be filled out by the owner after the office visit
   D. By identifying areas on the PLP for which environmental modifications are indicated

2. **Which statement best describes why it is important to consider individual preferences and patterns of behavior when considering possible home modifications?**
   A. Because socioeconomic conditions may determine what can be accomplished in the home
   B. Because each individual has specific needs that influence adaptation and usage of environmental features
   C. Because most people are eager to change their home environment when they realize it will allow them to age in place
   D. Because individual preferences and patterns of behavior determine level of care need

3. **Which inexpensive home modification tends NOT to increase levels of safety in the home?**
   A. Remove or secure loose throw rugs.
   B. Reframe doorway to accommodate wheelchair.
   C. Tie up or tape down electric cords.
   D. Install plug-in motion-sensing hallway night lights.

4. **Which of the following is NOT a primary domain of daily activity on the PLP?**
   A. Bathing, grooming, and dressing
   B. Utilitarian chores and tasks
   C. Mobility and connectedness
   D. Cooking, eating, supplements, and medications

5. **All of the following rank in the most prevalent home environment hazard(s) in older adults' homes EXCEPT:**
   A. Lack of grab bars
   B. Loose throw rugs
   C. Lack of no-slip tub mats
   D. Trip hazards such as unsecured electrical cords

ANSWERS TO PRE-TEST

1. A
2. B
3. C
4. B

ANSWERS TO POST-TEST

1. C
2. B
3. B
4. C
5. C

17

Family Caregiving

Deborah C. Messecar, PhD, MPH, RN, GCNS-BC

Carol Parker Walsh, JD, PhD

Allison Lindauer, RN, FNP

● **LEARNING OBJECTIVES**

1. Identify the key family caregiver characteristics that are associated with a high risk for strain, depression, and poor health in the caregiver.
2. Discuss components of a thorough assessment of the family caregiving situation.
3. Describe strategies for crafting interventions to support family caregivers of older adults.
4. Identify risk factors for elder mistreatment in a family caregiving situation.
5. Explain the screening process for elder abuse and neglect.

PRE-TEST

1. **Family caregiving can have a negative impact on a person's:**
   A. Physical and mental health
   B. Credit rating
   C. Ability to get life insurance
   D. Ability to manage stress

2. **Risk factors for increased feelings of strain or depression include all of the following EXCEPT:**
   A. Being female
   B. Being African American
   C. Reporting a poor relationship quality with the care receiver
   D. Not feeling prepared for the caregiver role

3. **Which characteristic of the *care recipient* is associated with higher risk for elder mistreatment?**
   A. Exhibits problematic behaviors
   B. Is financially secure
   C. Lives alone
   D. Has friends/ family near

CASE PRESENTATION 1: THE CAREGIVING PATIENT

Vernon is a 75-year-old African American, non–insulin-dependent diabetic with serious problems with hypertension who comes to your office for a repeat visit. His blood pressure has always been poorly controlled, but today he has called in and asked for a visit because he is often dizzy at home. The dizziness worries him because it affects his ability to care for his wife. She has had a stroke and is completely aphasic and bedridden. She requires total personal care and management of her feeding tube. They live in a modest house in a poorer part of the city. He has a daughter who lives in the city, but she works two jobs to support her family and has a hard time getting over to the house to give Vernon relief. When the visiting nurse makes visits to see his wife, her bed is always immaculately made, she is very well cared for and clean, and her skin is perfect without any breaks or tears. Vernon works many hours per week to ensure that all her needs are met. He tells the visiting nurse that he enjoys caring for his wife and takes pride in her well-being. Today, Vernon wants you to "fix him up" so he can get back home as soon as possible.

CASE PRESENTATION 2: A RELUCTANT CAREGIVER

Michelle Jones is the youngest of four children and the only one who still lives in the same city as her widowed father. She describes her relationship as very paternalistic without much love, only discipline. Her father, who recently suffered a stroke and is considered marginal for staying home by his provider, is expecting that Michelle will "move in and take care of me." He is being discharged today from the hospital. Michelle says she would feel awkward having to bathe and take care of her dad, and in addition she feels her relationship with him is so distant that she doesn't understand why she should have to be the caregiver at this time when she has her own problems to deal with. Adding to her difficulties, Michelle has three children of her own (ages 5, 7, and 16) who need her during the day and night.

● FAMILY CAREGIVING

For many older adults, being dependent on others for meeting daily needs due to functional impairments or chronic illness is a daily reality. Family caregivers provide a wide range of unpaid care to their chronically ill or functionally impaired older family members, partners, friends, or neighbors that exceed the support usually provided in family relationships.[1] The key difference between usual family care activities (such as preparing meals for a spouse) versus caregiving activities (such as bathing or dressing someone) is exceeding the bounds of what is normative or usual. Family caregiving has been formally defined as providing a broad range of unpaid care provided in response to illness or functional impairment for a chronically ill, disabled older adult family member or friend during any given year that exceeds the support usually provided in family relationships.[1-4]

Health care providers who focus only on family caregiving associated with the performance of tasks may fail to assess the full scope of the family caregiving role.[5,6] Family care activities include assistance with day-to-day activities such as bathing or feeding, illness-related care like administering medications and treatments, care management activities like arranging appointments, but also invisible aspects of care such as monitoring safety unobtrusively. Table 17–1 lists some examples of caregiving activities. As a rule, primary caregivers provide most of the everyday aspects of care (like Vernon), whereas secondary caregivers help out as needed to fill the gaps.[11-15] However, the range of the family caregiving role assumed and the intensity of care can vary widely from a very limited involvement such as protective caregiving by "keeping an eye on" an older adult who is currently independent but at risk, to full-time, around-the-clock care for a severely impaired family member. Depending on one's circumstances, caregiving can be potentially difficult, time-consuming work added on top of job and other family responsibilities (as Michelle fears) and making performance of these roles difficult.[2,16,17]

● TABLE 17–1 Examples of Caregiving Activities	
Day-to-day activities	Personal-care activities
	• Bathing
	• Eating
	• Dressing
	• Mobility
	• Transferring from bed to chair
	• Using the toilet
	IADLs
	• Meal preparation
	• Grocery shopping
	• Making telephone calls
	• Money management[2,7]
Illness-related activities	• Managing symptoms
	• Coping with illness behaviors
	• Carrying out treatments
	• Performing medical or nursing procedures that include an array of medical technologies[8]
Care management	• Accessing resources
	• Communicating with and navigating the health care and social services systems
	• Acting as an advocate[9]
Invisible aspects of care	• Protective actions caregivers take to ensure the older adults' safety and well-being without their knowledge[10]

Who provides family care? Currently, about 22.4 million households provide care for an older adult family member or friend.[18] Most caregivers are women, providing care to other women, but this demographic is changing as more men assume the caregiving role.[2,3] A broad range of family and informal caregivers provide care to older adults; many have their own unique challenges in delivering this care. Responses to caregiving and the types of care typically provided vary by gender, relationship to the care recipient, and ethnicity. For example, male caregivers differ from their female counterparts in that they are more likely to care for a male care recipient, to be working full time, and they on average provide fewer hours of care at a lower level of care,[2] while women, as in Michelle's case, are also more likely than men to say that they feel they did not have a choice in taking on this role (42% vs. 34%)[2]. Caregiving outcomes also differ between spouse caregivers who tend to be older and more frail, and non-spouse caregivers who are mostly adult children with other family responsibilities[19] like Michelle. For example, spousal caregivers have reported higher levels of depression than non-spouses.[20] The sandwich generation (a term coined by Miller in 1981[21] to describe adult caregivers caught in the simultaneous bind of providing care for their minor children and their aging parents) find themselves very stressed juggling the demands of work with multiple family responsibilities.[22] Trends indicate that many more women will occupy the parent-care role and thus become "women in the middle"[23] in the future.[13] Rates of caregiving also vary by ethnic group.[24] A notable trend among these caregivers, which Vernon exemplifies, is that ethnic minority caregivers provide more care[25,26] and report worse physical health than white caregivers.[26,27] Although caregivers are often talked about as if they were a single group, they actually differ considerably from one another in several important ways. Caregivers may not be fully aware of the many contextual circumstances that shape their caregiving experiences, but remember that you as the clinician can use this information to focus your assessment and intervention.

OUTCOMES OF CAREGIVING

Caregiver Burden, Stress, and Strain

Feeling burdened, distressed, or strained by the demands of caregiving is the most frequently reported outcome associated with caregiving, although this response is by no means universal. Each definition of caregiver burden, stress, and strain gives the clinician important clues about how individual responses to caregiving may vary even though the objective caregiving situation may seem to warrant a different response. For example, caregiver burden is defined as both the tangible, observable disruptions caused by caregiving such as demands on time, effort, and money and the less perceptible internal experience of negative feelings associated with caregiving.[28] Vernon actually does not report any burden caring for his wife, in spite of her heavy care needs, while Michelle is already anticipating a great deal of concern about becoming the primary caregiver for her father even though his needs are less than those of Vernon's wife. Caregiver stress is an internal response process caused by certain predisposing characteristics and resources of the caregiver and their primary stressors such as hardships and problems anchored in caregiving in combination with the secondary stressors to which they are exposed.[29] Michelle's complicated past history with her father probably makes it more likely that Michelle will experience a certain amount of intra-psychic stress if she has to assume his care. Caregiver strain has been defined as the felt difficulty in performing the caregiver role.[30,31] Vernon sees his caregiver role as a natural extension of his spouse and filial obligations, and he does not have the competing demands of employment and other family roles, while Michelle has many competing demands on her time with young children.

Given these nuanced definitions, it is easy to see why burden, stress, and or strain typically vary among different types of caregivers. While their objective situations may seem similar, often the appraisals or meanings that caregivers give to these stressors profoundly influence how much burden, stress, or strain they actually experience. Gender, familial relationships, co-residence, income, and ethnicity have all been associated with different levels of reported burden.[26,27,32-34] Several studies of ethnic minority caregivers in particular illustrate how, though their caregiving experiences objectively seem more difficult, their experience of burden and strain is less than for comparably stressed white caregivers. For example, in several studies African American caregivers reported experiencing less stress and depression and got more rewards from caregiving than their white caregiver counterparts.[26,27,32,33] Compared to white caregivers, non-white caregivers (1) were less likely to be a spouse and more likely to be an adult child, friend, or other family member; (2) reported lower levels of caregiver stress, burden, and depression; (3) endorsed more strongly held beliefs about filial support; and (4) were more likely to use prayer, faith, or religion as coping mechanisms.[35] Ethnic minority caregivers provide more care, use fewer formal services than white caregivers, and report worse physical health than white caregivers.[25-27]

Burden, stress, and strain are important to assess because research indicates that these outcomes lead to many other negative consequences for both the caregiver and the older adult.[34,36,37] Indeed, caregiving involves exposure to a long-term chronic stressor that produces disruption in family routines, psychological distress, psychological and physical morbidity, financial hardship, and work-related problems. The stress from this experience can be manifested through both physical and psychological illness in the caregivers.

Poor Health

Just being a caregiver puts an individual at increased risk for higher levels of stress and depression and lower levels of subjective well-being and physical health. Psychiatric health effects such as anxiety and depression are common, especially with dementia caregiving. Spouse caregivers who provide heavy care (36 or more hours per week) are six times more likely than non-caregivers to experience symptoms of depression or anxiety; for child caregivers the rate is twice as high.[38] Female caregivers, on average, provide more direct care and report higher levels of depression.[33] Spouse caregivers report higher levels of depression than non-spouse caregivers.[20,38] Hispanic and Asian American caregivers also report more depression.[20,26] However, several studies found that African American caregivers experience more satisfaction and less depression and get more rewards from caregiving than their white caregiver counterparts.[26,27,32,33] Less-educated caregivers also report more depression.[32,39]

In addition to mental health morbidity, family caregivers also experience physical health deterioration. Family caregivers have chronic conditions at more than twice the rate of non-caregivers.[2,4] Caregiving-related stress in chronically ill spouses is associated with a 63% higher mortality rate than non-caregiving peers.[40] Stress from caring for an elder with dementia has been shown to impact the caregiver's immune system for up to 3 years after caregiving ends.[41] Family caregivers experiencing extreme stress have also been shown to age prematurely. It is estimated that this stress can take as much as 10 years off a caregiver's life.[42] Ethnic minority caregivers provide more care, use fewer formal services, and report worse physical health than white caregivers.[25,26,42] A quantitative review by Vitaliano and colleagues[6] of 23 studies from North America, Europe, and Australia examined relationships of caregiving with several health outcomes. They consistently found across many studies that caregivers are at greater risk for health problems than are non-caregivers.

Rewards of Caregiving

Although early family caregiving research focused almost exclusively on negative outcomes of caregiving, clearly there are many positive aspects of providing care. Spouses can be drawn closer together by caregiving, which can act as an expression of love. Child caregivers can feel a sense of accomplishment from helping their adult parents. Caregivers often enumerate many perceived benefits of caregiving.[43-48] These can include the satisfaction of helping a family member, developing new skills and competencies, and improved family relationships. Clinicians may not be aware of the positive perspective on caregiving and focus on coping skills and stress management rather than facilitating the positive psychological factors. There are two very important reasons for exploring positive aspects of caregiving with the caregiver: caregivers want to talk about them, and these factors will be an important indicator of the quality of care provided to the care recipient. Clinicians need to encourage an increase in positive affect (ie, feelings such as gratitude, forgiveness, and the like) while at the same time working on decreasing negative feelings like depression, anxiety and guilt.

Clearly the relationship between caregiver load and burden, stress and strain, and health outcomes is complex and dynamic. As a child caregiver, Michelle is at higher risk for depression or anxiety, while Vernon is suffering from a number of chronic illnesses that may be exacerbated by the care he provides for his wife. The goal of interventions with caregivers will be to identify and address aspects of the caregiving situation amenable to modification. The possible targets for intervention will vary from one caregiver to another. Addressing aspects of caregiving that are strong predictors of burden, stress, and strain can help the clinician tailor his or her caregiver interventions.

● PREDICTORS OF INCREASED CAREGIVER BURDEN, STRESS, AND STRAIN

Lack of Preparedness

Given the complexity of the caregiving role, it is not surprising that most caregivers are ill prepared for the many responsibilities they face. Caregivers generally receive no formal instruction in their caregiving activities[2] and report that they are somewhat or not at all prepared for a variety of complex caregiving tasks such as managing medications, handling health insurance matters, or communicating with providers.[2,3] Stewart and colleagues reported that although health care professionals were a caregiver's main source of information on providing physical care, caregivers reported receiving no preparation on how to care for the patient emotionally or deal with the stresses of caregiving.[49] Lack of preparedness can greatly increase the caregiver's perceptions of strain, especially during times of transition from hospital to home,[30,31,43] and put caregivers at increased risk for mood disturbance outcomes.[50]

Caregivers may be reluctant to raise concerns about their lack of preparedness to the health care provider. They may connect lack of preparedness with being embarrassed about their own lack of understanding of the care recipient's condition, or they may simply not know what it is they don't know. For example, in Michelle's case, she may not realize that formal resources could be tapped to provide some of the personal care that she would be too embarrassed to perform. Vernon, while a very experienced caregiver, might be reluctant to admit there are aspects of his wife's care he is having difficulty with because this could raise concerns about his ability to provide care. Asking about preparedness, rather than waiting for caregivers to raise concerns, opens the door for the clinician to provide education, suggest new strategies, and refer resources to make caregiving easier. It also cues the caregiver to see the clinician as a resource and a partner in the provision of care for the older adult.

Poor Family Relationship Quality

One of the key differences between Vernon and Michelle's caregiving situations is the quality of the relationship between them and their actual or potential care receivers. A lack of mutuality (the positive quality of the relationship between caregiver and care recipient) is very predictive of future and sustained reported difficulty with caregiving.[51,52] Michelle has a distant relationship with her father now, and a history of a poor-quality relationship from childhood. This puts her at risk for experiencing more strain from caregiving than Vernon, who historically had a very high-quality relationship with his wife. This is true even though objectively, just looking at caregiving demands, Vernon's situation is far more difficult. That is because a poor quality of relationship can make caregiving seem more difficult even in situations where the objective caregiving situation (eg, hours devoted to caregiving, number of tasks performed) may seem less demanding.[30,31] Also, trouble in the caregiver–care recipient relationship causes more persistent problems. While the deleterious effects of lack of preparedness on caregivers in one study faded after 9 months, a poor relationship with the care receiver remained strongly related to the caregiver experience of strain.[30,31]

The link between objective caregiving demands (such as tasks), and a lack of mutuality and strain, is complex. Caregiving demand needs to be further contextualized by the amount of reported caregiving difficulty.[50,53] For example, objective demands may be low, but the caregiver's perceived difficulty with the demands can be high (Michelle and bathing her father). So it is important not just to ask what the caregiver is doing, but how much it bothers him or her to perform that task if at all, especially in situations where the relationship quality is already poor. At first glance, asking about the quality of the caregiver–care recipient relationship may not seem to be pertinent, and not nearly as important as verifying that the caregiver has key knowledge and understanding to perform delegated medical caregiving tasks. Many clinicians may also assume that there is nothing that can be done about a poor-quality relationship and hence are reluctant to broach the topic. However, it is important to realize how this background issue might complicate care and compromise its quality. Plus, ignoring these issues puts caregivers at risk. Troubled family relationships are linked with poor mental health outcomes for caregivers[54,55] and caregiver anger[50] (probably an underlying issue for Michelle). Structured questions to help the clinician explore with the caregiver his or her preparedness, mutuality, and strain will be presented as part of a systematic caregiver assessment.

Vernon's case study will be used to illustrate how the clinician can assess the caregiving situation, and use this targeted assessment to intervene. In Vernon's case, the caregiver is the patient being seen in the clinic. Assessment will include determining the magnitude of the negative consequences the caregiver may be experiencing and identifying aspects of the caregiving situation that may be amenable to intervention. Several assessment tools are introduced, as well as guidelines for selecting possible interventions. For some of these key areas, data about Michelle's case will be presented to contrast how her situation is so different from Vernon's. The assessment and intervention guidelines will then be applied primarily to Vernon's case, with only some areas including examples from Michelle's case.

• STRATEGIES FOR ASSESSMENT AND INTERVENTION

Caregiver Assessment

Assessing the caregiver involves asking about the caregiving context, the physical and mental health of both the caregiver and the care receiver, the caregiver's preparedness for providing care, and the quality of the relationship between the caregiver and the care receiver. Assessment focus may differ with caregiver experience, care setting and focus, persons involved in the care, and the acuity of the patient. The evaluation starts with an understanding that each caregiving situation is unique, and that some caregivers will be at more risk than others. Risk factors for poor caregiving outcomes identified in the evaluation should then be addressed in partnership with the caregiver.

Caregiving Context

Table 17–2 shows examples of questions that can be asked when taking a caregiver history, which can be very important in determining whether or not the caregiver has the basic resources and experience to provide care and identify some areas that could put the caregiver at risk for poor outcomes. Vernon is a spouse caregiver of an older adult with dementia and is therefore more at risk for depression and for problems with poor health. Caregivers who are spouses often have different issues with caregiving than do sons and daughters.[33,56] The duration of caregiving can give the clinician clues about whether or not the caregiver is new to the role and may be unprepared.[56] Vernon has been a caregiver for over 5 years and is very confident of his ability to provide care. However, he has been ignoring his own health for a very long period of time. Vernon is not employed, he is retired, but his social world has become very constricted with immediate family being his only social support. Vernon lives with his wife, but has no other family members close by to help. As a general

TABLE 17–2	Assessment of Caregiving Questions and Rationale
Risk Factor	**Assessment Questions**
Caregiving context	1. What is the caregiver's relationship to the care receiver—spouse, child, some other relationship?
	2. How long has the caregiver been caregiving?
	3. Is the caregiver employed?
	4. How many people live with the care receiver? Does the caregiver live with the care receiver?
	5. What is the home like? Are there many stairs? Is the bathroom accessible and safe? How difficult is it to get in and out of the home (for example, do the entry stairs have a railing, is the driveway steep?).
	6. Are financial resources adequate? Do the caregiver and care receiver have enough money to meet their needs?[6] Is the caregiver aware of resources he or she can use?
	7. What is the family's cultural background?
Caregiver's report of health and functional status of care recipient	1. Ask the caregiver to list the activities the care receiver needs help with, include both Activities of Daily Living (ADLs) and Instrumental Activities of Daily Living (IADLs).
	2. Does the care receiver have any cognitive impairment? If the answer is yes, ask if there any behavioral problems.
	3. Are there any mobility problems?
Caregiver preparedness for caregiving	Does the caregiver have the skills, abilities, and knowledge to provide the care receiver with the care that is needed? Use questions from the Preparedness for Caregiving Scale (Figure 17–1).
Quality of family relationships	Ask about the caregiver's perception of the quality of the relationship with the care receiver. Use questions from the Mutuality Scale (Figure 17–2).
Caregiver's physical and mental health status	1. How does the caregiver rate his or her health? Follow up with inquiries about the caregiver's various health conditions and symptoms.
	2. Is the caregiver depressed?
	3. Is the caregiver burdened, stressed, or strained by his or her caregiving responsibilities? Use the Caregiver Strain Index (CSI; Figure 17–3).

rule, in caregivers who live with the care receiver, stress is increased.[57] Vernon lives in a one-level, older home in a poorer part of the city. The home is over 60 years old. The interior is cramped but Vernon is making good use of the small home by putting his wife's hospital bed in the living room, which is the largest room in the house. Since she is entirely bedridden, the lack of accessibility of the bathroom is not as much of a problem. Vernon manages her elimination with adult diapers, which he changes. Vernon and his wife have enough money to meet their needs. As is typical for many African American families, they do not use very many formal services[26,27,58]—the only community service they are currently using is a home health nurse. Vernon reports very little to no strain from his caregiving. He views his caregiving as important and takes pride in his ability to provide care. So far the history indicates that Vernon, though his caregiving demands are high, has many strengths that he can draw upon in his caregiving.

Michelle has not yet taken on the caregiving role, but there are a couple of concerns that the context questions highlight. First, she will be a new caregiver; she has not taken on this responsibility before. Second, though not employed, she is a full-time mother of young children. Third, her father and/or his provider are suggesting that he needs a live-in caregiver, and she is not in a position to leave her own home to do this. Other questions need to be assessed about the care recipient's home (how disability-friendly is the home—is it even feasible for the care recipient to return to this home to live?), his financial resources (are there funds or resources that could be tapped to pay for some services, modify the existing home, or move to a new living situation?), and the cultural expectations that may be guiding Michelle's and her father's responses (feelings about filial obligation). The physical environment can create a situation where the care receiver is more dependent than they need be if accessibility is an issue.[6] Developing a list of resources is critical, as many caregivers may be unaware of resources in the community that they can use.[57] Different cultural groups have different risks and strengths with caregiving. Based on what is known from the literature, Michelle is probably less resilient to role strain and burden from caregiving than caregivers from other cultural groups.[27]

Caregiver's Report of Health and Functional Status of Care Recipient

This section of the caregiver assessment in Table 17–2 begins with outlining the caregiving demands. Even if the care receiver needs help with a given task, the caregiver may or may not be doing the activity for the caregiver; the task might be delegated, the care receiver may use equipment to get the task done, or the care receiver might hire assistance. The number of tasks that the care receiver needs help with indicates the level of functional impairment of the care receiver and the objective burden the caregiver must manage.[5,57] Vernon is providing total care—his wife cannot do any activities of daily living, nor can she manage instrumental activities of daily living. This means he is bathing, toileting, and feeding his wife, as well as being responsible for all of her instrumental needs—such as managing

finances, arranging transportation, and interacting with health providers on her behalf.

After making notes about what care is required, it is also helpful to ask about any cognitive impairment or mobility problems. Behavioral problems are particularly stressful for caregivers and can be very difficult to manage.[33,56] Vernon's wife is demented, is no longer able to speak, and is bedridden—so behavioral problems are not an issue. Vernon has to provide all of her care in the bed. She is bathed in bed by the home health aide a couple of times per week, and Vernon manages any spot bathing that is necessary between these visits. She does not get out of bed, so transfers are rare—but she must be turned and positioned frequently. The visiting nurse reports that her skin is intact and healthy.

Michelle currently is not providing any care, but depending on her father's cognitive and mobility status, his needs could be substantial. Mobility problems can create a host of difficulties with many activities of daily living and make caregiving more difficult.[30] This is a serious red flag indicating a need for more questioning and planning before Michelle assumes any caregiving responsibilities.

Caregiver Preparedness for Caregiving

Preparedness can be explored relatively easily by using the questions from the Preparedness for Caregiving Scale (Figure 17–1).[30,59-61] The scale poses eight questions that ask caregivers to rate how well prepared they think they are for caregiving. Some examples of the questions posed include: How well prepared do you think you are to take care of your family member's emotional needs? How well prepared do you think you are to get the help and information you need from the health care system? The clinician can interview the caregiver or ask the caregiver to complete the scale like a survey. The responses to the scale items can also be tallied and averaged for an overall score. If pressed for time, the clinician can simply ask overall, how well prepared the caregiver thinks he or she is to care for the family member, and then follow this with more specific questions if the response indicates preparedness is low. In Vernon's case, the items from the scale that he identifies as needing more help with including setting up services, handling emergencies, and getting help or information with the health care system.

In contrast, Michelle has answered that she is not at all prepared to take care of her father on any of the items listed on the preparedness scale. Michelle's case illustrates why this key component of the caregiving situation is so important to assess, instead of just assuming that the family can manage. Results like this indicate that perhaps an alternative living or care situation should be actively pursued for her father.

This is the area where the clinician can be so helpful in outlining a plan to either help the caregiver build his or her skills, or to identify situations that may call for an emergency social work referral to explore alternative living arrangements.

Quality of Family Relationships

To assess the quality of the family relationship you can use questions from the Mutuality Scale (Figure 17–2).[30] There are 15 questions that ask about the relationship between

---

YOUR PREPARATION FOR CAREGIVING

We know that people may feel well prepared for some aspects of giving care to another person, and not as well prepared for other aspects. We would like to know how well prepared you think you are to do each of the following, even if you are not doing that type of care now.

	Not at all prepared	Not too well prepared	Somewhat well prepared	Pretty well prepared	Very well prepared
1. How well prepared do you think you are to take care of your family member's physical needs?...	0	1	2	3	4
2. How well prepared do you think you are to take care of his or her emotional needs?..	0	1	2	3	4
3. How well prepared do you think you are to find out about and set up services for him or her?..	0	1	2	3	4
4. How well prepared do you think you are for the stress of caregiving?	0	1	2	3	4
5. How well prepared do you think you are to make caregiving activities pleasant for both you and your family member?............	0	1	2	3	4
6. How well prepared do you think you are to respond to and handle emergencies that involve him or her?	0	1	2	3	4
7. How well prepared do you think you are to get the help and information you need from the health care system?....................	0	1	2	3	4
8. Overall, how well prepared do you think you are to care for your family member?...	0	1	2	3	4

9. Is there anything specific you would like to be better prepared for? _____

_____

_____

_____

FIGURE 17–1. Preparedness for Caregiving Scale.

the caregiver and care receiver. Questions include: How close do you feel to him or her? How much does he or she express feelings of appreciation for you and the things you do? An overall score can be obtained by calculating the mean across all items, or the questions can be used in an open-ended interview format where the clinician then probes for more information and history about the relationship. This scale can also be completed via self-administration and then reviewed by the clinician with the caregiver (interview the caregiver apart from the care receiver). For this scale, there is not one item that asks about the relationship overall; instead, the items explore several key features of the relationship such as conflict, shared positive past memories, felt positive regard, and positive reciprocity between the caregiver and care receiver. The questions open the door for the clinician to probe in a gentle way the quality of the relationship. It also makes it okay for the caregiver then to raise

concerns about this sensitive, stress-producing aspect of caregiving and see the clinician as a support and partner for dealing with these issues.

Vernon had a hard time with about half of the questions on the Mutuality Scale, which assume that the care receiver is still able to talk and communicate. He answered them as he would have had his wife still been able to talk, as he felt that more accurately reflected the positive feelings he still held for her based on their history. What this means for the clinician is that Vernon's relationship with his wife is strongly positive, and will be a strength that Vernon can bring to the caregiving challenges ahead. In contrast, Michelle has responded negatively to all 15 items, indicating that there are serious relationship problems that could interfere with her safely assuming the caregiving role. If she does assume the role, the clinician should suggest several strategies that might help her with these feelings. One, a support group for caregivers could

YOU AND YOUR FAMILY MEMBER

Now we would like you to let us know how you and your family member feel about each other at the current time.

	Not at all	A little	Some	Quite a bit	A great deal
1. To what extent do the two of you see eye to eye (agree on things)?	0	1	2	3	4
2. How close do you feel to him or her?	0	1	2	3	4
3. How much do you enjoy sharing past experiences with him or her?	0	1	2	3	4
4. How much does he or she express feelings of appreciation for you and the things you do?	0	1	2	3	4
5. How attached are you to him or her?	0	1	2	3	4
6. How much does he or she help you?	0	1	2	3	4
7. How much do you like to sit and talk with him or her?	0	1	2	3	4
8. How much love do you feel for him or her?	0	1	2	3	4
9. To what extent do the two of you share the same values?	0	1	2	3	4
10. When you really need it, how much does he or she comfort you?	0	1	2	3	4
11. How much do the two of you laugh together?	0	1	2	3	4
12. How much do you confide in him or her?	0	1	2	3	4
13. How much emotional support does he or she give you?	0	1	2	3	4
14. To what extent do you enjoy the time the two of you spend together?	0	1	2	3	4
15. How often does he or she express feelings of warmth toward you?	0	1	2	3	4

FIGURE 17–2. Mutuality Scale.

give Michelle the opportunity to seek help from other caregivers in similar difficult situations. Counseling for Michelle might also be indicated—not because her responses to caregiving are abnormal, but to work through how she might decrease the intra-psychic stress she will experience from performing a difficult role. Plus the counselor could help Michelle set boundaries for what she will and will not do for her father—something that is difficult for most people to do on their own.

Caregiver's Physical and Mental Health Status

Assessment of the caregiver's physical and mental health status can be done with a single question that asks about the caregiver's perception of his or her health.[57] This should then be followed up with inquiries about various health conditions and symptoms.[57] Vernon acknowledges that his health is poor now, forcing him to come in for help. Vernon's complaints of dizziness need to be followed up on as well as the status of his diabetes. Any recommendations regarding changes in his treatment need to fit in with the restrictions in time and energy created by the heavy caregiving demands he must meet.

Ask caregivers if they think they are depressed. If they answer yes, screen further by using a depression instrument like the Center for Epidemiological Studies-Depression Scale (CES-D).[5,56,57] The CES-D is a good screening tool to use, as it has been used widely in intervention studies with a broad range of family caregivers. For each of the 20 items, participants rate its frequency of occurrence during the past week on a 1 point scale from 0 (rarely) to 3 (most of the time). Scores range from 0 to 60, with a higher score indicating the presence of a greater number and frequency of depressive symptoms. A score of 16 or higher has been identified as discriminatory between groups with clinically relevant and nonrelevant depressive symptoms.[62,63] Vernon says he is not depressed, he just doesn't feel that well because of the dizziness and tiredness, so in this instance the scale was not administered. Michelle denies any problems with either her physical or mental health.

Burden or strain can be assessed using the Caregiver Strain Index (CSI; Figure 17–3).[64,65] The CSI is a tool that can be used to quickly identify families with potential caregiving concerns. The tool can be easily completed by the caregiver via paper and pencil and then later reviewed, or can serve as an interview guide during the visit (again, interview the caregiver apart from the care receiver). Positive responses to 7 or more items on the index indicate a greater level of strain. In particular, a response of yes to "I feel completely overwhelmed" requires immediate follow-up by the clinician. Vernon's score of 2 on the CSI instrument is low. He answered affirmatively to only 2 items, that caregiving is sometimes a physical strain, and that it is somewhat confining. In contrast, Michelle has indicated that even as she anticipates the idea of caring for her father, she can identify a number of issues that are likely to cause her distress. This was apparent when the clinician interviewed her about taking her father home, and on the CSI, Michelle has scored 16. Michelle probably should not

Modified Caregiver Strain Index

Directions: Here is a list of things that other caregivers have found to be difficult. Please put a checkmark in the columns that apply to you. We have included some examples that are common caregiver experiences to help you think about each item. Your situation may be slightly different, but the item could still apply.

	Yes, On a Regular Basis = 2	Yes, Sometimes = 1	No = 0
My sleep is disturbed (For example: the person I care for is in and out of bed or wanders around at night)			
Caregiving is inconvenient (For example: helping takes so much time or it's a long drive over to help)			
Caregiving is a physical strain (For example: lifting in or out of a chair; effort or concentration is required)			
Caregiving is confining (For example: helping restricts free time or I cannot go visiting)			
There have been family adjustments (For example: helping has disrupted my routine; there is no privacy)			
There have been changes in personal plans (For example: I had to turn down a job; I could not go on vacation)			
There have been other demands on my time (For example: other family members need me)			
There have been emotional adjustments (For example: severe arguments about caregiving)			
Some behavior is upsetting (For example: incontinence; the person cared for has trouble remembering things; or the person I care for accuses people of taking things)			
It is upsetting to find the person I care for has changed so much from his/her former self (For example: he/she is a different person than he/she used to be)			
There have been work adjustments (For example: I have to take time off for caregiving duties)			
Caregiving is a financial strain			
I feel completely overwhelmed (For example: I worry about the person I care for: I have concerns about how I will manage)			

[Sum responses for "Yes, on a regular basis" (2 pts each) and "Yes, sometimes" (1 pt each)]

Total Score =

FIGURE 17–3. Caregiver Strain Index. Thornton M, & Travis SS. (2003). Analysis of the reliability of the Modified Caregiver Strain Index. *The Journal of Gerontology, Series B. Psychological Sciences and Social Sciences, 58(2), p. S129.* Copyright © The Gerontological Society of America. Reproduced by permission of the publisher.

become her father's primary caregiver unless she can receive adequate formal home services and counseling support from a medical social worker or other mental health professional.

Intervention

Studies of caregiver interventions, such as support groups, individual counseling, and education, confirm that there is no single, easily implemented, and consistently effective method for eliminating the stresses and or strain of being a caregiver.[56,57,66-68] However, that does not mean that interventions that use multiple strategies,[56,57,69] build caregiver skills,[56] and are tailored are most effective. Multicomponent interventions include a repertoire of various strategies that target different aspects of the caregiving experience. Tailored interventions are interventions that are crafted to match a specific target population, such as spouse caregivers of Alzheimer patients, and their specific caregiving issues and concerns identified through thorough assessment.[43,70] Collaboration or a partnership with the caregiver is also a key component of making the tailoring process more effective.[71] Suggested strategies for intervening are provided next.

Identify Skills Needed to Increase Preparedness

Some examples of the skills a caregiver may need to increase preparedness for the caregiving role include dealing with change, juggling competing responsibilities and stressors, providing and managing care, finding and using resources, and managing the physical and emotional responses to care. Michelle in particular is going to require some thoughtful help with deciding if it will be possible for her to help her father return to his home. This is probably a situation where a case manager or social worker should get involved to help Michelle sort out what she can and cannot do, and whether or not other resources or strategies can be used to supplement her limited availability. Skill-building interventions that include information about the care needed by the care receiver and how to provide it, as well as coaching on how to manage the caregiving role, are most effective.[33,56,72-74] In Vernon's case, we can take a look at the areas that he has identified as needing some additional skill preparation from the Preparedness Scale. But before designing any interventions, building rapport and mutual goal-setting will be needed.

Partner with the Caregiver

Prior to generating strategies to address the caregiver's issues and concerns, seek to understand what knowledge the caregiver already brings to the situation. Every family situation will be different, and interventions cannot be individualized without purposely collaborating with the caregiver.[31,58,71,75] The collaborative process can be started by asking Vernon about the items on the Preparedness Scale that he has indicated he does not feel totally confident of his ability to manage. For example, one area that Vernon does not feel as well prepared to handle is getting information or help from health care providers. This can be explored further to see what kind of problems he is experiencing, and what the barriers are to getting the help he needs. For Michelle, empathetic listening

to her worries and fears about the caregiving she is being asked to assume will help considerably with building trust and rapport that is going to be needed to plan for her father's care.

Identify the Issues the Caregiver Wants to Work on and Then Generate Ideas

Multiple suggestions should be generated, as a number of strategies may be needed to address one issue and or some suggestions will be unacceptable for one reason or another. Narrow, single-approach problem-solving doesn't tend to work well.[33,56,72] For example, Vernon has stated that one of his main problems with interacting with providers is that both he and his wife have so many medical problems that he often forgets to ask questions he had wanted to pose until after the visit. He also sometimes has difficulty with complex written instructions, such as the directions for operating the new pump for his wife's tube feeding, but is hesitant to complain when he receives then from either a provider or the visiting nurse. It helps at this point to explore with Vernon several ideas about what might help. Some possible suggestions for the first problem could include developing a list of questions ahead of a visit or phone call to a provider, and/or asking for a way to contact the provider for follow-up questions should they arise.

Michelle will probably need to focus initially on the care she can't provide and determine if there are alternative resources to provide that care. For example, if a certified nurse's aide could come to bathe her father two or three times per week, that might be enough to make the remaining caregiving tasks required manageable. However, if her father needs 7 day per week, 24-hour care, then strategy will be insufficient. This will probably be Michelle's first concern. Later, she may need to work on some of the issues in their relationship, but in the short term, the immediate discharge plan from the hospital will probably be where she wants to focus. However, we cannot assume that—it is important to check in with her to see what she thinks the priorities are.

Help the Caregiver Focus on His or Her Strengths and Potential Caregiving Rewards

Ask the caregiver to enumerate his or her perceived benefits of caregiving.[43] These can include the satisfaction of helping a family member, developing new skills and competencies, and improved family relationships. Strategize ways to increase the rewards. Incorporating pleasurable activities into the daily routine, or incorporating into some caregiving task something that is either fun or meaningful, are ways of enhancing caregiving.[76] In Vernon's case, emphasizing the high-quality care he is providing for his wife reinforces and supports the pride he takes in caring for her and will help encourage him to continue building his skills in the area that he and the provider have jointly identified for intervention. Even though at first glance it seems as if Michelle will not be able to find many rewards in caregiving, it is worthwhile to pose this question to her. Sometimes meeting a filial obligation, no matter how unfair the request may seem, can be very important for many people and they can derive satisfaction from this. The key point here is not to assume what a particular caregiver will or will not find rewarding, but to explore this openly with the caregiver and then build upon the responses.

Assist the Caregiver in Finding and Using Resources

Figuring out how the health care system works is one of the most difficult skills caregivers have to master.[43,73,77] Caregivers struggle when they have to translate a need that they have into a request for help from the health care system. Learning how to speak to providers, how to negotiate billing, request help with transportation, get the resources they need—all of these tasks can be overwhelming. Providers who can coach caregivers in this very important skill can save caregivers anguish and help improve outcomes for both the patient and the caregiver. For example, a tip sheet on how to prepare for the doctor's visit could be really helpful. Vernon has an organized list of medications, and questions that he prepares for his wife's visits that he developed with help from the visiting nurse—but has not thought to do this for his own visits. Michelle is really in need of obtaining more resources—she would clearly benefit from someone assisting her who is familiar with the myriad community resources, paid and unpaid—that could be used in this situation. It may not be realistic for her father to return home. An alternative living situation, whether permanent or temporary, might be required.

Help Caregivers Identify and Manage Their Responses to Caregiving

Caregiving is often associated with deterioration of the caregiver's health or significant depression.[54] In Vernon's case, his physical health is deteriorating rapidly and it has prompted his visit to the provider. However, Vernon sees no link between his caregiving duties and his deteriorating health. The only reason he has sought help is that his health problems are starting to interfere with his ability to provide care. To motivate Vernon to be more interested in his own self-care, help him see the association between good health and being able to continue providing care. Since he had identified getting help with obtaining services, this might provide an excellent opening to explore what services could ease Vernon's caregiving workload. Even though he doesn't resent providing such a high level of care, it is physically demanding. Generating strategies to take care of the caregiver is just as important as the strategies for caring for the care recipient. For Michelle, probably her greatest risk will be her mental health and well-being. This is where the suggestion for a caregiver support group or other counseling services might be the most benefit for her, rather than waiting until she is so stressed that she develops depression or other difficulties.

Use an Interdisciplinary Approach

Involving a team of other health professionals helps the nurse and family generate new ideas for strategies and brings a fresh perspective to the idea-generating process.[33,56,72-74] In Vernon's situation, a social worker could generate a number of suggestions on how to get more help and resources and might also be instrumental in counseling Vernon to accept this help. Even though he has been providing care for a long time, he could still benefit from a referral to occupational therapy, which might be able to teach him strategies to reduce the physical stress he endures in providing complete ADL care for his wife. Michelle could clearly benefit from either a social worker or a nursing case manager referral to help her sort through how care can be best managed for her father.

● KEY POINTS TO FAMILY CAREGIVING

The family caregiving situation is an important contextual variable that affects both the health and well-being of the care recipient and the caregiver. Your role as a provider is to assess this important domain as you consider and plan interventions for your patients who are care recipients. It is also important to consider how caregiving may be affecting the health status of your patients who are caregivers.

When do caregiving issues cross the line and become elder neglect, abuse, or mistreatment problems? Dramatic injuries or neglect don't pose an identification problem, but often problems with elder mistreatment are far more subtle and difficult to detect. This is especially true when the older adult has many chronic diseases, a history of falling, or is perhaps depressed or has other mental health issues that manifest themselves in self-neglect or a dispirited attitude. This next section of the chapter describes the problem of elder mistreatment and provides guidance on screening, assessment, and treatment.

CASE PRESENTATION 3: RISKING NEGLECT

Violet is a 78-year-old woman who moved to town 2 weeks ago from Arizona. She was moved by her son, Joe, so he can take care of her. She lived in a seniors-only housing complex in Scottsdale. One month ago, Violet's neighbors called Joe—they were concerned about her behavior. She was making excessive purchases (new car, new puppy), saying she was a New York socialite. Joe confirmed that his mother has a history of bipolar disorder. He arranged for her to move in with him. Now that she is here, she is very passive, and depends on Joe for everything, even cooking. Joe, a single man, works all day as a stockbroker. He likes to go out with his friends after work and feels Violet "cramps my style." Violet stays home all day. Joe states in your interview that Violet has never been a good mother. She is very "selfish" and they never had a good relationship. Joe realizes that she is more frail now and he needs to help her, but he also resents her. On top of the family stress, Joe is worried that she is now depressed. Since she has been in Joe's home she has fallen once (tripped over the cat). She "whines" constantly about missing her home and her aching back.

EMERGING PROBLEMS WITH NEGLECT OR ELDER ABUSE

Elder abuse or mistreatment is common, affecting approximately 500,000 persons older than 60 years per year. However, far fewer cases get reported and then substantiated by Adult Protective Services,[78] partly because elder mistreatment is so hard to define and detect.[79] Elder mistreatment includes an array of problems that includes neglect (by the caregiver and self-neglect), emotional and psychological abuse, physical abuse, and abandonment. An additional pattern of mistreatment noted in the literature is financial abuse or exploitation of the elder's resources.[80,81] Sexual abuse has also been added as a category of elder abuse.[82] Neglect accounts for 60% to 70% of all elder mistreatment reports made to Adult Protective Services and accounts for over 50% of all Adult Protective Services resources.[83]

Assessment or screening of mistreatment is difficult in older adults who are likely to have chronic conditions and geriatric syndromes that can look like or mask mistreatment. Screening for abuse may be difficult in a hurried or rushed primary care setting where the presence of the suspected abuser complicates the identification and management of mistreatment. As a result, elder mistreatment is often missed or unreported by clinical professionals who by some estimates only detect one in ten cases of mistreatment.[80,84]

ELDER MISTREATMENT SCREENING

Private offices and clinics and emergency departments are key clinical settings where screening for elder mistreatment in community settings should take place. Often in cases of elder neglect, emergency departments (EDs) are the first point of contact for victims.[85] In EDs and clinic settings, having a screening protocol in place makes screening for maltreatment more feasible for busy and rushed clinicians, who may not be comfortable identifying and reporting signs of abuse or neglect. A screening protocol helps clinicians systematically assess for and identify abuse. A protocol should include a list of risk factors for abuse, instruments to screen for abuse, and recommendations for intervention and reporting. Several instruments have been developed to help clinicians organize their assessment.

Nursing home mistreatment usually involves abuse by staff or by other patients. The predictors of abuse in nursing homes include (1) fewer beds in the facility, (2) for-profit status, (3) lower expenditures on providing care, (4) lower levels of education of staff, (5) younger staff with more negative attitudes toward older adults, (6) unlicensed staff, and (7) less experienced staff.[86] Surveys of staff found that providing education and opportunities to express pent-up frustration can help reduce abuse and minimize turnover.[87] Giving family caregivers the opportunity to talk about the caregiving situation could serve a similar function and will be part of the recommendations for assessment and intervention that will be offered in conjunction with the case study.

Risk Factors

Risk factors for abuse can be categorized by characteristics of the victim, the abuser, and the situation in which abuse occurs. Initially, researchers focused on identifying the risk factors of the individuals involved in the abuse. Victim characteristics of those more likely to be abused include being very old, female, in poor physical and or mental health with problematic behaviors, socially isolated, and dependent on a caregiver for most daily needs.[88] Abusers are typically care custodians or children of the abused who live with the victim and are financially dependent on the older adult.[88,89] Later research reviews identified the characteristics of caregiving situations that were problematic. Caregiving situations that put elders at risk for mistreatment include those where the older adult and caregiver live together, those that exceed the caregiver's ability to manage (for example, older adults with dementia), social isolation of the caregiver and older adult, a history of substance abuse or violence in the family or mental illness of the caregiver, and family conflict. Financial stress also increases vulnerability, particularly where there is financial dependency of the caregiver on the care receiver.[79] Patients who are depressed are at higher risk for self-neglect.[90]

The case study will be used to illustrate how the clinician can assess for possible neglect of the patient being seen in the clinic. Assessment will include determining the magnitude of the negative consequences the caregiver may be experiencing and identifying aspects of the caregiving situation that may be amenable to intervention. Several assessment tools are introduced, as well as several guidelines for selecting possible interventions. These assessment and intervention guidelines will then be applied to Violet's case.

Screening Guide

To adequately screen for mistreatment, the patient should be interviewed separately from the caregiver. Note any discrepancies in the information given. The questions in Table 17–3 are a synthesis of more extensive guidelines presented by Wagner and associates[91] (see Tables 18-4 and 18-5, pp. 324-325) and from the National Center on Elder Abuse.[82]

In Violet's case, there are a couple of warning signs that the caregiving situation may be problematic. The first is the self-reported poor-quality relationship between Violet and her son. Although he hasn't disclosed any childhood physical abuse, he may have been neglected or emotionally abused as a child and that can create a higher potential for abuse or neglect in this current situation. Assessing Joe's relationship quality with his mother using the Mutuality Scale could provide additional information, but even without that assessment, it is clear that the relationship quality is a problem. Second, both Violet and her son are now living in a household where there is stress and frustration as they adapt to living together for the first time in many years. What is Joe doing to cope with the added stress of making this transition? Does he need help? Would having a housekeeper during the day take some of the pressure off Joe? Is Violet living with him the best possible arrangement? Could Violet go to a senior center for the day?

● **TABLE 17–3** Screening Questions

Possible physical or emotional abuse:

   Are you afraid of anyone?

   Are you cared for by anyone who abuses drugs or alcohol?

   Are you cared for by anyone who was abused as a child?

   Do you live in a household where there is stress and/or frustration?

Possible sexual/physical abuse:

   Has anyone ever made you do things you didn't want to do?

   Has anyone ever touched you or tried to touch you without permission?

   Have you ever been tied down?

Possible neglect:

   Does anyone care for you or provide regular assistance to you?

   Are you alone a lot?

   Has anyone ever failed you when you needed help?

Investigate further if signs of:

   Bruising other signs of injury (physical or sexual abuse).

   Dehydration, malnutrition, poor hygiene, medication mismanagement (neglect).

Possible Financial Abuse:

   How do you manage your money?

   Changes in money handling or banking practice including adding new people on accounts or unexplained or unauthorized withdrawals or transfers or appearance of previously uninvolved family members (financial abuse).

Note any reports of being

   Physically mistreated in any way.

   Sexually assaulted or raped.

   Verbally or emotionally mistreated.

Note if a caregiver refuses an assessment of the older adult alone.

Another concern is the reported fall and any associated injuries. The examination for injury could offer the provider an opportunity to excuse Joe from the room and to examine Violet for bruising consistent with the reported fall. This would also give the provider a chance to explore with Violet her side of what is happening. It does sound like she is alone a lot, and that could be a real problem, especially if she is not safe in the home. Joe thinks she is depressed. Assess for this by interview, perhaps using a guide such as the CES-D. Depression puts older adults at greater risk for self-neglect.[90,92,93] Self-neglect has been described as a geriatric syndrome that is associated with increased mortality and possible functional decline. If self-neglect is a factor in Violet's situation, it may explain why she is falling more often. Ask her about any bruises and how she got them. Note any reports or signs of being mistreated, but also be suspicious of decline associated with the son's report of depression. Also, don't forget to ask if they need help with the cat. Is animal abuse a concern?

If abuse is suspected, it might be helpful to further assess the situation using a validated screening tool. The Fulmer Elder Assessment Instrument (EAI)[85,94,95] is a valid, reliable instrument designed to screen individuals who are suspect for four categories of abuse (Figure 17–4). The tool is considered highly sensitive but not very specific,[80] and has been tested for internal consistency and test-retest reliability.[96] The 41-item scale reviews signs, symptoms, and subjective complaints of elder abuse, neglect, exploitation, and abandonment. There is no "score." A referral to social services should be made if:

- There are signs of mistreatment without sufficient clinical explanation.
- The elder has made a complaint of mistreatment.
- The clinician believes there is high risk of probable abuse, neglect, exploitation, or abandonment.

Items that we might check for Violet on the EAI include being left alone in an environment that might be unsafe for extended periods, possible medication mismanagement (is she taking medications for her bipolar disorder?), and reports of depression by the caregiver that are validated by the patient's self-report and score on a depression screening instrument. Investigation of the bruising is imperative. In this case, the bruises are consistent with the reported fall and are confirmed by Violet as the cause of her injury. Cues or indicators of possible abuse by the caregiver include presenting a contradictory history, projecting blame on a third party, delaying care, over- or under-reacting to a given situation, refusing consent for further diagnostic care, or demonstrating symptoms of distress such as a loss of control or complaining continuously about problems that seem unrelated to the issue at hand.[97] None of these latter signs or indicators of abuse are present in Violet's situation. However, it appears that Violet is in a possibly unsuitable living situation that borders on neglect. Her caregiver is complaining of having a lot of stress taking care of Violet, and definitely needs help to sort out what the best course of action would be.

Intervention

A referral for social work should be made if there are any complaints of abuse, presentations of conditions or problems not consistent with what is being reported in the history, or other problems that trigger clinician suspicion of abuse or neglect. In Violet's case, offering a social work referral could be a particularly good place to start as the social worker can both address the adequacy of Violet's living situation while simultaneously exploring options with Joe to reduce his stress in providing care for Violet. Interdisciplinary collaboration can facilitate provision of services, referral for additional resources and counseling, and problem-solving about the current caregiving and living situation. The social worker can be particularly useful in helping the clinician decide if he or she needs to report suspected abuse. To report abuse, use the location-specific information for reporting abuse on website for the Center of Excellence in Elder Abuse and Neglect (http://65.110.72.145/elderabuse/eareporting.html). In some cases the patient may lack decision-making capacity. In Violet's case, if she did have impaired decision-making capacity and if concerns about Joe as her caregiver precluded asking him to make decisions for Violet, the provider or social worker could discuss financial management, conservatorship,

I General Assessment	Very Good	Good	Poor	Very Poor	Unable to Assess
1. Clothing					
2. Hygiene					
3. Nutrition					
4. Skin integrity					
5. Additional Comments:					

II Possible Abuse Indicators	No Evidence	Possible Evidence	Probable Evidence	Definite Evidence	Unable to Assess
6. Bruising					
7. Lacerations					
8. Fractures					
9. Various stages of healing of any bruises or fractures					
10. Evidence of sexual abuse					
11. Statement by elder re: abuse					
12. Additional Comments:					

III Possible Neglect Indicators	No Evidence	Possible Evidence	Probable Evidence	Definite Evidence	Unable to Assess
13. Contractures					
14. Decubiti					
15. Dehydration					
16. Diarrhea					
17. Depression					
18. Impaction					
19. Malnutrition					
20. Urine burns					
21. Poor hygiene					
22. Failure to respond to warning of obvious disease					
23. Inappropriate medications (under/over)					
24. Repetitive hospital admissions due to probable failure of health care surveillance					
25. Statement by elder re: neglect					
26. Additional Comments:					

IV Possible Exploitation Indicators	No Evidence	Possible Evidence	Probable Evidence	Definite Evidence	Unable to Assess
27. Misuse of money					
28. Evidence of financial exploitation					
29. Reports of demands for goods in exchange for services					
30. Inability to account for money/property					
31. Statement by elder re: exploitation					
32. Additional Comments:					

V Possible Abandonment indicators	No Evidence	Possible Evidence	Probable Evidence	Definite Evidence	Unable to Assess
33. Evidence that a caretaker has withdrawn care precipitously without alternate arrangements					
34. Evidence that elder is left alone in an unsafe environment for extended periods of time without adequate support					
35. Statement by elder re: abandonment					
36. Additional Comments:					

VI Summary	No Evidence	Possible Evidence	Probable Evidence	Definite Evidence	Unable to Assess
37. Evidence of abuse					
38. Evidence of neglect					
39. Evidence of exploitation					
40. Evidence of abandonment					
41. Additional Comments:					

VII Comments and Follow-up _____

_____

_____

_____

_____

_____

_____

_____

_____

> try this: Best Practices in Nursing Care to Older Adults
> from The Hartford Institute for Geriatric Nursing
>
> A SERIES PROVIDED BY
> **The Hartford Institute for Geriatric Nursing**
> EMAIL hartford.ign@nyu.edu
> HARTFORD INSTITUTE WEBSITE: www.hartfordign.org
> CONSULTGERIAN WEBSITE: www.ConsultGeriAN.org

FIGURE 17–4. Elder Assessment Instrument. *Adapted from: Fulmer, T., & Cahill, V.M. (1984). Assessing elder abuse: A study,* Journal of Gerontological Nursing, *10(12), 16–20; Fulmer, T. (2003). Elder abuse and neglect assessment.* Journal of Gerontological Nursing, *29(6), 4–5; Reprinted from* Journal of Emergency Nursing, *10(3), Fulmer, T., Street, S., & Carr, K. Abuse of the elderly: Screening and detection, pp. 131–140. Copyright 1984, with permission from* The Emergency Nurses Association.

guardianship, and/or protective court orders with Adult Protective Services.

For suspected caregiver neglect, assess possible underlying difficulties in assuming the caregiving role. The use of the Mutuality Scale and the Caregiver Strain Index was already highlighted in the prior case study. Joe's responses on the Mutuality Scale would indicate that the relationship quality is poor (his average score is 0.2, which is very low), and his score on the CSI is high (20). So Joe is a caregiver at risk. In addition, it would be important to assess if one of Joe's coping mechanisms with stress is increasing his drinking. If the caregiver has significant physical or mental health issues, it will interfere with his ability to provide adequate care. Caregivers who have substance abuse issues, serious depression, or unmanaged chronic health problems are more likely to provide substandard care.[98] Caregivers bearing a heavy load caring for care recipients with high activities of daily living and instrumental activities of daily living needs, or those who care for the cognitively impaired, are more at risk. Respite, and provision of resources for counseling and support groups, could help. Even if abuse is not suspected at this time, routinely screen for caregiver strain using appropriate tools (see "Caregiver Burden, Stress, and Strain" earlier in this chapter).

CONCLUSION

Elder mistreatment and self-neglect are significant clinical problems. Clinicians have an important role in screening for these issues during routine care visits. Any caregiving situation where the caregiver is overwhelmed presents special risks that should be assessed. The skilled and sensitive clinician observes for strain and intervenes in fragile situations. This fosters satisfying and comfortable lives for caregiver and receiver alike. These interventions can fundamentally alter the quality of life for patients and their families.

References

1. Schumacher K, Beck CA, Marren JM. Family caregivers: Caring for older adults, working with their families. *Am J Nurs.* 2006;106:40.

2. National Alliance for Caregiving (NAC) and the American Association for Retired Persons (AARP). Caregiving in the US. Washington DC; NAC/AARP; 2004.

3. Opinion Research Corporation (OPC). Attitudes and beliefs about caregiving in the US: Findings of a national opinion survey. Princeton, NJ; Opinion Research Corporation; 2005.

4. US Department of Health and Human Services (USDHHS). Informal caregiving: Compassion in action. Washington, DC; USDHHS; 1998.

5. Pinquart M, Sorensen S. Differences between caregivers and non-caregivers in psychological health and physical health: A meta-analysis. [see comment]. *Psychol Aging*. 2003;18:250-267.

6. Vitaliano PP, Zhang J, Scanlan JM. Is caregiving hazardous to one's physical health? A meta-analysis. *Psychol Bull*. 2003;129:946-972.

7. Walker A, Pratt CC, Eddy L. Informal caregiving to aging family members: A critical review. *Family Relations*. 1995;44:404-411.

8. Smith CE. A model of caregiving effectiveness for technologically dependent adults residing at home. *ANS Adv Nurs Sci*. 1994;17:27-40.

9. Schumacher KL, Stewart BJ, Archbold PG, et al. Family caregiving skill: Development of the concept. *Res Nurs Health*. 2000;23:191-203.

10. Bowers BJ. Intergenerational caregiving: Adult caregivers and their aging parents. *ANS Adv Nurs Sci*. 1987;9:20-31.

11. Cantor MH, Little V. *Aging and Social Care*. New York: Van Nostrand Reinhold; 1985.

12. Penning MJ. Receipt of assistance by elderly people: Hierarchical selection and task specificity. *Gerontologist*. 1990;30:220-227.

13. Stephens MAF, Franks MM. All in the family: Providing care to chronically ill and disabled older adults. In: Qualls SH, Zarit SH, eds. *Aging Families and Caregiving*. Hoboken, NJ: Wiley; 2009:45-60.

14. Sullivan MT. Try this: Best practices in nursing care to older adults. The Modified Caregiver Strain Index (CSI). *Am J Nurs*. 2008; 108:65-66.

15. Tennstedt SL, McKinlay JB, Sullivan LM. Informal care for frail elders: The role of secondary caregivers. *Gerontologist*. 1989;29:677-683.

16. MetLife Mature Market Institute and National Alliance for Caregiving. MetLife caregiving cost study: Productivity losses to U.S. business. New York: MetLife; July 2006.

17. MetLife Mature Market Institute. *Sons at Work: Balancing Employment and Eldercare*. New York: MetLife; June 2003.

18. National Family Caregivers Alliance. Random sample survey of family caregivers, 2000. Unpublished data.

19. Pinquart M, Sorensen S. Associations of caregiver stressors and uplifts with subjective well-being and depressive mood: A meta-analytic comparison. *Aging Mental Health*. 2004;8:438-449.

20. Pruchno RA, Resch NL. Mental health of caregiving spouses: Coping as mediator, moderator, or main effect? *Psychol Aging*. 1989;4:454-463.

21. Miller D. The "sandwich" generation: Adult children of the aging. *Social Work*. 1981;26:419-423.

22. Neal MBH, L.B. *Working Couples Caring for Children and Aging Parents*. Mahwah, NJ: Erlbaum; 2007.

23. Brody EM. "Women in the middle" and family help to older people. *Gerontologist*. 1981;21:471-480.

24. Weiss CO, Gonzalez HM, Kabeto MU, Langa KM. Differences in amount of informal care received by non-Hispanic whites and Latinos in a nationally representative sample of older Americans. *J Am Geriatr Soc*. 2005;53:146-151.

25. McCann JJ, Hebert LE, Beckett LA, et al. Comparison of informal caregiving by black and white older adults in a community population. *J Am Geriatr Soc*. 2000;48:1612-1617.

26. Pinquart M, Sorensen S. Ethnic differences in stressors, resources, and psychological outcomes of family caregiving: A meta-analysis. *Gerontologist*. 2005;45:90-106.

27. Dilworth-Anderson P, Williams IC, Gibson BE. Issues of race, ethnicity, and culture in caregiving research: A 20-year review (1980-2000). *Gerontologist*. 2002;42:237-272.

28. Zarit SH, Reever KE, Bach-Peterson J. Relatives of the impaired elderly: Correlates of feelings of burden. *Gerontologist*. 1980;20:649-655.

29. Pearlin LI, Mullan JT, Semple SJ, Skaff MM. Caregiving and the stress process: An overview of concepts and their measures. [See comment.] *Gerontologist*. 1990;30:583-594.

30. Archbold PG, Stewart BJ, Greenlick MR, Harvath T. Mutuality and preparedness as predictors of caregiver role strain. *Res Nurs Health*. 1990;13:375-384.

31. Archbold PG, Stewart BJ, Greenlick MR, Harvath TA. Clinical assessment of mutuality and preparedness in family caregivers to frail older people. In: Funk SG, Tornquist EM, Champagne MT, Wiese RA, eds. *Key Aspects of Elder Care*. New York: Springer; 1992.

32. Cuellar NG. A comparison of African American & Caucasian American female caregivers of rural, post-stroke, bedbound older adults. *J Gerontol Nurs*. 2002;28:36-45.

33. Gitlin LN, Belle SH, Burgio LD, et al. Effect of multicomponent interventions on caregiver burden and depression: The REACH multisite initiative at 6-month follow-up. *Psychol Aging* 2003; 18:361-374.

34. Hughes SL, Giobbie-Hurder A, Weaver FM, et al. Relationship between caregiver burden and health-related quality of life. *Gerontologist*. 1999;39:534-545.

35. Connell CM, Gibson GD. Racial, ethnic, and cultural differences in dementia caregiving: Review and analysis. *Gerontologist*. 1997;37: 355-364.

36. Gaugler JE, Kane RL, Kane RA, et al. Caregiving and institutionalization of cognitively impaired older people: Utilizing dynamic predictors of change. *Gerontologist*. 2003;43:219-229.

37. Hannum Rose J, Bowman KF, O'Toole EE, et al. Caregiver objective burden and assessments of patient-centered, family-focused care for frail elderly veterans. *Gerontologist*. 2007;47:21-33.

38. Cannuscio CC, Jones C, Kawachi I, et al. Reverberations of family illness: A longitudinal assessment of informal caregiving and mental health status in the Nurses' Health Study. *Am J Public Health*. 2002;92:1305-1311.

39. Buckwalter KC, Gerdner L, Kohout F, et al. A nursing intervention to decrease depression in family caregivers of persons with dementia. *Arch Psychiatr Nurs*. 1999;13:80-88.

40. Schulz R, Beach SR. Caregiving as a risk factor for mortality: The Caregiver Health Effects Study. [See comment.] *JAMA*. 1999; 282:2215-2219.

41. Kiecolt-Glaser JK, Preacher KJ, MacCallum RC, et al. Chronic stress and age-related increases in the proinflammatory cytokine IL-6. *Proc Natl Acad Sci USA*. 2003;100:9090-9095.

42. Arno PS. Economic Value of Informal Caregiving: 2004. Presented at the Care Coordination & the Caregiver Forum, Department of Veterans Affairs, National Institutes of Health, Bethesda, MD, January 25-27, 2006.

43. Archbold PG, Stewart BJ, Miller LL, et al. The PREP system of nursing interventions: A pilot test with families caring for older members. Preparedness (PR), enrichment (E) and predictability (P). *Res NursHealth*. 1995;18:3-16.

44. Boerner K, Schulz R, Horowitz A. Positive aspects of caregiving and adaptation to bereavement. *Psychol Aging*. 2004;19:668-675.

45. Cohen CA, Colantonio A, Vernich L. Positive aspects of caregiving: Rounding out the caregiver experience. *Int J Geriatr Psychiatry*. 2002;17:184-188.

46. Kramer BJ. Gain in the caregiving experience: Where are we? What next? *Gerontologist*. 1997;37:218-232.

47. Kinney JM, Stephens MA. Hassles and uplifts of giving care to a family member with dementia. *Psychol Aging*. 1989;4:402-408.

48. Murphy M, Bobele M, Gill S, et al. Is there more to caregiving than burden? *J Am Geriatr Soc.* 2006;54:S86.

49. Stewart BJ, Harvath T, Nkongho N. Role acquisition in family caregivers of older people who have been discharged from the hospital In: Funk SG, Tornquist EC, Wiese RA, eds. *Key Aspects of Caring for the Chronically Ill: Hospital and Home.* New York: Springer; 1993.

50. Schumacher KL, Stewart BJ, Archbold PG, et al. Effects of caregiving demand, mutuality, and preparedness on family caregiver outcomes during cancer treatment. *Oncol Nurs Forum.* 2008;35:49-56.

51. Croog SH, Burleson JA, Sudilovsky A, Baume RM. Spouse caregivers of Alzheimer patients: Problem responses to caregiver burden. *Aging Mental Health.* 2006;10:87-100.

52. Flannery RB Jr. Disrupted caring attachments: Implications for long-term care. *Am J Alzheimer's Dis.* 2002;17:227-231.

53. Schumacher KL, Stewart BJ, Archbold PG. Mutuality and preparedness moderate the effects of caregiving demand on cancer family caregiver outcomes. *Nurs Res.* 2007;56:425-433.

54. Mahoney R, Regan C, Katona C, Livingston G. Anxiety and depression in family caregivers of people with Alzheimer disease: The LASER-AD study. *Am J Geriatr Psychiatry.* 2005;13:795-801.

55. Mitrani VB, Lewis JE, Feaster DJ, et al. The role of family functioning in the stress process of dementia caregivers: A structural family framework. *Gerontologist.* 2006;46:97-105.

56. Sorensen S, Pinquart M, Duberstein P. How effective are interventions with caregivers? An updated meta-analysis. *Gerontologist.* 2002;42:356-372.

57. Pinquart M, Sorensen S. Gender differences in caregiver stressors, social resources, and health: An updated meta-analysis. *J Gerontol Series B Psychol Sci Soc Sci.* 2006;61:P33-P45.

58. Gitlin LN, Hauck WW, Dennis MP, Winter L. Maintenance of effects of the home environmental skill-building program for family caregivers and individuals with Alzheimer's disease and related disorders. *J Gerontol Series A Biol Sci Med Sci.* 2005;60:368-374.

59. Carter JH, Stewart BJ, Archbold PG, et al. Living with a person who has Parkinson's disease: The spouse's perspective by stage of disease. Parkinson's Study Group. *Mov Disord.* 1998;13:20-28.

60. Hudson PL, Aranda S, Hayman-White K. A psycho-educational intervention for family caregivers of patients receiving palliative care: A randomized controlled trial. *J Pain Symptom Manage.* 2005;30:329-341.

61. Silver HJ, Wellman NS, Galindo-Ciocon D, Johnson P. Family caregivers of older adults on home enteral nutrition have multiple unmet task-related training needs and low overall preparedness for caregiving. *J Am Dietetic Assoc.* 2004;104:43-50.

62. Radloff LS. The CES-D scale: A self-report depression scale for research in the general population. *Appl Psychol Meas.* 1977;1:385-401.

63. Radloff LST, L.Use of the CES-D with older adults. *Clin Gerontol.* 1986;5:119-136.

64. Thornton M, Travis SS. Analysis of the reliability of the modified caregiver strain index. *J Gerontol Series B Psychol Sci Soc Sci.* 2003;58:S127-S132.

65. Travis SS, Bernard MA, McAuley WJ, et al. Development of the family caregiver medication administration hassles scale. *Gerontologist.* 2003;43:360-368.

66. Knight BG, Lutzky SM, Macofsky-Urban F. A meta-analytic review of interventions for caregiver distress: Recommendations for future research. *Gerontologist.* 1993;33:240-248.

67. Toseland RW, Rossiter CM. Group interventions to support family caregivers: A review and analysis. *Gerontologist.* 1989;29:438-448.

68. Smith TL, Toseland RW. The effectiveness of a telephone support program for caregivers of frail older adults. *Gerontologist.* 2006;46:620-629.

69. Gallagher-Thompson D, Coon DW. Evidence-based psychological treatments for distress in family caregivers of older adults. [See comment.] *Psychol Aging.* 2007;22:37-51.

70. Horton-Deutsch SL, Farran CJ, Choi EE, Fogg L. The PLUS intervention: A pilot test with caregivers of depressed older adults. *Arch Psychiatr Nurs.* 2002;16:61-71.

71. Harvath TA, Archbold PG, Stewart BJ, et al. Establishing partnerships with family caregivers. Local and cosmopolitan knowledge. *J Gerontol Nurs.* 1994;20:29-35; quiz 42-43.

72. Acton GJ, Winter MA. Interventions for family members caring for an elder with dementia. *Ann Rev Nurs Res.* 2002;20:149-179.

73. Farran CJ, Gilley DW, McCann JJ, et al. Psychosocial interventions to reduce depressive symptoms of dementia caregivers: A randomized clinical trial comparing two approaches. *J Mental Health Aging.* 2004;10:337-350.

74. Farran CJ, Loukissa D, Perraud S, Paun O. Alzheimer's disease caregiving information and skills. Part I: Care recipient issues and concerns. *Res Nurs Health.* 2003;26:366-375.

75. Brodaty H, Green A, Koschera A. Meta-analysis of psychosocial interventions for caregivers of people with dementia. *J Am Geriatr Soc.* 2003;51:657-664.

76. Cartwright JC, Archbold PG, Stewart BJ, Limandri B. Enrichment processes in family caregiving to frail elders. *Adv Nurs Sci.* 1994;17:31-43.

77. Schumacher KL, Koresawa S, West C, et al. Putting cancer pain management regimens into practice at home. *J Pain Symptom Manage.* 2002;23:369-382.

78. National Center on Elder Abuse at the American Public Human Services Association. National Elder Abuse Incidence Study, 1998. Washington, DC: National Center on Elder Abuse at American Public Human Services Association; 1998.

79. Lachs MS, Pillemer K. Elder abuse. [See comment.] *Lancet.* 2004;364:1263-1272.

80. Fulmer T. Screening for mistreatment of older adults. *Am J Nurs.* 2008;108:52-59; quiz 59-60.

81. Fulmer T, Ashley J. Clinical indicators of elder neglect. *Appl Nurs Res.* 1989;2:161-167.

82. Abuse NCoE. Major types of elder abuse. Available at: http://www.ncea.aoa.gov/ncearoot/Main_Site/FAQ/Basics/Types_Of_Abuse.aspx. Accessed July 23, 2009.

83. Fulmer T, Paveza G, VandeWeerd C, et al. Dyadic vulnerability and risk profiling for elder neglect. *Gerontologist.* 2005;45:525-534.

84. Lachs MS, Williams C, O'Brien S, et al. Risk factors for reported elder abuse and neglect: A nine-year observational cohort study. *Gerontologist.* 1997;37:469-474.

85. Fulmer T, Paveza G, Abraham I, Fairchild S. Elder neglect assessment in the emergency department. *J Emerg Nurs.* 2000;26:436-443.

86. Pillemer KB-P, R. Helping and hurting: Predictors of maltreatment of patients in nursing homes. *Res Aging.* 1991;13:74-95.

87. Pillemer K, Hudson B. A model abuse prevention program for nursing assistants. *Gerontologist.* 1993;33:128-131.

88. Pillemer K, Finkelhor D. The prevalence of elder abuse: a random sample survey. *Gerontologist.* 1988;28:51-57.

89. Pillemer K, Moore DW. Abuse of patients in nursing homes: Findings from a survey of staff. *Gerontologist.* 1989;29:314-320.

90. Pavlou MP, Lachs MS. Self-neglect in older adults: A primer for clinicians. *J Gen Intern Med.* 2008;23:1841-1846.

91. Wagner L, Greenberg S, Capezuti E. Elder abuse and neglect. In: Cotter VT, Strumpf NE, eds. *Advance Practice Nursing with Older Adults: Clinical Guidelines.* New York: McGraw-Hill; 2002.

92. Abrams RC, Lachs M, McAvay G, et al. Predictors of self-neglect in community-dwelling elders. *Am J Psychiatry.* 2002;159:1724-1730.

93. Dyer CB, Pavlik VN, Murphy KP, Hyman DJ. The high prevalence of depression and dementia in elder abuse or neglect. *J Am Geriatr Soc.* 2000;48:205-208.

94. Fulmer T, Street S, Carr K. Abuse of the elderly: Screening and detection. *J Emerg Nurs.* 1984;10:131-140.

95. Fulmer T, Wetle T. Elder abuse screening and intervention. *Nurse Pract.* 1986;11:33-38.

96. Fulmer T, Guadagno L, Bitondo Dyer C, Connolly MT. Progress in elder abuse screening and assessment instruments. *J Am Geriatr Soc.* 2004;52:297-304.

97. Fulmer THM. Elder Mistreatment. In: Cassel RL, Cohen HJ, Larsen EB, Meier DE, eds. *Geriatric Medicine: An Evidence-Based Approach.* 4th ed. New York: Springer; 2003.

98. Beach SR, Schulz R, Williamson GM, et al. Risk factors for potentially harmful informal caregiver behavior. *J Am Geriatr Soc.* 2005;53:255-261.

POST-TEST

1. **Which of the following is FALSE about assessing mutuality?**
   A. Low mutuality is predictive of caregiver strain.
   B. Low mutuality is associated with poor preparedness.
   C. High mutuality reflects a high degree of regard between caregiver and care recipient.
   D. Changes in mutuality can occur over time.

2. **Nursing home abuse is associated with all of the following EXCEPT:**
   A. Younger staff in the facility
   B. Fewer beds in the facility
   C. Higher costs to provide care
   D. Higher use of unlicensed staff

3. **All of the following should prompt you to investigate further or be suspicious of elder mistreatment or neglect EXCEPT:**
   A. There are physical signs of injury but there is a plausible explanation.
   B. The patient reports being physically restrained.
   C. The patient reports being alone frequently.
   D. The caregiver will not let you interview the patient alone.

ANSWERS TO PRE-TEST
1. A
2. B
3. A

ANSWERS TO POST-TEST
1. B
2. C
3. A

18

Sexuality

Angela Gentili, MD
Michael Godschalk, MD

● LEARNING OBJECTIVES

1. Describe the effects of aging on sexuality and sexual function.
2. Discuss the evaluation and treatment of sexual dysfunction in older adults.
3. Identify methods to address inappropriate sexual behavior in the nursing home.
4. Describe the barriers that older gay, lesbian, bisexual, and transgender residents face in the nursing home environment.

PRE-TEST

1. **What is the most common cause of erectile dysfunction in aging men?**
   A. Drug side effects
   B. Neurologic
   C. Psychogenic
   D. Vascular

2. **In a patient with the sudden onset of erectile dysfunction and absent sleep-associated erections, what is the most likely etiology?**
   A. Drug side effects
   B. Neurologic
   C. Psychogenic
   D. Vascular

3. **A decrease in which hormone is most likely responsible for decreased sexual desire in older women?**
   A. Estrogen
   B. Progesterone
   C. Testosterone
   D. Thyroxine

SEXUAL FUNCTION AND DYSFUNCTION IN THE AGING MAN

CASE PRESENTATION 1: ERECTILE DYSFUNCTION

John, a 67-year-old man, comes to see you for a new patient visit. He is accompanied by Mary, his 65-year-old wife. They have been married for just 6 months and it is the second marriage for both of them. Mary has been your patient for many years and has convinced her husband to see you for a complete history and physical. John's past medical history is significant for hypertension, hyperlipidemia, and coronary artery disease status post MI and PTCA 2 years ago. A recent ECHO showed an ejection fraction of 55%. As part of the review of systems, you ask him if he has any concern regarding sexual function or dysfunction. He reports the gradual onset of the inability to achieve an erection stiff enough for penetration. He denies sleep-associated erections. He has not been able to have intercourse with Mary but has not mentioned this problem to any provider because he was too embarrassed to bring it up. He states that his libido is intact and he asks you if you can suggest anything to help him. His medications include atorvastatin, NPH insulin, aspirin, carvedilol, enalapril, isosorbide, and omeprazole.

Introduction

Sexual dysfunction among older men and women is relatively common and increases with increasing age as well as underlying co-morbidities. Unfortunately, many providers either believe that older persons are not sexually active or are not comfortable asking about sexual function in the clinical setting. Recognition of the scope of the problem and how to ask the appropriate questions, determine the etiology, and provide effective treatment can improve the quality of life for many older patients.

Studies show that older men are still interested in sex. In one survey, 90% percent of men aged 56 to 85 years reported good libido, but only one-third of these men could have sexual intercourse.[1] This inability to participate in sexual intercourse is primarily due to erectile dysfunction (ED). ED is defined by the NIH as the consistent inability to achieve and/or maintain an erection sufficient for satisfactory sexual activity.[2]

Effect of Aging on Sexual Function in Men

There are a number of changes that effect sexual function in older men. Libido may be diminished due to the age-related decline in testosterone levels. There is decreased penile sensitivity, making it more difficult to achieve and maintain an

erection. It takes longer to achieve orgasm—however, this may be beneficial in men with premature ejaculation. The duration of orgasm decreases and semen volume is reduced. Finally, the refractory period is prolonged and it may take several days before an older man is able to have another erection.[3] In addition, sexuality in older men is closely linked to health.[4] Physical illness (such as diabetes mellitus or prostate cancer) and treatment (medications, irradiation and surgery) frequently have a negative impact on sexual function.

Prevalence of Erectile Dysfunction

The prevalence of ED increases with aging. Data from the Massachusetts Male Aging Study show that almost 40% of men aged 40 years have ED; while over 60% of men aged 70 years report ED (Figure 18–1).[5] It is estimated that 20 to 30 million men in the United States and over 150 million men worldwide have ED. ED may be the most common chronic disease in older men.

Pathophysiology

Why is ED so common in older men? An erection is a complex event that requires the interaction of psychological, hormonal, neurologic, and vascular factors. Lifestyle choices and diseases that commonly occur with aging result in defects in these factors and predispose older men to develop ED.

The most common cause of ED is vascular disease. Vascular risk factors include diabetes mellitus, hyperlipidemia, hypertension, and smoking. There is such a strong association between vascular disease and ED that ED is thought to be a marker of future vascular events such as heart attack and stroke.[5]

Diabetes mellitus has a profound impact on sexual function. The risk of ED increases with the duration of the diabetes, with increasing levels of hemoglobin A_{1C}, and with age.[6,7] It is not unusual for ED to be the presenting symptom of diabetes.

The second most common cause of ED is neurogenic disease. Autonomic dysfunction impairs the parasympathetic-mediated vasodilatation needed for erection. This is frequently seen in diabetes and in Parkinson disease. It is also seen following pelvic injury or treatment of prostate cancer (prostatectomy or radiation therapy). Unfortunately, it is not unusual for diabetic men to have both vascular and neurogenic ED.

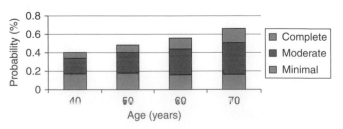

FIGURE 18-1. Erectile dysfunction by age.

Medications are the third most common cause of ED. The two groups of medications most likely to cause ED are the anticholinergics and antihypertensives. Anticholinergic medications such as diphenhydramine and the antipsychotics block the parasympathetic-mediated vasodilatation needed for erection. Antihypertensives such as β-blockers, thiazides, spironolactone, and clonidine also increase the risk of ED. Calcium channel blockers and ACE inhibitors do not seem to have a negative effect on erections.

The role of testosterone in erection is somewhat controversial. It is accepted that testosterone is important for libido; low testosterone levels are associated with decreased libido. However, some hypogonadal men are able to have erections, and the majority of men with ED are not hypogonadal. Animal studies suggest that testosterone is needed for erection. Testosterone may also improve the response to phosphodiesterase type 5 inhibitors in hypogonadal men.[8]

● **TABLE 18–1** Etiology of Erectile Dysfunction

	Onset	SAE
Psychogenic	Sudden	Present
Medication induced	Sudden	Absent
Organic	Gradual	Absent

tendon reflexes). Also during rectal exam the prostate should be examined for possible nodules. Finally, the shaft of the penis should be palpated for plaques (Peyronie disease).

Laboratory studies should include a lipid panel, hemoglobin A_{1C}, and total testosterone. The testosterone should be drawn between 8 and 10 AM. If it is low, the testosterone needs to be repeated and LH obtained. The results of the repeat testosterone and LH will help determine if further evaluation is indicated.

CASE PRESENTATION 1 (continued)

The physical exam is remarkable for an overweight male in no distress. He has bilateral mild gynecomastia, normal male escutcheon, and normal circumcised penis. Testes are normal size, but soft. Rectal tone is good. Prostate is moderately enlarged without nodules. Bulbocavernosal reflex is absent. The patient can stand up without difficulty. His gait is a little slow but steady and he does not use an assistive device.

Evaluation

Patients may be reluctant to volunteer information about sexual dysfunction and some physicians are uncomfortable asking patients about sexual function. The 5-item version of the International Index of Erectile Dysfunction (IIEF-5) may be used to overcome these barriers. The IIEF-5 is a self-administered questionnaire consisting of five questions about the patient's sexual function during the past 4 weeks.[9] Scores range from 5 to 25 (the higher the score, the better sexual function). A score of 21 or less suggests that the patient has erectile dysfunction. The IIEF-5 can be given to the patient by a nurse before he sees his provider. It is a useful tool to initiate the discussion about ED.

The most important part of the evaluation of sexual dysfunction is the history. The patient should be asked about libido, the onset (gradual or sudden), the presence or absence of sleep-associated erections (SAE), prior treatments and outcome, and medications (both prescription and over-the-counter). The onset of ED (gradual or sudden) and presence or absence of SAE can help determine if the etiology is psychogenic, medication induced, or organic (Table 18–1).

The physical examination of men with ED focuses on signs of hypogonadism (breasts, pubic and body hair, and testes), vascular (bruits and pedal pulses), and neurologic disease (rectal sphincter tone, bulbocavernosal reflex, and deep

CASE PRESENTATION 1 (continued)

Based on John's history of hypertension, hyperlipidemia, and coronary artery disease, you believe the most likely etiology of his ED is vascular disease. However, given the number and types of medications he is taking you can not rule out his medications as a contributing factor.

Treatment

The goal of treating ED is an erection that is stiff enough for penetration and lasts long enough for patient and partner satisfaction. The choice of treatment depends on the etiology. In patients with psychogenic ED, reassurance frequently works. If the problem persists, then referral for sex therapy may be needed. If the ED is drug induced, then the offending drug will need to be changed or eliminated (if possible). In patients with decreased libido and low testosterone levels, testosterone replacement (if there are no contraindications, such as prostate cancer, breast cancer, or prolactinoma) will improve their sex drive. However, most older men will have ED due to vascular or neurologic disease and the nonsurgical treatments include vacuum constrictive devices, phosphodiesterase inhibitors, intraurethral suppositories, and intracavernosal injection.

Vacuum constrictive devices (VCDs) have been around since the early 1900s. They consist of a plastic cylinder with a pump attached to one end and a rubber ring on the opposite end. The patient places the cylinder over his penis. He pumps out the air, creating a vacuum. The vacuum pulls blood into the penis, thereby making the penis hard. The rubber ring is slipped off of the cylinder onto the base of the penis and the cylinder is removed. The ring keeps the penis erect.

VCDs are a very effective treatment (about 70-80% success rate based on our experience) but require practice before attempting intercourse. Patients should be warned not to leave the ring on for more than 30 minutes since it acts like a tourniquet. Based on prices available online, vacuum constrictive devices cost about $300.

Yohimbine is an over-the-counter medication used to treat ED. It works by blocking presynaptic α-2 receptors. Studies have shown that it may increase penile blood flow and improve libido.[10] It is not FDA approved for ED. Our patients have reported poor results with yohimbine.

Stimulation of the penile nerve increases the activity of the enzyme nitric oxide synthase (NOS). NOS catalyzes the production of nitric oxide from L-arginine. Nitric oxide diffuses from the neuron into the smooth muscle cell and activates guanyl cyclase, which in turn produces cyclic GMP. Cyclic GMP promotes smooth muscle relaxation, vasodilation, and penile erection. Cyclic GMP is broken down by phosphodiesterase type 5 (PDE-5). The PDE-5 inhibitors (sildenafil, tadalafil, and vardenafil) improve erections by blocking the metabolism of cyclic GMP and thereby increasing smooth muscle relaxation and vasodilation (Figure 18–2).[8]

There are currently three approved PDE-5 inhibitors in the United States: sildenafil (Viagra), tadalafil (Cialis), and vardenafil (Levitra). These are oral medications with an onset of action of about 30 minutes. The half-life of sildenafil and vardenafil is about 4 hours; the half-life of tadalafil is about 17 hours. Sildenafil and vardenafil are taken "on demand"; tadalafil has both "on-demand" and daily dosing. The starting dose in older men is 25 mg for sildenafil, 5 mg for vardenafil, and 2.5 mg daily or 10 mg "on demand" for tadalafil. The starting doses should be decreased for men taking P450 inhibitors or with significant liver or kidney disease. The "on-demand" PDE-5 inhibitors cost about $15 per dose (prices obtained from Epocrates Rx). Daily tadalafil is around $5 per day.

The PDE-5 inhibitors are well tolerated. Side effects are related to smooth muscle relaxation and include headache, flushing, GERD, and rhinitis. In addition to inhibiting PDE-5, sildenafil has an inhibitory effect on PDE-6 (found in the retina) and may cause a transient disturbance in color vision (blue haze). Tadalafil also inhibits PDE-11 and may cause myalgia and backache. These side effects resolve with stopping the PDE-5 inhibitor. PDE-5 inhibitors should NEVER be given with nitrates. Nitrates promote vasodilation via producing nitric oxide. PDE-5 inhibitors potentiate the hypotensive effect of nitrates, resulting in hypotension and in some cases death.

There have been rare reports of sudden decrease or loss of vision (nonarteritic anterior ischemic optic neuropathy) and sudden hearing loss in men taking PDE-5 inhibitors.[11] A causal relationship with PDE-5 inhibitors has not been found. However, patients should be warned to stop PDE-5 inhibitor use and seek urgent evaluation for any sudden vision or hearing decrease or loss.

Another form of treatment is the transurethral administration of alprostadil (medicated urethral system for erection, or MUSE). Alprostadil (prostaglandin E1) increases cyclic AMP, which results in vasodilatation and erection. It is administered by using a plastic applicator to insert a suppository containing alprostadil into the urethra. Side effects include pain and prolonged erections (priapism). In our experience, it is effective in fewer than 50% of patients. The average dose costs about $31.

Intracavernosal injection (ICI) of alprostadil is the most effective treatment for ED. We have found it to be effective in 80% to 90% of patients. It is also the least popular treatment due to resistance to self-injection. ICI involves injecting a solution of alprostadil into the side of the penis. Side effects include pain, fibrosis of the penis, and priapism. Cost is about $22 per injection.

CASE PRESENTATION 1 (continued)

After the history and physical exam, you discuss treatment options with John and Mary. You explain that a VCD is probably the best initial treatment for him. Since it is not a medication there is no danger of drug–drug interactions. While easier to use than a VCD, PDE-5 inhibitors are contraindicated since he takes isosorbide. You educate the couple about sexually transmitted diseases and how older people are also at risk. The couple denies high-risk behaviors except having had other sexual partners before their marriage. You explain that the American College of Physicians recommends routine screening for HIV, as early identification and treatment can extend life in HIV-positive patients.[12] They both agree to have HIV testing.

At this point, Mary expresses her concerns about any treatment. Her objections boil down to the fear that he will have a myocardial infarction and die due to the exertion required for sexual intercourse.

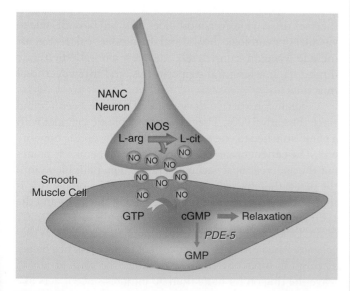

FIGURE 18-2. Steps involved in penile erection.

Fitness for Sexual Intercourse

The energy requirements from intercourse range from four to five metabolic equivalents (METs). This is about the energy it takes to climb two flights of stairs or to do heavy work around the house (moving heavy furniture, scrubbing floors). The amount of energy expended during intercourse is greater for the person on top compared to the person on the bottom. It is also greater after alcohol consumption and if the patient is involved in an extramarital relationship.[13] Patients with cardiovascular disease should be stratified to low, intermediate, and high risk according to the algorithm of the Princeton Consensus Conference.[14] Those at low risk can be treated for sexual dysfunction, while those at intermediate or high risk may need further cardiac evaluation. The following patients are considered at low risk and do not need cardiac testing:

- No symptoms and fewer than three major cardiovascular risk factors (excluding gender): age, hypertension, diabetes, cigarette smoking, dyslipidemia, sedentary lifestyle, family history of premature coronary artery disease. Personal history of cardiac disease is discussed separately.
- Controlled hypertension.
- Mild, stable angina pectoris.
- History of successful coronary revascularization.
- History of myocardial infarction more than 6 to 8 weeks previously in patients who are asymptomatic, do not have exercise-induced ischemia, or have undergone coronary revascularization.
- Mild valvular disease.
- Asymptomatic LV dysfunction (NYHA class I).

Intermediate-risk patients have three or more risk factors or their cardiac condition is uncertain and therefore needs further evaluation. High-risk patients are usually moderately to severely symptomatic and should not be sexually active until their cardiac condition is stabilized. For more details please see the Second Princeton Consensus Conference algorithm.[15]

CASE PRESENTATION 1 (continued)

In order to judge John's fitness for intercourse, you ask him about his functional status. John reports that he walks every day and can climb three to four flights of stairs without chest pain or shortness of breath. He denies any angina since his CABG and his blood pressure is well controlled. John is considered intermediate risk because he has three risk factors (age, hyperlipidemia, HTN), but he is asymptomatic during moderately intense physical activity; therefore he does not need stress testing. You consider him fit for intercourse and give him a prescription for a VCD.

● SEXUAL FUNCTION AND DYSFUNCTION IN THE AGING WOMAN

CASE PRESENTATION 1 (continued)

About 2 months, later Mary, John's 65-year-old wife, comes in alone for a routine office visit. She is in good health, has a history of hypertension, and takes an ACE inhibitor. She had a hysterectomy and bilateral oophorectomy at age 49 because of uterine fibroid tumors. You notice that she does not seem happy. When you ask if she has any problem or concern, she looks down and says that the VCD is working fine but she is not too enthusiastic about being sexually active again.

Introduction and Prevalence of Sexual Activity in Older Women

Several factors play an important role in the sexual response of older women, including changes that occur with menopause, cultural expectations, positive feelings for the partner versus relationship problems, rewarding past sexual experiences, chronic illnesses, and depression. Although the frequency of intercourse decreases with aging, sexuality remains important for older women. Among 545 women 65 to 74 years of age in the National Social Life, Health, and Aging Project (NSLHAP), 40% reported sexual activity with a spouse or partner in the previous year. Of those who were sexually active with a partner, 65% reported sexual activity at least 2 or 3 times per month. Among those women who had a spouse or other partner but had not been sexual active in the previous 3 months, 63% attributed the inactivity to the partner's physical health problems or limitations and 17% to their own health problems. Women in the oldest group (age 75-85) were less likely to have a partner and be sexually active: only 17% reported sexual activity with a spouse or partner in the previous year. Of note, the frequency of sexual activity did not decrease substantially among the oldest women: of those who were sexually active with a partner, 54% reported sexual activity at least 2 or 3 times per month (Figure 18–3).[4]

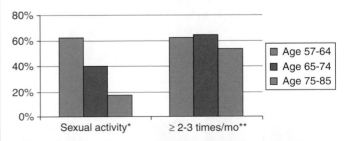

FIGURE 18-3. Prevalence of sexual activity in older women.
*Sexual activity with a partner in the previous 12 months among older female responders.
**Sexual activity at least 2 or 3 times a month among older women who were sexually active with a partner.

Changes in Sexual Function

The female sexual response cycle changes with aging. During the excitement phase, the clitoris may require longer direct stimulation, and there is decreased labial engorgement. Vaginal lubrication is reduced, although with increased foreplay and gentle stimulation, lubrication is usually adequate for intercourse. During the plateau phase, there is less expansion and vasocongestion of the vagina. During orgasm, fewer and weaker contractions occur, although older women can still achieve multiple orgasms. During the resolution phase, vasocongestion is lost more rapidly.[15] Despite these changes there is a high variability of sexual response in older women. According to a contemporary model of female sexual response, there is a circular relationship between sexuality and satisfaction. The four phases (excitement, plateau, orgasm, and resolution) can overlap and their sequence may vary.[16] In women desire does not always precede arousal. A woman may engage in sexual activity not because of sexual desire, but out of desire of intimacy or to increase her self-image (feeling attractive and loved). If the type and duration of stimulation is appropriate and she can stay focused, her arousal and sexual desire intensify. A positive experience increases her motivation for future encounters.[17] A lack of desire and sexual thoughts between and at the initiation of sexual encounters is common and does not imply a disorder; in fact, sexual thoughts and fantasies do not correlate with sexual satisfaction in women.

Menopause has a negative effect on sexuality due to a decline in serum estrogen concentration.[18] Younger age at menopause, severe hot flashes, and high vaginal pH are markers of increased vulnerability to sexual problems. The normal vaginal pH is 3.5 to 4.5; after menopause it increases up to 7.0 to 7.39. A pH higher than 5 increases the risk of urogenital atrophy and bladder infections.[19]

Sexual Dysfunction

In the NSLHAP, among women 65 to 74 years of age who were sexually active, the most common sexual problem were lack of interest in sex (38%), difficulty with lubrication (43%), sex not pleasurable (22%), and pain during intercourse (13%). A similar prevalence of sexual problems was present in the younger (57-64 years) and older (75-85 years) age groups (Figure 18–4). Women with poor self-rated health had a higher prevalence of these problems, and women with diabetes were less likely to be sexually active than those without diabetes.

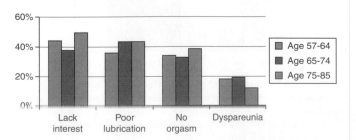

FIGURE 18-4. Prevalence of sexual problems in older women.

These sexual difficulties constitute a "dysfunction" only if they cause significant distress to the woman; so if lack of interest in sex is distressful to the partner but not to the woman, the woman cannot be classified as having sexual dysfunction.[20] Female sexual dysfunction is classified depending on whether the main problem is in one of these four areas: arousal, orgasm, desire, or pain.[13,16]

Estrogen replacement can improve vulvovaginal atrophy symptoms, but it has little effect on libido or sexual satisfaction. Libido is thought to be dependent on testosterone (even in women), rather than estrogen. The ovaries and adrenals are the main sources of androgens in women. The effects of female androgen deficiency were originally identified in women treated for advanced breast cancer with oophorectomy and adrenalectomy. When deprived of androgens, these women reported loss of libido.[21] As there are no normative data on plasma total and free testosterone in women and there is no well-defined clinical syndrome of androgen deficiency, The Endocrine Society does not recommend making a diagnosis of androgen deficiency in women.[22]

Evaluation

As for men, the most important part of the evaluation is the history, and careful questioning can detect problems that the woman might not otherwise volunteer. The most common reason clinicians fail to ask about sexuality is of lack of time.[23] Three simple questions are an effective screening[24]:

1. Are you sexually active?
2. Are there any problems?
3. Do you have pain with intercourse?

If the answers to number two and/or three are positive, further questioning is necessary to understand if the problem is mainly with arousal, desire, orgasm, or pain, or a combination of these areas. If the patient is not satisfied with her sexual life, clinicians should ask about duration and consistency of the problem; quality of the relationship; sexual communication between the couple; thoughts and emotions during sexual activity[25]; amount and adequacy of vaginal lubrication; and recent life events/stressors or previous negative experiences such as rape, child abuse, or domestic violence.

The medical history is important, as several chronic illnesses can cause sexual dysfunction, not only diabetes but any condition that causes debility, fatigue, poor function, and poor self-image (like rheumatic diseases and the presence of stoma or incontinence). After mastectomy for breast cancer, 20% to 40% of women experience sexual dysfunction, possibly because of disruption of body image, marital and family problems, spousal reaction, adjuvant therapy, or the psychologic impact of a breast cancer diagnosis. Coital urinary incontinence is often unreported; women should be questioned about it as it has a negative effect on sexuality.

Several medications can contribute to sexual dysfunction, including selective serotonin-reuptake inhibitors, antipsychotics, antihypertensives, antiestrogens, antiandrogens, narcotics, alcohol, and illicit/recreational drugs.[26]

Physical Examination and Laboratory Tests

Physical examination should include a pelvic examination, especially if the patient complains of dyspareunia (pain with intercourse).

Routine laboratory testing is not necessary to evaluate female sexual dysfunction. Testosterone levels do not correlate with sexual function.[27] Prolactin and TSH should be done only if there are symptoms that suggest possible abnormal levels.

CASE PRESENTATION 1 (continued)

Mary states before her husband started the VCD 2 month ago, she had not had intercourse for about 4 years because of the death of her first husband. Before her first husband died, she reports that they were having intercourse about twice a month and she did not have major problems; she was having adequate arousal and lubrication. Since she started being sexually active with John, they have brief foreplay, her lubrication is somewhat limited, and intercourse is painful. She experiences burning and stinging at the entrance of the vagina. The expectation of pain has decreased her ability to become aroused and her desire for sex. She denies feeling depressed or marital problems. She feels she has a good relationship with her husband but she has been reluctant to discuss the problem with him, because she is afraid that he will misinterpret it and think she is no longer attracted to him. Physical exam is remarkable for an overweight female in no distress. She has thinning of pubic hair. Vaginal exam shows that the vaginal mucosa is pale with few rugae. Petechiae are scattered throughout the mucosa, and there is an area of excoriation that is tender and bleeds easily. There is no cervix and the uterus is not palpated. Rectal tone is good. There are no rectal masses. Based on the history and physical exam, you diagnose postmenopausal vaginal atrophy.

Dyspareunia

Dyspareunia, defined as pain with intercourse, can be due to organic or psychological factors, or a combination of the two. As demonstrated in this patient, a woman may experience dyspareunia because of postmenopausal vaginal atrophy. With subsequent sexual encounters she anticipates pain, causing inadequate arousal with decreased lubrication. Because of this cycle, the woman continues to experience dyspareunia, which can continue even after treating the vaginal atrophy. The most common organic cause of dyspareunia is atrophic vaginitis due to estrogen deficiency. Other causes include lack of lubrication, vaginismus, localized vaginal infections, cystitis, Bartholin cyst, or improper angle of penile entry. Deep dyspareunia is pain from pelvic thrusting and can be due to the woman's position during intercourse, retroverted uterus, postoperative adhesions, pelvic tumors, endometriosis, pelvic inflammatory disease, ovarian cysts, or urinary tract infections.[28]

Treatment

Before discussing treatment, it is helpful to assess the patient's goals and agree upon reasonable expectations. Associated medical conditions should be addressed and medications reviewed to minimize sexual side effects.

Dyspareunia due to atrophic vaginitis and decreased lubrication responds well to topical or systemic estrogen therapy.[29-30] However, it is important to explain to the patient that complete restoration of vaginal tissue function may take up to 2 years.[31] A vaginal estradiol ring or tablet delivers low-dose estrogen locally with lower systemic absorption and risk of systemic side effect than vaginal estrogen.[32] If the patient is not a candidate for or does not want to use estrogen, water-soluble vaginal lubricants (eg, Replens, Astroglide, K-Y Jelly) are beneficial. Importantly, local stimulation through regular intercourse helps maintain a healthy vaginal mucosa. Longer foreplay allows more time for vaginal lubrication, just as older men often need longer and more direct stimulation to achieve an adequate erection.

Decreased libido may respond to a low-dose testosterone patch. In the last few years several randomized trials have demonstrated that a low-dose testosterone patch improved sexual desire in women with hypoactive sexual desire disorder and either surgically induced or natural menopause.[32-33] All women were taking systemic estrogens. Androgenic side effects like acne and hirsutism were uncommon and there was no decrease in HDL cholesterol as seen in studies with oral methyltestosterone. In a recent trial the testosterone patch was effective also in postmenopausal women who had hypoactive sexual desire and were not taking estrogens.[34] The side-effect profile (hair growth) was acceptable to the women and did not make them discontinue the medication. Although the testosterone patch seems effective, the trials mentioned were only 6 months long and there are no data about the long-term safety of the patch in women. The Endocrine Society clinical practice guideline on androgen therapy in women published in 2006 recommended against the generalized use of testosterone by women because of the concerns just outlined.[23] A 300-μg testosterone patch (Intrinsa) for postmenopausal women is available in Europe. In the US, testosterone for women is only available as oral methyltestosterone in combination with esterified estrogens and is FDA approved for moderate to severe vasomotor symptoms that are not improved with estrogens alone. The testosterone patch is not FDA approved for women. Further studies of the best dosage, delivery system, long-term efficacy, and safety of testosterone are underway.[35]

Studies of sildenafil for female sexual dysfunction yielded conflicting results. Large randomized trials showed no benefit.[36]

Treatment of urinary incontinence can improve sexuality, especially in patients with coital incontinence. When it is related to detrusor overactivity, it can be cured in about 60% of patients with an antimuscarinic agent.[37]

Psychologic issues, including depression, history of sexual abuse, and relationship problems, should be addressed and treated with antidepressants, psychotherapy, and marital therapy, as necessary. It is important to encourage the patient to start a discussion about her sexual needs and concerns with her partner.[38]

Finally, older women should receive education about male sexual aging in addition to female sexual aging. Otherwise, they might mistakenly attribute a partner's diminished erection and need for more genital stimulation to their own inability to arouse the partner.

CASE PRESENTATION 1 (continued)

Mary's main goal is to get relief from the dyspareunia. You discuss vaginal atrophy and how estrogens and regular intercourse are considered important to maintain a healthy vaginal mucosa. The patient agrees with trying the estradiol vaginal ring and lubricants during intercourse. As she asks whether a testosterone patch would help her. You explain that decreased testosterone level may contribute to decrease desire, especially after bilateral oophorectomy, but you do not think it is the case for her, as her main problem is dyspareunia that caused decreased desire for sex. Even if decreased desire were the main problem, you would not recommend the testosterone patch as it is not yet FDA approved because of lack of long-term safety data. You encourage her to have an open discussion with her husband. You recommend engaging in non–goal-oriented intimacy such as kissing and touching until she is able to achieve adequate lubrication. You offer to meet with both of them to discuss it further. You explain how a sex therapist can be helpful and how to locate one on the website of the American Association of Sex Educators, Counselors, and Therapists (www.aasect.org). She agrees to come back with her husband if things do not improve with the estradiol ring and lubricants. She does not think she will need a sex therapist but she appreciates the "Patient information: Sexual problems in women" that you printed for her from UpToDate.[39]

CASE PRESENTATION 2: SEXUAL BEHAVIOR IN THE NURSING HOME

As medical director for a local nursing home you are approached by the nursing supervisor during your weekly rounds regarding two situations that have been distressing to the nursing staff and that they were unsure how to handle. The nurses have noticed that Philip, a relatively new admission with underlying dementia of the Alzheimer type, has started making inappropriate comments to the female staff. One LPN became very upset when Philip made explicit sexual requests to her and disrobed in front of her. The nursing supervisor asks if you can give him a medication to control his sexual behavioral problem.

She also has another resident in the dementia unit who they are wondering how best to manage. Ron is a 72-year-old gay male and HIV positive. He has moderate dementia and is ambulatory. Every weekend his significant other of 30 years comes to visit and Ron shows his affection by kissing him and walking around hand in hand. The nursing staff and other family members feel the behavior is not appropriate for a nursing home.

● SEXUALITY IN THE NURSING HOME

Despite evidence to the contrary, the myth of older people as asexual beings still persists, especially in the nursing home setting where sexual needs of residents are frequently ignored. Sexual expressions are often considered behavioral problems that need to be suppressed. The need for love, touch, companionship, and intimacy continues in older age.[40] Most residents in a nursing home survey reported sexual thoughts and feelings but lacked the opportunity for sexual activity.[41] Nursing home residents are faced with multiple barriers to express their sexuality: lack of privacy, lack of a partner, staff and family members' attitudes, mental and physical illness, adverse effects of medications, feeling of being unattractive, erectile dysfunction in men, and dyspareunia in women.[42] The nursing home is designed to facilitate observation of the residents and the priority is to provide medical care, nutrition, hygiene, and a safe environment, rather than privacy for sexual activity. Both nursing home staff and family members come from varied cultural, moral, and religious backgrounds and may have negative views of sexuality in the residents.

Dementia can cause disinhibition and inappropriate sexual expressions like public masturbation, exposing, touching staff's or other resident's genitalia, and explicit sex talk. Some behaviors like public shedding of clothing and touching of genitals might be due to restlessness/agitation and stereotyped movements associated with dementia rather than sexual urges. If the inappropriate behavior is new, the resident should be evaluated for possible delirium. Medications like dopaminergic drugs can contribute to the behavior. Once medical conditions are ruled out, behavioral management should be attempted with redirection and distraction.

There are few data on pharmacologic management of inappropriate sexual behaviors in residents with dementia. There are mainly case reports and cases series. For men, serotoninergic drugs (especially SSRIs) are considered first choice, followed by antiandrogens (cyproterone acetate or medroxyprogesterone acetate), LHRH agonists, and estrogens.[43] Use of these medications for inappropriate sexual behavior is considered off-label.

Sexuality in the nursing home poses difficult legal and ethical dilemmas. On one side the nursing home should promote quality of life and autonomy, and sexual activity improves self-esteem and well-being. On the other hand the nursing home has a duty to protect the resident from harm during sexual activity, evaluate the risk of sexually transmitted diseases, and protect against sexual abuse if the patient is not capable of making decisions.

The medical director should make sure that the nursing home has a written medical policy that helps the interdisciplinary team create an individualized care plan that addresses sexuality. The American Medical Director Association has a policy on "Privacy and Sexuality" on its website that can be downloaded for free (http://www.amda.com).[44] This policy acknowledges the resident's right to privacy and that sexual activity conducted lawfully in private is protected. The interdisciplinary team together with the attending physician need to do a multidisciplinary assessment to include the resident's health status and presence of sexually transmitted diseases, mental health, risk of injury, marital rights, capacity to agree to sexual activity, risk of pregnancy, and effects on family and social relationships. The team also needs to take in account the caregivers' ethical, moral, and religious perspectives. The care plan is discussed and approved by the resident or responsible party and administration. Any off-label use of medications to modify sexual behavior must be approved by the medical director. The policy also addresses the importance of staff and family education and counseling. Several studies have shown that sexual sensitivity training of nursing staff improves attitudes. Patients and family education is also important; there is often the fear of litigation if families view sexual activities of residents as inappropriate.

Some nursing homes provide rooms for conjugal visits, in an effort to have a less asexual environment. After sexual activity has been approved by the interdisciplinary team as described above, these rooms can be reserved by couples and have a "Do Not Disturb" sign.

Gays, Lesbians, Bisexuals, and Transgender Residents in the Nursing Home

Although there are limited data on gays, lesbians, bisexuals, and transgenders (GLBT), it is estimated that they range from 5% to 10% of the general population and are as racially diverse as their heterosexual counterpart. As GLBT elders become frail, they have the same needs for public programs and assistance as heterosexual elders, but they are not eligible for the same benefits as married heterosexual couples. Social Security does not pay survivor benefits to same-sex partners and Medicaid does not protect the home when a same sex partner must spend down to become Medicaid eligible to pay for nursing home care. Even married same-sex couples are not considered spouses for Medicaid eligibility. Currently Massachusetts and Vermont are the only states that protect the jointly owned homes of married same-sex couples by using separate state funds to pay for the Medicaid long-term care benefits.[45]

GLBT elders often face prejudice and ignorance when they enter a nursing home. Lack of sensitivity for sexual activities is even stronger for homosexual expressions. The first form of discrimination is to treat all residents as if they were heterosexual without getting a sexual history on admission. Even if a sexual history is taken, GLBTs might choose not to disclose their sexual orientation or identity even if they were living "out of the closet" before entering the nursing home.

In a survey, GLBT individuals suspected that staff and residents of long-term health care facilities discriminate against GLBTs and felt they would have to hide their sexual orientation if admitted to a nursing home. They also felt that GLBT sensitivity training and possibly GLBT retirement facilities would be beneficial for older GLBTs.[46] Being "in the closet" has negative psychological and health effects for GLBTs. GLBTs become more isolated and depressed when they cannot talk about their lives and if they have to hide pictures or other signs of their identity for fear of discrimination. Even providers who feel compassionate toward their GLBT residents might not have the training necessary to know how to provide care in a culturally competent way and how to handle difficult situations, like when a heterosexual resident or other staff member makes homophobic comments regarding a gay resident.

There are organizations that provide GLBT cultural competence training. For example, Services and Advocacy for GLBT Elders (SAGE) in New York City offers "No Need to Fear, No Need to Hide: A Training Program for Healthcare Providers about Inclusion and Understanding of GLBT Elders." This curriculum includes a train-the-trainer module, a comprehensive training manual, and handouts for the staff on CD-ROM. It can be ordered by contacting SAGE at www.sageusa.org/programs/training.cfm. The Center for Applied Gerontology of the Council for Jewish Elderly (CJE) in Chicago produced "Understanding and Caring for Lesbian & Gay Older Adults: Frontline Worker Sensitivity Training System," an interactive, 1-hour curriculum for direct-care staff working with GLBT elders living at home and in institutional settings. An order form is at www.cje.net/Page.aspx?pid=249.

CASE PRESENTATION 2 (continued)

The interdisciplinary team meets to discuss sexuality in the nursing home. The team agrees to institute the AMDA policy. You explain to the team that a workup for acute delirium and medication review were negative, you could not find a reversible cause of Phillip's behavior, and that it is likely due to disinhibition from dementia. As his sexual behavior has been limited to comments and he has not touched any staff or other residents, it is agreed that medications are not yet needed and that the initial approach should be behavioral management. Caregivers are educated on the effect of dementia on disinhibition, are encouraged not to take the comments personally, and to redirect and distract the patient rather than getting angry and upset with him.

The team decides that Ron should be allowed privacy for visitation by his partner Jack and that the staff needs more training. The team meets with Jack, and explains that the nursing home now has a conjugal room that he can reserve to have some private time with Ron. They also inform him that the administration has agreed to provide GLBT sensitivity training to the staff. Jack appreciates being able to use the conjugal room; he was uncomfortable touching Ron in front of staff and other residents but did not want to push him away; he feared that with his dementia Ron would not understand why and would feel rejected. He also hopes that the GBLT cultural training will help the staff better understand and accept Ron's behavior and needs and make the nursing home more GLBT friendly.

CONCLUSION

Sexual function in older men and women is under-recognized and undertreated. As men and women age, they remain interested in sex. Providers should ask their older patients about sexual activity and offer treatment for sexual dysfunction. Nursing homes and other long-term care facilities need to be sensitive to the sexual needs of their residents. Treating sexual dysfunction improves quality of life for patients and is rewarding for providers.

References

1. Mulligan T, Moss CR. Sexuality and aging in male veterans: A cross-sectional study of interest, ability, and activity. *Arch Sex Behav.* 1991;20:17.

2. National Institutes of Health Consensus Panel. Impotence. NIH Consensus Statement 1992;10:1-33.

3. Meston C. Aging and sexuality. *West J Med.* 1997;167:285.

4. Lindau ST, Schumm LP, Laumann EO, et al. A study of sexuality and health among older adults in the United States. *N Engl J Med.* 2007;357:762.

5. Feldman HA, Goldstein I, Hatzichristou DG, et al. Impotence and its medical and psychosocial correlates: Results of the Massachusetts Male Aging Study. *J Urol.* 1994;1551:54.

6. Thompson IM, Tangen CM, Goodman PJ, et al. Erectile dysfunction and subsequent cardiovascular disease. *JAMA.* 2005;294:2996.

7. Rhoden EL, Ribeiro EP, Riedner CE, et al. Glycosylated haemoglobin levels and the severity of erectile function in diabetic men. *BJU Int.* 2005;95:615.

8. Bacon CG, Hu FB, Giovannucci E. Association of type and duration of diabetes with erectile dysfunction in a large cohort of men. *Diabetes Care.* 2002;25:1458.

9. Guay AT. Testosterone and erectile physiology. *Aging Male.* 2006;9:201.

10. Rosen R, Cappelleri J, Smith M, et al. Development and evaluation of an abridged five item version of the International Index of Erectile Dysfunction (IIEF-5) as a diagnostic tool for erectile dysfunction. *Int J Impot Res.* 1999;11:319.

11. Maggi M, Filippi S, Ledda F. Erectile dysfunction: From biochemical pharmacology to advances in medical therapy. *Eur J Endocrinol.* 2000;143:143-154.

12. Gorkin L, Hvidsten K, Sobel RE. Sildenafil citrate use and the incidence of nonarteritic anterior ischemic optic neuropathy. *Int J Clin Pract.* 2006;60:500.

13. Qaseem A, Snow V, Shekell P, et al. Clinical Efficacy Assessment Subcommittee, American College of Physicians. Screening for HIV in health care settings: A guidance statement from the American College of Physicians and HIV Medicine Association. *Ann Intern Med.* 2009;150:125-131.

14. Sainz I, Amaya J, Garcia M. Erectile dysfunction in heart disease patients. *Int J Impot Res.* 2004;16:S13.

15. Kostis JB, Jackson G, Rosen R, et al. Sexual dysfunction and cardiac risk (the second Princeton Consensus Conference). *Am J Cardiol.* 2005;96:313-321.

16. Masters WH, Johnson VE. Sex and the aging process. *J Am Geriatr Soc.* 1981;29:385.

17. Basson R. Women's sexual dysfunction: Revised and expanded definitions. *CMAJ.* 2005;172:1327.

18. Rosen RC, Barsky JL. Normal sexual response in women. *Obstet Gynecol Clin North Am.* 2006;33:515.

19. Kaiser FE. Sexuality in the elderly. *Urol Clin North Am.* 1996; 23:99.

20. Graziottin A. The aging woman. *JMHG.* 2006;3:326.

21. Kammer-Doak D, Rogers RG. Female sexual function and dysfunction. *Obstet Gynecol Clin North Am.* 2008;35:169.

22. Kaplan HS, Owett T. The female androgen deficiency syndrome. *J Sex Marital Ther.* 1993;19:3.

23. Wierman ME, Basson R, Davis SR, et al. Androgen therapy in women: An Endocrine Society Clinical Practice Guideline. *J Clin Endocrinol Metab.* 2006;91:3697.

24. Leonard C, Rogers RG. Opinions and practices among providers regarding sexual function: Do we ask the question? *Prim Care Update Ob Gyns.* 2002;9;218.

25. Plouffe L. Screening for sexual problems through a simple questionnaire. *Am J Obstet Gynecol.* 1985;151:166.

26. Basson, R. Sexual desire and arousal disorders in women. *N Engl J Med.* 2006;354:1497.

27. Carey JC. Pharmacological effects on sexual function. *Obstet Gynecol Clin North Am.* 2006;33:599.

28. Davis SR, Davison SL, Donath S, Bell RJ. Circulating androgen levels and self-reported sexual function in women. *JAMA.* 2005; 6;294:91.

29. Kaiser FE. Sexuality in the elderly. *Urol Clin North Am.* 1996;23:99.

30. Bachmann G, Lobo RA, Gut R, et al. Efficacy of low-dose estradiol vaginal tablets in the treatment of atrophic vaginitis: A randomized controlled trial. *Obstet Gynecol.* 2008;111:67.

31. Huang AJ, Yaffe K, Vittinghoff E, et al. The effect of ultralow-dose transdermal estradiol on sexual function in postmenopausal women. *Am J Obstet Gynecol.* 198:265e1, 2008.

32. Suckling J, Lethaby A, Kennedy R. Local estrogen for vaginal atrophy in postmenopausal women. *Cochrane Database Syst Rev.* 2006;4: CD001500.

33. Semmens JP, Tsai CC, Semmens EC, Loadholt CB. Effect of estrogen therapy on vaginal physiology during menopause. *Obstet Gynecol.* 1985;66;15.

34. Buster JE, Kingsberg SA, Aguirre O, et al. Testosterone patch for low sexual desire in surgically menopausal women: A randomized trial. *Obstet Gynecol.* 2005;105:944.

35. Braunstein G, Sundwall DA, Katz M, et al. Safety and efficacy of a testosterone patch for the treatment of hypoactive sexual desire disorder in surgically menopausal women: A randomized, placebo-controlled trial. *Arch Intern Med.* 2005;165:1582.

36. Simon J, Braunstein G, Nachtigall L, et al. Testosterone patch increases sexual activity and desire in surgically menopausal women with hypoactive sexual desire disorder. *J Clin Endocrinol Metab.* 2005;90:5226.

37. Shifren JL, Braunstein GD, Simon JA, et al. Transdermal testosterone treatment in women with impaired sexual function after oophorectomy. *N Engl J Med.* 2000;343:682.

38. Davis SR, van der Mooren MJ, van Lunsen RHW, et al. Efficacy and safety of a testosterone patch for the treatment of hypoactive sexual desire disorder in surgically menopausal women: A randomized, placebo-controlled trial. *Menopause.* 2006;13:387.

39. Shifren JL, Davis SR, Moreau M, et al. Testosterone patch for the treatment of hypoactive sexual desire disorder in naturally menopausal women: Results from the INTIMATE NM1 Study. *Menopause.* 2006;3:770. Erratum, *Menopause.* 2007;14:157.

40. Davis SR, Moreau M, Kroll R, et al. Testosterone for low libido in postmenopausal women not taking estrogen. *N Engl J Med.* 2008;359:2005.

41. Krapf JM, Simno JA. The role of testosterone in the management of hypoactive sexual desire disorder in postmenopausal women. *Maturitas.* 2009;63:213.

42. Basson R, McInnes R, Smith MD, et al. Efficacy and safety of sildenafil citrate in women with sexual dysfunction associated with female sexual arousal disorder. *J Womens Health Gend Based Med.* 2002;11:367.

43. Serati M, Salvatore S, Uccella S, et al. Female urinary incontinence during intercourse: A review on an understudied problem for women's sexuality. *J Sex Med.* 2009;1:40-48.

44. Weismiller DG. Menopause. *Prim Care.* 2009;36:199.

45. Shifren JL. Patient information: Sexual problems in women. *UpToDate.* www.utdol.com/online/content/topic.do?topicKey=wom_issu/5945. Accessed Sept. 11, 2009.

46. Hajjar RR, Kamel HK. Sexuality in the nursing home, part 1: Attitudes and barriers to sexual expression. *J Am Med Dir Assoc.* 2003;4:152-156.

47. Wasow M, Loeb MB. Sexuality in nursing homes. *J Am Geriatr Soc.* 1979;27:73.

48. Hajjar RR, Kamel HK. Sex and the nursing home. *Clin Geriatr Med.* 2003;19:575-586.

49. Guay DR. Inappropriate sexual behaviors in cognitively impaired older individuals. *Am J Geriatr Pharmacother.* 2008;6:269-288.

50. www.amda.com/tools/library/policymanual/cli-13.cfm.

51. Grant JM. *Outing Age 2010. Public Policy Issues Affecting Lesbian, Gay, Bisexual and Transgender Elders.* National Gay and Lesbian Task Force Policy Institute and Services & Advocacy for GLBT Elders (SAGE). November 23, 2009. Accessed at www.sageusa.org.

52. Jackson NC, Johnson MJ, Roberts R. The potential impact of discrimination fears of older gays, lesbians, bisexuals and transgender individuals living in small- to moderate-sized cities on long-term health care. *J Homosex.* 2008;54:325-339.

POST-TEST

1. Which of the following sexual problems is most common among older women?

A. Dyspareunia

B. Climaxing too quickly

C. Anxiety about performance

D. Lack of interest in sex

2. Which of the following is not FDA approved for the treatment of erectile dysfunction?

A. Intracavernosal injection of alprostadil

B. Sildenafil

C. Yohimbine

D. Transurethral administration of alprostadil

3. The energy requirement for intercourse is equivalent to which of the following activities?

A. Climbing two flights of stairs

B. Reading the newspaper

C. Running a 10K race

D. Watching television

ANSWERS TO PRE-TEST

1. D

2. A

3. C

ANSWERS TO POST-TEST

1. D

2. C

3. A

PART II

Interprofessional Geriatrics

19

Multi-Professional Team Care

Kathryn Hyer, MPP, PhD

Carol Babcock, MFT

Amanda H. Lucas, MSN, RN, ACNS-BC, CCRN

Larry E. Robinson, D Min, MFT

Lee A. Hyer, PhD

● **LEARNING OBJECTIVES**

1. Describe three models of geriatric interdisciplinary teams (geriatric assessment, primary care management, and nursing home diversion).
2. Differentiate team models by structure elements and team process.
3. Compare and contrast roles, training, and skills of major disciplines providing geriatric team care as well as disciplines that receive referrals from teams and provide services to patients and families across the continuum of care.
4. Explain the process of patient/team discussion to identify patient preferences and assure they are incorporated into the team's care plans.
5. Identify components of effective team meetings that enhance team communication and provide team management of patients.
6. Discuss approaches for conflict resolution within teams.
7. Discuss various stages in team development.

PRE-TEST

1. **Which of the following techniques has NOT been helpful in overcoming communication barriers within a health care team?**
   A. Confrontation
   B. Building trust inside team meetings
   C. Explaining one's beliefs about a care plan
   D. Assuming and deferring to one leader

2. **In an interdisciplinary team, treatment goals are determined by:**
   A. The physician
   B. The entire team

   C. Full-time members only
   D. Patient and family only

3. **Required elements of an interdisciplinary team include:**
   A. Formal leadership roles and overlapping skills among team members
   B. Fixed team roles that increase efficiency as the team improves performance
   C. Established goals, complementary skills, and mutual accountability
   D. Coordinated care provided within a hierarchical leadership

CASE PRESENTATION 1: GERIATRIC ASSESSMENT

You are the primary care provider for Mr. Thompson, an 83-year-old veteran who has an unscheduled visit in your office because he was discharged from the emergency department 2 days ago. He presented with complaints of acute shortness of breath at 6:30 AM on Saturday morning. Upon examination, you find Mr. Thompson is dehydrated and very weak. He seems confused. His wife complains that he hates the low-salt diet, keeps falling in the house, and cannot seem to keep straight which medications to take at what time of day. On examining the thick medical record you discover that this is his third emergency room visit for shortness of breath in 4 months. He was admitted 6 months ago with congestive heart failure and 7 months ago after falling in his bathroom and hitting his head. You note that his medications include regularly scheduled digoxin, furosemide, warfarin, metoprolol, albuterol MDI, and fluoxetine as well as trazodone as needed for sleep. He also takes Tylenol for joint pain. His wife complains that it is "difficult to care for him" and she spends all her time driving him to clinics at the VA on different days for multiple medical and laboratory appointments. She herself is increasingly having problems with everyday tasks, including medications, inactivity, and instrumental activities of daily living (IADLs).

After reviewing his record you recognize that this veteran has been admitted repeatedly for chronic conditions that require long-term management. This patient has multiple conditions, but you are uncertain if his medications need to be changed because they are ineffective or because the patient is taking the medications incorrectly. You wonder if the confusion is from dehydration; could it be dementia? His wife seems frustrated with the multiple clinic appointments. You know you cannot address all of the problems. You think that several specialists and different disciplines should probably assess him. Additionally, there are social service and coordination issues that must be considered.

You remember learning about a hospital program designed to help develop care management plans for geriatric patients with multiple conditions, including psychosocial issues. You refer him to a geriatric evaluation program and ask for an interdisciplinary health care team to perform multidimensional evaluation and to develop a plan of care.

● GERIATRIC EVALUATION AND MANAGEMENT PROGRAM (GEM)

Comprehensive geriatric assessment was developed during the 1930s by Dr. Marjory Warren in Great Britain. It migrated to the United States when the Veteran's Administration's Geriatric Research Education and Clinical Centers (GRECCs) established formal geriatric assessment programs in the 1970s. Because many disciplines were required to assess the patient's medical, psychological, social, environmental, and functional needs (ADLs and IADLs), from its inception comprehensive assessment required multiple professionals to work together to create a care plan. The team at minimum consists of a geriatrician, social worker, nurse, and pharmacist. Additional services that are frequently consulted include psychiatry, neuro- or gero-psychology, and rehabilitation services. The focus on multiple disciplines sharing information, debating priorities, and synthesizing recommendations into a single assessment is the foundation for multidisciplinary and team care. Studies have demonstrated that multidisciplinary assessment improves the process and outcome of clinical care by improving diagnostic accuracy, optimizing drug prescribing, assessing the home environment, identifying community resources, and addressing concerns of a caregiver.

Mr. Thompson appears to meet the targeted group of elderly patients who will most likely benefit from these services because he has complex medical, social, and behavioral conditions for which your routine clinic-based care has not been effective. He is frequently admitted to the hospital and emergency room and you have questions about how well he is adhering to your care plan. His wife seems distraught and you want to be certain she can continue to take care of him.

One week later, you receive a comprehensive assessment report and a note inviting you to review the findings with the team at its regularly scheduled meeting. You look at the care plan in amazement. The team has developed a comprehensive, detailed assessment providing you with insights into the family dynamics of Mr. Thompson, describing his home environment, summarizing his cognitive status, and recommending changes in his medication regime that will save him $40 month. You learn from the social worker about Mr. and Mrs. Thompson, their family support, and their finances, and there is a clear description of their well-kept, two-story home. The results of many tests of cognitive function from the psychologist are included along with cogent summaries, and the physical therapist has included assessments and recommendations on exercise for improving gait and balance. The pharmacist has reviewed all of the medications and recommended changes that will simplify administration as well as save money. The social worker has orders for you to sign for medical equipment (installation of grab bars in the shower, a new toilet seat, and a shower chair) and has arranged for a van to pick up Mr. Thompson for his appointments. The nurse will visit Mr. and Mrs. Thompson to develop a medication management regime by filling a weekly pill box that has labels for each day of the week and within each day has boxes for AM, noon, and PM medications. The nurse will work with the couple to be certain they understand how to fill the box and what to do if a medication is missed. The social worker has scheduled lab tests and specialist appointments to be coordinated on one day to avoid multiple trips to the VA. A dietary counseling session has been requested, and the social worker and dietician will visit with Mrs. Thompson to help her modify her menu to avoid a high-salt diet that worsens her husband's blood pressure and CHF symptoms.

You are accustomed to working alone, assessing information or having specialists provide specific information to you that you consider, and then you spend a great deal of time incorporating these into your care plan for the patient. You see that the core team is the medical director, nurse practitioner, RN case manager, social worker, pharmacist, psychologist, registered dietician, rehabilitation therapist (OT or PT), and program support assistant. The note indicates that additional services frequently consulted include psychiatry, neuropsychology, clinical nurse specialists, rehabilitation services, and home care. The geriatric assessment team has provided a table describing the practice role/skills, work environment, and education/training for all disciplines that routinely assess clients (Table 19–1). You want to be sure you understand the education and scope of practice of all the disciplines that were assembled to assess Mr. Thompson. You review Table 19–1 to familiarize yourself with the differences between nurse practitioners and clinical nurse specialists and remind yourself about the rehabilitation disciplines. The assessment team offers to provide more information to you if you request help. You are comfortable with the recommendation made by the team and decide to sign the orders. You keep the assessment unit number in your desk and vow to use them again for complicated patients.

● BACKGROUND

The Institute of Medicine report, *Retooling for an Aging America: Building the Health Care Workforce*, identifies three principles of how health care needs to be designed to care for older populations: Care needs to be addressed comprehensively; services need to be provided efficiently; and older persons need to be active partners in their own care.[1] Concerns about comprehensive and coordinated care have a long tradition but a short history. Comprehensive care began with comprehensive geriatric assessment (CGA) in the Veterans Administration. In 1984, Rubenstein and associates provided details from a randomized controlled trial of CGA at the Sepulveda Geriatric Evaluation Unit.[2] Like the case presentation, the staff at the inpatient unit of the VA unit worked across disciplines—social workers, nurses, geriatricians, psychiatrists, and others—to assess the medical, cognitive, social, and functional capacities of frail elders with complex medical conditions. The information gathered by these multiple providers was used to identify problems not previously recognized, develop treatment and long-term plans focused on the elder, and allowed elders and caregivers to be included in the process of developing goals of care and treatment plans. Part of the hospital stay involved teaching the patient and family how to manage the disease, improve function, and become involved in care. The outcomes of CGA were impressive. In comparison to patients with usual treatment, CGA patients had lower mortality rates, decreased nursing home placements, and improved functioning.

Katzenbach and Smith's definition of a team as "a small number of people with complementary skills who are committed to a common purpose, set of performance goals, and approach for which they hold themselves mutually accountable"[3] is a tenet of health care teams. Assessment teams, although large, still create a team work product. The assessment reflects the joint, real contribution of individual physicians, pharmacists, nurses, therapists, and social workers who provide insights about the patient, patient's needs, understandings of the disease process, and values. The care plan synthesizes the collective judgment of the team and the patient into a series of individual follow-up and coordinated activities.

Geriatric interdisciplinary care has evolved over the past 30 years, but it still differs from standard care because it focuses on elders with complex care needs that cannot be addressed by one provider; incorporates the perspectives of multiple providers into one integrated care plan that is aligned with the patient's goals; incorporates the elder and family into implementing the care plan; attempts to organize and facilitate services in the community on an ongoing basis; and focuses on the elder's functional status and quality of life. Teams outperform an individual provider when care is complex; no one individual has sufficient knowledge to assess or manage the problems; the care plan requires multiple providers and the patient needs to agree to and cooperate with the care plan implementation.

While "interdisciplinary" and "team care" practice are espoused as the standard for geriatric patients, how teams are structured (purpose of team, patients benefiting from type of team, setting in which the patient encounters the team, physical proximity of members, team size and composition, role of patient, duration/intensity of patient interaction with team, team outcome) and the processes teams use (leader of team, communication processes within teams, frequency and meeting regularity, role of team members, and audit of team outcomes) vary.

This chapter reviews team structure and team processes across three types of geriatric interdisciplinary teams: (1) geriatric evaluation teams, (2) primary care teams in managed care, and (3) Program for All-Inclusive Care for Elderly (PACE). Table 19–2 summarizes how each team varies by team structure and team process to reflect the purpose of the team. We will describe the primary care/team and the PACE program in patient vignettes that follow. First, however, we will briefly review the structure and processes of the geriatric evaluation team to define the elements of team structure and process. Regardless of team type, clinicians need to recognize how team structure and process facilitate the management of geriatric patients in various care settings.

● TEAM STRUCTURE

Team structure incorporates elements that create the purpose, goals, members, and rules and norms of the group. The first column in Table 19–2 describes the team structure of the geriatric evaluation unit that evaluated Mr. Thompson. The purpose of the team was to perform a comprehensive assessment. The strength of the inpatient team was developing

● TABLE 19–1 The Interdisciplinary Team

Discipline	Practice Roles/Skills	Practice Setting	Education/Training
Licensed Nursing			
Licensed Practical Nurse	Cares for people who are sick, injured, convalescent, or disabled under the direction of physicians and registered nurses. Measures and records vital signs, prepares and gives injections, monitors catheters, dresses wounds, collects samples for testing, and performs routine laboratory tests.	Most licensed practical nurses in hospitals and nursing care facilities work a 40-hour week, but because patients need round-the-clock care, some work nights, weekends, and holidays. They often stand for long periods and help patients move in bed, stand, or walk.	Most training programs, lasting about 1 year, are offered by vocational or technical schools or community or junior colleges. LPNs must be licensed to practice. Successful completion of a practical nurse program and passing an examination are required to become licensed.
Registered Nurse	RNs record patients' medical histories and symptoms, help perform diagnostic tests and analyze results, operate medical machinery, administer treatment and medications, and help with patient follow-up and rehabilitation. They also teach patients and their families how to manage their health.	Most RNs work in well-lighted, comfortable health care facilities. Home health and public health nurses travel to patients' homes, schools, community centers, and other sites. Hazards exist where an infectious disease, toxic compounds, solutions, and medications are present.	There are three major educational paths to registered nursing—a bachelor of science degree in nursing (BSN), an associate degree in nursing (ADN), and a diploma.
Advanced Practice Nurses	Core competencies include expert coach, clinical consultant, research knowledge, clinical and professional leadership, collaboration, patient and nurse advocacy. This category includes: Certified Registered Nurse Anesthetist (CRNA), Nurse Practitioner (NP), Clinical Nurse Specialist (CNS), Nurse Midwife.	Independently or in collaboration with physicians.	Graduate of a masters nursing program and most often nationally certified.
Nurse Practitioner	Orders and interprets diagnostic tests, diagnoses and treats acute and chronic conditions, prescribes medications and other treatments. Emphasizes health promotion and disease prevention.	Varied, including clinics, hospitals, emergency rooms, urgent care sites, private physician or NP practices, nursing homes, schools, colleges, and public health departments.	
Clinical Nurse Specialist	Three spheres of practice include providing direct care to patients, working to improve nursing outcomes through consulting, and improving systems organization-wide.	Clinicians defined by area of practice related to population (pediatrics, geriatrics, etc.), setting (critical care, emergency center, etc.), disease or medical subspecialty (diabetes, oncology, etc.), type of care (rehabilitation, etc.), and type of problem (pain, wounds, etc.).	
Psychosocial & Spiritual Support			
Social Worker	Assists patients with obtaining appropriate supportive resources in community that will improve quality of life. Provides counseling to individuals and families. Serves as an advocate for families by actively seeking benefits and services needed. Ensures appropriate referrals for suspected or actual abuse, neglect, or sexual assault.	Social workers usually spend most of their time in an office or residential facility, but they also may travel locally to visit clients, meet with service providers, or attend meetings.	A bachelor's degree in social work (BSW) is the most common minimum requirement to qualify for a job as a social worker. A master's degree in social work (MSW) is typically required for positions in health settings and is required for clinical work as well.
Psychologist	Studies the human mind and human behavior. Research psychologists investigate the physical, cognitive, emotional, or social aspects of human behavior. Psychologists in health service fields provide mental health care in hospitals, clinics, schools, or private settings	Varies by subfield and place of employment. Some have private practices, others are employed in schools, hospitals, nursing homes, and other health care facilities.	A doctoral degree is required for independent practice as a psychologist and generally requires 5 to 7 years of graduate study, culminating in a dissertation based on original research.
Medical Marriage and Family Therapist	Works with individuals and families with chronic or life-limiting illness. Using a biopsychosocial model, the therapist emphasizes education, family systems, and collaboration between therapist and health professionals to assist with complex problem-solving.	Private practice, hospice agencies, hospitals, rehabilitation facilities, counseling centers, prison systems, and mental health organizations.	A master's or doctoral degree is required. Also required is 500 family therapy contact hours under supervision. May work in hospital and government settings without licensure.
Chaplain	Provides pastoral visits with patients and family members at bedside. Offers spiritual support, counsel, and prayer with patients/families. Provides crisis interventions, (eg, emergency room, last rites); and arranges for leader in own faith.	Mainly present within hospital settings, including bedside, emergency room, ICU, and waiting areas.	Master's degree in theology, plus a minimum of 1 year of clinical supervision, is required. They can work in some settings without being fully certified.

(Continued)

TABLE 19–1 The Interdisciplinary Team (Continued)

Discipline	Practice Roles/Skills	Practice Setting	Education/Training
Ancillary and Rehab Services			
Pharmacist	Distributes prescription drugs to individuals. Advises patients as well as physicians and other health practitioners on selection, dosages, interactions, and side effects of medications. Pharmacists monitor the health and progress of patients to ensure the safe and effective use of medication.	Most pharmacists work in a community setting, such as a retail drugstore, or in a health care facility, such as a hospital, nursing home, mental health institution, or neighborhood health clinic.	Pharmacists must now receive a doctoral degree (Pharm.D.) Annual CEUs required range from 12 to 15 hours Residency/Advanced Training for 1-2 years after obtaining a PharmD may be completed to become a clinical specialist.
Occupational Therapist	Helps patients improve ability to perform tasks in living and working environments. Works with individuals who suffer from a mentally, physically, developmentally, or emotionally disabling condition. Improves upper body function and ability to perform activities of daily living.	Practices in rehabilitation centers, home health care services, acute care settings, and skilled nursing facilities.	A master's degree or higher in occupational therapy is the minimum requirement for entry into the field with a minimum of 6 months of field work; for OT assistant, an associate degree or OT assistant certificate is required with a minimum of 2 months of field work.
Physical Therapist	Provides services that improve or restore function and mobility, relieve pain, and prevent or limit permanent physical disabilities of patients suffering from injuries or disease. Restores, maintains, and promotes overall fitness and health.	Practice in hospitals, clinics, and private offices that have specially equipped facilities. They also treat patients in hospital rooms, homes, or schools.	A 4-year college degree in physical therapy is required to be eligible for the state exam; master's and doctoral degrees in physical therapy are available; 30 CEUs every 2 years are required.
Speech Therapist	Assesses, diagnoses, and treats speech, language, or swallowing difficulties, which may include inability to clearly produce speech, rhythm and fluency problems like stuttering, voice disorders, problems understanding and producing language, cognitive communication impairments, such as attention, memory, and problem-solving disorders, and swallowing difficulties.	Practices independently, in school systems, hospitals, rehabilitation hospitals, and skilled nursing facilities or through home health visits.	A master's degree and supervised clinical experience are required. If certified, 30 maintenance hours every 3 years are required.
Respiratory Therapist	Evaluates, recommends, and treats individuals with breathing or other cardiopulmonary disorders. Has advanced Asthma education. Performs diagnostic tests, and administer medications and interventions to improve oxygenation and ventilation. Skilled in bipap and ventilator start-up, management, and weaning. Inserts and monitors arterial lines. Skilled in attaining, maintaining, and managing the airway.	Hospitals, home health agencies, skilled nursing facilities, physician offices. Practicing under the direction of a physician.	An associate's degree is minimal entry education. Both bachelor's and master's degrees available.
Dietitian	Provides medical nutrition therapy to include planning, implementing, and monitoring the nutrition care of patients. This includes assessment of nutrition using data calculations, interpretation of nutrition status, and evaluation of nutrition care plans.	Usually work in clean, well-lighted, and well-ventilated areas, but some work in hot, congested kitchens.	A BS degree in food and nutrition and internship experience are required to be eligible for the RD exam; CEs are required (75 clock hrs every 5 years) to maintain registration; MS, PhD degrees are also available.

a comprehensive assessment with input from multiple perspectives. The team was efficient because each discipline operates in the hospital and was able to schedule assessments and interviews during his brief hospital stay. The number and scope of assessments were determined by your requests for information. The team knew its goal was to address the problems identified by you, the primary care doctor: reduce hospitalizations, improve the quality of care and life for Mr. T., reduce the stress on his wife, simplify the medication regime, and develop a workable care plan that you, as the primary care provider, could implement. You learned a great deal about Mr. T. through the assessment. The social worker established new contacts and services for your patient but the ongoing management still remains with you. The geriatric evaluation unit group did not have an ongoing relationship with Mr. Thompson; the care plan is the outcome. Teams are effective when members understand what they are trying to accomplish and agree on how to achieve the goals.

● TABLE 19–2 Geriatric Team Typology: Team Structure and Processes

Team Structure	Geriatric Evaluation	Primary Care Manager	Program of All-Inclusive Care for the Elderly
Purpose of team	Develop initial care plan based on comprehensive medical, cognitive, environmental, social and economic assessment	Manages complex chronic conditions (can include mental health diagnosis) of patients who are frequent users of inpatient or emergency room	Manage frail complex medical, cognitive, emotional, functional needs of community elders who are eligible for nursing home
Patients benefitting from type of team	Patients with multiple problems in many domains who require comprehensive assessment	Complex patients with multiple chronic conditions that are not well managed; many have mental health diagnoses	Frail elders who are nursing home eligible but wish to remain in community
Setting where team encounters patient	Hospital or intensive outpatient appointments	Primary care	Adult day care or other community-based setting
Physical proximity of team members	Team members work in same organization and generally work together	Team members are generally not assigned to work in same work space or area	Team members work in same area, generally see patients multiple times per week and share caseload
Team size and composition	Large team. Core team is generally MD, nurse, social worker, pharmacist, and therapists for assessment. Additional specialists provide consultation for specific issues	Small team; care manager (RN or mental health professional) works with patient and then is liaison with primary care provider	Largest team; members include professionals (primary care provider, nurse, social worker, therapists, pastoral counselors, dietary, activities staff) and paraprofessional workers (personal care aide or bus driver)
Role of patient on team	Provides information during assessments, adheres to care plan	Actively engaged in working with care manager on care plan	Engaged in care when possible; specify quality-of-life concerns and advance directives
Duration/intensity of patient interaction with team	One time/limited	Frequent interaction initially, home visit, RN/case manager is primary contact for all encounters	Daily or several times per week, ongoing management of all aspects of care
Team output	Care plan/recommendations for primary care provider	Agreed-upon care plan adjusted as patient needs change; coaching	Management and continual refinement of care plan
Leader of team	MD coordinated. May have shared leadership	Primary care provider	Shared responsibility
Communication process among members	One-time review, generally meeting includes most of team and patient together	Generally an electronic medical record (EMR) shared by all providers; case manager directly coaches patient; liaison between physician and patient; care manager writes in EMR	Electronic medical record (EMR) with input from members; team meets at one time on shared caseload; members meet together with routine reviews and ongoing changes as patient needs warrant
Meeting regularity and objectives	One-time assessment	Review as needed but generally care manager with primary care provider to manage if conditions change	Routinely scheduled frequent review; ongoing discussion of case and shared caseload
Role of team members	Fixed for assessment and learn to work with others to develop careplan	Case manager liaison with other members who are consulted	Input from direct care workers and all professional staff
Team outcome	Sort out issues and care plan developed	Maintain patient in the community and reduce inappropriate hospitalizations and ER visits	Maintain patient in home
Team audit: monitoring health care use and cost of patient population	Did primary care provider adopt plan? Were costs of care reduced because of better management of conditions?	Hospitalization rates and ER visits	Hospitalization rates, days of hospitalization, ER visits, nursing home placement rates

Within any team, performance depends both on individual members' competency and on the group's collective work. Teamwork requires discipline-specific clinical knowledge, skill, and the confidence to describe how the discipline skills advance the patient's care. Clinicians working in the geriatric evaluation unit trained in different disciplines but were familiar with one another because they have worked together for a long period, meet in one space routinely, and understand their roles in the development of the care plan.

● TEAM PROCESSES

Team process defines the way the team actually goes about doing its work. Team structure assumes that competent clinicians have the necessary skills and knowledge required and the team needs to agree on team interactions and work process. Elements generally include how the team communicates within the team and with others, what medical record formats capture decisions, how teams make decisions, how conflict is managed, and how the team evaluates its performance within the larger organization. Team types vary across settings, as Table 19–2 indicates, but effective teams are characterized by personal interactions that demonstrate trust, respect, and collaboration. The geriatric evaluation team had a common set of values and norms for operating and behaved as a cohesive unit. Team members were familiar with the skills and limits of other members because they work together. In well-functioning teams, members help one another, are alert to possible errors and problems, and combine their talents.

Team members are accountable to one another and agree to be held accountable for the team's performance. Regular team meetings facilitate effective teamwork and innovation. In non-team medical settings, leadership is pyramid shaped with a small number of decision-makers, generally physicians, at the top managing and controlling the work of others. A hierarchical structure does not promote discussion and participation in decision-making. If the physician dictates the care, the patient may not be part of the ongoing management of his or her own disease. Wagner argues that patient must be considered part of the team and agree to the care plan because the patient must agree to help manage the chronic condition.[4]

In teams, the organizational structure is often shaped like stars, circular networks, or spider webs. Decisions are made with free flow of information and substantive input from many providers and the patient or family. Leadership on teams requires preparation and keeping the meeting focused on the goals. Meetings that are not organized do not have clear purpose, and written records of formal agreements that are to be accomplished outside of the meeting process are rarely productive.

CASE PRESENTATION 2: PRIMARY CARE TEAM MODELS

You are an HMO primary care doctor. Mrs. Wu is your patient and she is constantly in your office needing medication adjustments because her blood pressure seems uncontrolled. Her daughter calls you distraught at least every month. You are concerned about her ability to remain in the community. She is a 77-year-old widow who lives alone in a two-story home in San Francisco. She has pulmonary disease, arthritis, hypertension, coronary artery disease, osteoporosis, and poor eyesight. She was admitted last year to a hospital with a slight myocardial infarction; she had a second admission with uncontrolled high blood pressure and was seen in the ER because of shortness of breath. She was placed in a short-term rehabilitation center (nursing and PT), and receives some home care services. Reports are that she may be cognitively compromised and has appeared depressed. She received two nursing visits and was counseled about medication management after her hospitalization for hypertension. She currently has eight medications but gets confused about what to take and when. Her daughter lives about 10 miles on the other side of town and is very upset about her mother's health and inability to manage her medications. The daughter worries about keeping her job because of time spent on her mother's care, especially issues related to taking her medications. The daughter also has two teenagers and a husband who complains about this expenditure of time. The family would like her to reside in an ALF (assisted living facility). Mrs. Wu is a retired teacher who has a pension and Social Security. Even with her HMO, she is making considerable out-of-pocket payments and she is worried that she does not have enough money to remain in her home.

The utilization review committee at your HMO is concerned about Mrs. Wu's hospitalizations and ER use. A new program has started and you have been asked if Mrs. Wu can be assigned a nurse care manager to help her understand her chronic disease and manage her care. You begin to learn about the program, which uses evidenced-based protocols to manage chronic diseases, and the special training the nurse-managers receive in this program.

● PRIMARY CARE TEAM MODELS

Improving care and reducing costs of chronic care for the 125 million American who have chronic conditions is important because 76% of Medicare expenditures in 2002 were spent on beneficiaries with five or more chronic conditions.[5] The system of chronic care for this family is fragmented, discontinuous, inefficient, difficult to access, unsafe, and expensive.[6] In the past decade, coordinated or integrated care as a best practice for older adults is increasingly recognized. We will discuss two models that have been preferred and accepted as best practice for holistic care.

As happens in usual care, Mrs. Wu is seen by myriad physicians, therapists, and nurses. Even though she is a member of an HMO, the doctors treating her in the hospital are not her primary care physicians. Her medications keep changing, different therapists have worked with her, and she is confused and dissatisfied with her experiences. The costs of her care are high because she is not adhering to the medications and does not seem to understand how to manage her condition or medications.

The primary care manager team is designed to help patients learn to manage their chronic conditions using a nurse or mental health counselor who works closely with the primary care physician to implement a treatment plan. In contrast to the larger geriatric evaluation team, the care manager and the physician work as a team and consult with specialists as needed. As Table 19–2 indicates, the primary care model team is smaller than the geriatric assessment and PACE team models; care managers have an ongoing relationship with a panel of clients in primary care and are less likely to have regular formal team meetings to review patients in a large interdisciplinary forum. Care managers do not necessarily work in the clinic close to the primary care physician. Communication among the primary care team, elder, and family is facilitated by a Web-accessible electronic health record that allows providers easy access to information whenever needed.

You learn your HMO has two chronic care manager models, Improving Mood Promoting Access to Collaborative Treatment for Late-Life Depression (IMPACT),[7] and Guided Care,[8] a program for chronic care diseases. Both manage older patients with complex needs. In IMPACT the care manager may be a nurse, social worker, or psychologist with specialized training in mental health. In a randomized controlled trial of 1801 patients across 5 states and 18 primary care clinics, IMPACT care-management clients compared to usual depression care clients had less depression, less physical pain, better functioning, higher quality of life, and greater satisfaction.[8]

In Guided Care, the program Mrs. Wu is eligible for, the care manager is generally a registered nurse assigned to 50 to 60 elders and teams of 2 to 5 primary care physicians. Early results of elders in Guided Care as compared to those in usual care rate the quality of their care highly[9]; patients have fewer hospital stays and emergency room visits, resulting in lower use and cost of expensive services.

You agree to the program, a nurse is assigned to you, and over the next few months you learn how to work with the care manager. First, the nurse visits Mrs. Wu in her home, conducts a comprehensive assessment, and develops a revised care plan that she presents to you. You and the nurse manager agree to the care plan and you are both assured it is evidence based. The care manager assigned to work with Mrs. Wu (the patient) and her daughter (the primary caregiver) will then educate Mrs. Wu and promote her self-management of medications and her diseases. The self-management includes development of specific patient goals by asking Mrs. Wu and her daughter to identify their highest priorities for optimizing her health and quality of life. Mrs. Wu wants to remain in her home and to have her daughter worry less about her. For Mrs. Wu's daughter, the priority is having Mrs. Wu learn how to take her daily medication at the times indicated in the pre-filled pill-box. Clearly, adhering to the medication regime is a priority for both Mrs. Wu and her daughter. The care manager helps Mrs. Wu create an action plan to take her medication on time and eat proper foods. The plan is displayed on her refrigerator to remind her and provides the care manager's phone number if she has questions or concerns.

The care manager monitors Mrs. Wu, coaches her to practice healthy behaviors, coordinates her transitions between hospital and ER if she needs that care, alerts you if Mrs. Wu is hospitalized or at the ER, educates and supports Mrs. Wu's daughter, and facilitates access to community resources. You learn there is a 15-hour course that Mrs. Wu can take that works with her to understand her diseases and refine her goals. The care manager interacts frequently (at least monthly) with Mrs. Wu and provides you, the physician, with ongoing reports of Mrs. Wu's progress. The care manager expedites visits to you or any other consultations as needed. The care manager also works directly with Mrs. Wu's daughter; she has disease management materials for her, allows her to access the materials Mrs. Wu has about the disease, and supports both Mrs. Wu and her daughter. The care manager helps Mrs. Wu and her daughter learn about transportation services Mrs. Wu can use to get fresh fruit and vegetables between the grocery shopping Mrs. Wu and her daughter do together. Mrs. Wu now attends a senior center for additional socialization. Mrs. Wu is

much better managed and she has not had an ER visit or hospitalization since the care manager was assigned. You have been careful to return the care manager's calls within a few hours when you have received a call about Mrs. Wu. You have learned about the home environment and the dynamics between Mrs. Wu and her daughter. The anxious calls from Mrs. Wu's daughter stopped as she became comfortable with the care manager. In fact, during your last clinic visit with Mrs. Wu the daughter volunteered that her stress level was lower and her last job performance was outstanding now that Mrs. Wu can adhere to the medication regime. The nurse manager carefully keeps the medical record updated and you are able to access Mrs. Wu's status at any time. The program is very effective in reducing hospitalizations and keeping Mrs. Wu's blood pressure managed. You are now comfortable about her ability to remain in the community.

● MULTIDISCIPLINARY TEAM TRAINING TOOLS

The John A. Hartford Foundation has a rich tradition of supporting geriatric education and multidisciplinary care planning. The foundation funded IMPACT and Guided Care and invested an additional $13 million in the Geriatric Interdisciplinary Team Training (GITT) program. Over 5 years of GITT, the project prepared medical students, geriatric nurse practitioner students, masters social work students, and doctoral-level pharmacy students, as well as graduate students in all the health care professions with the skills, knowledge, and attitudes to provide an interdisciplinary team care.[10] A key assumption is a well-functioning team is capable of achieving results with patients that individuals cannot achieve in isolation. An evaluation of the effectiveness of the health professions training indicated statistically significant improvement in geriatric team skills.[11]

In both primary care team models, care managers receive training on how to work with patients and how to work within the primary team model. Developing interdisciplinary skills to become an effective team member is essential; effective teams do not just happen or occur naturally; they require skills and training. Information on team skills for IMPACT can be found at http://impact-uw.org/about/research.html, and information on Guided Care managers can be found at http://www.guidedcare.org/nurse.asp.

In practice, GITT espouses the idea of an interdisciplinary model, where a group of different disciplines can assess and plan care in a collaborative manner, and where each discipline implements its independent plan as a contributing member of the group. Care is then interdependent, complementary, and coordinated. Leadership is determined as a function of the specific task at hand and the other professions involved. The GITT model provides training and guides for collaboration in care, for professions to work together for the planning, implementation/evaluation of care, to shared responsibility, and to recognize strengths of others with a high degree of respect for the health care recipient (www.GITTprogram.org).

More than just the medical treatment, there is holistic assessment and care of the patient's and family's spiritual, cultural, psychological, and social needs. Consistent with other team models, the primary care emphasizes the patient's living a full life based on the patient's definition of quality. Primary care teams also evaluate their ability to establish patient goals, have the patient achieve the specific goals, and, within their panel of patients as a population, to reduce hospitalizations and emergency care use. The evaluation system determines if the overall goals of the care management program create the outcomes expected for the intervention, by the team and for the program overall.

● CORE PROCESS MARKER: COMMUNICATION

The interdisciplinary team must communicate data constantly and do it well. Practically, communication regarding the patient's care is disseminated to the health care providers through personal phone calls, written documentation in the progress notes, and in the electronic record. The electronic documentation allows for continuity of the care itself (eg, using secure means such as Virtual Private Networks [VPNs] compliant with standards of the Health Insurance Portability and Accountability Act of 1996 [HIPAA]) and, importantly, the communication of patient and family concerns and the support and coping mechanisms necessary for care (eg, using patient portals such as Google Health or Microsoft HealthVault).[12]

This electronic database encourages collaboration because it captures all communications, interventions, and patient outcomes. It allows Internet-based access to staff whether in hospital or at an offsite location. An entry for each new patient is made by the staff and can be disseminated to the others via secure e-mail. If a patient had been seen during a previous admission, then a searchable function allows the next team member to easily become acquainted with previous contact and decisions. This system not only allows for tracking of the information discussed, but also discharge outcomes, progression of pain, and symptom management.

While still new, coordinated care and communication increasingly has included decision-support and point-of-care learning. This is learning that occurs at the time and place of a health professional–patient encounter. Point-of-care learning is most often distinguished by its context: the active encounter between the clinician and the patient in the health care site, at home, or elsewhere. During this process, information needs are identified, and the opportunity for clinician and patient education, clinical decisions, and patient management all intersect.

Point-of-care learning has several unique characteristics: it provides information based on needs identified during the clinical encounter; it employs evidence-based biomedical and other health-related literature and information resources; and it has the potential to provide an answer either at the time of the patient encounter or soon after. Further, point-of-care learning is seen as an important, and possibly necessary, subset of workplace learning. Point-of-care learning increasingly is considered a necessary component of individual and organizational quality improvement processes, linking point-of-care learning resources and activities to performance-level data.

● **TABLE 19–3** How to Run an Effective Meeting

1. **Create a Meeting Agenda.** A meeting agenda provides purpose, direction, and expectations to all the participants.

   All agendas should include:

   a. Meeting start time
   b. Meeting end time
   c. Meeting location
   d. Topic headings and expected leader for that topic
   e. Some topic detail for each heading
   f. Time allocation for each topic

2. **Establish roles prior to meeting or at start of meeting.** General meeting roles include facilitator/leader, timekeeper, and recorder.

   a. Leader is responsible for agenda, convenes and adjourns meeting, and facilitates discussion.
   b. Timekeeper reminds group about the amount of time each item is taking and works to keep group on task.
   c. Recorder summarizes agreements verbally and distributes a meeting record to all participants with decisions reached and the tasks participants have agreed to accomplish by specific dates.

3. **Establish agreement at beginning that the agenda meets participants' needs.** Get consensus that all will work to accomplish the tasks listed on agenda. Additional items can be added or deferred to another meeting date.

4. **Summarize meeting tasks assigned and obtain participant consent to work and timeframe established.** Modifications are made if needed.

5. **Evaluate meeting.** Participants provide feedback on the processes and outcomes of the meeting as part of a quality improvement process.

● RUNNING AN INTERDISCIPLINARY CARE TEAM MEETING

Running a team meeting is a key skill. Table 19–3 provides an outline of the elements of an effective team meeting. The meeting requires an agenda and the assignment of two additional roles: time keeper and recorder. A leader runs the meeting and must prepare an agenda beforehand, determine the time and place for the meeting, and provide a written record of who agreed to do what activities during the meeting. Meetings that are not organized, do not have clear purpose, and do not have a written record of formal agreements that are to be accomplished outside of the meeting process are rarely productive. Furthermore, productive teams monitor their performance over months and years by establishing team outcomes. Without clear goals and process measures, it is impossible to evaluate the performance of the team. As noted earlier, outcomes for primary care teams include reduction in ER use and hospitalizations and increased patient satisfaction with care.

CASE PRESENTATION 3: PACE

Mrs. Jones is a 92-year-old African American female who is presently under the care of her daughter and son-in-law in their home, where she has lived for the past 7 years. Medically, she is stable after being hospitalized for a cerebrovascular accident (CVA) and discharged to a nursing home for a short rehabilitation stay. The stroke left her in a wheelchair and she cannot transfer well but she was discharged home. The daughter worries that Mrs. Jones she does not seem "to be herself" and the PT who has made a few home visits reported she is not cooperating. Her caregivers are wondering if they need to seek placement in a nursing home, as the caregiver burden is starting to exceed what they can provide. Based on a recommendation from a friend, Mrs. Jones' family schedules an evaluation with a local Program for All Inclusive Care for the Elderly (PACE) program to see if she might be eligible. They inform her it will involve an intensive physical, medical and psychological evaluation, and then the PACE team will discuss her strengths, deficits, and potential eligibility for the program.

You, the family, are invited to a team meeting of the PACE program. The agenda is sent to you with the time, date, and place of the meeting. Mrs. Jones is the first patient on the agenda and the team requests you attend. You review the guidelines for meeting (Table 19–3) and are eager to attend the team meeting.

● PROGRAM FOR ALL INCLUSIVE CARE FOR THE ELDERLY

Program for All Inclusive Care for the Elderly is a program integrating Medicare and Medicaid financing and services for very frail elders who meet the state criteria to be in nursing homes. The typical PACE participant is older than 80 years and has an average of 8 acute and chronic medical problems such as heart disease, respiratory disease, and diabetes, and has 3.0 ADL (activities of daily living) dependencies such as walking, bathing, dressing, and toileting. To be eligible for PACE an individual must be 55 or older and certified by the state in which he or she resides as eligible for nursing home–level care.[13]

For families caring for an elderly individual needing long-term care services, the PACE model provides caregivers a broad range of services focused on keeping them at home and out of institutional settings. The IDT establishes the plan of care at enrollment. As with the hospital-based geriatric assessment team, the plan of care is developed by the IDT and is based on the individual discipline-specific assessment of each IDT member. Unlike the geriatric assessment team, once a person is enrolled as a PACE participant, care and services are coordinated on an ongoing basis by the PACE Interdisciplinary Team (IDT). The PACE team is larger than any of the other teams because it includes the aides helping with transport and all team members who have regular contact with members. PACE teams work with a defined caseload similar to primary care members but team members work together in close proximity and routinely review participants'

care plans. Participants and family members are active members of the care plan. The care plan is electronic and team members share the record as needed. The plan is modified based on changes in a participant's health condition or anticipated needs, but at least twice a year.

CASE PRESENTATION 3 (continued)

Team Meeting

8:00: The care manager calls the meeting to order and asks the team members to review the 55-minute meeting agenda. All agree and the meeting returns to the first case: Mrs. Jones. The social worker welcomes the family and Mrs. Jones to the care-planning meeting and asks each person to introduce himself or herself. The social worker then asks for a volunteer to be a timekeeper and someone else to record the team decisions and write up the meeting notes. Everyone is on time and appears ready to discuss Mrs. Jones and why PACE may be an appropriate program for her.

8:04: The nurse reports: Mrs. Jones lives at home. From all indications she had been declining and recently had a mild CVA. She was admitted to the local medical center. She was treated, discharged to a rehab unit for 3 weeks, and she is receiving some in-home care PT. She has a supportive daughter and son-in-law but Mrs. Jones is very difficult to care for at home. She requires help with most of her ADLs and anything that requires transfer. She is able to eat by herself. The nurse continues with a medical history: Diagnoses include diabetes, hypertension, obesity, peripheral neuropathy, a defibrillator, gastroesophageal reflux disease, hypothyroidism, congestive heart failure, and possible transient ischemic attacks.

8:07: Pharmacist: Mrs. Jones is on several medications, including the psychiatric meds sertraline and bupropion, and is on several pain medications including tramadol, hydrocodone/acetaminophen, and pregabalin. She is also diabetic. She has no history of alcohol abuse or tobacco use, and relates that her pain level is tolerable when she is seated and becomes a problem when she is trying to move about or is in PT. The patient has a long list of targets noted in the rehab center. They include functional rehabilitation, mood, falls, nutritional issues, dehydration, pressure ulcers, compliance with psychotropic medications, socialization, and diabetes.

8:12: Social Work provides her developmental history: The patient is a native of Georgia. She indicates that she had a positive upbringing and graduated from high school. She denies any milestone disruptions and relates positive stories about her upbringing. She married in the early 1950s, and was married to her husband for approximately 52 years, he having passed 7 years ago. He did not have a pension but did receive Social Security. She has been living with her daughter since this time because she could not maintain the apartment she lived in after her husband died. She has a very limited income from Social Security ($450/month) and is on Medicaid. She has three other children who live near her, as well as several grandchildren. One of her children is a problem to her as he does not visit and there have been reported quarrels. This has caused family strife. She feels supported by her other children. She has had problems being short with people, and having personal problems with some neighbors. Her children also see her as not being fully cooperative with them, her care, or health care professionals.

8:16: The psychologist welcomes you and indicates that the following tests were used for a cognitive assessment. Mrs. Jones was interviewed in her home by the case manager and also observed with her family. Cognitively she was sharp, gave no indication of word-finding problems, and was able to engage the conversation meaningfully. At times she was very assertive and defensive. She demonstrated a keen ability to recall dates and answer questions. She indicated that she does tear on occasion, but does not feel she is depressed. She indicates that she feels misunderstood. She does not appear to be anxious. She also denies this. There are no perceptual anomalies or delusionary thinking. She appeared reluctantly cooperative with the case manager and at times with her family. She does appreciate their assistance. She seems to have reasonable insight, as she is aware of her situation, but this can be strained when she is requested to comply. Her judgment then appears suspect.

Mrs. Jones has an estimated pre-morbid intelligence score above average, based on the WAIS-III Vocabulary (OPEI–V). A recent MMSE placed her score at 30/30. She is oriented and has a good understanding of her current condition and limits. She conversed as one facile with her situation, her family, the current situation, her malady, and her options. She also scored in the normal ranges on the cognitive domains of attention, visuospatial tasks, memory, executive functioning, as well as language. She was rated 0 on the Clinical Dementia Rating (CDR).

Emotional interviewer-based measures indicated that she is not depressed or anxious. Her MBMD was more revealing. This is less apt for dissimulation. She scored as one with minor or subclinical depression. Her MBMD is reflective too of concerns about functional deficits, pain sensitivity, and pessimism. She has a strong spiritual presence (see list below). Her basic personality is characterized by cooperative and respectful styles. Lifestyle markers of note include inactivity and eating. She is also fearful of falling and can be most controlling in her current situation. In effect, she appears to be one who has subclinical depression, is somewhat controlling, is fearful of functional decline (scared of falls), and is less able to tolerate her fears.

Stress moderators: Intrapersonal and extrapersonal characteristics that affect medical problems. They target cognitive appraisals, resources, and context factors.

Moderator	Weakness	Strength
Illness apprehension vs. Illness acceptance	X	
Functional deficits vs. Functional competence	X	
Pain sensitivity vs. Pain tolerance	X	
Social isolation vs. Social support		X
Future pessimism vs. Future optimism	X	
Spiritual absence vs. Spiritual faith		X

Treatment prognostics: Behaviors and attitudinal aspects that may complicate or enhance treatment efficacy.

Treatment Prognostic	Weakness	Strength
Interventional fragility vs. Interventional resilience		X
Medication abuse vs. Medication consciousness		X
Information discomfort vs. Information receipt		X
Utilization excess vs. Appropriate utilization		X
Problematic compliance vs. Optimal compliance		X

The timekeeper reminded the psychologist of the time. The MD then indicates that the team recommends the following plan of care.

MD: Our goal is to admit Mrs. Jones to our PACE program. We believe we will be able to provide an excellent level of care and to help all of you keep Mrs. Jones at home. We will monitor her blood pressure and lab values to be sure her hypertension and other medical conditions are well managed. The primary focus, however, will be her rehabilitation goals, because improving transfer will increase her ability to remain in the community. Targets for the intervention team include altering her mood (decreasing her depressive markers, such as crying), establishing a fall protocol, improving nutrition, having her handle pain with less anger, and engaging in activities. In general, they want her to be an active participant in her rehab program (including occupational therapy and physical therapy, which she will receive 4 days a week).

PT: Transfer and fear of falls: If the goal of transfer is to be achieved, Mrs. Jones must make considerable effort, as will the team. PT will work with Mrs. Jones and the team will encourage her to practice with her fear of falling. Gradual exposure to falling is the plan. In addition, the PT and Social Work will teach her how to slow down, breathe, and trouble shoot. The family will be encouraged to help Mrs. Jones practice this even when she is at home.

Social PACE Work: Mrs. Jones needs more socialization. At the program the staff will work with her to engage her in social hour, group exercise, and other things to increase her interaction with others. Because she will not seek out activities, it is important not to let her escape PT or other scheduled programs.

PT: She responds in a passive-aggressive manner that can be corrected with recognition or challenge. It is widely seen that she is not putting out sufficient effort for progress. People responsible for her care become easily frustrated. Efforts should be made to minimize this response. Again, we must remind the staff who work with her that a matter-of-fact attitude can be established and encouragement for effort provided.

Social Work: The plan includes your family involvement: You are told it is critical that you support the care plan and reinforce the ability of Mrs. Jones to stay in the community. You as the family must also adopt a matter-of-fact attitude to encourage Mrs. Jones to be independent when she is at home. The staff member will work with you and call you every 2 to 3 weeks to encourage reinforcement of independence.

Physician: For her depression care we will focus on behavior activation as well as control issues for her. If we assist with her interpersonal issues related to family and staff, her depression may resolve. Should it not, the team will reevaluate for psychiatric medications in 1 month.

Nurse: Do you as the family or Mrs. Jones have any questions?

Family: How will these services be paid? Mom has very little money.

Social Worker: Mrs. Jones is eligible for the program because she meets the criteria for nursing home placement and is already on Medicaid. We have done the assessments and she qualifies. If you agree, the team will pick her up at your home and deliver her back 4 days per week. During her time at the center she will receive medical care and her physical therapy. Any medications will also be included.

Family: You as a family are pleased that there will be one place for service and it seems that the care will be comprehensive. If Mrs. Jones leaves for the center, it will provide her with more services and reduce the work you have driving her to doctors' appointments and she should become more able to remain at home. Mrs. Jones is amenable to the staff and she is now open to becoming enrolled in PACE, attending their day program, and having the team organize her care. The PACE care plan will work directly with the rehab team at the center. You as the family will work to reinforce the rehab at home. Because Mrs. Jones will be at the day program, she will receive primary care from the nurse practitioner and geriatrician, and you also will be able to work with the psychologist and social worker as needed.

At 8:55 the team meeting is adjourned and you leave very pleased about this new program.

● TEAM DEVELOPMENT

Teams do not just emerge as functioning groups. The team provides information on a recursive, nonlinear basis, encouraging input and discussion. All components of the interdisciplinary process are necessary, but can vary considerably based on each individual situation. Interdisciplinary primary care is actually system care, involving many tentacles: the history and natural progression of the disease, understanding of the patient and family, recognition of transitions across settings over the course of illness, documenting to acute care staff the patient's preferences, and the ability of the care team to navigate the strong emotional response of patients and family. Patient needs are paramount; how team members flow in and out at determined points, using team technology, clinical acumen, and psychological reinforcements for this task requires coordinated team activity. As the care moves along a continuum from interventions that can remedy a condition to management to palliative and extended care, the number of team members grows.

Teams evolve and change as members enter and leave. The four phases of team development—forming, storming, norming, and performing—are defined in Table 19–4 and were initially described by Tuckman[14] as the necessary order for groups to develop. It is important that teams realize that teams move back and forth in these stages even after the "performing" stage is reached. Stages are important for members to recognize to understand team behavior and be more effective at moving teams to a higher level of performance. Teams change as members join and leave; teams should have a process to orient new members into the team culture, ground rules, and norms of operation. The second stage of teams, storming, allows members to share views and recognize that members have different views of work, the group, and patient care. Teams should recognize that conflict is critical for team development and performance. It is important for teams as they develop and become comfortable to avoid complacency and group-think. A key feature of good teams is the willingness of members to challenge one another and think independently. Team skills in stages two and three include active listening, probing to be certain you clarify issues, and responding constructively to views expressed by others.

In the norming stage, individuals on teams develop "processes" on how to work as a group. Standards for the team are established, including routine meeting times, ways to present cases, and how to disagree with one another. The team "rules" are developed. Oral and written communication methods will be established. Teams should discuss and agree to a standardized way to record information. Details about how the record should be constructed, what abbreviations are allowed, and who can add information or have access to data are the norms of the team. Medical records should be shared by all team members; if electronic, there should be protocols about how they can be accessed by any team member. Training on confidentiality and group process are additional norms that should be reviewed and agreed to by members.

By the fourth stage, teams are able to function as a high-performing unit. Members have become interdependent and they trust other team members. By this time members are motivated, positive about the team process, and knowledgeable about each other. A leader is almost always participatory rather than supervisory. Dissent is expected but it is expressed respectfully and always to advance the decision-making of the group. There is a willingness to learn from other disciplines and to expand knowledge about services that are routinely needed for effective care coordination. Ideally a team recognizes the interests and achievements of other team members. Team members are accountable to one another and to the group's performance standards over months and years. Role overlap is appreciated and members respect and solicit help from one another. When team members are committed to team process and content, the leadership functions are truly shared and mutual accountability is evident.

CONCLUSION

This chapter provides examples of collaborative care models of the one-time assessment team in a hospital-based setting, primary care management, and a community-based program caring for nursing home–eligible patients. Specifically, we outlined how interdisciplinary care can be provided for patients across the continuum and during transitions from community to hospital. If patients and families are encouraged to participate in their own care and manage their chronic condition, the patient is a member of the health care team. Care management models

---

● TABLE 19–4 Stages of Team Development

Stage 1: Forming is the first stage of team development. In this stage, individuals are trying to determine the purpose of the group and assessing others to determine motives, interests, and needs of the members of the team. Generally, members want to be accepted by others, will be courteous, and avoid conflict. Yet because individuals perceive themselves as independent of the group they are focused on themselves and not vested in the group. Serious issues, disagreement, and feelings are avoided. Members may want get to get to know one another, exchange some personal information, and make new friends. At this stage it is important that a clear agenda and expectations for the group performance be established. Directive management enables the team to establish its agenda and move to the next stage.

Stage 2: Storming is the second stage of team development. During this stage the team addresses how it wants to work and how decisions will be made as a group. Common issues include what leadership model the team will accept, how the team will function independently, and how as a team differences will be resolved (consensus or majority rule). Storming is necessary for growth and the establishment of a team where members are interdependent, rather than individuals working independently of one another. Storming generally is contentious and is difficult for members of the team who are averse to conflict. To move to the next stage, teams should be encouraged to be tolerant, listen to understand each team member's concerns, and create appropriate ways to respectfully disagree. Teams can get stuck in this phase if members with more power and prestige cut off discussion.

Stage 3: Norming is the third stage of team development. Team members know one another and work together in ways that make teamwork seem natural. Team members often work through this stage by agreeing on rules, values, professional behavior, shared methods, working tools, and even taboos. During this phase, team members begin to trust one another. Motivation increases as the team gets more accomplished. As team members trust one another and are comfortable with working relationships, group-think or a reluctance to disagree with the consensus may develop. Leadership is generally more participative than in forming or storming.

Stage 4: Performing is the fourth stage of team development. Teams function as a unit and work effectively. Team members have become interdependent and trust one another. Members are now competent in their independent roles, autonomous yet accountable to one another and the team. Disagreements are expected and encouraged but there is an agreed-upon method to disagree. Leadership is participatory and the team holds itself accountable for team performance goals.

Modified and adapted from Tuckman B. Developmental sequence in small groups. Psychol Bull. 1965;63:384-399.

work when complex patients participate in care and care managers and members of the team continuously provide support, education, and care. Through ongoing discussions, teams help patients learn about the natural progression of their illness and providers can elicit the preferences of patients. Preferences are then discussed, documented, and the goals of care are adjusted. If patients are complex and require help from multiple professionals, teams that are able to work together will develop care plans that are more coordinated and less fragmented. However, the ability to provide that care requires professionals to learn the skills of teams.

References

1. Institute of Medicine. *Retooling for an Aging America*. Washington, DC: National Academies Press; 2008.

2. Rubenstein LZ, Josephson KR, Wieland GD, et al. Effectiveness of a geriatric evaluation unit. A randomized clinical trial. *N Engl J Med*. 1984;311:1664-1670.

3. Katzenbach JR, Smith DK. *The Wisdom of Teams: Creating the High-Performance Organization*. New York: McKinsey & Co.; 1983.

4. Wagner EH. The role of patient care teams in chronic disease management. *BMJ*. 2000;320:569-572.

5. Bodenheimer T, Berry-Millett R. Follow the money: Controlling expenditures by improving care for patients needing costly services. *N Engl Med*. 2009;361:1521-1523.

6. Boult C, Karm L, Groves C. Improving chronic care: The Guided Care model. *Permanente J*. 2008;12: 50-54.

7. Unützer J, Katon WJ, Callahan CM, et al. Collaborative care management of late-life depression in the primary care setting: A randomized controlled trial. *JAMA*. 2002;288:2836-2845.

8. Unützer J, Katon WJ, Callahan CM, et al. Depression treatment in a sample of 1,801 depressed older adults in primary care. *J Am Geriatr Soc*. 2003;51:505-514.

9. Boult C, Reider L, Frey K, et al. Back to the future. Early effects of "Guided Care" on the quality of health care for multimorbid older persons: A cluster-randomized controlled trial. *J Gerontol Med Sci*. 2008;63A:321-327.

10. Fulmer T, Hyer K, Flaherty E. Geriatric interdisciplinary team training: Program results. *J Aging Health*. 2005;17:443-470.

11. Hyer K, Skinner JH, Kane R, et al. Using scripted video to assess interdisciplinary team effectiveness training outcome. *Gerontol Geriatr Ed*. 2003;24:75-92.

12. Wikipedia (online). Patient Portals. http:// en.wikipedia.org/wiki/Patient_portal. Accessed April 26, 2010.

13. Hirth V, Baskins J, Dever-Bumba M. Program of All-Inclusive Care (PACE): Past, present, and future. *J Am Med Dir Assn*. 2009;10: 155-160.

14. Tuckman BW. Developmental sequence in small groups. *Psychol Bull*. 1965;63:384-399.

POST-TEST

1. **Name the four sequential phases of team development.**
   A. Forming, storming, norming, performing
   B. Forming, norming, storming, performing
   C. Forming, storming, performing, leaving
   D. Forming, norming, storming, leaving

2. **Which of the following BEST captures the elements of team structure?**
   A. Frequency and regularity of physician-led team meeting
   B. Physical proximity of members, size of team, setting of team/patient encounters
   C. Audit mechanism for team outcomes and regular review of performance
   D. Purpose of the team, electronic medical record

3. **Which of the following best describes the elements of team process?**
   A. Communication processes, duration and intensity of patient/team interaction, establishment of meeting goals and objectives, and audit of team outcomes
   B. Team size, frequency and regularity of team meeting, physical proximity of team members, objectives, and audit of team outcomes
   C. Purpose of team, role of patient, communication processes, and audit of team outcomes
   D. Communication processes, frequency and regularity of team meeting, establishment of meeting goals and objectives, and audit of team outcomes

ANSWERS TO PRE-TEST

1. D
2. B
3. C

ANSWERS TO POST-TEST

1. A
2. B
3. D

20

Geriatric Consultation Services

Lisa M. Walke, MD

Maria Maiaroto, APRN

● **LEARNING OBJECTIVES**

1. Describe the objective and process of comprehensive geriatric assessment.
2. Compare and contrast geriatric consultation services, geriatric evaluation and management clinics, and geriatric evaluation units.
3. Explain the demonstrated benefits of a geriatrics-surgery co-management model of care.
4. Discuss the "ten commandments of effective consultation" and how they may be implemented.
5. Discuss the factors that influence the implementation of geriatric consultation services recommendations.

PRE-TEST

1. **Comprehensive geriatric assessment:**
   A. Is only beneficial when utilized in a hospital unit
   B. Focuses on the problems of robust older adults
   C. Seeks to identify and remediate the causes and effects of disability
   D. Is completed by the multidisciplinary team without input from the patient and/or caregivers

2. **The geriatric-surgery co-management model of care:**
   A. Has been utilized in several countries outside the United States
   B. Results in the duplication of services
   C. Does not improve outcomes for surgical patients
   D. Is effective even if communication between the disciplines is poor

3. **Which of the following is NOT a commandment of effective consultation?**
   A. Establish the urgency of the consult.
   B. Reflect in detail the data documented in the patient chart.
   C. Provide contingency plans and discuss their execution.
   D. Seek direct contact with the primary provider.

INTRODUCTION

Geriatric consultation services present the key principles of geriatrics care to non-geriatric primary providers via consultation. Similar to other consultation services, geriatric consultation services typically address a specific question presented by the requesting physician. However, unlike many other consultation services, geriatric consultation services utilize a multidisciplinary team approach similar to that employed on specialized geriatric units. While the specialties of the providers may vary across settings, consultation services uniformly include a geriatric physician and nurse (typically an advanced practice nurse); social workers, physical therapists, discharge coordinators, and clinical pharmacists may also be members of the team.

Geriatric consultation services are usually requested when an older adult is at risk for, or is experiencing, a condition that falls within the realm of geriatrics expertise. More specifically, geriatric consultation may be requested for persons with a geriatric syndrome (such as delirium, failure to thrive, or falls), a condition that increases in prevalence with age (such as dementia, decreased driving abilities, or polypharmacy), or for whom there are questions regarding the most appropriate living situation. Geriatric consultation is also increasingly being requested preoperatively for older surgical candidates. For these individuals, the goal is to identify and/or manage conditions that are present prior to surgery that may affect post-surgical outcomes. Regardless of the impetus for a geriatrics consultation request, the goal remains the same: to optimize outcomes through the utilization of a whole person, patient-centered approach.

Although the objective of geriatric consultation services remains constant across settings, the delivery of these services may vary substantially. Geriatric consultation may be provided in an ambulatory clinic, acute care facility, subacute facility, or in the home. Accordingly, the focus of geriatric consultation services may range from maintaining functional independence, to managing geriatric syndromes, to determining decision-making capacity. Moreover, geriatric consultation may be limited to a geriatrician acting alone or may involve multiple disciplines acting in concert; services may be provided in a single setting (such as a clinic) or wherever a need exists (via a mobile team).

COMPREHENSIVE GERIATRIC ASSESSMENT

A cornerstone of geriatric consultation services is the comprehensive geriatric assessment. Comprehensive geriatric assessment, as defined by the National Institutes of Health Consensus Conference on Geriatric Assessment Methods for Clinical Decision-Making, is a "multidisciplinary evaluation in which the multiple problems of older persons are uncovered, described, and explained, if possible, and in which the resources and strengths of the person are catalogued, need for services assessed, and a coordinated care plan developed to focus interventions on the person's problems."[1] More specifically, comprehensive geriatric assessment focuses on the "physical, psychosocial, and environmental factors" that influence the well-being of older adults.[2] Ideal candidates for comprehensive geriatric assessment are individuals who have compromised functional status and/or are at risk for functional decline or institutionalization.

The benefits of comprehensive geriatric assessment have varied according to site (hospital versus ambulatory clinic) and geriatrician role (primary provider vs. consultant); overall results of comprehensive geriatric assessment have been mixed. Some studies have demonstrated that older patients who receive care on specialized Geriatric Evaluation Units have improved outcomes compared with patients who receive "usual" care. In one study, older patients who were randomized to a geriatric evaluation unit lived longer, had better functional status, had higher morale, and utilized fewer acute care services compared with controls up to 1 year after randomization.[3] A multicenter study demonstrated improvement in health-related quality of life among older hospitalized patients who received care on an inpatient geriatrics unit.[4] One international meta-analysis demonstrated that comprehensive geriatric assessment positively affects mortality, physical and cognitive functional status, and living location.[5] Patients followed in an outpatient geriatric evaluation and management clinic for at least 1 year had improved health perceptions, lower medication use, greater social activity, and higher life satisfaction compared with persons receiving standard care.[6] These results were confirmed by a population-based study that demonstrated geriatric evaluation and management clinic participants had less functional deterioration, depression, health-related physical restrictions, and home health care service utilization than nonparticipants; these benefits persisted for up to 18 months after randomization.[7] Yet these studies also demonstrated no improvement in survival,[4] total number of hospitalizations,[6] or cost saving.[4,7]

GERIATRIC CONSULTATION SERVICES

Geriatrics consultation services seek to replicate the positive benefits demonstrated by geriatric evaluation units and geriatric evaluation and management clinics by utilizing similar methods. However, much like studies regarding specialized geriatric settings, geriatrics consultation services studies have demonstrated mixed results. Some investigations have shown geriatrics consultation services to be of no benefit compared with usual care.[8,9] Other studies have demonstrated improvements in mental status, lower medication utilization at discharge, and lower mortality for acute care patients[10,11]; temporary cognitive improvements[12] and decreased use of potentially inappropriate medications[13] have been demonstrated for ambulatory clinic patients.

GERIATRICS-SURGERY CO-MANAGEMENT MODEL OF CARE

In a co-management model, two services share responsibility and primary management for a panel of patients. Tasks such as note writing, medication ordering, and discharge paperwork are prospectively designated to one of the services in order to prevent tasks from being duplicated or inadvertently overlooked. Most importantly, frequent communication is essential if a co-management model is to be a success.

Various hospitals outside of the United States have utilized a combined geriatrics-surgery co-management care model for several years. In one study, a collaboration of surgeons and geriatricians in Japan used the functional and cognitive components of comprehensive geriatric assessment to predict which thoracic surgery patients were at highest risk for postoperative complications.[14] In several countries co-management between geriatrics and orthopedic surgery has resulted in reduced hospital complications, length of stay, readmission rates, mortality, cost, and acuity of care needs at discharge; better function, patient and provider satisfaction have also been demonstrated.[15] Recently some hospitals in the United States have implemented similar models.

Comprehensive geriatric assessment is a common component of co-management care models applied to patients scheduled for elective surgery. Additionally, several co-management studies have demonstrated improved patient outcomes when comprehensive geriatric assessment is utilized. In one investigation, older patients who had comprehensive geriatric assessment as part of a co-management model had shorter hospitalizations (11.5 vs. 15.8 days) and fewer delayed discharges (24.1% vs. 70.4%).[16] In another study, older hip fracture patients who were assessed by the geriatrics service within 24 hours of admission and subsequently co-managed by geriatrics and orthopedic surgery throughout the remainder of their hospitalization, had lower rates of delirium (relative risk = 0.64) and severe delirium (relative risk = 0.4) compared with patients who received usual care.[17] A different geriatrics-orthopedic co-management team demonstrated lower complication rates, lower readmission rates, decreased length of stay, and lower than expected mortality for their cohort of patients.[15] These investigations suggest that patient co-management may be an effective means to improve postoperative outcomes for older adults.

PRINCIPLES OF CONSULTATION

Not surprisingly, the relationship between consultant and primary physician is central to the effectiveness of any consultation service. Even the most comprehensive recommendations will be of no benefit to patients if they are not implemented by the primary team. In recognition of this fact, Goldman and associates published the "Ten Commandments for Effective Consultations" in 1983.[18] Their intent was to establish guidelines that would standardize and strengthen communications between internists and subspecialists. Salerno and colleagues recently updated the recommendations to ensure they remain pertinent for consultants today.[19] The revised commandments are listed in Table 20–1.

● **TABLE 20–1** Modified Ten Commandments for Effective Consultations

Commandment	Meaning
1. Determine your customer	As the requesting physician how you can best help them if a specific question is not obvious: they may want co-management.
2. Establish urgency	The consultant must determine whether the consultation is emergent, urgent, or elective.
3. Look for yourself	Consultants are most effective when they are willing to gather data on their own.
4. Be as brief as appropriate	The consultant need not repeat in full detail the data that were already recorded.
5. Be specific, thorough, and descend from thy ivory tower to help when requested	Leave as many specific recommendations as needed to answer the consult but ask the requesting physician if he or she needs help with order writing.
6. Provide contingency plans and discuss their execution	Consultants should anticipate potential problems, document contingency plans, and provide a 24-h point of contact to help execute the plans if requested.
7. Thou may negotiate joint title to thy neighbor's turf	Consultants can and should co-manage any facet of patient care that the requesting physician desires; a frank discussion defining which specialty is responsible for what aspects of patient care is needed.
8. Teach with tact and pragmatism	Judgments on leaving references should be tailored to the requesting physician's specialty, level of training, and urgency of the consult.
9. Talk is essential	There is no substitute for direct personal contact with the primary physician.
10. Follow-up daily	Daily written follow-up is desirable; when the patient's problems are not active, the consultant should discuss signing-off with the requesting physician beforehand.

IMPLEMENTATION OF RECOMMENDATIONS

Several investigations have explored the various components of the consultant–primary provider relationship in order to better understand the critical factors for compliance with recommendations. Interestingly, the components found to be associated with the implementation of geriatrics consultation services recommendations differ according to the level of training of the primary provider and the site of care. When collaborating with physicians-in-training, direct communication was shown to be associated with increased compliance with geriatrics recommendations.[20] Attending hospitalists were more likely to implement geriatrics recommendations that were entered electronically via a computerized provider order entry system. An electronic medical record used in a pilot investigation by Were and colleagues alerted hospitalists to review, modify, delete, or approve consultant orders. In their investigation, the implementation rate for recommendations improved significantly, from 59% to 78%, after the initiation of electronic consultant recommended orders.[21]

Outside of the hospital setting, the factors that prompt primary care providers to enact recommendations differ. Attending physicians providing care to community-dwelling older adults were more likely to implement geriatrics consultation services recommendations for patients enrolled in a health maintenance organization.[22] Recommendations labeled "most important" by the geriatric consultant were also more likely to be implemented by attending physicians in the community.[22] A similar study found that three physician-related factors—perceived potential legal liability if recommendations were ignored, estimated cost-effectiveness of the recommendation, and gender of the primary provider (eg, female)—were significantly associated with implementation of geriatric consultative service recommendations.[23]

Arguably, the determinants most critical to the implementation of geriatrics consultation services recommendations are patient preference and adherence. Patient request for the implementation of comprehensive geriatric assessment recommendations has been found to be the most significant predictor of primary physician compliance.[23] Additionally, patient–primary physician concordance has been shown to be a significant determinant of physician implementation of comprehensive geriatric assessment recommendations; concordance is also associated with higher patient adherence.[24]

● COST OF SPECIALIZED GERIATRICS CARE

Few studies have examined the cost of specialized geriatrics care. One study compared the cost of geriatric evaluation unit care with acute care for older patients and found geriatric evaluation unit care to be approximately $5000 less.[3] In another study, the cost of screening, testing, and professional services in an outpatient geriatric evaluation and management clinic was found to be $1350 per person.[7]

Geriatric consultants contribute to the care of older adults in a variety of settings. The cases that follow are representative of the role played and recommendations provided by geriatrics consultation services in both acute care and ambulatory care settings.

CASE PRESENTATION 1: A PUZZLING DIAGNOSIS?

Pertinent History

Mrs. M. is a 77-year-old woman who was admitted from the Emergency Department after being brought in by her nephew for evaluation of worsening fatigue. Her primary medical team is puzzled regarding her diagnosis, and is requesting a geriatrics consultation for a second opinion. Due to the urgent nature of the consultation request, you see Mrs. M. the morning after her admission.

You obtain the following information from Mrs. M. during your interview. Her energy level has been low for a few weeks. She and her husband used to be very active in the community until her husband's stroke 3 months ago. Now she rarely leaves the house except for her daily visits to her husband, who resides in a long-term care facility. She used to cook elaborate meals when her husband lived at home; since living alone, she has felt less motivated to do so. She has lost 10 pounds in the past 3 months. Her gait has become more unsteady. Last month she fell but did not sustain any injuries.

Physical Examination

Her vital signs are: blood pressure (BP) 124/76, heart rate (HR) 72 (supine), BP 100/70, HR 70 (standing), respiratory rate 16, temperature 98.8°F (37.1°C), height 66 inches (168 cm), weight 125 lbs (56.8 kg), body mass index 20.2. Her general physical examination is within normal limits. You instruct her on how to perform a Timed Get-Up-and-Go Test; she is unable to rise from her chair without the use of the armrests. Even with the use of the armrests, it takes her two attempts to rise. She ambulates with a normal stride length and cadence with mild path deviation. She takes multiple steps to turn and appears mildly unsteady. It takes her 15 seconds to walk 10 feet (3.05 m), turn around, and return to the chair without the use of an assistive device (normal is less than 10 seconds).

Testing

On laboratory testing her hematocrit and vitamin B_{12} levels are low-normal. On cognitive testing she recalled two out of three words on immediate recall. Her score on the St. Louis University Mental Status Exam[25] was 26 of a possible 30 points. Of note, she was able to draw a clock demonstrating the time of 10 minutes after 11 (11:10) with only minor deficits. She expressed depressive symptoms on 8 questions of the 15-item Geriatric Depression Scale.[26] Her score on the Mini-Nutritional Assessment[27] was 4 (maximum score is 14; a score ≤ 11 is concerning for malnutrition).

Assessment

Due to her change in sleeping habits, decreased socialization, lack of energy, and malnutrition you diagnose Mrs. M. with failure to thrive.

Recommendations

Since you were asked to provide a secondary opinion and not to co-manage Mrs. M. with the medical team, the decision whether or not to implement your recommendations will be made by the primary team, which consists of a resident, intern, and service attending. You recall that direct communication with physicians-in-training is associated with improved compliance with geriatrics recommendations. Therefore, you page the intern to discuss the following recommendations; they will also be placed in Mrs. M.'s chart. The recommendations section of your geriatrics consultation note follows:

1. Initiate treatment for depression. Serotonin selective reuptake inhibitors are first-line treatment for depression in older adults; it may take 4 to 8 weeks for their effects to be demonstrated. Antidepressants are a known contributor to falls. However, for Mrs. M. the benefits of antidepressant medication likely outweigh the risks. Recommend citalopram 10 mg daily. If more immediate results are desired, recommend adding methylphenidate 5 mg at 6 AM and 12 PM.

2. Gait instability/history of falls: Given the subjective history and objective gait assessment, further evaluation is warranted. Request physical therapy consultation for balance and gait assessment and lower extremity strengthening.

3. Malnutrition: In light of her history and Mini-Nutritional Assessment score, an intervention is appropriate. Request a nutritionist consultation for assessment of the appropriateness of nutritional supplementation.

4. Disposition planning: Treatment for depression, gait instability, and malnutrition will all likely need to be continued after her discharge from the hospital. Increased socialization when back in the community would likely be beneficial as well. Recommend: Mrs. M. and her nephew should visit the following senior centers to see which would be the best match for Mrs. M.

Thank you for this consult. We will continue to follow Mrs. M. with you. The geriatrics consultation service may be reached via pager or telephone number listed.

An outline of a full geriatrics consultation note can be found in Figure 20–1.

Reason for Consult:
History of Present Illness:
Past Medical History:
Medications:
Allergies:
Social History:
Geriatric Review of Systems:
Physical Examination:
Cognitive Assessment:
Pertinent Data:
Impressions:
Recommendations:

FIGURE 20–1. Sample geriatrics consultation note template.

Discussion

This case highlights the role of geriatrics consultation in an acute care setting. Using Goldman's ten commandments (Table 20–1) as a guide, we can break down the mechanics of this case. In this example, the role of the consultation service is clearly delineated; consultation is being requested to assist the primary team with the acute management of Mrs. M. Since Mrs. M. did not need imminent attention, this consult can be classified as urgent. Specific recommendations with contingency plans were provided but since comanagement was not requested, the actual implementation of the recommendations with be left to the discretion of the primary team. Personal interaction with the primary team was pursued as a means of clarifying any confusion regarding the recommendations and as a means of opening the lines of communication.

Since Mrs. M.'s condition is not emergent, her recommendations were listed in the order by which they could be initiated; recommendations that were future-minded (such as discharge planning) were included last. For persons with more urgent management issues, recommendations should be listed in the order of importance as determined by the expected onset of the desired effect.

Mrs. M. would likely only require daily follow-up for a short duration of time given the expected activeness of her issues. However, since the recommendations include the initiation of two new interventions (antidepressants and physical therapy), if these recommendations are followed, geriatric consultation services should remain actively involved until it is clear that Mrs. M. is tolerating these interventions without adverse effects.

CASE PRESENTATION 2: AN ISSUE WITH DRIVING
Pertinent History

Mr. Z. is an 85-year-old man who was referred to the geriatric consultation clinic for a driving evaluation at his daughter's request. Mr. Z. feels he is a good driver. He drives primarily on local roads during the day but does drive at night or on the highway "when the need arises."

A collaborative geriatric review of systems was performed privately with Mr. Z.'s daughter. Since she was concerned about his driving, she accompanied her father as he drove to the store. She observed that he drove below the speed limit, got angry at several other drivers, turned from inappropriate lanes, and wove between lanes of traffic without indicating. As such, his daughter has "passenger panic" and does not allow her children to ride with Mr. Z.

Review of systems reveals sensory deficits. Despite being prescribed glasses, Mr. Z. does not wear them while driving because he has "no difficulty seeing." He was diagnosed with sensorineural hearing loss several years ago but does not wear his hearing aids because they "itch." He also complains of frequent neck discomfort, which he attributes to arthritis. He has fallen twice in the past year, once after tripping over his dog and another time after slipping on an icy sidewalk.

Physical Examination

To further assess Mr. Z.'s ability to safely operate a motor vehicle, you complete the American Medical Association Assessment of Driving-Related Skills (ADReS) (Figure 20–2).[28] Apart from the deficiencies noted in the figure, other areas were within normal limits.

In addition you note the following physical findings. Vibratory sense: decreased at the ankles and toes. Mobility: mild bilateral upper extremity cogwheeling right > left.

Testing

Mini-Mental State Examination: 26/30 (minus 1 point for not knowing the day of week, minus 1 point on recall (he improved with cueing), minus 1 point on phrase repetition (dropped an "s" twice), minus 1 for design copying (drew two 4-sided objects with some overlap). On judgment testing when asked "If a ball rolled in front of your car, what would you be concerned about?" Mr. Z. replied "I would stop right away so I don't damage my car." Geriatric Depression Scale (GDS) score: 1/15.

Assessment

Objective testing suggests Mr. Z. has experienced mild cognitive decline and has executive dysfunction. The subjective history provided by his daughter combined with his objective testing support the need for a repeat driving evaluation.

Recommendations

Mr. Z.'s Mini-Mental State Examination score was of borderline significance (≤ 23/30 is significant) for correlating with a failed road test and the increased likelihood of having a first-time crash[29]; several additional components of his objective testing, including his judgment, were clearly deficient. As such, you discuss the following recommendations with the patient and his daughter. One, Mr. Z. should consider having a formal driver rehabilitation specialist on-the-road driving assessment to assess driving safety and whether he has rehabilitation potential. Two, if he performs poorly on his driving evaluation, the geriatric social worker

and driving rehabilitation specialist will help Mr. Z. and his daughter discuss transportation alternatives so that he may retain his independence. Three, Mr. Z.'s daughter and primary care physician should monitor Mr. Z. closely for signs of depression and isolation, if his license is eventually revoked.

Although initially resistant, after discussion with his daughter Mr. Z. agreed to proceed with a formal driving evaluation.

Discussion

Geriatric consultation services are frequently requested in an ambulatory clinic. When available, obtaining a collaborative history from an informed caregiver can be extremely useful, especially when topics that may make the patient defensive (such as driving abilities, question of poor safety awareness, possible depression) are discussed.

Referring back to Goldman's ten commandments of consultation (Table 20–1), this consult would be considered elective rather than emergent (meaning the patient is in imminent danger of suffering or causing harm) or urgent (meaning immediate treatment decisions are dependent upon Geriatrics input). Mr. Z. represents a case when geriatric consultation services are asked to assume the primary management for a specific issue or question. Nonetheless, direct communication with the primary provider is important to ensure the patient receives consistent information from all providers.

A follow-up appointment should be scheduled with patients and their family members shortly after the results of any recommended objective testing (such as on-the-road testing, neuropsychological testing, and radiologic evaluation) become available. This will assure that all parties—patient, caregivers, and providers—understand the additional information received and how that information will modify the previously discussed recommendations.

CASE PRESENTATION 3: RISK FOR DELIRIUM

Pertinent History and Physical Examination

Mr. V. is a 72-year-old man who is scheduled for an elective right hemicolectomy for colon cancer; his cancer was found during a routine colonoscopy. After the decision was made to proceed with a surgical resection, he is evaluated by the geriatric consultation service in the surgery preoperative clinic.

Mr. V. is asymptomatic with the exception of constipation. He has no functional limitations. He has at least two drinks with alcohol daily, usually with lunch and dinner. His physical examination is within normal limits.

Assessing Driving Related Skills (ADReS) Score Sheet

Patients's name: _Mr. Z_   Date: _____

1. **Visual fields**: Shade in any areas of deficit.

None

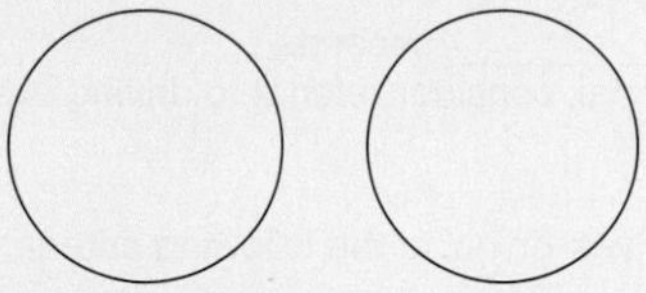

Patient's   L   R

2. **Visual acuity**: _20/40_ OU _20/30_ OS _20/40_ OD (right)
   Was the patient wearing corrective lenses? If yes, please specify: _No_
   If either eye acuity worse than 20/40, consider referral to ophthalmologist.

3. **Rapid pace walk:** _8_ seconds
   (>10 secs, abnormal and consider referral for driving evaluation and/or evaluation of gait disorder) Was this performed with a walker or cane? If yes, please specify: _____

4. **Range of motion:** Specify 'Within Normal Limits' or 'Not WNL,' If not WNL, describe.

	Right	Left
Neck rotation	Not WNL ~ 45°	Not WNL ~ 45°
Finger curl	Within normal Limits	Within normal Limits
Shoulder and elbow flexion	\\	\\
Ankle plantar flexion	Not WNL Slight ↓	Not WNL Slight ↓
Ankle dorsiflexion	Not WNL Slight ↓	Not WNL Slight ↓

Plan for any deficiencies (consider referral to OT/PT, address pain management, if indicated, and/or referral to driving clinic for vehicle modification)

5. **Motor strength:** Provide a score on a scale of 0–5.

	Right	Left
Shoulder adduction	5	5
Shoulder abduction	5	5
Shoulder flexion	5	5
Wrist flexion	5	5
Wrist extension	5	5
Hand grip	5	5
Hip flexion	4	4
Hip extension	4	4
Ankle dorsiflexion	4	4
Ankle plantar flexion	4	4

Plan for any deficiencies: (consider referral to OT/PT or driving clinic for vehicle modification)

FIGURE 20–2. American Medical Association Assessment of Driving-Related Skills (ADReS).

ADReS Score Sheet (continued)

Patients's name: _____ Mr. Z _____ Date: _____

6. **Trail-Making Test, Part B:** ___205___ seconds
(score greater than 180 secs abnormal, consider referral to driving evaluation clinic and/or work-up for cognitive/visual/motor impairment)

7. **Clock drawing test:** Please check 'yes' or 'no' to the following criteria.

	Yes	No
Only the numbers 1-12 are included (no duplicates or omissions)	✓	
The numbers are drawn inside the clock circle		✓
The numbers are spaced equally or nearly equally from each other		✓
The numbers are spaced equally or nearly equally from the edge of the circle	✓	
One clock hand correctly points to 2		✓
There are only two clock hands		✓
There are no intrusive marks, writing or hands indicating incorrect time		✓

(any abnormal elements consider referral to driving evaluation clinic and/or work-up for cognitive/visual/ motor impairment)

Assessment/Plan:

1) Mild cognitive decline
2) Mild to moderate executive dysfunction.
3) Safety/judgement may be impaired.

Recommend
1) Driving Rehab Evaluation

FIGURE 20–2. (Continued)

Trail-Making Test, Part B Patients's name: _Mr. Z_ Date: _____

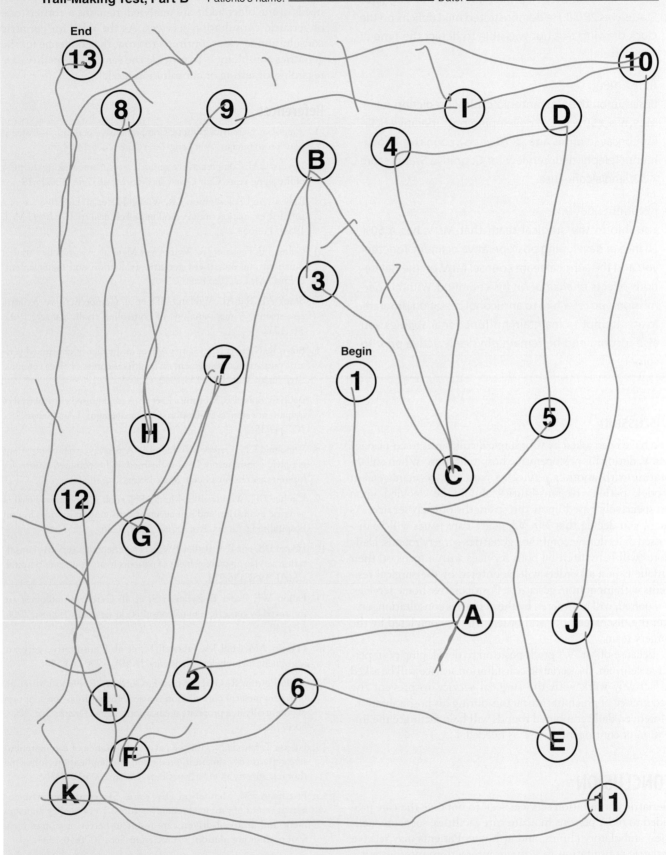

FIGURE 20–2. *(Continued)*

Testing

Mr. V.'s score on the Telephone Interview for Cognitive Status was 28/38. He demonstrated mild deficits on the clock drawing test but was able to depict the time of 1:45 correctly.

Assessment

Based upon the Marcantonio clinical prediction rule,[30] Mr. V. has a 50% risk of developing postoperative delirium because of his age (> 70 years), cognitive impairment (Telephone Interview for Cognitive Status score < 30), and alcohol use.

Recommendations

You inform the surgical team that Mr. V. has a 50% chance of developing postoperative delirium. Together you and the surgical team counsel Mr. V. on the deleterious effects of alcohol on his cognition. With his permission, you refer him to an alcohol cessation program. In an attempt to maintain his functional abilities you also recommend he remain physically active prior to surgery.

Discussion

You have been asked by your surgical colleagues to co-manage Mr. V. during his postoperative hospitalization. When collaborating with another service as part of a co-management model, patient responsibilities should be decided upon prospectively based upon the strengths of each service. As such, you decide that Mr. V.'s acute-care issues will be discussed daily during combined geriatrics-surgery rounds. Daily notes will be written by both services with a focus on their unique issues; all orders will be entered by the surgical residents with input from geriatrics. Postoperative home services, if required, will be ordered by the geriatrics consultation service; the discharge note and orders will be completed by the surgery team.

Because of Mr. V.'s predisposition to developing postoperative delirium, the geriatric consultation service will be asked to actively work with the surgical service to prevent the occurrence of precipitating factors during his hospitalization. Moreover, daily combined rounds will help facilitate the initiation of contingency plans as needed.

CONCLUSION

Geriatric consultation services seek to improve the care provided to older persons in acute care facilities, subacute facilities, ambulatory clinics, and at home. Patients may receive geriatric consultation in a single interaction, intermittently over a period of time, or daily as part of a co-management model of care. While geriatric consultation services are often provided by a multidisciplinary team, the consultation "team"

may also be limited to a single geriatric provider. Regardless of the setting or structure, comprehensive geriatric assessment, a process through which the physical and psychosocial needs of the older adult are analyzed, remains a cornerstone of geriatric consultation services. As the need for geriatric consultation services continues to grow, the challenge for the geriatrics consultant is to provide the same high-quality care regardless of setting or consultation model.

References

1. American Geriatrics Society. Comprehensive geriatric assessment position statement. *Ann Long-Term Care*. 2006;14:34-35.

2. Devons CAJ. Comprehensive geriatric assessment: Making the most of the aging years. *Curr Opin Clin Nutr Metab Care*. 2002;5:19.

3. Rubenstein LZ, Josephson KR, Wieland D, et al. Effectiveness of a geriatric evaluation unit: A randomized clinical trial. *N Engl J Med*. 1984;311:1664.

4. Cohen HJ, Feussner JR, Weinberger M, et al. A controlled trial of inpatient and outpatient geriatric evaluation and management. *N Engl J Med*. 2002;346:905.

5. Stuck AE, Siu AL, Wieland GD, et al. Comprehensive geriatric assessment: A meta-analysis of controlled trials. *Lancet*. 1993; 342:1032.

6. Burns R, Nichols LO, Graney MJ, et al. Impact of continued geriatric outpatient management on health outcomes of older veterans. *Arch Intern Med*. 1995;155:1313.

7. Boult C, Boult LB, Morishita L, et al. A randomized clinical trial of outpatient geriatric evaluation and management. *J Am Geriatr Soc*. 2001;49:351.

8. Winograd CH, Gerety MB, Lai NA. A negative trial of inpatient geriatric consultation: Lessons learned and recommendations for future research. *Arch Intern Med*. 1993;153:2017.

9. Kircher TTJ, Wormstall H, Muuler PH, et al. A randomised trial of geriatric evaluation and management consultation services in frail hospitalized patients. *Age Ageing*. 2007;36:36.

10. Hogan DB, Fox RA, Badley BWD, et al. Effect of a geriatric consultation service on management of patients in an acute care hospital. *CMAJ*. 1987;136:713.

11. Fallon WF, Rader E, Zyzanski S, et al. Geriatric outcomes are improved by geriatric trauma consultation service. *J Trauma*. 2006; 61:1040.

12. Epstein AM, Hall JA, Fretwell M, et al. Consultative geriatric assessment for ambulatory patients. *JAMA*. 1990;263:538.

13. Avila-Beltran R, Garcia-Mayo E, Gutierrez-Robledo LM, et al. Geriatric medical consultation is associated with less prescription of potentially inappropriate medications. *J Am Geriatric Soc*. 2008; 56:1778.

14. Fukuse T, Satoda N, Hijiya K, et al. Importance of a comprehensive geriatric assessment in prediction of complications following thoracic surgery in elderly patients. *Chest*. 2005;127:886.

15. Friedman SM, Mendelson DA, Kates SL, et al. Geriatric co-management of proximal femur fractures: Total quality management and protocol-driven care result in better outcomes for a frail patient population. *J Am Geriatr Soc*. 2008;56:1349.

16. Harari D, Hopper A, Dhesi J, et al. Proactive care of older people undergoing surgery (POPS): Designing, embedding, evaluating and funding a comprehensive geriatric assessment service for older elective surgical patients. *Age Ageing*. 2007;36:190.

17. Marcantonio ER, Flacker JM, Wright RJ, et al. Reducing delirium after hip fracture: A randomized trial. *J Am Geriatr Soc*. 2001;49:516.

18. Goldman L, Lee T, Rudd P. Ten commandments for effective communications. *Arch Intern Med*. 1983;143:1753.

19. Salerno SM, Hurst FP, Halvorson S, et al. Principles of effective consultation: An update for the 21st-century consultant. *Arch Intern Med*. 2007;167:271.

20. Allen CM, Becker PM, McVey LJ, et al. A randomized, controlled clinical trial of a geriatric consultation team: Compliance with recommendations. *JAMA*. 1986;255:2617.

21. Were MC, Abernathy G, Hui SL, et al. Using computerized provider order entry and clinical decision support to improve referring physicians' implementation of consultants' medical recommendations. *J Am Med Inform Assoc*. 2009;16:196.

22. Reuben DB, Maly RC, Hirsch SH, et al. Physician implementation of and patient adherence to recommendations from comprehensive geriatric assessment. *Am J Med*. 1996;100:444.

23. Maly RC, Abrahamse AF, Hirsch SH, et al. What influences physician practice behavior? An interview study of physicians who received consultative geriatric assessment recommendations. *Arch Fam Med*. 1996;5:448.

24. Maly RC, Leake B, Frank JC, et al. Implementation of consultative geriatric recommendations: The role of patient-primary care physician concordance. *J Am Geriatr Soc*. 2002;50:1372.

25. Tariq SH, Tumosa N, Chibnall JT, et al. Comparison of the Saint Louis University Mental Status Examination and the Mini-Mental State Examination for detecting dementia and mild neurocognitive disorder—A pilot study. *Am J Geriatr Psychiatry*. 2006;14:900.

26. Sheik JI, Yesavage JA. Geriatric Depression Scale (GDS): recent evidence and development of a shorter version. *Clin Gerontol*. 1986;5:165.

27. Guizog Y, Lauque S, Vellas BJ. Identifying the elderly at risk for malnutrition: The Mini Nutritional Assessment. *Clin Geriatr Med*. 2002;18:1.

28. Odenheimer GL. The physician's role in assessing driving skills of older patients. *Geriatrics*. 2006;61:14.

29. Sherman FT. Driving: The *ultimate* IADL. *Geriatrics*. 2006;61:9.

30. Marcantonio ER, Goldman L, Mangione CM, et al. A clinical prediction rule for delirium after elective noncardiac surgery. *JAMA*. 1994;271:134.

POST-TEST

1. **Among ambulatory care patients, geriatric consultation services is associated with which of the following?**
   A. Decreased use of potentially inappropriate medications
   B. Decline in cognitive function
   C. Remediable functional limitations
   D. Lower mortality

2. **Primary provider implementation of geriatric consultation services recommendations is positively associated with all of the following EXCEPT:**
   A. Use of a computerized order entry system
   B. Patient enrollment in Medicare
   C. Estimated cost-effectiveness of the recommendation
   D. Gender of the primary care provider

3. **Geriatric–orthopedic surgery co-management models of care are NOT associated with:**
   A. Lower rates of delirium
   B. Lower readmission rates
   C. Mortality rates less than ½ the expected
   D. Reduced patient–provider contact

ANSWERS TO PRE-TEST

1. C
2. A
3. B

ANSWERS TO POST-TEST

1. A
2. B
3. D

21

Perioperative Care of the Older Adult

James T. Birch, Jr., MD

Brian Leo, MD

Daniel Swagerty, MD, MPH

● **LEARNING OBJECTIVES**

1. Describe the impact and influence of the aging process on surgical risk and outcome.
2. Explain preoperative screening (cardiac, anesthesia, pulmonary, and neuropsychiatric) and how evaluation of each is important for risk stratification.
3. Compare and contrast high-, intermediate-. and low-risk procedures.
4. Discuss anticoagulation management in the preoperative period.
5. Describe assessment and management of the geriatric patient in the intra-operative and postoperative periods.

PRE-TEST

1. **Which of the following is the LEAST potent stand-alone risk factor for geriatric surgical patients?**

   A. Age

   B. Age-related physiologic changes

   C. Presence of chronic disease

   D. Functional status

2. **The leading cause of perioperative death in older adults is:**

   A. Falls/injury

   B. Infection

   C. Postoperative cardiac events

   D. Anesthesia complications

3. **Medications that should be discontinued within 7 days prior to elective surgery include all of the following EXCEPT:**

   A. Aspirin products

   B. Beta-blockers

   C. Estrogen

   D. Hypoglycemic agents

CASE PRESENTATION: EVALUATION OF A MASS

Mr. J.R. is a 78-year-old Hispanic male who presents to your Geriatric Medicine Clinic to establish care. He is asymptomatic and has no complaints of pain or discomfort. He is accompanied by his wife of 42 years.

He has a past medical history of hypertension, osteoarthritis, and COPD. Previous surgeries include appendectomy, inguinal hernia repair, ORIF left elbow, right knee replacement, bilateral cataract extraction, and intraocular lens replacement.

Current medications include lisinopril 20 mg PO daily for hypertension, hydrochlorothiazide 12.5 mg PO once daily for hypertension, calcium/vitamin D 600 mg/400 IU one tablet PO BID, ASA 81 mg PO once daily, and acetaminophen 500 mg 2 tablets up to TID PRN back and leg pain. He is allergic to sulfa drugs, penicillin, and latex.

He was last employed as a laborer for an automobile assembly plant, and is now retired for the past 12 years. He smoked cigarettes, 1.5 packs per day for about 40 years, and quit about 15 years ago. He admits consumption of alcoholic beverages socially but has negative responses to the CAGE questionnaire. J.R. is independent in all ADLs and IADLs; he pays the household bills and does handyman repairs as needed. ROS is negative except for occasional joint pain in hips and knees.

On examination, blood pressure is 134/72, pulse 76, respirations 20, temperature 98.2°F, and pulse oximetry 96% on room air. Other pertinent positive and negative physical findings include:

HEENT:	Bilateral arcus senilis, fair dentition; a few caries.
Neck:	No adenopathy, tenderness, rigidity, thyromegaly, or carotid bruits.
Lungs:	Clear to auscultation.
Heart:	Regular rhythm, with a grade II/VI systolic murmur in the pulmonic area; S4 gallop is present; PMI is nondisplaced.
Abdomen:	Mildly obese above plane, well-healed surgical scar in the left lower quadrant, smaller healed scar in the right lower quadrant; soft, no tenderness to palpation, no palpable masses or organomegaly; bowel sounds are normal.
Extremities:	8 × 5 cm, soft, nontender, slightly mobile mass at the distal-medial aspect of the proximal left lower extremity (above the knee). The distal border of the mass is nonpalpable. No other deformities or abnormalities noted. Peripheral pulses are normal. No edema.
Neurological:	Cranial nerves intact; speech is clear; no gait abnormality. Oriented to time, place, and person. No focal motor deficits.

The office visit assessment is:

- Large soft-tissue mass on proximal left lower extremity
- Hypertension—controlled
- Osteoarthritis
- COPD

Mr. J.R. is referred to an orthopedic surgeon for further evaluation of the mass on the right lower extremity. An MRI demonstrated a large lesion just deep to and involving a portion of distal sartorius. It appears to be well circumscribed without invasion into other tissues and does not have other characteristics suggestive of malignancy; it is felt by the radiologist most likely to be benign. A needle biopsy in the orthopedist's office under local anesthesia returns without any diagnostic cells. However, due to the large size of the lesion, the fact that according to the patient, the lesion has been enlarging, and concern by the surgeon of the possibility of a sarcomatous tumor, elective surgical removal of the mass is recommended.

● SURGERY AND AGING

Half of individuals over the age of 65 will have a major surgical procedure during their lifetime. Approximately one-third of the 44 million surgical procedures performed in the United States every year involve patients over the age of 65.[1] In hospitals, an estimated 40% of older adult patients are on surgical services. The fastest growing segment of the US population consists of those individuals over the age of 65, and is anticipated to represent 20% of the US population by the year 2030 (currently ~13%). Having knowledge of these trends, an increase in the number of older adults presenting for surgery should be anticipated along with an increase in the number of perioperative complications. However, age is less of a risk factor than the age-associated physiologic changes and the impact of chronic diseases.[2]

The physiology of the aging process makes the geriatric patient less able to compensate for perioperative stress, even when the patient is fit and without coexisting disease. Altered body composition, diminished kidney function, decreased enzyme activity, and decreased liver blood flow all contribute to changes in the pharmacokinetics of drugs. The volume of distribution of lipid-soluble drugs is increased because of the higher percentage of body fat and the lower albumin levels that occur with aging. Decreased protein binding, decreased total body water, and decreased cardiac output result in slower redistribution of drugs. There is also an increase in brain sensitivity to drugs.

Clearance is decreased as a result of the age-related decreases in hepatic blood flow, hepatic mass, and glomerular filtration rate. See Chapter 13 for considerations prior to prescribing medications.

Most healthy older adult patients have no noticeable alteration of baseline function in any number of systems. Cardiac and vascular stiffening, gradual decrement in numbers of cilia and ciliary function, stiffening of the thoracic cage, decreased thermoregulation, and a number of physiologic changes in the brain make hypotension, hypoxia, hypercarbia, low cardiac output, altered fluid regulation, postoperative pneumonia, and postoperative cognitive changes more likely to occur in the older population. The physiologic changes related to aging also make it more difficult for the patient to tolerate the inevitable shifts in intravascular volume that accompany surgical procedures. Surgical trauma shifts fluid into the extravascular compartment ("third spacing" of fluid). Inadequate volume replacement can cause hypovolemia and decreased cardiac output.

The aging process is extremely variable from person to person, and even within a person not all organ systems age at the same rate. Furthermore, older individuals may have one or several chronic conditions that might impact perioperative care either directly or indirectly through the medications used to treat those conditions. Close and meticulous attention to the special needs of the geriatric population will positively influence the quality of care that is given. Reduction of complication rates and mortality should be the goal of every practitioner who renders care to this vulnerable population.

● SURGERY IN THE ELDERLY AND COMPLICATION RATES

The increased rate of surgical complications in older adults correlates with prevalence of chronic disease and increased need for emergency surgery. Emergency surgery increases the complication rates two to four times in the elderly. Emergency surgery causes 7.8% mortality in patients at or over 90 years of age compared to 0.6% after elective surgery.[3]

The interaction of co-morbidities (eg, diabetes, heart disease, hypertension, chronic lung disease, and arthritis) and the inevitable physiologic changes that occur with aging combine to increase the perioperative complication rates in the elderly. The higher rates of complications typically occur with abdominal, thoracic, and aortic surgery. In a study of abdominal operations, the mortality rate for patients aged 80 to 84 years was 3%; it increased to 9% for patients aged 85 to 89; and it was even higher at 25% for patients older than 90.[4]

CASE PRESENTATION (continued)

The patient returns to your office about 2 weeks later for preoperative clearance. In the interim he has had pulmonary function tests performed, which show mild to moderate COPD. His arterial blood gas shows a room air oxygen of 94 mm Hg and no CO_2 retention. This time on exam, you notice he has an irregular heart rhythm. He is asymptomatic and denies chest pain, palpitations, diaphoresis, dyspnea, or decreased exercise tolerance. There are no other interval changes in the physical examination. An EKG done in the office demonstrates atrial fibrillation with a heart rate of 96/min. There are no ischemic changes on the EKG. He has never had a cardiac stress test or cardiac imaging. He is started on metoprolol 12.5 mg once daily and coumadin 5 mg daily with an INR scheduled in 1 week. Consultation with cardiology is requested for an echocardiogram, consideration for cardioversion of atrial fibrillation, and medical clearance for surgery.

● THE PREOPERATIVE PERIOD

Preoperative Care

Many older adults have Do-Not-Resuscitate (DNR) orders in place. Surgery should not be denied to patients with an existing DNR order.[2] There are institutions that might require suspension of DNR orders during surgery, operating under the premise that anesthesia is an iatrogenic condition and cardiac arrest in this situation has the potential to be reversed. Supporters of this approach argue that this is not the same as allowing a disease state to take its natural course. Of utmost importance is the fact that the primary care physician, the surgeon, the anesthesiologist, and the patient should collectively have a dialogue about how the DNR order is to be carried out during the perioperative period.[2]

Functional Assessment and Its Relationship to Surgical Outcomes

One can age without frailty or can be frail without being old. The concept of frailty is often associated with decreased muscle mass, weight loss with or without malnutrition or undernutrition, decreased strength, decreased exercise tolerance, slowed motor performance and longer reaction time, decreased balance and proprioception, altered gait, low physical activity, and vulnerability to stressors.[2] However, frailty does also include the decline in homeostatic regulatory mechanisms, which result in decreased functional reserve or the lack of homeostatic reserve to quickly respond to abrupt physiologic changes. There is still much to learn about the preoperative assessment of patients with varying degrees of frailty and how frailty directly impacts patient outcomes.[2] For more on frailty, please see Chapter 36.

Postoperative cardiovascular events are the leading cause of perioperative death. Older adult patients overall have decreased cardiovascular reserve, although the degree of deficit varies from one patient to another. However, the inability to exercise to a heart rate of at least 100 beats per minute has been associated with increased risk of both cardiac

METS	Activity
● TABLE 21–1	**Estimated Energy Requirements for Various Activities**
1	Sitting quietly, watching television, paying bills
2	Walking, less than 2.0 mph, level ground, cooking a meal
3	Loading/unloading a car, light to medium housework
4	Mowing the lawn, dancing, walking at 4 mph (6.5 km/h), moderate to heavy housework
5	Tennis, doubles
6	Skiing, downhill, moderate effort, general
7	Climbing hills with 0- to 9-pound load
8	Rock or mountain climbing
9	Running, cross country
10	Swimming laps, freestyle, fast, vigorous effort

● TABLE 21–2 **Clinical Predictors of Increased Perioperative Cardiovascular Risk (Myocardial Infarction, Heart Failure, Death)**

Major

Unstable coronary syndromes
- Acute or recent myocardial infarction[a] with evidence of important ischemic risk by clinical symptoms or noninvasive study
- Unstable or severe[b] angina (Canadian class III or IV)[c]

Decompensated heart failure

Significant arrhythmias
- High-grade atrioventricular block
- Symptomatic ventricular arrhythmias in the presence of underlying heart disease
- Supraventricular arrhythmias with uncontrolled ventricular rate

Severe valvular disease

Intermediate

Mild angina pectoris (Canadian class I or II)
Previous myocardial infarction by history or pathologic Q-waves
Compensated or prior heart failure
Diabetes mellitus (particularly insulin-dependent)
Renal insufficiency

Minor

Advanced age
Abnormal EKG (left ventricular hypertrophy, left bundle-branch block, ST-T abnormalities)
Rhythm other than sinus (eg, atrial fibrillation)
Low functional capacity (eg, inability to climb one flight of stairs with a bag of groceries)
History of stroke
Uncontrolled systemic hypertension

[a]*The American College of Cardiology National Database Library defines recent MI as greater than 7 days but less than or equal to 1 month (30 days); acute MI is within 7 days.*

[b]*May include "stable" angina in patients who are unusually sedentary.*

[c]*Campeau L. Grading of angina pectoris. Circulation. 1976;54:522-523.*

and pulmonary complications with surgery.[2] The general assessment of functional capacity is based on energy expenditure and is frequently expressed in METs (metabolic equivalents). Patients who are assessed as reaching a maximum of less than 4 METs are considered to have poor functional capacity. Those who can achieve ≥ 4 METs are assessed to have moderate or excellent functional capacity.[5,6] Table 21–1 lists METs expended based on physical activity.

Risk Stratification

Due to the multitude of physiologic changes that occur in older adults, there is a higher risk of perioperative complications. Cardiovascular problems, respiratory compromise, and neuropsychiatric changes represent the most common and most serious complications of surgical treatment of the older adult.[5] Likewise, preoperative screening and evaluation are important for risk stratification and placement of interventions that, whenever possible, might significantly reduce the risk of these complications as well as reduce perioperative morbidity and mortality. The strongest predictors of adverse cardiac outcomes (myocardial infarction [MI], congestive heart failure [CHF], and death) are also the presence or history of recent MI, uncompensated CHF, unstable ischemic heart disease, certain rhythm disorders, and severe valvular disease.[4]

Cardiac Risk Stratification

The American Heart Association and the American College of Cardiology have collectively developed a useful guideline for risk stratification of patients with known or suspected cardiac disease.[6] If there is no need for emergency noncardiac surgery, the patient is assessed as being in one of three groups of clinical predictors (major, intermediate, or minor) for cardiac complications based on the presence of cardiac symptoms, history of previous revascularization procedure, and history of noninvasive screening for coronary artery disease within the previous 5 years (Table 21–2).

Those with major clinical predictors will usually have non-emergent procedures delayed for coronary artery imaging studies or other treatment to reduce cardiac risks. Patients who are assigned the intermediate or minor clinical predictor categories are assessed according to the diagrams in Tables 21–3 and 21–4. Assessment of patients with intermediate and minor clinical predictors follows (with appropriate noninvasive or invasive coronary artery evaluation as indicated). However, more recently, based on retrospective surgical data and meta-analyses, it appears that the risk assessment as advocated by the American Heart Association and the American College of Cardiology, though helpful and accurate for assessing risk, probably results in too many patients going for coronary revascularization procedures prior to noncardiac surgery. The conclusion appears to be that perioperative revascularization does not benefit patients with stable CAD, whether single-vessel or multi-vessel CAD.[7]

As usual with somewhat conflicting recommendations, the clinician is left to use his or her best judgment as to what the most safe and appropriate course of action should be prior to subjecting the patient to noncardiac surgery.

There are also cardiac risks that are related to the type of surgery that is planned for the patient. Certain surgical procedures will cause a predictable amount of coronary and myocardial stress depending on the degree of hemodynamic stress involved with the noncardiac procedure. This is another risk category known as "surgery-specific risk."[6]

● **TABLE 21–3** Assessing Patients with Intermediate Clinical Predictors: ACC and AHA Guidelines for Cardiac Risk Screening[6]

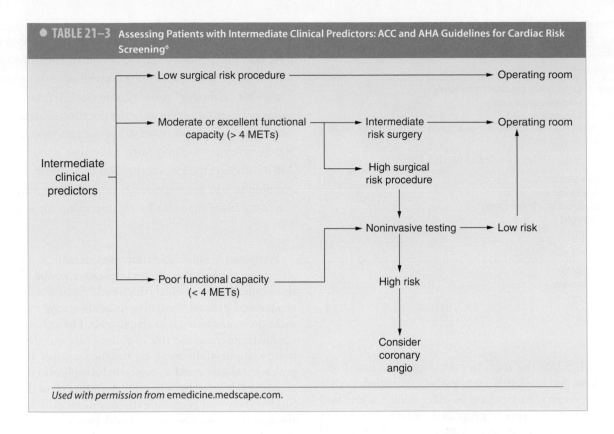

Used with permission from emedicine.medscape.com.

● **TABLE 21–4** Assessing Patients with Minor or No Clinical Predictors: ACC and AHA Guidelines for Cardiac Risk Screening[6]

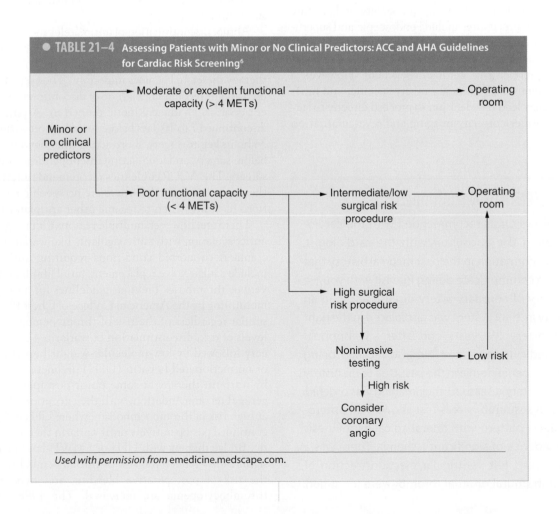

Used with permission from emedicine.medscape.com.

● **TABLE 21–5** Cardiac Risk Stratification for Noncardiac Surgical Procedures

High (Reported Cardiac Risk Often Greater Than 5%)
Emergent major operations, particularly in the elderly
Aortic and other major vascular surgery
Peripheral vascular surgery
Anticipated prolonged surgical procedures associated with large fluid shifts and/or blood loss
Intermediate (Reported Cardiac Risk Generally Less Than 5%)
Carotid endarterectomy
Head and neck surgery
Intraperitoneal and intrathoracic surgery
Orthopedic surgery
Prostate surgery
Low (Reported Cardiac Risk Generally Less Than 1%)
Endoscopic procedures
Superficial procedure
Cataract surgery
Breast surgery

Table 21–5 lists the risk categories organized into high, intermediate, and low levels. High-risk surgery includes major emergency surgery, particularly in older adults; aortic and other major vascular surgery; peripheral vascular surgery; and anticipated prolonged procedures associated with large fluid shifts and/or blood loss. Intermediate-risk procedures include intraperitoneal and intrathoracic surgery, carotid endarterectomy, head and neck surgery, orthopedic surgery, and prostate surgery. Low-risk procedures include endoscopic and superficial procedures, cataract surgery, and breast surgery. Following the steps associated with the risk factors provides a stepwise approach to preoperative cardiac assessment. However, a careful consideration of clinical, surgery-specific, and functional status may lead to a decision to proceed directly to surgery or to consider coronary imaging and revascularization procedures.

CASE PRESENTATION (continued)

Mr. J.R. follows up as recommended with the cardiologist. During the encounter with the cardiologist, he reveals information in the past medical history that he forgot to communicate during his visit with you. He has a history of coronary artery disease and had an angioplasty in 1989. A stent was also placed in the right coronary artery 2½ years ago after an abnormal nuclear medicine stress test. He also recalled being treated for hyperlipidemia in the past. Due to his history of coronary artery disease, further imaging was ordered. An exercise sestamibi stress test showed an antero-apical infarct pattern with lateral apical hypokinesis and no evidence of significant ischemia. There was a mildly reduced left ventricular ejection fraction of 45%. No intramural or atrial thrombi were identified.

An esophageal echocardiogram was not performed. He was subsequently started on diltiazem SR 240 mg once daily for ventricular rate control as well as a statin after his lipid panel results came back. Cardioversion was not performed because the duration of atrial fibrillation was unknown. Warfarin was continued and the dose adjusted to 3 mg once daily with a therapeutic INR. Although the clopidogrel was restarted by the cardiologist, you discontinued it to reduce the risk of an adverse bleeding event for his upcoming surgery.

Preoperative anticoagulation management is a considerable conundrum during the perioperative period. Although this subject has been widely discussed,[8–11] there are not many randomized clinical trials that provide strong evidence to make decision-making less complicated. Throughout the perioperative interval, the risk of thrombosis and thromboembolic complications must be weighed against the risk of prolonged bleeding and its associated complications. Bleeding is not considered to be as life-threatening as stent thrombosis. Studies show that premature discontinuation of antiplatelet therapy is the most significant independent risk factor for thrombosis of coronary artery stents (hazard ratio = 89.78).[8] Renal failure, lesions in arterial bifurcations, diabetes, and low cardiac ejection fraction are additional risk factors for stent thrombosis.

Abrupt discontinuation of antiplatelet therapy is not without consequences, as a rebound effect can occur, leading to a prothrombotic state. The timing of cessation of antiplatelet therapy therefore becomes important. The type of drug being used and its recommended time of discontinuation is dependent upon its pharmacokinetic properties. Aspirin should be discontinued 7 to 10 days before surgery, short-acting NSAIDs 24 hours before surgery, short-acting thienopyridines 24 hours before surgery, and long-acting thienopyridines 7 days before surgery. The ACCP guidelines recommend restarting aspirin the day after surgery, but there are no specific recommendations regarding when to resume other antiplatelet agents.

There are, however, multiple reasons for preoperative oral anticoagulation with anticoagulants like warfarin. The most common co-morbid conditions requiring anticoagulation include cardiac valve replacement, atrial fibrillation, and deep venous thrombosis. Previous guidelines for anticoagulation monitoring by the American College of Chest Physicians are similar regardless of the risk of thromboembolism.[11] For all levels of risk, discontinuation of warfarin 4 days before surgery followed by low-molecular-weight heparin (LMWH) or unfractionated heparin (UFH) preoperatively, followed by warfarin therapy at some point postoperatively, is the general recommendation, with the exception of the patient at high risk of thromboembolism, where UFH or LMWH are continued postoperatively until warfarin therapy is therapeutic. Bridge therapy with UFH or LMWH has been shown to significantly reduce the risk of thromboembolism, although the risk of postoperative bleeding and heparin-induced thrombocytopenia are increased. The 1998 ACC/AHA

● **TABLE 21–6** Updated Recommendations for Anticoagulation Management in the Perioperative Period

1. Discontinue warfarin 5 days before surgery for patients with INR between 2.0 and 3.0; discontinue 6 days before surgery for INR 3.0-4.5 (preoperative target INR less than 1.2).
2. Bridge therapy should be initiated with LMWH 36 hours after the last dose of heparin (enoxaparin 1 mg/kg or dalteparin 100 IU/kg SQ every 12 hours).
3. Last dose of LMWH to be given 24 hours prior to surgery (commonly discontinued 12 hours before surgery).
4. Discuss when to restart oral anticoagulation with the surgeon.
5. Resume the first dose of postoperative warfarin therapy 1 day after completion of surgery.
6. The prothrombin/INR should be monitored daily until the patient is discharged, and periodically after discharge until the INR is within the therapeutic range.
7. A complete blood cell count and platelet count should be done on days 3 and 7.
8. Discontinue LMWH when the INR is in the therapeutic range (2.0-3.0) for 2 consecutive days.

Source: ASA Physical Status Classification System (online). http://www.asahq.org/clinical/physicalstatus.htm. Accessed July, 2010.

● **TABLE 21–7** American Society of Anesthesiologists (ASA) Risk Assessment Classification

ASA Class I
A normal, healthy patient without organic, physiologic, or psychiatric disturbance (eg, healthy with good exercise tolerance)

ASA Class II
A patient with controlled medical conditions without significant systemic effects (eg, controlled hypertension or controlled diabetes without systemic effects, cigarette smoking without COPD, anemia, mild obesity, age younger than 1 year or older than 70 years, pregnancy)

ASA Class III
A patient with medical conditions with significant systemic effects, intermittently associated with significant functional compromise (eg, controlled congestive heart failure, stable angina, old myocardial infarction, poorly controlled hypertension, morbid obesity, bronchospastic disease with intermittent symptoms, chronic renal failure)

ASA Class IV
A patient with medical condition that is poorly controlled, associated with significant dysfunction and is a potential threat to life (eg, unstable angina, symptomatic COPD, symptomatic congestive heart failure, hepatorenal failure)

ASA Class V
A patient with a critical medical condition that is associated with little chance of survival with or without the surgical procedure (eg, multiorgan failure, sepsis syndrome with hemodynamic instability, hypothermia, poorly controlled coagulopathy)

ASA Class VI
A patient who is brain dead and undergoing anesthesia care for the purposes of organ donation

Source: ASA Physical Status Classification System (online). http://www.asahq.org/clinical/physicalstatus.htm. Accessed July, 2010.

guidelines for the management of valvular heart disease state the LMWH is not recommended for bridge therapy in the perioperative period. However, new data suggest that LMWH is the best choice being both safe and efficacious for perioperative bridge therapy in cases of cardiac valve replacement and atrial fibrillation.[8,9] The Fourth Annual Perioperative Medicine Summit updated the recommendations for anticoagulation management in the perioperative period, as shown in Table 21–6.[8]

It should also be noted that a 2003 systematic review concluded that major bleeding was a rare occurrence for individuals on oral warfarin for patients undergoing dental procedures, arthrocentesis, cataract surgery, upper endoscopy, or colonoscopy, and therefore no changes in warfarin therapy for these procedures are needed. Cessation of warfarin therapy for less than 5 days for minor outpatient procedures produced low rates of thromboembolism (0.75) and major bleeding (0.6%). A significantly higher risk of major bleeding was noted among patients who received bridge therapy with LMWH or UFH.[8]

As in many clinical situations involving the geriatric patient, the most appropriate approach to the perioperative management of anticoagulation and platelet therapy is to involve all members of the health care team, including the patient, to individualize clinical decisions based on all of the relevant medical conditions, medications, type of surgery, and risks of complications.[8,9] The risk reductions for bleeding and stroke are the most important considerations for a clinician. Both invasive and noninvasive methods of thromboembolism prevention have been introduced and are awaiting randomized trials.[10]

Anesthesia Risk Screening

The American Society of Anesthesiologists (ASA) has developed a system of physical status classification that is based entirely on the presence of significant organ system dysfunction and the severity of any functional impairment. It was not initially designed as a risk assessment tool or to predict surgical outcomes. Neither age nor type of operation is included in the ranking system. However, studies have demonstrated the ability of this tool to predict perioperative risk and outcomes better

than age alone. The classification system is a simple score that is easy to quantify using results from medical records review, patient history, and examination. No diagnostic testing is required. Subjective assignment to class II through V indicates an increased level of severity and increase postoperative mortality (< 1% in class 2, 25% in class 4).[14] The ASA classification, and examples of each class, are given in Table 21–7.

The choice of anesthesia that leads to the most favorable outcome with reduction in morbidity and mortality continues to be an area of study. Some of the verified benefits of regional anesthesia include lower incidence of postoperative DVT, decreased preoperative catecholamine levels, and decreased incidence of postoperative hypoxemia when compared with general anesthesia.[3]

Pulmonary Risk Screening

Age-related changes in the respiratory system reduce alveolar elasticity and increase chest wall stiffness, which predisposes older adult patients to atelectasis and decreased expiratory flow rates. These aged-related changes include reduced respiratory response to hypoxia by 50%, decreased ciliary function, reduced cough and swallowing function, decrease in bony thorax elasticity, loss of muscle mass, decreased lung parenchymal stiffness, impaired airway protective reflexes, and a decreased central nervous system responsiveness. Supine position, general anesthetic agents, and abdominal incisions also contribute to reduced functional residual capacity and increased airway resistance. Resulting hypoventilation and atelectasis may cause hypoxemia and pulmonary infection.

● **TABLE 21–8** Risk Factors for Pulmonary Complications in Older Adults

Impaired cognitive function
BMI $\leq 27 kg/m^2$, chest wall or upper abdominal incision
Smoking within the past 8 weeks/COPD
Age ≥ 60 years
Productive cough within 5 days of surgery
Diffuse wheezing within 5 days of surgery
FEV_1/FVC ratio less than 70%
$PaCO_2 > 45$ mm Hg
History of cancer
History of angina
ASA rating of class III or greater
Impaired neurologic status
Impaired cardiovascular status
Intravascular volume shifts
Incision length > 30 cm (11.8 in)
Incision approaching the diaphragm (upper abdominal and thoracic procedures)

Clinicians must identify older adult patients at high risk for respiratory decompensation to reduce the complication rate, even though there are no evidence-based guidelines for this process. Table 21–8 lists some of the many characteristics of older adults at increased risk for pulmonary complications. Risk of pulmonary complications is reduced by encouraging smoking cessation, adjunctive chest physiotherapy (deep breathing exercises, chest percussion, and incentive spirometry), antibiotics for infected sputum, and bronchodilators and steroids for bronchospasm.

Neuropsychiatric Risk Screening

The risk of a poor surgical outcome in older adults is significantly increased in the perioperative period by impaired cognitive status, especially in the presence of delirium or an acute confusional state. Delirium is defined as disordered cognitive function with disturbances in thinking, perception, and memory accompanied by waxing and waning in level of consciousness. The Confusion Assessment Method (CAM) is a validated screening tool and easy to administer. Its sensitivity is 81% and specificity 84%.

The incidence of postoperative delirium is 10% to 15% for persons over 70.[12] Preoperative factors that predispose to postoperative delirium include age 70 years or older, pre-existing cognitive impairment, limited physical function (including IADLs), history of alcohol abuse, abnormal serum electrolytes, abnormal glucose, hypoxia, sensory deprivation or overload (ie, pain), and high-risk surgical procedures (cardiac surgery, noncardiac thoracic surgery, abdominal aortic aneurysm repair, hip fracture repair, ophthalmologic surgery). Other independent precipitating factors are the use of physical restraints, malnutrition, respiratory insufficiency, dehydration, addition of more than three medications, and any iatrogenic event, such as nosocomial infection.

When preoperative risk factors are present, the physician can identify patients at greatest risk for developing delirium and management should focus on correcting fluid, electrolyte, and metabolic derangements and optimizing replacement of blood loss. Other strategies to reduce the risk of postoperative delirium include supplemental oxygen during surgery, discontinuation of high-risk medications, adequate nutritional

intake, mobilization out of bed on the first postoperative day, and treatment of severe pain.[12] For more on delirium please see Chapter 30.

CASE PRESENTATION (continued)

After J.R. was given the okay for surgery by cardiology his warfarin was discontinued 4 days prior to surgery. You discuss with J.R. and his wife the option of outpatient ambulatory surgery versus staying a day or two in the hospital after the procedure. You recommend that he be admitted for close monitoring due to his underlying coronary artery disease, COPD, and monitoring of his anticoagulation status. He is agreeable with that plan. On the day of the scheduled surgery J.R. is admitted to the hospital and started on enoxaparin at a dose of 1 mg/kg once daily. His preoperative INR is 1.3, his electrolytes are normal, and his heart rate, though still in atrial fibrillation, is under good control at 68.

● MEDICATION ISSUES

In addition to discontinuing antiplatelet and anticoagulant therapy, there are many other medications that need to be discontinued before surgery. A detailed medication review should be conducted well in advance of scheduled elective surgery and in the immediate preoperative period before emergency surgery. A few of the medications that should be discontinued at least 7 days prior to elective surgery are listed in Table 21–9.[13]

Patients on antiepileptics, antihypertensives, and cardiovascular drugs can take their morning dose with small sips of water before surgery. It is reasonable to consider reducing the dose or holding antihypertensive medications prior to surgery because of the risk of hypotension due to anesthesia as well as intravascular fluids shifts. Parenteral alternatives for some medications can be used until oral intake is resumed. Abrupt discontinuation of clonidine and beta-blockers should be avoided. Stable or controlled diabetics on insulin should receive half of their usual dose on the morning of surgery. Patients with chronic steroid use should receive stress coverage beginning the night before surgery and tapering to the usual maintenance dose of steroid after 3 to 5 days.

● **TABLE 21–9** Medications to be Discontinued within 7 Days Prior to Elective Surgery

- Any medications containing aspirin
- Estrogen products (oral contraceptives, hormone replacement therapy)
- MAO inhibitors
- Herbal medications and supplements such as echinacea, ginkgo biloba, garlic, ginseng, ma huang, St. John's wort, saw palmetto, and valerian
- Anticholinergics should be discontinued on the day of surgery
- Hypoglycemic agents should be discontinued the evening before surgery
- Taper off benzodiazepines before surgery

Beta-Blocker Therapy

Current studies suggest that beta-blockers reduce perioperative ischemia and may reduce the risk of MI and death in high-risk patients. Beta-blockers reduce ischemia by decreasing myocardial oxygen demand due to increased stress and catecholamine release in the perioperative period, and may help prevent and control arrhythmias. Beta-blockers should be started days or weeks before elective surgery, with the dose titrated to achieve a resting heart rate between 50 and 60 beats per minute. Class I recommendations exist if beta-blockers have been required in the recent past to control symptoms of angina or in patients with symptomatic arrhythmias or hypertension. Class II recommendations exist for the use of beta-blockers if the preoperative assessment identifies untreated hypertension, known CAD, or major risk factors for coronary disease. Acute withdrawal of a beta-blocker preoperatively can lead to substantial morbidity and even mortality. Beta-blockers should be continued in the perioperative period and continued throughout the hospital stay. There is a slight preference for beta-1 cardioselective beta-blockers (eg, metoprolol, esmolol), since they are less likely to cause adverse pulmonary and peripheral vascular effects; however, patients who are taking a nonselective beta-blocker (eg, propranolol) chronically do not need to switch to a beta-1 selective agent perioperatively.

Use of Antibiotics

Surgical site infections remain a significant contributor to postoperative morbidity and mortality. Among other interventions, appropriate administration of prophylactic antibiotics has been shown to decrease the risk of perioperative infections. The goal of prophylactic antibiotic administration is to decrease the risk of contamination of the wound from skin flora in the case of clean procedures, and to add coverage for organisms that are anticipated to contaminate the surgical field, as in open bowel procedures. The National Surgical Infection Prevention Project guideline recommends prophylactic antibiotics be given within 1 hour before incision (2 hours with the use of vancomycin/fluoroquinolone) and discontinued within 24 hours after the end of surgery to prevent the emergence of resistant bacteria associated with the use of prolonged prophylactic antibiotic therapy.[15]

● LABORATORY TESTS

Preoperative testing of the geriatric patient involves maintaining a balance between ordering tests that are necessary and avoiding those that are unnecessary, some of which can add expense and possibly create delays for a needed procedure. The purpose of all preoperative testing is to identify systemic, organ, and other functional deficits that are unknown and to correct, modify, or determine the severity of known medical conditions in order to reduce the risk of perioperative morbidity and mortality. Of equal importance is the retrieval of as much pertinent information as possible for the purpose of obtaining informed consent.

Preoperative testing of the geriatric patient should first include a thorough history and physical examination. A detailed review of all medications should be conducted as thoroughly as possible including prescription, over-the-counter, and alternative medicines. Other investigations should include laboratory testing with appropriate blood tests, x-rays, EKG, cognitive assessment, and nutritional assessment. All of the tests described in the next sections are considered appropriate for preoperative testing.[1]

Blood Tests

Complete Blood Count (CBC)

It is important to know the baseline hemoglobin of a patient before surgery. A hemoglobin level of 9 to 10 g/dL (90-100 g/L) is considered the minimum level needed to approve a patient for surgery with reasonable safety. Some procedures are associated with more blood loss than others, and this should be taken into consideration preoperatively. Having several units of blood on standby preoperatively is prudent for procedures where intraoperative blood loss can be severe. Severe anemia will cause tissue hypoxia that might affect intraoperative and/or postoperative outcomes.

If identified, anemia needs to be evaluated with appropriate testing of iron metabolism, folate, and vitamin B_{12} levels. Endoscopies should be delayed when urgent or emergent surgery is necessary and can be scheduled later in the postoperative period. The WBC count is important for identifying a myeloproliferative disorder. Specific workup is determined by the type of abnormality. The platelet count can be useful for the same purpose and should be done in patients who complain of having a history of easy bruising or spontaneous or prolonged bleeding. Platelet counts above 100,000 μL (1×10^9/L) are generally safe for surgery.

Blood Chemistry

An electrolyte panel is recommended for patients older than 60 years. It should also be considered for patients who have hypertension on diuretic therapy to evaluate for electrolyte abnormalities that can easily be corrected during the preoperative period. Furthermore, assessment of renal function by measurement of the BUN and creatinine, and then calculation of the GFR by the Cockcroft–Gault equation or the Modification of Diet in Renal Disease (MDRD) study equation, should be considered paramount for the prudent use of medications throughout the perioperative period.

The aging kidney decreases in size along with the decreases in nearly all other aspects of physiologic function of the kidney. Fluid resuscitation needs to be monitored closely. Anesthesia and all medications might require dosage adjustments due to the associated decline in renal function that accompanies aging. Do not assume that a normal serum creatinine indicates normal renal function in older adults, particularly in small, underweight patients.

Several studies have highlighted the importance of measurement of serum albumin preoperatively. There is a fourfold higher rate of postoperative pulmonary complications in patients with a serum albumin level less than 3.6 mg/dL (36 g/L).[16] Serum albumin levels lower than 3.5 mg/dL

(35 g/L) have also been demonstrated to be an important predictor of 30-day perioperative morbidity and mortality in the National VA Surgical Risk Study as well as in many other studies of the hospitalized older patient.

Urinanalysis (UA)

An urinanalysis should not be routinely ordered even though asymptomatic bacturia is common in older adults, as it is not cost-effective. If the patient reports symptoms, it can be performed preoperatively.

Nutritional Assessment

Though not necessary for healthy older adults, particularly when evaluating them for low-risk interventions or most outpatient procedures, consideration for a thorough nutritional assessment should be done for older patients with frailty, malnutrition, weight loss, or low body mass. Particularly for patients in whom delayed recovery will likely lead to poor outcomes such as hip fracture repair and most intra-abdominal procedures, a nutritional assessment can improve recovery. Unfortunately, though data on nutritional interventions are scarce and often show minimal to no benefit, particularly in non-malnourished patients, nutritional interventions are still a worthwhile endeavor for those patients at high risk.

EKG

An EKG is not recommended in asymptomatic patients undergoing low-risk noncardiac procedures regardless of patient age.[8]

Decisional Capacity and Informed Consent

An assessment of decisional capacity is required for obtaining informed consent or refusal for a surgical procedure. It is not necessary for a patient to be completely cognitively intact or intact at all times for consent to be legal. For example, some patients may present with short-term memory loss, but this does not always preclude them from having decisional capacity. They may very well be able to judge the necessity or appropriateness of having a surgical procedure depending on their ability to understand the complexity and the risks. Other patients have "sundowning" in the latter portion of the day, but might be lucid at other times. Ideally, the care team will use an interdisciplinary approach to assess the decisional capacity of a patient. Mental status testing can be done to help, but the score should not be used to determine capacity to make decisions, as this is a poor surrogate for decision-making capacity. In the presence of severe cognitive deficits or if the patient is otherwise unable to provide consent, the individual holding durable power of attorney (DPOA) provides the consent. If there is no DPOA, then the guardian, spouse, children, and siblings (usually in that order, but depending on state law) are given the information to provide informed consent for a recommended procedure. Communication should also include potential complications and goals of care. Requirements for obtaining consent vary from state to state.

Informed consent is critical to planning and delivery of quality of care, an important aspect of clinical documentation,

and a potential target of liability. It is also an ethical obligation. Old age, fewer years of education, and delirium impair or prevent adequate informed consent. In these cases, surrogate consent may be necessary. For more on decision-making capacity please see Chapter 10.

● THE INTRAOPERATIVE PERIOD

Judicious Fluid Replacement

In older adults, the ability to maintain homeostatic levels of fluids is reduced, and the margin between too little and too much fluid is relatively narrow. There are hormonal changes that occur in response to the tissue injury associated with surgery. These changes create a predisposition to extravascular fluid accumulation, which increases the risk of iatrogenic events related to intravenous fluid replacement. Overexpansion of the extracellular compartment from excess isotonic fluid administration may be dangerous because cardiopulmonary reserves are also limited in the elderly. Conversely, intravascular volume depletion can lead to acute renal tubular injury, which is also to be avoided in the perioperative period.

Initially, the amount of IV fluids can be estimated, but fluid administration should be adjusted to optimize blood pressure, pulse, and urine output (which are closely monitored). Central venous pressure, daily weights, and urine output measurements help determine fluid requirements. Enough fluids are given to replace insensible fluid losses and measured or estimated external losses and to produce a urine output of 0.5 mL/kg per hour, or about 30 mL/hr.

When external losses are minimal, fluid requirements are usually 1500 to 2500 mL for 24 hours. However, more fluid may be needed if third-space sequestration of fluids is excessive (eg, because of a distended bowel or inflammation of subcutaneous tissues due to burns). Careful monitoring of fluid volume status is imperative to prevent the common postoperative occurrence of volume overload. IV flow rates should be adjusted according to any changes in the patient's condition.

The following guide is recommended to assist with calculation of fluid requirements[5]:

1. Estimate the intracellular volume as a percentage of body weight:
   - 25% to 30% for men aged 65 to 85 with weight 40 to 80 kg
   - 20% to 25% for women aged 65 to 85 with weight of 40 to 80 kg
2. Estimate the daily metabolic requirements per liter of intercellular volume (without acute stress and situations that will affect salt and water balance) as follows: water 100 mL, energy 100 kcal, protein 3 g, Na^+ 3 mmol, K^+ 2 mmol.

Example

A 75-year-old woman who weighs 60 kg has 12 L (60 kg × 20%) of estimated intracellular volume. The maintenance requirement for water would be 1.2 L (100 mL of water per L of volume, so 100 mL/L × 12 L = 1.2 L/day) and the IV flow rate would be 50 mL/hr (1200 mL/24 hours).

Type of Anesthesia

Factors influencing the choice of anesthetic technique are numerous and complex, but when both regional and general anesthetics are appropriate, the choice is usually guided by the consideration of the type of procedure being done, the depth of anesthesia needed, and which has the highest likelihood to produce the most favorable outcome. Initial small, randomized trials showed that regional anesthetics had some benefits for pulmonary and cardiac outcomes.[17] Local anesthesia, with epidural and spinal techniques, has been demonstrated to reduce blood loss, reduce thromboembolic risk, and improve cardiovascular outcomes. There is also evidence that inhaled and intravenous anesthetic medications can affect the inflammatory response either positively or negatively.[17] The relationship between general anesthetics, inflammation, and long-term outcomes is an area of active interest and research, but mechanisms remain to be defined.

CASE PRESENTATION (continued)

After an assessment by the nurse, social worker, and physician, the geriatrics team believes that J.R. is able to consent for the procedure. He understands the risks and benefits of the procedure and is able to repeat and discuss them with the staff. Written informed consent is obtained, and after receiving a report of a safe INR of 1.3, J.R. is taken to the operating room for excision of the mass on the proximal left lower extremity. The procedure is performed under general anesthesia. Reported blood loss is recorded as "minimal." There are no intraoperative or immediate postoperative complications. The patient is transported to the recovery room in stable condition.

After demonstrating alertness and stabilization of vital signs, he is taken to the medical ward for observation. He has postoperative orders written that include oxycodone-acetaminophen 5/325 mg one tablet every 4 hours as needed for pain and docusate sodium 100 mg daily. All preoperative medications are continued. His warfarin is written to restart on postoperative day 1 and he is to continue enoxaparin for now.

On postoperative day 1, J.R. wakes from sleep in the early morning and is noted by the nurses to be exhibiting mild confusion and complaining of excruciating pain. His surgeon is called, who advises giving 5 mg of morphine IV now and increasing the oral narcotic to 2 tablets every 4 hours as needed. Three hours later, the patient's pain had subsided satisfactorily and the mild confusion resolved. The postoperative course is otherwise uneventful and he is discharged home later that afternoon.

Written instructions are provided that he is to continue all medications as previously ordered, including the narcotic as well as taking an additional laxative while on the pain medication. He is given an appointment with his primary care physician for coagulation monitoring in 1 week. The same instructions are communicated to his wife, along with a printed list of discharge instructions. He is to return to the surgery clinic in 5 days for wound inspection, and sooner if bleeding or other drainage soils the wound dressing. An emergency contact number is provided in his written instructions.

• THE POSTOPERATIVE PERIOD

Pain Management

Pain management is a crucial aspect of perioperative care. Depression, anxiety, fear, fatigue, and cognitive impairment can all affect the perception of pain. The assessment and treatment plan for pain management should be individualized, and it should be reassessed and modified frequently based on the patient's response.

The oldest-old and cognitively impaired patients appear to be at highest risk for undertreatment of pain, which could result in the development of postoperative delirium. Studies have documented that old age is associated with less aggressive pain treatment and the resulting stress may worsen survival rate. Inadequate pain management for several major surgeries can precipitate decreased lung volumes that eventually lead to lobar atelectasis, pneumonia, or respiratory failure.[1]

Most postoperative pain will require therapy with narcotic analgesia.[18] The risk of addiction to opioids is small when used for acute pain syndromes. Patients with intact cognition should be considered for patient-controlled analgesia (PCA), which has been shown to provide significantly better pain relief and lower risk of postoperative confusion than intramuscular narcotic dosing. More recent evidence is inconclusive regarding and beneficial impact on postoperative pulmonary complications rates with the use of PCA.[1]

Postoperative patients should be directly questioned about their pain at frequent intervals (not less than every 2 to 3 hours for the first 24 hours). Pain medication should be scheduled and given at regular intervals, with additional doses available for breakthrough pain.

Estimation of creatinine clearance should always be formed when dosing analgesics in the older adult. A bowel regimen should also be ordered that consists of the combination of a stimulant laxative and a stool softener or osmotic agent. A stool softener alone does very little to prevent constipation in patients who are receiving regular doses of narcotic analgesics, as narcotic medications interfere with normal peristalsis.

Meperidine and propoxyphene should be avoided because of toxic metabolite accumulation and the increased likelihood of adverse drug interactions. To avoid the risk of acetaminophen toxicity, the total dose should not exceed 4 g per 24-hour period, and a more conservative approach would be not to exceed 3 g in older patients with normal liver function. Nonsteroidal anti-inflammatory medications are best avoided because of increased risk of nephrotoxicity, fluid retention, and gastric irritation.

Patients who are unable to communicate effectively and have pain should be given standing orders for narcotic analgesics, with guidelines as to when to hold the medications, combined with frequent assessment of medication by visual analog pain scale or other visual or indirect symptom-based pain assessment tool. Nonpharmacologic therapies, such as ice packs, heating pads, massage, and relaxation techniques, are also useful adjuncts to therapy.

Postoperative Infections

In addition to the surgical site, the other most common types of postoperative infection are those involving the urinary tract (UTI) and the lungs (pneumonia).[2] Diminished immune function in older adults is the most common predisposing factor. Prolonged catheterization is the primary vector for UTI, and aged patients are more likely to be catheterized due to problems with mobility, medication side effects, and pre-existing incontinence.[2] Early removal of catheters and general avoidance of catheterization whenever possible are important steps that can prevent and reduce UTIs and UTI-associated complications. Symptoms of UTI can be very subtle and might initially present as confusion or delirium.

Next to cardiovascular events, pneumonia is a leading cause of postoperative mortality in the elderly. In the postoperative period, early mobilization, pulmonary toilet including encouraging deep breathing, and incentive spirometry are useful to prevent this complication. Nasogastric tubes, immobility, and dementia are factors that increase the risk of pneumonia.

Delirium and Postoperative Cognitive Dysfunction (POCD)

Delirium (see "Neuropsychiatric Risk Screening" earlier in the chapter) occurs in 10% to 50% of older adults who have surgery and is associated with increased morbidity and mortality. There are multiple causes, but it is often related to infections, medications, cardiorespiratory disorders, sensory deprivation, limited reserve capacity, and metabolic derangements.

Treatment of delirium should be aimed at removing or treating reversible causes and putting environmental safeguards in place to prevent harm. Haloperidol is usually the first drug of choice but many people avoid its use due to concerns of extrapyramidal effects. The atypical antipsychotic agents can also be given, but there are current concerns

about the increased risk of sudden death with their use. Whenever medications are necessary for management of delirium, they should be used sparingly and cautiously to prevent adverse events. One must remember to "start low and go slow." Benzodiazepines should be used primarily in patients suspected of having delirium tremens associated with alcohol withdrawal.

Physical restraints can increase the risk of injury and should be avoided as much as possible when managing the delirious patient. Treatment should also involve the presence of family members, caregivers, or the assistance of trained hospital personnel who can provide 24-hour observation until the patient is stabilized.

Although it is tempting to blame anesthetic drugs for the majority of cases of postoperative delirium, there has been no proven correlation between the two.[2] Some studies suggest that preoperative treatment with low-dose haloperidol in high-risk patients reduced the duration and severity of delirium in elderly patients who had hip surgery, but did not decrease the incidence.[12]

Postoperative Cognitive Dysfunction

Postoperative cognitive dysfunction (POCD) was previously associated with cardiac surgery, especially coronary artery bypass graft procedures. Although the syndrome has long been recognized, it still goes unrecognized by many because it is not always obvious. In POCD, there is a deterioration of intellectual function presenting as impaired memory or concentration (impairment ranges from mild forgetfulness to severe cognitive dysfunction resulting in loss of independence). The cause is not well understood, but there is the "functional cliff" theory that suggests that at some point along the continuum of progressive cognitive decline that normally occurs with aging, the patient comes very close to a point that can be considered cognitive impairment or early dementia. There is then an increased vulnerability to physiologic insults such as the anesthesia or mild trauma associated with surgery, which pushes the patient over into impaired functioning.[19]

The diagnosis of POCD must include a newly recognized decline in at least two areas of cognitive functioning that persists for at least 2 weeks after surgery. The diagnosis can also be corroborated with neuropsychological testing or noting evidence of greater memory loss than one would expect due to normal aging. Preoperative neuropsychological testing can facilitate early detection of POCD in patients undergoing elective procedures. The duration can range from weeks to several months to being permanent.

A recent study found cognitive dysfunction to be common in adults of all ages at hospital discharge following major noncardiac surgery. However, 3 months after surgery, 12.7% of patients aged 60 or older continued to have POCD, which was more than twice the rates noted in young and middle-aged groups.[12] Some of the predisposing factors that have been identified include advanced age, metabolic problems, lower educational level, and previous cerebral vascular accident. POCD has also been documented in patients with none of these predisposing factors. POCD is different from delirium in that it is often associated with the wearing off of anesthesia.

Mobility and Venous Thromboembolism Risk Reduction

Any acute illness or surgery can cause a significant decline in strength and mobility. Immobility can have deleterious effects on multiple organ systems including the skin, cardiovascular system, lungs, musculoskeletal system, gastrointestinal system, and genitourinary system.[2] It also contributes to negative nitrogen balance, which can aggravate malnutrition. Older adult patients are also more likely to be on prolonged bed rest in the postoperative period due to underlying frailty, debility, and other mobility problems. Pressure ulcer risk is extremely high postoperatively, especially in patients who have hip fracture. Immobility also increases the risk for osteoporosis as it increases the rate of bone resorption, which has been documented by both biopsy and biochemical markers in previous studies.[2]

Ambulation and other forms of mobilization and exercise that are initiated early in the postoperative period can help patients gain strength and prevent frailty.[12] It is purported by many that early ambulation prevents venous thromboembolism (VTE); however, there are no documented studies in support of this opinion. There is also no evidence that forcing an unhealthy person to walk helps prevent VTE. Early ambulation is definitely good hospital care and encouragement should continue, but considering it as VTE prophylaxis is unfounded. Walking might be considered a good marker of health, and most healthy persons are less likely to develop thromboses.[12]

Prophylaxis for DVT should be considered in all older adult patients undergoing a surgical procedure. Patients who have been determined to be at high risk for DVT and a low risk for bleeding should receive therapeutic anticoagulation postoperatively.[20] External compression devices, which are worn on the lower extremities, are also another option and can be worn before, during, and after surgery. They are recommended for patients who are at high risk for bleeding. However, compliance with these devices is frequently poor so that careful monitoring to optimize adherence cannot be over-emphasized.

A number of recommendations for the use of aspirin in VTE prophylaxis have been purported. However, there is no evidence-based approach for use of aspirin in VTE prophylaxis. Moreover, there is a greater absolute increase in bleeding complications compared to the absolute reduction in episodes of symptomatic deep venous thrombosis.[12] Aspirin is not recommended for DVT prophylaxis by the American College of Chest Physicians (ACCP).

The American College of Chest Physicians (ACCP) Guidelines on antithrombotic and thrombolytic therapy for specific orthopedic procedures are widely available (http://chestjournal.chestpubs.org/content/133/6_suppl/67S.full.pdf+html) and evidence based. These comprehensive guidelines address many other surgical procedures that are common in older adults and are highly recommended for review by any practitioner providing care to surgical patients.[21]

Postoperative Nutrition

Appetite and caloric intake typically decrease in the older patient so that early, aggressive nutritional support should be given to patients preoperatively who have evidence of malnutrition. Preoperative testing for folate and B_{12} deficiencies are appropriate in patients with a history of alcohol consumption, and supplements should be considered in the postoperative period regardless of the results of serologic testing.

Malnutrition can contribute to frailty, but there is no strong evidence for benefits of supplemental nutrition, with the exception of meta-analyses of nutritional intervention studies that did demonstrate improvement in mortality risk and decreased morbidity (ie, pressure ulcers) in hospitalized elderly. Those who will likely gain the most benefit are patients who are 75 years of age or older and noted to be malnourished in the preoperative evaluation.[12] Assessment tools should include the body mass index (BMI), serum albumin, and prealbumin. A BMI less than 18.5 kg/m² is an indicator of malnutrition.[1] Low serum albumin has been associated with poor outcomes in the postoperative and post-hospitalization periods leading to increased morbidity and mortality.[5]

Nutritional support becomes very important in the postoperative period due to the energy demands associated with wound healing. Supplemental oral feedings, tube feedings, or total parenteral nutrition may be given, depending on the patient's condition. If anorexia or dysphagia makes oral feeding difficult, but gastric and intestinal motility and absorption are normal, enteral feedings may be given by continuous drip. In such cases, the enteral route is preferable to the parenteral route because it causes fewer complications, costs less, and may have a trophic effect on the intestine. Total parenteral nutrition can be used when intestinal motility or absorption is abnormal.

The Diabetic Patient

Maintenance of glycemic control in the diabetic older adult is of paramount importance during all intervals of the perioperative spectrum. Management strategies are also variable depending on where the patient is in the timeline. Intensive glycemic control reduces the risk of infectious complications and may also reduce mortality in critically ill patients. Three different levels of physiologic insulin replacement need to be managed: basal insulin, prandial insulin, and supplemental insulin replacement. Goals of therapy should include avoidance of hypoglycemia. The American Association of Clinical Endocrinologists and the American Diabetes Association collectively recommend using insulin therapy for target blood glucose less than 180 mg/dL (10.0 mmol/L) in critically ill patients and less than 140 mg/dL (7.8 mmol/L) in noncritically ill patients.

The postoperative change to subcutaneous insulin can begin 12 to 24 hours before discontinuing intravenous insulin by initiating basal insulin replacement plus supplemental rapid-acting insulin. When the patient begins oral intake of food, prandial insulin can be started. Postoperatively, this transition can be complicated due to wide variation in the amount of oral intake, physiologic and environmental stresses, and increased insulin resistance. However, it is recommended that exclusive use of supplemental sliding-scale regular insulin in the hospitalized patient should be abandoned.[12]

Discharge/Transitions of Care

Physicians can significantly aid older adult surgical patients by anticipating and planning for care transitions. It is important to understand how the older adult will get help when he or she returns home. Watching a patient transfer, walk, and perform activities of daily living will help guide choices about appropriate discharge destination and home services that would be required to maximize a safe transition. Physical and occupational therapists can assist with such assessments during hospitalization. Careful review of diagnoses with the older adult and/or caregiver is important. A verbal or written summary of the hospital course is also very helpful.

A medication review is essential for a safe discharge transition, including what specific medications should be taken at home and which of the prehospital medicines should be discontinued. Comprehension of any special instructions about dosing and timing of medication should be verified as well as an assessment of the patient's or caregiver's ability to properly administer medications.

It is also useful to make sure that there is understanding among older adult patients and caregivers regarding the basics of managing the disease(s), special treatments, and the need for follow-up appointments. When being transferred to another health care facility, it is very useful to facilitate the transition by communicating directly with the next care provider, because ongoing care of geriatric patients is generally very complex, especially for those patients who are being discharged to another institutional setting. For more on health care transitions please see Chapter 22.

SUMMARY

Perioperative care of the older adult requires vigilance and careful attention to the ongoing evaluation of multiple organ systems while assessing and preventing risks of perioperative complications and mortality. All health care providers of older adults share the responsibility of reducing their risks and maximizing their recovery when they become surgical patients.

High-quality postoperative care involves close monitoring and intervention for infection, cardiorespiratory problems, reducing DVT risk, delirium, and detection of POCD. Facilitation of safe transitions of care during the postoperative period is equally as important as the care rendered during the earlier phases of treatment.

The use of multidisciplinary teams can maximize the ability to provide the type of comprehensive care that is needed for the management of the complex care the older adult patient often requires, especially following operative procedures. With greater understanding and research of aging physiology, it is possible to improve perioperative morbidity and survival.

Finally, assisting patients and families with goals of care should not be ignored. When older adult patients and their families have been fully informed of their disease process and the options for treatment, the patient should be respected for the option to not have any surgical procedure. However, it should be emphasized to all that *age* is but a minor risk factor for complications. The sum of the physiologic effects of comorbid illnesses plays a much more influential role in perioperative mortality.

References

1. Jaffer AK (ed.). Perioperative management. *Clin Geriatr Med.* 2008; 24:573-738.

2. Beliveau MM, Multach M. Perioperative care for the elderly. *Med Clin North Am,* 2003;87:273-289.

3. Liu LL, Wiener-Kronish JP. Perioperative anesthesia issues in the elderly. *Crit Care Clin.* 2003;19:641-656.

4. Ersan T. Perioperative Management of the Geriatric Patient. http//emedicine.medscape.com; Dec. 2007.

5. Landefeld CS, Palmer R, Johnson MA, et al. *Current Geriatric Diagnosis and Treatment.* New York: McGraw-Hill; 2004:45-51.

6. Eagle KA, Guyton RA, Davidoff R, et al. ACC/AHA Guideline Update for Perioperative Cardiovascular Evaluation for Noncardiac Surgery—Executive summary. *JACC.* 2002;39:542-553.

7. Chopra V, Flanders SA., Froehlich JB, et al. Perioperative practice: Time to throttle back. *Ann Intern Med.* 2010;152:47-51.

8. Jaffer AK. Perioperative management of warfarin and antiplatelet therapy. *Cleveland Clin J Med.* 2009;76:S37-S44.

9. Jaffer AK. Anticoagulation management strategies for patients on warfarin who need surgery. *Cleveland Clin J Med.* 2006;73(suppl): S100-S105.

10. Ezekowitz MD. Anticoagulation interruptus not without risk. *Circulation.* 2004;110;1518-1519.

11. Dunn AS. Perioperative management of patients on oral anticoagulants: A decision analysis. *Med Decis Making.* 2005;25:387-397.

12. Palmer RM. Perioperative care of the elderly patient: An update. Proceedings of the Perioperative Medicine Summit. *Cleveland Clin J Med.* 2009;76:S16-S21.

13. Spine Institute of New York, Beth Israel Medical Center. Surgery Instructions: Pre-Operative Patients. www.spineinstituteny.com/ instructions.surgery.html. Retrieved May 15, 2009.

14. Richardson JD, Cocanour CS, Kern JA, et al. Perioperative risk assessment in elderly and high risk patients. *J Am Coll Surg.* 2004;199:133-144.

15. Arora VM, McGory ML, Fung CH. Quality indicators for hospitalization and surgery in vulnerable elders. *JAGS.* 2007;55:S347-S358.

16. Qaseem A, Snow V, Fitterman N, et al. Risk assessment for and strategies to reduce perioperative pulmonary complications for patients undergoing noncardiothoracic surgery: A Guideline from the American College of Physicians. *Ann Intern Med.* 2006;144:575-580.

17. Parker BM. Anesthetics and anesthesia techniques: Impacts on perioperative management and postoperative outcomes. Proceedings of the Perioperative Medicine Summit. *Cleveland Clin J Med.* 2006; 73(suppl):S13-S17.

18. Perioperative care. In: Colleen Christmas, Peter Pompei, (eds.). *Geriatrics Review Syllabus.* 6th ed. Dubuque, Iowa: Kendall/Hunt Publishing Company; 2006.

19. Souders JE, Rooke GA. Perioperative care for geriatric patients. *Ann Long-Term Care.* 2005;13:17-29.

20. Mood GR, Tang WHW. Perioperative DVT Prophylaxis. www. emedicine.medscape.com/article/284371/. Retrieved May 15, 2009.

21. Geerts WH, Pineo GF, Heit JA, et al. Prevention of venous thromboembolism. *Chest.* 2008;133(suppl):381S-453S.

POST-TEST

1. **Which of the following is a recommended preoperative diagnostic/laboratory test in older adults?**
   A. Urinalysis
   B. Serum albumin
   C. ECG
   D. Liver function tests

2. **All of the following are drugs to be avoided for pain management in the postoperative period EXCEPT:**
   A. Meperidine
   B. Propoxyphene
   C. NSAIDs
   D. Morphine

3. **Prophylaxis for DVT should be considered for:**
   A. All older adult patients undergoing surgical procedures
   B. Only patients with higher risk for its development
   C. Patients who cannot take aspirin
   D. Frail patients

ANSWERS TO PRE-TEST

1. A
2. C
3. B

ANSWERS TO POST-TEST

1. B
2. D
3. A

22

Discharge Planning and Transitional Care

Erin L. Cooper, MD

William L. Lyons, MD

● **LEARNING OBJECTIVES**

1. Explain why unplanned transitions are an important and costly problem in the geriatric population.
2. Identify patients at high risk for poor outcomes after a transition.
3. List the key components of an effective discharge summary.
4. Describe strategies to improve the transitional care of elders.

PRE-TEST

1. **Which of the following BEST illustrates why geriatric transitional care is challenging?**

   A. Older adults require more time to review discharge instructions and medication changes.

   B. Older adults have multiple co-morbid conditions and medications that require ongoing management.

   C. Older adults have longer lengths of stay, making the discharge summaries more complex.

   D. Older adults have more difficulty following instructions, and as a result are admitted to the hospital more often.

2. **Medical errors in older adults that occur after hospital discharge are most commonly related to which one of the following?**

   A. Medications

   B. Incomplete work-ups

   C. Missed lab results

   D. Poor communication

3. **Which of the following is most TRUE regarding follow-up after hospital discharge?**

   A. Patients are more likely to follow-up if they make the appointment themselves.

   B. Patients are more likely to follow-up if it is with a provider they know.

   C. Patients are more likely to follow-up if the hospital provider emphasizes the importance of the visit.

   D. Patients are more likely to follow-up if the appointment is made for them before they leave the hospital.

CASE PRESENTATION: ANTICIPATING TRANSITIONS

Mrs. G. is a 76-year-old, community-dwelling, Japanese American woman. You are seeing her in the emergency department after a fall at home, after slipping in the bathtub, which resulted in a right hip fracture. Her medical problems include hypertension, chronic atrial fibrillation, macular degeneration, and osteoporosis. You are able to retrieve her medication list from her primary care physician's electronic health record, since that practice is part of the hospital system, and you review these medications with her. Her medications include lisinopril 10 mg daily, warfarin 2 mg daily, calcium 600 mg twice daily, vitamin D 1000 international units daily, gingko biloba supplement 120 mg daily, and a multivitamin daily. She lives at home with her husband and English is their second language. They have two children, including a daughter who lives nearby and who, by Mrs. G.'s report, is quite attentive. Mrs. G. is independent in all ADLs and IADLs as well as being the primary caregiver for her husband, who has early dementia and other chronic medical problems. She wishes to have full medical treatment for anything that may arise, including resuscitation in the case of cardiac or pulmonary failure.

On exam, her temperature is 97.4°F (36.3°C), heart rate is 84 beats/min and irregular, blood pressure is 126/72 mm Hg, and respirations are 16/min. She is having mild discomfort due to the fracture. Laboratory data reveal a hemoglobin of 10.2 g/dL (102 g/L), protime of 29 seconds, INR (international normal ratio) of 2.5, and normal electrolytes and creatinine.

You ask her who can take care of her husband while she is in the hospital, and she says that if you can find her a telephone she will call her daughter, who can probably help out for a few days. You engage the social worker to see if a home health aide can also be provided to lessen the burden on the daughter as well.

In addition to your usual admission orders, you hold her warfarin, write for a small dose of oral vitamin K to reverse her anticoagulation, and stop her gingko biloba, in anticipation of her hip surgery. You also order physical and occupational therapy, and ask social work to start an evaluation for discharge planning options and have dietary come by to ask Mrs. G. about her food preferences as well as to perform a nutritional assessment. Finally, you call her primary care physician's office and leave a message with the answering service that Mrs. G. has been hospitalized with a hip fracture and to please notify her physician.

BACKGROUND

Older adults have complex medical needs, often requiring care in various settings, with frequent transitions between them. Transitional care is defined as "a set of actions designed to ensure the coordination and continuity of healthcare as patients transfer between different locations or different levels of care within the same location."[1] Each change in setting—home to emergency department, emergency department to medical floor, medical floor to operating room, hospital to skilled nursing facility, skilled nursing facility to home—requires not only a physical transition for the patient, but a transition in all aspects of his or her medical management. New providers, different nurses, medication changes, new expectations for self-care, and importantly, opportunities for errors, accompany each transition.

Unplanned transitions are a common and costly problem in geriatrics. After hospital discharge, 20% of older adults will be readmitted to the hospital within 30 days and nearly two-thirds of patients will return to the hospital within 1 year.[2] These unplanned readmissions are estimated to cost Medicare over $17 billion every year.[2] Additionally, as patients move into and out of the hospital they are at increased risk for medical errors. One study found that over half of patients had at least one unintended medication discrepancy after hospital admission.[3] About 20% of patients experience an adverse event in the month following hospital discharge.[4,5] Over two-thirds of these events are related to medications, and many of them could have been prevented. One study examining the significance of errors after hospital discharge found that almost half of all patients experienced a medical error (medication discrepancy, test that was not followed up, or a workup recommendation that was not completed) in the 3 months following discharge.[6] Importantly, patients who had a workup that was not completed were six times more likely to be readmitted to the hospital. In this way, poor transitional care may further lead to increased health care utilization, including additional office visits, emergency department visits, and hospitalizations.

HEALTH SYSTEM CHALLENGES

Health system characteristics present challenges for providers of transitional care. Increased awareness of these characteristics will help you anticipate and address potential problems during the discharge process.

Discontinuity

As health care continues to become more specialized, the same provider rarely cares for a patient across multiple settings. Hospitalists now commonly care for patients in many hospital systems, with primary care providers focusing their efforts in the clinic or other outpatient settings. This trend has been evidenced by a steady decline in outpatient-to-inpatient continuity over the past 10 years.[7] This loss of continuity may have a more significant impact on geriatric patients, who often have multiple chronic illnesses, which require ongoing management and coordination of care. As you discharge patients from the hospital, keep the primary provider in mind and remember to communicate the hospital course and discharge plans to him or her to improve continuity and ensure any ongoing medical needs will be addressed. In addition to sending the formal discharge summary, this can be accomplished by a brief phone call to the primary provider's office or through electronic or facsimile transfer of the discharge plans and instructions on the day of discharge.

Sending Facilities

Hospitals and hospital providers are charged with the responsibility of caring for the acutely ill and seeing them safely to the next level of care (home, skilled nursing facility, or other facility). Economic pressures on hospitals have led to shorter lengths of stay and patients being discharged more quickly than in the past, many still with ongoing medical needs. Hospital pharmacy formularies may require medication substitutions when a patient is admitted, increasing the risk for medication discrepancies at the time of discharge.[8] Occasionally, a particular hospital may be at or over capacity, forcing patients to be diverted to a different hospital and a new set of providers, with another disruption in continuity.[9]

Additionally, hospital culture often keeps the main focus on the medical problem at hand, the workup, diagnosis, and treatment. Patient goals, functional status, and psychosocial needs often take a back seat to the more pressing medical issues. These other factors play an important role in discharge planning and if not considered, may increase the risk of readmission. In the case of Mrs. G., she is the primary caregiver for her husband. As you plan for her discharge and rehabilitation needs, one major issue to consider is who will assume the care of her husband while she recovers. In the short term her daughter will help, but if she returns to caring for him too soon, she may risk another injury and rehospitalization.

Characteristics of Receiving Facilities

At the time of hospital discharge, patients may be transferred to a variety of care facilities. Rehabilitation facilities, skilled nursing facilities, and home health agencies are generally separate from the hospital, with different providers and different medical records systems. With hospitals discharging patients as soon as medically stable, these receiving facilities may have patients transferring to them in the evenings or on weekends when staffing is lower, and supplies and medications may not be readily available. Different facilities have different capabilities. Some skilled nursing facilities may not have a registered nurse on site overnight or on the weekends, with the majority of patient care carried out by nursing assistants. Most facilities do not have a pharmacy on site and have to request medications and supplies once the orders are received from the hospital. Many communicate with providers using a fax machine, which is often slow, and do not have access to the electronic medical records from the hospital. Taken together, these factors present challenges that must be considered at the time of patient transfer, to assure that all care needs will be met when the patient arrives. One strategy is to send your discharge orders and instructions to the receiving facility the day before the patient is discharged. This allows the facility adequate time to review the orders and obtain all supplies and medications necessary before the patient arrives.

Economic Challenges

Transitional care is labor intensive and requires a large amount of time spent on communication and patient education and counseling. Although there is a growing appreciation of the importance of skillful transitional care, the lack of financial incentives for hospitals to prevent readmissions and for clinicians to coordinate care and oversee transitions slows the process of improvement. Payment for patient education and coordination of transfers and discharges could appropriately compensate clinicians for the time required to provide quality transitional care.[9–11]

CASE PRESENTATION (continued)

After ensuring that Mrs. G.'s medication orders are complete, you call the orthopedist who will be performing her hip repair surgery. You ask him to consider options that might improve her leg function more quickly such as a hemiarthroplasty as opposed to a dynamic screw or intramedullary nail if that is what is indicated. You also ask him to discuss anesthesia options with the anesthesiologist, as you feel that she may be at moderate risk for delirium and you would like to prevent this complication if at all possible. You tell the orthopedist that you will manage all of her medications and pain control after the surgery and ask him only to write orders specifically related to the surgery. You also ask him, in his postoperative orders, to specify for the physical therapists how soon and what type of therapy can be started.

• PATIENT-SPECIFIC CHALLENGES

Geriatric patients, as compared to younger adults, present unique challenges when it comes to transitional care. For example, in the case of Mrs. G., her hip fracture and resultant surgery will require a stay in a skilled nursing facility (an extra transition before she is able to return home); she has several chronic medical problems and medications that will require ongoing follow-up with a health care provider after she leaves the hospital; she may experience delirium after her surgery, which could impair her ability to understand and remember medical instructions; and she has an elderly husband with dementia and will need to rely on others (her children, friends, or professionals) to support her during her recovery.

Specific patient characteristics (Table 22–1), including recent hospitalization, the use of five or more prescription medications, and difficulty with activities of daily living (Table 22–2), can be useful in identifying those patients who may be at increased risk for poor transitional outcomes.

● **TABLE 22–1** Risk Factors for Complicated Transitions

- Older age
- African American race
- Medicaid enrollment
- Low socioeconomic status
- Fair to poor self-assessment of health
- Living with non-relatives
- More than 2 chronic illnesses
- More than 5 prescription medications
- ED visit or hospitalization in prior 12 months
- Longer length of hospital stay
- Reason for hospitalization (DRG)[a]
- Discharge to a skilled nursing facility
- Impairment of activities of daily living

[a]*Diagnosis-related group. Diagnoses most commonly associated with rehospitalization include heart failure, psychoses, vascular surgery, chronic obstructive pulmonary disease, pneumonia, gastrointestinal problems, hip or knee surgery, major bowel surgery, and cardiac stent placement.[2]*

Source: Data from Jencks et al.,[2] Aliyu et al.[33] Bernheim et al.[34] and Kind et al.[35]

Although most of the risk factors identified in Table 22–1 cannot be modified or prevented, they can be easily identified. Once you recognize one or more of these risk factors in a hospitalized patient you can adjust the discharge plan to optimize the transition. For example, when caring for an older patient with low income who feels her health is poor, a hospital social worker can be consulted to determine if the patient qualifies for financial assistance in obtaining medications or treatments, offer information on community meal assistance (eg, Meals on Wheels), and ask about transportation availability to and from follow-up appointments. For another patient with recurrent congestive heart failure exacerbations, taking 12 medications with declining functional abilities, a thorough review of his medications by the health care provider and/or clinical pharmacist can be helpful in identifying unnecessary medications or alternative dosing to simplify the schedule and improve compliance. A referral to a home health agency after discharge would provide a visiting nurse to check weight, blood pressures, and medications, and assess for signs of worsening illness in the vulnerable period following hospitalization.

In the next sections we will discuss other patient-specific challenges and offer strategies for meeting these patient needs.

Co-Morbidity

Multiple co-morbid illnesses are common in the geriatric population. The natural result is that our patients often see multiple providers and take many medications, increasing the chances for miscommunication and medication discrepancies. Given the long lists, and frequent changes, patients may be unprepared to give a full medication history at the time of hospital admission, or they may be unable to do so because of acute or chronic cognitive impairment (delirium or dementia, respectively). When admitting a patient to the hospital, it is important to gather information from family members or the patient's community pharmacy if necessary, to confirm that the medication list is accurate. Communication with the patient's outpatient health care provider may provide additional information regarding prior disease management, social needs, and discharge planning.

In addition, elderly patients often have illnesses that require skilled nursing care or home health care (eg, hip fracture or congestive heart failure). Involving the social worker early in the hospital stay provides adequate time for the patient and family to choose an appropriate facility.

Social Support

Older adults may have a family member or friend who acts as an informal caregiver. This person may be consulted to help with decision-making, will require education regarding ongoing care, and should be provided with support during the stressful time of transitions, just as the patient is.[12] Hospital nurses should be providing the caregiver with education on any activities they will be assuming after discharge, including wound care, dressing changes, and medication administration. The caregiver should be given a list of signs to watch for, indicating worsening illness, and should have instructions on what types of diet and activities are acceptable for the patient to maintain. The social worker can be very helpful in identifying any patient needs that will not be met by the caregiver and can provide referrals to agencies that can help (eg, home health agency or community resources).

In many cultures, including Chinese, Japanese, other Asian groups, Latino, and African American, the value of filial piety is important and may need to be considered at the time of hospital discharge. Filial piety comes from the Chinese principle that children should love and respect their parents, and in modern culture this may manifest as an unstated expectation that family members will care for their elders. This may prevent some families from utilizing help from home health agencies, bath aides, or in many cases, skilled nursing care or nursing home placement. In these cases, a more detailed assessment of informal support and the abilities of the caregivers may be required.

Not all seniors have an informal support network to assist them with transitions. Certain groups, including seniors who live alone, recent immigrants, and lesbian, gay, bisexual, and transgender (LGBT) seniors, may have little support available to them.[12] Special attention should be paid to these groups at the time of discharge to assure their needs will be met once they return home. Issues to think about include planning for transportation to follow-up appointments and assessing the patient's level of independence with activities of daily living (Table 22–2). If needed, arrangements should be made for appropriate support services prior to discharge, for example home health care, a bath aide, or transportation.

● **TABLE 22–2** Activities of Daily Living (ADLs) and Instrumental Activities of Daily Living (IADLs)

ADLs	IADLs
Toileting	Cooking
Bathing	Doing household chores
Dressing	Shopping
Grooming	Managing finances
Eating	Using the telephone
Transferring (eg, moving from the bed to the chair, or from the chair to the toilet)	Managing medications
	Driving or managing transportation

Another group that may not receive adequate formal support services are "near poor" seniors, or those whose income is too much to qualify for assistance but not enough to cover necessary treatments, such as help with setting up medications or a visiting nurse to check weekly weights and vital signs. Social work may be able to provide information on community resources available to assist seniors with these types of needs.

caregiving responsibilities she has and that her wish is to return home to the caregiving role as soon as possible. Finally, you tell her that she was on warfarin for chronic atrial fibrillation, which was held for her surgery but that has now been resumed, and that an INR should be obtained a day or two after arriving in the rehabilitation facility.

CASE PRESENTATION (continued)

You stop by the room of Mrs. G. the morning following her right hip total arthroplasty. She doesn't remember you and is asking to speak to her mother, who passed away years ago. You recognize that she is delirious, likely due to the effects of anesthesia and postoperative pain medications. You note that she is on a good bowel regimen, but the nursing staff report that she has not had a bowel movement since admission. You adjust her pain medications and add another laxative, which gives good results by that afternoon.

In the days that follow, Mrs. G.'s delirium improves, her pain is controlled, and she is able to participate fully with the therapists and is reported to be making very good progress. Her daughter and her husband have assumed the care of Mrs. G.'s husband while she continues to recover. Plans are made for her transfer to a local skilled nursing facility for rehabilitation. As you prepare the transfer paperwork, Mrs. G.'s nurse informs you that she has been having difficulty ordering food using the hospital menu and admitted to the nurse that she has some difficulty reading and writing in English.

As the nurse reviews the written discharge instructions with Mrs. G, she remembers that she has some difficulty reading English. To be sure that Mrs. G. understands what to expect at the skilled nursing facility, the nurse reviews with her the course of her hospitalization as well as the plan for therapy and her recovery, and asks Mrs. G. to "teach-back" the information reviewed. The social worker comes in to reassure Mrs. G. that her husband is being well taken care of and that the rehabilitation facility is going to focus not only on her rehabilitation but also the use of proper techniques to use in the care of her husband so that she minimizes the risk of any injury to herself. You call the rehabilitation facility and ask to speak to the physician. You tell her about Mrs. G., that she had a fall with hip surgery but that she is doing well now. You inform her that her postoperative course was complicated by a mild delirium that has resolved, and that she may be sensitive to pain medications and is prone to constipation. You tell her of the

Health Literacy

As in the case of Mrs. G., some older adults may have difficulty reading or understanding medical instructions due to hearing or vision impairment, cognitive impairment, or inadequate health literacy.

"Health literacy" has been defined by the National Institutes of Health as the "degree to which individuals have the capacity to obtain, process and understand basic health information and services needed to make appropriate health decisions." Limited literacy affects approximately 90 million adults in the United States and is especially prevalent in the elderly population.[14] Lower reading ability among the elderly is multi-factorial and is related not only to chronic diseases, cognitive impairment, and education level but also to age-related declines in information processing.[13] Because of this, patients with inadequate literacy may have difficulty not only with reading but also with oral and written communication.[14] These limitations may be exacerbated at the time of a transition, when the setting is unfamiliar and important medical information is often presented in written format using medical jargon. Without adequate understanding of these changes in their care, adhering to recommendations is more difficult for patients, increasing the likelihood for complications and readmission.

In everyday practice, health care providers can take simple steps to improve the health literacy of their patients. Speaking more slowly, avoiding medical jargon, and using technological aids such as audiovisual materials can improve patients' understanding of medical conditions.[14,15] Adoption of a standard method for confirming patient comprehension, such as the "teach-back" approach, is another suggestion. For example, after instructing a patient on how to use a new medication, the provider should ask the patient to repeat back the instructions, and if the patient is unable to do so, the provider can then adjust the teaching method to assure understanding.[14] For more on health literacy please see Chapter 11.

Cultural Considerations

The geriatric population in the United States is becoming more ethnically and culturally diverse, and by 2050 it is estimated that 25% of older adults will be from an ethnic minority group. Regardless of ethnic group, patients and their caregivers report inadequate communication and education at the time of hospital discharge.[12] Providing patient education handouts and discharge materials in a patient's native language and the use of interpreters to assist with discharge counseling and education are important steps you can take toward a safe and successful transition.

Other racial and ethnic disparities exist and should be considered in the transitional care of some groups. Elderly black and Latino patients are less likely to have Medicare part B coverage compared to whites, and thus may have fewer outpatient visits or less follow-up for their chronic medical conditions.[16] Fewer outpatient visits and subsequent worse self-management of chronic conditions increases the risk for complications and hospital readmissions. Blacks and Latinos are also more likely to be readmitted than whites, even after correction for socioeconomic, demographic, or clinical factors, and these differences are more prominent among the elderly.[17]

Another subtle cultural factor to consider is the shift in roles that older patients are expected to undergo during transitions. While hospitalized or in skilled nursing facilities elderly patients often assume a passive role, depending on others for medication management and administration, daily needs such meals or bathing, and assistance or supervision with other activities. Then, upon the transition home they are suddenly expected to take on a much more independent role, not only in their previous responsibilities but also in self-management of their medical condition, and they are often left ill prepared.[8,9,18] Part of our role as health care providers should be to empower patients to take a more active role in their health care, especially around the time of a transition. Encouraging patients to be involved in the treatment plan (offering treatment options to choose from), and to assert their preferences during discharge planning (preferred time and date for follow-up), may help them feel more prepared for the next steps in their recovery.

CASE PRESENTATION (continued)

After a successful rehabilitation stay at the skilled nursing facility, Mrs. G. is ready to return to her home. Her discharge medications include lisinopril 20 mg daily, calcium 600 mg twice daily, vitamin D 1000 international units daily, warfarin 3 mg daily, omeprazole 20 mg daily, a multivitamin daily, and acetaminophen 1000 mg three times a day. She is to continue with outpatient physical therapy and needs to have lab work drawn in 1 week to check her protime. She is informed of the changes in her medications and doses, and has a follow-up appointment scheduled with her primary care provider for the following week and another appointment with orthopedic surgery in 2 weeks. Written instructions are provided as well. An updated medication list and problem list is sent to both her primary care provider and her orthopedist. A brief phone call to her regular doctor confirms that he is aware of what has transpired as well as the changes in her medications, with a recent INR that was therapeutic and that her gait function is with a wheeled walker.

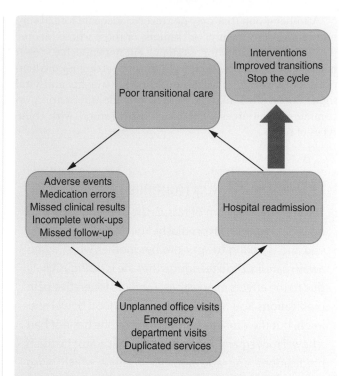

FIGURE 22–1. Consequences of poor transitional care.

Several days after her discharge to home the hospital pharmacist makes a follow-up phone call to see if she is experiencing any medication side effects. She mentions that she is feeling very unsteady on her feet when she gets up at night to go the bathroom. The pharmacist discovers that she is taking 20 mg of lisinopril twice a day, instead of once a day as ordered. The pharmacist notifies her primary provider and home health is ordered for a home safety evaluation and blood pressure checks. Her blood pressure is found to be running between 86 and 100 mm Hg systolic and her walker is now adjusted too high for her height. As a result, her lisinopril is decreased and her walker is adjusted to the proper height. Home health aides are coming now three times per week to assist Mrs. G. with her caregiving of her husband, and her daughter still helps out quite often. When asked how she is doing, Mrs. G. replies that considering that she broke her hip, she is quite pleased with her progress and says she will work hard to "get rid of this walker" (Figure 22–1).

Unfortunately the consequences of poor health care transitions are vast and vary from minor to life threatening. In the next section we will discuss techniques and procedures to ensure transitions are more likely to be successful and ensure optimal outcomes.

STRATEGIES FOR SUCCESSFUL TRANSITIONS

A number of researchers[19-22] have studied the effects of various transitional care innovations in randomized trials of patients being dismissed from hospital. Although the studies differed in the populations considered (for example, in one[20] subjects were not exclusively elderly, and another[22] enrolled only those with heart failure) and in the philosophical focus of the intervention (Coleman and associates aimed to coach their subjects to acquire transitions-related self-management skills, rather than to be passive recipients in the process[19]), these scholars have demonstrated that changes in hospital practices can reduce the risk of readmission. These interventions were multifactorial and typically incorporated one or more of the following ingredients:

- Coordination of the discharge (ie, identifying post-discharge needs and arranging for them, making appointments with physicians and other services, resolving transportation and other logistical problems).
- Educating patients about their discharge diagnoses and treatment plans, as well as how to recognize signs of clinical worsening and what to do.
- Medication reconciliation, ensuring that medications were at the correct dose, had an indication for use, and that any changes in medications were accounted for.
- Assuring transfer of crucial information (ie, in the form of a discharge summary) to follow-up providers.
- Some manner of contact with the patient at home after discharge (eg, nurse visit, pharmacist telephone call).

Medication Reconciliation

The medication list should be a key point of focus at the time of a transition because such a high proportion of adverse events surround medications. When preparing a patient for discharge, the health care provider should compare the discharge medications with the medication list at the time of admission. Differences should be carefully checked for errors and, once verified, should be made clear to the patient to avoid confusion.

Medication reconciliation between the patient and a health care professional, often a nurse or pharmacist, provides an opportunity to review changes to the previous medication regimen and to highlight new medications. During this process, the nurse or clinical pharmacist should provide the patient and caregiver with a paper copy of the discharge medications. The names of the medications, indications, dosage, schedule, and potential side effects should be reviewed. Special mention should be made of any dosage or schedule changes, new medications, or previous medications that have been discontinued. Medication reconciliation is also a good time for the patient and his or her caregiver to voice any questions and for the health care team to assess understanding and identify issues that may hinder compliance.

The discharging health care provider should also provide a detailed medication reconciliation in the discharge summary, making the changes clear to the next provider assuming care of the patient. A separate section titled "Discharge Medications" should appear in the discharge summary and state the name, dosage, route, schedule, and indication for each medication. Any previous medications that were stopped during admission should be listed as such. The following is an example of a medication reconciliation from a sample discharge summary (Figure 22–2).

Patient Name: Mrs. G.
Medical Record Number: 12345678
Date of Admission: 1-1-10
Date of Discharge: 1-9-10
Attending Physician: Ralph Brown, MD
Referring Physician: Susan Green, MD
Resident Physician: Sally White, MD
Discharge Diagnoses:
   Right hip fracture after a fall at home
   Delirium, post-operative, worsened by narcotic pain medications
   Osteoporosis
   Atrial fibrillation, chronic, on anticoagulation with warfarin
   Hypertension
   Macular degeneration
   Gastroesophageal reflux
   Inadequate health literacy, English is second language, preferred language is Japanese
Procedures Performed during Admission:
   Right hip total arthroplasty on 1-3-10
Consultations during Admission:
   Dr. Harold Smith—orthopedic surgery
Hospital Course:
   Mrs. G. is a 76-year-old woman who was admitted to the hospital on 1-1-10 after tripping on a throw rug in her bathroom, which resulted in a fall and a right-sided hip fracture. Please see the dictated history and physical from that date for additional information about her admitting physical examination and laboratory data.

1. *Right hip fracture*: On admission her INR was 2.5. Warfarin was held, and on 1-3-10 was 1.4 and orthopedic surgery proceeded with right hip total arthroplasty. Her post-operative course was complicated by delirium (see #2 below). By postoperative day #3 she was able to participate fully with therapy and her course progressed normally. On the day of discharge she was ambulating 50 feet with a walker and 1 person assist.
2. *Delirium, post-operative*: Mrs. G. experienced post-operative delirium, thought to be due to anesthesia and narcotic pain medications. In the days following her surgery, narcotic medications were weaned and pain was controlled with acetaminophen 1000 mg TID. Her delirium improved and on the day of discharge she was at her baseline normal mental status.
3. *Osteoporosis*: Calcium and vitamin D supplementation were continued without change.
4. *Atrial fibrillation, chronic, on anticoagulation*: Warfarin was held on admission, in preparation for surgery. It was restarted the day after surgery and INR on the day of discharge was 2.1. Goal INR is between 2 and 3. Heart rates were controlled throughout admission ranging 65-80.
5. *Hypertension*: Blood pressures were elevated post-operatively and lisinopril was increased to 20 mg daily. This achieved better control with systolic blood pressures less than 140 mmHg.
6. Gastroesophageal reflux: Mrs. G. has symptoms of reflux during her hospital stay and was started on omeprazole.
Discharge Medications:
1. Lisinopril 20 mg po daily, for hypertension—THIS IS A NEW DOSE—previous dose 10 mg daily
2. Calcium 600 mg po twice daily, for osteoporosis
3. Vitamin D 1000 international units po daily, for osteoporosis

---

FIGURE 22–2. Sample hospital discharge summary.

4. Warfarin 3 mg po daily, for atrial fibrillation—THIS IS A NEW DOSE—previous dose 2 mg daily
5. Multivitamin, one tablet po daily, for macular degeneration
6. Acetaminophen 1000 mg po three times a day, for pain—THIS IS A NEW MEDICATION
7. Omeprazole 20 mg po daily, for reflux—THIS IS A NEW MEDICATION

Gingko biloba supplement, 120 mg po daily WAS STOPPED during admission due to surgery

Discharge Instructions: Mrs. G. will be transferred to Shady Acres Skilled Nursing Facility for rehabilitation. Dr. Anthony Black will follow her there. She is to resume her previous diet (general). She is a one assist for ambulation and uses a walker. She will be followed by physical and occupational therapy at the skilled nursing facility. If she experiences easy bruising, bleeding, worsening pain or confusion, please contact Dr. Ralph Brown at 555-1234.

Follow-Up Appointments: With primary care physician, Dr. Green on 2-1-10 at 10 a.m. If she continues to require skilled nursing care at that time, please reschedule appointment for 1 week after her discharge from Shady Acres. Follow-up with Dr. Smith in orthopedic surgery on 2-7-10, with x-rays of the right hip to be done at the hospital before the appointment.

Laboratory Studies: INR to be drawn on 1-12-10. No laboratory or imaging studies are pending from her hospital stay.

Goals of Care/Code Status/Surrogate Decision-Maker: Mrs. G.'s son John lives nearby and is her durable power of attorney for health care. John's cell phone in 555-1111. Mrs. G. continues to desire treatment for her medical conditions and does want full efforts made in the event of a cardiac or pulmonary arrest (Full Code).

Functional Status at Transfer: Mrs. G. is at her baseline cognitive function, which is normal, with no deficits. She now ambulates with a walker and requires assistance with transfers, bathing, toileting, and dressing.

Dictated by: Sally White, MD, pager 555-0000
CC: Susan Green, MD, Anthony Black, MD

FIGURE 22–2. *(Continued)*

Discharge Medications

1. Lisinopril 20 mg by mouth daily, for hypertension—THIS IS A NEW DOSE—previous dose 10 mg daily
2. Calcium 600 mg by mouth twice daily, for osteoporosis
3. Vitamin D 1000 international units by mouth daily, for osteoporosis
4. Warfarin 3 mg by mouth daily, for atrial fibrillation—THIS IS A NEW DOSE—previous dose 2 mg daily
5. Multivitamin, one tablet by mouth daily, for macular degeneration
6. Acetaminophen 1000 mg by mouth three times a day, for pain—THIS IS A NEW MEDICATION
7. Omeprazole 20 mg by mouth daily, for reflux—THIS IS A NEW MEDICATION

Gingko biloba supplement, 120 mg by mouth daily, for memory, WAS STOPPED during admission, due to surgery.

Information Continuity

Unfortunately, patients often do not understand their discharge diagnoses, medications, or symptoms of worsening illness. This can make adhering to recommendations more difficult. In one survey of patients ready for discharge, less than half could identify their diagnoses and 72% could not name their medications.[23] Patients and their caregivers have

a better understanding of discharge instructions when material is provided in both verbal and written format.[24] At the time of discharge to home, patients need discharge instructions and a medication list provided in everyday language, and they need adequate time and opportunity to ask questions about their discharge plans before they leave the hospital.[25]

Coleman and colleagues have called for a change of mind-set surrounding hospital discharge, with a shift in thinking from that of a "patient discharge," something that has a definite end point, to that of a "patient transfer" with ongoing care.[10] Keeping this in mind as providers implement transitions, key items that should be considered include the site of the "transfer," what level of care the patient will receive there, who the next provider will be, and what information needs to be transmitted to support the ongoing care. Communication between providers is an essential component of this task.

One of the most important ways that a transferring provider can communicate to the receiving provider is through the discharge summary. Patients are often discharged from the hospital with test results pending, new medication regimens, and further work-up recommendations and follow-up appointments needed for ongoing medical problems. An effective discharge summary communicates these needs in addition to other information about the hospital course to the receiving provider. See Figure 22–2 for a sample discharge summary.

As it happens, discharge summaries are available for the first follow-up visit less than one-third of the time.[26,27] Even when these important documents do arrive in time, they are often too long and contain unnecessary information, making it difficult to find the important points needed.[25,28] Ideally, the discharge summary should be available to the primary provider within 24 hours of discharge. This is important not only for the first follow-up appointment, but also for any phone calls the provider may receive from the patient or family regarding discharge instructions, new symptoms, or other questions. If completion and transmission of the discharge summary within 24 hours is not possible, a brief phone call from the hospital team to the primary provider ensures continuity.[29] Some have also recommended a brief transfer form that can be filled out at the time of discharge and transmitted immediately to the primary care provider for review.[30] Some groups, including the Society for Hospital Medicine, also advocate for including the name and 24-hour contact information of the hospital physician in the discharge summary and patient discharge instructions, giving the patient and receiving provider a way to contact the hospital physician for questions in the vulnerable period immediately after discharge.[31]

Standardized Discharge Summary Components

Keeping a discharge summary brief and to the point is often a challenge, especially when caring for complex patients, but doing so is important so that a time-pressured next provider will be able to pull out the key points and recommendations easily. Although not every provider will agree on what he or she wants in a discharge summary, there is some consensus regarding the most important points to include. Primary care physicians agree that the main diagnosis, pertinent physical

● **TABLE 22–3** Key Points to Be Included in a Discharge Summary

✓ Reason for hospitalization
✓ Main diagnosis and secondary diagnoses
✓ Brief hospital course—best organized by problem, not chronologically
✓ Main findings and test results
✓ Procedures and treatments performed
✓ Discharge destination and provider
✓ Anticipated problems and recommendations
✓ Condition at discharge—including functional and cognitive status
✓ Reconciled medication list with specific changes noted
✓ List of unresolved medical issues, pending studies
✓ Education provided to patient/caregiver
✓ Follow-up appointments—primary care and subspecialty
✓ 24/7 callback number of hospital provider
✓ Resuscitation status/goals of care

Source: Data from Louden[29] and Halasyamani et al.[31]

The next major section in the discharge summary is the "Hospital Course." This key component is often the largest part of the document and all too often contains unnecessary information commonly listed in chronological order, making it difficult to pull out the key points. Our sample discharge summary (Figure 22–2) shows this section organized by problem or diagnosis and parallels the "Discharge Diagnoses" section. Each numbered item details one problem and highlights the major events and treatments that occurred during the hospital stay. Daily lab results, vital signs, and physical exam findings generally are not included. Items that were not addressed or "treated" during the hospital course, such as Mrs. G.'s macular degeneration, do not need to be listed in this section.

In addition to the reconciled medication list, discussed previously, the remaining key components of the discharge summary include the discharge instructions, follow-up appointments and labs or imaging, and any test results that remain pending at the time of discharge. We also advocate for including a section detailing the patient's goals of care and code status and a review of functional status (physical and cognitive) at the time of discharge. This information often proves very useful for the next provider, who may not have any previous experience with the patient for comparison. Refer to Figure 22–2 for examples of these components.

findings and test results, discharge medications with changes specifically noted, follow-up information, and patient and family education are "must have" items.[27,28] In addition, other groups have looked at this problem and published communications detailing what data elements are most important to communicate to the next provider.

Table 22–3 lists many of the items that providers feel are important components of a complete discharge summary. In the first major section, "Discharge Diagnoses," notice that the first item listed is the primary diagnosis and reason for admission. Placing this at the top of the list makes it easy for the reader to quickly identify what led to the hospitalization. Also notice that the primary diagnosis has a brief statement included with it to explain that this hip fracture was a result of a fall at home, highlighting a key piece of information from the history. The other diagnoses listed include Mrs. G.'s chronic medical conditions, but also included are delirium and inadequate health literacy. Affective (ie, depression), behavioral (ie, delirium), functional (ie, inability to ambulate independently), and social problems (ie, inadequate health literacy and caregiving for her husband) are important components that should be included in this section of the discharge summary. A new health care provider assuming the care of Mrs. G. can get a very quick, yet thorough picture of her health conditions by reading this list.

Discharge Diagnoses

Right hip fracture after a fall at home
Delirium, post-operative, worsened by narcotic pain medications, possible narcotic pain medication sensitivity
Osteoporosis
Atrial fibrillation, chronic, on anticoagulation with warfarin
Hypertension
Macular degeneration
Gastroesophageal reflux
Inadequate health literacy, English is second language, preferred language is Japanese
Caregiver to her husband who has early dementia

Follow-Up

In a recent analysis of Medicare beneficiaries, of all the patients with an unplanned readmission to the hospital in the first 30 days after discharge, 50% had not been seen by a primary provider.[2] Given the high risk of readmission in the early postdischarge period, some have argued that all elderly patients should have a follow-up appointment within 2 weeks after discharge.[25] Follow-up appointments should be made before the patient leaves the hospital, and the time to follow-up should be based on the patient's medical problems and risk of worsening condition, with the highest-risk patients being seen by a primary care provider within days after discharge and lower-risk patients allowed a later follow-up date within 2 weeks.[25,31,32]

Table 22–4 provides a list of practical tips for successful transitions.

● **TABLE 22–4** Tips for Successful Transitions

✓ Provide brief discharge communication, verbal or written, on the day of discharge to the next provider; send full discharge summary when available.
✓ Involve the primary provider in discharge planning, if possible.
✓ Complete medication reconciliation at the time of discharge, indicate dose changes, medications stopped, and new medications added—communicate to patient and next provider.
✓ Assess for unmet outpatient needs and consider additional services if indicated.
✓ Arrange for follow-up before the patient is discharged.
✓ Patient education prior to discharge targeting main diagnoses, red flags of worsening illness, medication changes, follow-up appointments, and provider contact information.
✓ Provide patient materials in both written and verbal form.
✓ Consider cultural factors, language, and health literacy.
✓ Encourage patient and caregiver participation in decision-making and take patient preferences into account.

Source: Data from Kripalani et al.[25]

SUMMARY

Quality transitional care is an important component of good medical care. Providers must actively involve patients and their caregivers in decision-making surrounding transitions and prepare them for the next step to come. Communication between providers is essential in preventing errors and improving patient safety during transitions. Patient transitions should be standardized and formalized, with the sending team of providers being responsible and available to the patient until the receiving team takes over care in the next setting. Provider collaboration, consideration of patient preferences, effective patient education, and awareness of the challenges surrounding changes in care settings provide the framework for improved transitional care (Figure 22–2).

References

1. Coleman EA, Boult C, American Geriatrics Society Health Care Systems Committee. Improving the quality of transitional care for persons with complex care needs. *J Am Geriatr Soc.* 2003;51:556-557.

2. Jencks SF, Williams MV, Coleman EA. Rehospitalizations among patients in the Medicare fee-for-service program. *N Engl J Med.* 2009;360:1418-1428.

3. Cornish PL, Knowles SR, Marchesano R, et al. Unintended medication discrepancies at the time of hospital admission. *Arch Intern Med.* 2005;165:424-429.

4. Forster AJ, Clark HD, Menard A, et al. Adverse events among medical patients after discharge from hospital. *CMAJ.* 2004;170:345-349.

5. Forster AJ, Murff HJ, Peterson JF, et al. The incidence and severity of adverse events affecting patients after discharge from the hospital. *Ann Intern Med.* 2003;138:161-167.

6. Moore C, Wisnivesky J, Williams S, McGinn T. Medical errors related to discontinuity of care from an inpatient to an outpatient setting. *J Gen Intern Med.* 2003;18:646-651.

7. Sharma G, Fletcher KE, Zhang D, et al. Continuity of outpatient and inpatient care by primary care physicians for hospitalized older adults. *JAMA.* 2009;301:1671-1680.

8. Coleman EA. Falling through the cracks: challenges and opportunities for improving transitional care for persons with continuous complex care needs. *J Am Geriatr Soc.* 2003;51:549-555.

9. Coleman EA, Berenson RA. Lost in transition: Challenges and opportunities for improving the quality of transitional care. *Ann Intern Med.* 2004;141:533-536.

10. Coleman EA, Fox PD. One Patient, Many Places: Managing health care transitions, part I: Introduction, accountability, information for patients in transition. *Ann Long-Term Care.* 2004;12:25.

11. Snow V, Beck D, Budnitz T, et al. Transitions of Care Consensus Policy Statement American College of Physicians-Society of General Internal Medicine-Society of Hospital Medicine-American Geriatrics Society-American College of Emergency Physicians-Society of Academic Emergency Medicine. *J Gen Intern Med.* 2009;24:971-976.

12. Graham CL, Ivey SL, Neuhauser L. From hospital to home: Assessing the transitional care needs of vulnerable seniors. *Gerontologist.* 2009;49:23-33.

13. Baker DW, Gazmararian JA, Sudano J, Patterson M. The association between age and health literacy among elderly persons. *J Gerontol B Psychol Sci Soc Sci.* 2000;55:S368-S374.

14. Paasche-Orlow MK, Schillinger D, Greene SM, Wagner EH. How health care systems can begin to address the challenge of limited literacy. *J Gen Intern Med.* 2006;21:884-887.

15. Baker DW, Gazmararian JA, Williams MV, et al. Functional health literacy and the risk of hospital admission among Medicare managed care enrollees. *Am J Public Health.* 2002;92:1278-1283.

16. Harris MI. Racial and ethnic differences in health insurance coverage for adults with diabetes. *Diabetes Care.* 1999;22:1679-1682.

17. Jiang HJ, Andrews R, Stryer D, Friedman B. Racial/ethnic disparities in potentially preventable readmissions: The case of diabetes. *Am J Public Health.* 2005;95:1561-1567.

18. Coleman EA, Smith JD, Frank JC, et al. Development and testing of a measure designed to assess the quality of care transitions. *Int J Integr Care.* 2002;2:e02.

19. Coleman EA, Parry C, Chalmers S, Min SJ. The care transitions intervention: Results of a randomized controlled trial. *Arch Intern Med.* 2006;166:1822-1828.

20. Jack BW, Chetty VK, Anthony D, et al. A reengineered hospital discharge program to decrease rehospitalization: A randomized trial. *Ann Intern Med.* 2009;150:178-187.

21. Naylor MD, Brooten D, Campbell R, et al. Comprehensive discharge planning and home follow-up of hospitalized elders: A randomized clinical trial. *JAMA.* 1999;281:613-620.

22. Rich MW, Beckham V, Wittenberg C, et al. A multidisciplinary intervention to prevent the readmission of elderly patients with congestive heart failure. *N Engl J Med.* 1995;333:1190-1195.

23. Makaryus AN, Friedman EA. Patients' understanding of their treatment plans and diagnosis at discharge. *Mayo Clin Proc.* 2005;80:991-994.

24. Flacker J, Park W, Sims A. Hospital discharge information and older patients: Do they get what they need? *J Hosp Med.* 2007;2:291-296.

25. Kripalani S, Jackson AT, Schnipper JL, Coleman EA. Promoting effective transitions of care at hospital discharge: A review of key issues for hospitalists. *J Hosp Med.* 2007;2:314-323.

26. van Walraven C, Seth R, Austin PC, Laupacis A. Effect of discharge summary availability during post-discharge visits on hospital readmission. *J Gen Intern Med.* 2002;17:186-192.

27. Kripalani S, LeFevre F, Phillips CO, et al. Deficits in communication and information transfer between hospital-based and primary care physicians: Implications for patient safety and continuity of care. *JAMA.* 2007;297:831-841.

28. O'Leary KJ, Liebovitz DM, Feinglass J, et al. Outpatient physicians' satisfaction with discharge summaries and perceived need for an electronic discharge summary. *J Hosp Med.* 2006;1:317-320.

29. Louden K. Creating a better discharge summary: Is standardization the answer? *ACP Hospitalist.* Published online March 2009. http://www.acphospitalist.org/archives/2009/03/discharge.htm. Accessed July, 2010.

30. Balaban RB, Weissman JS, Samuel PA, Woolhandler S. Redefining and redesigning hospital discharge to enhance patient care: A randomized controlled study. *J Gen Intern Med.* 2008;23:1228-1233.

31. Halasyamani L, Kripalani S, Coleman E, et al. Transition of care for hospitalized elderly patients—Development of a discharge checklist for hospitalists. *J Hosp Med.* 2006;1:354-360.

32. Coleman EA, Williams MV. Executing high-quality care transitions: A call to do it right. *J Hosp Med.* 2007;2:287-290.

33. Aliyu MH, Adediran AS, Obisesan TO. Predictors of hospital admissions in the elderly: Analysis of data from the longitudinal Study on Aging. *J Natl Med Assoc.* 2003;95:1158-1167.

34. Bernheim SM, Spertus JA, Reid KJ, et al. Socioeconomic disparities in outcomes after acute myocardial infarction. *Am Heart J.* 2007;153:313-319.

35. Kind AJ, Smith MA, Frytak JR, Finch MD. Bouncing back: Patterns and predictors of complicated transitions 30 days after hospitalization for acute ischemic stroke. *J Am Geriatr Soc.* 2007;55:365-373.

POST-TEST

1. **You are caring for an 81-year-old woman admitted to the hospital for community-acquired pneumonia. During the course of her hospital stay you discover that she lives alone. Which of the following is most important to assess before she leaves the hospital?**

   A. Is she able to complete her activities of daily living (ADLs) independently, and if not, who is available to help her?

   B. Is she able to drive her car, and if not, who is available to help her?

   C. Is she able to walk 500 feet unassisted, and if not, who is available to help her?

   D. Is she able to balance her checkbook independently, and if not, who is available to help her?

2. **Which of the following patients is at the HIGHEST risk of hospital readmission?**

   A. An 84-year-old woman who lives alone, has hypertension and macular degeneration, and takes two chronic medications

   B. An 84-year-old woman who lives with her husband, has hypertension, diabetes mellitus and coronary artery disease requiring three hospital admissions in the past year, and takes five chronic medications

   C. An 84-year-old man who lives with his son, has hypertension and peripheral vascular disease, needs to go home on oxygen for a chronic obstructive pulmonary disease (COPD) exacerbation, and takes five chronic medications

   D. An 84-year-old man who lives with his son, has hypertension and diabetes mellitus, fell and broke his hip requiring a skilled nursing facility (SNF) stay, needs help with bathing and dressing, and takes five chronic medications

3. **Which of the following is the best step to take when discharging a patient, knowing that your discharge summary will NOT reach the primary care provider right away?**

   A. Ask the hospital nurse to call the office and leave a message notifying the provider of the patient's discharge.

   B. Tell the patient that your discharge summary will not be available immediately and ask the patient to bring a copy of his or her discharge instructions to the follow-up appointment.

   C. Make a brief telephone call to the primary provider on the day of discharge to give an update on the patient's condition and treatment plan and to provide your contact information in case of further questions.

   D. Fax a copy of all hospital notes to the primary provider for review before the patient's follow-up appointment.

ANSWERS TO PRE-TEST

1. B
2. A
3. D

ANSWERS TO POST-TEST

1. A
2. D
3. C

23

Advanced Illness Care and Elders at the End of Life

Maura Brennan, MD

Mayu Sekiguchi, MD, MPH

Julie McCole Phillips, MD

● **LEARNING OBJECTIVES**

1. Describe the challenges in caring for frail elders with advanced illness.
2. Discuss the role of the palliative care and hospice teams in relief of suffering or improving quality of life.
3. Delineate appropriate circumstances for the involvement/consultation of palliative care and hospice teams.
4. Discuss the process for breaking bad news to patients and families.
5. Discuss the difficulty in approaching and determining prognosis.
6. Explain the pros and cons regarding artificial food and hydration at the end of life.
7. Describe the process and physiology of dying.
8. Discuss guidelines and dosage of opiate and non-opiate medications to relieve pain and minimize side effects.
9. Describe barriers to opiate use.

PRE-TEST

1. **Which of the following accurately defines the term "pseudo-addiction"?**

    A. Patients pretend to be addicted to opiates to secure more of the drugs.

    B. Patients are lethargic and confused for other reasons but are thought by health care professionals to be overmedicated with opiates.

    C. Patients' family members are addicted to opiates and divert the patients' pain medications.

    D. Patients exhibit "drug-seeking" behavior solely because they have not had their pain controlled and no longer request escalating treatment once appropriate analgesia is provided.

2. **Which of the following is correct regarding home hospice services?**

   A. Hospice emphasizes quality of life for patients and family rather than focusing on life-prolonging therapies.

   B. The majority of patients in hospice have cancer.

   C. Hospice patients must have a "do not resuscitate" order and may not be re-hospitalized.

   D. If patients survive more than 6 months they are automatically discharged from hospice.

3. **Which of the following is NOT true about bereavement?**

   A. Most bereaved individuals do not require treatment for their grief.

   B. Integrated grief is normal.

   C. Longer time in hospice is associated with higher incidence of complicated grief in survivors.

   D. Poor concentration, difficulty sleeping, and physical symptoms may persist for months after a major loss.

4. **"Difficult conversations" explore prognosis and expectations, break bad news, or seek to clarify the goals of care. Which of the following statements about them is TRUE?**

   A. Culture and ethnicity have little impact on these discussions, which are deeply personal in nature.

   B. In order to fully respect patients autonomy it is best to discuss life-changing diagnoses and information with patients alone prior to including families.

   C. Patients with dementia should not participate in these discussions because they will forget the details.

   D. Most patients wish to know their diagnoses and options but a small minority prefer to defer all difficult discussions to loved ones and should be permitted to do so.

● INTRODUCTION

In the early 1900s, life expectancy in the United States was approximately 50 years of age. There were no antibiotics and treatments were limited. The focus was on "caring" and not "curing"; clinicians strove to promote comfort and alleviate illness-related suffering.

Subsequent technologic advances have greatly affected disease trajectories. Mortality rates have declined due to scientific advances and improvements in living standards and preventive medicine. At present life expectancy at birth for both sexes in the United States is 78 years. Death in modern times is more protracted and complex than in the pre-industrial era. Most Americans now die of complications related to chronic, debilitating, and life-limiting illnesses. They suffer a lengthy series of losses punctuated by intermittent crises. Eventually this culminates in a more rapid terminal functional decline.[1]

Worldwide, cancer, cardiovascular diseases, or chronic respiratory diseases cause six out of every ten deaths.[2] The mortality patterns in developing countries reflect women's high risk of death during pregnancy and childbirth as well as the prevalence of infectious diseases (eg, AIDS, tuberculosis, malaria). As the world's population ages and global deaths related to tobacco use and HIV infection rise, the need for assiduous palliative care becomes more urgent.

Each country faces unique challenges. In the United States, roughly four out of five adults would prefer to die at home, yet only about 20% do so. Almost two-thirds die in acute-care hospitals and one in five ends life in a nursing home. Sadly, care for people with advancing illness is often suboptimal. Family members of patients who die in hospitals and nursing homes identify many unmet needs for symptom management and are distressed by poor physician communication. They also feel unsupported emotionally and believe that their dying loved ones are not always treated respectfully.[3]

In more developed nations, the geographic dispersion of families, the entry of women into the workforce, and high divorce rates have all led to fewer family caregivers for patients when illness advances. The resultant need for institutionalization has dramatically altered our experience with death and dying, which some even say has become "sanitized." Professionals now commonly care for the dying and prepare the body for cremation or burial. This deprives loved ones of the final gestures of love and respect once regarded as instrumental in the bereavement process.

The hospice/palliative care movement seeks to address these challenges. The National Consensus Project for Quality Palliative Care states:

> The goal of palliative care is to prevent and relieve suffering and to support the best possible quality of life for patients and their families, regardless of the stage of the disease or the need for other therapies. . . [It] expands traditional disease-model medical treatments to include the goals of enhancing quality of life for patient and family, optimizing function, helping with decision-making and providing opportunities for personal growth . . . incorporating psychosocial and spiritual care according to patient/family needs, values beliefs and culture(s).[4]

CASE PRESENTATION 1: A FAMILY MEETING

You are evaluating Mr. Jorge Feliciano, age 75 years, for his fourth hospital admission for congestive heart failure. He is the beloved patriarch of his family. He lost his wife shortly after immigrating to the United States from Mexico and raised their two small daughters alone. His past medical history includes his first heart attack when he was in his 50s and three others that followed over the years. He underwent coronary artery bypass surgery twice, as well as two angioplasties with stenting, but ultimately developed left ventricular failure with an ejection fraction of 24%, in addition to chronic kidney disease from type 2 diabetes. An automated internal cardiac defibrillator was placed upon the recommendation of his cardiologist approximately 1 year ago. He reports he is taking his medications faithfully, but more recently has been having more medication-related side effects.

He says he used to enjoy walking around his assisted living complex but increasingly has had to stop at every bench along the way to catch his breath. This decline culminated in orthopnea and now his fourth admission in as many months. His daughter is requesting a family meeting. You discuss Mr. Feliciano's situation with him as well as remind his family of an earlier conversation you had with them regarding considering a transition to palliative care or hospice. He and his family say they are now ready for hospice and arrangements are made to return home with a hospice evaluation scheduled.

● FAMILY MEETINGS

Family meetings require careful planning and thought. Clinicians must carefully review the medical record and possible treatment options and discuss expectations and the goals of the meeting among themselves beforehand. This will avoid "mixed messages" and limit patient and family distress. The meeting should occur in a quiet, private place with everyone seated within reach of tissues. Following introductions, the patient and loved ones ought to be asked what they understand about the situation and how much they wish to know. Bad news is "any news that adversely and seriously affects an individual's view of his or her future."[5] It may be helpful to fire an initial "warning shot" such as "I'm afraid I have some bad news for you today." The information should then be conveyed in short sentences that avoid medical jargon. Identification and empathic acknowledgement of the emotions experienced demonstrates the physician's caring. The meeting usually ends with a summary and review of the plan.[6,7]

● HOME-BASED PALLIATIVE CARE

Almost 60% of those receiving home hospice services in the United States have nonmalignant advanced illnesses such as end-stage heart, lung, liver, or kidney disease or neurodegenerative diseases (dementia, amyotrophic lateral sclerosis, or Parkinson disease). About 10% simply enroll in hospice with "debility" (ie, multifactorial, rapidly declining function with decreased food intake and weight loss).[8] Medicare offers a hospice benefit for those whose prognosis appears to be 6 months or less; there are established guidelines for hospice admissions for most major terminal illnesses.[9] Each person is unique, however, and hospice staff can help determine if enrollment is appropriate. The "6-month rule" and rigid criteria often delay access to needed services. Palliative Medicine consultants should become involved much earlier in the trajectory; they can assist with a holistic, patient- and family-centered approach to care even while the patient continues to pursue life-prolonging and curative therapies.

CASE PRESENTATION 1 (continued)

Jorge Feliciano Asks about Prognosis

After having his symptoms under better control with your management and hospice care, Mr. Feliciano decides that he does not want cardiopulmonary resuscitation if his heart stops and he does not want his defibrillator to restart his heart either, so his defibrillator is turned off.[10] His cardiologist understood that it was becoming more difficult for Mr. Feliciano to continue to come to her office and sensitively acknowledged this. She told Mr. Feliciano she was honored to have been his doctor. "I'll really miss hearing your stories; I have greatly admired your courageous spirit." Mr. Feliciano appreciated this gesture and thanked her for her dedication and good care over the years. It was a meaningful exchange for them both.[11] At the end of the meeting, he had one more question: "Doctor, how much time do you think I have left to live?"

● PROGNOSTICATION

The question of "How much time do I have?" is one of the most important yet daunting questions asked of the medical professional. If patients and families understand how much time remains, they can make rational decisions about whether to spend it with family or in estate planning, funeral arrangements, or other practical issues. It also can alter treatment plans greatly, ensuring that choices are based on likely outcomes rather than hoped-for results that may be unrealistic.

Despite its importance, many providers struggle to respond to questions about prognosis. A number of factors can assist with prognostication. Declining functional status usually precedes death. Additionally, symptoms such as anorexia, weight loss, dysphagia, dyspnea, and delirium portend shortening survival.[12]

When estimating survival, physicians tend to overestimate by a factor of three.[13] This has many repercussions and is one of the reasons why people are often referred to hospice late; this limits support and care from trained staff at this difficult time. The hospice Medicare benefit in the United States provides home-based services for 6 months with recertification and continued care thereafter in increments of 2 months if the person continues to have a poor prognosis. In 2008, the median length of stay for hospice patients was only 21.3 days, although the average length of stay increased slightly to 69.5 days.[8] In fact, 35.4% of hospice patients died or were discharged within a week of enrollment.[8]

Balancing hope with realism can be a challenge.[14] In discussing prognosis, it helps to acknowledge that no one can say precisely how much time is left and that each person is unique. However, based on how the person has been feeling and the usual course of the illness, it is generally possible to give a sense of whether the time frame is hours to days, days to weeks, or weeks to months. Parameters that suggest improvement or progressing decline can be identified in advance (such as energy level, functional status, and response to treatments), and the provider can revise prognostic estimates as the clinical situation evolves.

CASE PRESENTATION 1 (continued)

Prior to Mr. Feliciano's discharge home, you review his medications, and only those contributing to comfort are continued. You try an opioid for dyspnea with good effect. (See "Treating Pain with Opioids" later in the chapter for more details.) With his symptoms under better control, the home-based palliative care team was able to work with him to identify unfinished business including "things that might be left unsaid or undone" if time were shorter than he wished. He and his family were told how phrases beginning with "please forgive me, I forgive you, thank you, and I love you"[15,16] can sometimes promote healing. The hospice psychologist catalyzed a family meeting to encourage dialogue and connectedness.[17] The family, including Mr. Feliciano's grandchildren, gathered around him to speak about his illness and its impact, their worries, his life story, and their relationships. Tears were shed but laughter was also shared as the family celebrated this great man's life and healed some past hurts.

Mr. Feliciano was sorry that he would miss his granddaughter's wedding the next autumn. The hospice team arranged for her to come to his home in her wedding gown. A hospice volunteer trained in therapeutic letter writing helped Mr. Feliciano put down on paper some words of wisdom and a blessing to be read at the celebration. Mr. Feliciano was pleased with the letter and took pride in passing on his "Ethical Will" or statement of values, wisdom, hopes and advice.[18] Two months later he died peacefully at home with both daughters at his bedside. The reading of Mr. Feliciano's letter at his granddaughter's wedding was a moving part of the ceremony.

● THE INTERDISCIPLINARY TEAM

The interdisciplinary team is at the heart of the hospice and palliative medicine approach. It differs from the traditional multidisciplinary team in which the physician makes all decisions and other services are invited in as consultants. The interdisciplinary team collaborates to devise a coordinated care plan, enhances teamwork, and ideally decreases the stress of caring for the dying. Team composition varies with available resources and patient/family needs. Medicare regulations, however, require that a minimum of four core team members meet to review each person's care at least every 2 weeks. The participants must include a nurse, physician, social worker, and pastoral or other counselor. Some organizations also include a bereavement coordinator, volunteers, and therapists (music, speech, physical, etc.). The viewpoints of many professionals with differing backgrounds prevent "medicalization" of the meeting and promote wide-ranging discussion that includes the emotional, spiritual, and psychological needs of patients and their loved ones.

CASE PRESENTATION 2: FREDERICK JOHNSON'S BATTLE WITH LUNG CANCER

Mr. Frederick Johnson is a 66-year-old, right-handed, African American gentleman who had served in the Marines during the Vietnam War. Five months ago you diagnosed an inoperable right apical lung cancer after Mr. Johnson presented with cough and an unusual fullness in his right supraclavicular fossa. He underwent a CT-guided biopsy of the lung mass and then was referred to oncology, which recommended palliative chemotherapy. More recently he has developed a significant amount of pain that is affecting his daily activities. While his vitals are being taken in triage at the VA clinic, when the nurse administers the standard analog pain scale, which she does for every veteran, he rates his pain as 9 out of 10 in his right shoulder and describes intermittent shooting pains down his right arm.

● DIAGNOSING AND ASSESSING PAIN

A thorough pain assessment is critical; this should include the location, character, frequency, and any alleviating and/or exacerbating factors. There are three main categories of pain:

somatic, visceral, and neuropathic. Somatic pain (eg, from arthritis, bone metastases, or a fracture) tends to be a constant, dull aching that worsens with movement. Visceral pain is usually a deeper ache or twisting cramp that is less well localized. It can be caused by tumor infiltration or compression or distension of thoracic or abdominal organs. This pain may be referred to a cutaneous site distant from the source of the pain. Neuropathic pain results from tumor compression or invasion of nerves, nerve roots, or the spinal cord; surgical trauma; chemotherapy-induced neuropathies; or sequelae from radiation.

A variety of pain scales exist. These include numeric scales, visual analog scales, and drawn faces expressing the range from comfort to distress. Self-report should be used whenever possible. Many studies have shown that observers often underestimate patients' pain. Clinicians must understand that people suffering from chronic pain do not present the same way as those with acute pain. Chronic pain may simply manifest itself as decreased functional status, anxiety, or depression and can interfere with sleep, appetite, and concentration.

It is essential to fully assess pain and other symptoms for people with advancing illnesses. One validated tool is the Memorial Symptom Assessment Scale,[19] which evaluates 32 physical and psychological symptoms as well as the associated intensity, frequency, and level of distress. The Brief Pain Inventory is another easily understood, self-administered questionnaire.[20] Similar instruments exist to evaluate pain in vulnerable patients who are nonverbal or cognitively impaired.[21]

Once the patient has rated the pain, the provider must identify and analyze the various factors affecting the pain experience to tease out which may respond to additional medications or escalating doses. Each person has unique prior experiences and neurophysiologic responses to pain. Other physical symptoms (nausea, constipation, etc.), emotional pain, and existential or spiritual suffering as well as the perceived meaning of the pain all impact the "total pain" experienced by the sufferer.

CASE PRESENTATION 2 (continued)

Mr. Johnson's Pain

When you see Mr. Johnson in clinic he complains that his handgrip on the right has weakened, he now has difficulty opening jars, and more recently he has been dropping items. Just moving his arm brings on intense pain that wakes him from sleep. He reports difficulty concentrating, feels like he is more irritable, and his appetite is poor and he has lost 10 lb (4.5 kg) in the last 2 months. When you examine him, you note decreased range of motion due to pain and muscle atrophy in the C7-T1 distribution. You think that he might have developed a right brachial plexopathy causing severe neuropathic pain. You discuss your findings with Mr. Johnson and recommend he start on an oral opioid and oral steroids. When your nurse calls him 3 days later he reports that he has experienced significant relief with better range of motion and thinks he will be able to proceed with his chemotherapy.

● TREATING PAIN WITH OPIOIDS

Occasionally, for mild pain, non-opioid medications such as nonsteroidal anti-inflammatories suffice, at least initially. More often, especially in advanced illness, an opioid is required for adequate analgesia or to address refractory dyspnea. In general, one starts with a dose titration period using a short-acting medication. Care must be taken if the medication selected has a non-opioid moiety attached such as acetaminophen. Acetaminophen manufacturers impose a ceiling dose to avoid liver toxicity which thereby limits the usefulness of such combination medications for constant moderate to severe pain. Short-acting medications provide relief within an hour, but this same rapid rise in peak plasma concentration can result in adverse effects such as sedation and confusion. The duration of relief is brief; pain may recur prior to the next dose. This "peak and trough effect" from shifting plasma levels is undesirable and "around-the-clock" dosing every 4 hours is burdensome; patients may awake in severe pain at night as drug levels fall.

Thus, for patients who are not actively dying, one commonly finds the dose of immediate-release opioid that optimally controls the pain and then converts it to an equivalent dose of a longer-acting opioid. The short-acting formulation should remain available for breakthrough pain and generally is ordered at 10% to 15% of the total daily dose. For example, if the patient takes oral sustained-release oxycodone 40 mg twice a day, the breakthrough dose should be 10 mg of immediate-release oxycodone for intermittent pain that occurs despite the more even basal control provided by the longer-acting drug. Oral immediate-release opioids usually reach peak effect in an hour; thus, rescue doses can be taken hourly if needed. Clearly, if frequent breakthrough doses are required, the regimen should be readjusted. Usually, this includes a corresponding upward titration in the dose of the longer-acting opioid.

● OPIOID SELECTION

Morphine is metabolized by the liver into several active metabolites that are then largely cleared by the kidney. If there is significant renal impairment, morphine-6-glucuronide can accumulate and cause neurotoxicity including sedation, delirium, and myoclonus. Hydromorphone, oxycodone, fentanyl, or methadone are reasonable alternatives in the setting of chronic kidney disease. However, long half-life opioids such as methadone are very challenging to titrate and monitor. Methadone is particularly difficult to use since cross-tolerance is unpredictable and the risk of QT prolongation and arrhythmias is real. (Cross-tolerance refers to changes in receptor affinity for chronically used opioids. Calculated "equianalgesic" doses must be decreased when rotating opioids in opioid-tolerant patients to avoid overdose.) Methadone is a useful drug but should only be prescribed by very experienced clinicians.

The least invasive, safe route is the best approach to analgesia. The oral route is always preferred if feasible. The transdermal route is an option (though admittedly a more expensive one) for those who are unable to reliably take oral medications. Fentanyl is available in a patch that is applied every 2 to 3 days. The subcutaneous reservoir of medication initially builds up over almost a day; there can be significant variation in bioavailability. Due to the long half-life, rapid titration is impossible so fentanyl patches should not be used in a pain crisis that needs dose-finding. Transmucosal formulations of the highly lipophilic fentanyl are available for buccal use as rapid-onset alternatives for breakthrough or movement-induced pain.

Liquid concentrates of opioids can be useful. They are not well absorbed buccally or sublingually; most of the medication probably eventually makes it way to the back of the mouth and is swallowed. Clearly, a person with dysphagia or somnolence will be unable to take more than a milliliter or two without increasing the risk of aspiration, so this route has limited use in these settings.

Parenteral opioids may be appropriate for select patients. The relative potency of oral to intravenous or subcutaneous medication can vary considerably from person to person, so doses must be carefully monitored and adjusted. When intravenous access is not feasible or desired, subcutaneous infusions provide basal pain or dyspnea control along with bolus capacity.

OPIOPHOBIA

Patients, loved ones, and even some health care professionals share a number of fears ("opiophobia") and misconceptions about opioids. This confusion can result in a reluctance to use them. It is critical for medical professionals to fully comprehend the concepts of tolerance, dependence, addiction, and pseudo-addiction.

Tolerance is an expected physiologic response to chronic use of an opioid and likely involves changes at the receptor level. Tolerance is actually desirable since as patients acclimate to the drugs the somnolence, nausea, and even respiratory depression that may accompany opioid use abates. Tolerance develops quite slowly, if at all, to the decreased gut motility that results in constipation. For this reason, it is critical to simultaneously prescribe laxatives. Patients sometimes worry that tolerance will develop to the analgesic benefit of opiates and may try to "save" the drugs for a time of future desperation when the suffering is intolerable and refractory to treatment. In fact, the need for escalating doses of opioids usually is due to disease progression (or less commonly, rising emotional distress) rather than true analgesic tolerance.

If a patient takes opioids chronically, physical dependence will develop and abrupt discontinuation or administration of an opioid antagonist will result in physiologic withdrawal. Patients should be reassured that this is not unique to opioids and does not represent an addiction. Abrupt discontinuation of a beta-blocker causes rebound tachycardia but nobody says that patients are "addicted" to metoprolol! Addiction is characterized by a psychological dependence resulting in aberrant behaviors to procure the medication even in the absence of symptoms warranting its use. When opioids are appropriately prescribed for patients with cancer pain, true addiction is exceedingly rare.

Pseudo-addiction describes the situation when undertreatment of pain causes an individual to exhibit what appears to be "drug-seeking behavior." Once the pain is properly relieved, however, the behavior ceases. Clinicians must carefully access and manage pain to avoid erroneously stigmatizing and labeling patients as "addicts" when the problem is really suboptimal prescribing.

ADJUVANT MEDICATIONS

Adjuvant medications have a primary indication other than pain relief but also offer analgesic benefit in certain conditions. They are often utilized to improve relief in refractory cases or to be "opioid sparing," that is, to reduce untoward side effects of opioids by allowing a lower dose. Among others, classes of adjuvants include corticosteroids, antidepressants (especially the heterocyclics), alpha-2-adrenergic agonists, anticonvulsants, and radiopharmaceuticals. In general, adjuvants are less reliable and effective analgesics, may carry a higher burden of side effects, and have a slower therapeutic onset than opioids. Usually prescribers should first optimize the dosing of the opioid and then weigh the pros and cons of adding adjuvant therapy if pain control is inadequate and further escalation of opioids is limited by side effects. Polypharmacy is a problem; careful scrutiny of potential risks and benefits prior to initiation of an adjuvant is important, as is intermittent reassessment to ensure ongoing need.

CASE PRESENTATION 2 (continued)
Frederick Johnson's Hospitalization

Mr. Johnson has done well for several months but now his disease has progressed. Unfortunately, neither you nor his oncologist discussed home hospice with him. One evening, he becomes acutely dyspneic and a concerned neighbor calls emergency medical services. Mr. Johnson has no documentation of his code status or advance directives at home or in his records at the Veterans Administration Hospital. When the ambulance arrives he is almost intubated. He is evaluated in the emergency room, stabilized on a noninvasive positive pressure mask, and admitted to the intensive care unit (ICU) for treatment of a post-obstructive pneumonia.

Mr. Johnson improves and then subsequently has a discussion with the ICU team about his goals of care and advance directives. He decides that he does not want his care to include mechanical ventilation. Based on his wishes and discussion with the ICU team he is transferred to the Veterans Affairs inpatient hospice unit. Despite what appears to be good pain and dyspnea control, the hospice team notes he is restless and upset. They come to the conclusion that he may be suffering from emotional pain.

ADVANCED DIRECTIVES

Complications predictably arise as illnesses advance. The clinical realities and the goals of care determine the optimal response. It is crucial to define and document choices beforehand to guide care when inevitable decompensations occur. A number of tools promote discussion of advance directives.

One popular document is the living will called "Five Wishes."[22] This easy-to-use booklet was introduced in 1997 and has been translated into 23 languages. It meets the legal requirements of an advance directive and provides patients with a way to document health care proxies and specific emotional, spiritual, and medical wishes. The last "wish" allows the patient to detail preferences regarding organ donation, anatomic gift, and burial or cremation arrangements. The person can even record how he or she would like to be remembered.

The MOLST (Medical Order for Life Sustaining Treatment) form[23] is a standardized order form that complements advance directives. It is completed by the physician based on a conversation with the patient or designated decision-maker. It details goals and preferences with regard to cardiopulmonary resuscitation, artificial hydration, future hospitalizations, and antibiotic use. It accompanies the patient through all health care setting transitions to ensure his or her wishes are known and respected.

As early as feasible, health care providers should suggest that patients consider, discuss, and document preferences and values. In the setting of advancing illness, certain complications are fairly common, such as post-obstructive pneumonia in lung cancers, and should be anticipated and discussed. Infections, including aspiration pneumonia, may well prove to be the "terminal event" of an incurable disease. In that situation many patients would forego acute hospitalization and intravenous antibiotics. In other cases, a time-limited trial of treatment with antibiotics may be desired. It is always important to keep the "big picture" in mind and help patients and loved ones understand all the pros and cons of available interventions.

Colon and ovarian malignancies may result in bowel obstruction. Again, wise reflection and careful discussion are required to balance benefits and drawbacks and ensure that therapy reflects patient wishes. Sometimes, palliative surgery or a venting gastrostomy is appropriate. If the cancer is advanced and a decision is made against surgery, pharmacologic treatment often can provide relief and spare patients the discomfort of nasogastric tubes. Typically, subcutaneous infusions of opioids, anti-emetics, and antispasmodics are used. Intravenous corticosteroids may reduce inflammation and swelling and ease suffering. The costly somatostatin analogue, octreotide, can be used subcutaneously as well if a person with a proximal obstruction has refractory symptoms.

PSYCHOLOGICAL, SOCIAL, AND SPIRITUAL ASSESSMENTS

A comprehensive person-centered approach to care requires emotional and spiritual assessments. It helps to learn what has been important to the ill person. Determining how the patient finds meaning and purpose can be instrumental in coping. A number of tools explore the role of spirituality in a person's life. The HOPE acronym offers a framework to address the sources of **H**ope, the role of **O**rganized religion for the person, personal spirituality and **P**ractices, and the **E**ffect that these have on medical decision-making.[24] Alternatively, a simple question such as "Are you at peace?" may serve to open up this discussion.[25]

CASE PRESENTATION 2 (continued)

Mr. Johnson's Death

Mr. Johnson is an agnostic but deeply spiritual man. The chaplain and psychologist spend time offering caring presence[26] to him and discover that he had unresolved grief around experiences during the Vietnam War. A tailored healing ceremony promoting self-forgiveness results in a greater sense of peace for him. He tells the social worker on the team that he loves music and once had played the drums. The recreational therapist compiles meaningful and memorable songs for him to listen to in his room. He slowly declines over the next few days. When swallowing becomes difficult, a subcutaneous infusion is adjusted to maintain optimal control of his symptoms and he passes away peacefully. As his flag-draped body leaves the unit, staff and saluting veterans respectfully gather in the hall. A light on the unit was lit for 3 days in his honor. The staff later remember him fondly at their quarterly memorial service.

DIAGNOSIS

CASE PRESENTATION 3: MRS. SUGIHARA, THE DIAGNOSIS

Sumi Sugihara met her husband in Tokyo in 1947. Dan was a Japanese American interpreter on General MacArthur's staff. After they returned to the United States Sumi raised their daughter, Nancy, and worked in the library. Sumi also taught flower arranging and calligraphy and volunteered with the Buddhist temple's ladies' auxiliary. After Dan's death Sumi moved in with Nancy. Sumi's only medical problems were hypertension and a depression that followed Dan's death. When Sumi was 75 her gait and handwriting changed and she could no longer teach calligraphy. She fell several times, so Nancy took her to the doctor. While Sumi was getting her blood drawn, Dr. Rosen told Nancy that her mother had Parkinson disease. Nancy was dismayed and said, "My grandfather had Parkinson disease and couldn't walk or eat at the end. Please don't tell Mom she has Parkinson disease. The news will kill her."

Cultural Differences, Family Expectations, and the Disclosure of Bad News

Cultural norms range widely on disclosing threatening diagnoses to patients. Different societies place varying weight on autonomy, justice, benevolence, and nonmaleficence. The Anglo-American tradition emphasizes individual rights and autonomy. Many Latin, African, and Asian cultures stress benevolence and the need to protect the sufferer. When this approach predominates in a society (like the Japanese) that values a consensual approach to decision-making and avoidance of overt conflict, families often request nondisclosure.[27] The resulting conflict can drive a wedge between the physician and family at precisely the time when the patient requires the support of both. The clinician needs superb sensitivity and skill to communicate effectively in this emotion-laden situation. Each individual is unique and family relationships are complex. Not everyone in a given society conforms to dominant social standards but it helps to anticipate common expectations and responses. The clinician should also remember that the Western emphasis on self-determination remains the minority view in the world today.

Stressing the patient's "right" to know can be counterproductive. It helps to explain that the patient usually knows that something serious is wrong and may be relieved finally to have an explanation for what is happening. Disclosing the diagnosis also allows the patient to speak openly about feelings and fears and thus can actually help loved ones support the patient. Most families understand that physicians cannot lie to their patients. It is critical for loved ones to hear what is said and to be reassured that the patient will not be "forced" to hear unbearable information.

It is usually best to have the family present when breaking bad news. The doctor can begin by asking the patient what he or she thinks is wrong. Frequently this resolves the problem, as it becomes apparent that the patient has either already guessed the diagnosis or is worried about an even worse outcome. If that is not the case, the doctor should ask the patient how he or she prefers to approach complicated medical situations. Would the patient like to discuss the

diagnosis and therapy directly or would the patient rather cede care plan decisions to the family? The overwhelming majority of older patients prefer to be directly involved in treatment choices but they usually also wish to have loved ones and physicians involved in a "shared" decision-making approach.[28] If the patient asks for the information and the family is present to offer support and see the physician's caring and sensitive manner, the "culture clash" between the clinician's obligation to disclose and the family's desire to protect can be averted. However, if the patient prefers to delegate decision-making to the family, that choice must be respected.

CASE PRESENTATION 3 (continued)

Sumi Sugihara: Progressing Disease

Sumi already knew she had Parkinson disease and told Dr. Rosen so in Nancy's presence. The doctor sustained hope by stressing the availability of new medications; she told Sumi that she hoped to improve her gait so she still could teach flower arranging and read weekly to the children at the library. Dr. Rosen began Sumi on oral carbidopa-levodopa, and Sumi did well initially but over time her symptoms worsened. She stopped driving; dressing and eating were hampered by tremor and stiffness. She rarely left the house and was self-conscious about her appearance. Her drug regimen was complex; she took pills four times daily and often had side effects such as nausea, bowel problems, and disturbed sleep.

When Sumi was 81 years old, Nancy told Dr. Rosen that her mother was forgetful and "lacked common sense." Sumi was found by Dr. Rosen to have moderate dementia related to her Parkinson disease. It was past time to clarify the goals of care. Dr. Rosen suspected Sumi might soon decompensate and decided to broach the issue of cardiopulmonary resuscitation. Dr. Rosen also worried about Nancy, who had recently retired to care for her mother. She looked tearful and exhausted.

● ADVANCED CARE PLANNING, CARDIOPULMONARY RESUSCITATION, AND SPECIAL CHALLENGES IN DEMENTIA

As the population ages, the number of elders with dementia will skyrocket. Dementia presents special challenges for palliative care in general and advanced care planning in particular. Dementia sufferers struggle with complex information, forget agreed-upon plans, and lack normal coping mechanisms. Loved ones must be involved in all discussions. As grown children assume decision-making for aging parents, the role reversal can be jarring for both, but if the challenge is not confronted, the result will be missed opportunities and delays in appropriate goal setting. The patient's personality and remaining strengths determine his or her ability to participate in complex discussions. Encouraging the patient to express goals will clarify the patient's grasp of medical realities and demonstrate his or her reasoning. Frequently, the patient can voice values but needs the help of family for complicated decisions such as the desirability of cardiopulmonary resuscitation, hospitalization, feeding tubes, or surgery.

Physicians delay conversations about goals of care for a variety of reasons. Doctors often have little training in holding "difficult discussions" and usually overestimate patients' likely survival. They may be pressed for time, unwilling to admit that the disease is "winning," or simply wish to avoid the personal pain that results from upsetting a patient. It is very difficult to overcome these barriers even in well-supported research settings.[28]

Clinicians must be kind but frank and specific about the patient's situation. Asking "If your heart stops do you want the doctors to restart it with shocks and chest compressions?" is not useful. Very few people would choose to remain dead if given another realistic option. One recent study showed that older inpatients greatly overestimated the success rate of resuscitation attempts and only 11% could accurately identify two components of cardiopulmonary resuscitation.[29] The clinician should stress that he hopes to keep the patient well for a long time but that it is best to plan for all eventualities and carefully explain what is involved. The thoughtful physician will not refrain from offering information about likely outcomes. It is unethical to pressure patients and families into accepting a choice favored by the doctor. It is also unkind to deny patients the benefit of professional advice and experience when they request it.

● CAREGIVER STRESS

Caring for chronically ill elders at the end of life is daunting and exhausting. In the last year of life informal caregivers provide an average of 43 hours weekly of direct care.[30] Many caregivers become socially isolated, fail to take care of their own health, deplete their financial resources, or become depressed. These caregivers even have a higher mortality rate themselves.[31,32] Clinicians should be alert for signs of caregiver stress. Loved ones may feel less guilty and be more willing to accept help if reminded that they must stay well to continue to care for their ill relatives. Support groups, practical help, medical care for the stressed loved ones, and respite stays can ease the strain. Frail elders battling chronic, advancing illness live and die within the cocoon of their families and support groups. Thoughtful clinicians will evaluate the needs of caregivers as well as patients. Despite the inherent difficulties, most caregivers remain committed to serving their suffering relatives and report real rewards in meeting these personal responsibilities well.[30]

CASE PRESENTATION 3 (continued)
Sumi Sugihara's First Hospitalization

Dr. Rosen asked Sumi and Nancy if they had seen resuscitation attempts on television. She told them that in real life they only succeeded about 18% of the time.[33] She gently informed them that Sumi's chances for survival would be much worse in view of her advanced age, other medical problems, and the low likelihood that a code would stem from a witnessed arrhythmia (which would have had a better chance of success). She also told them that chronically ill elders with memory problems often had a worse quality of life even if they did live. Sumi hadn't appeared to be listening but suddenly quoted a Buddhist proverb about the moon (a symbol of enlightenment) rising to light the way out of a swamp for a lost soul. Nancy sensed Sumi was ready to accept death and signed a "Do Not Attempt Resuscitation" order.

A month later, while Sumi was on her way to the bathroom, she tripped and fractured her right hip. After surgery she developed an agitated delirium. A consulting geriatrician, Dr. Acosta, noted that her antidepressant had been stopped on admission because it was not on the hospital formulary; she suspected serotonin withdrawal syndrome. Sumi was still receiving hydrochlorothiazide despite poor intake; she was in pain, dehydrated, and had a fecal impaction. A new intern in training had ordered prochlorperazine suppositories for nausea and oral benztropine for tremor. Dr. Acosta noted these mediation changes and resumed the citalopram and stopped the prochlorperazine and benztropine due to their anticholinergic side effects. Sumi was given IV fluids, treated for pain, and disimpacted. She improved but did not regain her prior cognitive level and was transferred to a subacute facility.

● TRANSITIONS AND ERRORS

Frail elders frequently have multiple transfers between sites of care; in the 6 months prior to death, the average Medicare patient has 2 to 5 transitions and a host of different physicians.[34] Few primary care doctors still round in the hospital or visit patients at home or in nursing facilities. Hospitalists do not see patients after discharge, and often shift multiple times during a given acute stay. This increases the likelihood of errors and missing information due to the numerous "baton passes." The frequent transitions also decrease the probability that goals of care will be addressed, since nobody knows the patient well. Caregivers may be uncertain about the content of previous discussions or unaware of recent medical events. All are busy and tempted to defer difficult discussions to the next site of care. Finally, patients and families may feel unmoored without a consistent, trusted provider to guide choices. It is more difficult to shift goals of care if vulnerable elders and their loved ones are unsure of the commitment and expertise of constantly changing professional caregivers.

HAZARDS OF HOSPITALIZATION: DELIRIUM AND COGNITIVE DECLINE

Chronically ill elders with diminished reserves are high risk to suffer the hazards of hospitalization. Chief among these is delirium. Compassionate and thorough physicians adopt a tripartite approach. They search for and treat underlying causes, alleviate suffering, and strive to prevent further complications such as functional decline, skin breakdown, malnutrition, aspiration, and falls. Delirium often leaves a legacy of loss. Even a year after an episode of delirium, elders have higher rates of mortality, nursing home placement, and functional and cognitive decline.[35,36] Full recovery is particularly rare for patients with advanced dementia. Evaluation and management decisions must adjust as the likelihood of meaningful and lasting reversibility recedes.

It is imperative to relieve these patients' suffering. Physicians may be afraid to treat pain with opiates for fear of triggering delirium and worsening outcomes. A recent trial of analgesia in older patients undergoing hip and knee surgery demonstrated that the judicious use of opiates decreased acute and chronic pain, improved function, and shortened length of stay. The study did not explicitly assess the occurrence of delirium, but it is unlikely that function and comfort would have improved if there had been a rise in delirium.[37] Suboptimally treated pain can precipitate delirium, but delirious patients also sometimes express confusion as generalized pain. Pain and delirium often coexist. At times, even experienced professionals may be unsure if agitation is the result of pain, delirium, or a combination of both. Alternating or combined trials of analgesics and antipsychotics may be required.

Scant data support the drug treatment of delirium. Even less is known to guide choices for frail, delirious elders at the end of life. The current standard of care is to select an antipsychotic based on the degree of sedation desired, existing co-morbidities (such as Parkinsonism), and available routes of administration (some drugs have no intravenous formulations). Most frequently haloperidol is used. For elders with dementia, antipsychotics increase mortality and rehospitalizations over a 30-day period. (In one recent study the number needed to harm varied with antipsychotic class and nursing home residence, but ranged from 1 in 9 to 1 in 26.)[38] Nonetheless, these patients are struggling with a degenerative brain disease, so relief of suffering is paramount. Antipsychotics should be prescribed at the lowest effective dose, and tapered and stopped as soon as symptoms abate.

OTHER HAZARDS: CONSTIPATION, FUNCTIONAL DECLINE, FALLS, MALNUTRITION, INCONTINENCE, SKIN BREAKDOWN

For the elder with progressing debility, hospitalization frequently results in dehydration and malnutrition. Patients often have "nothing by mouth" orders prior to procedures and due to concern about potential aspiration. Water pitchers may be across the room, familiar foods are unavailable or the wrong temperature, and careful hand feeding is scarce on busy inpatient units. Little attention is paid to toileting; new incontinence and constipation are prevalent. Patients often have bed rest orders and harried staff may not adhere to prompted ambulation and bathroom schedules. Lines, catheters, bedrails, and an unfamiliar environment further increase the risk of deconditioning, falls, skin breakdown, and new incontinence. (Please see Chapters 28 and 29 on hospital-based care for further discussion.)

CASE PRESENTATION 3 (continued)

Sumi Sugihara: The Subacute Unit

Sumi was more confused and spoke and ate less. She was courteous and cooperative but made little progress ambulating. There were many per diem staff due to budget cuts and summer vacations; no one got to know Sumi well. Dr. Rosen knew that she had been hospitalized for a hip fracture and went to rehabilitation but she had no idea how she was doing or what her plan of care was. The hospital discharge summary did not mention her dementia and reported that her delirium had resolved. On admission, the nurse practitioner asked Sumi if she wanted cardiopulmonary resuscitation and hospital readmission if she became critically ill. Sumi forgot what Dr. Rosen had said about likely outcomes and replied, "I guess so if the doctors think I need it." (Nancy was out of town for a wedding and not present.) A week later, Sumi choked eating lunch and developed pneumonia. Oral antibiotics failed and she returned to the hospital. In the ER, Sumi was hypoxic and developed ventricular tachycardia. By the time Nancy arrived, Sumi had been defibrillated for ventricular tachycardia and intubated; she was sedated in the intensive care unit with vasopressors, antiarrhythmics, fluids, and antibiotics running.

DYSPHAGIA

Swallowing disorders occur in 7% to 22% of older adults. Dysphagia can result from behavioral or age-related sensorimotor problems or new pathology. The prevalence rises to 40% to

50% in long-term care residents.[39] Up to 70% of those with advanced dementia have dysphagia.[40] Patients with late-stage Parkinson disease, amyotrophic lateral sclerosis, and other neurodegenerative diseases universally develop dysphagia. The result is dehydration, malnutrition, weight loss, and aspiration pneumonias. Family members need help in understanding that these are not distinct problems but predictable consequences of the primary illness. Unless professional caregivers clarify this, family members will not readily grasp the link between episodic decompensations and the progressing underlying brain disease.

DISCONTINUITIES IN INFORMATION

In addition to frequent medication errors, information about patients' diagnoses, abilities, and care plans are often lost during transitions in care. Boockvar and associates found a disturbing dearth of documentation on cognition in a study of transfers between nursing homes and acute care. About one-third of the transfer documents failed to mention cognition; most of these patients were demented.[41] The implications are profound. Caregivers at the new site of care cannot determine if the patient has an "altered mental status" because the baseline is unknown. This may result in overlooking a new delirium (a medical emergency) or an unwarranted return to the hospital when the patient is really unchanged. The economic and clinical magnitude of this slipshod documentation likely is profound.

INTENSIVE CARE

CASE PRESENTATION 3 (continued)

Sumi: Intensive Care

The family gathered; Sumi's brother flew in from Tokyo. Nancy was conflicted; her mother was resuscitated "by mistake" and now might survive but she was bloated, sedated, and in restraints. Tubes, lines, and equipment were everywhere. Nancy was afraid to touch her. Dr. Acosta, the geriatrician, who was also certified in palliative medicine, was re-contacted to assist with the situation. She quickly realized that the family was not ready to consider discontinuing technical support given the rapid changes in the past few days. They felt Sumi deserved "a chance." Dr. Acosta suggested they reassess her progress in a few days. She worked with the intensivists to devise a plan for analgesia, sedation, skin care, less restrictive restraints, a visit by a Buddhist minister, and ongoing family support. Sumi improved and was extubated but remained weak and confused and was unable to swallow more than a few mouthfuls of food or fluid. After an emotional meeting with

Dr. Acosta, Nancy decided not to place a feeding tube. Sumi's brother disagreed, feeling that his sister couldn't be "left to starve." Dr. Acosta was physically and psychologically drained after the 90-minute meeting. That evening, she practiced relaxation techniques and planned a trip with her husband. Sumi was transferred to a nursing home known for good end-of-life care.

INTENSIVE CARE IN THE FINAL MONTHS OF LIFE

Although most Americans would prefer to die at home, about 20% expire during or after a stay in intensive care units, often following a decision to discontinue life-sustaining treatments. An even higher number spend some of their last weeks in critical care settings.[42,43] Elders should not be denied access to intensive care strictly on the basis of age. A growing body of evidence suggests that age alone is a poor predictor of critical care outcomes. A recent revision of the Mortality Probability Model revealed that elders who lacked other risk factors had a remarkably low mortality rate (2% vs. 14% overall, $p < 0.001$). In fact, patients in their 90s who lacked other risk factors and were admitted emergently to the ICU were more likely to survive than similar patients in their 50s with risk factors.[44] Nonetheless, frail, malnourished, bed-bound elders with advanced dementia or metastatic cancers are frequently admitted despite the virtual certainty of poor outcomes. This reflects American politics and culture and an unspoken belief that it should always be possible to prevent death if the medical establishment tries hard enough. Physicians are often unwilling to discuss mortality before a crisis; the lack of a consistent caregiver and discontinuities across sites of care heighten the problem, making good communication and advanced care planning even less likely.

A group of compassionate and thoughtful critical care and palliative medicine practitioners have begun to transform the approach to these patients by incorporating palliative principles into intensive care protocols. A variety of models have been developed. These range from intensive education of staff and incorporation of palliative principles into critical care protocols, to mandated family meetings, palliative care consultation, or the incorporation of a palliative medicine specialist into the critical care team. Families were more satisfied with care, patients were more comfortable, and length of stay in intensive care was shorter.[45-49]

ARTIFICIAL FOOD AND HYDRATION AT THE END OF LIFE

Agonizing decisions about the provision of artificial food and hydration are frequent dilemmas for families of patients at the end of life. Physicians and loved ones alike may feel that ensuring adequate nutrition differs fundamentally from other medical procedures and is ethically required. Cultural values and family histories impact choices. Food and drink are symbols of welcome and caring everywhere. It is hard not to "nourish" the mother who cooked thousands of meals and loaded the table with the family's favorite foods at every holiday. Evidence is equivocal on whether feeding tubes prolong life. They do not improve function or prevent aspiration for dementia patients.[50-54] Quality of life may be worse with feeding tubes and intravenous lines. Patients lose one of their last pleasures—tasting small amounts of favored foods—and caregivers spend less time interacting with them. Confused patients may pull at tubes, causing injury and necessitating restraints. Inserting and maintaining lines and tubes cause discomfort. Data on treating dehydration in dying adults are limited; some studies report less delirium and myoclonus at the end of life with hydration, and others document increased edema and more dyspnea from respiratory secretions. No rigorous studies have been done in dying dementia patients.[55]

Comfort needs will be met if the mucosa and lips are kept moist and patients are offered sips and bites as desired. It may help families to recall times they were ill themselves when they weren't hungry. Explaining that patients at the end of life often similarly lose their appetite can ease guilt and aid decision-making at a difficult time.[39] Since feeding tubes and intravenous hydration may increase the burden of suffering without a clear benefit there is no ethical requirement to provide them. Foregoing artificial food and hydration at the end of life is not tantamount to euthanasia.

SELF-CARE FOR PROFESSIONAL CAREGIVERS

Doctors and nurses frequently physically and emotionally withdraw from dying patients. Death may be seen as a professional failure; practitioners often feel helpless. Clinicians sometimes wish to insulate themselves from the sadness of the patient and family—physicians tend to focus on work-related tasks and use intellectualization as a defense mechanism. The impending death may raise painful thoughts about their own mortality or remind them of past or future losses of their own loved ones.

Professionals must recall that there is honor and skill in performing this difficult work well; there is much to contribute even when death is near. Those who care for the dying must "take their own pulses" and be attentive to their own needs to avoid burnout and compassion fatigue. It helps to share the emotional and caregiving work with other team members. Sumi's story illustrates the importance of team-based care. In the last weeks of her life, she was cared for by nurses, a Buddhist minister, physicians, nursing assistants, physical therapists, a social worker, and family. These people from different backgrounds and disciplines made crucial contributions and supported each other through this challenging and valuable work.

CASE PRESENTATION 3 (continued)
Approaching Death in the Nursing Home
Sumi was given a private room dedicated to the dying, she slept much of the time and took only sips of fluid. The nursing home physician, Dr. Gupta, discontinued most of her medications. He used intravenous formulations or highly concentrated elixirs and suppositories. A few days later, Sumi became restless and called for her dead husband and mother. Dr. Gupta knew that antipsychotics could worsen her Parkinsonism, but Sumi could not walk, swallow, or reliably communicate any longer. He doubted she would live more than a few days and diagnosed terminal delirium. He scheduled 2.5 mg of orally dissolvable olanzapine every 6 hours and ordered 1 mg of sublingual lorazepam as needed. Sumi calmed. Her family was determined she would not die alone. They took turns keeping a bedside vigil. A tape recording of Buddhist monks chanting the sutras played in the background; Sumi's brother pinned an amulet on her pillow from the Asakusa Kannon Temple in their old Tokyo neighborhood. Nancy tucked a family photo from the early years of Sumi's marriage into the pocket of her mother's hospital gown.

TERMINAL DELIRIUM

Terminal delirium is an irreversible, acute confusional state in the final days of life that occurs in up to 88% of dying patients. Morita and associates[56] found one or more potential etiologies in 93% of cases. The most frequent causes included fluid imbalance (42%), hepatic failure (29%), medications (25%), hypoxia (16%), and electrolyte imbalance (13%). Distressing diagnostic testing to define "causes" is unkind and unhelpful in the face of imminent death. At that point, an exclusively palliative approach to delirium is needed. All clinicians caring for these patients must be able to clearly and empathetically communicate this situation to loved ones; this is a crucial, high-level professional skill.

DEATH IN THE NURSING HOME

Entry into a nursing home is a seminal event for patients and their loved ones. It forces a clearer recognition of the stage of the disease and highlights ongoing losses. This symbolic and emotionally laden moment of transition provides an important opportunity to gently readdress goals. One study showed that a 15-minute discussion at admission about prognosis and goals not only improved family members' satisfaction with care but also decreased suffering at the end of life for dementia patients.[57] With the aging of the population and the dispersal of American families, an increasing number of elders die in nursing homes. For the oldest Americans, nursing homes are the most common site of death.[58] The majority of American nursing homes have some affiliation with a hospice provider (76% in 2000[59]), yet most nursing home residents still die without hospice support. (Nationwide only 22% of all hospice enrollees in the United States die in nursing homes.[8])

CASE PRESENTATION 3 (continued)

Sumi: The Last Day

Nancy nervously asked Dr. Gupta what to expect—she had never seen anyone die. He described the changes preceding death. He told Nancy that the eyes and mouth might not close, the body would cool, the limbs would "mottle," and the pattern and quality of the breathing change. Respirations might become noisy. He assured her this did not indicate suffering. He explained that there might be a loss of sphincter control and asked her to let the staff know if she saw any restlessness or evidence of pain or twitching. Dr Gupta also stressed what Nancy could still do to help her mother—mouth and skin care, comforting words and touch, positioning, and caring presence. Early the next morning, Nancy heard lengthening gaps in Sumi's respirations. As Sumi took her last breath Nancy told her mother goodbye and thanked her for all she had done. She promised never to forget her and to tell all Sumi's greatgrandchildren about her life.

After the death, Nancy was dazed and couldn't concentrate. There were intermittent paroxysms of grief. She was touched to get a sympathy card from Dr. Rosen; the ritual of the Buddhist memorial services in the first months was comforting. The first holidays were difficult but Nancy went back to work, focused on her family, and was able to surmount her loss. The birth of a new grandchild 6 months after Sumi's death restored Nancy's joy in life and taught her to laugh again.

● THE DYING PROCESS

Although most Americans would prefer to die at home, few actually do so. Most end their lives in hospital wards, nursing homes, emergency rooms, and intensive care units; families may not witness the process and moment of death. Even many elders have not seen another person die. Relatives do not know what to expect; they have no sense of what is normal as death nears. They look to physicians to point out expected mileposts, model how to interact with the dying, and offer guidance on ways to help their loved ones in their last days. Clinicians can help by outlining the common physical and neurocognitive changes at the end of life. This will ease fears and allow relatives to feel more in control. It is critical to honor the central role of families by assisting them to care for their loved ones to the end.

As life ebbs, blood pressure drops, the body cools, and the skin appears pale and feels clammy. The extremities may show signs of hypoperfusion first with "mottling" of the skin. Urine output declines and ceases and muscles slacken. Eyes may not completely close and the mouth often drops open. Respirations become more erratic; at various times there may be Kussmaul or Cheyne-Stokes type patterns. At the end, apneic pauses lengthen interrupted by brief agonal breaths. Throat muscles relax, swallowing is lost, and secretions pool above the larynx. When the breath passes through this fluid layer, noisy respirations result. Lay people call this a "death rattle" and may interpret this as suffering. If the family is distressed and the risk of hyperactive delirium is low, a scopolamine patch, oral atropine drops, or intravenous glycopyrrolate all decrease secretions (the later crosses into the brain less readily and has fewer central nervous system side effects).

In the days before death, people usually appear to gradually detach from their surroundings and become progressively more stuporous. They sleep much of the time, cease eating and drinking, become incontinent, rarely communicate, and may not even move in bed. Families need to understand this is inherent to the dying process and not a withdrawal from loved ones, a failure of character, or "giving up."

Hearing and touch are probably the last senses lost. Families and clinicians who care for the dying believe that patients may respond to a voice or a caress until just before the moment of passing. A primitive fear of the unknown or the sense that patients are too fragile to be touched may prevent family members from showing affection. They may feel more comfortable touching and speaking to their loved ones if physicians show them how to do so by smoothing hair over a forehead, gently placing a hand on a shoulder, or saying a few words even to unconscious patients in the family's presence.

Clinicians can help families find ways to serve the dying. Loved ones can moisten mucosa and eyes with saline, assist with repositioning, massage limbs, or range joints to minimize disturbance pain. They can play favorite music, pray or read to patients, and provide the calm that flows from a caring presence, a held hand, or a word of love. Families also can monitor for signs of suffering and alert staff if treatments need adjusting. These tasks are likely to promote comfort. Even if patients remain unaware, the demonstrations of devotion will help families meet their emotional responsibilities, bring them peace, and decrease the risk of complicated bereavement. These are the people that the patient loved; helping them through this ordeal is one final way that clinicians can serve their patients.

An unfortunate minority take a rockier path to death with agitated delirium, overt suffering, restlessness, and even seizures. Myoclonus is an early warning sign. Prompt action must be taken to prevent this progression or the patient will be denied a peaceful end and families will carry the memory of the witnessed suffering through the remainder of their own lives. This can result from a buildup of opioid metabolites (such as 3- and 6-glucuronides); rotating to a different analgesic may resolve the problem. A trial of fluids also can be considered, although this may worsen peripheral edema and tracheal secretions. Alternatively, the addition of benzodiazepines will prevent seizures although the level of consciousness will predictably decline.

Proportional palliative sedation refers to the use of the minimum amount of sedatives required to relieve suffering.[60] Deliberate sedation with the goal of unconsciousness may be warranted if death is imminent and suffering cannot otherwise be relieved. The patient/next of kin should agree that alleviating the distress warrants the loss of awareness. Most palliative care experts believe that terminal sedation is justified by the principle of "double effect." In other words, the physician provides a treatment (in this case sedation) to relieve refractory suffering although death may be hastened as an unintended consequence.[61] Physicians must reflect carefully on the complex ethical issues involved and act accordingly.

● BEREAVEMENT

A frail elder's death is often preceded by a lengthy period of direct care by family members. During this time caregivers may experience "anticipatory grieving" with symptoms very similar to acute grief. This allows some psychological preparation and the development of coping skills in advance of the death.[62] After the loved one dies, surviving caregivers must find a new focus for their lives. Grief requires real work and the passage of time.

Emotions are complex and bereaved family members often fear they are "going crazy." There is usually a mixture of sadness, anger, denial, disbelief, guilt, helplessness, fear, and confusion. Somatic symptoms typically include sleep and appetite changes, difficulty concentrating, nausea, and fatigue. Each individual has a unique response to loss; it is difficult to define "normal" grief.[63] Survivors may think they hear the deceased loved one's voice or feel his or her presence. People need reassurance that these responses are normal. Depending on coping mechanisms, the nature of the relationship, and manner of death most bereaved people successfully move through the normal stages of grief over 6 months to a year. They transition into "integrated grief" and learn to live without their loved one. Life may never be the same and the deceased is not forgotten but a new sense of identity and meaning is found and the bereaved returns to the world more fully. Most do not require treatment for their grief. It is important for a clinician to understand the normal range of responses to bereavement since a subset of survivors suffer from pathologic grief and require treatment.

About 10% of survivors suffer depressive symptoms that reach the level of complicated grief. This rises to 20% for dementia caregivers following the death of their loved ones.[64] Complicated grief is preoccupying, disabling, and interferes with function and quality of life. It may manifest as major depression, substance abuse, delayed mourning, or a complete absence of emotions with an inability to experience normal grief reactions. Caregiver counseling, assistance with the burdens of care, and treating caregiver depression prior to the demise can decrease the risk of complicated grief. Bradley and associates found that caregivers of patients enrolled in hospice for less than 4 days before death had more major depression a year later compared to those with longer enrollments.[65] Thus, earlier hospice referrals and the 12 months of post-death support may further reduce the risk of depression for family. Bereaved relatives usually are deeply grateful to physicians who contact them to ask how they are coping with the loss. This is the final gift that clinicians can give their patients—to help those who survived them—and is a mark of true excellence in care.

References

1. Lunney JR, Lynn J, Foley DJ, et al. Patterns of functional decline at the end of life. JAMA. 2003;289:2387-2392.

2. World Health Statistics. Geneva, Switzerland: WHO Press; 2009.

3. Teno JM, Mor V, Welch LC, et al. Family perspectives on end-of-life care at the last place of care. JAMA. 2004;291:88-93.

4. National Consensus Project for Quality Palliative Care. Clinical Practice Guidelines for Quality Palliative Care. 2nd ed. 2009. http://www.nationalconsensusproject.org.

5. Buckman R. Breaking bad news: Why is it still so difficult? BMJ. 1984;288:1597-1599.

6. Baile WF, Buckman R, Lenzi R, et al. SPIKES—A six step protocol for delivering bad news: Application to the patient with cancer. Oncologist. 2000;5: 301-311.

7. Quill TE, Arnold RM, Platt F. "I wish things were different": Expressing wishes in response to loss, futility and unrealistic hopes. Ann Intern Med. 2001;135:551-555.

8. National Hospice and Palliative Care Organization. NHPCO Facts and Figures: Hospice Care in America. National Hospice and Palliative Care Organization; October 2009.

9. Stuart B. Medical guidelines for non-cancer disease and local medical review policy: Hospice access for patients with diseases other than cancer. Hospice J. 1999;14:139-154.

10. End of Life/Palliative Education Resource Center. Fast Fact #112. www.eperc.mcw.edu.

11. Back AL, Arnold RM, Tulsky JA, et al. On saying goodbye: Acknowledging the end of the patient-physician relationship with patients who are near death. Ann Intern Med. 2005;142: 682-685.

12. Glare PA, Sinclair CT. Palliative medicine review: Prognostication. J Palliat Med. 2008;11:84-103.

13. Vigano A, Dorgan M, Buckingham J, et al. Survival prediction in terminal cancer patients: A systematic review of the medical literature. Palliat Med. 2000;14:363-374.

14. Back AL, Arnold RM, Quill TE. Hope for the best, and prepare for the worst. Ann Intern Med. 2003;138:439-443.

15. Byock I. The Four Things That Matter Most: A Book about Living. Tampa: Free Press; 2004.

16. Murphy NM. The Wisdom of Dying: Practice for the Living. St. Petersburg, FL: Element Books; 1999.

17. Grassman D. Peace at Last: Stories of Help and Healing for Veterans and Their Families. St. Petersburg, FL: Vandamere Press; 2009.

18. Gessert, et al. Ethical wills and suffering in patients with cancer. J Palliat Med. 2004;7:517-526.

19. Portenoy RK, et al. The Memorial Symptom Assessment Scale: An instrument for the evaluation of symptom prevalence, characteristics and distress. Eur J Cancer. 1994;30:1326-1336.

20. Daut RL, Cleeland CS, Flanery RC. Development of the Wisconsin Brief Pain Questionnaire to assess pain in cancer and other diseases. Pain. 1983;17:197-210.

21. Warden V, Hurley A, Volicer L. Development and psychometric evaluation of the Pain Assessment in Advanced Dementia (PAINAD) Scale. J Am Med Dir Assn. 2003;4:9-15.

22. Five Wishes. www.agingwithdignity.org. Accessed September 6, 2009.

23. MOLST. www.compassionandsupport.org. Accessed September 6, 2009.

24. Anandaraja G. Spirituality and medical practice: Using the HOPE questions as a practical tool for spiritual assessment. Am Fam Physician. 2008;63:81-88.

25. Steinhauser K, Voils C, Clipp E, et al. Are you at peace? One item to probe spiritual concerns at the end of life. *Arch Intern Med.* 2006;166:101-105.

26. Yoder G. *Companioning the Dying: A Soulful Guide for Counselors and Caregivers.* Fort Collins, CO: Bereavement Publications; 2005.

27. Tanabe MKG. Older Japanese-Americans in doorway thoughts. In Adler R, Kamel H, eds. *Cross-Cultural Health Care for Older Adults.* Vol. 1. Sudbury, MA: Jones & Bartlett; 2004.

28. Covinsky KE, Fuller JD, Yaffe K, et al. Communication and decision-making in seriously ill patients: Findings of the SUPPORT project. The Study to Understand Prognoses and Preferences for Outcomes and Risks of Treatments. *J Am Geriatr Soc.* 2000; 48(suppl):S187-S193.

29. Heyland DK, Frank C, Groll D, et al. Understanding cardio-pulmonary resuscitation decision making perspectives of seriously ill hospitalized patients and family members. *Chest.* 2006;130:419-428.

30. Wolff JL, Dy SL, Frick KD, Kasper JD. End-of-life care: Findings from a national survey of informal caregivers. *Arch Intern Med.* 2007;167:40-46.

31. Etters L, Goodall D, Harrison BE. Caregiver burden among dementia patient caregivers: A review of the literature. *J Am Acad Nurs Pract.* 2008;20:423-428.

32. Schultz R, Beach S. Caregiving as a risk factor for mortality: The caregiver health effects study. *JAMA.* 1999;282:2215-2219.

33. Ehlenback WJ, Barnato AE, Curtis JR, et al. Epidemiologic study of in-hospital cardiopulmonary resuscitation in the elderly. *N Engl J Med.* 2009;361:22-31.

34. Teno JM, Mitchell SL, Skinner J, et al. Churning: The association between health care transitions and feeding tube insertion for nursing home residents with advanced cognitive impairment. *J Palliat Med.* 2009;12:359-362.

35. McAvay GJ, Van Ness PH, Bogardus ST, et al. Older adults discharged from the hospital with delirium: 1-year outcomes. *J Am Geriatr Soc.* 2006;54:1245-1250.

36. Kiely DK, Marcantonio ER, Inouye SK, et al. Persistent delirium predicts greater mortality. *J Am Geriatr Soc.* 2009;57:55-61.

37. Morrison RS, Flanagan S, Fischberg D, et al. A novel interdisciplinary analgesic program reduces pain and improves function in older adults after orthopedic surgery. *J Am Geriatr Soc.* 2009;57:1-10.

38. Rochon PA, Normand SL, Gomes T, et al. Antipsychotic therapy and short-term serious events in older adults with dementia. *Arch Intern Med.* 2008;168:1090-1096.

39. Easterling CS, Robbins E. Dementia and dysphagia. *Geriatric Nurs.* 2008;29:275-285.

40. Feinberg MJ, Ekberg O, Segall L, Tully J. Deglutition in elderly patients with dementia: Findings of videofluorographic evidence and impact on staging and management. *Radiology.* 1992;183:811-814.

41. Boockvar KS, Fridman B, Marturano C, et al. Ineffective communication of mental status information during care transfer of older adults. *J Gen Intern Med.* 2005;20:1146-1150.

42. Angus DC, Barnato A, Linde-Zwirble WT, et al. Use of intensive care at the end of life in the United States: An epidemiologic study. *Crit Care Med.* 2004;32:638-643.

43. Curtis JR, Rubenfeld GD. Improving palliative care for patients in the intensive care unit. *J Palliat Med.* 2005;8:840-854.

44. Higgins TL, Teres D, Copes WS, et al. Assessing contemporary intensive care unit outcome: An updated Mortality Probability Admission Model (MPM$_0$-III). *Crit Care Med.* 2007;35:827-835.

45. Ray D, Fuhrman C, Stern G, et al. Integrating palliative medicine and critical care in a community hospital. *Crit Care Med.* 2006;34(suppl):S394-S398.

46. Treece PD, Engelberg RA, Shannon SE, et al. Integrating palliative and critical care: Description of an intervention. *Crit Care Med.* 2006;34(suppl):S380-S387.

47. Curtis JR, Treece PD, Nielsen EL, et al. Integrating palliative and critical care: Evaluation of a quality-improvement intervention. *Am J Resp Crit Care Med.* 2008;178:269-275.

48. Billings JA, Keeley A, Bauman J, et al. Merging cultures: Palliative care specialists in the medical intensive care unit. *Crit Care Med.* 2006;34(suppl.):S388-S393.

49. Byock I. Improving palliative care in intensive care units: Identifying strategies and interventions that work. *Crit Care Med.* 2006; 34(suppl):S302-S306.

50. Finucane TE, Bynum JP. Use of tube feeding to prevent aspiration pneumonia. *Lancet.* 1996;348:1421-1424.

51. Peck A, Cohen CE, Mulvihill MN. Long-term enteral feeding of aged demented nursing home patients. *J Am Geriatr Soc.* 1990;38: 1195-1198.

52. Mitchell SL, Kiely DK, Lipsitz LA. Does artificial enteral nutrition prolong the survival of institutionalized elders with chewing and swallowing problems? *J Gerontol A Biol Sci Med Sci.* 1998;53: M207-M213.

53. Murphy LM, Lipman TO. Percutaneous endoscopic gastrostomy does not prolong survival in patients with dementia. *Arch Intern Med.* 2003;163:1351-1353.

54. Kaw M, Sekas G. Long-term follow-up of consequences of percutaneous endoscopic gastrostomy (PEG) tubes in nursing home patients. *Dig Dis Sci.* 1995;40:920-921.

55. Good P, Cavenagh J, Mather M, Ravenscroft P. Medically assisted hydration for adult palliative care patients. *Cochrane Database Syst Rev.* 2009:2.

56. Morita T, Tei Y, Tsunoda J, et al. Underlying pathologies and their associations with clinical features in terminal delirium of cancer patients. *J Pain Symptom Manage.* 2001;22:997-1006.

57. SE Engel, Kiely DK, Mitchell SL. Satisfaction with end-of-life care for nursing home residents with advanced dementia. *J Am Geriatr Soc.* 2006;54:1567-1572.

58. Gruneir A, Mor V, Weitzen S, et al. Where people die: A multilevel approach to understanding influences on site of death in America. *Med Care Res Rev.* 2007;64:351-377.

59. Miller SC, Mor V. The opportunity for collaborative care provision: The presence of nursing home/hospice collaborations in the U.S. states. *J Pain Symptom Manage.* 2004;28:537-547.

60. Quill TE, Lo B, Brock DW, Meisel A. Last-resort options for palliative sedation. *Ann Intern Med.* 2009;151:421-424.

61. Billings JA. Recent advances: Palliative care. *BMJ.* 2000;321:555-558.

62. Worden JM. *Grief Counseling and Grief Therapy: A Handbook for the Mental Health Practitioner.* 4th ed. New York: Springer; 2009.

63. Bonanno GA, Kaltman S. The varieties of grief experience. *Clin Psychol Rev.* 2001;21:705-734.

64. Schulz R, Boerner K, Shear K, et al. Predictors of complicated grief among dementia caregivers: A prospective study of bereavement. *Am J Geriatr Psychiatry.* 2006;14:650-658.

65. Bradley EH, Prigerson H, Carlson MD, et al. Depression among surviving caregivers: Does length of hospice enrollment matter? *Am J Psychiatry.* 2004;161:2257-2262.

POST-TEST

1. Which of the following is LEAST helpful in assessing prognosis for frail elders with advanced disease?
   A. Functional status
   B. Dyspnea
   C. Weight loss
   D. Age

2. Hospitalizations and multiple transitions in sites of care present a variety of hazards for vulnerable older adults in the last months of life. These include all the following EXCEPT:
   A. Delirium
   B. Frequent hip fractures
   C. "Lost" care plans, diagnoses, and advance directives
   D. Functional decline

3. Which of the following is FALSE about the optimal use of opiates?
   A. Breakthrough or rescue opiates are usually prescribed at 10% to 15% of the total daily dose of long-acting opiates.
   B. Morphine is the opiate of choice for patients with advanced, oliguric renal failure.

C. Methadone should only be prescribed by experts due to unpredictable cross-tolerance, half-life, and the risk of QT prolongation.
   D. Patients usually become tolerant to the side effects of opiates such as lethargy in about a week but do not acclimate to constipation, so laxatives should be ordered with initiation of opiate therapy.

4. Which of the following statements about the last hours of life is NOT correct?
   A. Myoclonic twitching is virtually inevitable and should be expected prior to death.
   B. Noisy respirations occur when the ability to swallow is lost and secretions pool above the larynx.
   C. Most patients become progressively more lethargic and stuporous in the days and hours before death.
   D. As perfusion fails, the body cools, and the limbs begin to "mottle."

ANSWERS TO PRE-TEST

1. D
2. A
3. C
4. D

ANSWERS TO POST-TEST

1. D
2. B
3. B
4. A

24

Home Care

Peter Boling, MD

Rachel Selby-Penczak, MD

● **LEARNING OBJECTIVES**

1. Identify patients for whom house calls are the best option to receive medical care.
2. Describe the basic tools and skills necessary to make house calls.
3. List several ways in which a clinician can incorporate home visits into other daily practice routines.
4. Name the potential team members, services, and other providers that make delivering quality home care possible.
5. Explain when home care is not the best or safest option for patient, caregiver, or health care provider.

PRE-TEST

1. **Which of the following patients would MOST benefit from house calls?**

   A. An ambulatory 94-year-old with moderate dementia who requires cueing for self-care

   B. A 72-year-old paraplegic patient who needs a care van to attend hemodialysis three times a week

   C. A 79-year-old patient with diabetes and hypertension who is confined to bed and chair following a stroke 2 months ago

   D. An 85-year-old patient with osteoarthritis whose pain is managed with narcotic analgesics and walks with a walker

2. **Which member of the home care team provides the majority of daily care to homebound patients?**

   A. Unpaid caregivers such as spouses, children, and siblings

   B. Home health aides

   C. Physicians, nurse practitioners, and physician assistants

   D. Nurses and therapists from home health agencies

3. **Which of the following services is currently NOT yet possible to deliver in the home?**

   A. Sleep studies

   B. X-rays

   C. Magnetic resonance imaging (MRI) studies

   D. Doppler ultrasound exams

● HOUSE CALLS

Until the mid-20th century, most health care in the United States was provided in the home. House calls still invoke the image of a physician on horseback, black bag in hand, visiting an ailing patient lying in bed, and giving simple "low-tech" treatments. In addition to gratitude, payment might have been chickens, eggs, or other bartered services.

As technology, transportation, and economies evolved, medical care changed. House calls declined and patients received care in clinics or hospitals. With increased medical sub-specialization, attention to productivity dominated and house calls in the United States came to be seen as a rare, charitable service to long-standing, bed-bound, and dying patients. US clinicians have shied away from house calls due to lack of familiarity, perceptions that this is no longer normative behavior, concern about safety, time conflicts, and reimbursement. Yet in Europe, Canada, Russia, India, and other countries, house calls are still routine.[1]

As the US population rapidly ages, with 20% expected to be 65 years and older by 2030, health care delivery will have to change. Though the rate of new disability is slowly dropping, the aggregate number of ailing people who cannot easily "go to the doctor" will rise rapidly. Without house calls, the emergency room (ER) is a common point of access, and hospitalization often results. This sort of emergent care may "solve" a crisis, but will ultimately fail. These complex patients enter a revolving door of repeat hospitalizations and ER visits, and even institutionalization, while the system fails to deal with the chronic nature of the multiple interacting diseases they have accumulated. The emergency response strategy is more expensive both in dollars and in quality of life while patients and physicians are frustrated by fragmented care and wish for "a better way."

In addition to being better for patients and families, house calls offer providers a unique opportunity to accurately assess the patient and give comprehensive care. Home visits provide insight that might otherwise go unrecognized. These encounters provide time for caregiver education, observation of how patients manage their many medications, and identification of services and equipment to preserve or restore health. House calls offer opportunities to prevent injury and promote safety plus a glimpse of daily socioeconomic choices that families face. Clinicians practicing in the familiar settings of a clinic or hospital are expected to design treatment plans to meet patients' needs at home. Without knowing the home environment, these clinicians are at a disadvantage.

The basic medical history and physical is the same wherever it is performed. Yet, when on their own turf, patients and caregivers are more relaxed and more readily open up. Competing noise from family members or pets adds challenges but yields important insight. The home setting encourages patient and caregiver participation in formulating and carrying out care plans. In the end, they are the most important participants in the health care "team" and they are crucial to ultimate success.

The cases in this chapter illustrate how to organize and deliver home-based medical care, how to develop and use extended interdisciplinary teams, how to manage post-acute and transitional care, and what to do when staying at home is no longer safe.

CASE PRESENTATION 1: THE GRANTS

Beverly and Frank Grant are long-time office patients who have lived in the same house for five decades. Their three grown children have their own families out of state, but the Grants still savor holiday visits with their 10 grandchildren.

At 79, Beverly is a retired nurse and avid gardener. She enjoys lunching with lifelong friends, playing cards, and swapping stories. Since retirement 10 years ago, she and Frank often travel overseas with their church group. Despite hypertension, type II diabetes, and osteoarthritis, Beverly is robust. Frank, now 84, still glows when he sees his beautiful wife, constantly amazed by her energy and ability to "keep things running like clockwork" despite pain in her hands and knees.

A retired mechanic, Frank was always physically active. He enjoys tinkering in his workshop which is now limited by glaucoma. He takes arthritis pain medication plus a statin. Last year, a car accident aggravated his back pain and Frank was diagnosed with spinal stenosis. He now needs a walker. Inactivity led to gaining 30 lbs (13.6 kg); at 240 lbs (109 kg), getting around is difficult. Beverly, a slight woman, looks at his 6-foot frame and jokes there is "more of him to love." Aging gracefully has become difficult.

The Grants are usually prompt, but today they are late. The electronic medical record (EMR) shows a recent refill of Beverly's lisinopril but you notice a cancelled appointment 3 months ago. Twelve patients later, a typical busy afternoon ends and the Grants were a no-show. Concerned, you give them a call.

After pleasantries about their first great-grandchild, you ask if everything is o.k. and hear uncharacteristic hesitation. Apologetic and tearful, Beverly says that Frank stopped driving and needs her help even to get dressed. His pain and immobility prevent most of their preferred social activities. Caregiving aggravates her arthritis. She sleeps poorly. She won't leave Frank alone because "he has always been proud and strong. I think he will hurt himself trying to get up while I'm out." Friends have brought groceries and sat with Frank so she can run her most important errands.

The children advised their parents to move closer to family, but the Grants do not want to be a burden. They considered assisted living but decided "things were not that bad yet." Apologizing again, Beverly says someone agreed to drive them to your office today but Frank was too weak to descend the steps. Exhausted, they fell asleep and forgot to cancel. She badly wanted to be seen since Frank visited a local ER 2 weeks ago after a hard fall. He had labs and x-rays and was told "nothing is wrong" but he remains weak. She wants to reschedule next week once they "get their strength back."

You recall seeing an article about homebound elders and realize that a house call is the answer: less burdensome for them and more insightful for you. Reviewing your schedule you decide to see the Grants en route to the office early tomorrow.

● PATIENT SELECTION FOR HOUSE CALLS

The Grants are typical of many elders. They have led fulfilling lives despite chronic conditions until a new burden disrupted the balance. Beverly remains self-sufficient but feels the brunt of caregiving, which conveys risk for personal decline. Studies have shown increased depression, uncontrolled hypertension, and even early mortality when comparing stressed caregivers to others.[2] Beverly puts her loved one first. She misses medical appointments, does necessary but strenuous work that negatively impacts her health, and gives up social activities that she values. She is tied to the home by concern for her husband's safety, but is not homebound.

Frank now depends on Beverly to safely get around the house, needs help with basic activities of daily living such as bathing, dressing, and transferring, cannot leave home without great burden on him and others, and rarely attends social functions.

Thus Frank meets the operational definition of "homebound" in Chapter 7 of the Medicare Benefit Policy Manual that lists coverage criteria for skilled home health agency care under Medicare Part A. These criteria are important for physicians to know. However, these strict criteria are not required for Medicare Part B home visits by physicians or nurse practitioners. Medical providers still need a good reason for seeing a patient at home rather than the office, and should document that reason. Clearly Frank is eligible for a medical home visit and he may also qualify for home health agency care.

● SCHEDULING CHRONIC VERSUS URGENT AT-HOME CARE FOR HOME-BOUND PATIENTS

All clinicians want to provide quality medical care. However, this can pose a dilemma in an era of productivity and efficiency. Your office schedule has 25 patients per day, leaving time for little else. Yet you wonder if other patients like the Grants have trouble coming to the office. Your staff helps you learn that 20 patients with visits in upcoming months have become frail and fallen through the cracks. You are happy to help the Grants, but now wonder how to balance the needs of these others with those of your office and personal life. This need not be overwhelming.

After getting comfortable by making a few home visits at the beginning or end of the day you might schedule one or two half days per week for home visits. In a larger group this can be organized so that someone is always doing mobile care, and office staff overhead can be proportionately reduced. Some clinicians eventually stop office or hospital practice and concentrate exclusively on home visits. Others start there.

Factors to consider include patient location in respect to the clinician's home or business, geographic concentration of patients for efficiency (apartment buildings), neighborhood safety, resources such as nurse practitioners and physician assistants, and coordination with home health agencies. Visit scheduling is easy in a small practice; patients and caregivers are flexible and grateful though some still have unique needs like a bedfast patient who cannot answer the door, and whose working caregiver's schedule may dictate your itinerary. As the home care practice grows, and if you add providers or provide urgent care, scheduling grows more complex. The American Academy of Home Care Physicians (aahcp.org) offers useful tools to help with these issues.

The Grants' situation is urgent. Frank's fall, weakness, and dependence on Beverly must be addressed promptly to prevent bad outcomes. When you see him, along with blood pressure, lung, and cardiovascular issues, you will look for factors contributing to his fall and decline (pain, medications, environmental risks, cognition) and focus your plan on functional recovery. Some conditions like high cholesterol can wait.

● CORE MOBILE MEDICAL TEAM MEMBERS

Care for homebound patients may involve multiple individuals. In the simplest scenario, it suffices for a physician to periodically visit stable, less dependent patients. In complex situations home medical care may "take a village."

The most important team members are always the patient and unpaid caregiver(s). Unpaid caregivers provide about 80% of the care that a homebound individual receives. Ideally, patients and caregivers are engaged, active participants, willing to learn and collaborate with clinically trained providers. A patient who left school after fifth grade can become expert in managing his or her own care. Conversely, a person with advanced degrees may be a weak link if unavailable, unwilling, or unable to participate.

Selection of mobile team members depends on your practice. The authors' clinical team is a hospital-supported house calls practice (275 patients) staffed by nurse practitioners, physicians, a social worker, and clerical staff. Nurse practitioners and physicians manage their own patients, make visits independently, and cover during absences. All members meet weekly and discuss all hospitalized patients plus difficult clinical problems. This provides opportunity for consultation and mutual education. Group members request home visits from one another for "second opinions" and advice. At this academic center, group members also educate learners (medical, nurse practitioner and pharmacy students, residents, and fellows) who join in visits and team meetings. The social worker provides telephone and in-person consultation as needed.

In some programs, drivers or medical technicians travel with clinicians to enable more efficient use of travel time and help with vital signs, medication review, ordering equipment, or drawing blood. There is a balance between cost and efficiency that the practice must consider during program design.

OFFICE SUPPORT FOR THE CORE HOUSE CALLS TEAM

Office support models vary as do the clinical teams. Clinicians in an office setting who incorporate a few home visits rely on existing staff to take messages, do scheduling, triage phone calls, and assist with pharmacy requests. Compared to office practice, the support staff shrinks as house call programs grow, and staff roles change. There are more phone calls and more forms from home health agencies and equipment companies, but fewer claims to file or office systems to maintain. Overhead and costs shift to provider time during transit, mobile testing, triage, and routing. Providers are usually in the field. Patients' bedrooms and living rooms are exam rooms. When phone calls and paperwork are not completed in the home, the car may be a makeshift "mobile office." Others prefer charting and doing paperwork at a desk and have a base for these activities plus storage for paper charts and other documents. As electronic health records increase in practicality, the paperwork will lessen and work efficiency may increase.

In some practices a nurse triages calls, provides telephone advice for non-urgent matters, coordinates urgent clinician visits, contacts home health agencies or mobile x-ray companies, and calls in prescription refills. The ratio of mobile clinicians to office staff varies with the volume, clinical model, and acuity of patient illness.

To start with, you will see the Grants at home and ask your office staff to identify other patients who may be helped by home-based medical care. How this will pan out is uncertain, but you are excited by the new roads that your practice may take.

THE "BLACK BAG"

In anticipation of visiting the Grants tomorrow morning, you visit your supply closet this late afternoon and pack up some equipment. You don't need much equipment for a basic house call, but you must bring everything that you may need.[1] A soft, durable bag with multiple pockets works well. One with wheels is even better. A small fishing tackle box is useful for blood-drawing supplies. In a more advanced practice, portable scales, an oximeter, point-of-care testing devices, and a portable EKG machine may be useful (Table 24–1).

Those who still use paper records usually need a copy of the chart (not the original), with the medication and problem lists, a progress note template, prescription pad, and key phone numbers (home health and hospice agencies, mobile x-ray companies, equipment supply companies). In an organized house call program you should have a packet for new

TABLE 24–1 House Call Bag Contents	
Basic Model	**Advanced Care Model**
Stethoscope	Scale
BP cuff with several sizes of cuffs	Oximeter
Oto-ophthalmoscope	I-STAT (point-of-care chemistry)
Reflex hammer	Glucometer
Thermometer (digital, with covers)	EKG machine
Gloves (sterile, nonsterile)	Spirometer
Hemoccult slides and jelly	Infusion equipment
Reflex hammer	
Tape measure	
Nail clippers (robust, for toenails)	
Scalpel, scissors, forceps	
Gauze and tape	
Syringes, needles, specimen tubes	
Marking pen, labels	
Foley catheter	
Sharps container	

patients, including an introduction to the program, names and contact numbers for office and staff, policies for regular and acute visits, affiliations with hospitals or other providers, telephone and after-hours availability, charges for services, and consent to treat forms.[3]

Low Tech or High Tech

Advances in technology make possible home x-rays, ultrasound, venous Doppler studies, sleep studies, electrocardiograms, 24-hour EKG monitoring, and overnight pulse oximetry. The portable I-STAT device uses drops of blood obtained from a finger stick to determine chemistry, hemoglobin, pH, cardiac markers, and INR values within 2 minutes.[4] Though each point-of-care lab test itself costs much more than a comparable test run in huge batches at commercial labs, the cost of a provider's time to obtain and transport specimens more than balances that difference. These devices require calibration and are regulated (CLIA—Clinical Laboratory Improvement Amendments). Point-of-care devices may be costly for a solo practitioner but many large organizations now use them. Also, patients on chronic warfarin therapy who need frequent monitoring are eligible for Medicare coverage of this type of device for personal use.

Electronic health records (EHR) and laptop computers are useful and many providers are moving quickly in that direction. The ability to share important medical information and maintain continuity can be critical as the homebound patient traverses sites of care. Wireless Internet access and slow upload and download speeds sometimes impact the pace of EHR adoption.[4]

Handheld devices such as personal digital assistants (PDAs), Palm Pilots, smart phones, BlackBerries, and I-Phones are frequently used to enable use of resources such as Geriatrics at Your Fingertips, ePocrates, Fast Facts, MedMeister/iSilo, and Mobile Merck Medicus. GPS (Global Positioning System) devices reduce the need for paper maps.

Ventilators, parenteral nutrition, and intravenous therapies like antibiotics and fluids can be prescribed for patients who need "home hospital" care. Although the home has historically been a less technologically advanced setting, high-tech care is now safe and often preferred by patients and families. With reliable caregivers and paid services to provide acute care at home, families are less stressed[5] and more satisfied,[6] patients can be kept more comfortable, and they have fewer hospital-acquired complications such as delirium[7] and functional decline.[8] Since your brick-and-mortar office has an EHR system, you grab your laptop and head out the door with basic blood-drawing equipment and a blood pressure cuff in your "black bag" and important phone numbers in your PDA.

• PRACTICAL MOBILE PRACTICE ISSUES

Travel time during house calls is not reimbursed separately by Medicare nor is it a defined part of the visit cost in the Medicare fee schedule, and homebound patients with multiple medical and social issues are usually more complex than office patients. Efficiency is enhanced by concentrating visits geographically. Still, the number of patients seen is half that seen in a typical office during an equivalent period.[1] Volume also depends on visit type. New patients, post-hospital visits, complex social situations, and patients with multiple active issues all take more time than following up on hypertension or diabetes. Numbers vary, but average home care clinicians see about five patients per half day.[1]

Transportation is typically by car, but may include taxi, bus, subway, bicycle, or even on foot in urban settings. Where needed, safety policies minimize provider risk. During travel, charts must be kept secure to protect sensitive patient information. Clean supplies must be kept separate from dirty supplies to prevent contamination and meet Joint Commission standards if you are seeking accreditation.

Like office-based peers, house call clinicians must pay attention to their business, stay on task, keep overhead down, and keep moving. Comparing Medicare reimbursement rates for house calls with other sites of care (hospital, office, nursing home), it helps that payments per home visit are greater, but the margins in fee-for-service Medicare for house call practices are still thin. Mindful scheduling of patients and following appropriate billing practices including use of prolonged service and care management codes when appropriate can help to ensure a successful practice. Multi-provider groups may also be able to reduce office overhead as the house calls practice grows.

Most home visits are made by primary care providers, but specialists need not be excluded. Given the medical complexity of the patients, specialist input may be needed. Consider a bedfast diabetic Medicare patient with a foot ulcer that you think may need revascularization to prevent amputation. You seek a vascular surgery consult. The patient cannot sit, and ambulance transport will cost $1000, which is not covered by Medicare. The surgeon may order imaging studies (another trip) and a follow-up appointment. The visits are physically burdensome and out-of-pocket cost for transport may be $3000 without other coverage (eg, from Medicaid, which will cover transportation costs for outpatient appointments). If the surgeon would consult and follow up at home either in person or via telemedicine it would save two trips.

Hospital-based house calls programs may be partially funded by a medical center. These programs contribute to a hospital's fiscal success in several ways: hospital admissions, reduced institutional costs through early discharge and more efficient inpatient care, help with transitions for high-risk patients; referrals for specialists and outpatient diagnostic testing; and good community public relations. These programs also have a role in educating learners at multiple levels.[9-10]

Concierge practices are increasingly popular. These clinicians opt out of Medicare for at least 2 years and may not bill Medicare during that time. Patients are charged an annual membership fee and billed directly for services. Concierge services are thus only available to those with higher incomes.

You need after-hours coverage for your homebound patients, and patients should know what to expect. The authors inform all new house calls patients that clinicians make visits during weekday daylight hours and provide after hours and weekend telephone coverage, but a patient may need to use the emergency room after hours if a situation cannot be resolved by phone or wait until the next business day.

CASE PRESENTATION 1 (continued)

The Visit

At 7:30 AM you are greeted by a slightly disheveled Beverly Grant. Though embarrassed by her appearance, she is very grateful and welcomes you. Frank is sleeping in his recliner. On a nearby table are a bottle of Darvocet from his ER visit and an empty Advil bottle. Quickly folding rumpled sheets on the sofa, Beverly says Frank almost fell again last night. His back was hurting so he slept where he was most comfortable. "I was afraid to leave him, so I stayed on the sofa. Around 3 AM, he needed to pee. Knowing I was tired, he did not call me. I woke just as he was sliding and pushed a step stool under his bottom to keep him from hitting the floor. Somehow we got him back in the chair. Now he says his hip hurts."

While you wash your hands, Beverly wakes Frank. He initially thinks you are his eldest son, but is quickly reoriented. His back pain slowly increased this past year, but is much worse since his fall and radiates down his legs. He has taken Advil every 6 hours without relief, but "muddled through" by walking less. He started the Darvocet last week when the pain got so bad he could not sleep. Since then he has slept on and off day and night and hardly eaten. He feels a need to urinate but only a little comes out. Though he denies constipation his last bowel movement was 4 days ago. Smiling weakly he jokes, "I tell Beverly to put me out to pasture, but she won't hear of it."

Frank is afebrile. His pulse is regular at 96 and respirations are 16 per minute. Blood pressure is 110/60, slightly below his baseline. He appears uncomfortable and cannot reposition himself in the chair. Mucous membranes are dry. Heart and lungs are unremarkable. His abdomen is protruberant and firm. He has gained weight since your last encounter and your exam is limited by his position in the recliner. As you consider how to move him to the bed for a better exam you spot a wheelchair in the corner. Frank says, "My buddy Carl brought that yesterday after our failed attempt to drag my carcass to your office; it was his wife's but she died." With Beverly's nursing experience and your brawn, you get Frank into bed. He has hypoactive bowels sounds, distention, and mild suprapubic tenderness. Rectal tone and prostate are normal. There is much firm stool in the vault. There is no spinal tenderness, but you note discomfort over the right greater trochanter. There is pain with internal hip rotation but no deformity. Pulses are intact and you are pleasantly surprised by 4+/5 muscle strength in his lower extremities.

● WHEN TO STAY FOCUSED AND WHEN TO COVER ALL BASES

Providers who make home visits find that they uncover more clinical problems and do so more efficiently than they do in the office. Research on low-income, functionally impaired patients who enrolled in the GRACE program, which provided comprehensive geriatric assessment by nurse practitioners who reported back to primary care providers, showed that among intervention patients, the home visitors far more often uncovered and addressed depression, incontinence, and gait problems in patients with falls when compared with control subjects.[11]

CASE PRESENTATION 1 (continued)

There are urgent concerns involving the Grants today. The chief complaint is pain, but you are considering dehydration, muscle weakness, caregiver burnout, depression, inappropriate medications, urinary infection, metabolic abnormalities, fecal impaction, and delirium. Safety is an issue for both husband and wife. The Grants are overwhelmed and you start to feel the same. Recalling the Grants' preference to avoid hospitals, you make a plan. The first question is: Can the workup safely be done at home? His slightly low blood pressure, borderline tachycardia, and mucous membranes suggest dehydration, yet his vital signs

are stable, he is taking oral fluids, and he has an attentive caregiver. You want to rule out urinary tract infection, fecal impaction, and a right hip fracture even though his exam is not classical. Frank's pain needs to be managed better and Beverly needs help, at least short term. These issues require immediate attention. Other concerns remain. Could weight gain and constipation reflect hypothyroidism? Are physical decline and dependence making him depressed? Cholesterol and vitamin D status and preventive cancer screening can wait. You draw blood for a metabolic profile, blood count, and TSH. Frank is continent, but with concern about possible urinary retention, you catheterize his bladder and obtain a few teaspoons of amber urine. You manually assist Frank to have a bowel movement and see prompt improvement in his abdominal exam.

After educating the Grants about Darvocet side effects including delirium, urinary retention, and constipation you advise them that the best way to dispose of the remaining pills is to remove all identification from the pill bottle, empty the pill bottle, and mix those tablets with coffee grounds or other undesirable trash in a sealed plastic bag and dispose of this in the garbage.[12] You also recommend avoiding nonsteroidal anti-inflammatory drugs (NSAIDs) like Advil due to potential for edema, hypertension, intestinal bleeding, and renal injury. You write instructions for acetaminophen (500 mg) four times daily plus low-dose oxycodone and arrange for a pharmacy to deliver enough pills for twice-daily scheduled and "as-needed" dosing. You inform the couple that oxycodone is an opiate but is better tolerated in the elderly and has fewer side effects than Darvocet. You prescribe a good bowel regimen and increased fluids, ask about depression, and make a note to inquire further when his pain is controlled and labs are back.

It is 8:30 AM and you will be late for your office session. The Grants are grateful in more ways than you know. Beverly understands that she is not alone. She knows to call your office with concerns and what to do if urgent problems arise. Although lengthy, you know the visit was worthwhile. Seeing the situation first-hand provided more insight in less time than could have been achieved in the office. Any other strategy would have required ambulance transport to an ER. Frank would not meet inpatient criteria and would be sent home. Your hour saved the system and the Grants thousands of dollars and likely avoided further misdirected care. You plan to call Beverly later today to see how things are going and arrange to return within the week for a follow-up visit.

This visit was necessarily comprehensive. Other visits focus on a few selected issues. As in all medical encounters, patient history, a physical exam, and the expertise of the clinician, together dictate the scope of the visit.

• WHEN TO SEEK HELP: THE EXTENDED HOME CARE TEAM

Complex medical, functional, and social issues often require an extended team including home health or hospice agencies. Home health agencies provide skilled nursing, aide services, physical, occupational, and speech therapies, and social work. Medicare covers this care if a physician certifies that the patient is homebound and has a skilled need that can be safely met with intermittent services. A patient need not be bedridden, but must have a physical or psychiatric condition that prevents leaving home without considerable, taxing effort: the patient cannot "leave their place of residence except with the aid of: supportive devices such as crutches, canes, wheelchairs and walkers; the use of special transportation; or the assistance of another person; or if leaving home is medically contraindicated."[13] Home health agency services now average only 19 visits per patient enrolled in a 60-day episode. Visit numbers have dropped dramatically in the past decade since agencies are paid prospectively for 60 days of care (episodes) rather than by the visit. Physicians may need to advocate for patients if they see home care episodes or in-home rehab services ending too soon while skilled needs still exist.

Skilled services by nurses include patient education, wound care, medication management, and technical work related to various ostomies and infusion devices. Nurses can draw blood as long as this is not the only reason for the home care referral, fill pill boxes, hang IV fluids, manage catheters, and give shots. They assess patients for clinicians and teach patients and families, giving them the tools to monitor and manage chronic illnesses such as diabetes, hypertension, and heart failure independently.

Home health aide services can be provided within a Medicare Part A episode; while not licensed to give medications, administer tube feedings, do wound care, or provide other skilled services, they are invaluable. They help with activities of daily living (ADLs), do light housework, shopping, or meal preparation, and may accompany patients to appointments. For patients with Medicaid, long-term care insurance, or funds to pay for the service, personal care aides can be placed in the home for 8 or more hours per day.

Need for physical therapy (PT) qualifies a patient for skilled care, and a Medicare home health care episode can be initiated with a nursing, physical therapy, or speech therapy order. Therapy involvement results in higher payments for the episode. PT and occupational therapy enable functional recovery and home safety. Medical providers should recall that agencies receive a fixed 60-day payment in one of about 80 categories and must manage their visits and care plan within that framework

Agencies that provide the services mentioned are usually not directed by the home medical providers but they are vital to an extended interdisciplinary team. In the best practices, medical groups and home health agencies coordinate efforts routinely.

In all of these arrangements, insurance coverage and financial assets affect the options. For instance, a patient may have Medicare and be eligible for skilled services at home, but because the patient's assets exceed poverty level, he or she may not qualify for a Medicaid home heath aide, yet may be unable to pay for such services out of pocket (~$17/hr).

• CARE TRANSITIONS AND HOME CARE

Most individuals are free of serious chronic illness until their final years of life. When they are failing, in the span of a year you may find multiple hospitalizations. Even then, most care is delivered by informal caregivers at home. These patients, with numerous medical problems and high acute-care use, risk further decline and absorb most of the health care dollars. Currently the clinicians who manage such patients in the hospital are usually not on their primary care team. And, while inpatient providers may do an excellent job in the hospital, they often do less well when initiating post-hospital care, which is unfamiliar territory. Detailed information about the inpatient stay is often lacking, limited, or late, making it difficult for the primary care provider to "pick up the ball."

Caregivers and patients often leave hospitals with unanswered questions and a poor understanding regarding the medications and treatments needed to avoid returning to the hospital. Poor communication, discontinuity, and medical instability combine to cause repeat hospitalization and further downhill spirals.

This is the zone of transitional care into which many chronically ill primary care patients often fall. In the absence of established house call programs for continuity at home, care models using nurse practitioners and other case managers promote safe and timely transfer of patients from one level of care to another (eg, acute to subacute) or from one setting to another (eg, hospital to home).[14] The focus is on improving post-hospital outcomes for high-risk, high-cost patients, and research shows that the more effective models are interdisciplinary and involve face-to-face communication rather than relying on phone calls.[15] The next case describes a typical scenario; additional discussion on transitional care can be found in Chapter 22.

CASE PRESENTATION 2: FLORENCE JONES

Mrs. Jones is an 80-year-old woman with degenerative joint disease, hypertension, type II diabetes mellitus, and renal insufficiency. Widowed for 5 years, she has been living alone and able to maintain an active, satisfying lifestyle with help from family and friends. A few hours after returning home from a dinner outing, she develops facial flushing, diaphoresis, and vomiting. Thinking that she has food poisoning she phones her son Henry to bring diet ginger ale to settle her stomach. He arrives 30 minutes later to find his mother severely short of breath and lethargic and calls 911.

Florence has an acute myocardial infarction. Catheterization shows high-grade coronary disease that leads to emergent bypass surgery of three vessels. Surgery goes well but she develops MRSA (methicillin-resistant *Staphylococcus aureus*) bacteremia from a saphenous vein harvest site infection. She requires an insulin drip plus dialysis for acute kidney injury due to prolonged hypotension while septic. Her muscles are weak from ICU myopathy.

Two weeks later she is improving. Creatinine returned to baseline (1.6 mg/dL [141 μmol/L]) but she is still too weak for inpatient rehabilitation. Discharge planners recommend skilled nursing facility rehabilitation where she will get the remaining 2 weeks of IV vancomycin. Because of a bad nursing home experience when her husband died, Mrs. Jones refuses and insists on going home. The discharge planner calls a family meeting. Her son is on summer break from his teaching job and offers to have Florence live with his family temporarily. Medicare will cover home nursing, IV therapy (except the

medicine that is now covered by Medicare part D), and physical and occupational therapy. In addition to hanging antibiotics, the nurse can teach patient and family about peripherally inserted central catheter (PICC) line care, wound care, and diabetes management. Florence now needs insulin. She is too weak to transfer. Her Social Security income is above the Medicaid threshold so she will need to pay extra for a home health aide. Serving as her hospitalist, you are concerned about short-term medical follow-up. You ask Gloria Reynolds, the transitional care nurse practitioner, to bridge the gap until Florence can get back to her primary doctor.

● TRANSITIONAL CARE TEAM

Staffing for some transitional care (TC) programs includes advanced practice nurses with physician support, similar to a house calls team. These TC teams assume interim management duties, seeing the patient and coordinating with inpatient physicians, home health agencies, and outpatient physicians. At Virginia Commonwealth University Health System (VCUHS) in Richmond, the TC team has two experienced nurse practitioners (NPs) who are comfortable managing complex patients. Once consulted by an inpatient team, the NPs read the chart and meet the patient, families, and doctors. They help with discharge planning, and suggest what equipment, services, and education are needed. The NP then visits the patient at home for 4 to 6 weeks, provides clinical care and family support, and coordinates care until the patient can return to the office. The NPs provide detailed notes about the transition period and may attend the first clinic visit. They give the primary care clinician information that is otherwise hard to get, establish continuity, and lower repeat hospitalizations by half or more if patients are selected well.[16] In addition, a randomized controlled clinical trial in which acutely ill patients deemed eligible for hospital admission were cared for in the home using advanced home care resulted in greater patient satisfaction, less delirium, and less functional decline.[17]

● SKILLS REQUIRED TO CARE FOR "HOSPITAL-AT-HOME" OR TRANSITIONAL CARE PATIENTS

The skill set for TC clinicians is extensive. They manage challenging patients with multiple co-morbidities and many medications plus complex devices. They should know hospital regimens and be comfortable providing them in the home. They need strong interpersonal skills to work with patients, families, and home health agencies that are grappling with serious illness and end-of-life issues. They must also correspond with and obtain clinical support from inpatient and outpatient physicians. Knowing ventilator and tracheostomy care is important if patients require such technology, but access to specialists by phone can substitute. They must also know community resources.

CASE PRESENTATION 2 (continued)

Gloria is reassuringly capable. She suggests that while Florence is in the hospital, nursing staff begin teaching and observe Henry's ability to do PICC line and wound care, operate the glucometer, and give insulin. She asks physical therapy to instruct Henry on transfer techniques, and helps order a hospital bed, bedside table, and bedside commode that will be delivered to Henry's home before discharge. Gloria confirms follow-up plans and reviews the medicines to weed out hospital-specific items and avoid wasting time on prior authorization for drugs not on the patient's Medicare Part D plan. Gloria suggests bowel and pain regimens and tells the team which pharmacies deliver. She helps select a home health agency that can meet Mrs. Jones needs.

On the day of discharge, Gloria calls Henry's home to see how things are going. Delighted to be out of the hospital, Henry reports that "Mom indulged in a bowl of ice cream for lunch but her pre-dinner sugar is 450 (25 mmol/L)." Gloria tells him how to adjust the regular insulin. She asks Henry to recheck the sugar in 3 hours, call her if it remains above 300 (16.7 mmol/L), and tells him that she will visit in the morning.

• CASELOAD

Due to acuity and instability, transition patients need more frequent visits and support than typical house call patients. For example, high-risk patients followed by Naylor and colleagues[14] received an average of 4.5 NP visits in 4 weeks after hospital discharge. An NP's caseload in this role may be as low as 10 patients. Since the VCUHS transitional care program started in 2000, more than 450 complex patients have been managed successfully. The return on this investment is large. In multiple studies by Naylor and colleagues, total health care savings are about 50%, and at VCU using historical controls, estimated hospital costs were 65% lower 6 months after enrollment compared with pre-enrollment data.[18] To generate more revenue and avoid clinician burnout, at VCU we keep a mix of intensive transitional care and chronic care patients in each provider's panel.

CASE PRESENTATION 2 (continued)

At Henry's home the next morning, Gloria finds the entire household asleep. Henry apologizes, saying "Mom was up all night with diarrhea, so we are worn out." Florence easily arouses but seems uncomfortable. She complains of vague stomach discomfort and a sore bottom. Exam shows a temperature of 100.8°F (38.2°C), hyperactive bowel sounds, mild abdominal distention, and nonspecific tenderness. Lungs are clear and oxygen saturation is 99% on room air. Her leg wound is unchanged, with slight serosanguinous drainage and early granulation tissue. Her briefs are wet. She has non-blanching erythema on her sacrum that is new. Her PICC site is not inflamed.

Henry feels guilty for not changing his mother earlier or getting her on the commode during the night. He fears that the celebratory bowl of ice cream aggravated her lactose intolerance, causing the diarrhea. Gloria gently reassures him and explains that with the home health agency she will help him. She watches him accurately check his mom's blood sugar and they review the sliding scale. She reconciles the discharge medications with Mrs. Jones pre-hospital bottles, confirming that both Mrs. Jones and her son understand the changes. Armed with knowledge of the hospital course, which included broad-spectrum antibiotics, Gloria has another idea about the diarrhea.

Suddenly, Mrs. Jones says, "I have to go right now." Gloria sees Henry struggling to get her on the commode and helps. Gloria collects a stool specimen in a sterile urine cup to test for *Clostridium difficile* toxin. Noting several young grandchildren running downstairs to the kitchen, Gloria talks about techniques to limit spread of organisms like MRSA and *C. difficile* to others in the household.

MRSA colonization is prevalent in the community, found in 8% of older patients who were screened when admitted to a French hospital.[19] Inpatient staff members take extensive precautions to prevent MRSA being passed from one patient to the next by staff[20]; however, there is no evidence that measures like gowns and isolation are needed at home. While there is no evidence of danger to healthy members of the household, colonization is common and clinical impacts are possible for others in the community who have weakened immunity. Therefore, reasonable precautions such as good hand washing techniques, donning of gloves when handling bodily fluids, proper disposal of patient waste and soiled dressings, and separate washing of patient linens and clothing are appropriate when drug-resistant organisms are involved.[21]

CASE PRESENTATION 2 (continued)

While Henry gives his mother insulin and gets her breakfast tray, Gloria draws blood for a complete metabolic profile and CBC. She instructs Mrs. Jones to drink more fluids and confirms that both mother and son know the signs and symptoms of both hypo- and hyperglycemia and how to treat them. After answering questions from both patient and caregiver, Gloria emerges from the home almost 2 hours after arriving.

En route to her next visit, Gloria drops the STAT samples at the lab and calls the home health agency to confirm that nursing will hang the IV vancomycin and instruct the family on wound care, and that physical therapy will teach the son transfer techniques. Gloria is thankful that her next three appointments are patients whom she knows well and who are less complex. She plans to return to her office by mid-afternoon, follow up unresolved issues, and call the Jones family to see how their day went.

At 2 o'clock Gloria receives an urgent page from her office to call Henry Jones, who reports, "Mom still has diarrhea and she is very weak. She has not had much to eat or drink all day, but her blood sugar is still over 300. The home health nurse called to say she is on her way, but I am thinking of bringing Mom back to the hospital." He reports Mrs. Jones is awake and alert but tired. Gloria asks him to wait briefly while she checks the morning's lab results. With her laptop, she accesses the hospital EMR through a secure website and notes a newly elevated white count of $15 \times 10^3/\mu L$ (15×10^9/L) plus a BUN of 30 mg/dL (10.7 mmol/L) and creatinine of 2.2 mg/dL (194.5 μmol/L) suggesting dehydration. The stool contains *C. difficile* toxin.

C. difficile toxin is found on the first test in about 80% to 90% of confirmed cases but with a range of sensitivity from 65% to 95%,[22] which underlines the importance of knowing how your lab works, and may require two or three tests for definitive diagnosis in patients with the condition to avoid false negatives. Some authors also suggest use of different testing methods for the second test in a given patient.[23]

Gloria calls Henry to revise the care plan and has the home infusion company deliver half-normal saline IV bags. She gives the home health nurse orders on rate of administration and tells her that the pharmacy will deliver metronidazole (500 mg every 8 hours).[24] Tired and concerned, Henry is relieved to know that the diagnosis is made and there is a solution that will avoid another hospitalization with all of the attendant risks.

Gloria spent 3 hours taking care of Mrs. Jones. Billable services include the home visit, prolonged service time, and care plan oversight, but these will not fully cover the cost. Is this worth it? Being at home is preferred by patients and caregivers. Henry is dedicated and willing to learn; he will succeed given support.

As a provider, keeping the patient at home is rewarding. Mrs. Jones already has two antibiotic-resistant organisms and would run additional risks if re-hospitalized. Soon, the hospital may also be accountable for costs of re-hospitalization.[25] Gloria's time investment saves Medicare thousands of dollars and helps the health system have a bed free for another patient.

In general physicians are involved to a limited degree during immediate post-hospital and home health agency care, and more than one-third of patients have no direct physician contacts in this critical post-acute period.[26] This gap in care management led to the creation of "transitional care" teams, and several studies now report as much as 50% savings from such teams' impact on post-hospital readmission rates. These include intensive models such as the nurse practitioner–based strategy described in our example, and less intensive coaching models that have a somewhat smaller and perhaps less durable but still significant and meaningful effect.[27] Those planning health policy and considering transitional care models must still grapple with the ongoing care to those patients who are still too immobile for office-based care when "transitional care" ends. We would argue that house calls are the only realistic answer.

● WHEN CARE AT HOME IS NOT THE BEST OPTION

Whether it is safe to continue treating a patient at home extends beyond purely medical issues. Inadequate heating or cooling, rodents and bugs, lack of electric power or running water, absent phone access, unsafe neighborhoods, and insufficient food or medications can impact care. These factors are usually unknown to physicians in a clinic or hospital, but quickly recognized in the home. Community resources resolve some of these issues but some socioeconomic problems are challenging to uncover and fix.

What Constitutes an Unsafe Home Environment?

Patients with an intense desire to remain in their homes may lack insight into the extent of their own needs, lack capability to recognize decline, or have insufficient vision, hearing, mobility, or cognition to manage alone. Cogent patients admit to being in conditions that are suboptimal, yet refuse to change. These "social" cases are most frustrating to health care providers, but patients are free to make what others may consider poor choices if the risk is reasonable and they understand it.

Beyond environmental problems, elders are at risk for abuse or neglect. Abuse brings to mind physical wounds or suspicious fractures, but may also be psychological or economic. Caregivers' financial needs may put patients at risk. A caregiver may not provide the frequent continence care and dressing changes needed to heal a bedsore, yet refuse nursing home placement because they need the patient's Social Security check. These motives can involve even well-meaning caregivers. Consider Pamela Sneed.

CASE PRESENTATION 3: PAMELA SNEED

Mrs. Pamela Sneed has been a house call patient for years. Despite severe osteoarthritis that limits mobility, pernicious anemia, and mild cognitive impairment, she has managed on her own, saying she "would rather die than be in a nursing home." You have noted slow progression to dementia but she has remained safe enough with help from close friends, a daughter who visits, and a home health nurse who gives her a monthly vitamin B_{12} shot. Now you find a kitchen burner on while Pamela has no recall of cooking. Other clues lead you to broach the subject of memory and safety. She admits to being more forgetful and agrees it would be nice for someone to live with her and keep an eye on things. Pamela convinces her daughter Judy to move back home. However, Judy must work to cover the bills, so Mrs. Sneed is still unsupervised during the day.

While this might be considered neglect, it is unintentional. Judy is well meaning and changed her life to care for her mother. The least disruptive step would be to call the home health agency social worker who could arrange for an aide to stay with the patient or find a local adult day care center for the hours that the daughter works.

HELPFUL RESOURCES

Communities provide a variety of resources for elders at risk. Hospital social workers maintain a list of services. Websites such as Eldercare.gov sponsored by the Department of Health and Human Services help "find local agencies in every U.S. community that can help older persons and their families to access home and community-based services like transportation, meals, home care and caregiver support services." Note that in less populous areas those services may be located at some distance. Area Agencies on Aging located throughout the United States have a wealth of information on eldercare resources. Houses of worship may assist with transportation, shopping, cleaning, or home repair. Organizations will build ramps or make free, safety-related structural renovations. Meals on Wheels can be critical to a patient with limited access to food. Health-watch devices help to alert emergency responders.

HOW TO CHANGE THE DYNAMIC

The home care clinician has unique opportunities to directly observe the complex factors that affect a patient's daily life, yet social issues must be approached judiciously. Fear of being judged may stop a patient or caregiver from speaking openly. The best clinicians will ultimately fail if the clinicians' goals differ from those of patients and caregivers. One may plan a complex antihypertensive regimen to prevent a stroke but the patient may worry about the impact on caregivers' time or finances. Flexibility and willingness to ask about concerns of patient and caregivers are vital.

The best way to change the dynamic is to earn trust. Sometimes this takes time. It is instinctual for patients and caregivers to take a defensive position if they feel their choices being scrutinized. When trying to change a care plan, first acknowledge the caregiver's previous good work. Listen and ask questions in a compassionate, nonjudgmental fashion. Simple statements like "Please tell me what is most important to you" let people know that you value their opinions; they may then be more willing to consider other options. Some patients and families find comfort knowing that you have experienced similar situations yourself. It is essential to let patients know that you are interested in their goals, religious and cultural preferences, financial worries, prior health care experiences, and emotional ties.

This work can be more difficult when patients cannot speak for themselves or when multiple caregivers are involved. Identifying the primary decision-maker is the first challenge. This caregiver may then also be influenced by other family members or close contacts. Clinicians easily get caught in family disputes. It helps to focus on the patient as your priority. A family meeting with all involved parties is usually beneficial. Ask about previous health care experiences; this may shed light on caregivers' decisions. All parties must be allowed to voice opinions to reach consensus or overcome conflict.

Most states have a legal hierarchy for decision-makers when an incapacitated patient has no previously declared power of attorney. When there are multiple potential decision-makers, it is wise to have the family choose one person as the lead contact. This may not be the person providing the daily care, which can add tension if the parties disagree. Social work help is often valuable at this juncture.

Ultimately, remember that a successful clinician must have willing participation by patients and caregivers in a plan of care. This will take you far.

JUDGING ADEQUACY OF FAMILY SUPPORT

Although a full discussion of caregivers and caregiving can be found in Chapter 17, the topic is so important to home care that is also bears mentioning here. Many factors determine whether a family is providing adequate support. Care for a loved one can be burdensome, given the physical and emotional strain, economic impact, and needed sacrifices. Caregivers like Mrs. Grant ignore their own health, and physical efforts needed to turn or transfer a bed-bound patient may cause injury and exhaustion. Anxiety and depression occur; many caregivers are isolated from social supports. Daughters like Judy may quit work and face financial crisis rather than seem uncaring. Clinicians must put patients first, but helping patients requires helping caregivers with encouraging words and services, and sometimes you should propose an alternate strategy.

Some families simply cannot cope. Monitoring blood sugar is easy for some but impossible for others. Caregivers who have done well for years fail to handle a new problem like urinary incontinence. Clinicians must notice signs of inadequate care both subtle and obvious. Pressure ulcers can mark either terminal decline or inadequate turning. Weight loss can reflect a thyroid disorder, depression, or cancer, or may result when a caregiver does not take time to feed a disabled patient, or the home lacks nutritious food.

Do not be led astray by assumptions based on socioeconomic status. Affluent families provide inadequate care if they are unable to fill in when a paid home health aide cancels at the last minute. Conversely, caregivers with meager resources provide excellent care in the most complex and difficult situations imaginable.

Often you find yourself in shades of gray. Clinicians must avoid being judgmental or imposing their own values. With a nonthreatening manner, observe interactions between patient and caregivers, investigate medical conditions that may contribute, and pay attention to patient preferences. Then, only after doing a comprehensive assessment can a clinician offer a sound opinion about adequacy of care. It helps to discuss the most difficult situations with colleagues because it is not easy to resolve these complex cases.

If you decide that care is insufficient, you must tell the patient and caregiver of your concerns and offer options. Patient and caregiver response to a balanced clinical opinion, plus willingness to engage in discussion, accept help, and modify their approach is often the best guide regarding the viability of continued care at home.

● WHO IS RESPONSIBLE AND WHEN TO CALL ADULT PROTECTIVE SERVICES (APS)

If social work support was not available to help with Mrs. Sneed, contact with Adult Protective Services (APS) would be necessary. Clinicians are legally required to report when abuse or neglect is suspected, and in some states penalties can be imposed for failure to do so.[28] Patient self-neglect and abuse or neglect by caregivers are all reportable. Each state has requirements that clinicians must know, and in most states health care workers—including home health nurses and aides, therapists, social workers, and physicians—are mandated reporters. APS must then take and investigate reports, assessing decision-making capacity and risk. Often patients are found capable of decisions but are making poor choices; this limits the options for APS, which can include emergency in-home personal care, institutional placement, legal or law enforcement action, guardianship, and housing, social, financial, and medical interventions.

In general, abuse or neglect involves "intentional actions that cause harm or a serious risk of harm to a vulnerable elder by a caregiver or person who stands in a trust relationship with the elder, or failure by a caregiver to satisfy the elder's basic needs or to protect the elder from harm."[29] When seeing shades of gray, health care workers should know that an APS report often is not a punitive action but a way to get needed help. Reports are anonymous; unless malicious intent is proven, the reporter is safe from legal action. Even so, APS reports are perceived in a negative light by some families and reporters must keep that in mind. The National Center for Elder Abuse website has information about state laws and resources.[30]

● WHEN MAKING A HOME VISIT IS UNSAFE FOR THE PROVIDER

Homebound patients live in all types of settings and neighborhoods. It is natural for a home care provider to worry when he or she enters an unclean, cluttered, or chaotic environment, or to feel safe in affluent homes that are actually less safe than they seem. Clinicians must understand the environment and take steps to maintain their own safety.

In general home care is safe; patients and their families are grateful and clinicians are safe even in urban housing projects. When there are overt warning signs such as physical or verbal abuse to a patient or direct threats to the provider by an agitated or intoxicated caregiver, the clinician should leave, call law enforcement, and file an APS report once out of harm's way. Clinicians have a duty to protect the patient but must protect themselves first. Although a rare necessity, law enforcement can accompany a clinician into the home of a patient in immediate risk.

Most situations are less overtly risky. A provider may still need intuition. Suspicion of heavy drug or alcohol abuse is an example. Such environments can be unpredictable, and may warrant APS referral or termination of services with a referral to other options for care even if these are limited to the emergency room.

Structural damage (rotten floors or ceilings) can also, though rarely, put clinicians at risk for injury. This may require immediate APS referral to get the patient in a safe living situation until repairs are made. Likewise, aggressive animals can pose a risk; this is often remedied by calling ahead.

Some house call programs have procedures to promote provider safety: traveling in pairs, limiting visits to daylight hours, not carrying medications that have street value, dressing in a manner that does not draw attention, carrying a cell phone, and informing the office of their daily schedule. It is wise to include a statement in the initial new patient agreement for "permission to treat" that clinicians will not practice in situations that infringe on their personal safety and this may lead to termination of care.

SUMMARY

As the US population ages and numbers of immobile persons increase, the demand for home visits will continue to rise. Technological advances have leveled the playing field, blurring boundaries between what is possible in medical offices, hospitals, and the home. Home visits provide high quality-medical care to complex patients who may otherwise go without consistent medical attention. For patients and families, house calls are often a preferred way to obtain medical care. Patients are more comfortable and at ease with their providers, who in turn can directly observe the many factors that potentially alter clinical outcomes. Clinicians who make house calls have expressed professional satisfaction from their careers and enjoy the opportunity to spend more time with patients.

Easing transitions from hospital to home and managing patients who are chronically immobile with timely response when they are ill can avoid unnecessary readmissions and lead to cost savings for our health care system. With increased awareness and training, and anticipated government attention to encouraging care models of this sort, we hope to see a broad renewal of interest in house calls.

References

1. Kao H, Conant R, Sorian T, McCormick W. The past, present and future of house calls. *Clin Geriatr Med.* 2009;25;19-34.

2. Coe NB, Van Houtven CH. Caring for Mom and neglecting yourself? The health effects of caring for an elderly parent. *Health Economics.* 2009;18:991-1010.

3. American Academy of Home Care Physicians. Practice Management Frequently Asked Questions. aahcp.org.

4. Gresham CB, Boling PA. New diagnostic and information technology for mobile medical care. *Clin Geriatr Med.* 2009;25:93-107.

5. Leff B, Burton L, Mader S, et al. Comparison of stress experienced by family members of patients treated in Hospital at Home with that of those receiving traditional acute hospital care. *J Am Geriatr Soc.* 2008;56:117-123.

6. Leff B, Burton L, Mader S, et al. Satisfaction with Hospital at Home care. *J Am Geriatr Soc.* 2006;54:1355-1363.

7. Leff B; Burton L, Mader S, et al. Hospital at Home: Feasibility and outcomes of a program to provide hospital-level care for acutely ill older patients. *Ann Intern Med.* 2005;143:798-808.

8. Leff B, Burton L, Mader S, et al. Comparison of functional outcomes associated with Hospital at Home care and traditional acute hospital care. *J Am Geriatr Soc.* 2009;57:273-278.

9. Hervada-Page M, Fayock KS, Sifri R, Markham FW. The home visit experience: A medical student's perspective. *Care Manage J.* 2007; 8:206-210.

10. Boling PA, Willett RM, Gentili A, et al. The importance of "high valence" events in a successful program for teaching geriatrics to medical students. *Gerontol Geriatr Higher Ed.* 2008;28:59-72.

11. Counsell SR, Callahan CM, Clark DO, et al. Geriatric care management for low-income seniors: A randomized controlled trial. *JAMA.* 2007;298:2623-2633.

12. US Department of Health and Human Services, US Food and Drug Administration. How to Dispose of Unused Medicines, http://www.fda.gov/ForConsumers/ConsumerUpdates/ucm101653.htm.

13. Home health services. *Medicare Benefit Policy Manual.* Chapter 7.

14. Naylor MD, Brooten D, Campbell R, et al. Comprehensive discharge planning and home care follow-up of hospitalized elders. *JAMA.* 1999; 281:613-620.

15. Sochalski J, Jaarsma T, Krumholz HM, et al. What works in chronic care management: The case of heart failure. *Health Affairs.* 2009; 28:179-189.

16. Boling PA. Care transitions and home health care. *Clin Geriatr Med.* 2009;25:135-148.

17. Leff B, Burton L, Mader SL, et al. Hospital at Home: Feasibility and outcomes of a program to provide hospital-level care at home for acutely ill older patients. *Ann Intern Med.* 2005;143: 798-808.

18. Smigelski C, Hungate B, Holdren J, et al. Transitional model of care at VCU Medical Center—6 years' experience. *J Am Geriatr Soc.* 2008;65(suppl):S197.

19. Lucet JC, Grenet K, Armand-Lefevre L, et al. High prevalence of carriage of methicillin-resistant *Staphylococcus aureus* at hospital admission in elderly patients: Implications for infection control strategies. *Infect Control Hosp Epidemiol.* 2005;26: 121-126.

20. Clock SA, Cohen B, Behta M, et al. Contact precautions for multidrug resistant organisms: Current recommendations and actual practice. *Am J Infect Control.* 2009;1-7.

21. McGoldrick M, Rhinehart E. Multi-drug resistant organisms in home care and hospice: Prevention and control. *Home Healthcare Nurse.* 2007;25:580-586.

22. Eastwood K, Else P, Charlett A, Wilcox M. Comparison of nine commercially available *Clostridium difficile* toxin detection assays, a real-time PCR assay for *C. difficile* tcdB, and a glutamate dehydrogenase detection assay to cytotoxin testing and cytotoxigenic culture methods. *J Clin Microbiol.* 2009;47:3211-3217.

23. Peterson LR, Robiccsek A. Does my patient have *Clostridium difficile* infection? *Ann Intern Med.* 2009;151:176-179.

24. Pawloowski SW, Warren CA, Guerrant R. Diagnosis of acute or persistent diarrhea. *Gastroenterology.* 2009;136:1874-1886.

25. The Patient Protection and Affordable Care Act. Detailed summary. http://dpc.senate.gov/healthreformbill/healthbill05.pdf. Accessed on November 27, 2009.

26. Wolff JL, Meadow A, Boyd CM, et al. Physician evaluation and management of Medicare home health patients. *Med Care.* 2009;47:1147-1155.

27. Coleman EA, Parry C, Chalmers S, Min SJ. The care transitions intervention: Results of a randomized controlled trial. *Arch Intern Med.* 2006;166:1822-1828.

28. Abbey L. Elder abuse and neglect: When home is not safe. *Clin Geriatr Med.* 2009;25;47-60.

29. Lachs MS, Pillemer K. Elder abuse. *Lancet.* 2004;364:1263-1272.

30. National Center for Elder Abuse. http://www.ncea.aoa.gov/NCEAroot/Main_Site/Index.aspx.

POST-TEST

1. A 75-year-old woman is confined to home with emphysema, heart failure, kidney disease, and gout. She was recently hospitalized twice and was discharged home 1 week ago with new medications. Previously, she could walk to her bathroom; now she requires help from her family to stand and transfer to a bedside commode. She has Medicare Part A and Part B, plus Medicaid coverage under which she auto-enrolled in Medicare Part D. Which of these is NOT reimbursed under her insurance coverage?

   A. Home health agency visits for skilled nursing

   B. Travel time for a physician making home visits

   C. Hospital bed and wheelchair

   D. In-home physical and occupational therapy visits by home health agency

2. Under which of the following circumstances should a home care provider call adult protective services?

   A. When a normally attentive caregiver forgets to check his or her loved one's blood sugar before administering insulin and causes hypoglycemia

   B. When a clinician disagrees with the medical choices being made by a patient who has the capacity to understand the risk of his or her decisions

   C. When a family cannot come to agreement on the medical options available for a patient who is unable to make decisions

   D. When a caregiver does not purchase necessary medications for a patient while spending Social Security check monies on their own clothing

3. Of the following factors, which is the MOST important key to success when providing medical care to a homebound patient?

   A. Having a pharmacy that is willing to deliver medications to the home

   B. Having a patient and/or caregiver who is willing to learn and collaborate with clinically trained providers

   C. Having a good health insurance plan

   D. Having a home health agency available to provide skilled nursing, therapy, and aide services

ANSWERS TO PRE-TEST

1. C
2. A
3. C

ANSWERS TO POST-TEST

1. B
2. D
3. B

25

Long-Term Care

Daniel Ari Mendelson, MS, MD, FACP

Robert M. McCann, MD, FACP

● **LEARNING OBJECTIVES**

1. Compare and contrast housing options for older adults.
2. Discuss the characteristics for determination of necessity for long-term care.
3. Identify and describe goals of care based on a patient's functional status, medical conditions, and preferences.
4. Discuss the practical, cost-effective approach to evaluating and managing common geriatrics syndromes in the long-term care (LTC) setting.
5. Describe Medicare/Medicaid coverage in long-term care.

PRE-TEST

1. The approximate percentage of nursing home residents that require assistance with five activities of daily living is:
   A. 5%
   B. 15%
   C. 35%
   D. 50%

2. Cardiopulmonary resuscitation leads to full recovery (pre-arrest functional status) for approximately what proportion of LTC residents who suffer an unwitnessed cardiac arrest?

   A. < 1%
   B. 5%
   C. 10%
   D. > 25%

3. The most common co-morbid condition found in LTC residents is:
   A. Chronic obstructive pulmonary disease
   B. Congestive heart failure
   C. Dementia
   D. Significant renal insufficiency

● INTRODUCTION

Long-term care (LTC) is a broad term covering the scope of diverse health care and social facilities and services that provide rehabilitative, restorative, custodial, and/or ongoing skilled nursing care in a variety of settings to patients or residents in need of ongoing medical care and/or assistance with activities of daily living (ADLs). Long-term care facilities include skilled nursing facilities and nursing homes (NHs), rehabilitation facilities, inpatient behavioral health facilities, long-term chronic care hospitals, assisted living facilities, and nontraditional facilities such as community hospices and religious retirement homes. LTC also includes the Program of All-inclusive Care for the Elderly (PACE), long-term home health care programs through home care agencies, Medicaid community waiver programs, continuing care retirement communities, naturally occurring retirement communities, and other formal and informal programs.[1,2] Many of these facilities or programs will enroll residents on the basis of levels of impairment in the instrumental and basic activities of daily living (IADLs/ADLs). Increasing dependence in basic ADLs is associated with an increase risk of placement in a facility providing greater levels of care and loss of independent living.[2,3]

The next sections describe some of the different types of LTC facilities or delivery modalities.[4]

Assisted Living Facilities

Assisted living facilities (ALFs) are for those who need some help with IADLs but otherwise are fairly independent and wish to live on their own as much as possible. Typical assistance in an ALF might include management of medications, help with bathing, provision of meals, and laundry services. Such facilities are an intermediate step between living completely independently and living in a NH.

Continuing Care Retirement Communities

Continuing care retirement communities (CCRCs) are like little towns that may include apartments, small houses, assisted living areas, and NHs. CCRCs offer different levels of care along a continuum. The appeal of these communities is that older adults can move in when they are healthy and independent and enjoy access to health care, recreation, social, and other activities, and if their health declines they can move to different parts of the community with escalating levels of service available based on the needs of the resident.

Home Care

Home care includes services provided within recipients' homes by community nursing agencies. Some agencies offer enough services in combination with adult day care, home health aides, or other programs in order to allow otherwise NH-appropriate patients to stay at home. This is sometimes referred to as long-term home health care program (LTHHCP) or community long-term care (CLTC). The Program of All-inclusive Care for the Elderly (PACE) is another provider of community care in which participants requiring a nursing home level of care

instead attend a day health center where all of their medical needs are addressed in a congregate setting but in the evenings and on weekends they are back in their own homes.

Hospice Care

Hospice care is for those who are not expected to live more than 6 months. Hospice is designed for patients at the end of life where symptom management and quality of life are the main goals. Program eligibility and services are tightly regulated by Medicare for hospice care in the United States. Hospice care may be provided at homes or in NHs, hospitals, etc.

Nursing Home

NHs are for older adults who need more nursing care and generally have an impairment such they require moderate to total dependence in at least two ADLs. Under Medicare, an NH may be utilized for short-term rehabilitation following a hospitalization for an acute illness (eg, heart attack) or injury (eg, a broken hip); following this short-term stay, patients transition back to home or remain in long-term care settings under different payment arrangements. (Medicare with a few exceptions does not cover long-term supportive care.) For "long-term" long-term care, NHs are utilized by impaired, dependent older adults who, due to financial, social, or intensity of care needs, require an environment in which 24-hour care from skilled professionals is available. Nursing home care tends to be the most expensive type of long-term care, with annual costs ranging from $50,000 to over $100,000 per year.

Personal Care/Rest Home/Boarding Home

Personal care homes (aka "rest homes") are for those who need some help but who also can do most things for themselves. Personal care homes tend to be smaller, often family run, with a limited number or residents, perhaps as few as 5 to as many as 15. They are geared for older persons who enjoy shared meals and the social aspect of small group living.

Retirement Community

Retirement communities usually contain apartments, rooms, or small homes that do not require much upkeep. This type of setting might be appropriate for older adults who would like to minimize the need for upkeep of a home or garden with routine services such as lawn service and maintenance provided by the community employees. The living quarters usually come with capabilities for adaptive equipment to be installed with relative ease or may have universal wheelchair access for all rooms.

LTC Financing and Organization

LTC is expensive. NH care ranges from about $50,000 to more than $100,000 per year in the United States.[5] LTC insurance has developed specifically to cover the costs of LTC services, most of which are not covered by traditional health insurance or Medicare. These include services in the home, such as assistance with ADLs, as well as care in a variety of facility and community settings.[1,4] LTC insurance can be cost-prohibitive, but can be beneficial for individuals with at least moderate incomes who have financial assets they wish to protect. Older adults who meet criteria for being classified as "poor" or "indigent" can usually qualify for Medicaid, which is the major public payer for NH or other LTC. Older persons who are neither poor nor covered by private LTC insurance are effectively "self-insured," and have to directly pay for care until they "spend down" their assets and are eligible for Medicaid. Placement in an NH may be delayed while eligibility for Medicaid or other payment sources are identified. Often LTC services are augmented by unpaid or unreimbursed support from family, friends, or other caregivers. In fact, a great proportion of long-term, supportive care is "informal," and in fact the level and quantity of "formal" LTC needed or utilized is determined by the relative availability of informal care. For example, permanent NH placement is often the result of having long-term dependency needs while living alone.

As noted earlier, Medicare covers skilled care in a skilled nursing facility (SNF) under certain conditions, for a limited time. Skilled care is provided by nursing or rehabilitation staff for patient management, observation, and evaluation purposes. Examples of skilled care include changing sterile dressings, providing IV antibiotics, and physical therapy. It is delivered in a Medicare-certified SNF. Medicare covers certain skilled care services that are needed daily on a short-term basis (up to 100 days).[6] Medicare will cover skilled care only if all of the following conditions are met:

1. The older adult has Medicare Part A (Hospital Insurance) and has coverage days remaining in his or her current benefit period.
2. The older adult has a qualifying stay, generally defined as 3 consecutive days (72 hours) or more, in an acute hospital. The eligible older adult must enter the SNF within a short time (generally 30 days or less) of leaving the hospital, and require skilled services related to the hospital stay. If after leaving the SNF, the older adult re-enters the same or another SNF within 30 days, another 3-day qualifying hospital stay is not required to get additional SNF benefits. This is also true if the patient stops getting skilled care while in the SNF and then starts receiving skilled care again within 30 days.
3. The patient's doctor has decided and ordered daily skilled care. It must be given by, or under the direct supervision of, skilled nursing or rehabilitation staff. If the older adult is in the SNF for skilled rehabilitation services only, the care is considered daily care even if these therapy services are offered just 5 or 6 days a week.
4. The facility in which these skilled services are received has been certified by Medicare.
5. The older adults needs these skilled services for a medical condition that was treated during a qualifying 3-day hospital stay or started while receiving Medicare-covered SNF care. An example would be if a patient is in the SNF because she had a stroke, and she develops an infection that requires IV antibiotics.

Medicaid is a state and federal government program that pays for certain health services and NH care for older and disabled people with low incomes and limited assets. In most states, Medicaid also pays for some long-term care services at home and in the community. Who is eligible and what services are covered and available vary from state to state and even within states. Most often, eligibility is based on income and personal resources (assets like a home).[7] Unlike under Medicare, the recipient of Medicaid-paid LTC is not required to have skilled nursing needs, and benefits continue for as long as the recipient has care needs and limited financial resources. The value of assets that determines a person's eligibility for Medicaid benefits is determined by each state and varies widely. Generally, the private pay rates for nursing homes far exceed the Medicaid rates in a given community. Thus, NHs budget for a certain mix of private pay and Medicaid reimbursements to meet their financial goals. With population aging, the portion of each state's budget that funds Medicaid LTC is growing rapidly. It is not uncommon in many states that > 50% of the Medicaid budget is consumed by long-term care expenses.

Determining which LTC setting is best for any individual can be daunting. The most appropriate setting will depend on personal and caregiver preferences and characteristics, availability of family or other caregivers, community resources, financial resources, service needs, prognosis, health status, and other factors. What works in one community for one individual will not necessarily work elsewhere or for another. Often decisions about LTC are made following an acute hospital stay or rehabilitative NH stay; both hospitals and NHs have social workers or discharge planners who help patients and families determine the best discharge or LTC plan for them. Many communities have local, regional, or state LTC offices or elderly assistance programs that can help identify the best options. Home care agencies have social workers on staff as well.

In addition to nursing and rehabilitative services, medical services are also usually provided in NHs. These services are rendered by attending physicians, consulting physicians, nurse practitioners, physician assistants, and clinical nurse specialists under the guidance and supervision of a medical director. The medical director is responsible for overseeing the quality improvement program, employee health program, and insuring the overall quality of medical care each resident receives. Most NHs have an "open" medical staff model in which any community medical providers who wish to care for residents may do so. There is a substantial trend toward specialization in NH care, and some NHs are developing a "closed" staff model wherein only a few well-qualified and credentialed providers care for the residents. The open model allows for continuity of care between the NH, hospital, and community, while the closed model favors specialized care.[6,8-11]

LTC facilities vary in the types of services that they provide. Some smaller NHs only provide assistance with ADLs and basic nursing and medical management equivalent to custodial care. Most offer at least basic rehabilitative services. The majority of NHs provide basic podiatric, dental, optometric, diagnostic, hospice, and psychiatric services.[3] Other, usually larger, NHs may offer a variety of services and specialty care approaching nearly a hospital level. Advanced services sometimes offered include specialized dementia care, neurobehavioral care, ventilator and assisted ventilation care, advanced wound care, brain injury rehabilitation, respiratory rehabilitation, cardiac rehabilitation, intravenous fluids, intravenous antibiotics, other intravenous therapies, dialysis, bariatric care, and acute hospice care. Services may vary based on local regulations and reimbursement as well as type of practice.

CASE PRESENTATION: NURSING HOME ADMISSION

Mrs. S. is an 87-year-old woman who is being admitted to an LTC facility today from her home. Her son and daughter-in-law have come from out of town to help her move. Mrs. S. has late-stage Alzheimer-type dementia. Her most recent Mini-Mental Status Exam score was 8/30; she exhibits word-finding difficulties, and speaks only in partial sentences. She also has osteoarthritis with joint disease affecting her ability to ambulate, essential hypertension, hyperlipidemia, and urinary incontinence with occasional fecal incontinence. Her husband had been her primary caregiver in a local independent senior living community. He passed away suddenly 4 weeks ago from a myocardial infarction.

Initially, the family tried to keep the patient in her own home with additional services including formal and informal caregivers and a personal emergency response system. Despite these services, Mrs. S. continued to decline, experiencing confusion, falls, weight loss, and more frequent episodes of incontinence. Her family became increasingly worried by their mother's decline and weary from responding many times in the day and night to the alerts triggered from her emergency response bracelet. After being turned down by several ALFs, they reluctantly decided upon NH placement for Mrs. S. with the guidance of the local office for the aging.

Besides assistance for incontinence care, Mrs. S. requires supervision for wandering and dispensing of medications. She needs assistance with bathing. She requires "cueing" (verbal direction) for dressing, and needs hands-on assistance with laces, zippers, and buttons. She requires meal preparation and set-up, but feeds herself with cueing. She is independent with transfers and ambulation, but has had falls, so far without injury.

Mrs. S. does not have LTC insurance, but she has a modest pension from her husband. Her savings consist of the remaining proceeds from the prior sale of their home and her husband's life insurance policy. Mrs. S. is fortunate to have sufficient funds to pay for at least 2 years of NH care before she will need to apply for Medicaid.

According to the 2004 National Nursing Home Survey, there were 1.5 million NH residents in 16,100 facilities.[3] This means about one in 200 Americans lives in a NH.[3,12] There will be around 3 million NH residents by 2050.[13] Approximately half of persons admitted for LTC at a skilled nursing facility have dementia.[14] About 60% of NHs are for-profit, private institutions. More than 45% of NH residents are over age 85 years, 85% are white, and women outnumber men five to two. About half of residents are admitted from a hospital or other health care facility. Prior to being admitted to NHs, about a third of all residents have had at least one reported fall in the previous 6 months, and one-third of new residents have bowel and/or bladder incontinence.[3]

Many individual and caregiver characteristics factor into whether a person becomes a long-term care resident. The biggest predictors are: impairment in ADLs (particularly three or more); cognitive dysfunction; and prior NH use.[15-17] Caucasians are more likely to use NHs than African Americans or Hispanics, and it is uncertain whether this is due to socioeconomic or cultural differences.[15,16] Losses of social supports or caregiver stresses are also predictors of NH placement for individuals with dementia.[15-20] Fewer than 2% of NH residents have no ADL impairment; more than 50% are impaired in all ADLs.[3]

CASE PRESENTATION (continued)

Mrs. S. had an advance directive filled out 8 years ago, when she was first diagnosed with dementia, indicating that her husband was her primary health care agent, and her daughter, who died 5 years ago from breast cancer, as her alternate agent. A durable power of attorney had also been completed naming her husband and son. No other directives were noted; these documents had been received at admission and placed in the chart.

Sixty-five percent of patients in NHs have some form of an advance directive.[3] Unfortunately, these directives are often not specific about wishes, incomplete, or not up to date, such as in this case. About 20% of Americans die in an NH, and this number is rising.[21,22] In fact, the pattern of increasing deaths in institutions is being seen worldwide.[22-24] Having an advance directive, understanding residents' preferences with regard to life-sustaining treatments, and improving the end-of-life experience are increasingly important for the quality of NH care.[25-28] All patients, including those living in NHs, have a right to express their advance directives and to expect that the directives will be followed.

The Patient Self-Determination Act (PSDA) of 1991 required that patients of health care institutions reimbursed by Medicare or Medicaid be informed of their rights to participate in medical decisions and to use advance care plans.[29]

CASE PRESENTATION (continued)

Eight weeks after her admission, Mrs. S.'s roommate was diagnosed with influenza A. Mrs. S. had not received the influenza vaccine in the community because her husband's death coincided with the time her primary care provider was administering the vaccine. The staff vaccination rate in her facility was about 50%. Her aide, who had a child at home with influenza, was not vaccinated due to fear of needles. The aide came to work with "a cold" because she had used all of her sick time, and could not afford to lose any salary. Mrs. S. and her roommate were restricted to their room and placed on droplet precautions.

Influenza vaccination for patients and staff of LTC facilities significantly reduces morbidity and mortality for patients.[30-32] Barriers to vaccination and preventing sick staff from coming to work, as illustrated in this case, can be daunting.[33-35] Hand washing and adherence to isolation precautions are essential but challenging in all health care facilities.[36,37] Prophylaxis with antiviral agents is costly, less effective in frail older patients, and not without side effects, such as delirium, nausea, and dizziness.[37]

CASE PRESENTATION (continued)

Mrs. S. was started on influenza prophylaxis with amantadine 100 mg by mouth daily; the dose was reduced due to her age, frailty, and renal dysfunction. Mrs. S. experienced dizziness, orthostasis, anorexia, and hallucinations 2 days after she began taking the amantadine. A nurse practitioner from her primary care doctor's office evaluated her on the fourth day and ordered a complete blood count, urinalysis, and electrolyte profile. The staff was also instructed to encourage fluid intake.

Our patient suffered some of the common side effects of antiviral treatment. While the workup ordered was reasonable, the abrupt change in the patient's condition after the introduction of amantadine should have prompted consideration of stopping the antiviral medication. She is at significant risk of falling and becoming dehydrated, which now represents the greatest risk to her continued well-being. It is also important to take renal function into account, as renal function declines predictably with age, when deciding upon an appropriate dose of the influenza antiviral agents.[37-39]

CASE PRESENTATION (continued)

A complete blood count showed a normal white cell count with slight excess in lymphocytes and slightly decreased red cell count. Urine was dark and concentrated; the urinalysis demonstrated leukocytes, epithelial cells, and bacteria. Electrolyte profile had moderately elevated blood urea nitrogen and minimally elevated creatinine. Mrs. S. did not have fevers, rigors, diaphoresis, dysuria, change in frequency or incontinence, or any flulike symptoms. She was still confused, weak, anorectic, falling, and not taking much fluid.

Staff was again instructed to push fluids, and levofloxacin 250 mg per day by mouth was started for presumed urinary tract infection. At 2:00 AM on the sixth day after starting influenza prophylaxis with amantadine, the resident was found to be more confused with decreased level of consciousness at the side of her bed. Her vital signs at the time demonstrated a low blood pressure, tachycardia, and a normal temperature. The doctor was called and she was sent to the emergency department for evaluation.

The most likely cause of this patient's decline remains medication-induced delirium and dehydration. Both amantadine and fluoroquinolones are associated with confusion in the elderly.[38-40] Frail institutionalized elders have an extremely high prevalence of asymptomatic bacteriuria and pyuria. Several studies have demonstrated that treating asymptomatic urinary tract infections is of no benefit in this population, and there may be harm in overtreating, as occurred for our patient. When making the decision to obtain a urinalysis and/or culture, one must keep in mind that there is a high likelihood that a positive urine culture may not reveal the cause of a sudden decline or fever in a patient living in an NH.[41-43] When residents with dementia develop agitation or delirium, it is common for staff to send a urine sample for analysis and culture, which often is positive for the growth of bacteria. Patients will often be treated with antibiotics in this situation, because nurses and clinicians relate the positive urine culture to the behavior being exhibited by the patient. While this may sometimes be correct, often the agitation represents a worsening of the underlying illness, or a need to adjust the environment of care for the patient, or how caregivers are approaching the patient. Concentrating just on the treatment of a "urinary tract infection" and not the environment of care will lead to suboptimal care. Another problem with frequent antibiotic use in NHs is the propensity of organisms to develop antibiotic resistance that has become a serious problem in the United States with the emergence of some bacteria that are resistant to all antibiotics.[41,42]

Adequately hydrating patients in the NH can be time consuming and difficult to track. Most NHs are not equipped to deliver intravenous fluids; however, hypodermoclysis, the subcutaneous infusion of fluids, may represent an alternative way to provide hydration without sending the patient to the hospital.[44,45] Another consideration in our patient, given her advanced dementia, would be to meet with the family and consider directing therapies toward comfort and symptom control, and not necessarily toward life-prolonging measures. Given the time of night, the patient's signs and symptoms, and the lack of a clear advance directive limiting hospital transfers, management in an acute setting became the most likely option.

CASE PRESENTATION (continued)

Mrs. S. was admitted to the hospital for acute mental status changes, dehydration, and urinary infection. In the rush to send her to the hospital, the facility neglected to call her son. The emergency department attempted to call the expired husband and daughter, both of whom were listed on the advance directive sent from the NH, and thus had no immediate knowledge of the patient's wishes or preferences.

Mrs. S. was given intravenous fluids; amantadine was discontinued, and oseltamivir was started. Urine culture from the NH was now complete and showed contamination with mixed bacterial flora, so antibiotics were discontinued. Mrs. S.'s only neurologic findings were confusion with lethargy. Despite the lack of focal neurologic findings or evidence of head trauma, a CT scan of the brain was ordered to rule out "intracranial pathology."

While waiting for the scan, Mrs. S. almost fell off the gurney due to confusion, but an aide bringing another patient to the waiting area saw her trying to get up and was able to redirect her. Ultimately, the scan was done and showed generalized loss of volume, prominent sulci, and white matter changes without any acute disease.

Initially, Mrs. S. failed a swallowing evaluation and was not allowed to have anything other than medications by mouth. The speech pathologist wrote a comment about considering alternate forms of nutrition either temporarily or perhaps indefinitely. After 3 days, she was nearly back to baseline and was able to take oral nutrition with assistance and returned to the nursing facility.

Unfortunately, this downward spiraling of events is not uncommon, and highlights several areas that merit discussion. First, the hospital poses inherent hazards to these patients, such as increasing falls risk, resistant infections, exacerbation of delirium, and other iatrogenic, avoidable insults.[46,47] Second, transferring a patient to another facility

often results in the loss of important information—in this case, family contacts—that can result in patient harm.[48] Lastly, feeding problems occur in a majority of patients with advanced dementia, and often herald a patient who is entering the final weeks to months of life. The greatest use of feeding tubes in the United States occurs in patients with advanced dementia. Feeding tubes have not been shown to decrease aspiration, prolong life, or improve comfort in patients with advanced dementia. There is also a growing concern that the use of feeding tubes in LTC settings may represent a more inexpensive way to feed patients than careful hand feeding.[49-54]

CASE PRESENTATION (continued)

Three days after returning to the NH, Mrs. S. developed copious, foul-smelling, watery diarrhea. A stool sample was positive for *Clostridium difficile* toxin. She was started on metronidazole 250 mg every 6 hours by mouth and moved to a private room. After 2 days, she would not take any food, and staff was having trouble getting Mrs. S. to take fluids and medications, including the metronidazole. She was weak and exhibited mild agitation. Her primary care doctor evaluated her and thought the anorexia was due to metronidazole-induced nausea; she was switched to vancomycin 125 mg every 6 hours by mouth to complete a 14-day course. Clinically, she developed signs and symptoms of recurrent dehydration and acute renal insufficiency; however, with careful hand feeding and hypodermoclysis, the staff was able to avoid sending her back to the hospital for hydration. The diarrhea resolved and her appetite improved.

Quinolone antibiotics have recently been associated with a higher incidence of virulent *Clostridium difficile* colitis.[55] Antibiotic use in the NH should be deliberate and thoughtful in order to avoid complications of antibiotic use like this.[55-58] Because of emerging metronidazole resistance, increasing *C. difficile* virulence, and metronidazole toxicity in the frail elderly, oral vancomycin should be considered for first-line therapy in select NH patients.[59,60] For mild cases, metronidazole and vancomycin are equally effective, but metronidazole is much less costly.[61] Hand washing remains one of the most important measures to prevent the transmission of *C. difficile* as well as other resistant infections. Thorough cleaning of the room is also important to eliminate the *C. difficile* spores.[57,62,63] Some facilities use ultraviolet light treatments, which are toxic to the spores of the bacterium (unpublished data). Contact precautions may be important to minimize spread, but can be associated with negative outcomes as a result of isolation and decreased care.[64,65]

CASE PRESENTATION (continued)

Mrs. S. lost 15 lbs (6.8 kg) or more than 10% of her body weight during her first 3 months at the NH. She was seen by the nutritionist and given liquid supplements between meals and during medication administration. Her son and daughter-in-law came for a visit and were upset that Mrs. S. seemed so frail since she had moved into the NH. The son was also angry that he was not called when Mrs. S. was admitted to the hospital the previous month.

The nurse practitioner, social worker, and nurse manager met with the family and reviewed the patient's clinical issues and stated that further functional decline was inevitable as her dementia progressed. The team particularly addressed the fact that when patients with dementia develop infections and eating problems, it reflects a worsening of the illness and portends a very poor prognosis.

A recent study confirms that when patients with advanced dementia develop febrile episodes, pneumonia, or problems eating, they have a 60% to 70% chance of dying in the next year. These findings are illustrated in Figures 25–1 and 25–2.[49]

The same study noted that in the final months of life, symptoms such as pain, agitation, and coughing from aspiration are common and expected events. Preparing families for these likely events ahead of time can be very useful in helping to develop and carry out effective and compassionate goals of care.[49]

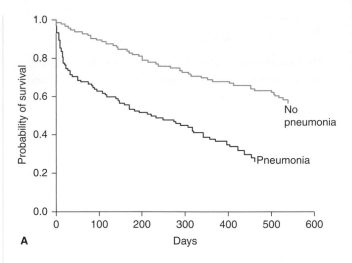

A

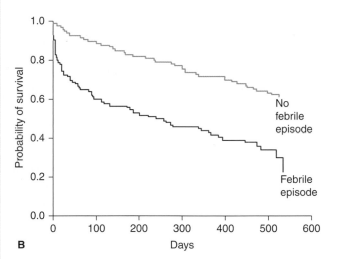

B

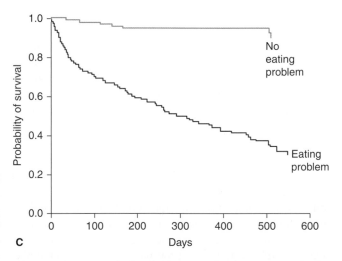

C

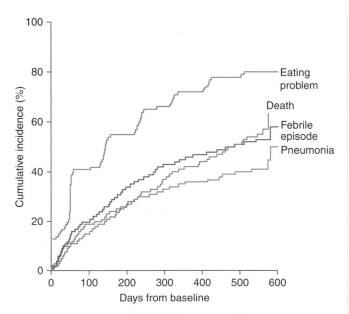

FIGURE 25–1. Overall mortality and cumulative incidences of pneumonia, febrile episodes, and eating problems among nursing home residents with advanced dementia. Overall mortality for the nursing home residents during the 18-month course of the study is shown. The residents' median age was 86 years, and the median duration of dementia was 6 years; 85.4% of residents were women.

FIGURE 25–2. Survival after the first episode of pneumonia, the first febrile episode, and the development of an eating problem. Panel A shows the results of the survival analysis for pneumonia, Panel B the results for a febrile episode, and Panel C the results for an eating problem. The red line in each panel shows survival after development of these complications. The blue line in each panel shows the estimated survival before the complication developed or in its absence (for residents in whom the complication never developed). All curves are presented in median age (85 years), median duration of dementia (6 years), and distribution according to sex (85.4% women).

The increasing use of nurse practitioners, physician assistants, and advanced practice nurses has been shown to improve the quality of care in NHs and the satisfaction of patients and their families. On-site providers also decrease hospitalizations for NH residents.[66-68] Facilitating communication between the care team, the LTC resident, and the family is important for resident and family satisfaction and insuring that residents' preferences are elicited and honored.[25,69,70] Having a clear understanding about the natural history of dementia and its terminal nature is important in guiding patients and families through choices.[49] Explaining to residents and caregivers the clear burdens and unclear benefits of artificial feeding and hydration can prevent the use of burdensome and often ineffective therapies.[51,52,54]

Advance directive discussions should include both values as well as preferences for specific therapies, such as resuscitation and artificial feeding and hydration. Physician Orders for Life Sustaining Treatments (POLST) forms are an actionable way to document a resident's preferences for specific therapies and can be useful initiating a meaningful conversation about goals and prognosis.[71] POLST was initiated in Oregon and has since been adopted in an increasing number of states. POLST allows physician-specific orders about resuscitation, ventilation, artificial feeding and hydration, antibiotics use, and other specific therapies to be issued.

Acute renal failure and chronic renal insufficiency are common in the NH. A recent study demonstrated that most NH patients who accept a trial of dialysis die within 1 year and have a significant decline in functional status.[72] For these very frail residents, dialysis may not be better than best medical management.[73] Given the increasing use of dialysis by residents of NHs, it may be appropriate to include preferences about dialysis with other advance directive discussions.

Swallowing difficulties are common in the NH and are often a sign that a patient is failing. Feeding via a gastrostomy tube is invasive and is not necessarily better than careful hand feeding, which is often the preferred way to try to maintain nutrition for a frail resident.[52-54] Pressure ulcers are a common complication for residents who are failing, and are also considered a major quality indicator for NHs. Skin is best maintained by reducing pressure, maintaining nutrition, and keeping the skin clean and dry where possible.[74-76] Unfortunately, not every pressure ulcer is avoidable in patients who are dying.

It is important to note that it is not unusual that part of the success in caring for Mrs. S. was due to her relationship with her nursing aide. Nurses and nursing aides or assistants provide almost all of the direct care to NH residents. The nursing staff is organized and managed by a nursing director. It cannot be overstated how important the quality and attention of the nursing staff is to each resident.[77]

respiratory distress with respiratory rate up 30 breaths per minute, hypoxia with oxygen saturation initially of 75% on room air, visible anxiousness, tachycardia to 110 beats per minute, and increased confusion. She responded to oxygen, gentle oral pharyngeal suctioning, mouth care, an albuterol nebulizer treatment, and 5 mg of morphine concentrate sublingually; she became much more comfortable. The nurse practitioner and family met and decided to continue a conservative care plan with best management at the NH. The attending physician, who had spoken with the nurse practitioner prior to the family meeting, also agreed.

It is possible to successfully manage an aspiration event in the NH by acting quickly. The main goal for this patient is to keep her comfortable. Opioids act on brainstem receptors to alleviate dyspnea. Opioid concentrates are absorbed through the oral mucosa, are low volume, relatively rapid acting, and are very useful to alleviate dyspnea in situations like this. Clearing secretions and oral contents with mouth care and gentle suctioning can help. Respiratory treatments may also be helpful.[78,79]

CASE PRESENTATION (continued)

Mrs. S. was sleepy but comfortable with no oral intake for the rest of the day, but was much better the next day. She continued to have an aspirating event once or twice per week that was handled similarly, and each time appeared comfortable after receiving morphine. She continued to lose weight, and her albumin dropped to 2.6 mg/dL (26 g/L). The primary care doctor reviewed the patient's condition, prognosis, and preferences with the son at the next follow-up. They agreed that comfort remained the main goal, and decided to continue the present plan of care, and not order any further diagnostic tests. Hospice care at the NH was offered and accepted.

Although more than one in five Americans die in an NH and 25% of Americans die under the care of hospice, many fewer NH residents receive hospice services at the time of their death. At least 76% of American NHs have a contract with a hospice and could provide hospice services.[25,80]

CASE PRESENTATION (continued)

The hospice nurse evaluated the resident the next day and spoke with the nursing staff and then met with the family. The hospice plan of care was reviewed and coordinated with the NH staff and primary care doctor. Everyone agreed that the focus of Mrs. S.'s care would be quality of life and symptom management. It was assumed that she would eventually develop a serious infection as part of the syndrome of adult failure to thrive and end-stage dementia with cerebral vascular disease and dysphagia. No antibiotics or artificial fluids would be used, and she would not be transferred to the hospital unless it was necessary for her to be comfortable. No lab tests or studies would be ordered if not needed to evaluate her comfort. In addition to concentrated liquid morphine for respiratory distress or pain, low-dose liquid concentrated haloperidol as needed for distressing delirium or nausea, and lorazepam as needed for anxiety or insomnia were prescribed. Senna was prescribed to prevent opioid- and dehydration-induced constipation, as well as bisacodyl suppositories or tap-water enemas as needed.

As an antipsychotic, low-dose haloperidol has frequently been used for delirium. While haloperidol has not been proven to be useful for nausea and vomiting in palliative care patients, there are many case reports, and there is good evidence for effectiveness in non-palliative care patients. The anti-emetic effect is thought to be through antagonizing dopamine receptors. Haloperidol is inexpensive and readily available in several forms.[81,82] Constipation is a serious side effect of opioids and is not relieved by tolerance. Constipation is an important cause of nausea, vomiting, and anorexia for many nursing patients, and should be aggressively managed.[83,84]

CASE PRESENTATION (continued)

After 4 more weeks of steady decline, Mrs. S. developed dyspnea, fever, diaphoresis, and hypoactive delirium. She was kept comfortable with the medications, low-flow oxygen, and cool compresses. Her son and daughter-in-law arrived and the hospice nurse visited to support them and the NH staff. She remained sleepy and unresponsive, and died comfortably the next morning.

The family received ongoing bereavement support from the hospice chaplain, social worker, and nurse over the next year. The aide who had become close to the patient also received support. The director of nursing asked the hospice agency to provide a bereavement in-service for the facility, and that was arranged. A follow-up satisfaction survey from both the NH and hospice indicated that the son and daughter-in-law were quite pleased with Mrs. S.'s end-of-life and NH care. Her total time at the NH was about 9 months.

• INNOVATIONS IN LONG-TERM CARE

LTC has changed considerably in the last decade, and will likely continue to as our population ages. As ALFs develop more capabilities to care for frail, medically complex persons, patients entering LTC will have more complicated medical issues, more advanced dementia, and will likely require more medical and nursing interventions. Skilled nursing rehabilitation is also likely to become more important as a way of maximizing patients' function, allowing them to return to the community. The goals of care in these patients will be different from those residents who will live at the facility for the remainder of their lives.

While there is a trend toward more medicalization of LTC, there are several programs emphasizing an environment that optimizes residents' independence and quality of life through culture change and facility adaptations to create a more home-like atmosphere. Programs like the Eden Alternative and the Pioneer Movement have had a worldwide impact, improving the lives of people living in LTC facilities.[85,86] The vision statement of the Pioneer Movement is to create "a culture of aging that is life-affirming, satisfying, humane, and meaningful."[86] Other programs, like the Program of All-inclusive Care for the Elderly (PACE), utilize adult day centers to provide cost-effective medical care and socialization for frail older persons who wish to remain living in the community.[87]

CONCLUSION

The cost of LTC in the United States is considerable. In 2005, $206.6 billion was spent on LTC in the United States, with 70% coming from Medicare and Medicaid.[88] This does not include care provided by informal caregivers in the community, such as family and friends. These costs also do not include lost productivity or opportunity costs. For every person residing in an NH, there are five equally frail persons living in the community. The lifetime risk of using NH care is at least 46% and rising dramatically.[88] There is an imperative that we develop environments of care that emphasize quality of life and are cost-effective for our vulnerable elders.

Once most individuals need LTC, priorities often center around quality time with family and friends, not suffering, autonomy, and not being a burden on their families. Length of life is rarely the main concern, and this is especially true if the LTC resident is not meeting any of these four core goals. It is therefore critical that medical assessments and interventions center on the LTC patient's goals and that the benefits of any care appropriately outweigh the burdens. As this perspective is not universal, it is important to individually assess patient values and goals and to document them in the medical record.

NH care is complicated and challenges medical staff, so individuals providing care in LTC settings should be vested and develop proficiency in caring for these patients. Providers need to see a sufficient number of LTC patients to obtain and maintain sufficient skills. Regulatory issues and payment issues add to the complexity of caring in these environments.

It is likely that future models of care will hold providers responsible for the quality and costs of caring for patients across the spectrum of care settings. This will decrease the financial incentives of nursing homes to send patients to the hospital, where Medicare pays for costs incurred there. Large, integrated delivery systems are likely to include hospitals, nursing homes, visiting nurse services, and specialty and primary care physicians, who will be paid a set amount of money to care for a population of patients in the community. In such systems, the financial incentives will be in place to keep people living in the least restrictive environments, hopefully resulting in improved quality, satisfaction, and value. These systems are highly dependent on integrated and coordinated interdisciplinary care. The tremendous costs of LTC in an aging population and proportionately declining workforce will be one of the greatest challenges of the next century.

References

1. National Clearinghouse for Long Term Care. 2008. Available from: http://www.longtermcare.gov/. Accessed March 7, 2010.
2. Understanding LTC Basics. 2008. Available from: http://www.longtermcare.gov/LTC/Main_Site/Understanding_Long_Term_Care/Basics/Basics.aspx. Accessed March 7, 2010.
3. Jones AL, Dwyer LL, Bercovitz AR, Strahan GW. The National Nursing Home Survey: 2004 overview. Vital Health Stat. 2009;13:1-155.
4. Long term care definition. A Website for Utah Caregivers. 2008. Available from: http://ucare.utah.gov/what_is_ltc.html. Accessed March 7, 2010.
5. What Does Long-Term Care Cost in Your State? 2009. Available from: http://www.aarp.org/families/caregiving/state_ltc_costs.html. Accessed March 15, 2010.
6. Medicare.gov. Your Medicare Coverage. 2009. Available from: http://www.medicare.gov/coverage/Home.asp. Accessed March 7, 2010.
7. Medicare.gov. Long-Term Care. 2009. Available from: http://www.medicare.gov/longTermCare/static/home.asp. Accessed March 15, 2010.
8. Katz PR, Karuza J, Intrator O, Mor V. Nursing home physician specialists: A response to the workforce crisis in long-term care. Ann Intern Med. 2009;150:411-413.
9. Stall R. The physician's role in long-term care culture change. J Am Med Dir Assoc. 2009;10:587-588.
10. Jacob D. Roles and responsibilities of attending physicians in skilled nursing facilities. J Am Med Dir Assoc. 2003;4:231-243.
11. AMDA. About AMDA: Medical Director Roles and Responsibilities. 2006. Available from: http://www.amda.com/about/roles.cfm. Accessed March 7, 2010.
12. US Census Bureau. Annual Estimates of the Resident Population for the United States, Regions, States, and Puerto Rico: April 1, 2000 to July 1, 2008 (NST-EST2008-01). Washington, DC: USCB Population Division; 2008.
13. The future supply of long-term care workers in relation to the aging baby boom generation. Report to Congress, 2003.

14. Magaziner J, German P, Zimmerman SI, et al. The prevalence of dementia in a statewide sample of new nursing home admissions aged 65 and older: Diagnosis by expert panel. Epidemiology of Dementia in Nursing Homes Research Group. *Gerontologist.* 2000; 40:663-672.

15. Gaugler JE, Duval S, Anderson K, Kane R. Predicting nursing home admission in the U.S.: A meta-analysis. *BMC Geriatr.* 2007;7:13.

16. Yaffe K, Fox P, Newcomer R, et al. Patient and caregiver characteristics and nursing home placement in patients with dementia. *JAMA.* 2002;287:2090-2097.

17. Hatoum HT, Thomas SK, Lin SJ, et al. Predicting time to nursing home placement based on activities of daily living scores: A modelling analysis using data on Alzheimer's disease patients receiving rivastigmine or donepezil. *J Med Econ.* 2009;12:98-103.

18. Gaugler JE, Yu F, Krichbaum K, Wyman J. Predictors of nursing home admission for persons with dementia. *Med Care.* 2009;47:191-198.

19. Buhr GT, Kuchibhatla M, Clipp EC. Caregivers' reasons for nursing home placement: Clues for improving discussions with families prior to the transition. *Gerontologist.* 2006;46:52-61.

20. Banaszak-Holl J, Fendrick M, Foster N, et al. Predicting nursing home admission: Estimates from a 7-year follow-up of a nationally representative sample of older Americans. *Alzheimer Dis Assoc Disord.* 2004;18:83-89.

21. Flory J, Young-Xu Y, Gurol I, et al. Place of death: U.S. trends since 1980. *Health Aff* (Millwood). 2004;23:194-200.

22. Gruneir A, Mor V, Weitzen S, et al. Where people die: A multilevel approach to understanding influences on site of death in America. *Med Care Res Rev.* 2007;64:351-378.

23. Gomes B, Higginson IJ. Where people die (1974-2030): Past trends, future projections and implications for care. *Palliat Med.* 2008; 22:33-41.

24. Ahmad S, O'Mahony MS. Where older people die: A retrospective population-based study. *QJM.* 2005;98:865-870.

25. Levy C, Morris M, Kramer A. Improving end-of-life outcomes in nursing homes by targeting residents at high-risk of mortality for palliative care: Program description and evaluation. *J Palliat Med.* 2008;11:217-225.

26. Flacker JM, Kiely DK. Mortality-related factors and 1-year survival in nursing home residents. *J Am Geriatr Soc.* 2003;51:213-221.

27. Goldberg TH, Botero A. Causes of death in elderly nursing home residents. *J Am Med Dir Assoc.* 2008;9:565-677.

28. Levy CR, Fish R, Kramer A. Do-not-resuscitate and do-not-hospitalize directives of persons admitted to skilled nursing facilities under the Medicare benefit. *J Am Geriatr Soc.* 2005;53: 2060-2068.

29. Castle NG, Mor V. Advance care planning in nursing homes: Pre- and Post-Patient Self-Determination Act. *Health Serv Res.* 1998;33:101-124.

30. Lemaitre M, Meret T, Rothan-Tondeur M, et al. Effect of influenza vaccination of nursing home staff on mortality of residents: A cluster-randomized trial. *J Am Geriatr Soc.* 2009;57:1580-1586.

31. Hayward AC, Harling R, Wetten S, et al. Effectiveness of an influenza vaccine programme for care home staff to prevent death, morbidity, and health service use among residents: Cluster randomised controlled trial. *BMJ.* 2006;333:1241.

32. Shugarman LR, Hales C, Setodji CM, et al. The influence of staff and resident immunization rates on influenza-like illness outbreaks in nursing homes. *J Am Med Dir Assoc.* 2006;7:562-567.

33. Gavazzi G. Influenza vaccination for healthcare workers: From a simple concept to a resistant issue? *Aging Clin Exp Res.* 2009;21:216-221.

34. Nace DA, Horrman E, Resnick N, Handler S. Achieving and sustaining high rates of influenza immunization among long-term care staff. *J Am Med Dir Assoc.* 2007;8:128-133.

35. Hutt E, Radcliff TA, Liebrecht D, et al. Associations among nurse and certified nursing assistant hours per resident per day and adherence to guidelines for treating nursing home-acquired pneumonia. *J Gerontol A Biol Sci Med Sci.* 2008;63:1105-1111.

36. Mitka M. Hand washing, a key anti-flu strategy, often neglected by health care workers. *JAMA.* 2009;302:1850-1851.

37. Mossad SB. Influenza in long-term care facilities: Preventable, detectable, treatable. *Cleve Clin J Med.* 2009;76:513-521.

38. Hota S, McGeer A. Antivirals and the control of influenza outbreaks. *Clin Infect Dis.* 2007;45:1362-1368.

39. Burch J, Paulden M, Conti S, et al. Antiviral drugs for the treatment of influenza: A systematic review and economic evaluation. *Health Technol Assess.* 2009;13:1-265, iii-iv.

40. Slobodin G, Elias N, Zaygraikin N, et al. Levofloxacin-induced delirium. *Neurol Sci.* 2009;30:159-161.

41. Juthani-Mehta M. Asymptomatic bacteriuria and urinary tract infection in older adults. *Clin Geriatr Med.* 2007;23:585-594, vii.

42. Nicolle LE. Asymptomatic bacteriuria: Review and discussion of the IDSA guidelines. *Int J Antimicrob Agents.* 2006;28(suppl): S42-S48.

43. Nicolle LE. Asymptomatic bacteriuria in the elderly. *Infect Dis Clin North Am.* 1997;11:647-662.

44. Turner T, Cassano AM. Subcutaneous dextrose for rehydration of elderly patients—An evidence-based review. *BMC Geriatr.* 2004;4:2.

45. Rochon PA, Gill S, Litner J, et al. A systematic review of the evidence for hypodermoclysis to treat dehydration in older people. *J Gerontol A Biol Sci Med Sci.* 1997;52:M169-M176.

46. Friedman SM, Mendelson D, Bingham K, McCann R. Hazards of hospitalization: Residence prior to admission predicts outcomes. *Gerontologist.* 2008;48:537-541.

47. Fernandez HM, Callahan K, Likourezos A, Leipzig R. House staff member awareness of older inpatients' risks for hazards of hospitalization. *Arch Intern Med.* 2008;168:390-396.

48. Cheng HY, Tonorezos E, Zorowitz R, et al. Inpatient care for nursing home patients: An opportunity to improve transitional care. *J Am Med Dir Assoc.* 2006;7:383-387.

49. Mitchell SL, Teno J, Kiely D, et al. The clinical course of advanced dementia. *N Engl J Med.* 2009;361:1529-1538.

50. Teno JM, Fenf Z, Mitchell S, et al. Do financial incentives of introducing case mix reimbursement increase feeding tube use in nursing home residents? *J Am Geriatr Soc.* 2008;56:887-890.

51. Lacey D. Tube feeding, antibiotics, and hospitalization of nursing home residents with end-stage dementia: Perceptions of key medical decision-makers. *Am J Alzheimers Dis Other Demen.* 2005;20: 211-219.

52. Tuya A, Teno J. Feeding tubes for nursing home residents with advanced dementia: How to approach feeding tube decisions. *Med Health RI.* 2008;91:33-34.

53. Finucane TE, Christmas C, Leff BA. Tube feeding in dementia: How incentives undermine health care quality and patient safety. *J Am Med Dir Assoc.* 2007;8:205-208.

54. Mitchell SL, Buchanan J, Littlehale S, Hamel M. Tube-feeding versus hand-feeding nursing home residents with advanced dementia: A cost comparison. *J Am Med Dir Assoc.* 2003;4:27-33.

55. Weiss K. Clostridium difficile and fluoroquinolones: Is there a link? *Int J Antimicrob Agents.* 2009;33(suppl):S29-S32.

56. Mills K, Nelson AC, Winslow BT, Springer KL. Treatment of nursing home-acquired pneumonia. *Am Fam Physician.* 2009;79:976-982.

57. Richards CL Jr. Infection control in long-term care facilities. *J Am Med Dir Assoc.* 2007;8(suppl): S18-S25.

58. Regal RE, Pham CQ, Bostwick TR. Urinary tract infections in extended care facilities: Preventive management strategies. *Consult Pharm.* 2006;21:400-409.

59. McFarland LV. Update on the changing epidemiology of *Clostridium difficile*-associated disease. *Nat Clin Pract Gastroenterol Hepatol.* 2008;5:40-48.

60. Makris AT, Gelone S. *Clostridium difficile* in the long-term care setting. *J Am Med Dir Assoc.* 2007;8:290-299.

61. Zar FA, Bakkanagari SR, Moorthi KM, Davis MB. A comparison of vancomycin and metronidazole for the treatment of *Clostridium difficile*-associated diarrhea, stratified by disease severity. *Clin Infect Dis.* 2007;45:302-307.

62. Malani PN. Infection control in long-term care facilities: The need for engagement. *J Am Geriatr Soc.* 2009;57:569-570.

63. Smith PW, Bennett G, Bradley S, et al. SHEA/APIC Guideline: Infection prevention and control in the long-term care facility. *Am J Infect Control.* 2008;36:504-535.

64. Morgan DJ, Diekema DJ, Sepkowitz K, Perencevich EN. Adverse outcomes associated with contact precautions: A review of the literature. *Am J Infect Control.* 2009; 37:85-93.

65. Kirkland KB, Weinstein JM. Adverse effects of contact isolation. *Lancet.* 1999;354:1177-1178.

66. McAiney CA, Haughton D, Jennings J, et al. A unique practice model for nurse practitioners in long-term care homes. *J Adv Nurs.* 2008;62:562-571.

67. Mezey M, Burger SG, Bloom HG, et al. Experts recommend strategies for strengthening the use of advanced practice nurses in nursing homes. *J Am Geriatr Soc.* 2005;53:1790-1797.

68. Intrator O, Fend Z, Mor V, et al. The employment of nurse practitioners and physician assistants in U.S. nursing homes. *Gerontologist.* 2005;45:486-495.

69. Rich SE, Gruber-Baldini A, Quinn C, Zimmerman S. Discussion as a factor in racial disparity in advance directive completion at nursing home admission. *J Am Geriatr Soc.* 2009;57:146-152.

70. Finucane T. Disparities in late-life planning and treatment. *J Am Geriatr Soc.* 2009;57:1320.

71. Meier DE, Beresford L. POLST offers next stage in honoring patient preferences. *J Palliat Med.* 2009;12:291-295.

72. Kurella Tamura M, Covinsky K, Chertow G, et al. Functional status of elderly adults before and after initiation of dialysis. *N Engl J Med.* 2009;361:1539-1547.

73. Carson RC, Juszczak M, Davenport A, Burns A. Is maximum conservative management an equivalent treatment option to dialysis for elderly patients with significant comorbid disease? *Clin J Am Soc Nephrol.* 2009;4: 1611-1619.

74. Vickery K. CMS issues pressure ulcer guidelines. *Provider.* 2005; 31:19-20.

75. Wipke-Tevis DD, Williams D, Rantz M, et al. Nursing home quality and pressure ulcer prevention and management practices. *J Am Geriatr Soc.* 2004; 52:583-588.

76. Baier RR, Gifford D, Lyder C, et al. Quality improvement for pressure ulcer care in the nursing home setting: The Northeast Pressure Ulcer Project. *J Am Med Dir Assoc.* 2003;4:291-301.

77. Temkin-Greener H, Zheng N, Cai S, et al. Nursing home environment and organizational performance: Association with deficiency citations. *Med Care.* 2010;48:357-364.

78. Waldrop DP, Kirkendall AM. Comfort measures: A qualitative study of nursing home-based end-of-life care. *J Palliat Med.* 2009;12:719-724.

79. Qaseem A, Snow V, Shekelle P, et al. Evidence-based interventions to improve the palliative care of pain, dyspnea, and depression at the end of life: A clinical practice guideline from the American College of Physicians. *Ann Intern Med.* 2008;148:141-146.

80. Han B, Tiggle RB, Remsburg RE. Characteristics of patients receiving hospice care at home versus in nursing homes: Results from the National Home and Hospice Care Survey and the National Nursing Home Survey. *Am J Hospice Palliat Med.* 2007;24:479-486.

81. Perkins P, Dorman S. Haloperidol for the treatment of nausea and vomiting in palliative care patients. *Cochrane Database Syst Rev.* 2009;2:CD006271.

82. Abernethy AP, Zhukovsky D. Palliative care pharmacotherapy literature summaries and analyses. *J Pain Palliat Care Pharmacother.* 2009;23:426-432.

83. Messinger-Rapport BJ, Thomas D, Gammack J, Morley J. Clinical update on nursing home medicine: 2009. *J Am Med Dir Assoc.* 2009;10:530-553.

84. Kapoor S. Management of constipation in the elderly: Emerging therapeutic strategies. *World J Gastroenterol.* 2008;14:5226-5227.

85. The Eden Alternative. Improving the lives of the Elders and their Care Partners. 2009. Available from: http://www.edenalt.org/. Accessed March 7, 2010.

86. Pioneer Network. Culture Change in Long-Term Care. 2010. Available from: www.pioneernetwork.net. Accessed March 7, 2010.

87. National PACE Association. Home. 2002. Available from: http://www.npaonline.org. Accessed March 7, 2010.

88. Spillman BC, Lubitz J. New estimates of lifetime nursing home use: Have patterns of use changed? *Med Care.* 2002; 40:965-975.

POST-TEST

1. **Asymptomatic bacteriuria (positive urine culture without any signs or symptoms of infection) in LTC patients:**

   A. Is always treated with broad-spectrum antibiotics to avoid developing sepsis

   B. Is common and does not require further follow-up or treatment

   C. Is a result of dehydration and will improve with oral fluids

   D. Is a major cause of delirium and treatment should be considered

2. **Sources of payment for custodial LTC services include all of the following EXCEPT:**

   A. LTC insurance

   B. Medicaid

   C. Medicare

   D. Self-pay (private pay)

3. **What percent of Americans will ultimately spend some time in a nursing home?**

   A. < 10%

   B. 10-20%

   C. 30%

   D. > 40%

ANSWERS TO PRE-TEST

1. B
2. A
3. C

ANSWERS TO POST-TEST

1. B
2. C
3. D

26

An Approach to Assessing and Ordering Physical Therapy

Jonathan W. Donley, PT, DPT, M Ed, ATC

● **LEARNING OBJECTIVES**

1. Describe the appropriate assistive device(s) based on the needs and ability of the patient.
2. Discuss strategies for overcoming resistance to using assistive devices.
3. Identify some of the more common assistive devices and explain their applications and limitations.

PRE-TEST

1. **Which assistive device is the best choice to prescribe for an individual living independently at home with some decreased standing balance, but who continues to be active in the outdoors and has not reported any falls in the last 3 months?**

   A. Straight or offset cane

   B. Quad cane

   C. Rolling walker

   D. Transport wheelchair

2. **Which of the following is NOT a concern for most seniors using an assistive device?**

   A. Becoming a target for crime

   B. Feeling assistive devices aren't a good way to prevent falls

   C. Appearing to be losing their independence

   D. Physical size of the device

3. **Which of the following is LEAST helpful when considering prescription of an assistive device?**

   A. Needs/goals of patient

   B. Previous level of functioning

   C. Ability to use device properly

   D. Time the patient will use the device

CASE PRESENTATION: PAIN AFFECTING FUNCTION

Mrs. Dolly is an 86-year-old Caucasian female seeking a consult for low back and leg pain. She reports her pain is chronic, spanning over the past 24 years, with increasing intensity over the past 6 months. She complains of intermittent periods of "shooting" pain down her right leg with a constant sensation of localized paresthesia over the anterolateral lower right leg and foot. Her past medical history includes osteoporosis, decreased 25 OH-D, osteoarthritis, mild spinal stenosis of the lumbar L2-4 region, presbycusis, and presbyopia. She is 5 feet (1.52 m) tall and weighs 91 lbs (41.3 kg). She reports her walking distances have decreased from once around the block (1/4 mile, 400 m) to staying within household distances because she fatigues quickly walking outside and has increasing pain with activity. Walking, especially downhill, standing for a prolonged time, or any activity requiring extension of her spine also increases her pain. Sitting or leaning forward will alleviate severity of symptoms.

Her previous levels of activity include attending church one to two times per week, grocery shopping while using a buggy for support, and eating weekly Sunday dinner with her daughter's family. She states she loved "delivering meals on wheels to the elderly." Her hobbies include being outside and working with her husband doing gardening activities, requiring the ability to walk on various uneven surfaces and bending down to plant and weed the flower beds. She has not participated in outside gardening since her back and leg pain has increased over the past 4 months.

She reports her legs are getting weaker, and because she tires quickly she is becoming more limited with her endurance. When inquiring about her use of ADs, she stated she intermittently uses a wooden cane that belonged to her father and a quad-base cane she uses "when I'm going outside because it helps keep my balance better and I can lean on it if I get tired or my back starts tightening up." She will only use the cane around the house and usually only if her pain is really severe, and will not take it to church or the grocery store.

Her social history includes three healthy children (now adults) and eight grandchildren, and she lives with her husband, Frank, in a two-story house. There are nine steps into the front entry of the home with no handrails. Her bedroom is on the main floor, as is the master bathroom. Her bathroom includes a standard-height toilet and tub/shower combination requiring an approximate 12-inch (30.5-cm)-high step into the tub to bathe. There are no grab bars installed. In the living room is a large wooden bench with a thin cushion where she has been sleeping for the past several weeks because she states, "this is the only place where I can get my back comfortable for sleeping."

● BACKGROUND

Mrs. Dolly is similar to other older persons who experience ranging levels of decline in functional ability due to increased levels of pain from multiple various pathologies.[1] There is a positive correlation between increasing age and increasing rate of assistive device (AD) usage.[2] In the United States and Scandinavia, at least 20% of the population over age 70, and approximately half the population by age 75, uses ADs.[3,4]

When choosing an AD to minimize or relieve symptoms or impairments, patients often self-select based on what they feel to be important, obtain information from many sources, or take advice from their friends who have similar experiences using ADs. They will sometimes seek prescriptions from physicians or allied health professionals for an AD, based on advertising, personal experience or their best guess.

An AD is defined as any product, instrument, strategy, service, and practice used by people with disabilities and older people, specially produced or generally available, to prevent compensate, relieve, or neutralize the impairment, disability, or handicap, and improve the individual's autonomy and quality of life.[5] The most commonly known ADs are observed in general use, such as canes and walkers. Canes are the most commonly used AD in the United States, with more than 4 million users (approximately 15% of all AD use), followed by walkers, used by more than 1.5 million.[3,6] However, thousands of different ADs are employed to enhance a person's ability to perform Activities of Daily Living (ADLs) and Instrumental Activities of Daily Living (IADLs).

CASE PRESENTATION (continued)

Primary Care Physician Consult

A consultation for physical therapy was requested by Mrs. Dolly's physician. Mrs. Dolly's goals were: (1) getting rid of her pain, (2) going back to her previous activity levels, and (3) remaining at home without having to depend on her husband. She is afraid her husband may injure himself if he assists her with mobility.

The primary care physician lists the following symptoms on the referral: (1) back pain with radiation increased with activity, (2) decreased mobility, and (3) increased risk for falling. The diagnoses underlying these symptoms are degenerative arthritis, spinal stenosis, and back pain with radiculopathy. During the physical therapy evaluation, Mrs. Dolly momentarily breaks down and cries at her frustration and states she feels her situation will not get better, and that the increased pain and her decreased physical abilities are starting to concern her about her risk of losing her independence. Together the physical therapist and Mrs. Dolly form a plan of care. The first steps are to prescribe conservative treatment of physical (physio)therapy for 4 weeks to decrease pain, strengthening exercises, and an AD prescription. Ms. Dolly is scheduled for a follow-up appointment with her regular doctor to reassess her condition in one month.

• USE OF ASSISTIVE DEVICES

One of the most common reasons to use an assistive device is for reduction of pain with movement. By reducing weight-bearing on one or both legs, ADs may alleviate or reduce pain.[7] Another common reason is to improve overall mobility and allow for increased respiratory and muscular endurance.[7,8]

Because mobility impairment is significantly associated with functional decline, ADs may improve the quality of the patient's life in a cost-effective way, promote mobility and independence by enabling the patient, reduce the risk or assistance from caregivers, and reduce risk factors associated with falling.[3,4,9-16] The use of ADs allows opportunities to enable, not disable, people. There are also psychosocial benefits of increased mobility by using ADs as older persons can maintain their occupational skills.[17]

CASE PRESENTATION (continued)

Physical (Physio)Therapy Assessment

Mrs. Dolly was consulted for low back pain with radiculopathy into her right leg. The therapist reviewed her medical record, with the recorded information being confirmed by Mrs. Dolly. Standardized tests were administered, including the Berg Balance Test, in which her balance was tested sitting, standing, and during transfers. Her results from the 14-item assessment totaled 41. Higher scores indicate better performance. Because Mrs. Dolly is at elevated risk for falling, it is determined that she would benefit from an AD to improve balance and decrease risk of falls. Scores < 45 indicate a greater risk of falls. The Berg Balance Test suggests the following actions for these scores:

Score	Action
> 50	Normal, no AD needed
47-49.6	Consider using a cane outdoors
44-46.5	Cane or a walker for both indoors and outdoors
26.7-39.6	Should use a walker at all times

Because Mrs. Dolly's score is between intervals, she may benefit at times from the walker to help reduce weight-bearing through her extremities and back, and at least a cane both indoors and outdoors.

Mrs. Dolly also performed a Timed Get-Up-and-Go screen. Her ability to quickly get out of an armchair and walk (3 meters) and return to the chair was 24 seconds (normal is less than 10 seconds). This screen also identifies her as being at increased risk for falling. Mrs. Dolly also performed a gait velocity test, where she walked a timed 10-meter distance, resulting in a gait speed of 0.5 m/sec. A score of less than 1 m/sec also indicates a risk for falling.[15,18] This test also served as a gait assessment, revealing decreased step length, decreased cadence, a narrow base of support with occasional scissoring of her legs, increased double leg stance time, and consistent watching of the floor during ambulation with a forward flexed trunk. During the test, Mrs. Dolly hit the marker cones and demonstrated difficulty when trying to identify obstacles. All of these tests were performed without the use of an AD.

Her neurologic assessment revealed 2+ patellar and Achilles reflexes bilaterally. She reported decreased sensation in her right leg over the L3-L5 dermatomes. Manual muscles testing demonstrated her strength was grossly 4/5 in her left and 3+/5 in her right lower extremities. She stated she was tired after the walking activities and her pain scores increased to 9/10 pain. After 10 minutes of resting seated in a chair, her pain decreased to 6/10. A Falls Efficacy Scale was administered, indicating she had a fear of falling as established by her score of 80. A score of greater than 70 indicates a fear of falling.[19]

Her social history and previous levels of functioning were documented, and inquiry into any assistive devices she owns or uses was made. She stated she had and sometimes uses a quad cane or wooden straight cane. The therapist asked her if she brought them with her, and she replied, "No, I don't always need them."

The therapist asked if she would consider using some other ADs, but Mrs. Dolly politely declined because she felt they were mostly used by disabled people; she stated, "Those just get me one step closer into the old-folks home. I don't want people to think I am weak or my children to start talking to me about how I may be too old to live in my home."

INDICATION TO USE ASSISTIVE DEVICES

This patient has several characteristics that would indicate assistive devices are warranted for use in ADLs. These include decreases in balance reflected in her Berg scores, vision impairment as evidenced by hitting the cones, sensation impairment of the lower extremities including the feet, gait disturbance, weakness, decreased endurance, needing assistance to perform ADLs, weight-bearing reduction of extremities, and the patient's increased fear of falling. Other indications for AD use not applicable to Mrs. Dolly include:

Acute trauma
Recent surgery
Need to protect vulnerable limbs
Neuropathy
Episodes of functional incontinence due to decreased mobility and transfers[1,7,9,20-22]

Mobility aids increase the patient's base of support and thereby allow greater range of center of mass movement to be tolerated with less stability.[23,24] One of the components of balance is vision. At least 15% of persons over the age of 65 have visual impairments.[1] There are associated risks of falling with decreased vision. ADs provide additional stability when encountering obstacles, including when the obstacles are unseen. Another factor indicating ADs use is the sensation of paresthesia. The inability to have confident sensory touch of one's foot may inhibit the ability of firm foot placement.

Prescription of ADs should also include consideration when evaluating strength and respiratory endurance. Decreased lower extremity strength, balance deficits, gait deficits, and cardiovascular diseases are well-documented risk factors for falling.[14] These may lead to lower extremity disabilities that are important predictors of functional loss in community-dwelling elderly.[9]

ADs can lead to physiologic benefits such as prevention of osteoporosis and cardiorespiratory deconditioning, as well as enhanced circulation by increased venous return, thereby decreasing risk of blood clots and improving renal function.[8] In addition to the physiologic benefits of using ADs, there is also a psychological benefit that may be underestimated by health care providers.

Rehabilitation and ADs may be used to address issues of depression in a population with loss of physical activity and perceived inability to be mobile.[10] In Sweden, the use of ADs led to reduction in perceived difficulties with daily activities by 42%.[11]

The timing of an AD prescription may have great impact on the patient's overall mobility. Use of an AD should begin when routine activities are being reduced or eliminated. When regular activities are becoming difficult for a patient to perform, assessment of the cause and nature of the activity modification should be performed immediately. There are associated morbidities with decreased mobility. Often, the first signs will include becoming sedentary. Resistance to getting out of bed or extended sleeping or frequent napping beyond a person's normal routine should be considered an alert. Other signs may include decreased personal hygiene with infrequent bathing and smell of body odor, which may be associated with fear of falling in the shower. One may also observe odors of urinary or fecal incontinence, due to physical inability to get to the bathroom because of arthritic pain, decreased strength, or decreased endurance.

CASE PRESENTATION (continued)

Assistive Device Consultation

After the initial physical therapy evaluation, the therapist and Mrs. Dolly reviewed the results and addressed some concerns. Together they created and wrote down Mrs. Dolly's therapeutic goals: to decrease her pain, to return to gardening, to dress herself without help or fear of falling, and to walk around her neighborhood with her husband.

The therapist and Mrs. Dolly then discussed the plan for strength training, balance training, gait training, and fall education/prevention. Both parties agreed until the therapist raised the topic of ADs, specifically the use of a rolling walker and cane. Mrs. Dolly resisted the suggestion that she use an AD. She repeated her intention of remaining independent and not wanting her family to think she was incapable of being mobile. She stated she thought walkers and canes probably could help, but really they were for people who were disabled. She also did not want to become a conspicuous target for criminals.

BARRIERS TO USING ASSISTIVE DEVICES

The patient's understanding and willingness to adopt ADs into daily routines are critical for compliance. The prescribing provider must work with the patient to identify goals, and base any prescription on the current situation and impairments. In conjunction with the patient's goals, providers will frequently find patients often have unrealistic expectations or need help to prioritize their goals, such as saying, "I'd like to walk" when the patient hasn't been ambulatory for 2 months and the therapist recognizes that the first goal might be to work on balance and then strength followed by transfers and finally ambulation.[1] Goals may include increasing function, decreasing impairments, and/or optimizing psychological components of adaptation: for example, increasing independent mobility, endurance, ambulation, transfer ability, strength, balance; decreasing pain and paresthesia; increasing socialization with friends and family; or decreasing fear of falling. Functional goals may include return to a baseline following some acute change, or improvement upon previous levels to achieve age-normative function. Some patients have adapted over time to their functional loss and do not consciously realize impairments exist.[1] Others may be unaware of physical impairments because of cognitive decline.

Prescription of ADs to patients with cognitive impairment should include several safety assessments. Training with the AD needs to be performed during every treatment, as repetition of proper use is important to prevent events such as falls. Generally, frail older persons with cognitive impairment use fewer and are less satisfied with ADs than frail elderly patients not cognitively impaired. Early intervention of device use is important for patients at risk for cognitive decline. Cognitive limitation is a more important predictor of AD non-use than dissatisfaction than with training and support.[25]

Overcoming barriers to successful AD use starts with acknowledgment of the patient's goals and concerns. In our case, Mrs. Dolly's goals and concerns were to be independent and safe. One technique to facilitate adoption of devices is to ask the patient to try a few devices in the health care setting. Two important factors in prescribing ADs are to give proper instructions and proper fitting. After patients have tried the device, ask them if they feel they can walk better, have better balance, or feel less likely to fall. Patients must perceive a need if an AD is to be tried and successfully used.[1] By allowing the patient to conclude that the device has benefits, acceptance of the device may be increased.

Mrs. Dolly's concerns can be addressed by explanation that ADs will increase her ability to master situations, especially evident with increased safety and reduction of effort in ADLs, implying a reduced handicap.[4] Using ADs can increase older adults' confidence and feeling of safety, resulting in increased levels of activity and independence.[12,26]

Many seniors share the concerns of Mrs. Dolly, and her hesitation to use ADs is familiar. Patients support the use of ADs by perception of external safety, internal safety, and respect and perception of weakness or losing independence.[27] Seventy percent of seniors report having mobility or health issues that reduced quality of life due to a physical limitation and increased risk of falling. Of these seniors, 63% reported they had fallen in the last year, and though most felt that ADs were a good way to prevent falls, almost half did not use an AD.[28]

One reason seniors refrain from adopting ADs is the perception that ADs make them appear disabled. In a Canadian study, approximately one-third of seniors polled believed ADs made them appear old and frail, indicating loss of independence.[28] Assurances that ADs can prolong independence for community dwellers should be given often, and include pointing out improvement of function using ADs during therapy sessions or health care provider visits. Security is also a primary concern for the older population. Two-thirds of seniors believed AD use was a threat to their security, making them targets for crimes. Seniors should be informed that in most countries, including Canada and the United States, people age 65 and older are the least likely age group to be targeted for crimes.[28,29]

CASE PRESENTATION (continued)
Compliance Consult of Assistive Devices

After the evaluation of Mrs. Dolly's impairments, the therapist reviewed the results with acknowledgment and understanding by Mrs. Dolly. Reflecting back on her recorded goals and reluctance to use ADs, the therapist encouraged Mrs. Dolly to complete the Perceived Consequences of the Use of Assistive Devices Scale. Items in this instrument include "Using ADs, I can do things independently and I don't need help; perception of other people thinking she is old and sick; she can go faster; easier; a sense of security; and if friends and family would visit anymore." By addressing these items and previous concerns, Mrs. Dolly stated she would consider using ADs. The therapist was concerned that her "consideration to use the device" would not translate into using the device; he continued the conversation to explain some general information and the implementation of the device.

● SELECTION OF DEVICES

Several studies have revealed that many patients have inadequate information on ADs and their proper use.[30] Common misunderstandings of AD use include on which side to use a cane, the height a device should be for ambulating, how to use wheel locks, the ability to push, and not picking up rolling framed walkers to advance them. ADs are evolving technologies and are not yet fully successful in the geriatric market.[31] Patients may not be aware of available ADs despite having positive perceptions. The decreased compliance rate of ADs is mostly attributed to lack of training.[3]

The health care provider needs to identify the primary and secondary settings in which the person will be using the device and the purpose of the device.[32] A community dweller will most likely require multiple devices for different settings; a senior living in a nursing home with level, even surfaces may need only one. AD purposes include balance, weight-bearing reduction, rehabilitation from acute trauma such as a total knee replacement, and ADs used for personal ADLs.

When selecting an AD, the least restrictive device should be chosen, realizing that prescriptions for more than one device may be needed, as one device may not fit all situations. The device(s) selected may only be needed for short-term use, but decisions should be made on the patient's current status. As mobility and impairments change, reassessments will be needed to consider prescription to a less restrictive or more robust device to maintain safety and achieve set goals.

Most devices can be set to the size of the patient. The physical size or weight of an AD itself may be challenging.[7] A bariatric walker that is wider and heavy duty to support the large amount of weight for a heavier patient but is issued to a thin, frail elderly woman will be equally as difficult and dangerous to use as an obese patient trying to use a narrow walker. ADs are a risk factor for falls in part because of the precipitating decline that necessitated use of an AD and/or incorrect AD use contributes to an adverse event.[7]

Training sessions with the AD(s) are mandatory and critical for compliance and safety. A device should never be given to a patient or patient's caregiver without the appropriate training and fitting on the patient himself or herself.

CASE PRESENTATION (continued)

Assistive Device Prescription

On her next visit, Mrs. Dolly brought to the therapist her father's wooden cane she occasionally used, as well as her quad cane. Mrs. Dolly stood with the cane in her right hand, with the top handle approximately at the level of her iliac crest. She then demonstrated walking with the cane, continuing to keep it in her right hand as she advanced her right leg. When the therapist asked her if she thought the cane was too tall for her, she replied, "Well, Daddy was a tall guy, does it matter?" The therapist then asked her to demonstrate walking with the quad cane. The cane was set at approximately the same height as the wooden straight cane. She continued to keep the cane in her right hand; however, now she would stop walking, advance the cane, then walk up to the cane, then repeat the cycle.

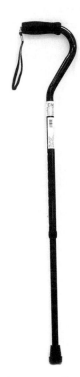

FIGURE 26–1. Offset cane.

● CANE PRESCRIPTION

The therapist first determined the primary purpose initially was for balance-related issues. Selection of a cane is usually the first choice as it gives good support while walking and is usually prescribed for people who have mild to moderate impairments.[32] Canes are generally wood, plastic, or metal, easy to use and relatively inexpensive.

A straight or offset cane with a single tip is usually the first AD of choice for balance purposes. The offset cane—sometimes referred to as the "question mark or crooked cane"—has an added benefit that the cane allows for the force to be in line with the shaft of the cane and hand, instead of at an angle as with the typical hook-shaped cane (Figure 26–1). The offset cane is prescribed more often because of the ease of applying different grips. Grips can be interchanged on some of these models more easily than on others. Grip selection is often more of a personal preference, but can be important when prescribing a device to someone with hand or wrist weakness or pathologies such as carpal tunnel disease or arthritis in the hands. In these cases, a foam or ergonomic grip can be applied to keep correct position of the wrist or add comfort to the hand. Alternatively, a platform may be installed to support the wrist. Also consider a gutter crutch, or use of a cane such as the StrongArm crutch (Figure 26–2).

When using only one cane, it should be held on the opposite side of the weak or involved extremity. If a cane is used solely for balance and no impairments to a single extremity are present, it is acceptable for the patient to put the cane in the hand with which they are more comfortable carrying the device.

Mrs. Dolly's most affected side is her right and she incorrectly uses the cane in her right hand, as many people initially do. The cane should be placed in the opposite hand of the involved extremity, advancing the cane and involved leg forward followed by the uninvolved leg.[33] In her case, the cane should be placed in her left hand, so when she is advancing her right leg, her left arm advances holding the cane and providing a wider base of support to increase stability.

The second problem with Mrs. Dolly using her father's cane is that it is too long for her. ADs requiring the use of the hands for ambulation devices should place so that the device

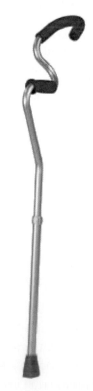

FIGURE 26–2. StrongArm cane.

handgrip is at the level of the wrist when the arm is at a relaxed position. This level is approximately the same level as the greater trochanters of the femur, and will allow for approximately 20 degrees of elbow flexion. The importance of proper cane height is that if the cane is too long, work is increased, and it is harder to pick up and advance the cane. If the cane is too short, shifting weight to one side unevenly will occur, which may perturb one's balance.

When a patient is using a previously used device, the ferrules should be inspected. The ferrule is the rubber tip, though in colder, icy climates a removable ice pick may be installed. The ferrule provides traction to the device. Periodic inspection should be performed to the ferrules of all ADs.

One feature added to single-point canes is a flange, or a clamp-like device, that allows the cane to be rested or affixed to a surface such as a tabletop. An Internet search for "cane holder" will illustrate some of these devices. Even with such an add-on, providers need to check that the patient is able to retrieve the device from the floor safely in the likely event it will fall.

Another option that may be considered but is not often implemented in geriatrics is the use of two single-point canes for bilateral impairments. Many times this strategy is seen in the acute younger population, generally with amputation or neuropathology with only mild to moderate impairment.

The use of a tripod or quad cane is indicated if a patient appears unsteady or wobbles with single-point canes. Tripod canes tend to be more self-selected. They are bulky, but have a seat that some desire. The quad cane has the benefits of being able to provide more support than a standard cane, because it distributes force to a wide base over four extension feet. This also allows the cane to stand upright when not used.

This cane had been set to the same height as Mrs. Dolly's other cane, because that is what she was used to using, even though it was an improper fit. In addition, Mrs. Dolly stated initially that she liked to use the cane outdoors on the uneven ground for better stability and she was able to lean on it when she was tired. Both of these assumptions by Mrs. Dolly are incorrect and place her at risk for falling.

Quad canes are best used in level, uncluttered settings. Because the cane has the four extensions at the base, applying the feet to irregular surfaces increases the fall risk and compromises safety if they are not evenly distributed over a level surface such as uneven ground. Planting one of the feet off the edge of the surface can result in tipping, especially during weight transfer. When using the cane inside, the areas should be clutter free, as more space is needed to allow for clearance of the wide base. During ambulation, it is important to fit the cane to the right or left side of the body, as the one side of the base of the cane will protrude out, as identified by the arrow in Figure 26–3. The shaft of the cane is to remain closer to the patient. By reversing sides and using incorrectly, the wide base portion may protrude closer to the leg, causing a tripping hazard during ambulation. The wide base also may pose a problem on stairs. Patients may have to turn the base 90 degrees to allow the cane to fit on the stairs. This should be reinforced and practiced before allowing a person to use this device. Failure to turn the device on steps with narrower treads may result in only one or two of the ferrules contacting

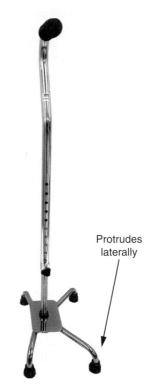

Protrudes laterally

FIGURE 26–3. Right-hand quad cane.

the step. This may cause the cane to be displaced, tipping forward or backward depending on whether the patient is going up or down stairs.

● STAIR TRAINING

When training a person on stairs, teaching the phrase "up with the good, down with the bad" will be needed to be repeated and reinforced frequently, until the act of ambulating stairs with an AD has become an integrated motor pattern. To help people remember, clarification that "good people go up to heaven and bad people go down" may help them remember as well. In this example, good refers to the persons' strong leg and the bad leg would be the weaker or involved leg. The AD should be used in conjunction with the "bad" or involved leg.

In Mrs. Dolly's case, her left leg would be the stronger leg. Ascending the stairs, she would have her cane in the left hand and would most likely walk up the right side of the stairs so her right arm would be able to use a handrail if available. She would first step with her left leg, followed by advancement of the cane in her left hand and then her right leg. Many people with impairment will demonstrate this "step-to" where the involved leg is only stepping to the tread of the same level of the good leg. A goal would be to advance her gait pattern to a reciprocal stepping pattern, where Mrs. Dolly's right leg would advance to the tread on the stairs above the level of her other leg.

Descending stairs is the opposite of ascending. The person should first advance the cane to the lower step followed by the involved leg and lastly the uninvolved or good leg should be lowered. The sequence is repeated. Many people will note that going down the stairs is more difficult than going up.

The caregiver may also be instructed to assist by standing behind the patient when ascending the stairs and in front of the patient when going down stairs. Instructions to "always be below the person on stairs" may assist caregivers in remembering their appropriate position.

● WALKING FRAME PRESCRIPTION

Mrs. Dolly does not currently use a walker; however, there are indications for such a prescription. In her history, she stated she would go to the grocery store and use a "buggy" (shopping cart) to lean on during her trip. Using a shopping cart is similar to people who use a walker, allowing for weight reduction of the lower limbs, which is an important benefit for patients with weakness, injury, or joint pain in the lower extremities as well as generalized weakness, debilitating conditions, or poor balance control.[31-34]

Her Berg Balance Scale score also indicates use of a walker, and reflects her decreased endurance. When choosing a walker, determination of the ability of the patient to use the walker in her environment should be given first consideration. The most common choices will be between a rigid frame or no-wheeled walker (Figure 26–4), a two-wheeled walker (Figure 26–5), or a four-wheeled walker, with variations in size, color, and accessories (Figure 26–6). Three-wheeled walkers do exist, but are not common.

A standard walker with no wheels has the advantages of being lighter, folding flatter than wheeled walkers, providing a large, stable base, and costing less than other walkers. This is an ideal choice for those with significant balance impairment, including those with significant forward-flexed

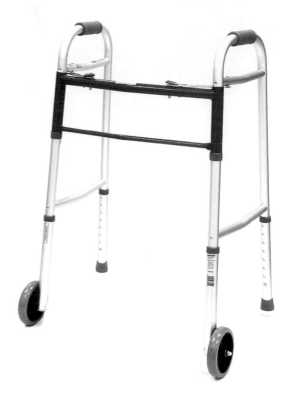

FIGURE 26–5. Two-wheeled rolling walker.

postures. The use of this device requires repetitive lifting and placing the walker in front of the patient's center of mass, resulting in increased fatigue compared to walkers using wheels. Patients with weak upper extremities or shoulder and cervical pathology may find it difficult to use.

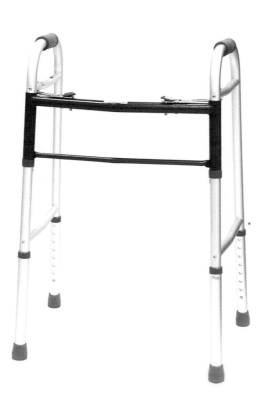

FIGURE 26–4. Rigid-frame walker.

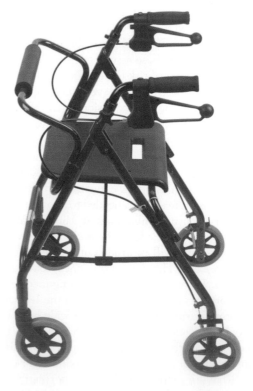

FIGURE 26–6. Four-wheeled rolling walker.

In addition, those with certain neurologic conditions such as Parkinson disease would not benefit from using this walker, as there is an increased incidence of freezing when compared to using a wheeled walker.[35]

Mrs. Dolly's evaluation revealed weakness in her extremities in addition to her balance impairments. She demonstrated a mild to moderate forward-flexed posture secondary to her spinal stenosis and wedging of vertebrae due to osteoporosis, and because the process of repetitive lifting would potentially increase her low back and leg pain and she already fatigues quickly, a rolling walker is a better choice.

The decision to prescribe a two-wheeled versus a four-wheeled walker is based on safety and environment. Sometimes, both may be indicated. Two-wheeled walkers can be used both inside and outside. They are ideal for indoor environments because they are less bulky and more stable than four-wheeled walkers. The wheels on two-wheeled walkers come in various sizes and positions. Larger wheels (4-5 in, 10-13 cm) allow for continuous movement on slightly uneven terrain. Objects like pebbles or small-thickness thresholds may retard smaller wheels more easily, allowing displacement of the walker and creating an increased fall risk. Mounting of the wheels is also an important consideration. The smaller-diameter wheels are usually placed in line with the front post of the walker. This is appropriate for narrow environments. Larger-wheeled walkers will be mounted on the outside of the front post, though occasionally people will mount on the inside of the post. Inside mounting can increase tripping hazard if the foot makes contact with the wheel during ambulation. Also, notable tracking problems with the wheels out of alignment on the inside increases resistance while pushing the walker. These walkers do not have wheel locks common on other devices.

The rear post on two-wheeled walkers will have rubber feet. These provide additional stability. Some patients may feel the resistance of these feet is not desirable. Other external devices may be mounted to the rear post, including commercially purchased sliders, a type of plastic shaped as a flat plate with a curled front. The more popular method is to cut slits in tennis balls and place one ball on each post. Other accessories that can be mounted to the top or cross bars include trays, bags, and small-ledged seats. Use of accessories should be carefully considered with respect to the patient's ability to safely use the device with the additional bulk, or ability to transfer to and from an object that has the ability to slide.

The prescription of a four-wheeled walker should be given to more mobile patients, especially those who plan to be active outdoors. The four-wheeled walker is the bulkiest of all the framed walkers, weighs the most, and is the least stable. This walker is ideal for those who have large enough space inside their home environment and wish to traverse ground outside.

These walkers often come with seats and other accessories. They almost always have wheel locks and usually have large levers to allow patients to use gross motor movements to engage and disengage them. The locking mechanisms can be confusing to those with dementia, who may attempt to push the device when the wheel locks are engaged.

For patients with only minimal to moderate balance impairment, up to moderate visual impairment, and adequate cognition to safely work the device, these walkers will allow for faster ambulation and enable sitting when needing to rest. The four wheels also make traversing even or uneven ground easier.

Whichever walker is prescribed, the walker handles should be placed at the level of the greater trochanter or the level of the wrist when the arm is relaxed by the side of the body. There are also associated weight limitations for these devices, and the person's weight should be provided when ordering the device.

Walking patterns for the device will depend on the weight-bearing status for each leg. Instructions for full weight-bearing on both legs should sequence the walker to advance the walker first, then one leg, then the other. For partial weight bearing, or when one extremity is involved, sequencing should be advancing the walker first, next advancing the involved lower extremity, followed by the uninvolved lower extremity, then repeat.[30]

> ## CASE PRESENTATION (continued)
> ### Summary
> Mrs. Dolly was prescribed a new offset cane and a four-wheeled walker. She received AD training each time she came for her physical therapy appointment. By evaluating her ability and needs, and assessing her environment, a prescription to improve her mobility and maintain her independence was achieved. By listening to her concerns and identifying her goals, she adopted the use of the devices into her normal daily routine.

CONCLUSION

The appropriate application of an AD requires the health care professional to consider not only the deficit to which the device is being applied but also the social and environmental considerations that may impact the use of the device. The therapist must balance the ease of use, acceptability, cost, amount of education/training the user will require, and environmental factors that might impede the proper adoption of the device as well as the patient's own goals as they relate to his or her function. Only with consideration of all these factors can successful use and implementation to best benefit the patient occur.

References

1. Wasson JG. The prescription of assistive devices for the elderly. *J Gen Intern Med.* 1990;5:46-54.

2. Russell JH. Trends and differential use of assistive technology devices: United States, 1994. *ADV Data.* 1997;13:1-9.

3. Roelands MV. Awareness among community-dwelling elderly of assistive devices for mobility and self-care and attitudes towards their use. *Soc Sci Med.* 2002;54:1441-1451.

4. Sonn U. Longitudinal studies of dependence in daily life activities among the elderly: Methodological development, use of assistive devices and relation to impairments and functional limitations. *Scand J Occup Ther.* 1995;2:41.

5. Jensen, L. *Go For It!* European Commion. www.siva.it/research/eustat/index.html. 1999.

6. Laplante MH. Assistive technology devices and home accessability features: Prevalence, payment, needs and trends. Advanced Data from Vital Health Statistics. Hyattsville, MD: National Center for Health Statistics; 1992:217.

7. Bateni HM. Assistive devices for balance and mobility: Benefits, demands, and adverse consequences. *Arch Phys Med Rehabil.* 2005;86:134-145.

8. Jaeger RY. Rehabilitation technology for standing and walking after spinal cord injury. *Am J Phys Med Rehabil.* 1989;68:99-116.

9. Mahoney JE. Use of an ambulation assistive device predicts functional decline associated with hospitalization. *J Gerontol A Biol Sci Med Sci.* 1999;54:83-88.

10. McDonnall, M. Risk factors for depression among older adults with dual sensory loss. *Aging Ment Health.* 2009;13:569-576.

11. Nordenskiold U. Questionnaire to evaluate the effects of assistive devices and altered working methods in women with RA. *Clin Rheumatol.* 1998;17:6-16.

12. Aminzadeh F. Exploring seniors' views on the use of assistive devices in fall prevention. *Public Health Nurs.* 1998;15:297-304

13. Demers L. A conceptual framework of outcomes for caregivers of assistive technology users. *Am J Phys Med Rehabil.* 2009;88:645-658.

14. American Geriatric Society, British Geriatrics Society, and American Academy of Orthopaedic Surgeons: Guideline for the Prevention of Falls in Older Persons. *J Am Geriatr Soc.* 2001;49: 664-672.

15. Fritz S. White Paper: "Walking Speed: the Sixth Vital Sign." *J Geriatr Phys Ther.* 2009;32:1-4.

16. Roelands R. A social-cognitive model to predict the use of assistive devices for mobility and self-care in elderly people. *Gerontologist.* 2002;42:39-50.

17. Kraskowsky L. Factors affecting older adults' use of adaptive equipment: review of the literature. *Am J Occup Ther.* 2001;55:303-310.

18. Montero-Odasso M. Gait velocity as a single predictor of adverse events in healthy seniors aged 75 years and older. *J Gerontol A Biol Sci Med Sci.* 2005;60:1304-1309.

19. Tinetti MR. Falls efficacy as a measure of fear of falling. *J Gerontol.* 1990;45:239.

20. Bennett L, Murray MP, Murphy EF, Sowell TT. Locomotion assistance through cane impulse. *Bull Prosthet Res.* 1979;38-47.

21. Engel J. Walking cane designed to assist pertial weight bearing. *Arch Phys Med Rehabil.* 1983;64:386-388.

22. Brand R. The effect of cane use on hip contact force. *Clin Orthop.* 1980;181-184.

23. Joyce B. Canes, crutches and walkers. *Am Fam Physician.* 1991;43:535-542.

24. Tagawa Y. Analysis of human abnormal walking using a multi-body model: joint models for abnormal walking and walking aids to reduce compensatory action. *J Biomech.* 2000;33:1405-1414.

25. Nochajski S. The use and satisfaction with assistive devices by older persons with cognitive impairments: A pilot study. *Top Geriatr Rehabil.* 1996;12:40-53.

26. Tinetti M. Fear of falling and low self-efficacy: A case of dependence in elderly persons. *J Gerontol.* 1993;48:35-38.

27. Greta H. Elderly women's way of relating to assistive devices. *Technol Disabil.* 1999;10:161-168.

28. Public Health Agency of Canada. Go for it! A guide to choosing and using assistive devices, 2007.

29. U.S. Department of Justice: *Bureau of Justice Statistics.* From http://www.ojp.usdoj.gov/bjs/glance/vage.htm. 2006 September.

30. Mann W. Assistive Devices used by home-based elderly persons with arthritis. *Am J Occup Ther.* 1995;49:810-820.

31. Rehabilitation Engineering and Assistive Technology Society of North America (RESNA). *Assistive Technology Workbook.* (R. P. Publisers, Ed.) Washington, DC: www.resna.org. 1990

32. Pain H. *Choosing Assistive Devices: A Guide for Users and Professionals.* Philadelphia, PA: Jessica Kingsley Publishers; 2003.

33. Rothstein J. *The Rehabilitation Specialist Handbook.* Philadelphia, PA: FA Davis Co.; 1998.

34. Minor M. Patient care skills. *Norwalk.* 1995;494.

35. Cubo E. Wheeled and standard walkers in Parkinson's disease patients with gait freezing. *Parkinsonism Relat Disord.* 2003;10:9-14.

POST-TEST

1. Where should the grip of an offset cane be placed when the arm is relaxed to the side of the patient?
   A. Iliac crest
   B. Wrist
   C. Forearm
   D. Elbow

2. Which device is best recommended for a patient who has just had a surgical operation on the right lower extremity and has been restricted to partial weight-bearing status?
   A. Straight or offset cane
   B. Quad cane
   C. Rolling walker
   D. Transport wheelchair

3. When using a cane on the stairs with a person who has right knee pain, the proper sequence for ascending the stairs is:
   A. Step up with the left leg first, then the cane in the left hand, then the right leg.
   B. Step up with the left leg first, then the cane in the right hand, then the right leg.
   C. Step up with the right leg first, then the cane in the left hand, then the left leg.
   D. Step up with the right leg first, then the cane in the right hand, then the left leg.

ANSWERS TO PRE-TEST

1. A
2. B
3. D

ANSWERS TO POST-TEST

1. B
2. C
3. A

27

Integrating Technology into Older Adult Living

Eun-Shim Nahm, PhD, RN

Barbara Resnick, PhD, CRNP, FAAN

● **LEARNING OBJECTIVES**

1. Explain different types of available technology-based interventions.
2. Describe specific cases where technology-based interventions can be applied.
3. Discuss user requirements for assessments before implementing technology-based interventions.
4. Identify and explain issues and limitations in using technology-based interventions.

PRE-TEST

1. **Which of the following technology usability factors would reflect a preference of older adults?**

   A. Web pages with a large font size and sophisticated functions

   B. Printed version of step-by-step operational guidelines

   C. Preset timing for use without adaptation

   D. Error pop-up with every phase of use

2. **Glucose tracking is a good example of which remote health management system?**

   A. Telehealth

   B. Telemedicine

   C. eHealth

   D. Telemonitoring

3. **Ms. Tunner is using an electronic personal health record (PHR) provided by a health insurance service. Who would be allowed access to this PHR?**

   A. Authorized health care providers

   B. The health insurance services of the older adult

   C. Wife/husband of the older adult

   D. Children out of the geographic area

● INTRODUCTION

CASE PRESENTATION 1: TECHNOLOGY IN ACTION

Alicia Jones, a 78-year-old widowed female, climbs out of bed but notices that she does not feel "quite right." She checks her blood sugar, which is 225 mg/dL (12.5 mmol/L) and notes this is quite high for her. On the way to the bathroom she stumbles but catches herself. She eats a small breakfast and wonders what is wrong. Fortunately for her, her home is equipped with a smart home monitoring system. As she was checking her blood sugar these results were wirelessly sent to the home hub and then relayed to her physician via an Internet link. In addition, the system reported, based on floor sensors and motion sensors, that she almost fell and that she had been up three times that night to the bathroom, her usual being once. The nurse practitioner in the office is alerted to these results and calls Ms. Jones to get more history and ask her to come to the office for a visit. Later that morning, in the doctor's office, she is found to have a urinary tract infection and is provided with treatment and instructions.

While remarkable advances in modern health care during the last century have improved longevity, growing numbers of older adults are living with chronic conditions and are experiencing diminishing cognitive function. Currently, more than 90 million Americans live with chronic illnesses,[1,2] and dementia has become a significant health problem among older adults.[3,4] In addition, family members in today's society are often dispersed geographically, and older couples or single older adults living alone face challenges with obtaining appropriate "care" at home.

Current information and communication technology (ICT) has transformed individuals' paradigms of life style, and the concepts of distance and time have changed significantly. Communication and data exchanges among people in other states or other countries can be easily made over the Internet using both text and audio, as well as video functions. ICT has also changed health care delivery, offering great potential to assist older adults maintain healthy and independent lives in the community.[5-7] While adoption of ICT among older adults has been slower as compared to younger generations who grew up with information technology, older adults in recent years have become the fastest-growing ICT adopters. In 2010, 38% of American adults age 65 and older were online. A Pew Internet survey in 2008 reported that approximately half of adults between the ages of 50 and 64 and 26% of those 65 and older in the United States have home broadband access.[8] In addition, 62% of American

adults used mobile devices to perform some digital activities in 2007.[8] As the advancement of ICT accelerates in society, the potential to use this technology for health care will grow exponentially.

The importance of technologies in health has been recognized nationally, noticeably since the *To Err Is Human*[9] report was published. This importance has resonated with the Obama administration, which called for a $10 billion-a-year investment in Health Information Technology (HIT) over 5 years.[10] This national agenda has significant implications for current health care professionals who care for older adults and their caregivers, as they must capitalize on the opportunity to develop and implement technologies to help older adults maintain a high quality of life in their later years. This chapter will focus on current ICT technologies, as well as those that are actively under development, that can be integrated into older adults' daily lives to assist in their ability to live independently and maintain their health when their cognitive functions start to decline. The intent of this chapter is to introduce applicable technologies in caring for older adults and their caregivers, rather than focusing on technical or developmental aspects of those technologies.

The technologies integrated into older adults' lives can be effective only when they are usable. Otherwise, they would add an unnecessary burden to these individuals. As compared to younger generations, older adults have unique usability requirements for technologies due to age-related changes. It is important that health care professionals and technology developers understand and assess those aspects to properly develop/configure systems to meet the needs of the older adult users. The scientific discipline concerned with these aspects is human factors, and this chapter starts with a brief overview of human factors and usability issues in older adults.

● HUMAN FACTORS AND USABILITY

Technologies have great potential to make positive changes in people's everyday lives. At the same time, the impact can be negative. Sometimes, products or programs may not function as they were originally envisioned and consequently yield untoward outcomes.[11,12] The problems could be human related, machine related, or often the result of combined effects. The developer's understanding of typical user needs and characteristics is critical in making technologies useful. For instance, many younger online users prefer Web pages with lots of "bells and whistles" and sophisticated functions. Those Web pages, however, may not be user-friendly for many older adults who have limited Web experience and unique design needs. Most older adults prefer simple Web pages with a large font size and specific color scheme.[13-15] As shown in this example, different user groups may have different user requirements for the same technology. The match between technologies and users is more critical in health care technology because it can influence the safety of individuals.

Human Factor Issues in Older Adults

The terms "human factors" and "ergonomics" are often used interchangeably and are both related to engineering psychology. The principles of ergonomics include the optimization of machine design for human operation. The goal of selection and training is to obtain the best performance possible from people within machine design limitations.[16] Human factors, which encompass the four disciplines of engineering, psychology, sociology, and computer science, are associated with anything that affects users' performance with the system (eg, hardware, software, or other products).[3] In developing technologies used for older adults, developers need to consider age-related changes, including changes in sensory, perceptual, cognitive, psychomotor, and other physical abilities (more specific changes are explained in detail in Chapters 3, 8, and 34).[18]

For instance, older adults may experience changes in visual acuity[19] and visual fields.[20] They also may have some decline in short-term or working memory (the ability to process information while maintaining intermediate thoughts).[15,21] The major changes in psychomotor functions in the aging process are a slower response speed and weakening motor coordination and dexterity.[15] Some chronic health conditions prevalent in older adults, such as arthritis and/or stroke, often contribute to the weakening psychomotor response and increase risk for injuries (eg, falls). In addition to the consideration of these age-related changes, the design of the products should match the older adult's mental map.[11]

Usability of Technologies

Usability of a product depends on what users are trying to accomplish, as well as the developers' specific objectives for the product.[22,23] The term "usability" applies to all aspects of a product with which a user might interact.[22] Nielsen suggested five usability attributes: (1) learnability, (2) efficiency, (3) memorability, (4) error prevention, and (5) satisfaction.[22] For older adults, however, it may be more proactive to provide a means to compensate for diminished working memory (eg, a printed version of simple step-by-step guidelines).

User requirements for usability vary depending upon products and users. A product that is usable by a certain group may be unusable by another. For instance, currently many online health resources are available to older adults. Although many older adults use computers and the Web, the majority of them are still unfamiliar with the most recent Web technologies (eg, web blogs) or do not have the technological configuration to support those. Thus, assessment of specific user requirements must be completed a priori to the development or purchase of a program. The infrastructure of technology-based health interventions must be configured to accommodate the majority of their target population. In addition, testing of the product usability is also critical. Detailed explanations of testing methods are beyond the scope of this chapter and can be found in other references.[22-24]

TECHNOLOGIES TO HELP COMMUNITY-DWELLING OLDER ADULTS MANAGE AND IMPROVE HEALTH

CASE PRESENTATION 2: TECHNOLOGY IN THE COMMUNITY

Mary Jackson (M.J.) is a 70-year-old female who has lived alone in a single two-story house after her husband passed away 5 years ago. She was recently discharged from the hospital after an acute exacerbation of congestive heart disease. Additional co-morbid conditions include hypertension, osteoporosis, and type II diabetes. At home, she monitors her blood glucose daily (q AM) and has been instructed to call her primary health care provider when her blood glucose is over 200 mg/dL (11.1 mmol/L). She takes Glyburide 2.5 mg daily. In addition, she takes hydrochlorothiazide 25 mg daily to control blood pressure, Boniva (Ibandronate) monthly for osteoporosis, and a multivitamin. Although she is independent in all activities of daily living, she has had multiple falls over the past few years and sustained a hip fracture 2 years ago. M.J. is now status post right hemiarthroplasty. She has a daughter and a son, both of whom live out of state. The children call her frequently and attempt to schedule visits quarterly.

This scenario depicts several chronic health conditions that many older adults are experiencing within community settings. These conditions can be particularly difficult for older adults because they require constant monitoring and management, as well as significant life style changes (eg, diet, exercise), and adherence to multiple medications. Medical regimens to control these conditions can be complex and require ongoing reinforcement and oversight to best optimize outcomes. Unfortunately, many older adults also experience some decline in cognitive function, which could affect adherence to these regimens. Several health care technologies are now beginning to be used to help these older adults optimally manage their chronic conditions at home.

Remote Health Management Systems

Telehealth technologies have advanced rapidly since the late 1960s.[25,26] The scope and practice of care delivered remotely varies a great deal among different settings. Various terminologies have been used to describe such practice. The most frequently used terminologies are telemedicine, telehealth, eHealth, and telemonitoring (Table 27–1).[27-35] Telemedicine has the longest history and is defined as the provision of health care services and education over a distance using telecommunication technology.[28] Telehealth is a broader term

● TABLE 27–1	Terminology
EHealth	All forms of electronic healthcare delivered over the Internet[27,29,30]
EHR	Electronic health record
Ergonomics	The principles of ergonomics include the optimization of machine design for human operation; the goal of selection and training is to obtain the best performance possible from people within machine design limitations[2]
GPS	Global positioning system
HIT	Health information technology
Human factors	Human factors, which encompass the four disciplines of engineering, psychology, sociology, and computer science, are associated with anything that affects users' performance of the system (eg, hardware, software, or other products)[17]
ICT	Information and communication technology
Mental map	A person's personal point of view or perception of his or her own world
PHR	Personal health record
Telehealth	The integration of telecommunication systems into the practice of health promotion, as compared to telemedicine, which is more focused on medical treatment[27]
Telemedicine	The provision of health care services and education over a distance using telecommunication technology[28]
Telemonitoring	A type of telecommunication technology that uses monitoring devices (eg, blood pressure or glucose monitoring devices)[27,31]
Usability	All aspects of a product with which a user might interact[22]; it concerns whether a product is "usable" by users

that includes the integration of telecommunication systems into the practice of health promotion, as compared to telemedicine, which is more focused on medical treatment.[27] EHealth, a more recent terminology, incorporates all forms of electronic health care delivered over the Internet.[27,29,30] Telemonitoring is a type of telecommunication technology that uses monitoring devices (eg, blood pressure or glucose monitoring devices; Figure 27–1).[27,31]

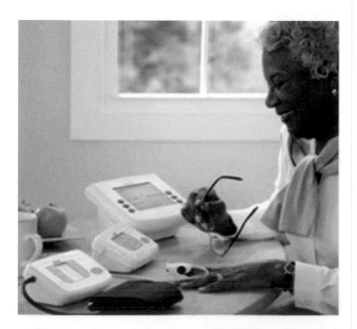

FIGURE 27–1. Glucose measurement incorporating telemonitoring. (From http://www.medicalphillips.com/main/products/telehealth/products/devices.wpd.)

● SEVERAL TECHNOLOGY-BASED INTERVENTIONS MAY BE HELPFUL TO M.J.

Telehealth Management Programs

Nurse-managed telehealth programs can assist older adults in managing chronic illnesses, such as heart failure (HF) or diabetes (DM), at home.[7,31] Various systems are already in the commercial market, including weight, blood pressure, glucose, and EKG monitoring devices, as well as pulse oximetry. Most recent devices are wireless, using Bluetooth technology. The measurements are gathered through a hub in the older adult's home and transmitted to the designated service providers.

For instance, when M.J. was discharged, her doctor recognized that she lived alone and was becoming more forgetful. She is at high risk for readmission due to her heart condition and her fluctuating blood glucose levels. Thus, Dr. Smith, M.J.'s primary physician, recommended that M.J. register for the telehealth clinic that is supervised by a nurse practitioner. Once M.J. registered for the program, the hospital staff brought the following wireless devices to M.J.'s home: a weight scale, blood pressure cuff, wrist bands to record electrocardiogram (EKG) rhythm strips, a glucometer, and a telehealth station. The telehealth station serves as a hub to gather data from all devices and to send the information to the nurse practitioner in the clinic using a telephone line. This station is also equipped with a two-way videophone function.

When M.J. takes her weight, blood pressure, and other measures as prescribed, the monitoring devices display values on the monitoring screen, as well as via sound, so that M.J. knows her measurements. The nurse practitioner (NP) reviews the data transmitted to her screen, and if needed, she calls M.J. and gives specific instructions to manage her symptoms. M.J. can also send a message to her NP if she needs to talk to her. If the measurements are not transmitted to the NP as prescribed, the NP calls M.J. to remind her to take her measurements and to ensure that she is alright.

M.J.'s children, who live out of state, are concerned about M.J.'s condition and wish to participate in managing her health. With M.J.'s approval, her children may also have access to a telehealth station and review their mother's health data. The caregiver's telehealth station can assist children in motivating their parents. Specifically, children can use information from the telehealth station to provide feedback to their parents about how they are doing. M.J.'s children feel much more comfortable knowing their mother's current health status and about their ability to be more actively involved in their mothers' care and well-being.

Medication Management Systems

In M.J.'s case, her primary physician and children were concerned about adherence to her medication schedule, because M.J. sometimes forgets to take her medication due to her memory problems. Currently, various medication management systems are available, from something as simple as a

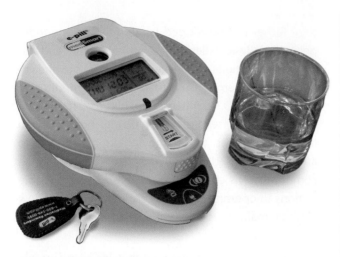

FIGURE 27–2. Smart pillbox. (Courtesy e-pill® Medication Reminders at www.epill.com, 1-800-549-0095.)

plastic compartment for daily medications to more sophisticated computerized programs. For older adults who are becoming more forgetful, "smart" medical management boxes can be helpful. Functions available on these systems vary. For instance, some pill boxes can store a day's worth of medications and alarm (eg, beep, vibrate) to notify the person when it is time to take medications. These boxes can be purchased in drugstores at a low cost. More sophisticated systems can store and dispense medications for a longer period of time, and medication dispensers can be remotely monitored by a service provider.[32] Some new and innovative technologies are also under development. For instance, the "Electronic Pill Pet" developed by Massachusetts Institute of Technology's AgeLab has incorporated the concept of "toy" in a "smart" pill box.[33] One major limitation of these systems is that monitoring can be done only for medication retrieval, missing the information about actual medication ingestion (Figure 27–2).

In M.J.'s case, when Dr. Smith prescribed telemonitoring devices he also recommended a "smart" medication box, which stores a monthly supply of medications and dispenses the medications at scheduled times. This system reminds M.J. of the times to take medications using a programmable music or human voice reminder. The system alarms 15 minutes prior to the time medications are to be taken. M.J.'s children take turns stocking medications monthly in the pillbox and keep track of medication dispenses. Medication dispenses are recorded and transmitted to the designated child's telehealth center. If M.J. misses a dose of a medication, the system reminds M.J. and alerts her designated child. Initially, M.J. thought the "talking" medication box was annoying, but over time she indicated that she felt this reminder was very useful.

Emergency Medical Alert System

M.J. has fallen multiple times in the past 2 years. She already fractured her hip a year ago. At that time, the accident happened while she was shopping with her friend, and M.J. received prompt medical treatment. Although M.J. recovered

quickly and now can function without a cane, her children worry about recurrent fractures, especially at home while no one is around. Currently, many older adults are using emergency alert system services. Different companies offer various levels of services. When older adults or their caregivers are shopping for a service provider, they need to prepare a list of considerations, including support coverage hours and whether the service provider has its own monitoring center.[34]

M.J.'s friend, who is using this type of service from a company, highly recommended her service. M.J.'s children investigated the company's reputation, considered service options, and decided to use the service. Now M.J. wears a pendant (a wrist band is also an option) that has an alert button with a two-way communication system. During an emergency, she can just press the button and start talking. Throughout the house, two-way hands-free speaker phones are mounted with a panic button. Once she presses the alert button, the speaker phone will be activated and she can then start talking to the service. The service then will contact a designated response team (eg, ambulance). Both M.J. and her children feel much safer with this system.

Personal Health Record System and Health Portals

A personal health record (PHR) system can be especially helpful for older adults who are living with multiple chronic illnesses and taking many medications, because all health-related information can be systematically stored in a secure system. Depending on the product, family members can access the system to help older adults manage their health. In addition, when family members are living out of state and the older adults experience an emergency situation, the PHR can serve as a critical resource, providing the older adult's health information.

The HIMSS Personal Health Record Steering Committee defines an electronic personal health record (ePHR) as follows:

> A universally accessible, layperson comprehensible, lifelong tool for managing relevant health information, promoting health maintenance, and assisting with chronic disease management via an interactive, common data set of electronic health information and e-health tools. The ePHR is owned, managed, and shared by the individual or his or her legal proxy(s) and must be secure to protect the privacy and confidentiality of the health information it contains. It is not a legal record unless so defined and is subject to various legal limitations.[35]

The technology architectures of PHRs vary, including a stand-alone PHR device (eg, a card embedded with a computer chip) and Web-based programs. Some programs can be integrated with electronic medical record systems and some may be managed by individual users. Maintenance of health data security and privacy are important issues in PHRs, and the systems should have rigorous authentication processes as well as the policies and procedures. In particular, older adults may need to allow proxies and other health care providers to access their PHRs. Thus, the systems must have clear policies and procedures to cover these aspects.

Web-based PHRs can be particularly helpful for older adults and their caregivers, especially when the caregivers live far away.[36,37] An older adult can give a designated caregiver access to the PHR, and the caregiver can help the older adult manage his or her health. These PHRs can facilitate communication among health care providers, older adults, and caregivers. If the older adult is not familiar with using computers or is having difficulty using a keyboard due to other health issues, alternative input technologies are available such as touch screen or voice recognition systems.

Some health care providers offer health portals to their enrollees. For instance, *MyHealtheVet* (MHV)[38,39] is a national Web portal for veterans and Veterans Affairs (VA) employees health benefits and services.[39] The Web portal provides access to the PHR, various health resources (eg, health information or links to federal and VA benefits and resources), as well as online prescription refill. Other private providers such as Kaiser Permanente[40] also offer such health portals.

M.J.'s family realized that her private insurance group offers a Web-based PHR to their enrollees. After further follow-up, M.J.'s daughter decided that she would help M.J. enroll in the PHR program and maintain the health record. Fortunately, M.J.'s PHR is integrated with the hospital's electronic health record (EHR) system. Using the PHR, M.J. and the designated caregivers can maintain medication lists, view permitted laboratory results, and communicate with their care providers. Additionally, M.J.'s private insurance company offers a health Web portal of which the PHR is a component. The health Web portal offers the following functions: scheduling outpatient appointments, prescription renewal, and health learning centers.

Although M.J.'s daughter lives out of state, she knows exactly what is going on with M.J.'s health on a daily basis and assists M.J. in managing her health care services. In addition, she communicates with M.J.'s health care providers more frequently and conveniently. MJ had not used computers before and was not familiar with a keyboard. Fortunately, the health portal is accessible via a touch screen. M.J.'s children installed a touch screen computer and showed her how to use it. In particular, her grandson developed written step-by-step instructions, placed them next to the computer, and agreed to be available to assist his grandmother with this technology whenever necessary. Now, M.J. often turns the computer on and reads health information. She has also learned to do simple Internet searches. When she has specific questions, she uses an Ask-the-Doc function to forward her health inquiries. She usually receives a response within 72 hours.

• TECHNOLOGIES TO ASSIST OLDER ADULTS WITH COGNITIVE DECLINE

CASE PRESENTATION 3: TECHNOLOGY IN FUNCTIONAL DECLINE

James Darby (J.D.) is a widower and it has been 2 years since he started using telemonitoring programs to manage his diabetes. J.D.'s children have noticed that their father has developed trouble with some independent daily activities such as paying his bills and taking his medication regularly. Sometimes J.D.'s telehealth nurse has to remind him to use his telemonitoring devices. When J.D.'s children visited him, they found that he had some bruises and cuts on his leg and arm due to falls. J.D. is very resistant to moving out of his home to a more supervised setting such as an assisted living community. His children investigated some possible options to optimize their father's safety and yet allow him to remain in his own home.

In this scenario, J.D. has started showing cognitive, physical, and functional decline yet he is living alone. This situation represents many current older adults' family situations. Adult children often have their own families and have moved out of state. As older adults continue to age, they are likely to lose their spouse and may experience cognitive deterioration in addition to physical frailty. These situations increase the risk of injuries such as falls or burns in the home setting, and place them at risk for poor nutritional intake, exacerbation of medical problems due to a lack of adherence to medications, social isolation, and depression.[41-44] Despite these potential risks, many older adults are reluctant to relocate nearer to their children because they do not want to leave their friends and the familiar place where they have lived for many years. For these individuals, remaining in their home environment is important in optimizing their quality of life. Several technology-based programs can be used to assure their safety while they live independently at home.

Home Automation ("Smart Home") Technologies

Recent advancements in home automation ("smart home") technologies can help older adults with mild cognitive deterioration maintain safety at home (Figures 27–3 and 27–4).

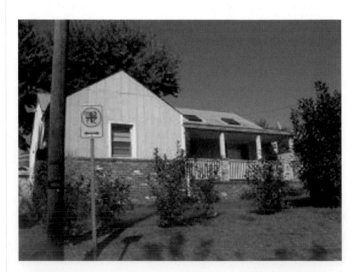

FIGURE 27–3. Smart homes. (Source: http://marc.med.virginia.edu/projects_smarthomemonitor.html.)

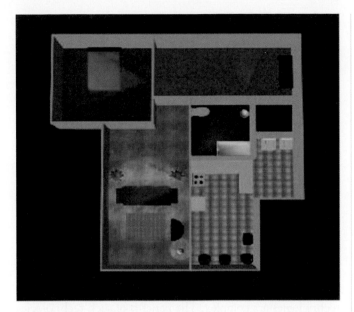

FIGURE 27–4. In-home monitoring system. (Source: http://marc.med. virginia.edu/projects_smarthomemonitor.html.)

Smart home technology is a broad term that refers to the incorporation of various information and communication technologies in living quarters. Homes can be equipped with different types of sensors, audio- and video technologies, and other assistive devices connected to a remote service site(s).[6,45]

In J.D.'s scenario, the family was able to locate a retirement community where each older adult can own his or her single home in a well-maintained campus and if needed, the community provides "smart home" technologies to protect its residents' safety in their home environment.[46-48] When J.D. and his children decided that J.D. would move in, they had a team meeting with the facility staff, including a nurse practitioner, physical and occupational therapists, facility manager, and social worker. The team made the decision to include the following smart home technology services:

- Motion sensors in the living area: Strategically placed sensors protect each individual's privacy while monitoring residents' activities.
- Floor carpet sensors: To detect falls.
- Sensors in the pantry and refrigerator doors: To ensure the older adults' daily meal consumption.
- Reminder board (memory board): A computer screen embedded in the wall to remind the resident of important plans/activities for the day. The frequency and reminder mode (eg, voice only, text only, or both) can be programmed as needed.
- Medical emergency alert system: This service is directly provided by the retirement community center.
- Telehealth systems: For J.D., this included the ongoing use of his own current medication management system and the telehealth program he used to manage his diabetes.
- The house is equipped with Internet access, touch screen computer interface, enabling J.D. to continue to use his own Web-based PHR provided by his private health insurance provider. J.D. and his family included the nurse practitioner in the facility as a provider and gave her limited access to J.D.'s PHR.

The following technologies were also available but J.D.'s current health condition did not yet make them necessary:

- Sink and bathtub monitors: This system monitors the water level of the sinks and the bathtubs. When a preset water level is reached, the system automatically turns off the water.
- The time of day voice reminder: The program provides messaging through voice units distributed around the house
- The stove monitor: This system monitors the stove and turns it off if smoke or gas is detected.
- Global Positioning System (GPS): GPS technology (eg, GPS shoes[49]) can provide older adults with mild cognitive impairment simple directions to help guide them when walking outdoors. GPS technology can also help caregivers rescue the older individual by providing information about his or her location at any point in time.[49,50]

UPCOMING TECHNOLOGIES

Technology-Based Games

The use of technology-based games (eg, video, computer, or online games) for health is an emerging research field.[51,52] Limited studies have found some positive effects of video-based games designed to improve health, especially for children (eg, increased energy expenditure).[53-55] Recently, older adults have also started using technology-based games, and some retirement communities have adopted those games, the most popular of which is the Nintendo Wii.[56] Effects of those games on health outcomes, however, still need investigation.

Researchers have been pilot testing the use of technology-based games to assess cognitive functions and to delay or even reverse cognitive decline. For instance, Jimison and associates[57] developed a computer game that has embedded assessment algorithms for various aspects of cognition. The monitoring of the user's performance over time allows the early detection of cognitive decline. Some other studies also have shown some limited effects of word games in assessing older adults' verbal fluency or card games to assess short-term memory and working memory.[57,58] Games also have been used for cognitive training for older adults.[57,59-61] Prior findings have shown that specific cognitive skills can be trained in older adults. The issue, however, has been that training of those specific skills did not seem to transfer to other cognitive abilities.[59,62] More recent studies have shown that use of selected methodologies (eg, training of reasoning skills or use of individualized feedback using individualized-scenario driven games) transfers to other functions, such as activities of daily livings (ADLs) or executive control functions or memory processes of older adults.[62,63] For more on cognitive training see Chapter 3.

Robotic Personal Assistants

Robotic technology is an exciting field that can integrate various aspects of assistive technologies and telehealth.[64-67] The levels of sophistication and the purposes of robots vary, such

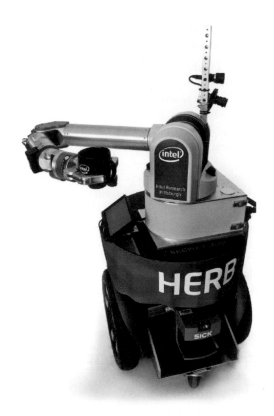

FIGURE 27–5. HERB (home exploring robotic butler). (Source: http://www.ri.cmu.edu/research_project_detail.html?type=publication&project_id = 639&menu_id=261.)

as HERB,[65] designed to assist older adults or persons with disability to maintain independence and healthier lives, or robot pets, the purpose of which is to provide psychosocial support (Figure 27–5).[67]

Robots designed as a personal assistant for older adults can incorporate various functions. They can assist older adults doing chores overcoming barriers, such as moving objects or doing laundry. Some other important functions can also be included, such as telemonitoring devices or memory aids reminding older adults of important tasks. More important, these robots can permit more realistic tele-presences (as compared to two-way videophones) and social interactions. Robots can be programmed to express their emotions depending on specific social context. The levels of help functions can be set based upon older adults' physical condition, and the robot's movements can be also monitored. These features will offer older adults the ability to maintain independent living in a safe environment.

ETHICAL ISSUES WITH TECHNOLOGY USE

CASE PRESENTATION 4: PRIVACY AND TECHNOLOGY

Patricia Kennedy lives in a continuing care retirement community (CCRC). Her health deteriorates, and additional assistance is needed to maintain her safety in her apartment. Currently, she lives in an apartment where the hallway has embedded video cameras for safety purposes. She also has a NurseBot that helps her manage her own health without a live-in caretaker. She expressed concerns that the video cameras on the hallway were intrusive and invaded her privacy. She also indicated that she did not need NurseBot and she wanted to continue to manage her own chores in her home.

Home automation may use various types and levels of technologies. For instance, monitoring of activities can be done using sensors, audio devices (eg, in bathrooms), or video cameras that are more obtrusive than sensors.[9,68] Although these technologies can help older adults maintain independent lives without risking their safety, ethical aspects of these assistive technologies are complex. The benefits of such technologies should be weighed against potential issues that may arise with their use. For instance, some technologies automatically perform many tasks that are helpful for keeping older adults cognitively stimulated and engaged and may ultimately increase their dependency on the technologies. If voice reminders constantly remind older adults of their schedules, they may not even try to remember things on their own, or they may not remember to turn off faucets if the system stops them automatically. Sometimes older adults may feel a loss of autonomy, if the technologies in their homes perform tasks according to the program set by others instead of their own preferences.

The potential benefits and detriments of these technologies must be carefully weighed in accordance with each individual's situation. Prior research has indicated that older adults vary with regard to their attitudes about use of technologies such as smart homes.[47,69] Some older adults addressed concerns about those technologies.[69] Others who tried such technologies reported that the need for safety could override the privacy issue.[47] In some cases, older adults' decreased cognitive abilities may hinder them from recognizing privacy issues; however, the issue still exists. In addition, the concept of and expectations for privacy may differ for individuals with different ethnicity and culture and must be assessed before selecting/configuring technology-based interventions. One of the resolutions of this ethical dilemma would be early preparation through discussions of these issues with older adults while they are still able to make such decisions.

CONCLUSION

Considering fast-growing modern technologies and the increasing number of older adults, more ICT-based health management programs and assistive technologies will be incorporated into older adults' living. Currently, collaborative efforts are being made between academia, aging organizations, and large corporate laboratories such as Intel[70] and GE[71] to facilitate a move toward a more integrated technological era associated with the care of older adults. In developing and implementing technologies, developers and providers must consider older adult users' unique design needs to ensure those technologies are indeed helping older adults without adding additional stress. Furthermore, technologies must connect all individuals involved in care of older adults (eg, older adults, family members, and health care providers). Development and delivery of these technologies are quite costly and must be addressed at the policy level to support more active research and development, as well as to ensure provision of such technologies for underserved older adults. At the same time, some other issues, such as ethical issues or measurement of cost-effectiveness, must be carefully evaluated.

References

1. Centers for Disease Control and Prevention. Chronic Disease Overview. Available at: http://www.cdc.gov/nccdphp/overview.htm. Accessed August 3, 2007.

2. Agency for Healthcare Research and Quality. Designing Healthcare Systems That Work for People with Chronic Illnesses and Disabilities. Available at: http://www.ahrq.gov/news/ulp/ulpchrn.htm. Accessed August 4, 2007.

3. Alzheimer's Association. 2009. Alzheimer's Disease Facts and Figures. Available at: http://www.alz.org/national/documents/report_alzfactsfigures2009.pdf. Accessed June 25, 2009.

4. Lyketsos CG, Colenda CC, Beck CT, et al. Position statement of the American Association for Geriatric Psychiatry regarding principles of care for patients with dementia resulting from Alzheimer disease. *Am J Geriatr Psychiatry*. 2006;14:561-572.

5. Resnick B, Galik E, Nahm ES, et al. Problems with adherence in the elderly; dementia/mild cognitive impairment. In: Shumaker SA, Ockene JK, Riekert KA, eds. *The Handbook of Health Behavior Change*. 3rd ed. New York: Springer; 2008:519-535.

6. Demiris G, Oliver DP, Dickey G, et al. Findings from a participatory evaluation of a smart home application for older adults. *Technology Health Care*. 2008;16:111-118.

7. Weintraub AJ, Kimmelstiel C, Levine D, et al. A multicenter randomized controlled comparison of telephonic disease management vs automated home monitoring in patients recently hospitalized with heart failure: SPAN-CHF II trial. Paper presented at the 9th Annual Scientific Meeting of the Heart Failure Society of America, September 18-21, 2005; Boca Raton.

8. Rainie, Lee. Pew Internet and American Life Project. Available at http://www.pewinternet.org/~/media//Files/Reports/2010/PIP_December09_update.pdf. Accessed July 21, 2010.

9. Kohn LT, Corrigan JM, Donaldson MS, eds. *To Err Is Human: Building a Safer Health System*. Washington, DC: National Academy Press; 2000.

10. US Government. White House: Issues—Technology. Available at: http://www.whitehouse.gov/issues/technology/.

11. Norman D. *The Design of Everyday Things*. New York: Basic Books; 2002.

12. Charness N, Schaie KW, eds. *Impact of Technology on Successful Aging*. New York: Springer; 2003.

13. Nahm ES, Resnick B, Covington B. Development of theory-based, online health learning modules for older adults: Lessons learned. *CIN: Computers, Informatics, Nursing*. 2006;24:261-268.

14. Nahm ES, Resnick B. Development and testing of the Web-Based Learning Self-Efficacy Scale (WBLSES) for older adults. *Ageing Int*. 2008;32:3-14.

15. Fisk AD, Rogers WA, Charness N, et al. *Designing for Older Adults: Principles and Creative Human Factors Approaches*. Boca Raton: CRC Press; 2004.

16. Proctor RW, Vu KPL, eds. *Handbook of Human Factors in Web Design*. Boca Raton: CRC Press; 2004.

17. Cacciabue PC, Cacciabue C. *Guide to Applying Human Factors Methods*. London: Springer; 2004.

18. Mead SE, Lamson N, Rogers WA. Human factors guidelines for Web site usability: Health-oriented Web sites for older adults. In: Morrell RW, ed. *Older Adults, Health Information, and the World Wide Web*. Mahwah, NJ: Erlbaum; 2002:89-107.

19. Fozard JL. Vision and hearing in aging. In: Birren KWS, ed. *Handbook of the Psychology of Aging*. 3rd ed. New York: Academic Press; 1990:150-170.

20. Ball K, Owsley C, Beard B. Clinical visual perimetry underestimates peripheral field problems in older adults. *Clin Vis Sci*. 1990;5:113-125.

21. Craik FIM, Salthouse TA, eds. *The Handbook of Ageing and Cognition*. Mahawah, NJ: Erlbaum; 2000.

22. Nielsen J. *Usability Engineering*. San Diego: Morgan Kaufmann; 1993.

23. Dix A, Finlay J, Abowd G, Beale R. *Human-Computer Interaction*. 3rd ed. London: Prentice Hall; 2003.

24. Nahm ES, Preece J, Resnick B, Mills ME. Usability of health Web sites for older adults: A preliminary study. *CIN: Computers Informatics*. 2004;22:326-334, 343.

25. Strehle EM, Shabde N. One hundred years of telemedicine: Does this new technology have a place in paediatrics? *Arch Dis Child*. 2006;91:956-959.

26. Murphy RLH, Bird K. Telediagnosis: A new community health resource. Observations on the feasibility of telediagnosis based on 1000 patient transactions. *Am J Public Health*. 1974;64:113-119.

27. Maheu M, Whitten P, Allen A. *E-health, Telehealth, and Telemedicine*. San Francisco: Jossey-Bass; 2001.

28. Barnason S, Zimmerman L, Nieveen J, et al. Impact of a home communication intervention for coronary artery bypass graft patients with ischemic heart failure on self-efficacy, coronary disease risk factor modification, and functioning. *Heart Lung*. 2003; 32:147-158.

29. Effertz G. Telemedicine 101: Using a business case for telehealth: A model for persuading decision makers. *Telemedicine Information Exchange*. April 18, 2005. Available at: http://tie.telemed.org/articles/article.asp?path=telemed101&article=businessCase_geffertz_tpr04.xml. Accessed October 10, 2005.

30. Aldred H, Gott M, Gariballa S. Advanced heart failure: Impact on older patients and informal carers. *J Adv Nurs*. 2005;49:116-124.

31. Trief PM, Teresi JA, Eimicke JP, et al. Improvement in diabetes self-efficacy and glycaemic control using telemedicine in a sample of older, ethnically diverse individuals who have diabetes: The IDEATel project. *Age Ageing*. 2009;38:219-225.

32. MedSignals. MedSignals. Available at: https://www.medsignals.com/default.aspx. Accessed June 15, 2009.

33. AgeLab T. Pill Pet. Available at: http://web.mit.edu/agelab/projects_wellness.shtml#1. Accessed March 1, 2007.

34. LifeStation Inc. 11 Crucial tips you need to know when choosing a medical alert system. Available at: http://www.lifestation.com/how_choose.php. Accessed June 10, 2009.

35. The HIMSS Personal Health Record Steering Committee. HIMSS Personal Health Records Definition and Position Statement. Available at: http://www.himss.org/content/files/PHRDefinition071707.pdf. Accessed June 15, 2009.

36. Ball MJ, Smith C, Bakalar RS. Personal health records: Empowering consumers. *J Healthcare Info Manage*. 2007;21:76-86.

37. Tang PC, Ash JS, Bates DW, et al. Personal health records: Definition, benefits, and strategies for overcoming barriers to adoption. *J Am Med Informatics Assoc*. 2006;13:121-126.

38. United States Department of Veterans Affairs. MyHealthe Vet: Overview. Available at: https://www.myhealth.va.gov/mhv-portalweb/anonymous.portal?_nfpb=true&_pageLabel=aboutMHVOverview&_nfls=false. Accessed September 3, 2008.

39. United States Department of Veterans Affairs. MyHealtheVet. Available at: https://www.myhealth.va.gov/mhv-portal-web/anonymous.portal?_nfpb=true&_nfto=false&_pageLabel=mhvHome. Accessed June 25, 2009.

40. Collmann J, Cooper T. Breaching the security of the Kaiser Permanente Internet patient portal: The organizational foundations of information security. *J Am Med Informatics Assoc*. 2007;14:239-243.

41. Iliffe S, Kharicha K, Harari D, et al. Health risk appraisal in older people. 2: The implications for clinicians and commissioners of social isolation risk in older people. *J R Coll Gen Pract*. 2007;57:277-282.

42. Horton KJ. Falls in older people: The place of telemonitoring in rehabilitation. *J Rehabil Res Dev*. 2008;45:1183-1194.

43. Wong P, Choy VY, Ng JS, et al. Elderly burn prevention: A novel epidemiological approach. *Burns*. 2007;33:995-1000.

44. Koskinen S, Joutsenniemi K, Martelin T, Martikainen P. Mortality differences according to living arrangements. *Int J Epidemiol*. 2007;36:1255-1264.

45. Helal A, Mokhtari M, Abdulrazak B. *The Engineering Handbook of Smart Technology for Aging, Disability and Independence*. Hoboken, NJ: Wiley-Interscience; 2008.

46. Demiris G, Hensel BK. Technologies for an aging society: A systematic review of "smart home" applications. *Yearbook Med Informatics*. 2008:33-40.

47. Courtney KL, Demiris G, Rantz M, Skubic M. Needing smart home technologies: The perspectives of older adults in continuing care retirement communities. *Informatics Prim Care*. 2008;16:195-201.

48. Adlam TD, Orpwood RD. Taking the Gloucester Smart House from the Laboratory to the Living Room. Work in Progress Bringing Smart House Technology for People with Dementia to Its Intended Users. Paper presented at the 3rd International Workshop on Ubiquitous Computing for Pervasive Healthcare Applications, Naha City, Okinawa, Japan; 2004.

49. Associated Press. GPS Shoes Make Tracking Kids, Elderly Easier. Available at: http://www.foxnews.com/story/0,2933,251122,00.html. Accessed March 1, 2007.

50. Global Action on Aging. Targeting Elderly Needing Help by GPS. Available at: http://www.globalaging.org/elderrights/world/2005/gps.htm. Accessed March 1, 2007.

51. The Serious Games Initiative. SeriousGames. Available at: http://www.seriousgames.org/index.html. Accessed January 30, 2010.

52. Robert Wood Johnson Foundation. Games for Health. Available at: http://www.rwjf.org/pr/product.jsp?id=29171. Accessed January 30, 2010.

53. Deutsch JE, Borbely M, Filler J, et al. Use of a low-cost, commercially available gaming console (Wii) for rehabilitation of an adolescent with cerebral palsy. *Phys Ther*. 2008;88:1196-1207.

54. Graf DL, Pratt LV, Hester CN, Short KR. Playing active video games increases energy expenditure in children. *Pediatrics*. 2009;124:534-540.

55. Lanningham-Foster L, Foster RC, McCrady SK, et al. Activity-promoting video games and increased energy expenditure. *J Pediatr*. 2009;154:819-823.

56. Snider M. Wii finds home in retirement communities, medical centers. *USA Today*, May 15, 2008.

57. Jimison HB, Pavel M, Bissell P, McKanna J. A framework for cognitive monitoring using computer game interactions. *Medinfo*. 2007;12:1073-1077.

58. Jimison H, Pavel M, Le T. Home-based cognitive monitoring using embedded measures of verbal fluency in a computer word game. Conference Proceedings: Annual International Conference of the IEEE Engineering in Medicine & Biology Society, 2008:3312-3315.

59. Ball K, Berch DB, Helmers KF, et al. Effects of cognitive training interventions with older adults: A randomized control trial. *JAMA*. 2002;288:2271-2281.

60. Schmall V, Grabinski CJ, Bowman S. Use of games as a learner-centered strategy in gerontology, geriatrics, and aging-related courses. *Gerontol Geriatr Ed*. 2008;29:225-233.

61. Cameron B, Dwyer F. The effect of online gaming, cognition and feedback type in facilitating delayed achievement of different learning objectives. *J Interact Learn Res*. 2005;16:243-258.

62. Basak C, Boot WR, Voss MW, Kramer AF. Can training in a real-time strategy video game attenuate cognitive decline in older adults? *Psychol Aging*. 2008;23:765-777.

63. Willis SL, Tennstedt SL, Marsiske M, et al. Long-term effects of cognitive training on everyday functional outcomes in older adults. *JAMA*. 2006;296:2805-2814.

64. Boissy P, Corriveau H, Michaud F, et al. A qualitative study of in-home robotic telepresence for home care of community-living elderly subjects. *J Telemed Telecare*. 2007;13:79-84.

65. Srinivasa S, Ferguson D, Helfrich C, et al. HERB: A home exploring robotic butler. *Autonomous Robots*. 2010;28:5-20.

66. Tsai TC, Hsu YL, Ma AI, et al. Developing a telepresence robot for interpersonal communication with the elderly in a home environment. *Telemed J E-Health*. 2007;13:407-424.

67. Tamura T, Yonemitsu S, Itoh A, et al. Is an entertainment robot useful in the care of elderly people with severe dementia? *J Gerontol Series A Biol Sci Med Sci*. 2004;59:83-85.

68. Chen J, Kam AH, Zhang J, et al. Bathroom Activity Monitoring Based on Sound. Paper presented at Third International Conference on Pervasive Computing, Munich, Germany, 2005.

69. Demiris G, Rantz MJ, Aud MA, et al. Older adults' attitudes towards and perceptions of "smart home" technologies: A pilot study. *Med Informatics Internet Med*. 2004;29:87-94.

70. Intel Corporation. Intel's Proactive Health Lab. Available at: http://www.intel.com/healthcare/hri/pdf/proactive_health.pdf. Accessed June 25, 2009.

71. SeniorNet. IBM and SeniorNet Unlock the World Wide Web for Millions More Users. Available at: http://www.seniornet.org/php/default.php?PageID=6583&Version=0&Font=0. Accessed March 1, 2007.

POST-TEST

1. **What kind of technology can be embedded in a patient's home to monitor older adults' falls that is usually acceptable to the elder?**
   A. Video camera
   B. Laser beam
   C. Carpet sensors
   D. Robots

2. **Before implementing technology-based interventions, which aspect of the user requirements is NOT generally assessed?**
   A. User's technology competency
   B. User's support by family
   C. User's perception of privacy and security toward the technology to be used
   D. User's preference for the intervention

3. **Ms. Jones lives independently in her retirement community and loves to walk. Although she manages to live independently, sometimes she gets lost when she goes for a walk. Which approach would be most helpful for Ms. Jones in order to remain healthy and safe?**
   A. Recommend she move to an assisted living place.
   B. Request that a staff member accompany her whenever she goes out for a walk.
   C. Embed a video camera on the hallway of her apartment so that the staff knows when she goes out and when she comes back.
   D. Have her use a global positioning system, so that when she gets lost the staff from the retirement center can help her.

ANSWERS TO PRE-TEST

1. B
2. D
3. A

ANSWERS TO POST-TEST

1. C
2. B
3. D

28

Interprofessional Management of the Complex Acute Surgical Patient

Mihaela S. Stefan, MD

Gladys L. Fernandez, MD

● **LEARNING OBJECTIVES**

1. Explain the role of geriatric medical consultants in optimizing the patient for surgery and evaluating prognosis.
2. Describe the unique geriatric considerations that influence mortality and morbidity in surgical outcome.
3. Define decision-making capacity and delineate consent and decisions that need to be made by individuals other than the patient.
4. Describe hazards of hospitalization in the elderly, including delirium, and the role of multidisciplinary approaches towards preventing these hazards.
5. Discuss transition of care within the hospital system and at discharge, including readmission risk in older adults.

PRE-TEST

1. **Which of the following factors related to surgical management of the geriatric patient does NOT contribute to increased mortality rates in this population?**

   A. Female gender

   B. Emergency surgical procedure

   C. Presence of polypharmacy

   D. Two or more involved family members

2. **Which of the following statements regarding informed consent is MOST correct?**

   A. Decision-making capacity is a prerequisite for providing informed consent or refusal.

   B. The treating physician makes the final judgment regarding decision-making capacity.

   C. A patient whose short-term memory is compromised may not provide consent for any suggested intervention.

   D. The formal requirements for binding power of living wills and durable power of attorney are universal and do not vary from state to state.

INTRODUCTION

The elderly represent approximately one-eighth of the US population, but they account for more than 25% of trauma and critical care resources.[1] By the year 2030, one in five people in the United States will be over age 65, while one out of four elderly individuals will be older than 85 years of age.[2] In this context, the preoperative evaluation of geriatric surgical patients is becoming more and more an important part of surgical practice in the 21st century. More elderly patients have surgery, and sicker patients are being considered to be eligible for surgery than in previous decades. Frail and elderly patients have medical issues that general surgeons are not uniformly trained to identify and address, such as impaired cognition, dementia, delirium, multiple co-morbidities, polypharmacy, depression, frequent falls, decreased nutrition, and social problems.[3] Many patients have associated co-morbid medical problems, which ideally should be managed concomitantly with the surgical issue(s).

Preoperative evaluation of elderly patients offers a prime opportunity for comprehensive geriatric assessment, and the medical or geriatric consultant can be instrumental in preparing the elderly patient for surgery, with the goal of preventing, identifying, and treating surgical or hospital-associated complications. It is important to understand the risk of coexisting disease, emergency presentations, and physical and cognitive function and their role in perioperative morbidity and mortality. Recent studies have shown that age is less predictive of operative mortality than is the presence of coexisting disease.[4] In addition, emergency procedures have been noted to be associated with higher mortality risk than in other age groups.[5] Changing views on timing of surgery for the elderly are turning toward early surgical intervention rather than later whenever possible, due to the nature of perioperative risk.[6] Delaying surgery just because of the patient's age is not consistently supported in the literature at the present time.[2] Ensuring that an early multidisciplinary team approach is sought during the course of patient care, from optimization of cardiopulmonary status to nutritional condition and multiple other factors in the preoperative and postoperative period, is critical for optimal outcomes.

To provide effective surgical care to this population one needs to understand the effect of aging on the anatomy, physiology, and psychology of the individual patient. Compared to patients younger than 65, older patients tend to have more co-morbidities, require longer hospital stays, exhibit higher risks of hospital-associated complications, and have higher re-hospitalization rates.[7] Many have preexisting cardiac, pulmonary, metabolic, endocrine, and neurologic states that may have an effect on perioperative outcomes. They are at higher risk for specific perioperative complications such as delirium, falls, pressure ulcers, infections, and iatrogenic complications. Caretakers involved with these patients need to be very cognizant of these perioperative risks in order to implement preventive strategies as well as monitor for the development of these problems. The literature suggests that careful assessment and management preoperatively and postoperatively are key factors in improving morbidity and mortality, and some institutions have developed medical–surgical co-management teams that care for complex patients in the perioperative setting.[8-12] The Co-management Geriatric Fracture Center implemented at Highland Hospital, New York demonstrated that using standardized geriatric evidence-based protocols resulted in shorter lengths of hospital stay, lower readmission rates, lower complication rates, and lower mortality for patients with hip fractures.[13] The co-management model between orthopedic surgeons and geriatricians is used in the United Kingdom, New Zealand, and Europe, but much less so in the United States.[8,14,15] Specialized acute-care geriatric units with environmental enhancement suitable for elderly patients have revealed improved patient outcomes without increasing costs.[16]

With the development of the hospitalist movement in the United States, hospitalists have become more involved in the perioperative care of surgical patients and medical co-management has become an important aspect of inpatient medicine. In a national survey in 1999, 44% of hospitalists reported that they were the primary physician for surgical patients.[17] The limited number of geriatricians in the United States, relative to the number of older patients with surgical problems, means that other health care professionals will have to be trained in geriatrics in order to provide optimal care for the elderly. The use of hospitalists as consultants for elderly surgical patients can be a valuable method of applying the principles of geriatric management in patient care, if the hospitalist has the geriatric training, knowledge, and skills to implement these specialized models of care.

CASE PRESENTATION: DECISIONAL CAPACITY IN AN OLDER TRAUMA PATIENT

Mr. Julio Mendes is a 78-year-old Hispanic male who is brought to the hospital by ambulance after being involved in a motor vehicle collision. The emergency medical technician report noted that the vehicle had significant front-end damage and the patient was found unrestrained in the driver's seat, awake but mildly confused. The patient reported driving at low speed in the downtown area and somehow losing control of his car and hitting a tree. You are part of the trauma team evaluating this patient. When you begin assessing the patient, you note that he is slightly disoriented and vague in his responses. His English is limited. His son arrives and reports that his father has had chills and a productive cough for the past 3 to 4 days and has not had much to eat or drink in days. He has been tired and has spent most of his time in bed. However, today he felt better and decided to go see his primary care physician.

Mr. Mendes has a history of hypertension, non–insulin-dependent diabetes mellitus, chronic atrial fibrillation, osteoarthritis, and hearing loss (for which he wears bilateral hearing aids). His medications include hydrochlorothiazide, lisinopril, atorvastatin, metformin, warfarin, metoprolol, and a multivitamin. His wife died 7 months ago, and after her death he moved from North Carolina to this area to live with his only son. His apartment is on the second floor and he goes up and down the stairs many times in the day without complaining of any chest pain or shortness of breath. The son does mention that his father has seemed forgetful lately and has lost approximately 10 pounds over the last 6 months.

Upon evaluation, the patient appears thin and frail and is moaning in pain. Vital signs include blood pressure (BP) 110/60 mm Hg, heart rate (HR) 102/min, temperature (T) 100.2°F (37.8°C), oxygen saturation (O_2 Sat) 93% on room air, and body mass index (BMI) 17 kg/m². The physical exam is remarkable for contusions over the left temporal region, poor dentition, bilateral cerumen impaction with no hearing aids in place, decreased breath sounds at the right base with dullness to percussion, slight tenderness to palpation over the left lower costal margin at the 11th and 12th rib levels anteriorly, irregularly irregular heart rhythm, abdomen with mild tenderness at the left upper quadrant and hypoactive bowel sounds, without rebound or guarding, Glasgow Coma Score (GCS) of 14 (with orientation to self and place, but only partially to time), and decreased hearing.

Laboratory studies are remarkable for white blood cell count (WBC) of 17,040 cells/mm³, hemoglobin (Hb) of 11.4 g/dL (114 g/l), serum sodium (Na+) of 148 mEq/L (148 mmol/L), blood urea nitrogen (BUN) of 28 mg/dL (9.99 mmol/L), creatinine (Cr) of 1.5 mg/dL (114.39 μmol/L), blood glucose of 243 mg/dL (13.76 mmol/L), albumin (Alb) of 2.7 g/dL (27 g/l), international normalized ratio (INR) of 2.8, and ethanol (EtOH) level of 0 mg/dL.

Chest radiograph reveals a possible right lower lobe consolidation; no fractures, hemothorax, or pneumothorax. Electrocardiogram reveals atrial fibrillation at a rate of approximately 100/min. CT of the abdomen and pelvis reveals a mild to moderate lower-pole splenic laceration without evidence of other injury. CT scan of the head and cervical spine, as well as plain films of the left wrist and ankle, are all negative for acute injury.

The trauma team decides that the patient may need a splenectomy if hemodynamic instability develops further after volume resuscitation and anticoagulation reversal. The team decides to manage him via close observation in a monitored ward for 1 to 2 days while optimizing his medical conditions. The surgical team informs the patient that he may need to have surgery if he deteriorates and asks him to sign consent for the possible laparotomy. During this request for consent, the patient repeatedly states, "I don't understand you" with a confused look on his face. The surgeon decides that the patient likely does not have optimal decision-making capacity and asks the son to sign the consent. In response, the son states "my father usually makes his own decisions" and refuses to sign the surgical consent.

BACKGROUND

In recent years, multiple task force mandates from a variety of leading organizations in health care have published critical information regarding the fact that outcomes in health care depend on effective team performance for all patients. These governing bodies include the Institute of Medicine (IOM), the Association for Healthcare Reform and Quality (AHRQ), the Joint Commission for Assessment of Healthcare Organizations (JCAHO), the World Health Organization (WHO), and others in specialty areas of medical, nursing, and ancillary health care. The authors of this chapter emphasize the magnitude of the importance of these principles for management of the geriatric population, whereby minimal error, breaks in communication, or seemingly unimportant factors may account for large differences in outcomes, often to the detriment of the patient.

SPECIAL CONSIDERATIONS IN ELDERLY PATIENTS

In addition to the characteristic changes that take place with aging, the frequent progression of noteworthy disease states can have a profound impact on an elderly person's response to injury and stress. Awareness of concomitant disease states is vital to the appropriate management of the injured elderly, and an aggressive search for such information is essential.

This information will influence management strategies, as well as aid in planning care. Cardiovascular diseases, diabetes mellitus, liver disease, malignancy, pulmonary disease, renal disease, and neurologic compromise are common conditions encountered in this population which must be assessed and understood in order to optimize perioperative care.[10] Cognitive, functional, and psychosocial impairments also greatly influence management strategies provided by health care teams.

CASE PRESENTATION (continued)

The trauma team asks the geriatrician to help evaluate the patient for decision-making capacity.

When examining the patient, the geriatrician notices that he has cerumen impaction and he lacks his hearing aids. The cerumen is removed after lavaging the ear canal with a syringe and warm water, and the patient is provided with his hearing aids. Because the patient's English is very limited, a Spanish interpreter has been asked to assist the surgeon in explaining the procedure. The geriatrician performed a cognitive evaluation using the MiniCog and the patient had a score of 3 and a normal clock drawing test, both of which lead to the conclusion that he is not demented. Questioning both the son and patient about his physical function revealed that he was able to do all his ADLs as well as driving and shopping for groceries.

After the patient is provided with his hearing aids and assisted by a Spanish interpreter, he is informed about the risks and benefits of surgery in simple and clear language and he agrees to consent for possible surgery. Under these additional circumstances, he was able to communicate his choice, demonstrate understanding of the information given about the medical condition, appreciate the risks and benefits of the procedure, and was able to discuss the options with the surgeon.

Lack of clear comprehension regarding the needs of elderly patients by teams without geriatric training plays a significant role in the excess morbidity and mortality in elderly trauma and surgical patients.[18] Often, the medical consultant follows the well-known preoperative guidelines for cardiac and pulmonary risk stratification and medication adjustment, and ignores specific assessments and prevention factors important for the geriatric patient. (Please see Chapter 21 for further details.) The goal of preoperative assessment in an elderly patient is to identify factors associated with increased risk of specific complications related to procedures and tailoring of the management plan for the elderly. The preoperative assessment for an elderly patient should include cognitive, functional, and nutritional assessment, as well as review of

psychosocial factors and advance directives. These are often as important as the physiologic major organ system testing and evaluations that most preoperative patients are subjected to.

Cognitive Status

Cognitive impairment is common in patients older than age 70 and is a risk factor for developing delirium postoperatively.[19] Elderly patients should be assessed for their cognitive abilities at baseline prior to surgery, as it will serve as a prognostic indicator as well as make it easier to detect delirium if it appears. Unfortunately, there are no validated tools for assessing cognition in the acute hospital setting. Most health care providers use the MiniCog Assessment instrument, which combines a three-item recall test with a clock-drawing test that can be administered in about 3 minutes, does not require any special equipment, and is relatively uninfluenced by level of education or language.[20] Our patient was assessed for cognitive impairment, but this should be done with the help of a Spanish translator. If head injury had been a confounding injury in this trauma setting, this baseline assessment might not be reliable. Caretakers also need to be aware of the effects of analgesics and other medications, as well as hemodynamic and ventilatory factors, endocrine states, and metabolic conditions that may impair cognitive abilities when preparing to make such assessments. (For more in-depth information about cognitive assessment please see Chapters 3, 30, and 31.)

Functional Status

The functional assessment should document activities of daily living (ADLs) which include toileting, feeding, dressing, grooming, physical ambulation, and bathing, as well as instrumental activities of daily living (IADLs), which include telephone use, shopping for groceries, transportation, meal preparation, housework, and handling of finances. These functional assessments should be made at or near time of admission, and are also very important for discharge planning. (For more details on functional assessment please see Chapter 7.)

Frailty, which is seen more often in elderly adults, places them at increased risk of adverse events such as death, disability, and institutionalization. In the Cardiovascular Health Study published in the United States in 2001, 7.3% of women over age 65, and 4.9% of men over 65, were frail, with frailty being especially common in those over 80 years of age.[21-24] As a result of aging, physiologic reserve of every organ system declines and the capacity to compensate under stress decreases as well. (See Chapter 36 for more on frailty and functional decline.)

Nutritional Status

Nutritional status is a key factor related to the perioperative course. Poor nutrition can complicate the postoperative course, resulting in poor wound healing, prolonged intubation, and extended hospitalization.[25] This patient has a BMI of 17 kg/m^2 and his albumin is 2.7 (27 g/L), both of which indicate that he is probably seriously malnourished. Hypoalbuminemia increases the risk of pulmonary complications and correlates with increased mortality and increased rates of readmission.[26,27] Efforts should be made to avoid long periods of "nothing by mouth" before surgery. A dietician should be consulted for appropriate recommendations, and in our patient a full dietary assessment and initiation of high-calorie foods would be appropriate.

Psychological Status

This patient should be assessed for depression by the Geriatric Depression Scale (GDS) short form, as depression is very frequent in hospitalized patients. The GDS is an easy-to-use, well-recognized instrument to diagnose depression.[28] In the case scenario presented here, it was noted that this patient's wife died only 7 months ago, and thereafter he moved from his home to live with his son. Patients with depression are noted to have longer hospital stays and experience worse hospital outcomes. Psychosocial assessments and evaluation of mental status, mood, and psychiatric conditions may be required during this hospitalization. (For more on depression please see Chapter 37.)

Co-Morbidities

Mr. Mendes' risk of developing cardiovascular complications is low because he had good functional status (prior to hospitalization he was able to climb a flight of stairs, which is equivalent to 4 METs). Diabetes mellitus is the only cardiac risk factor that increases his risk of perioperative cardiovascular complications. He has a mild increased risk of perioperative stroke because the anticoagulation required reversal and cessation due to his injuries and inherent surgical bleeding risks. His other co-morbid risk factor is his malnutrition, which puts his ability to deal with the stress of hospitalization as well as a possible surgery in a significantly compromised condition.

It is wise to adequately prepare an elderly patient for surgery, but unwise to defer surgery simply on the basis of age, especially in the case of urgent and emergent conditions, as multiple studies have noted that age is a less important independent risk factor for surgical outcomes than other factors noted earlier.[5,6] As noted in a comprehensive review by Souders and Rooke, studies that factor co-morbidities into analyses indicate that age primarily increases operative risk via an interaction with co-morbid disease, and that age alone is not an independent predictor.[27] As such, it is evident that the need for expert consultant care in co-morbid states of the elderly patient may be a vital component of outcome measures in this population.[9] Unnecessary delay at intervention may result in aggravation of the inciting condition, as well as exacerbate complications related to preexisting conditions. Early consultation, efficient optimization of conditions in the preoperative and postoperative period, effective communication, and multidimensional understanding of the numerous factors essential to patient care, as noted earlier, are critical to affecting perioperative risk. Families are often concerned about the

risk of surgery; however, it is imperative that the medical team inform them that they should be more concerned about the risks of the postoperative period. Souder and Rooke's review of perioperative care for the geriatric population revealed that morbidity and mortality rates are doubled in the first 24 hours after surgery and are tenfold higher over the first postoperative week.[4]

● DECISION-MAKING AND MEDICAL CONSENT

Obtaining informed consent before performing any procedure is the responsibility of the treating physician, who should explain the nature of the problem, the proposed intervention, the alternative approaches, and the risks and benefits of the procedure. Assessment of patient decision-making capacity to consent to treatment is imperative before turning to surrogate decision-makers. (For more in-depth discussion about how to assess medical decision-making capacity, please see Chapter 10.) There is a preconceived notion that elderly, frail adults are not capable of making their own decisions, and often medical personnel seek alternatives to obtaining informed consent from the patient before it is indicated.[29] Prior to deciding that this patient cannot make a decision about surgery or treatment, one needs to identify if there is any cause to remediate. The patient in this case had limited English proficiency and a Spanish interpreter was utilized to translate the assessment of comprehension and decision-making capacity. He also had hearing impairment and he should have working hearing aids in place. The interpreter is an important member of the team when managing a patient who does not speak English or who has limited proficiency in the language. More information needed to be obtained from the son regarding the patient's baseline cognitive status and what he meant by stating that "my father makes his own decisions" and additionally, what type of decisions the patient really makes. In addition, one must consider social and cultural circumstances that may arise due to varying ethnic and/or heritage principles with respect to hierarchy, parental roles, and issues of respect. Understanding cultural norms and socio-ethnic behavioral principles regarding discussions being addressed in patient care, such as in this case, are important to keep in mind. In addition, obtaining a detailed social history is critical in evaluating his baseline function and social situation as well as obtaining information from his primary care physician that may shed light on family dynamics, pre-hospitalization status, and discussions about advanced directives.

The decision-making capacity of this patient should be assessed by the treating physician. When there is uncertainty or conflict, a psychiatry or geriatric consult should be requested. Psychiatric consultation may also be useful for a patient with mental illness or impaired judgment. Up to 25% of inpatient psychiatry consults are called for assessing patient's competence for treatment-related decisions.[30] In addition, inclusion of social services, chaplaincy services, and occasionally an expert in medical ethics may be required in order to assist with patient and family discussions regarding prognosis and expectations for meaningful recovery.[31] It is always prudent to consider early consultation with experts in ethics and social services to help the entire health care team with difficult decisions. It is only with the assistance of multiple experts in vital areas that an appropriate approach can be led toward making decisions critical to patient care.

CASE PRESENTATION (continued)

The patient is evaluated by a medical consultant, who concludes that he has a low cardiovascular risk for surgery and intermediate risk for perioperative pulmonary complications. Metformin, hydrochlorothiazide, and warfarin are on hold and metoprolol is increased to control his heart rate. Ceftriaxone and azithromycin are started for a possible community-acquired pneumonia. Fresh frozen plasma and vitamin K are used to reverse anticoagulation in preparation for surgery. The hospitalist asks to be re-consulted if new problems arise and recommends the need for nutritional consultation and social work assessment for discharge planning as well.

On the afternoon of hospital day 2, Mr. Mendes develops abdominal distension, increased pain, and hypotension and is taken emergently to the operating room for a splenectomy. The surgical team informs the medical consultant of this turn of events and the medical consultant agrees to follow the patient after surgery. The surgery for splenectomy was uneventful and the patient returned to the surgical ward after a brief period of time in the post-anesthesia care unit. Postoperatively, he was maintained on intravenous fluids, perioperative antibiotics, and intravenous morphine for pain control. A Foley urinary catheter had been inserted for assessment of volume status and he was provided with an incentive spirometer for pulmonary toilet and sequential compression devices for deep venous thrombosis prophylaxis.

On the morning of hospital day 4 (postoperative day 2 status post surgery), Mr. Mendes' son exits from the patient's room upset because he arrived to find his father in restraints, his breakfast tray untouched, and his father agitated and not recognizing him. During the previous night, the patient had repeatedly tried to get out of bed and pull out his intravenous lines and his urinary catheter. He had been calling for his dead wife. The patient was uncooperative with any blood draws and did not take any medications by mouth.

From the chart notes you find out that the patient was lethargic on postoperative day 1. He received morphine intravenously at a dose of 4 mg on five occasions for pain and has not had a bowel movement since

admission. Overnight, he also received intravenous injections of diphenhydramine 12.5 mg for sleep and lorazepam 1 mg twice due to agitation. Orders for medications had been noted to be duplicated and/or contradicting in several areas of the patient's chart from various sources. Upon review of the postoperative course, the surgical and medical team agree to discuss the patient's progress to date in detail, review feedback on a daily basis, and proceed with a multidisciplinary approach to care, but with only the primary admitting team writing any orders into the chart based on all recommendations. In this manner, all input and care is directed by a single leading group composed of several experts in the necessary designated patient care areas vital to this case. Mr. Mendes' medications are streamlined, the duplicate orders are deleted, the diphenhydramine and lorazepam are discontinued, and he is given a scheduled laxative after two enemas result in good stool output.

● HAZARDS OF HOSPITALIZATION

This patient has an acute confusional state known as delirium and the following factors should be considered to be contributing or causing the confusion: recent anesthesia, pain, narcotics, anticholinergic medications, benzodiazepines, constipation, unmasked dementia, depression, hearing impairment, sleep-cycle disturbance, electrolyte disturbances, hypoglycemia, ethanol withdrawal, urosepsis from a urinary tract infection (the Foley catheter is still in place), postoperative cardiac ischemia, anemia, hypotension, hypoxia, or pneumonia. Upon review of his postoperative course, it is evident, as is noted in most states of confusion and delirium in the elderly, that the cause is multifactorial. Delirium complicates hospitalization of older patients in 25% of inpatients, and the incidence ranges from 5.1% to as high as 52.2% after noncardiac surgery.[19] The 1-year mortality rate for patients with delirium has been reported to be 35% to 40%.[32] Delirium prevention should begin in the preoperative period, and all patients older than 65 years should be screened for risk factors for postoperative delirium. Prevention of delirium should engage the nurse, the family member, geriatrician, physical therapist, and other health care providers.

Despite being one of the most frequent postoperative complications for elderly patients, the lack of assessing cognitive function at admission is an important reason for missing the diagnosis of delirium when it appears later. Preexisting dementia is a major factor for developing delirium in the hospital.[33] Without timely diagnosis, management is delayed or suboptimal. There are three main types of interventions for delirium: general geriatric approaches, nursing care, and family interventions. Involvement of the geriatric team (geriatrician, geriatric nurse, hospitalist with geriatric training) can prevent or decrease the risk of postoperative delirium.[34] Some of the interventions are nonpharmacologic and require active nursing participation: orientation protocols, nonpharmacologic protocols for sleep, noise reduction, provision of visual and hearing aids, and removal of indwelling catheters. Presence of family members is very important in preventing delirium, and the family should be considered part of the patient care team. The family should be updated daily regarding the medical condition and should be asked to stay with the elderly patient as much as possible because it will aid with reorientation and decrease the anxiety caused by the new and unfamiliar environment. For the elderly patient, the risk of delirium should be assessed in the preoperative consultation period and a multicomponent strategy should be implemented to reduce the patient's risk of developing delirium. The family should be informed about the vulnerability and risks of their loved one to develop delirium. Another person who should be involved in minimizing the vulnerability and susceptibility of the patient to postoperative delirium is the rehabilitation specialist. Physical and occupational therapy should be involved in patient care soon after surgery because early mobilization and activity is another measure that can decrease the risk of developing delirium.[34,35]

The nursing staff needs to understand the susceptibility of the elderly patient for delirium and how important nonpharmacologic approaches are for prevention and treatment. Restraints should be avoided at all costs, and alternative pharmacologic and nonpharmacologic strategies to manage the agitated or delirious patient should be implemented. In a randomized control study of patients with hip fractures, Marcantonio and associates demonstrated that a multi-component strategy that involved a multidisciplinary team with a geriatrician was able to prevent one case of delirium for every five patients seen.[35] While geriatric consultation is not available in all institutions, the recommendations in the study are evidence-based, proactive, and practical interventions. A "delirium room" model with dedicated beds, trained staff, and interdisciplinary rounds demonstrated that elderly patients with delirium could be treated with nonpharmacological measures and without physical restraints in most cases.[36] In a prospective, controlled clinical trial of 850 hospitalized patients 70 years or older, Inouye[34] demonstrated that an intervention strategy consisting of standardized protocols for management of the main risk factors for delirium (cognitive impairment, sleep deprivation, immobility, visual and hearing impairment, and dehydration) resulted in a significant reduction in the number and duration of episodes of delirium. (For more on delirium see Chapter 30.)

Hospitalized elderly patients can develop iatrogenic complications that may or may not be related to the initial diagnosis. These can prolong hospitalization and cause significant decline in functional status. Many of the risk factors for these hazards can be identified and addressed, and there is evidence that the incidence of these complications can be reduced.[34,37] The most important identified risk factors are sensory impairment (decreased hearing and vision), incontinence, polypharmacy, malnutrition, depression, immobility, falls, and sleep problems.[37] Some of the hazards are risk factors for developing another complication, the most important being delirium, which can result in falls, incontinence, and pressure ulcers. Decreasing the incidence of these hazards requires a multidisciplinary team approach or at a minimum a clinician skilled at risk assessment. Prevention of some hazards is discipline-specific, whereas others require that all members of the team be aware of the risks. Some of these hazards are considered in the nursing purview, such as orienting to day and time, and informing the patient what his or her plan of care is and when tests will be performed, but the physician cannot address them if he or she is not made aware. After surgery, patients often have limited dietary intake, in addition to often having been without oral intake for a period preoperatively. As such, they are often in a negative nitrogen balance state in the perioperative period. Insufficient nutrition can result in malnutrition, infection, increased risk of pressure ulcers, delay in wound healing, and delayed recovery.[38] A Cochrane review on dietary supplements showed a small decrease in mortality, in undernourished persons, and small but consistent weight gain but no effects on length of stay, clinical outcomes, or improvement in function in elderly hospitalized patients at risk or suffering from malnutrition.[39] A dietary consultant can assess the patient's needs and guide the nutritional interventions (eg, nutritional supplements) that will most benefit the patient. In the case of Mr. Mendes, the dietician recommended high-calorie foods and a supplement between meals.

Another risk factor of morbidity and mortality in the perioperative period is immobility. After surgery, patients may be placed on bed rest for extended periods; they may have limited mobility due to pain, or be inadvertently immobilized through chemical or physical restraints. Just a few days of bed rest will result in loss of muscle mass and strength and will require long periods of rehabilitation because efforts at reconditioning take much longer than the time needed for deconditioning.[22] For an elderly patient, 1 day of rest results in loss of up to 5% of muscle strength, and an increase in the risk of falls.[37] Falls alone are known to be a leading cause of morbidity and mortality in elderly patients, and several studies have revealed that early mobilization of patients can prevent complications and lead to improved functional recovery post-discharge.[40] Immobility is also a risk factor for pressure ulcers, increase in vasomotor instability, and bone demineralization.[41]

CASE PRESENTATION (continued)

By day 4 post-splenectomy, Mr. Mendes' cognition has improved, his pain is well controlled on small amounts of oral analgesics, and he is out of bed to a chair, but his diet remains quite poor. Physical therapy evaluated him today and found that he is able to transfer with the assistance of one person. The son states that his father is almost back to his baseline but "not quite." He appears alert, oriented to person and place, but not to the date. On physical exam, the incision site is healing well without any signs of infection and he has good bowel, bladder, and respiratory function.

The case manager calls a meeting with the primary team, physical therapist, geriatrician, and nurse and they discuss plans for discharge and transition of care issues.

TRANSITION OF CARE AND DISCHARGE PLANNING

At this point we should assess whether the patient is back to his or her baseline functional status and the geriatric functional assessment prior to hospitalization should be reviewed using the activities of daily living (ambulating, transferring, feeding, dressing, bathing, toileting) as well as instrumental activities of daily living (cooking, shopping, medication use, telephone use, transportation, paying bills, and housekeeping). The documentation of ADL/IADL is more frequently done by the admitting nurse or by the physical therapist than other health care providers. For the patient to be discharged to home, the health care team needs to ensure that he or she is close to baseline functional status, has the resources to manage at home, and that any safety issues are addressed prior to going home.

Physical therapy and occupational therapy play a critical role in achieving this goal and they should be consulted as soon as possible with the goal of preparing the patient to go home. Physical therapy will evaluate the patient's gait and mobility, will help the patient improve strength, and will recommend the appropriate assistive devices for ambulation. Occupational therapy will evaluate the patient for the ability to complete activities of daily living and may perform a home visit to assess the need for grab bars, elevated toilet seats, or other safety items.

The discharge planner needs to be consulted early in the hospitalization to assure a smooth transition of care from the hospital to home or to a rehabilitation unit. The patient's living situation and social support should be clarified. We should also recognize what individualized interventions and services are needed for the patient in order to go home and be safe and independent. (For more on transitional care see Chapter 22.)

CASE PRESENTATION (continued)

By postoperative day 5 the delirium has completely resolved and the patient's son wants to take him back home. The case manager is concerned to have the patient home alone for 8 hours daily when the son is at work and suggests short-term rehabilitation. However, Mr. Mendes' wife was in a nursing home and sustained a fall with multiple complications leading to her death. Because of this incident, the patient and his family insist on having him back home and are agreeable to having someone at home with him 24 hours a day for the first week after his discharge.

Optimally all team members should participate in the discharge planning process, and this process should begin early in the hospitalization. It is important to remember that the patient is the decision-maker. A family meeting should include the patient, patient's spouse or family member, surgeon, geriatrician or medical consultant, discharge planner, physical therapist, and nurse at a minimum. Other supportive family members should also be included in this meeting if they are cited as individuals who will assist in the patient's transition back to home life. The patient and family should be presented with the options and facilities available (nursing home/skilled nursing facility, transitional care unit, acute rehabilitation, and home with services), how insurance coverage will affect this discharge plan, and what resources are available if he or she goes home. Many patients prefer to go to back to their familiar surroundings, and physicians should honor this preference with the appropriate support if possible.

Optimizing Discharge Planning

A multidisciplinary approach to the treatment and rehabilitation of the surgical elderly that begins at the time of hospital admission is important in ensuring that optimal discharge standards are met. Home care agencies, spouses, and family members play an integral role in allowing patients to return home and to a productive life.[42] In other words, minimization of readmission risk begins with awareness and coordination at the time of admission. Lack of coordination of care is common after hospital discharge, and there are multiple studies that have documented this.[43] When a patient is discharged from the hospital, the primary care physician is frequently not aware of the hospitalization, discharge summaries do not include accurate information, or the primary caretaker does not have access to the discharge summary record.[44] Forty-eight percent of patients who received a new medication in the hospital reported not getting information about the side effects of the drug,[45] and 47% of patients were unable to repeat the physician instructions, demonstrating a lack of clarity provided by the physician.[46] There is evidence that detailed preparation of the patient and family with a "discharge coach" and timely follow-up with the primary care physician reduces rehospitalization.[47] Patient and family education on the discharge plan that includes medications, diet, activity prescriptions, knowledge of the warning signs and how to respond, is very important in decreasing the risk of readmission. A comprehensive discharge summary has to be transmitted to the physician accepting responsibility of care and be available to all those involved in post-discharge care. An early follow-up visit with the primary care physician a few days after hospitalization is very important to decrease the patient's risk of readmission.

So how might this all work in an ideal situation? Let's look at the case and see what could have been done better. At the time of admission Mr. Mendes was living alone and was residing in a second-floor apartment. His social network included one son who lives in the area. He was independent in all activities of daily living as well as transportation and shopping.

Later we found out that he did not want to go to a nursing home for rehabilitation at any cost. His social work problem list might look like this:

Problem	Action Item
1. Second-floor apartment, possible mobility concerns	Consider gait function prior to discharge.
2. Limited social network, one son who works	See if other family or friends in the area.
3. Refusal to go to nursing home rehab	Evaluate resources for home therapy, and possible home aid, no need for PPD placement for nursing home.
4. Lack of transportation	Consider driver safety evaluation, look into transportation alternatives.

Subsequently his medical team would try to address these problems as well as call and update his primary care provider as to his condition, medical diagnoses and treatment in the hospital, what medication changes occurred, including stopping the warfarin for his surgery, as well as arranging post hospital discharge follow-up in a timely manner. With a proper assessment of his resources and his current functional status as well as weighing his preferences a mutually agreeable discharge plan can be developed that addresses his needs as well as communicates with his regular physician what has transpired and what he will need in the near future.

CONCLUSION

The geriatric population presents differences in physiology and complexity of care at a multitude of levels. Outcome goals aimed at reduced morbidity and mortality make the comprehensive and multidisciplinary approach toward elderly patients necessary. A meticulous preoperative assessment and preparation for surgery is essential. Thorough assessment and detailed management of the postoperative conditions prevalent in this population must also be at the forefront of care. The vulnerable elderly patient with multiple medical co-morbidities is best served by collaboration among health care providers with skills in geriatric care and requires aggressive, team-based, interdisciplinary and multidisciplinary care to best ensure optimal outcomes for this patient population.

References

1. MacKenzie EJ, Morris JA Jr, Smith GS, Fahey M. Acute hospital costs of trauma in the United States: Implications for regionalized systems of care. *J Trauma.* 1990;30:1096-1101; discussion 1101-1103.

2. Liu LL, Leung JM. Perioperative Complications in Elderly Patients. in the *Syllabus on Geriatric Anesthesiology.* http://www.asahq.org/clinical/ geriatrics/perio_comp.htm. Accessed July 21, 2010.

3. Hardin RE, Le Jemtel T, Zenilman ME. Experience with dedicated geriatric surgical consult services: Meeting the need for surgery in the frail elderly. *Clin Interv Aging.* 2009;4:73-80.

4. Souders J, Rooke G. Perioperative Care for Geriatric Patients. *Ann Long Term Care.* 2005;6:1524-1530.

5. Khoja JR GD, Gupta M, Nagar RC. Evaluation of risk factors and outcome of surgery in elderly patients. *J Ind Acad Geriatr.* 2008;1.

6. Caron JL. Surgery in the elderly patient: A time for reappraisal. *Can J Surg.* 1996;39:94-95.

7. Barlow AP, Zarifa Z, Shillito RG, et al. Surgery in a geriatric population. *Ann R Coll Surg Engl.* 1989;71:110-114.

8. Vidan M, Serra JA, Moreno C, et al. Efficacy of a comprehensive geriatric intervention in older patients hospitalized for hip fracture: A randomized, controlled trial. *J Am Geriatr Soc.* 2005;53: 1476-1482.

9. Fisher AA, Davis MW, Rubenach SE, et al. Outcomes for older patients with hip fractures: The impact of orthopedic and geriatric medicine cocare. *J Orthop Trauma* 2006; 20(3): 172-178; discussion 179-180.

10. Elliot JR, Wilkinson TJ, Hanger HC, et al. Collaboration with orthopaedic surgeons. *Age Ageing.* 1996;25:414.

11. Elliot JR, Wilkinson TJ, Hanger HC, et al. Collaboration with orthopaedic surgeons. *Age Ageing.* 1996;25:259.

12. Elliot JR, Wilkinson TJ, Hanger HC, et al. The added effectiveness of early geriatrician involvement on acute orthopaedic wards to orthogeriatric rehabilitation. *NZ Med J.* 1996;109:72-73.

13. Friedman SM, Mendelson DA, Kates SL, McCann RM. Geriatric co-management of proximal femur fractures: total quality management and protocol-driven care result in better outcomes for a frail patient population. *J Am Geriatr Soc.* 2008;56: 1349-1356.

14. Thwaites JH, Mann F, Gilchrist N, et al. Shared care between geriatricians and orthopaedic surgeons as a model of care for older patients with hip fractures. *NZ Med J.* 2005;118:U1438.

15. Zuckerman JD, Sakales SR, Fabian DR, Frankel VH. Hip fractures in geriatric patients. Results of an interdisciplinary hospital care program. *Clin Orthop Relat Res.* 1992:213-225.

16. Kresevic DM, Counsell SR, Covinsky K, et al. A patient-centered model of acute care for elders. *Nurs Clin North Am.* 1998;33: 515-527.

17. Lindenauer PK, Pantilat SZ, Katz PP, Wachter RM. Hospitalists and the practice of inpatient medicine: Results of a survey of the National Association of Inpatient Physicians. *Ann Intern Med.* 1999;130:343-349.

18. Boyd CM, Landefeld CS, Counsell SR, et al. Recovery of activities of daily living in older adults after hospitalization for acute medical illness. *J Am Geriatr Soc.* 2008;56:2171-2179.

19. Dasgupta M, Dumbrell AC. Preoperative risk assessment for delirium after noncardiac surgery: A systematic review. *J Am Geriatr Soc.* 2006;54:1578-1589.

20. Borson S, Scanlan JM, Watanabe J, et al. Simplifying detection of cognitive impairment: Comparison of the Mini-Cog and Mini-Mental State Examination in a multiethnic sample. *J Am Geriatr Soc.* 2005;53:871-874.

21. Fried LP, Tangen CM, Walston J, et al. Frailty in older adults: Evidence for a phenotype. *J Gerontol A Biol Sci Med Sci.* 2001; 56:M146-M156.

22. Gill TM, Allore H, Guo Z. The deleterious effects of bed rest among community-living older persons. *J Gerontol A Biol Sci Med Sci.* 2004;59:755-761.

23. Gill TM, Allore H, Holford TR, Guo Z. The development of insidious disability in activities of daily living among community-living older persons. *Am J Med.* 2004;117:484-491.

24. Gill TM, Allore HG, Holford TR, Guo Z. Hospitalization, restricted activity, and the development of disability among older persons. JAMA. 2004;292:2115-2124.

25. Schiesser M, Kirchhoff P, Muller MK, et al. The correlation of nutrition risk index, nutrition risk score, and bioimpedance analysis with postoperative complications in patients undergoing gastrointestinal surgery. Surgery. 2009;145:519-526.

26. Corti MC, Guralnik JM, Salive ME, Sorkin JD. Serum albumin level and physical disability as predictors of mortality in older persons. JAMA. 1994;272:1036-1042.

27. Gibbs J, Cull W, Henderson W, et al. Preoperative serum albumin level as a predictor of operative mortality and morbidity: Results from the National VA Surgical Risk Study. Arch Surg. 1999;134:36-42.

28. Sheikh JA, Gambhir YK. Analysis of the truncation schemes for the physical boson states with Dyson's description. Phys Rev C Nucl Phys. 1986;34:2344-2347.

29. Eiseman B. Surgical decision making and elderly patients. Bull Am Coll Surg. 1996;81:8-11, 65.

30. Farnsworth MG. The impact of judicial review of patients' refusal to accept antipsychotic medications at the Minnesota Security Hospital. Bull Am Acad Psychiatry Law. 1991;19:33-42.

31. Rix TE, Bates T. Pre-operative risk scores for the prediction of outcome in elderly people who require emergency surgery. World J Emerg Surg. 2007;2:16.

32. Demeure MJ, Fain MJ. The elderly surgical patient and postoperative delirium. J Am Coll Surg 2006. 203:752-757.

33. Williams-Russo P, Urquhart BL, Sharrock NE, Charlson ME. Postoperative delirium: Predictors and prognosis in elderly orthopedic patients. J Am Geriatr Soc. 1992;40:759-767.

34. Inouye SK. A practical program for preventing delirium in hospitalized elderly patients. Cleve Clin J Med. 2004;71:890-896.

35. Marcantonio ER, Flacker JM, Wright RJ, Resnick NM. Reducing delirium after hip fracture: A randomized trial. J Am Geriatr Soc. 2001;49:516-522.

36. Weeks SK. RAP: A restraint alternative protocol that works. Rehabil Nurs. 1997;22:154-156.

37. Creditor MC. Hazards of hospitalization of the elderly. Ann Intern Med. 1993;118:219-223.

38. Costarelli V, Emery PW. The effect of protein malnutrition on the capacity for protein synthesis during wound healing. J Nutr Health Aging. 2009;13:409-412.

39. Milne AC, Potter J, Vivanti A, Avenell A. Protein and energy supplementation in elderly people at risk from malnutrition. Cochrane Database Syst Rev. 2009;2:CD003288.

40. Hoenig HM, Rubenstein LZ. Hospital-associated deconditioning and dysfunction. J Am Geriatr Soc. 1991;39:220-222.

41. Lindgren M, Unosson M, Fredrikson M, Ek AC. Immobility—a major risk factor for development of pressure ulcers among adult hospitalized patients: A prospective study. Scand J Caring Sci. 2004;18:57-64.

42. Kauder D. The geriatric puzzle. Assessment challenges of elderly trauma patients. JEMS. 2000;25:64-66, 68-70, 72-74.

43. Coleman EA, Boult C. Improving the quality of transitional care for persons with complex care needs. J Am Geriatr Soc. 2003;51:556-557.

44. Kripalani S, Jackson AT, Schnipper JL, Coleman EA. Promoting effective transitions of care at hospital discharge: A review of key issues for hospitalists. J Hosp Med. 2007;2:314-323.

45. Schoen C, Osborn R, Huynh PT, et al. Taking the pulse of health care systems: Experiences of patients with health problems in six countries. Health Aff (Millwood). 2005 (suppl Web Exclusives); W5:509-525.

46. Schillinger D, Piette J, Grumbach K, et al. Closing the loop: Physician communication with diabetic patients who have low health literacy. Arch Intern Med. 2003;163:83-90.

47. Jack BW, Chetty VK, Anthony D, et al. A reengineered hospital discharge program to decrease rehospitalization: A randomized trial. Ann Intern Med. 2009;150:178-187.

POST-TEST

1. **Which of the following is TRUE regarding postoperative immobility in the elderly?**

   A. One day of bed rest results in 5% loss of muscle strength.

   B. An order of bed rest should be routinely placed for all patients for day one postoperatively.

   C. Physical therapy should be avoided in frail patients.

   D. Early mobilization predisposes a patient to falls.

2. **When assessing perioperative risks in the elderly surgical patient, which of the following is MOST important relative to good outcomes?**

   A. Age-adjusted renal function

   B. Anesthesia airway assessment

   C. Multidisciplinary approach assessment

   D. Surgeon procedural statistics

3. **Which of the following increases the risk of pulmonary complications and correlates with increased mortality and increased rates of readmission?**

   A. Cognitive impairment

   B. Hypoalbuminemia

   C. Depression

   D. Frailty

ANSWERS TO PRE-TEST

1. D
2. A
3. B

ANSWERS TO POST-TEST

1. A
2. C
3. B

29

Interdisciplinary Team Care of the Older Adult with Cancer

Cathy C. Schubert, MD

Heather Riggs, MD

● LEARNING OBJECTIVES

1. Delineate current issues and challenges in the care of older adults with cancer.
2. Describe the unique impact of geriatric syndromes on the older adult with cancer.
3. Discuss important considerations for older adults that can impact cancer treatment decisions.
4. Describe the role of the geriatric interdisciplinary team in the care of the older adult with cancer.

PRE-TEST

1. **Which member of the interdisciplinary team is most likely to focus attention on the issues that may affect the day-to-day personal physical functioning of the patient?**
   A. Geriatrician
   B. Geriatric nurse
   C. Social worker
   D. Dietician

2. **Which of the following is LEAST appropriate to use to assess nutritional status in the outpatient setting?**

   A. History of weight loss
   B. Mini Nutritional Assessment
   C. Body mass index
   D. 72-hour calorie count

3. **A vital indicator of the patient's prognosis is:**
   A. Functional status/decline
   B. Cognitive impairment
   C. Socioeconomic status
   D. Social isolation

CASE PRESENTATION 1: A RECURRENCE OF CANCER

Mrs. T. is a 92-year-old African-American female with no significant past medical history other than bladder cancer treated 5 years ago with simple tumor resection who presents to the emergency room with gross hematuria for 24 hours. She recently moved to the United States from Haiti to live with her daughter because of need for assistance with instrumental activities of daily living, but had been in her normal state of health until this acute episode. Urinalysis showed numerous red and white blood cells. The emergency room provider gave her a prescription for an antibiotic for a possible urinary tract infection, and the nurse gave the patient's daughter the phone number for the local urology office to call for an appointment. When the daughter called that office the next day, she was given an appointment in 3 weeks as the first available.

Over the next few days while on the antibiotic, Mrs. T. developed nausea and vomiting and decreased her oral intake as a result. She soon became dizzy when standing and then fell while ambulating to the bathroom. Her daughter brought Mrs. T. back to the emergency room, where she was found to be dehydrated and hypotensive. She was admitted to the hospital for rehydration. Once she was hemodynamically stable, urology was consulted. Cystoscopy was pursued and revealed several small tumors in the bladder and a large bleeding tumor close enough to the bladder outlet that impending obstruction was a concern. The urologist placed an indwelling Foley catheter. After the cystoscopy, the urologist met with Mrs. T. and her daughter to review the results, explaining that her bladder cancer had returned and that she needed surgical intervention and further localized chemotherapeutic treatment. However, Mrs. T. declined such aggressive measures. Since Mrs. T. was now medically stable, the ward nurse instructed the patient and her daughter in how to care for the indwelling catheter, and Mrs. T. was discharged home later that day with the phone number for an internal medicine practice with which to establish primary care. When the daughter called the practice, she was told their first available new patient appointment was in 2 weeks.

Once home, the patient found it difficult to ambulate with the catheter, so Mrs. T. began to spend most of her time in a chair or in bed. She continued to have hematuria. One week later her nausea and vomiting returned, so she and her daughter again returned to the emergency room. The patient was again dehydrated,

so she was given intravenous fluids, a prescription for prochlorperazine, and sent home. At home, the daughter dutifully administered the prochlorperazine, which helped the nausea but also made Mrs. T. somnolent and confused.

When Mrs. T. arrived for her first appointment with the internist the following week, he found a cachectic, lethargic older lady who could not even stand when he tried to assist her from her wheelchair and whose catheter bag was full of dark red urine and clots of blood. He had her urgently admitted to the hospital. Unfortunately, Mrs. T. went into cardiac arrest that evening. As her code status had not yet been discussed with the patient or her daughter, she was resuscitated and moved to the intensive care unit on a ventilator and vasopressor support. When the daughter arrived, she tearfully explained to the critical care physician that her mother would not have wanted such aggressive measures. She asked that the vasopressors be stopped and that the ventilator be removed. After a lengthy discussion with the daughter, the critical care specialist complied. Mrs. T. died a few hours later.

CASE PRESENTATION 2: CO-MORBIDITY AND CANCER

Mr. P. is a 75-year-old Caucasian male who was referred to the geriatric clinic for a comprehensive geriatric assessment by his oncologist after having recently been diagnosed with stage II non–small-cell lung cancer. Prior to that diagnosis, he had been having progressive fatigue and weight loss for the previous 3 months along with a 1-month history of cough productive of blood-tinged sputum. Mr. P. had a complicated medical history, including coronary artery disease with recent cardiac stent placement, hypertension, type 2 diabetes with peripheral neuropathy and renal insufficiency, peripheral vascular disease, severe chronic obstructive pulmonary disease requiring home oxygen at 2 liters, and a history of prostate cancer treated with brachytherapy and ongoing androgen-deprivation therapy. He was taking 14 medications, including 2 different proton-pump inhibitors and a benzodiazepine as needed for sleep. Mr. P. was widowed, living alone, and had no children. He quit smoking 1 year ago but had a 100 pack-year history. After retiring from the Army 15 years ago, he worked part-time driving cars for an auto auction house until 2 months ago, when his fatigue and weakness forced him to cease. He remained independent in all activities of daily living (ADLs) and instrumental activities of daily living (IADLs), but he acknowledged that it was taking increasing amounts of energy and time to complete these tasks.

On examination, Mr. P. was ill-appearing but in no acute distress. He was edentulous, and lung examination revealed diminished breath sounds bilaterally with prolonged expiratory phase. His strength was equal and intact throughout, but he had to push up on the arms of the chair to stand. Once upright, he was steady on ambulation but did touch the chairs and table frequently for support as he walked. His Mini Mental Status Exam score was 29/30, but his Geriatric Depression Scale score was 8/15. His lab work was significant for a creatinine level of 1.7 mg/dL (150.3 μmol/L), albumin of 2.9 g/dL (29 g/L), and hemoglobin of 9.5 g/dL (95 g/L). His PET/CT scan showed a left perihilar tumor with multiple enlarged mediastinal lymph nodes with increased metabolic activity along with extensive fibrotic interstitial changes in the lung parenchyma.

His radiation oncologist planned to initiate definitive radiation treatment for Mr. P.'s lung cancer, and he was asking for the geriatric consult team's assistance in managing Mr. P. and his complex issues.

OVERVIEW OF CANCER IN OLDER ADULTS

Aging Population Means More Cancer

The population of the United States and other industrialized nations is aging rapidly. Since 60% of cancers and 80% of cancer deaths occur in the 12% of the population who are age 65 and older,[1] the burden of cancer is going to increase as the population ages.

Aging and cancer appear to go hand in hand when one considers that a longer life span results in more exposure to carcinogens and an accumulation of mutations at the cellular level. These mutations can result in the activation of oncogenes and in the suppression of the cell's antiproliferative, or tumor suppressor, genes. On the other hand, aging also brings about a progressive decrease in the length of telomeres and in telomerase activity and an activation of the P14 gene, which produces an inhibitor of cell proliferation. These latter changes may actually be protective against developing some neoplasms. Behavior of some malignancies changes with age.

Overall, these genetic and cellular changes over the lifespan seem to increase the older adult's risk of developing cancer. In addition, they also may account for why some malignancies behave differently in older adults than in younger patients. For example, acute myelogenous leukemia and ovarian cancer in older adults are less responsive to

currently available chemotherapy regimens, so survival is decreased compared to younger populations. On the other hand, breast cancer in older adults tends to exhibit more indolent behavior, and lung cancer is more likely to present in early, more treatable stages.[2]

The Burden of the Unknown

Currently, care of the older adult with cancer is especially challenging because of a paucity of evidence-based medicine on which to base treatment of such patients. Only one-fifth of subjects enrolled in phase II clinical trials are older adults[3]; they tend to be excluded from such trials because of co-morbidity, frailty, and other such geriatric issues. In addition, the medical centers that offer the comprehensive cancer care that includes input from interdisciplinary geriatric teams from which many older adults would most benefit are few and far between.

GERIATRIC SYNDROMES AND THEIR IMPACT ON MANAGEMENT OF MALIGNANCY

Homeostenosis

Caused by the natural changes of aging as discussed in Chapter 2, homeostenosis is the slow but progressive loss of organ reserve needed to maintain physiologic homeostasis when the body is stressed. With time, the body declines in its ability to function well in the environment and to tolerate the challenges of illness and disease. Clinically, homeostenosis manifests as a blunted and sometimes insufficient response to stressors. In the case of Mrs. T., for example, even though she had no known co-morbid conditions other than her bladder cancer, her advanced age and borderline baseline functional status were indicative of enough homeostenosis that she was unable to tolerate relatively simple stressors such as an indwelling catheter or prochlorperazine with its sedating and anticholinergic side effects.

Co-Morbidity

Co-morbidity is defined as the extent of physical and psychological disease that is present in a patient in addition to the disease for which treatment is being considered. Like homeostenosis, a high burden of co-morbidity causes the body to have less physiologic reserve. Mr. P. from the second case may seem on first glance to be an extreme example of the degree of co-morbidity many older adults with cancer can manifest. However, Medicare data from the United States show that 65% of adults aged 65 and older have at least two or more chronic medical diseases,[4] meaning that Mr. P. is really not all that unusual.

Concomitant disease burden is important because, in patients with malignancy, higher co-morbidity is associated with worse survival than in patients with fewer pre-existing illnesses. On the other hand, studies looking at co-morbidity's impact on treatment tolerance have had conflicting results, so more research needs to be done in this area.

Another consequence of high co-morbid burden is the polypharmacy that often accompanies it. As discussed more fully in Chapter 32, 29% of adults age 70 or older take five or more prescription medications daily, and the average number of medications being prescribed to older adults per year has almost doubled in the last decade.[5] As in our case with Mr. P., increasing numbers of prescriptions increase the likelihood of pharmacologic duplication (two proton pump inhibitors) and inappropriate medication use (the benzodiazepine for sleep). In addition, the physiologic changes of aging (decreasing muscle mass reducing the volume of distribution for water-soluble drugs; an increasing percentage of fat raising the volume of distribution for fat-soluble medications; decreasing renal and hepatic clearance capabilities) coupled with polypharmacy also cause an increased risk of adverse drug reactions in older adults. Unfortunately, little formal research has been done up to this point that specifically measures the impact of polypharmacy on tolerance or efficacy of cancer therapy, but the changes of aging certainly make it a concern to be considered when caring for the older adult with cancer.

Cognitive Issues

Dementia and delirium are discussed more fully in Chapters 31 and 30, respectively. Notably, in studies of older adults with cancer where the patients were screened for cognitive impairment, 25% to 50% of them screened positive.[6] While a positive screen simply means the patient needs further workup for causes of cognitive decline and does not actually diagnose dementia, those numbers are nonetheless clinically concerning. Cognitive impairment can have profound impact on the older adult with cancer as it impacts decision-making capacity, ability to comply with therapy and remember appointments, and ability to recall and recognize signs of toxicity. While no studies have been published as yet concerning morbidity or mortality of older adults with concurrent cognitive impairment and cancer, in the general geriatric population, having dementia is associated with a higher risk of death. Cognitive condition in cancer is also becoming increasingly important because with advances in cancer treatment and its tolerability, more and more cancer care is moving to the outpatient setting. With this shift, patients or their caregivers are taking on care roles previously filled by medical professionals. Thus, recognizing and accounting for cognitive impairment in the older adult with cancer is increasingly paramount to successful treatment.

In studies of older adults with cancer requiring hospitalization, 14% to 40% have been found to have delirium. As in the general geriatric population, delirium in older patients with malignancy prolongs their hospital stay, increases their morbidity, and has a poorer overall prognosis. Studies of the causes of delirium in elderly cancer patients reveal that it is most often multifactorial. The most common contributors to the mental status changes are medications; systemic infections; metabolic dysfunctions such as hyponatremia, hypoxia, and renal failure; and central nervous system lesions including brain metastases and cerebrovascular accidents.[7]

Malnutrition and Unintentional Weight Loss

As described in Chapter 35, in community-dwelling older adults, the prevalence of overt malnutrition is low, at only 2%. However, at least one-fourth of community-dwelling elders are at high risk of developing malnutrition, especially in the setting of acute illness. In fact, when older adults are ill and hospitalized, the prevalence of malnutrition quickly rises to an average of 24%.[8] Thus, for many older adults such as our case with Mr. P., malnutrition or at least depleted nutritional stores may already be present at the time of cancer diagnosis. This is concerning because it contributes to homeostenosis and explains why weight loss and poor nutritional status are associated both with poorer response to cancer therapy and with decreased survival.

Depression

Studies that have examined older adults with cancer and depression have been limited. This is in spite of the fact that patients with malignancy face several stressors that increase their risk for psychiatric disorders, including grief about current or anticipated loss of function, fear of death, social isolation during treatment, and concern about the future of their loved ones. Even the prevalence of depression in cancer patients remains poorly understood; estimates in studies range from 3% to 38%.[9] However, in spite of the paucity of evidence, depression is important because it may be associated with worse survival in cancer. In addition, depression has been proven to increase the risk of functional decline over time, and depressed patients utilize more health care resources than patients who are not depressed. Most of all, depression and other psychiatric issues need to be considered when treating the older adult with cancer because relief of suffering is of paramount importance when considering cancer care. Depression is discussed more fully in Chapter 37.

Functional Decline

Functional status at baseline and during the course of cancer treatment has long been recognized as a vital indicator of the patient's prognosis. In fact, functional status predicts survival, risk of chemotherapy toxicity, and risk of postoperative morbidity and mortality in older adults with cancer. Oncologists have traditionally used either the Karnofsky Performance Scale[10] or the Eastern Cooperative Oncology Group Scale[11] to describe and categorize a patient's functional status (see Tables 7–10 and 7–11). In older patients, however, these scales tend to under-detect functional impairment. In our case of Mr. P., for example, his oncologist rated him with an ECOG of 0 because he was still maintaining his self-care activities independently. However, on more detailed questioning, it was obvious that Mr. P. was teetering on the edge of no longer being able to complete more strenuous IADLs such as his housework and grocery shopping.

As described in Chapter 36, much research has been done in general geriatrics using IADLs and ADLs as measures of function, and some early work using these scales has been accomplished in geriatric oncology. In older adults with non–small-cell lung cancer, for example, pretreatment IADL ability correlated with survival.[12] Needing assistance in IADLs was associated with increased risk of toxicity from chemotherapy in older females with ovarian cancer[13] and with increased risk of postoperative complications in older adults whose cancer was being treated surgically.[14] Less is currently known about impact of ADL dependence on cancer outcomes because most studies thus far have been conducted in the outpatient arena where patients are less ill. However, it is significant that a chart review of patients admitted to an Oncology Acute Care for Elders unit revealed that 45% of them required assistance in their ADLs.[15]

As discussed earlier, homeostenosis associated with aging contributes to a gradual but progressive decline in the older person's ability to function in the environment and to tolerate stresses such as illness. While an older adult such as Mr. P. may be managing to maintain function at baseline, the rigors of cancer treatment can be a significant insult to the body. Unless care is taken to prepare the older adult physically, socially, and emotionally as much as possible for such a stress, functional decline, medical decline, and even death in some cases may be the result.

Socioeconomic Issues

In many cases in the United States, older adults are retired from the workforce and are living off their savings and/or Social Security payments. Thus they often have a fixed amount of money with which to pay their monthly expenses. Health insurance may be prohibitively expensive for older adults, especially if they have multiple co-morbidities. Because of these issues, older adults in the United States are often reliant on Medicare to pay the majority of their health care costs. However, cancer treatment is becoming increasingly complex and expensive as new regimens are developed, and some of the burden of these costs is being shifted to patients as cancer treatment moves increasingly to the outpatient arena. This economic challenge may quickly overwhelm the finances of the typical older adult with cancer. In fact, low-income older adult cancer patients spent 27% of their income on out-of-pocket medical expenses in one study.[16] In addition, as discussed in Chapter 17, if an informal caregiver is necessary for the older adult with cancer, the duties of caregiving unfortunately may also have a negative impact on the family's financial status. In the United States, informal caregivers spend an average of 10 hours per week in the care of cancer patients of all ages.[16] This is a financially significant amount of time if the caregiver is taken away from formal employment and thus is not earning any income.

Older adults are often also at risk of social isolation. Sometimes their spouses and close friends have died or are too frail themselves to be available as potential caregivers. In addition, with the increasing mobility of our society, an older adult's children or other family members may not be nearby or available to help care for them. Older adults may also have functional issues that impair their ability to drive, and many areas of the United States have little or no mass transportation available as alternative options. For example, in our second case, Mr. P. was at high risk of becoming socially isolated because of being a childless widower who no longer worked or had many activities outside of his home. In addition, because of his illness, he was in danger of becoming too frail to be able to drive any longer.

Because of these socioeconomic issues, as cancer treatment is increasingly being provided in outpatient sites, older adults with cancer are among those at highest risk of being unable to comply with a treatment regimen due to transportation issues, lack of caregivers for assistance, or lack of monetary resources to afford the treatments. This may begin to explain why social isolation is associated with increased risk of mortality in older adults with cancer.

Frailty

While frailty is still a poorly defined syndrome in terms of our physiologic and scientific understanding of its etiology and mechanisms, most practitioners recognize its signs and symptoms when confronting it in clinical practice. Patients, or sometimes their caregivers, will complain of weight loss, generalized weakness and fatigue, inactivity, and decreased food intake. In terms of clinical signs, evidence of sarcopenia, osteopenia, deconditioning, and balance and gait abnormalities are usually present; patients may also have low albumin and blood urea nitrogen if blood levels are checked.

To further visualize frailty and its impact on a patient's clinical course and overall prognosis, frailty is present when homeostenosis has so depleted a patient's physiologic reserves that even the most minor of physical stresses causes severe compromise. The case of Mrs. T. is a good example, where a few hours of nausea and vomiting caused her to need an emergency room visit and hospital admission for hypotension and falls. In many cases, frailty can best be visualized as "end-stage homeostenosis." Many questions remain about frailty, however. For example, is frailty a reversible clinical condition, or can the downward spiral not be mitigated once it begins? Is frailty a consequence of aging at the cellular level? If so, what are the substances, such as interleukins or cytokines, causing this aging? Frailty is the focus of much research interest currently, so hopefully answers will begin to emerge in the near future. (For more on frailty see Chapter 36.)

Older adults with malignancy often develop a specific type of frailty called cancer cachexia. Though often attributed to the burden of the tumor consuming energy and nutrients in preference to the rest of the body, it can even develop in patients whose cancer seems to be responding to active treatments such as radiation or chemotherapy. This has usually been explained as being due to the severe toxicity associated with cancer treatments; in the future, as new treatments are developed that more closely target the malignancy and cause less systemic toxicity, it will be interesting to observe if there is a change in the prevalence of cancer cachexia.

● QUESTIONS TO CONSIDER IN THE GERIATRIC ONCOLOGY PATIENT

When an older adult is initially diagnosed with malignancy, it is important to consider the five questions given next when considering the treatment plan.

Is the Patient Going to Die with or of Cancer?

An older adult who has been diagnosed with a fairly aggressive malignancy, such as colon cancer or lung cancer, will likely have a better prognosis and life expectancy if that patient undergoes some form of cancer treatment. Intervention for more indolent cancers, such as prostate cancer or chronic lymphocytic leukemia, however, may cause more harm than benefit to the patient in some cases if the patient has other co-morbid conditions that are more likely to result in death. In our case of Mr. P., he certainly had multiple chronic medical conditions and overall was an extremely ill man. However, since his other co-morbidities were clinically stable, an aggressive malignancy like lung cancer would most likely cause his death and thus should be considered for treatment.

Is the Patient Likely to Suffer Complications of Cancer?

While cancer treatment is seldom without risks and toxicity of its own, the benefit of avoiding the complications of untreated cancer often outweighs those risks. In our case of Mrs. T., having palliative surgery to reduce the tumor burden in her bladder may have helped her avoid a chronic indwelling Foley catheter and the ongoing blood loss from hematuria. Quality of life for both her and the caregiver daughter might have been improved during the last days of Mrs. T.'s life. For Mr. P., treatment with palliative radiation will likely decrease pain and breathing symptoms he would develop if the cancer continued to grow, and reduce his risk of worsening hemoptysis/bleeding if the tumor were to invade his pulmonary vasculature.

Is the Patient Able to Tolerate Treatment?

A basic tenet of geriatrics is to consider each patient individually, as older adults are the most heterogeneous patient population and numerical age often has little relation to the patient's actual health status. This concept of customized treatment becomes especially important in the older adult with malignancy. Obviously, a 70-year-old man who is bedbound with severe dementia is not going to survive the rigors of induction chemotherapy for acute myelogenous leukemia. However, an 86-year-old woman who lives independently and is active in her community would likely be a candidate for surgical treatment and chemotherapy for her gastric cancer. In the case of Mr. P., while he was considered medically inoperable because of his co-morbid conditions, radiation therapy for his lung cancer offered him a good chance for an improved quality of life and prolonged survival with minimal toxicity.

Are There Reversible Conditions Impacting the Patient's Ability to Tolerate Treatment?

Clinical trials in geriatric oncology show that older adults can often tolerate the same rigorous treatment regimens as younger patients if care is taken to address their co-morbidities and geriatric syndromes. Thus, the National Comprehensive Cancer Network,[17] the International Society of Geriatric Oncology,[18] and other oncology organizations recommend that all adults age 70 and older who have been diagnosed with a malignancy undergo a comprehensive geriatric assessment as part of their cancer treatment plan. The purpose of such an assessment is to detect geriatric syndromes such as polypharmacy, depression, malnutrition, and socioeconomic deficiencies early in the disease course so that they may be addressed prior to their interfering with successful treatment of the malignancy. As will be discussed in detail, in the case of Mr. P., an assessment by the geriatric interdisciplinary team revealed multiple geriatric issues that needed intervention.

Is the Intent of Treatment Curative or Palliative?

In much of oncology, the stage of the cancer and the treatments available for that cancer determine whether it can be cured. For example, lung cancer that is detected prior to metastasis may be surgically resected and thus cured. In older adults, however, factors discussed earlier, such as degree of homeostenosis, geriatric syndromes, and overall functional status, must also be considered in addition to the cancer stage and risk of treatment toxicity. In essence, we must also "stage the age" of the patient in addition to staging the cancer when considering treatment options. The most effective way to perform this assessment of an older adult is using an interdisciplinary team to perform a comprehensive geriatric assessment.

● ROLE OF THE INTERDISCIPLINARY TEAM IN CARE OF THE COMPLEX OLDER ADULT CANCER PATIENT

The areas of specialty of the members of an interdisciplinary team often vary from medical center to medical center and in some cases from patient to patient. At a minimum, the team performing a comprehensive geriatric assessment for an older adult with cancer should include a geriatrician, a nurse with training in geriatrics, and a social worker who is knowledgeable of resources available to older adults. In many cases, nutritionists, pharmacists, and rehabilitation therapists can also be beneficial additions to the team. Each team member has a defined role in the evaluation, and all are equally important and vital to best care of the older adult with malignancy. One example of the structure and roles of a geriatric interdisciplinary team is described below, though the specifics of how each patient is evaluated may vary from team to team or even from case to case.

Geriatric Nurse

The geriatric nurse often focuses attention on the issues that may affect the day-to-day personal physical functioning of the patient. When performing a geriatric review of systems during the initial assessment, the nurse queries the patient about any issues with skin, vision, hearing, dentition, bowel habits, continence, nutrition, and cognition. Because patients and their families sometimes may be unaware or in denial of cognitive issues, it is beneficial for the nurse also to include screening for memory problems as part of his or her assessment, such as the Mini Mental Status Examination[19] or the six-item screener.[20] As older adults with malignancy are also at risk of weight loss and malnutrition, having the nurse complete formal nutritional screening such as the Mini Nutritional Assessment (MNA)[8] can also detect unrecognized issues. As discussed further in Chapter 35, the MNA is a quick and easy tool that can both screen and then further assess elderly patients who are either at risk for or are already malnourished. The nurse should also review how the patient accomplishes instrumental activities of daily living and basic activities of daily living. However, because older adults may minimize difficulties they are having accomplishing these on self-report, including a performance-based assessment of function such as the Timed Up and Go[21] or Gait Speed tests can also be revealing. In the case of Mr. P., the geriatric nurse discovered he was having considerable difficulty with constipation and that he had difficulty chewing meats because of his lack of teeth. He had had issues with urinary incontinence since his prostate cancer treatment several years before, but he now was having trouble obtaining his continence supplies because he was too fatigued to get to the pharmacy where he usually bought them. She also found that he was eating cold cereal with milk for breakfast and lunch and then heating up a frozen pre-made meal for dinner because he "didn't feel like cooking just for one anymore."

Social Worker

The role of the social worker on the interdisciplinary team is to focus on issues that impact how the patient can function in the environment, including how the patient maneuvers through the pursuit of cancer treatment. The social worker inquires about marital status, living arrangements, and other local family support that is available to the patient. Asking about religious practices may reveal further available social supports for the patient while also bringing up any religious beliefs that may impact cancer treatment decisions. Questions about financial status and insurance allow the social worker to prepare for need of assistance with prescription medications, transportation, and other supportive programs. In cases where a caregiver is involved, it is of paramount importance to screen for and address caregiver stress to ensure the best care and safety for that patient in the future. Finally, the social worker should also screen the patient for depression or other mood disorder using an instrument such as the Geriatric Depression Scale.[22] In the case of Mr. P., the social worker's assessment revealed that he was quite isolated with almost no social support, would have no transportation if Mr. P. became unable to drive himself, and suffered from depression of at least moderate severity.

Geriatrician

The geriatrician's primary roles are to assess the patient's medical needs and to serve as the leader of the interdisciplinary team (the latter is discussed later in the chapter).

To define the patient's medical issues, the geriatrician usually performs a comprehensive history and physical examination. Because of the co-morbidity of many older adults, the geriatrician should make special note of the prescribed and over-the-counter medications the patient is taking; whenever possible, the patient should be encouraged to bring all medication bottles to each visit for review. A thorough medical review of systems and a comprehensive physical examination can help detect any smoldering symptoms or medical issues that are at risk for being missed or neglected during the heavy focus on the patient's malignancy and its acute treatment. For Mr. P., the geriatrician's assessment discovered that he was taking duplicate medications (two proton pump inhibitors) and a benzodiazepine, which is a class of medications generally to be avoided in the older adult population. He also appeared quite ill on exam and was obviously teetering on the edge of becoming frail as a result of his medical illnesses.

Nutritionist

As discussed already, many older adults are at risk of developing malnutrition, especially when they become acutely ill. In the case of malignancy, underlying malnutrition may impact how well the patient is able to tolerate treatment and how well he or she recovers from it. When malnutrition is present or even suspected in an older adult with malignancy, a nutritionist can be of great service to the patient. Such a specialist can make recommendations for maximizing intake of protein and other nutrients vital to restoring the nutritional state. In addition, when nausea or poor appetite related to the cancer treatment is a problem, the nutritionist can give the patient or caregiver advice such as eating small, frequent meals and instructions on how to improve food palatability.

Pharmacist

Since older adults are often at risk of polypharmacy due to their co-morbid conditions, having the input of a pharmacist with training in geriatrics and/or oncology is invaluable. Older adults may have some degree of renal impairment and have less vigorous hepatic blood flow, so they are already at increased risk of adverse drug reactions at baseline. When treatment of malignancy is also in the picture, the risk for drug interactions and adverse reactions may be even higher because of the chemotherapeutic agents the patient is receiving. Thus, having the input of an expert in pharmacology is helpful for minimizing the risk of adverse drug reactions.

Rehabilitation Specialists

Older adults with malignancy may present with baseline functional issues such as difficulty walking due to knee osteoarthritis or deconditioning as a consequence of the acute illness. In addition, generalized fatigue can be a prominent symptom in malignancy, and the rigors and side effects of cancer treatment can often exacerbate its severity. Physiatrists, physical therapists, and occupational therapists can often make recommendations for exercises and assistive devices to improve the patient's functional ability. In cancer patients, rehabilitation experts can also educate the patient in energy-conserving techniques that will help alleviate the fatigue and ensure that the older adult has the energy necessary to complete important tasks and activities of daily life.

Interdisciplinary Team Rounds

After each member of the geriatric interdisciplinary team assesses the older adult with malignancy, the team then gathers together to present and discuss their findings. The geriatrician presents the patient's medical history and details of the malignancy. The nurse and the social worker then discuss their findings while the team makes note of relevant issues that have been found. The geriatrician then presents the positive results of the physical exam and leads the team in developing a list of problems found in the patient and then the team jointly develops a plan for how they may be addressed.

When the geriatrician, nurse, and social worker met for the interdisciplinary team rounds for Mr. P., the clinical picture that quickly emerged was of a chronically ill elderly gentleman with lung cancer who was at high risk of becoming frail as a result of his co-morbidities, malnutrition, depression, and social isolation. While his radiation oncologist wanted to initiate palliative radiation treatment of his lung cancer, Mr. P. seemed likely to respond poorly because of these other "geriatric" issues.

The geriatrician discontinued one of the proton pump inhibitors and initiated a gentle laxative for Mr. P.'s constipation. She then conferred with the pharmacist for further recommendations. The pharmacist provided advice on how to safely wean the bedtime benzodiazepine while adding an antidepressant to help with Mr. P.'s mood and insomnia but that was at low risk for interacting with his other medications. As an additional measure against insomnia, the nurse educated Mr. P. on how better to maintain his sleep hygiene. She also arranged for the nutritionist to see Mr. P. later that day. The social worker made arrangements for Mr. P.'s incontinence supplies to be delivered by mail to his home. She also facilitated enrolling him in community resources for transportation and increasing Mr. P.'s socialization. The geriatrician referred him to outpatient physical therapy for strengthening and balance and to see if he could benefit from an assistive device for ambulation.

The nutritionist who saw Mr. P. later that day teamed up with the social worker to have provided home-delivered meals that he would be able to chew. She also recommended a multivitamin and some liquid supplements that could quickly and easily improve his caloric, nutrient, and protein intake. When Mr. P. saw the physical therapist a few days later, she instructed him in several exercises to improve his leg strength and sense of balance and also fitted him with a four-prong cane. The therapist also provided a tub chair and education on energy-saving techniques to help combat Mr. P.'s fatigue.

Importance of Inter-Specialty Communication in the Care of Older Adults with Cancer

Because older adult patients can have high levels of both medical and psychosocial complexity, the importance of communication between the providers caring for them cannot be overstated. Efficient and effective communication improves the quality of patient care by reducing duplication of efforts and errors while also streamlining the process of care for the patient. The geriatric interdisciplinary team should communicate their concerns and plans for treatment to the oncologist and to the primary care provider. Likewise, as the patient's treatment for malignancy goes forward, all groups should continue to update one another of any major events.

Mr. P. began his palliative radiation treatment for his lung cancer soon after his geriatric evaluation. His cough improved fairly quickly, though he did have some skin erythema and mild discomfort at the radiation site. By the time he was completing his radiation treatments a few weeks later, his appetite had improved and he was gaining some weight. He was ambulating well with his four-prong cane and had become involved in a cancer support group and some social activities at the senior center near his home. His mood was upbeat and he was sleeping well at night. While he still fatigued easily with exertion, he had sufficient energy to maintain his independence in all IADLs and ADLs and also pursue some activities that he enjoyed.

Transitioning to Hospice Care

In some cases, older adults with malignancy may not respond to treatment or may find themselves unable or unwilling to tolerate the complications and side effects of that treatment. When this occurs, their medical providers need to have honest and open discussions with the patient and family/caregiver about prognosis and the disease course they can expect when active treatment is stopped. In general, the goals of care at this time shift from that of curative to palliative and often comfort care. In these cases, enlisting the assistance of a hospice team can often be helpful as such a team has special training and experience in symptom palliation and other supportive measures for the patient and the family. Even if the patient is no longer receiving active treatment, however, it is still important for the oncologist, geriatrician, or primary care provider to remain involved in the case to ensure that the patient's medical needs are met and to provide support to the hospice team as they care for the patient.

Mr. P. continued to do well for 4 months after completing his radiation. One day, however, he began to have pain in his left thigh. It was worse on ambulation but also present at rest. He mentioned this pain during his routine visit with the geriatrician 2 days later. Concerned, the geriatrician checked an x-ray of the left hip and femur, but no abnormalities were seen. She allowed Mr. P. to return home after his visit but then contacted his oncologist to discuss this symptom. The oncologist called Mr. P. and asked that he undergo a bone scan to evaluate his leg pain further. Unfortunately, the bone scan revealed new metastatic disease in Mr. P.'s left femur and also in his ribs and spine. Mr. P. then underwent palliative radiation to the painful metastatic lesions on his femur with good relief of his symptoms. When that was completed, because he knew he was not a candidate for more aggressive treatment, Mr. P. decided that he wanted to transition to hospice care. The geriatric social worker made that referral and also helped Mr. P. arrange for a hired caregiver to be with him in his home for several hours daily. With the assistance of hospice, Mr. P. died peacefully in his home 2 months later.

● SURVIVORSHIP

Cancer treatment has made rapid and wonderful advances in the past couple of decades. Malignancies that were uniformly fatal in the past are now curable; those that cannot be cured can in many cases at least be changed into something of a chronic disease. This recent success in treating cancer is creating an especially unique population of older adults: cancer survivors. While these patients are at risk for or may already have common medical co-morbidities such as hypertension, diabetes, and coronary artery disease just like their cohorts, their history of successfully treated cancer may add additional layers of complexity to their care.

While a recurrence of the original cancer is always a concern, these older adults also need routine screening for other malignancies (mammogram, colonoscopy, pap smear, etc.) as part of their usual medical care. In addition, their medical providers need to be aware of potential late effects of the cancer treatment, such as lymphedema, bone loss, fatigue, and neuropathy. Some cancer survivors report symptoms of memory impairment, a complaint occurring commonly enough to be termed "chemo brain." While a definitive study proving chemo brain's existence has not yet been published, memory symptoms are distressing and worrisome to the patient, and the provider needs to be prepared to evaluate and address these issues.

While the concept of cancer survivorship care is still in its infancy, interdisciplinary team care of the older adult cancer survivor is an area that deserves further study. Comprehensive geriatric assessments have been shown to decrease morbidity, improve function, and decrease risk of institutionalization in the general geriatric population. As more and more older adults survive cancer in the future, it will be interesting to evaluate formally what positive impact the geriatric interdisciplinary team can have on these patients as well.

References

1. Ries LAG, Harkins D, Krapcho M, et al. *SEER Cancer Statistics Review, 1975–2003*. Bethesda: National Cancer Institute; 2006.

2. Carreca I, Balducci L, Extermann M. Cancer in the older person. *Cancer Treat Rev*. 2005;31:380-402.

3. Lewis JH, Kilgore ML, Goldman DP, et al. Participation of patients 65 years of age and older in cancer clinical trials. *J Clin Oncol*. 2003;21:1383-1389.

4. Wolff JL, Starfield B, Anderson G. Prevalence, expenditures, and complications of multiple chronic conditions in the elderly. *Arch Intern Med*. 2002;162:2269-2276.

5. Qato DM, Alexander GC, Conti RM, et al. Use of prescription and over-the-counter medications and dietary supplements among older adults in the United States. *JAMA*. 2008;300:2867-2878.

6. Extermann M, Hurria A. Comprehensive geriatric assessment for older patients with cancer. *J Clin Oncol*. 2007;25:1824-1831.

7. Tuma R, DeAngelis LM. Altered mental status in patients with cancer. *Arch Neurol*. 2000;57:1727-1731.

8. Guigoz Y. The Mini Nutritional Assessment review of the literature—what does it tell us? *J Nutr Health Aging*. 2006;10:466-487.

9. Kadan-Lottick NS, Vanderwerker LC, Block SD, et al. Psychiatric disorders and mental health service use in patients with advanced cancer. *Cancer*. 2005;104:2872-2881.

10. Karnofsky DA, Burchenal JH. The clinical evaluation of chemotherapeutic agents in cancer. In: MacLeod CM, ed. *Evaluation of Chemotherapeutic Agents*. New York: Columbia University Press, 1949:196.

11. Oken MM, Creech RH, Tormey DC, et al. Toxicity and response criteria of the Eastern Cooperative Oncology Group. *Am J Clin Oncol*. 1982;5:649-655.

12. Maione P, Perrone F, Gallo C, et al. Pretreatment quality of life and functional status assessment significantly predict survival of elderly patients with advanced non-small-cell lung cancer receiving chemotherapy: A prognostic analysis of the multicenter Italian lung cancer in the elderly study. *J Clin Oncol*. 2005;23:6865-6872.

13. Freyer G, Geay JF, Touzet S, et al. Comprehensive geriatric assessment predicts tolerance to chemotherapy and survival in elderly patients with advanced ovarian carcinoma: A GINECO study. *Ann Oncol*. 2005;16:1795-1800.

14. Audisio RA, Ramesh H, Longo WE, et al. Preoperative assessment of surgical risk in oncogeriatric patients. *Oncologist*. 2005;10: 262-268.

15. Flood KL, Carroll MB, Le CV, et al. Geriatric syndromes in elderly patients admitted to an oncology-acute care for elders unit. *J Clin Oncol*. 2006;24:2298-2303.

16. Cross ER, Emanuel L. Providing inbuilt economic resilience options: An obligation of comprehensive cancer care. *Cancer* (suppl). 2008;113:3548-3555.

17. Balducci L, Cohen HJ, Engstrom PF, et al. Senior adult oncology clinical practice guidelines in oncology. *J Natl Comp Cancer Net*. 2005;3:572-590.

18. Extermann M, Aapro M, Bernabei R, et al. Use of comprehensive geriatric assessment in older cancer patients: Recommendations from the task force on CGA of the International Society of Geriatric Oncology (SIOG). *Crit Rev Oncol Hematol*. 2005;55: 241-252.

19. Folstein MF, Folstein SE, McHugh PR. Mini-mental state: A practical method for grading the cognitive state of patients for the clinician. *J Psychiatr Res*. 1975;12:189-198.

20. Callahan CM, Unverzagt FW, Hui SL, et al. Six-item screener to identify cognitive impairment among potential subjects for clinical research. *Med Care*. 2002;40:771-781.

21. Podsiadlo D, Richardson S. The timed "Up & Go": A test of basic functional mobility for frail elderly persons. *J Am Geriatr Soc*. 1991;39:142-148.

22. Almeida OP, Almeida SA. Short versions of the geriatric depression scale: A study of their validity for the diagnosis of a major depressive episode according to ICD-10 and DSM-IV. *Int J Geriatr Psychiatry*. 1999;14:858-865.

POST-TEST

1. **The most common clinical manifestation of homeostenosis is:**
   A. Hypotension and tachycardia
   B. Delirium
   C. Blunted and sometimes insufficient response to stressors
   D. Gait instability and falls

2. **Which of the following is NOT a known contributor to carcinogenesis in older adults?**
   A. Activation of oncogenes
   B. Activation of the P14 gene

   C. Suppression of antiproliferative genes
   D. Exposure to carcinogens

3. **Which of the following is NOT associated with poorer survival/prognosis in older adults?**
   A. Cancer cachexia
   B. Co-morbidity
   C. Dementia
   D. Depression

ANSWERS TO PRE-TEST

1. B
2. D
3. A

ANSWERS TO POST-TEST

1. C
2. B
3. A

PART III

Geriatric Syndromes and Important Issues

30

Delirium

Franklin S. Watkins, MD

Jeff D. Williamson, MD, MHS

● **LEARNING OBJECTIVES**

1. Define delirium and distinguish it as a disorder.
2. Identify common etiologies/risk factors for the development of delirium.
3. Discuss preventive strategies to reduce the incidence of delirium.
4. Describe strategies to treat symptoms of delirium, focusing on nonpharmacologic interventions.
5. Explain the impact of delirium in increasing patient morbidity, mortality, and health care expenditures.

PRE-TEST

1. **For the diagnosis of delirium to be established, all of the following signs must be present EXCEPT:**
   A. Acute change in mental status
   B. Fluctuation in the course of the patient's mental status
   C. Inattention
   D. Verbal responsiveness

2. **The most common presentation of delirium is:**
   A. Hypoactive
   B. Hyperactive
   C. Mixed
   D. It depends upon the setting

3. **Nonpharmacologic interventions for delirium include:**
   A. Physical restraints for safety
   B. Eliminating vital signs
   C. Presence of family member
   D. Darkened room

CASE PRESENTATION: ALTERED MENTAL STATUS

E.M. is an 82-year-old Caucasian female, who resides in a local assisted living facility because of slowly declining physical function as well as needing help managing her medicines. She is admitted to your hospital. Her past medical history includes two-vessel coronary artery disease status-post stenting, chronic atrial fibrillation, pacemaker placement for sick sinus syndrome, hypertension under good control on an ACE inhibitor, diabetes mellitus without complications, osteoarthritis limiting her mobility, and chronic insomnia most nights of the week. You are asked to evaluate her by a referring colleague after her admission to the hospital last night with complaints of "altered mental status." Approximately 2 days prior to admission, she developed signs of confusion and decreased energy for which she had been referred to the emergency room. In addition, on the day of admission, she had fallen in her room at her assisted living facility, which resulted in a left distal radius fracture (which was discovered after her exam revealed a painful, swollen left wrist). She was also found to have a fever of 103°F (39.4°C) on presentation.

INTRODUCTION AND OVERVIEW

Delirium is a common, serious, and often unrecognized complication of age-related chronic and acute conditions. The diagnosis of delirium is a medical emergency and is often complicated by the lack of early recognition of its presenting symptoms by clinicians. *Delirium*, often confused with dementia, is acute in onset, characterized by a fluctuating course, can be preventable, and is almost always reversible (unless it leads to death); while *dementia* is a chronic, irreversible, progressive disease with sometimes minor fluctuations in cognition and attention. Additional symptoms and signs differentiating delirium and dementia are given in Table 30–1. Other nomenclature used for delirium includes acute confusional state and altered mental status.

EPIDEMIOLOGY

As many as one-third of elderly patients admitted to the hospital experience symptoms of delirium,[1] and the incidence of delirium increases with age. Both the severity of the medical illness and the burden of co-morbidity (as seen in our case example) increase the likelihood of developing delirium in the geriatric population. Previous studies have found delirium to occur in 15% to 53% of geriatric patients postoperatively, and between 50% and 80% of patients requiring intensive care.[2,3] While delirium is commonly associated with hospitalization and severe medical illness, it also occurs frequently in

● **TABLE 30–1** Differentiating Delirium from Dementia

	Delirium	Dementia
Onset	Abrupt	Insidious
Duration	Hours to days, even weeks	Months to years; slow progression
Attention	Impaired—fluctuates	Disease-stage dependent
Neurologic assessment	Variable: may be able to perform complex tasks such as counting backward or have short-term recall ability	Unable to perform complex tasks
Alertness	Fluctuating, reduced Three subtypes: hyperactive, hypoactive, mixed	Varies with disease stage but generally constant
Speech	Incoherent, disorganized, rambling	Little fluctuation
Communication	Understands written and spoken word at times, but variable	Often limited ability to process written or spoken word

the outpatient and, in particular, the long-term care (nursing home and assisted living) settings. Importantly, just as with other preventable complications, delirium is associated with a significantly increased risk of mortality both in the hospital and the posthospital convalescence setting.

ASSOCIATED HEALTH CARE COSTS

With increasing life expectancy, many national health care systems are experiencing fiscal crises with intensified pressure to appropriately allocate health care resources for all patients. Identifying best practices for efficient resource allocation is especially important in the aging populations of developed and developing nations. Delirium is not only prevalent in hospitalized and recently discharged older adults, but it is also a potent risk factor for increasing the cost of care through prolonging length of hospital stay and increasing the need for inpatient rehabilitation and long-term nursing home placement.[4] Coupled with the increasing life expectancy in many nations, the annual cost of preventable illness-associated delirium is high. Recent US data from a study evaluating the medical costs incurred 1 year after hospital discharge in patients age 70 and older demonstrated that the increased cost was between $16,000 and $64,000 for persons experiencing delirium versus no delirium. Despite these greater expenditures, patients with delirium experienced reduced survival.[5]

PROGNOSIS

Patients who develop delirium are at increased risk for other adverse medical outcomes. In the general geriatric population, delirium is associated with a ten-fold increased risk of in-hospital mortality, and three- to five-fold increased risk of other nosocomial complications.[6] These same patients are also found to be at greater risk for requiring nursing home placement at discharge. Further studies have found that delirium is associated with poorer physical functional recovery and an increased risk for death up to 2 years after hospital discharge.[6] In the critical care setting, the development of delirium during ICU admission is associated with a three-fold increased risk of mortality at 6 months, prolonged hospital length of stay, and a ten-fold higher incidence of cognitive impairment at discharge.[7]

● CLINICAL PRESENTATION AND CLASSIFICATION

Although the clinical presentation typically exhibits substantial heterogeneity, delirium is usually classified into three groups:

- Hypoactive
- Hyperactive
- Mixed (both hypoactive and hyperactive)

This heterogeneity in the presentation of delirium often results in the diagnosis being missed, and although the diagnosis is overlooked in all forms of delirium, it is most frequently misdiagnosed or under-diagnosed in patients with the hypoactive form of delirium.[8] Due to the patient's intermittent confusion, it is imperative to obtain additional medical history from persons who are familiar with the patient's baseline level of cognition, interaction, and medical history. These individuals include family members, caregivers, nursing staff from the patient's nursing facility, or any other informant who is familiar with the patient's usual level of interaction and cognition.

Numerous methodologies have been developed to assist in the identification and diagnosis of delirium. Unlike other neurologic diagnoses that frequently rely on criteria outlined in the *Diagnostic and Statistical Manual of Mental Disorders*, 4th edition (DSM-IV), delirium is more often diagnosed through use of bedside screening tools, such as the Confusion Assessment Method (CAM).[9] The CAM is easy to apply in the clinical setting and consists of five criteria that are evaluated to be either present or absent. For the diagnosis of delirium to be established, all three of the following signs must be present: (1) an acute change in mental status, (2) fluctuation in the course of the patient's mental status, and (3) inattention. Additionally, one of two additional criteria must be met: disorganized thinking or altered level of consciousness. An advantageous feature in the use of the CAM is that it does not require verbal responsiveness and can be used by clinicians and nursing staff in patients with significantly altered levels of consciousness.

While the CAM is useful in the diagnosis of delirium, it must be used in the context of the patient's medical history and in coordination with other assessments of the patient's cognition, including the Folstein Mini-Mental State Examination. Once the diagnosis of delirium is determined, a thorough examination of the patient's health status, including rapid assessment for the two most common etiologies of delirium—medication changes and infectious etiologies—should be undertaken as guided by the patient's history.

Hypoactive Delirium

While the agitated, confused, and sometimes aggressive patient is usually the more widely and easily recognized example of delirium, the hypoactive form of delirium is the most common presentation. Because patients with hypoactive delirium often lack the "classic" hallmarks of delirium, a high degree of suspicion for delirium should be undertaken when evaluating a patient who is hypoactive. Patients presenting with this form of delirium are often described as "lethargic," "confused," or as presenting with "altered mental status." The most common feature of hypoactive delirium is psychomotor retardation or decreased overall movement. Those with hypoactive delirium, however, will still manifest symptoms of inattention, disorganized thoughts, and acuity in the onset of symptoms.

Hyperactive Delirium

The presentation of a patient with hyperactive delirium is generally characterized by "agitation" or appearing "delusional." Typically, these patients will present with psychomotor agitation, which involves unintentional, purposeless movements often associated with the complaint of anxiousness. Other symptoms often demonstrated in patients with hyperactive delirium are alterations in the sleep cycle, delusions or hallucinations. As previously noted, the diagnosis of hyperactive delirium is often easier to recognize relative to those presenting with the hypoactive form. Patients presenting with psychomotor agitation are often at increased risk for receiving interventions that prolong or worsen their underlying delirium, such as the use of physical restraints or psychotropic medications to control the symptoms of delirium, while evaluation for the underlying cause of the delirium is either neglected or significantly delayed.

Mixed Delirium

Often, patients with delirium may present with a fluctuating course of symptoms, alternating between symptoms consistent with hypoactive delirium and those consistent with hyperactive delirium. In this presentation, the diagnosis and management of the patient are challenging, and delirium may erroneously be attributed to an underlying psychiatric disorder.

CASE PRESENTATION (continued)

As part of your evaluation, you call the patient's daughter, who lives in the same city. She reports that E.M. has no prior history of dementia or any history of cognitive impairment. She has, however, had a long history of recurrent urinary tract infections. As far as she knows, her mother has not had a history of falling.

When you perform your initial evaluation, you note that she appears lucid and is able to tell you that her current fall resulted from her "legs buckling." She experienced no dizziness or chest pain with her fall. When you speak to the patient's nurse, she provides additional history that the nurse on duty last night reported that EM was up much of last night screaming, "You get out of here." She evidently was very agitated and could not be calmed down by any of the staff.

Your exam reveals her blood pressure is 112/74, heart rate is 92, temperature is 99°F (37.2°C), and respiratory rate is 22. Her mucous membranes are slightly dry, her heart rhythm is irregularly irregular though rate-controlled, and her lungs have prominent bibasilar crackles on auscultation. Her left wrist is now in a cast, her fingers are warm, and her sensation is intact. Her neurologic exam reveals spontaneous movement of all four extremities, and her cranial nerves are intact. She is oriented to person only (not to place, setting, or time), and there was no evidence of head trauma with her fall.

Her medication list includes digoxin 0.25 mg daily, metoprolol 50 mg daily, atorvastatin 40 mg daily, lisinopril 40 mg daily, glipizide 20 mg daily, clopidogrel 75 mg daily, zolpidem 10 mg at night as needed for insomnia, and two recent additions: haloperidol 5 mg as needed for agitation and lorazepam 2 mg IV as needed for agitation.

● RISK FACTORS

As with most geriatric syndromes, the development of delirium is most commonly a multifactoral process and rarely will a single explanation be found to explain the onset or the severity of all of the patient's delirium-related symptoms. Medication side effects and infectious etiologies are the two most common causes of delirium. However, environmental factors, altered sensory perception, and the contributions of underlying medical co-morbidities are often important factors in the severity and persistence of delirium. Risk factors for delirium may be divided into two broad categories: intrinsic risk factors, which often cannot be changed, and extrinsic risk factors, which can be altered or eliminated. These risk factors are given in Table 30–2.

Intrinsic Risk Factors

Intrinsic risk factors are conditions that predispose an older patient to the development of delirium. Often, these risk factors are not modifiable. Examples of intrinsic risk factors for delirium include age, underlying cognitive impairment, and chronic co-morbidities. In our case, EM has risk factors of age and a number of chronic co-morbidities. From the history provided by her daughter, your patient does not have underlying cognitive impairment. Some intrinsic factors are, however,

● **TABLE 30–2** Risk Factors for Delirium

Intrinsic Risk Factors	
Age	
Cognitive impairment	
Medical co-morbidity	
Severity of illness	
Surgical intervention	
Sensory impairment (hearing, visual, etc.)	

Extrinsic Risk Factors	
Classes of Risk Factors	Examples
Pharmacologic	Overmedication, withdrawal syndromes, medication interactions
Infectious	Urinary tract infections, pneumonia
Neurologic	Stroke, subdural hematoma, seizure
Cardiac	Arrhythmia, myocardial infarction, CHF exacerbation
Renal/Urologic	Renal failure, urinary retention
Metabolic	Dehydration, electrolyte abnormalities, hypoxia
Endocrine	Hypothyroidism, hyperthyroidism, hypoglycemia, hyperglycemia

modifiable to some extent and include sensory impairments, specifically decreased visual and auditory acuity. Examples of approaches to modifying these risk factors include encouraging the patient to use his or her own eyeglasses when hospitalized or the use of large print to communicate. Similar to use of these strategies in persons with decreased visual acuity, the use of the patient's own hearing aids or providing a voice amplifier may help with communication and orientation in the patient with poor hearing.

Special emphasis must be placed on determining the pre-delirium cognitive function of each patient undergoing delirium evaluation. In this case, E.M.'s cognitive history was obtained by calling her daughter; however, similar information probably could have been obtained from her assisted living facility. The high prevalence of underlying dementia in combination with new cognitive declines in patients experiencing acute delirium makes a reliable determination of baseline cognitive function difficult and it is often not possible when relying on the patient alone. The cognitive deficits may be similar in persons with either dementia or delirium, and therefore involving caregivers (family, others) in obtaining the patient's history is critical in order to avoid misdiagnosing the patient as having only dementia or some other chronic syndrome of cognitive impairment. Again and most importantly, underlying cognitive impairment is itself a major risk factor for delirium, and both diagnoses many times coexist in the same patient.

Extrinsic Risk Factors

The majority of modifiable risk factors for the development of delirium are extrinsic. The identification of these risk factors in patients and implementation of interventions aimed at modification of these risk factors has been shown to decrease the incidence of delirium and to improve important patient outcomes. However, if prevention has not succeeded, prompt assessment and treatment of new-onset delirium through systematic accounting for each underlying potential cause of delirium should be implemented in an effort to reverse the effects of delirium on patient morbidity, mortality, and length of hospital stay. Common examples of extrinsic risk factors (listed in Table 30–2) include inappropriate Foley catheter use and medication side effects (eg, an inadequate pain control regimen postoperatively). The next sections describe in more detail the range of extrinsic risk factors associated with delirium and address approaches to risk reduction.

Pharmacologic Risk Factors

Medication-related adverse effects are the most common cause of delirium. While many medications are associated with development of delirium, three general categories of medication use are most commonly linked to its development. These categories include (1) medications known as being "high risk" for incident delirium in the elderly, (2) under/overutilization of medications with an established indication for symptom relief in the elderly (especially pain), and (3) in hospitalized patients, precipitous withdrawal of medications regularly used in the outpatient setting prior to admission. Useful tools have been developed for the identification of medications associated with a high risk for adverse events such as delirium. Perhaps the most widely known of these lists is the Beers criteria, a helpful guide for clinicians in safe medication management in older adults.[10] In both inpatient and outpatient clinical encounters, a thorough review of medications using the Beers list or a similar list is of paramount importance to clinicians to eliminate potential causes of delirium. Many electronic medical records now provide this safety feature. The medication review should focus not only on the patient's current prescription medications, but also include investigation for any recent additions or recently discontinued medications, as well as a review of over-the-counter medications. Additionally, this history should include an assessment of current alcohol intake or use of medications in which abrupt discontinuation could lead to a withdrawal syndrome (such as benzodiazepines or narcotics). If significant alcohol intake or medications with the potential for a withdrawal syndrome are identified, appropriate medical strategies to prevent withdrawal should immediately be implemented.

Table 30–3 describes the classes of medications that, though often useful and even necessary in clinical practice, are associated with a significantly increased risk of incident delirium. Psychotropic medications are by far those most commonly associated with the development of delirium due to their effective penetration across the blood–brain barrier. Medications in this category include antipsychotic medications (both atypical and typical), benzodiazepines, narcotics, and antidepressants. Also important are medications with anticholinergic properties, such as those commonly used to treat urinary incontinence. These medications have repeatedly shown an association with alteration in mental status consistent with delirium.[11] However, many other medication classes, such as antibiotics, cardiovascular agents (some antihypertensives and statins), or endocrine agents (steroids) have been associated with delirium. For outpatients or patients admitted with acute delirium, medication review must include over-the-counter medications. Many common over-the-counter medications contain substances associated with delirium, such as diphenhydramine, which may lead to symptoms of confusion and increase other risks, such as the risk of falls. In summary, a full review of the patient's medication list must be undertaken in every patient with new-onset delirium.

● TABLE 30–3 Medication Classes Increasing the Risk of Delirium
Antipsychotic medications
Antidepressants
Benzodiazepines
Opioid analgesics
Over-the-counter medications (eg, diphenhydramine)
Sedative-hypnotic sleeping aids
Medications for urinary incontinence

CASE PRESENTATION (continued)

Upon review of E.M.'s medication list, you are concerned not only about the recent medication additions but also the medications she has been on long term. You ask the clinical pharmacist to help you determine how E.M.'s medications might have contributed to her delirium.

Medication List

Digoxin 0.25 mg daily

Metoprolol 50 mg daily

Atorvastatin 40 mg daily

Lisinopril 40 mg daily

Glipizide 20 mg daily

Clopidogrel 75 mg daily

Zolpidem 10 mg at night as needed for insomnia

Haloperidol 5 mg as needed for agitation

Lorazepam 2 mg IV as needed for agitation

Your list of potential offending drugs is substantial. Digoxin at a dose of 0.25 mg per day is often too high a dose for the geriatric patient (0.125 would be preferable) and can be associated with confusion, somnolence, headaches, and visual disturbances. If her oral intake has been poor, then glipizide may have caused hypoglycemia, which can certainly cause fluctuations in mental status. You don't know how long she has been on the zolpidem, but as this medication is centrally acting and given her unknown tolerability to these agents, you already have three drugs on the list that may be contributing to her condition. The recent additions of both haloperidol and lorazepam are troubling to both you and the pharmacist, as they have the potential to prolong her condition and likely will not help resolve the delirium.

You agree to adjust the dose of her digoxin, check the digoxin level, review her recent labs to evaluate her renal function and blood glucose measurements, and discontinue the haloperidol and lorazepam. You also will call the facility to find out how long she has been on the zolpidem and whether it has been effective.

Infectious Risk Factors

Infectious etiologies of delirium are also frequently encountered in the evaluation of a patient with delirium. The clinician should have a low threshold for suspicion of an infection as the primary cause leading to delirium in the geriatric patient. Often these patients present with no fever or other systemic signs or symptoms of infection (see Chapter 9 on atypical disease presentations). Urinary tract infections and respiratory infections (eg, pneumonia) are the most commonly seen infections leading to delirium, though numerous other sources of infection, such as an abdominal abscess, must also be considered. Although rare in comparison to other infections, bacterial and viral meningitis frequently present alterations in mental status as the initial symptom of infection, and in persons without an obvious source for their delirium and a normal brain scan or nonfocal neurologic exam, a lumbar puncture to evaluate for evidence of meningitis or other central nervous system infectious etiologies may be warranted.

Neurologic Risk Factors

Acute neurologic events may present with onset of confusion and an altered level of consciousness. Cerebrovascular accidents (either acute or subacute in presentation) should be considered first on the differential diagnosis for a patient presenting with confusion and a focal neurologic deficit. Neuroimaging of the brain, via either magnetic resonance imaging (preferred for acute stroke) or CT scan of the brain, may be used to determine whether an acute stroke has occurred. In patients with a recent fall, intracranial bleeding, such as a subdural hematoma, should also be considered. Seizure disorder should also be considered in the differential diagnosis of a patient presenting with confusion, as the postictal state after seizure frequently presents with confusion and lethargy. For patients without a known seizure history and in whom there is a clinical suspicion for seizure disorder, an electroencephalogram (EEG) should be obtained to evaluate for this potential etiology of delirium.

Cardiac Risk Factors

In the geriatric population, atypical presentation of a myocardial infarction may be associated with confusion without the classic history of chest pain or chest pressure. This presentation may, in particular, be seen in patients with dementia or underlying cognitive impairment, due to the inability to adequately describe the typical underlying symptoms. Additionally, perception and interpretation of pain may be altered in geriatric patients due to other co-morbidities, and their presentation for myocardial infarction may more commonly present as the "silent myocardial infarction."[12] Furthermore, exacerbation of underlying cardiac disease, such as exacerbations of congestive heart failure or development of arrhythmias, may lead to dysregulation in oxygen delivery with subsequent hypoxia and confusion.

Renal and Urologic Risk Factors

Patients presenting with acute renal failure will often have associated altered mentation or frank confusion. Disruption in the clearance of nitrogen and other metabolic products leads to mild confusion which may progress to lethargy and either hypoactive (more frequently) or hyperactive delirium. Additionally, patients with urinary retention may develop acute confusion which can rapidly improve after the retention is alleviated. This has been termed "cystocerebral syndrome," though the full mechanism behind this entity leading to delirium is poorly understood.[13]

Metabolic Risk Factors

Probably the most common metabolic abnormality associated with delirium is dehydration with its associated hypernatremia. Dehydration also predisposes the geriatric patient to other potential causes of delirium, such as fecal impaction. Preventing dehydration has been shown to decrease rates of delirium.[14] Furthermore, acute confusional states can be seen with electrolyte abnormalities, such as hypercalcemia (which can be seen in malignancies and endocrine abnormalities) and hyponatremia (which can occur with a syndrome of inappropriate antidiuretic hormone, SIADH).

Endocrine Risk Factors

Disturbances of the endocrine system can occur that lead to delirium and should be considered based upon the patient's history, exam, and initial lab work. Both severe hypothyroidism (sometimes referred to as myxedema coma) and hyperthyroidism (often called thyroid storm) may also lead to delirium. Hyperparathyroidism, with its associated hypercalcemia, can also present with acute confusion when calcium levels become significantly elevated. Abnormalities in adrenal function, including adrenal insufficiency, may present with altered mental status. Additionally, both hypoglycemia (common in "brittle" diabetics or aggressive diabetes management) and hyperglycemia (as seen in cases of diabetic ketoacidosis and hyperosmolar hyperglycemia) can present with significant alterations in mental status.

● ADDITIONAL DIFFERENTIAL DIAGNOSIS

Although delirium occurs more commonly than almost every form of new-onset psychiatric disorder in the geriatric population (especially in the setting of an acute medical illness), underlying psychiatric causes should be considered in patients presenting with confusion. However, all potential underlying causes of delirium should be evaluated prior to making the diagnosis of an underlying psychiatric illness. Once again, the history is a key contributor to differentiating delirium and psychiatric illness, with psychiatric illness typically developing more slowly and delirium typically being relatively acute in onset. In patients with hypoactive delirium, underlying or concurrent depression should be considered. However, evaluation for depression should take place only after other causes have been ruled out, unless history from the patient's caregivers is consistent with an underlying major depressive disorder. Since patients with hyperactive delirium often present with psychomotor agitation or hallucinations, these patients are often misdiagnosed as having an underlying psychiatric disorder, and are frequently referred for psychiatry consultation in the hospital setting. While the possibility of underlying bipolar disorder, mania, or schizophrenia exists, the diagnosis of primary psychiatric etiology should only be made after the initial evaluation and elimination of other potential etiologies of delirium and altered mental status. If psychiatric illness is felt to be the diagnosis, consultation with or referral to a geriatric psychiatrist should be undertaken.

• PREVENTIVE STRATEGIES

As previously established, many risk factors for delirium in the hospital setting may be identified and eliminated. Even in instances where the patient has irreversible (or intrinsic) risk factors, such as requiring care in an intensive care unit, modification of the treatment environment and the therapeutic plan will often reduce the incidence in the development of delirium. Independent baseline risk factors for the development of delirium have been identified in the hospitalized geriatric patient. These risk factors included cognitive impairment, visual impairment, high blood urea nitrogen/creatinine ratio, and severe illness.[15] Identification of these risk factors in an older patient should prompt the clinician to consider the patient at high risk for delirium. Additionally, precipitating risk factors for the development of delirium during hospitalization have also been identified and include use of physical restraints, malnutrition, use of a bladder catheter, addition of more than three medications, and any iatrogenic event.[16] Each of these risk factors is considered modifiable or preventable and would be amenable to prevention strategies, which further emphasizes the need for effective preventive strategies at all levels of clinical training and hospital settings.

Strategies to prevent the development of delirium should especially focus on reducing medication and infectious causes of delirium. Periodic review and elimination of all unnecessary medications is critical to delirium prevention in both the inpatient and outpatient setting. Vigilance in reducing infection-related delirium risks includes practices such as avoiding inappropriate use of Foley catheters and their associated iatrogenic urinary tract infections. Foley catheters should only be used when there is a clear indication (ie, when treating urinary retention, in early evaluation of patients with acute renal failure, in patients early in the postsurgical course, or in cases where the patient is in the terminal stages of life and catheter use is primarily for comfort), and should be

discontinued immediately when their use is no longer indicated. Other strategies to prevent infection-related delirium include the use of incentive spirometry to decrease the incidence of pneumonia and early mobilization to prevent functional decline and the associated risk of infection from immobility.

Preventive interventions focused on addressing six known risk factors have demonstrated a decreased incidence of persistent delirium at hospital discharge. These interventions included early mobilization of patients, addressing visual and hearing impairment through environmental modifications, implementing strategies to prevent sleep deprivation, preventing dehydration, and implementing reorientation and other cognitive exercises that engage patients with known cognitive impairment during their hospital stay. These interventions reduced the incidence of delirium most effectively in patients with two or more of the six identified risk factors.[14]

Because delirium is a frequent complication in hospitalized older adults, an additional strategy for prevention is education of the patient, family, and caregivers at the time of admission regarding the risk for, and warning signs of, the development of, delirium. Family and caregivers, along with nursing staff, often provide critical early observations of change in patient behavior that is a harbinger of impending delirium. Many of the interventions noted (for example, reorientation and the use of visual and hearing assistive devices) can be delivered with the assistance of family members. Additionally, the symptoms associated with delirium may cause significant distress for the patient, patient's family, and caregivers, both professional and informal. This discussion establishes a partnership between the health care team, the patient, and the patient's family for the express purpose of prevention, early detection, and treatment of delirium.

Recommended Initial Workup of Delirium

Laboratory and imaging orders should be based upon the differential diagnosis formulated from a thorough history and physical examination. In a patient whose history and physical examination do not point to an obvious delirium etiology, Table 30–4 provides a guideline regarding the utility of initial laboratory testing and imaging in the patient with delirium.

• TABLE 30–4 Routine Laboratory and Imaging Recommendations for Initial Workup of Delirium[a]

Test	Conditions Evaluated
Complete blood count (CBC)	Leukocytosis (infectious marker)
Basic metabolic profile (BMP)	Electrolytes, renal function, dehydration
Urinalysis (UA)	Urinary tract infection, dehydration
Chest x-ray	Respiratory infections, CHF exacerbation
Electrocardiogram (ECG)	Arrhythmias, myocardial injury
Urine drug screen	Intoxications
Neuroimaging (CT scan or MRI)[b]	Stroke, subdural hematoma

[a]Further testing should proceed from results of these tests as well as clinical suspicion based on the patient's history and physical examination.
[b]If the above tests are negative and/or if focal neurologic deficit is found on examination.

Recommended tests include a complete blood count to evaluate for leukocytosis that may indicate infection; a basic metabolic profile to evaluate for electrolyte abnormalities, renal function, and dehydration; a urinalysis and chest x-ray to evaluate for the more common infectious etiologies for delirium (UTI and pneumonia); an electrocardiogram to evaluate for arrhythmias or myocardial infarction; and a urine drug screen to evaluate for occult substance abuse/misuse etiologies. Neuroimaging via CT or MRI should be considered if the other recommended tests do not identify an obvious source for delirium or in the setting of either a focal neurologic deficit on exam or high clinical suspicion for intracranial abnormalities (such as cerebrovascular accident or subdural hematoma).

CASE PRESENTATION (continued)

You review E.M.'s chart and notice a urinalysis that appears to have been overlooked. The urine is noted to be dark with a specific gravity of 1.025 as well as 4+ bacteria, 3+ white blood cells, and positive leukocyte esterase. Blood cultures obtained at the time of admission have remained no growth. Your patient's laboratory work reveals a white blood cell count of $15 \times 10^3/\mu L$ ($15 \times 10^9/L$) with neutrophil predominance. Her electrolyte panel reveals mild hypernatremia with a sodium level of 148 mEq/L (148 mmol/L), a BUN of 31 mg/dL (11.1 mmol/L), and a creatinine of 0.9 mg/dL (79.6 μmol/L). Her glucose on arrival was 186 mg/dL (10.3 mmol/L) and subsequent glucose values have all been above 100 mg/dL (5.55 mmol/L), and her digoxin level is at a therapeutic level of 1.5 ng/mL (1.92 nmol/L). Cardiac enzymes are negative.

Her EKG is unchanged in comparison to previous EKGs from outside the hospital. Her chest x-ray demonstrates bibasilar atelectasis. A head CT obtained in the emergency room showed mild atrophy, but no evidence for stroke or other acute changes.

The BUN to creatinine ratio is suggestive of a prerenal state, which confirms what you saw on exam, so you give E.M. a fluid bolus as well as increase her IV rate for a few hours. In addition, you start an IV antibiotic for her urinary tract infection.

● MANAGEMENT OF DELIRIUM

Even the most systematic approach to delirium prevention strategies is often insufficient to prevent delirium. As with prevention strategies, the management of delirium is also often multifactorial and multidisciplinary, requiring effective coordination and communication by the entire medical team and the family. In general, management of delirium can be broadly classified into two categories—nonpharmacologic and pharmacologic interventions.

Nonpharmacologic Interventions

Often the very medications clinicians use to treat the symptoms of delirium may actually worsen or prolong its course. For this reason, nonpharmacologic interventions are preferred as first-line treatment in patients with delirium. These interventions are geared toward decreasing or eliminating the extrinsic risk factors associated with the development of delirium as well as in decreasing the intensity and length of delirium symptoms. Nonpharmacologic interventions are typically focused on patient-centered interactions and modifications of the hospital environment.

The medical environment should be optimized to facilitate adequate sleep in the evenings. Examples of environmental modifications include minimizing assessment of vital signs overnight in clinically stable patients, moving the timing of phlebotomy to avoid early morning awakenings, and reducing or eliminating noise from hospital staff activities. Methods to improve the patient's sensory environment are also recommended, particularly for persons with decreased visual acuity (eg, large clocks in the room, orientation boards, and large numbers on the telephone surface) and auditory acuity (voice amplifiers as well as using a voice in communication that is slow, calming, and appropriate for the level of hearing loss).

Family members, caregivers, and the clinical staff of the hospital are critically important members of the care team in terms of both communication and promoting patient safety for the patient with delirium. Patients can manifest symptoms ranging from mild symptoms (such as disorientation to time) to more severe cases of altered environmental perceptions (such as hallucinations, which can be threatening to the patient). Reassurance of safety, redirection of the patient's attention toward nonthreatening subjects, engaging the patient in conversation and other cognitive tasks tailored to their interests, and maintaining the patient's interaction throughout the day (minimizing both understimulation and overstimulation) are all effective methods for reducing the patient's anxiety and psychomotor symptoms related to delirium. Additionally, if the presence of family members is noted to help calm the patient, asking family members to spend the night with the patient may help improve sleep quality and minimize symptoms.

Physicians and clinical staff should avoid interventions proven to increase the risk of delirium or exacerbate existing delirium. This includes the use of physical restraints or medications (so-called "chemical restraints") used to treat the symptoms of delirium but not the underlying cause, such as antipsychotics, except in specific conditions (outlined later). Use of such approaches may unintentionally increase the severity or duration of the patient's symptoms. In addition, medications used for valid purposes in the treatment of a patient's underlying medical illness (narcotics after surgery, anti-emetics, etc.) may have the unintended consequences of increasing the risk, severity, and duration of delirium.

The use of physical restraints has, fortunately, significantly declined in the hospital and community care settings. Restraints have been repeatedly shown to increase agitation, increase the risk of injury and death, and contribute to the prolongation of delirium.[14,17] Physical restraints should be used only for a very short term (minutes to a very few hours) in the most severe cases of psychomotor agitation, where there is significant risk of physical injury to the medical staff or patient. Even in the ICU, restraint use should be limited to settings where removal of life-supporting devices could prove fatal. If physical restraints are used, they should be used after exhausting all other possible options, and the indication for their use should be evaluated frequently throughout the day to insure that the restraints are being used for the least amount of time possible.

Pharmacologic Interventions

While nonpharmacologic interventions are by far the preferred method of treatment for delirium, the intensity of the patient's symptoms may sometimes require a brief treatment with medications to decrease the patient's agitation and prevent harm to the patient or staff while evaluating for the underlying causes of the patient's delirium. The current evidence base for the use of medications in the treatment of delirium demonstrates no truly "safe" medication to be used in the treatment of delirium. The medications used to treat delirium often have a significant side effect profile and can increase the risk of adverse outcomes in patients due to their sedative properties. The geriatric patient is especially susceptible to the harmful effects of these medications due to age-related changes in drug metabolism and underlying medical co-morbidity. Thus, a careful review of the patient's medical history should occur when deciding to use a medication for symptomatic treatment and, when absolutely necessary, medications should be started at the lowest dose possible and subsequently titrated up in dose, if needed and tolerated by the patient. In the setting of a physically violent patient or those where life-sustaining instruments are at risk of being removed by the patient (such as central lines or endotracheal tubes), the benefit of a short course of sedating medications likely exceeds the risks. However, medications to attempt to treat the symptoms of delirium should not be used in instances where patients are simply causing a "disruptive" environment or are requiring "too much attention" through increased ancillary supervision.

Antipsychotics are the drug class that has been best studied in the symptomatic treatment of delirium. Antipsychotics can be divided into two classes: typical and atypical. Atypical antipsychotics are often used initially, given their decreased anticholinergic characteristics and more rapid clearance from the body in comparison to typical antipsychotics; however, the evidence base for their use in delirium is limited.[18] The typical antipsychotic most often used in the symptomatic treatment of delirium is haloperidol (Haldol). When using antipsychotics in the elderly, a clinician should start with the lowest possible dose of the medication (eg, 0.5 mg of haloperidol). An increase in the dosage should be considered only after reevaluating the patient and after other nonpharmacologic measures have been attempted, and medications should be used for the shortest duration possible to achieve symptom control.

Few studies have examined the effectiveness of atypical antipsychotics in the symptomatic treatment of delirium, and the side effect profile associated with antipsychotics makes it crucial for the clinician to carefully consider the necessity of the medication and weigh the risk/benefit profile to the situation. Extrapyramidal symptoms such as motor restlessness or tardive dyskinesia may result from antipsychotic use. Additionally, antipsychotic medications may lead to an increased risk of falls due to both sedative effects as well as potential alterations in muscle tone. Finally, cardiac abnormalities, including torsades de pointes, can be seen due to prolongation of the QT interval. Due to the increased cardiac risk, patients initially placed on antipsychotics likely benefit from cardiac monitoring. Use of antipsychotics should be strongly reconsidered and avoided, if possible, in patients with an extensive cardiac history and should not be used in patients with a prolonged QT interval at baseline.

The other class of medications frequently used in the symptomatic treatment of delirium is benzodiazepines. However, these medications should not be used as first-line pharmacologic treatments unless there is a contraindication to antipsychotic use. This is due to the risk for increased sedation and potential to intensify the patient's underlying mental status changes with the use of these medications. In addition, there is the risk of a paradoxical reaction in which the agitated behavior can worsen with increasing doses of benzodiazepines. In these circumstances, the agent should be stopped immediately. If used, benzodiazepines with short half-lives, such as oxazepam or lorazepam, should be used to avoid prolonged sedation. There are certain disease states where benzodiazepines may be indicated for initial use in the symptomatic treatment of delirium, such as in patients with known QT prolongation or a significant cardiac disease history, patients with Parkinson disease, or those patients with Lewy body dementia with superimposed delirium. The latter two classes of patients may react more favorably to benzodiazepines, as antipsychotics may increase the patient's muscle tone and worsen mobility. Finally, patients with alcohol or benzodiazepine withdrawal syndromes should be treated with benzodiazepines to prevent the life-threatening complications from these withdrawal states.

To reiterate, nonpharmacologic interventions should always be pursued in the initial treatment plan for patients presenting with signs and symptoms of delirium. Nonpharmacologic interventions, including family and staff education about symptom interpretation and management, environmental modification, increased supervision from ancillary staff, and family sitting with the patient, should all be strongly considered prior to the initiation of pharmacologic interventions or physical restraints. If pharmacologic treatment or physical restraints are required, clinician assessment and frequent reassessment are warranted. If pharmacologic treatment or restraints are felt to be necessary, clear and complete documentation of the reason for their requirement, risk/benefit discussion with family, plan for addressing the patient's delirium, and subsequent discontinuation of these agents should be documented in the patient's chart.

CASE PRESENTATION (continued)

A geriatrics team meeting was held to discuss the optimal management for E.M. A number of recommendations were developed. Your social worker contacted the patient's daughter and asked her, if possible, to stay with her mother in the hospital for the next evening. A bedside chair that reclined to accommodate sleep was requested for the patient's room. The nursing staff recommended stopping the 2 AM vital signs as well as switching her IV medications and fluids to oral as soon as possible. The pharmacist said that she would again review all of E.M.'s medications to see if there remained any that may still be contributing to her condition as well as prescribe a suitable antibiotic that would provide adequate coverage in oral form. The therapy staff indicated that they would perform a functional assessment and, if needed, they would work with social work on a short-term rehabilitation placement.

Over the next few days E.M. improved remarkably and was able to return home with outpatient therapy provided through her assisted living facility.

CONCLUSION

Delirium is a common, though serious, medical emergency, given its association with adverse outcomes including functional decline, increased morbidity, and increased mortality. However, as delirium is a potentially preventable geriatric syndrome, interventions focused on the prevention and early detection of signs and symptoms of delirium are critical. Evaluation of all older patients, but particularly those with significant risk factors for delirium, is essential in optimizing patient outcomes. Particular emphasis should be placed on frequent evaluation of the patient's medication profile and evaluation for possible infectious etiologies. Treatment of delirium should focus on treating the underlying cause, if possible, and implementing nonpharmacologic interventions, centered on a multidisciplinary approach to patient care.

References

1. Sumner AD, Simons RJ. Delirium in the hospitalized elderly. *Cleve Clin J Med.* 1994;61:258-262.

2. Inouye SK. Delirium in older persons. *N Engl J Med.* 2006;354:1157-1165.

3. Pisani MA, McNicoll L, Inouye SK. Cognitive impairment in the intensive care unit. *Clin Chest Med.* 2003;24(4):727-737.

4. McAvay GJ, van Ness PH, Bogardus ST, et al. Older adults discharged from hospital with delirium: One year outcomes. *J Am Geriatr Soc.* 2006;54:1245-1250.

5. Leslie DL, Marcantonio ER, Zhang Y, et al. One-year health care costs associated with delirium in the elderly population. *Arch Intern Med.* 2008;168:27-32.

6. Marcantonio ER. Delirium. In: *Geriatrics Review Syllabus.* 6th ed. New York: American Geriatrics Society; 2006.

7. Ely EW, Shintani A, Truman B, et al. Delirium as a predictor of mortality in mechanically ventilated patients in the intensive care unit. *JAMA.* 2004;291:1753-1762.

8. Young J, Inouye SK. Delirium in older people. *BMJ.* 2007;334:842-846.

9. Inouye SK, van Dyck CH, Alessi CA, et al. Clarifying confusion: The Confusion Assessment Method. A new method for detection of delirium. *Ann Intern Med.* 1990;113:941-948.

10. Fick DM, Cooper JW, Wade WE, et al. Updating the Beers criteria for potentially inappropriate medication use in older adults: Results of a US consensus panel of experts. *Arch Intern Med.* 2003;163:2716-2724.

11. Han L, McCusker J, Cole M, et al. Use of medications with anticholinergic effect predicts clinical severity of delirium symptoms in older medical inpatients. *Arch Intern Med.* 2001;161:1099-1105.

12. Gregoratos G. Clinical manifestations of acute myocardial infarction in older patients. *Am J Geriatr Cardiol.* 2001;10:345-347.

13. Blackburn T, Dunn M. Cystocerebral syndrome. Acute urinary retention presenting as confusion in elderly patients. *Arch Intern Med.* 1990;150:2577-2578.

14. Inouye SK, Bogardus ST Jr, Charpentier PA, et al. A multicomponent intervention to prevent delirium in hospitalized older patients. *N Engl J Med.* 1999;340:669-676.

15. Inouye SK, Viscoli CM, Horwitz RI, et al. A predictive model for delirium in hospitalized elderly medical patients based on admission characteristics. *Ann Intern Med.* 1993;119:474-481.

16. Inouye SK, Zhang Y, Jones RN, et al. Risk factors for delirium at discharge: Development and validation of a predictive model. *Arch Intern Med.* 2007;167:1406-1413.

17. Evans D, Wood J, Lambert L. Patient injury and physical restraint devices: A systematic review. *J Adv Nurs.* 2003;41:274-282.

18. Lonergan E, Britton AM, Luxenberg J, Wyller T. Antipsychotics for delirium. *Cochrane Database Syst Rev.* 2007;2:CD005594.

POST-TEST

1. **A precipitating risk factor for the development of delirium is:**
   A. Change in diet
   B. Adding a new medicine
   C. High blood pressure
   D. Physical restraint

2. **Prevention interventions for delirium include all of the following EXCEPT:**
   A. Prevent sleep deprivation
   B. Careful fluid restriction
   C. Early mobilization
   D. Family and caregiver education

3. **All of the following are extrinsic risk factors for delirium EXCEPT:**
   A. Inadequate pain management
   B. Presence of a Foley catheter
   C. Underlying cognitive impairment
   D. Fecal impaction

ANSWERS TO PRE-TEST

1. D
2. A
3. C

ANSWERS TO POST-TEST

1. D
2. B
3. C

31

Dementia

Loren S. Greenberg, MS, MD

● **LEARNING OBJECTIVES**

1. Identify signs of cognitive impairment.
2. Discuss the differential diagnosis of cognitive impairment and the key features of each type.
3. Describe the components and process of patient evaluation when cognitive impairment is suspected.
4. Compare and contrast major types of dementia in terms of pathology, risk factors, and presentation.
5. Describe behavioral and clinical strategies used to treat patients with dementia.

PRE-TEST

1. **Patients with early dementia most commonly present with which symptom?**
   A. Complaints of loss of memory
   B. Evidence of depression
   C. Marked decline in social skills and inability to relate to others
   D. Difficulty with attention

2. **Which of the following demonstrates mild cognitive impairment?**
   A. Mini-Mental State Exam score of less than 24 but greater than 20
   B. Positive Mini-Cog
   C. Diagnosis of mild dementia but is still able to live independently
   D. Memory difficulties but is independent in activities of daily living

3. **Which of the following is TRUE when treating patients with dementia who experience agitation?**

   A. Neuroleptics are shown to be safe and effective in treating agitation in dementia.
   B. Trying to redirect aggressive behavior usually creates further agitation.
   C. Typical antipsychotics should be used over atypical antipsychotics.
   D. Increasing environmental stimuli may reduce agitated behavior.

4. **Which of the following is appropriate patient counseling for risk of developing Alzheimer dementia?**
   A. Mild cognitive impairment is not a likely risk factor for Alzheimer dementia.
   B. Reducing vascular risk factors may reduce the risk of Alzheimer dementia.
   C. Onset of depression early in adulthood is predictive of dementia and therefore should be treated.
   D. Patients should be tested for the ApoE4 gene as its presence is reassuring for reduced risk.

INTRODUCTION

Dementia is an acquired syndrome of decline in multiple cognitive abilities, including memory, severe enough to interfere with daily function. The current estimated prevalence of dementia is more than 13% of the population aged 71 and older.[1] Alzheimer dementia alone affects about 13% of the population in the United States aged 65 and older,[1,2] which is equivalent to over 5.3 million people. The number of older adults with dementia is expected to explode worldwide as the population ages and lifespan increases.

Dementia has a tremendous physical, emotional, and financial impact on the patient, the family, and society. Those suffering from dementia will experience increased mortality, loss of function and independence, as well as psychological disturbances and social isolation. In 2006, Alzheimer disease was the sixth leading cause of death in the United State and contributed to 11.2% of all years lived with disability, higher than that from stroke, musculoskeletal disorders, heart disease, and cancer.[2]

CASE PRESENTATION: MILD MEMORY CHANGES

E.P. is a 75-year-old retired high school math teacher who comes to your geriatrics practice for evaluation of her general medical problems. She feels well and has no symptoms. E.P. has hypertension, mild intermittent asthma, and osteoporosis. She reveals that her T score was −3.0. She takes quinipril, lovastatin, albuterol, and risedronate. She brings her medications and is able to tell you accurately the names of her medications and the doses. Her social history reveals that she lives alone and is independent in all of her daily activities including managing her own finances. She takes public transportation and took two buses to come to your office. She recently gave up driving, stating that she no longer needed the car as she has moved into a new retirement community that offers many group trips. She does not have children but has many friends. She had smoked about 10 pack-years and stopped "many years ago." As part of the routine initial visit, you ask about her memory. She initially denies any difficulties but on further questioning reveals that she has been having difficulty remembering the names of new people she is meeting in the retirement community. She comments, "I was always so good with names." She admits to receiving a late notice for an electric bill, but thinks that she never received the original bill. Additionally, she missed a dental cleaning because she forgot the appointment but attributes this to her busy schedule. When asked about depression, E.P. states that she is in good spirits and enjoys her new blossoming social life. E.P.'s only involved family member, her nephew, confirms that she is not having difficulty caring for herself although she seems to forget some important details of their conversations at times.

THE EVALUATION OF COGNITIVE IMPAIRMENT

Suspecting Impairment

Possible cognitive impairment may come to the attention of a health care provider through the report of an informant (family, friends, caregivers), through screening for cognitive impairment, or less often through patient self-report of memory problems. Cognitive impairment along with loss of insight often makes self-awareness of impairment and therefore self-report unlikely. Informants should be asked specifically about impairment as this is often not reported due to lack of understanding of the significance of the problems.

The health care provider should observe for clues for cognitive impairment, especially if the patient comes alone, as in the case of E.P. Patients may forget appointments or have difficulty coordinating transportation. They may have difficulty articulating their concerns, prior history, or medications, or may not seem to comprehend fully the plan of care. Often when asked simple questions, the patient with cognitive impairment may turn to an accompanying caregiver for answers. If there is any suspicion based on observation or screening, further history should be sought from informants. In E.P.'s case, she was articulate and knowledgeable about her medical history and medications, not causing much suspicion for impairment except for possible forgetfulness on self-report.

Screening

Screening for impairment using cognitive testing in all older patients is controversial. The US Preventive Services Task Force Guidelines recommend limiting screening to patients in whom there is a suggestion of cognitive impairment based upon clinical observation or concern expressed by patients, family, friends, or caregivers.[3] ACOVE (Assessing Care of Vulnerable Elders) recommends screening for all "vulnerable elderly," defined as those who are in poor health and have difficulty with activities of daily living.[4] The American Geriatrics Society recommends screening in populations at risk for cognitive impairment or dementia, although these populations are not clearly defined.

The History

The evaluation for early dementia should begin by asking the patient and informant questions about a decline in memory, difficulties in performing daily activities, or changes in personality, behavior, or mood (Table 31–1).

TABLE 31–1 Clues to Suspecting Dementia

Memory Decline	Psychiatric Symptoms
Disoriented to time	Depression
Inability to learn new information	Anxiety
Repetitive conversation	Agitation
	Paranoia, delusions
	Misinterpretation of auditory/visual stimuli

Decline in Other Cognitive Domains	Personality Changes
Language (word finding, conversational skills)	Apathy/loss of prior interests
Reasoning/problem solving/ planning	Social withdrawal
Judgment	Hostility
Calculation/abstraction	Disinhibition (inappropriate friendliness, explosiveness)
Visuospatial skills/spatial orientation	
Ability to follow/understand conversation	
Skills for complex tasks	

Decline in Performance of Daily Activities	Behavior
Instrumental ADLs decline first (eg, handing bills)	Self-neglect
	Restlessness
	Sleeping more during day than night

Questions about memory include whether or not the patient is frequently having difficulty remembering details of recent personal activities, repeating or forgetting conversations, forgetting appointments or bills, misplacing items, leaving the stove on, or getting lost. Patients with very mild cognitive impairment may be able to self-report problems with memory, as in the case of E.P. Forgetting names is new for her and may be a cause for concern. Although her missing an occasional bill or appointment does not necessarily indicate cognitive impairment, in the context of new forgetfulness, further evaluation is indicated.

Questions about daily activities should address difficulties performing usual home, work, or social activities, as well as prior hobbies and interests. It is important to ask who handles responsibilities such as finances and shopping, as caregivers may have assumed the patient's responsibilities, concealing the patient's impairment. Identifying the reason that the family member has taken over a task may be revealing. For example, financial management may be delegated to a family member after the patient has made repeated mistakes in bill payments. The physician should explore whether EP really gave up driving because she no longer needed to drive, or because she was having difficulty driving.

Finally, a complete medical history, including medical problems, physical and psychiatric symptoms, medications, and social history, is important as this may reveal factors that may be interfering with cognition. A history of prior strokes should always be elucidated, as the evidence of prior strokes may no longer by apparent on exam. Questions about other risk factors for dementia (discussed later in this chapter) including a family history may reveal factors that increase your index of suspicion for dementia.

Differential Diagnosis of Cognitive Impairment

Complaints of memory loss are very common in older adults and can cause the patient or family a great deal of distress. Often, patients who complain about memory loss will not have dementia, particularly when symptoms are mild, vary in type or nature, and are not confirmed by others. Aside from dementia, the differential diagnosis of memory difficulties includes *changes of normal aging, mild cognitive impairment, delirium,* or *depression.* In addition, medications, systemic illness, pain, illicit drugs, alcohol, sleep deprivation, or stress can interfere with cognition.

Cognitive changes that are associated with *normal aging* do not significantly impact daily function. An evaluation that does not reveal a pathologic cause for cognitive changes is reassuring to the patient (see Chapter 3).

Depression is in the differential diagnosis of dementia when it presents with cognitive impairment, often known as "pseudodementia" (Chapter 37). Therefore, screening for depression is an important part of the evaluation of cognitive impairment. The cognitive deficits associated with depression tend to be most evident in tasks requiring effort or sustained attention.[5] Treating depression may at least partially reverse the impairment, although depressed patients are at higher risk for dementia later, and thus need to be monitored. Fortunately, depression was not a concern for E.P.

Delirium (Chapter 30) should be considered in the evaluation of cognitive impairment as well. In delirium, patients have an acute onset and rapid decline in cognition, as well as difficulty with attention compared with patients with dementia, who tend to have a slowly progressive course with spared attention until late in the disease. Table 31–2 highlights some differences.

Finally, *mild cognitive impairment* (MCI) should be considered when evaluating changes in mentation. MCI refers to cognitive impairment beyond that anticipated with normal aging, but that does not meet the criteria for dementia and does not interfere with activities of daily life.[5,6] The definition and distinction between normal aging, MCI, and early dementia are controversial. In general, a diagnosis of MCI should only be made after careful neuropsychological testing conducted by a skilled neuropsychologist with experience in dementia and MCI evaluations. There are various types of MCI, but amnestic MCI is most commonly described.

TABLE 31–2 Comparison of Dementia with Delirium

Dementia	Delirium
Gradual onset/progressive	Abrupt onset (hours or days)
Generally irreversible	Generally reversible
Relative stable	Hour-to-hour variability
Attention intact early on	Inattention prominent early
Preserved social interaction until late	Impaired social interaction
Word-finding difficulties	Incoherent or illogical language
Consciousness level intact until late	Altered level of consciousness (hyperalert or hypoalert)

The Mayo criteria for amnestic MCI are most commonly used in research.[7] The Mayo criteria define MCI as memory impairment, preferably corroborated by an informant and by cognitive testing, with preserved general cognitive function and intact activities of daily living. Whether or not MCI interferes with activities of daily life is controversial. Patients may experience interference with complex activities or social or work function, although not to the extent that someone else needs to assume a function for them.[6]

Individuals with amnestic MCI are at high risk for developing Alzheimer dementia. Statistics on conversion to Alzheimer dementia vary widely probably due to the lack of uniformity applied to the clinical criteria for MCI. The most recent studies show conversion rates as varying from 6% to 25% per year and 11% to 64% after 2 years; however, the consensus appears to be that almost all amnestic MCI patients will eventually convert over to Alzheimer disease. Conversely, population studies have shown that up to 44% of patients with MCI (all types) were estimated to return to normal a year later.[5,6,8]

The definition of MCI is expanding to include other categories. Amnestic multiple-domain MCI is memory loss plus impairment in at least one other domain, such as executive function. Non-amnestic single-domain MCI is impairment in one cognitive domain without memory loss. Finally, non-amnestic multiple-domain MCI is impairment in multiple cognitive domains without memory loss. MCI without memory impairment is less likely to convert to Alzheimer dementia but may be a prodrome of other types of dementia.[6]

Evidence of memory difficulty by E.P.'s history and impairment in recall on testing without obvious significant impairment in her daily activities makes MCI a possibility for her.

Dementia, commonly defined by the DSM-IV criteria,[9] is memory impairment plus impairment in at least one other cognitive domain. These cognitive deficits must cause significant impairment in social or occupational functioning, represent a significant decline from a previous level of functioning, and not be due to another cause such as delirium.

DSM-IV includes four possible involved cognitive domains:

- *Agnosia*: The inability to recognize and identify objects despite intact sensory function
- *Aphasia*: The impairment of language despite intact hearing and motor components of speech
- *Apraxia*: Difficulty executing skilled learned motor activities despite intact motor function and memory of the performance
- *Impairment in executive function*: Impairment in planning, sequencing, organizing, reasoning, or abstracting

The DSM-IV criteria may not be accurate in diagnosing dementia where impairment in other cognitive domains predominate,[10] such as inattention, spatial ability, calculation, or self-awareness. For example, attention deficits may be greater than memory impairment in Parkinson disease dementia.[11]

The fact that E.P. could accurately discuss the details about her medical history, easily coordinates her transport to her appointment by two buses, continues to socialize, and functions well independently, makes dementia less of a concern at this time.

CASE PRESENTATION (continued)

On physical examination, E.P. has an "upbeat" affect and is well dressed. Her examination reveals a blood pressure of 170/80 mm Hg but is otherwise unremarkable, including a normal gait and neurologic examination. She is articulate in discussing current events and answers simple math problems. She scores 28/30 on the Mini-Mental State Exam with two points lost on delayed recall. She accurately draw the numbers in the face of a clock and places the hands correctly to 10 minutes after 11, but both hands are the same length. You adjust her blood pressure medications and order lab work.

Physical Examination

The physical examination may provide further clues to the existence of dementia or suggest an etiology of dementia. Observation of disheveled appearance may be suggestive of cognitive decline. A thorough general examination may provide evidence of illness causing delirium. A complete neurologic examination should be performed looking for focal deficits, gait abnormalities, or findings specific to potential dementing disorders. Focal neurologic finding may be due to prior strokes or space-occupying lesions, for example. Parkinsonism, such as rigid gait and cogwheeling, may suggest Parkinson disease or dementia with Lewy bodies. E.P.'s physical exam only revealed hypertension—a risk factor for both Alzheimer and vascular dementia—but did not demonstrate evidence of strokes or other neurologic problems.

As part of the physical examination, cognition should first be assessed informally, followed by more formal tests described later. Short-term memory may be assessed by asking a patient to remember a short story or discuss current events. Difficulty with word finding, or use of vague terms and speech that is superficial in content, may represent aphasia. Agnosia may be tested by asking the patient to name various objects in the room. Apraxia may be elicited by asking the patient to pantomime how to use tools, such as "show me how you comb your hair." Impairment in executive function is difficult to test in isolation as it integrates many of the other cognitive skills needed to organize and execute plans. It is best evaluated by exploring how the patient completes real-life tasks such as balancing a checkbook or cooking. Tests of everyday mathematical skills may provide some information about executive function. For someone with a high level of education and intelligence, there would need to be a significant amount of cognitive decline before impairment is detected during this brief evaluation. E.P., who is a retired math teacher, would not be expected to have difficulty in basic math at this stage.

Formal Cognitive Testing

Many cognitive tests can be used for either screening or further evaluation of cognitive impairment. Only a few of these tests will be described here. Choice of test may depend on the situation, the amount of time available, language and level of education of the patient, as well as the severity of dementia suspected. Clinicians often screen with tests designed for rapid administration followed by more comprehensive testing if cognitive impairment is suspected. This may be done by combining a few different brief tests, each addressing different areas of cognition. At least one should include tests of memory. Patients should be tested on more than one occasion, as other transient factors such as effort, illness, or stress may interfere.

The Mini-Mental State Examination

The Mini-Mental State Examination (MMSE)[12] is one of the most widely used tests of cognition. It is a 30-point test that examines a range of cognitive functions. A score of less than 24 points suggests cognitive impairment. The MMSE score must be interpreted with caution as the score may be affected by factors other than cognitive ability, such as age, ethnicity, education, language, and motor and sensory deficits.[13] It may miss early dementia, especially in patients who are highly educated or have high baseline intelligence. E.P. scored a 28 and therefore had a negative MMSE. On the other hand, for a person with a high education level for whom a score of 30 out of 30 may be expected, the loss of 2 points may be sufficient reason to continue to monitor the patient closely. Her difficulty with delayed recall did reveal objective short-term impairment and supports at least the diagnosis of mild cognitive impairment. Alternatively, a low score does not necessarily diagnose cognitive impairment or differentiate between the etiologies of impairment. One literature review calculated the mean likelihood ratio (LR) for dementia for a positive result on the MMSE to be 6.3, while the likelihood ratio for dementia when memory loss was reported from an informant was 6.5. The likelihood ratio of a negative result was 0.19.[5] Once dementia is diagnosed, the MMSE may be a good tool for evaluating dementia severity and documenting subsequent decline.

The Mini-Cog

The Mini-Cog[14] has become popular because of the ease of administration and the lack of effect of language and education on scoring. It combines a three-item recall test with a clock-drawing test. The Mini-Cog asks the patient to remember three words. The clock-drawing test is then used to distract the patient prior to asking the patient to recall the three words. This involves asking the patient to put the numbers in the face of a clock either on a blank sheet of paper or in a large circle already drawn on the page and asking the patient to draw the hands set to a specific time. "10 minutes after 11 o'clock" is often used to differentiate abstract from concrete thinking, as the 2 on the clock face is symbolic for 10 minutes after the hour. Although E.P. had a negative Mini-Cog, it is concerning that the length of the hands that she drew were not varying appropriately in length. Figure 31–1 shows some examples of abnormal clocks that may be drawn by patients with dementia.

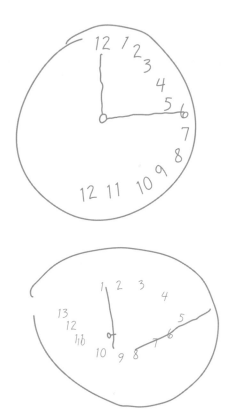

FIGURE 31–1. Clock drawing in patients with dementia.

Short Portable Mental Status Questionnaire

The Short Portable Mental Status Questionnaire (SPMSQ)[15] is a similar to the MMSE but takes education into account in the scoring. It is comprised of 10 questions encompassing orientation, memory, calculation, and personal history. The advantages of the SPMSQ include ease of administration, generally taking 5 minutes or less to administer, but test results must be adjusted for level of education.

Category Fluency Testing

Category Fluency is one test of language fluency. The patient is asked to name as many animals or grocery items as possible in one minute. One study demonstrated that less than 12 items is always abnormal.[16] The number score can also be used to monitor progression.

One large limitation for most brief cognitive tests is the lack of sensitivity for detecting early dementia in highly educated patients. More comprehensive tests such as the Montreal Cognitive Assessment and the Modified Mini-Mental State Exam may be more sensitive in this population, but require ample time for testing.[5,13] Other brief tests such as the Hopkins Verbal Learning Test are promising[5] but need further testing in the primary care population.

● DIAGNOSIS OF DEMENTIA

The diagnosis for dementia is one of clinical judgment. The diagnosis can be made when a combination of the history and cognitive testing demonstrates that a patient has a decline in multiple areas of cognition that is severe enough to cause a decline in a previous level of function. Physical exam, laboratory testing, and imaging may provide additional information to support to the diagnosis and identify potentially reversible causes and dementia subtype.

Laboratory Testing

The American Academy of Neurology (AAN) recommends screening for vitamin B_{12} deficiency and hypothyroidism in patients with cognitive impairment. Complete blood count, electrolytes, glucose, renal, and liver function tests may be considered but there is no clear evidence regarding their utility. These tests may identify abnormalities that are actually causing delirium or other contributory factors to cognitive impairment. Screening for syphilis is not recommended unless there is a high clinical suspicion for neurosyphillis.

Imaging

The AAN recommends a noncontrast CT or MRI of the brain in all patients with cognitive impairment. The American Geriatrics Society makes no specific recommendations on routine neuroimaging. However, its recommendations emphasize situations in which the yield may be higher with neuroimaging, such as young age of onset of cognitive impairment (less than 60), rapid deterioration, severe symptoms at the onset, or focal neurologic signs. Possible stroke history, as well as predisposing conditions for brain pathology such as metastatic cancer or the use of anticoagulants, should prompt neuroimaging as well. For most routine workups of cognitive dysfunction suggestive of Alzheimer disease, it is reasonable to forgo neuroimaging. Some clinicians perform imaging if risk factors for atherosclerotic disease are present. The finding of silent cerebrovascular disease may help assist in determining how modifiable risk factors should be treated.

Positron emission tomography (PET) scanning may be suggestive of dementia, but its clinical utility is still an area of ongoing investigation.

CASE PRESENTATION (continued)

One month after the initial visit, E.P. returns for a follow-up. You review her laboratory testing, which does not have any remarkable findings, to explain her difficulty with memory. You explain that although she likely has some short-term memory loss, you do not believe that she has dementia, but would like to follow her closely. One year later, the social worker at her retirement community calls because E.P.'s friends have started reporting concerns about her memory. She recently started having difficulty keeping up with conversations and often needs to be reminded about the dates and venues of outings. E.P. comes back to the office accompanied by a friend who was concerned that E.P. would not make it to the appointment. The friend states that E.P. seems to be very forgetful lately. E.P. protests, saying, "My memory is perfect." You note that E.P. is having some difficulty with word finding. The MMSE is repeated and she scores 28/30 again, losing 2 points on recall. Her clock drawing is unchanged from the last time. Given this significant decline in function was noticed by her friends, but lack of obvious decline on office testing, you refer E.P. for neuropsychological testing. This testing revealed significant deficits in delayed recall and in visual spatial reasoning. Based upon her significant memory difficulties plus a second area of cognitive impairment, she was diagnosed with likely mild Alzheimer dementia. After discussion about the risks, benefits, and limitations of cognitive enhancers, E.P. decides that she would like to try donepezil. You also decide that her blood pressure should be controlled more aggressively to slow the further decline of E.P.'s memory.

Neuropsychological Testing

Neuropsychological testing is an extensive evaluation of cognition, mood, personality, and behavior conducted by a licensed clinical neuropsychologist. Testing may take several hours but be quite useful when the diagnosis of cognitive impairment is unclear.

Referral may be useful when either the history or brief office testing is suspicious for dementia but neither is significant enough to make a diagnosis, or when a highly suspicious history is not corroborated by testing. Testing may help confirm a diagnosis that is difficult to make in cases of early dementia in a highly educated patient or may identify another diagnosis such as depression or mild cognitive impairment. Alternatively, the anxious patient or caregiver may be relieved to find out the patient's cognitive changes may be normal age-related changes.

More formal testing may also be warranted when office testing suggests cognitive impairment not confirmed by informant history, representing inadequate recognition of cognitive impairment by the family or simply unavailability of corroborating informants. Alternative explanations include a low level of education or a learning disability, an acute confusional state, or a psychiatric disorder in a patient without real cognitive decline.

● ETIOLOGY OF DEMENTIA

Although there are many subtypes of dementia (Table 31–3), the major ones in the elderly include:

- Alzheimer dementia
- Vascular dementia and mixed dementia
- Lewy body dementias
- Frontotemporal lobe dementia
- "Reversible dementias"

TABLE 31–3 Classification of Dementia

Cortical	Associated with Infection
Alzheimer	Viral (HIV and associated syndromes)
Frontotemporal lobe (Pick disease)	Spirochetal (neurosyphillis, Lyme disease)
Mixed	Prion (Creutzfeld-Jakob disease)
Vascular	**Structural/Potentially Reversible**
Multiinfarct (cortical and lacunar)	Normal-pressure hydrocephalus
Biswanger disease	Chronic subdural hematoma
Mixed	Brain tumor
Lewy-Body Associated	**Other Potentially Reversible**
Dementia with Lewy bodies	Thyroid deficiency
Parkinson disease dementia	Vitamin B_{12} deficiency
Progressive supranuclear palsy	Other metabolic/nutritional
	Medication/drugs
Toxin Associated	**Genetic**
Chronic alcohol/Korsokoff syndrome	Huntington chorea
Heavy metal poisoning	

Alzheimer dementia is the most frequent type of dementia, comprising about 70% of all cases of dementia in those aged 71 and older. The proportion of cases of dementia attributable to Alzheimer disease increases with age. Vascular dementia accounts for approximately 17% of cases of dementia. All other dementia subtypes account for the remaining 13%.[1,2] As there is evidence that many of those with dementia actually have multiple etiologies,[18] these statistics are based on the most predominant dementia for each patient.

Alzheimer Dementia

Pathophysiology

Alzheimer disease is a progressive neurodegenerative disorder caused by the destruction of acetylcholine-secreting neurons in the neocortex and hippocampus. The pathologic hallmark is deposits of an insoluble protein called beta amyloid (neuritic plaques) and the hyperphosphorylated protein tau (neurofibrillary tangles). Abnormal accumulation of the proteins cause destruction of neurons in these regions.[19]

Risk Factors

The most important risk factor for Alzheimer dementia is older age. The prevalence of Alzheimer dementia rises from 0.6% to 0.8% at age 65, to 11% to 14% at age 85, and to 36% to 41% at age 95.[9] Family history is another important risk factor. A meta-analysis shows that inheriting the ApoE4 variant of the ApoE gene increases the risk of Alzheimer dementia threefold. Having two APOE4 genes increases the risk 15 times.[19] Head trauma, low level of education, and reduced mental and physical activity late in life may also be risk factors for Alzheimer dementia. Risk factors for vascular disease, such as diabetes, hypertension, hyperlipidemia, and prior strokes, have been linked to Alzheimer dementia, in addition to vascular dementia and all-cause dementia individually.[5,19,20] This suggests a pathogenic role for vascular disease in AD (this will be discussed later).

Clinical Presentation

Alzheimer dementia is characterized by a gradual onset and slowly progressive cognitive decline.[9] It is a diagnosis of exclusion in that there must be an absence of focal neurologic deficits and findings specific for other dementia subtypes. Additionally, the deficits should not be explainable by other central nervous system conditions (eg, cerebrovascular disease), systemic conditions (eg, hypothyroidism), or substance abuse. Imaging is not needed to diagnose Alzheimer dementia if the patient follows a typical course.

Although the symptoms of AD and the rate of progression vary from person to person, the general course of progressive decline is somewhat predictable. Based on the FAST (Functional Assessment Staging) scale,[21] in mild or early-stage AD dementia, the loss of memory for recent events is typically the most prominent finding, while remote memory remains intact. The patient may have decreased ability to remember names, recent events, or recently read material. Aphasia occurs early, and is often manifested as problems with word finding or in circumlocution—the use of many words to describe simple thought. Loss of visuospatial skills is sometimes very prominent at presentation and may lead to difficulty navigating in unfamiliar environments and frequent misplacement of objects. Decline in executive function is often subtle and evident only in demanding situations. Difficulty in situations such as planning dinner for guests or managing finances may be perceived by others as motivational problems. Subtle personality changes may occur before memory impairment is noticed. These changes range from apathy and social disengagement to disinhibition or even hostility. While social withdrawal may be due to apathy, it may also be attributable to the feeling of insecurity in facing increasingly challenging situations. Apathy may be difficult to distinguish from depression, which can also occur early. While personality may subtly change, social skills remain preserved until late in the course of the disease; therefore, changes such as increased hostility occurring in the context of socially appropriate situations should raise the concern for another type of dementia such as Lewy body or frontotemporal dementia.

In moderate dementia, loss of more remote memory begins. Patients may be unable to recall important details from the past such as the name of their high school. They may lose knowledge for personal details such as their current address but usually continue to retain knowledge about themselves such as their name, birth date, and names of family members. Disorientation (to date, time, and place), apraxia and agnosia, as well as a more significant loss of executive function emerge.[16,22,23] Patients have trouble with simple arithmetic and choosing proper clothing for the season. Eventually, patients become unable to carry out even simple tasks like buttoning a shirt.

In moderately severe dementia, patients may begin to forget aspects of personal history, such as names of family members, but usually they remember their own name. They may make errors such as putting pajamas over daytime clothes and need assistance in dressing. They may begin to have urinary and fecal incontinence and need help with the details of toileting such as wiping and flushing. Psychiatric changes may be prominent such as suspiciousness, delusions, and hallucinations, along with behavioral changes such as agitation, repetitive behaviors (hand wringing), and wandering.

In the late stages of dementia, patients often need complete assistance with all activities including eating. Speech becomes unrecognizable except for occasional words or phrases. Eventually loss of motor function results in trouble swallowing, walking, speaking, and even sitting up, smiling, and holding the head up.[2,23]

According to the Alzheimer's Association, people with Alzheimer disease die an average of 4 to 6 years after diagnosis, although this can range from 3 to 20 years.[2] Difficulty swallowing and immobility lead to complications that hasten death such as aspiration pneumonia, urinary tract infections, infected pressure ulcers, pulmonary emboli, malnutrition, and fall-related injuries. AD seems to decrease survival rate even in the absence of specific complications, although the mechanism of death has not been defined fully. The inability to cope with stressors such as cardiac disease may hasten death from any co-morbid illness.

Vascular Dementia

Vascular dementia is most commonly caused by one of three mechanisms. It may be caused by one or more large infarcts, which are usually cortical but sometimes subcortical. An accumulation of multiple small, subcortical infarcts (lacunes) can also cause dementia. Finally, severe white matter disease secondary to hypertension, known as Biswanger disease, may be responsible. Not everyone with cerebrovascular disease develops vascular dementia. Risk factors for developing vascular dementia in the context of cerebrovascular disease may include severity of the stroke, diabetes, hypercholesterolemia, atrial fibrillation, and hypertension. Diabetes seems to double the risk of vascular dementia while LDL in the highest quartile triples the risk.[20,24-26]

The classic definition of vascular dementia as defined by DSM-IV criteria[9] is dementia with evidence of cerebrovascular disease judged to be etiologically related. Evidence of cerebrovascular disease may be either focal neurologic signs and symptoms or signs of disease on neuroimaging.

Vascular dementia was classically diagnosed when there was evidence of an abrupt onset of cognitive decline, presumably caused by a stroke, followed by a stepwise progression of disease. This means that there is a period of stability or even improvement in cognition after the first decline, followed by another sudden decline with the next stroke. This picture is most often seen when there are large strokes, most often accompanied by focal deficits. When a clinically apparent stroke occurs followed shortly by cognitive decline, the diagnosis of vascular dementia is easy. The classic thinking was that the stroke had to occur no more than 6 months prior to the cognitive decline for vascular dementia to be diagnosed.[24] Current thinking is that cognitive decline may occur much later than 6 months post stroke, making the relationship between the two less obvious. Additionally, the progression of dementia caused by the accumulation subcortical infarcts and Biswanger disease is often more subtle and may be difficult to distinguish from Alzheimer dementia or mixed

dementia. Subcortical infarcts and Biswanger disease may be clinically silent, making the temporal relationship between the disease and dementia even more unclear, although subcortical infarcts may present with subtle deficits such as imbalance.

It is difficult to distinguish vascular dementia from other types of dementia superimposed on cerebrovascular disease. Cognitive findings consistent with vascular dementia may help with the diagnosis but there is often significant overlap in cognitive features between various types of dementia. Cognitive features in vascular dementia associated with large strokes are specific to the areas affected. A cortical infarct in the left parietal lobe may cause aphasia, apraxia, and agnosia as in AD, but it is often accompanied by focal deficits. Subcortical infarcts may present with prominent personality and mood changes as well as emotional lability. They may have accompanying gait disturbances and unsteadiness. The feature that most readily distinguishes vascular dementia from AD is that the language and personality disturbances, psychomotor retardation, and bradyphrenia (slowness of thought) are often much more prominent then memory disturbances. In Alzheimer dementia, the memory loss is most prominent except sometimes very early in the process. Bradyphrenia may be difficult to distinguish from actual memory loss,[24] but if the person with bradyphrenia is given time, he or she will often be able to retrieve the memory.

Interaction between Alzheimer Dementia and Vascular Disease

The interaction between Alzheimer dementia and vascular disease is complicated. One may have a combination of both Alzheimer disease and vascular dementia, known as mixed dementia. Alternatively, one may have Alzheimer disease superimposed on vascular brain disease that is not severe enough to alone cause dementia. It is now believed that this superimposed vascular disease may speed up the progression of the Alzheimer disease, causing a synergistic rather than an additive effect on cognitive decline.[25]

Lewy Body Dementias

Lewy body dementias (LBDs) include dementia with Lewy bodies (DLB), Parkinson disease with dementia (PDD), and progressive supranuclear palsy (PSP). LBDs share the pathologic hallmark of Lewy bodies, deposits of the protein alpha-synuclein in brain cells.[27]

The core features of LBDs include abrupt fluctuations in cognitive function and persistent, well-formed hallucinations, usually visual in someone with parkinsonian motor symptoms. Although the progression of the dementia is gradual, the fluctuation around each new baseline is wide and abrupt and may appear like delirium. The most important issue that makes an accurate diagnosis of LBDs important is that those with LBDs may have non–dose-related life-threatening reactions to antipsychotics, including features of neuroleptic malignant syndrome, irreversible worsening of parkinsonian symptoms and impaired consciousness.

DLBs and PDD are the most common LBDs. LBD most commonly refers to dementia with Lewy bodies, which is more common than PDD. As clinical differences between the two dementias are often subtle, the diagnosis is made based on the "the 1-year rule." If the onset of cognitive symptoms occurs within 1 year of the onset of motor symptoms, the diagnosis of DLB is more likely. If cognitive decline occurs more than a year after the onset of motor symptoms, PDD is more likely.[11,28] This timing may be difficult to establish, especially when there is superimposed Alzheimer or vascular dementia.[11,27]

The differences in clinical features may be more quantitative than qualitative.[27] In DLBs, cognitive fluctuations,[27] psychotic features, and severe reactions to neuroleptics are usually more prominent than in PDD.[11,28,29] In Parkinson disease with dementia, the motor symptoms such as tremor, slowness of movement, gait abnormalities, and cogwheeling occur early and are more prominent than in DLB. In DLBs, motor symptoms are usually symmetric with an absence of tremor and respond less robustly to levodopa therapy.[11,27,28]

Distinguishing cognitive features of LBDs include the prominence of inattention, bradyphrenia, executive dysfunction, and visual spatial difficulties, which may be more profound than memory loss[10,11] and more prominent than in AD. A normal clock would make LBD less likely.[28,30] In contrast to AD, language is usually preserved.

Progressive supranuclear palsy is an uncommon LBD. The cognitive and motor features are similar to DLB, but the downward gaze abnormality is distinctive.

Frontotemporal Lobe Dementia

Frontotemporal lobe dementia (FTLD) is less common in the geriatric population than the prior subtypes. The age of onset is usually between the ages of 45 and 65, but ranges from 21 to 85 years old. Forty to fifty percent of those with FTLD have a positive family history.[31,32]

FTLD is caused by frontal and temporal lobe atrophy that results in profound loss of social skills along with marked changes in personality and behavior preceding or predominating over cognitive decline.[31] Features range from disinhibited or compulsive behaviors (eg, compulsive eating or hypersexuality), inappropriate social conduct, and aggression, to apathy, loss of empathy, and poor hygiene. There may be deficits in executive function and language while memory and visuospatial skills remain relatively preserved.[31,32]

"Reversible" Causes of Dementia

Although previously referred to as "reversible dementia," treatment for these dementias may not fully reverse dementia and may only prevent further decline. Clues to these dementias include subjective cognitive complaints, age younger than 60, and acute presentation.

Metabolic and nutritional causes, especially hypothyroidism and B_{12} deficiency, should be considered but are often only contributory to another type of dementia. Neurologic deficits should prompt a search for structural brain disorders such as tumors or normal pressure hydrocephalus (NPH).

The classic triad of NPH is dementia, "magnetic gait," and incontinence. Ventriculoperitoneal shunting may partially reverse the dementia. Neurosyphillis, which is now uncommon, may be suspected in the setting of prior syphilis infection and neurologic findings such as dysarthria or psychosis.

Medication toxicity or acute drug use can cause easily reversible dementia-like syndromes, and therefore should always be considered. Psychotropics, sedative-hypnotics, opioids, drugs with anticholinergics side effects, and alcohol are the biggest offenders.

● COMPREHENSIVE APPROACH TO THE MANAGEMENT OF DEMENTIA

As there is no current cure for most dementia syndromes, the most valuable management focuses on safety, quality of life, and co-morbid illnesses and symptoms.

General Goals of Management

Safety

Safety is a concern for even those with mild dementia, and concerns may vary by environment (Chapter 16). Patients who live alone are at the highest risk for self-neglect, environmental injuries, injury from falls, medical crisis, and getting lost.

Self-neglect may be due to apathy, cognitive dysfunction, or physical impairment. There should be a periodic assessment of the ability of the patient to carry out daily function by talking to caregivers, neighbors, and friends. The health care provider should look for signs of self-neglect such as uncontrolled medical problems, missed appointments, weight loss, and unkempt appearance.

A home safety evaluation and a fall assessment should be done to assess risk of injury (Chapter 34). Measures such as teaching a patient to use a microwave early in his or her disease process while learning is still possible, in order to prevent fire from a stove, may decrease environmental hazards. Fall prevention strategies should be instituted, including taping rugs, providing grab bars and assistive devices, as well as addressing visual disturbances.

Medication errors may be reduced by pre-arranging medications in pill boxes and having caregivers or family members remind the patient to take his or her medication. Similarly, providing a system to remind patients of appointments will reduce the chance of a medical crisis. Medical alert services may help patients who are in crisis and cannot get to the phone. Communication of the medical plan with family or caregivers is essential.

A tendency to wander, memory loss, and spatial impairment can lead to getting lost. Adequate supervision is needed once the patient begins to show signs of disorientation to place. Registration in the Alzheimer's Association Safe Return program or similar programs should be considered.

As need for assistance with activities of daily living and home supervision increases, family, case managers, and home care programs become vital. More supportive environments such as assisted living or long-term care facilities may be necessary.

Driving

Driving must be addressed early, as even mild dementia is associated with an increased accident rate. All older patients who drive should be screened for warning signs that cognitive impairment may be interfering with driving. Informants should be asked about these warning signs, which may include frequent damage to the car or garage, tickets for moving violations, poor judgment, near misses, driving at inappropriate speeds, getting lost in familiar areas, family members expressing concern, and frequent horn honking from other drivers.

The legal requirement to report a patient to the Department of Motor Vehicles (DMV) when driving is suspected to be impaired varies from state to state, but physicians should refer the patient to the DMV when the physician feels the patient is no longer safe. Recommendations by a health care provider to stop driving should be based on severity of the dementia or a demonstration of impaired driving competence as reported by the informant. Some experts recommend that anyone with dementia refrain from driving while others believe that it is safe for someone with mild dementia to drive when accompanied by a competent driver. All patients with dementia, however mild, who continue to drive, should be referred to centers that evaluate driving ability with neuropsychological and road testing.

Advance Planning

As dementia progresses, patients will lose the ability to manage finances and ability to comprehend their own medical care. Patients will need to be assessed for decision-making capacity (Chapter 10) for various decisions repeatedly over the disease course, as this capacity will vary depending on the decision that needs to be made, the stage of the disease, day-to-day fluctuations, and delirium. Advance directives should be discussed early while patients can still make their wishes known. A living will is one type of advance directive that addresses the patient's goals of medical care, including whether or not the patient would want cardiopulmonary resuscitation. Additionally, the patient should be encouraged to appoint a guardian over finances and health care (health care proxy).

Psychosocial Support

Patients with dementia often experience social isolation due to changes in social skills and loss of the cognitive ability to converse with peers, as well as the loss of ability to arrange, remember, and access social situations. This may lead to depression, anxiety, self-neglect, reduced food intake, and even aggressive behavior. It is essential to provide a venue for socialization and psychosocial support within the living environment of the patient (Chapter 16). For patients in the community, senior centers, or adult day care centers and with more advance disease, provide a variety of group activities. Assisted living environments provide group dining and other group activities. Activities such as music, reading, and reminiscence therapy may be performed in all environments and may help older adults cope with the stressors of dementia.

Caregivers

Caregiver stress (Chapter 17) often goes unrecognized. The increasing levels of supervision and personal care that patients with dementia require, as well as their changes in behavior and personality, require a large time, financial, physical, and emotional investment. This may impact the caregiver's health, relationships, employment, and finances, often leading to anxiety and depression, as well as the feeling of being overwhelmed, which sometimes results in elder abuse. Elder abuse must be looked for and addressed.

In-home or facility-based respite care can provide caregivers with free time for self-care, socializing, and sometimes even travel. Support groups may provide psychological support and education such as tips for dealing with behavioral disturbances and improving patient function to ease the burdens of caregiving. Respite and support groups can be located with the assistance of social services or through the Alzheimer's Association.

Psychiatric Symptoms

Neuropsychiatric Symptoms

Neuropsychiatric symptoms (NPS) in patients with dementia generally refer to disruptive behaviors such as screaming, restlessness, or physical aggression, often labeled as "agitation." Other disruptive symptoms referred to under this category are behaviors such as wandering, hoarding, and repetitive questioning. NPS may be the most emotionally difficult and even dangerous aspect of dementia for caregivers and health care providers. They may be one of the crucial factors leading to long-term care placement.[33] These behaviors may be caused by a "catastrophic reaction," or being overwhelmed by stressors due to the loss of coping skills and the inability to express it.[33] There is a tendency to try to treat them with antipsychotics, as this is an easy approach, but there is no evidence supporting this use for many types of behaviors and this may even be harmful.[34]

Behavioral Interventions

The best clinical research to date in the behavioral treatment of NPS supports identifying potential underlying causes of behavioral symptoms.[34] Addressing stressors such as unmet needs (hunger, comfort), pain, sleep deprivation, delirium, illness, adverse medication effect, emotional stress (anxiety, depression), or environmental triggers (over- or under-stimulation) may be efficacious in reducing disruptive behaviors, such as screaming, resisting care, and aggression. Environmental triggers of agitation should be identified and removed. Complex tasks should be broken down into simple steps to reduce being overwhelmed by challenges. Fear or paranoia caused by memory lapses (eg, misplacement of wallet causing belief that someone stole it) can lead to agitation and may respond to reality orientation.[33] Other NPS such as wandering may be due to boredom and may respond to increasing daytime activities.

Behaviors that occur without an obvious cause may be addressed by specific techniques such as redirecting patients, removing reinforcing rewards (eg, stop providing attention for inappropriate behaviors), delivering rewards for appropriate behaviors, and providing a calm environment and well-structured routines. In a meta-analysis, educating caregivers in behavioral interventions reduced at least one behavior that caregivers identified as problematic.[34] Although research in nonmedical techniques is evolving, approaches such as reducing stress in living environments (noise, distractions, etc.), bright light therapy, exercise, aroma therapy, music, massage, and pet therapy may be efficacious in treating NPS, and are extremely safe to implement.[33,34]

Individualizing treatment may need to be creative. One such attempt was reflected in a study of "person-centered bathing."[35] Patients in a long-term care facility with moderate dementia received baths that were tailored to each individual's preference. Aggression was less in the "person-centered bathing" than in usual or towel bathing.

Although agitation that is refractory to behavioral interventions may require medication, there is currently no evidence indicating the effectiveness of medications to target other NPS such as wandering, hoarding, repetitive questioning, withdrawal, and social inappropriateness. These respond best to behavioral techniques.

Pharmacologic Approaches

Medication should target specific psychiatric syndromes when identified as potentially responsible for the agitated behavior (Table 31–4). For example, antidepressants treat both depression and anxiety, which may be responsible for symptoms such as repetitive vocalizations or pacing.[36] Antipsychotics may be useful for delirium or psychotic symptoms that are resulting in physical aggression or resisting caregiving.

Antipsychotics are the most frequently used medication for agitated symptoms in dementia but should be reserved for patients whose problems persist after behavioral approaches were attempted and psychiatric disorders were addressed. Antipsychotics for this purpose are an "off-label" use due to unclear efficacy and adverse side-effect profiles. Most of the clinical trials of these drugs addressed NPS outcomes only as a group, rather than as individual symptoms. A Cochrane Review comparing the typical antipsychotic haloperidol with placebo concluded that only aggression was improved, but not agitation as a whole. Atypical antipsychotics may have better efficacy but side effects are still problematic and include increased risk of stroke.[36]

All antipsychotics need to be used with caution (see Chapter 30). The FDA issued a black box warning regarding increased mortality from antipsychotics secondary to cerebrovascular and cardiovascular events, as well as pneumonia.[36,37] The risk may be greater in typical antipsychotics than atypical antipsychotics.[37] Additionally, typical antipsychotics are associated with a high rate of extrapyramidal side effects and cognitive decline in the elderly. Atypical antipsychotics may have a lower risk of extrapyramidal effects, but a higher risk of anticholinergic side effects including somulence, gait disturbances, orthostatic hypotension, urinary retention, and constipation.[36] As discussed previously, LBDs are especially prone to severe side effects. If it is absolutely necessary, only the lowest dose of atypical antipsychotics should be used in LBD.

Trials have shown small but statistically significant benefit of cholinesterase inhibitors (described later in this chapter) in the treatment of NPS in dementia, but the clinical significance is questionable.[36] Given the safe side-effect profile, a trial of cholinesterase inhibitors is worthwhile, especially in Lewy body dementia. Rivastigmine is the most well studied in LBD.[27,36] There is some evidence that selective serotonin selective uptake inhibitors (SSRIs), such as citalopram, may be somewhat efficacious in treating the NPS of dementia,[36] including the symptoms of disinhibition and impulsivity in FTLD.[31] Benzodiazepines should be avoided for NPS, especially for long-term management. They may lead to increased confusion, falls, and may paradoxically increase agitation in patients with dementia.[36]

TABLE 31–4 Medications Used in Symptomatic Treatment of Dementia

Medication	Usual Dose (Geriatric Population)	Uses	Side Effects
Typical Antipsychotics Haloperidol	Doses for agitation: 0.5-1.0 mg bid	Delirium, psychosis; sometimes used for agitation in dementia, but most successful with aggression only	Extrapyramidal side effects, cognitive decline, and increased mortality from cerebrovascular and cardiovascular events and pneumonia
Atypical Antipsychotics Olanzepine Risperdal Quetiapine	Doses for agitation: 2.5 daily to bid 0.25-1.0 mg bid 25-100 mg daily (often divided bid)	Same as typical antipsychotics	Anticholinergic side effects (somulence, gait disturbance, urinary retention, EPS) less common than the typical antipsychotics; increased mortality as with typical antipsychotics (but may be lower)
Cholinesterase Inhibitors Rivastigmine Donepezil Galantamine	3-6 mg bid 5-10 mg bid 8-12 mg bid	Cognitive enhancers Rivastigmine possibly effective in NPS in LBD	Mild diarrhea, nausea, or vomiting; less common: nightmares, agitation; rare: bradycardia
NMDA Receptor Antagonist Memantine	Start 5 mg daily and titrate to 10 mg bid	Cognitive enhancer	Dizziness, increased confusion, or hallucinations with dose escalation
Serotonin Selective Reuptake Inhibitors Citalopram Sertraline	20-40 mg daily 50-100 mg daily	Antidepressant. Effective for generalized anxiety Citalopram possibly effective in NPS in FTLD	Nausea, somulence, insomnia, nervousness, hyponatremia; less likely: serotonin syndrome

Other Symptoms

Depression. The treatment of depression in those with dementia is important, as depression may worsen cognition, cause NPS, impair the quality of life, and be dangerous to the health of the patient (Chapter 37). Recognition of depression may be a challenge in patients with dementia because they are less likely to express symptoms. Anhedonia, or loss of interest, in depression may be difficult to differentiate from the apathy that occurs with dementia. Both anhedonia and apathy cause withdrawal from social activities and from prior interests, but—in apathy—the patients are not distressed by this and do not have other features of depression. The treatment of depression often requires medication, while apathy often only requires reassuring the family and continuing to engage the patient.

Sleep Disturbances. Day-night reversal of sleep occurs commonly in AD and may be disturbing to both the caregiver and the patient. It increases nighttime disturbances such as vocalizations and wandering, and may be dangerous (eg, causing falling, getting lost, turning on a stove). Treatment depends on restoring the normal circadian rhythm through adequate exposure to sunlight, stimulating activities, and exercise during the day and avoiding these activities within a few hours of bedtime.

Insomnia is also frequent early in the course of dementia. Sleep deprivation increases the risk of delirium, falls, and agitated behavior, as well as worsening of cognition. Typical causes of insomnia in patients with dementia include poor sleep hygiene, pain, anxiety, depression, caffeine, or medication side effects. Cholinesterase inhibitors may cause nightmares, and should be considered in the differential diagnosis of insomnia. The treatment plan should address the underlying cause, encourage good sleep hygiene, and provide relaxation techniques such as a warm bath before bed. A light snack and avoiding fluid intake right before bed may prevent awakenings due to bedtime hunger and need to urinate. Severe sleep disturbances may benefit from medication when other methods failed.

Treatment of Cognitive Impairment

General Management

Because the benefit of current available medications for cognitive enhancement is controversial, modifying the rate of cognitive decline by treating vascular risk factors is especially important in Alzheimer dementia, vascular dementia, and mixed dementia.[25] The best evidence so far is in the control of systolic hypertension and hyperlipidemia.[6,25] Minimizing other factors that can interfere with cognition such as certain medications (eg, anticholinergic medications), sleep deprivation, and psychiatric disturbances can improve daily cognitive functioning. Other treatment goals should focus on helping patients cope with memory impairment, such as using memory reminders (eg, leaving notes on the refrigerator to remind a patient that he or she already ate).[33]

Cognitive Enhancers

The medications most widely used for cognitive enhancement are cholinesterase inhibitors and N-methyl-D-aspartate receptor (NMDAr) antagonists (Table 33–4). Cholinesterase inhibitors are FDA approved for use in patients with Alzheimer dementia only, although studies may indicate utility in vascular dementia and LBDs.[25,27] NMDAr inhibitors are approved for moderate to severe AD, but have also shown efficacy in vascular dementia. There are few studies demonstrating efficacy of cognitive enhancers in other types of dementia, and they have not been effective in the prevention of progression from MCI to dementia.[6]

Cholinesterase Inhibitors

Cholinesterase inhibitors increase the amount of the neurotransmitter acetylcholine in the synapse of neurons in the hippocampus and neocortex. Its beneficial effect on cognition is thought to be due to increasing the acetylcholine in areas of degeneration of acetylcholine-secreting neurons.[19]

Cochrane Reviews find that cholinesterase inhibitors have a moderate symptom-modifying effect in those with Alzheimer disease and are generally well tolerated, but demonstrate this effect only in about 10% more people taking the active drug over placebo.[22] One Cochrane Review of 10 randomized double-blinded placebo-controlled clinical trials showed that treatment with the cholinesterase inhibitors donepezil, rivastigmine, or galantamine for 6 months produced improvement in cognitive function, on average, −2.7 points over placebo on a 70-point scale (Alzheimer Disease Assessment Scale-Cognitive Subscale, or ADAS-COG), and a 1.4-point benefit on the MMSE. The biggest benefit was in those with mild to moderate AD. Although the treatment group withdrew 11% more often (29% vs. 18%) than the placebo group, this was most often for only minor adverse events such as nausea, vomiting, and diarrhea.[38]

Similar results were noted in an earlier meta-analysis of 22 randomized control trials, which estimated that the efficacy of cholinesterase inhibitors over placebo varied from −1.5 to −3.9 points on the ADAS-Cog (ie, like "turning back the clock" about 6 to 12 months at best). The authors argue that this falls below the 4 points that an expert panel from the FDA propose as a minimally clinical important effect.[39] As many clinicians would argue that most of these studies demonstrate a responder rate between 10% and 30%, it is possible that cholinesterase inhibitors have a more robust effect on the subgroup of responders. Side effects consisted mainly of diarrhea, nausea, vomiting, weight loss, and dizziness.

There is some evidence of efficacy of cholinesterase inhibitors in vascular dementia, but data are limited in quantity and quality. A Cochrane Review of galantamine in vascular dementia demonstrated an improvement over placebo (−2.3 on the ADAS-COG) in only one of two studies.[40] The review of donepezil was similar.

Although cholinesterase inhibitors seem to have cognitive benefits in terms of test scores, this may not translate into clinically meaningful benefits such as time to institutionalization or progression of disability in ADLs.[25] Additionally, there appears to be no neuroprotective function or slowing of disease progression. Once the medication is removed, cognitive test results are the same as placebo. As the side effects of cholinesterase inhibitors are relatively mild and well tolerated, they are often worth a trial. Additionally, more disturbing but less common CNS side effects have been reported such as insomnia, agitation, nightmares, and panic. Rare but more worrisome is the potential for cardiovascular side effects including bradycardia, dizziness, and syncope.

NMDA Receptor Antagonists

Memantine, an NMDA receptor antagonist, blocks abnormally increased glutameric activity seen in Alzheimer disease and cerebrovascular disease. Glutamate, the major excitatory neurotransmitter in the brain, is important for learning and memory when released intermittently during appropriate activity. Under abnormal conditions of sustained release, glutamate can impair learning and cause neurotoxicity. It is theorized that blocking glutamate during abnormal release can prevent cell death and enhance learning.[19]

Most studies of memantine in Alzheimer dementia included patients with moderate-to-severe disease. Two 28-week trials involving such patients (MMSE 3-14) found a beneficial effect of memantine alone or in addition to donepezil. The first study demonstrated better outcomes for memantine over placebo on scales of cognitive activities used in daily living, global outcome, and behavior.[41] For example, on the Severe Impairment Battery (SIB), a 100-point scale, there was a benefit of 6.1 points. The benefit was 0.7 points on the MMSE. Although the benefits were only modest, the dropout rate was actually lower for memantine than for placebo. In the second trial, memantine combined with donepezil demonstrated a 1.6-point benefit on the SIB scale over placebo combined with donepezil.[42] Despite the theoretical rationale for neuroprotective properties of memantine, current trials are too short to assess if the drug has any disease-modifying effects.

There is evidence of benefit of memantine in vascular dementia. In a 28-week trial of patients with mild to moderate vascular dementia (MMSE 12-20), there was improvement of memantine over placebo of 2 points on the 70-point ADAS-Cog. Those with moderate dementia (MMSE < 15 points) seem to benefit the most.[43]

The side effects of memantine seem to be fewer than those of cholinesterase inhibitors. Dizziness is the most common side effect of memantine. Confusion and hallucinations are reported at a lower frequency and usually occur during initiation or dose escalation.[44] The medication should be started at the lowest dose, and titrated to the maximum dose. Each new dose should be maintained for a week prior to titration and if confusion develops, the dose should be dropped back to the prior dose.

Using Cognitive Enhancers

The use of cognitive enhancers is controversial given the lack of evidence for disease modification, questions of clinically meaningful benefit to patients and caregivers, as well as potential costs. Because these medications are generally well tolerated, some clinicians find a trial to be worthwhile, especially in those who are independent and trying to maintain their level of independence.

The evidence would suggest giving a cholinesterase inhibitor for mild-to-moderate AD or vascular dementia, and using memantine, either alone or in combination with a cholinesterase inhibitor, for moderate to severe dementia. Although immediate cognitive improvement might not be seen with the start of cognitive enhancers, there should be slowing of decline on cognitive testing if the medications are having a beneficial effect. If after 6 months to a year, the rate of cognitive decline is rapid (more than 1-2 points on the MMSE), stopping the medication should be considered.

● FUTURE DIRECTIONS

The future direction for treatment of the cognitive impairment of dementia will likely be more targeted to the disease process and disease modification. Promising research in the treatment of Alzheimer disease focuses on the use of inhibitors of the enzymes (beta and gamma secretases) responsible for the formation of beta amyloid plaques, and inhibitors of the enzymes (tau kinases) responsible for hyperphosphorylation of the tau protein in the production of neurofibrillary tangles.[19] More specifically targeted and efficacious agents should have the additional benefit of pushing clinicians to diagnose dementia earlier and more accurately.

Overall, Alzheimer and other dementias are devastating illnesses, which are increasing in frequency in the Western world. The burden on families, caregivers, and health systems will be substantial and will present challenges to health professionals who are mostly trained to treat acute illness. Though early recognition and treatment are perhaps less important now, recognition of the earliest signs of the onset of a dementing illness will be imperative as disease-modifying agents become available.

References

1. Plassman BL, Langa K.M, Fisher GG, et al. Prevalence of dementia in the United States: The aging, demographics and memory study. *Neuroepidemiology*. 2007;29:125.

2. Alzheimer's Association. *Alzheimer's Disease: Facts and Figures*. 2009. www.alz.org.

3. *Screening for Dementia: Recommendations and Rationale*. US Preventive Services Task Force, June 2003.

4. ACOVE Investigators. Introduction to the assessing of vulnerable elders. 3. Quality Indication Measurement Set. *J Am Geriatr Soc*. 2007;55(suppl):293.

5. Holsinger T, Deveau J, Boustani M, Williams J. Does this patient have dementia? *JAMA*. 2007;297:239.

6. Gouthier S, Reisberg B, Zaudig M. Mild cognitive impairment. *Lancet*. 2006;367:1262-1270.

7. Petersen RC, Stevens JC, Ganguli M, et al. Practice parameter. Early detection of dementia: Mild cognitive impairment (an evidence-based review). Report of the Quality Standards Subcommittee of the American Academy of Neurology. *Neurology*. 2001;56:1133.

8. Morris JC, Storandt M, Miller JP, et al. Mild cognitive Impairment represents early-stage Alzheimer's disease. *Arch Neurol.* 2001; 58:397.

9. American Psychiatric Association. *Diagnostic and Statistical Manual of Mental Disorders.* 4th ed. Text revision. Washington, DC: APA Press, 1994.

10. Knopman DS, Dekosky ST, Cummings JL, et al. Practice parameter: Diagnosis of dementia (an evidence-based review). Report of Quality Standards Subcommittee of the American Academy of Neurology. *Neurology.* 2001;56:1143.

11. Dubois B, Burn D, Goetz C. Diagnostic procedures for Parkinson's disease dementia: Recommendation from the Movement Disorder Task Force. *Mov Disord.* 2007;22:2314-2324.

12. Folstein MF, Folstein SE, McHugh PR. Mini-Mental State: A practical method for grading the cognitive state of patients for the clinician. *J Psychiatr Res.* 1975;12:189.

13. Kerwin D. How to prevent a delayed Alzheimer diagnosis. *J Fam Pract.* 2009;58:9.

14. Borson S, Scanlan J, Brush M, et al. The mini-cog: A cognitive "vital signs" measure for dementia screening in multi-lingual elderly. *Int J Geriatr Soc.* 2000;15:1021.

15. Pfeifer E. Short Portable Mental Status Questionnaire. *JAGS.* 1975;10:433.

16. Weiner M, Neubecker K, Bret M, Hynan, L. Language in Alzheimer's disease. *J Clin Psychiatry.* 2008;69:1223.

17. Rosen WG, Mohs RC, Davis KL. A new rating scale for Alzheimer's disease. *Am J Psychiatry.* 1984;141:1356-1364.

18. Schneider JA, Arvanitakis Z, Bang W, et al. Mixed brain pathologies account for most dementia cases in community-dwelling older persons. *Neurology.* 2007;69:2179.

19. Blennow K, De Leon M, Zetterberg H. Alzheimer's disease. *Lancet.* 2006;368:387.

20. Shadlen M, Larson E. Risk factors for dementia. *Up to Date.* Version 17.1. http://www.uptodate.com/patients/content/topic.do?topicKey=~ZcncVEHyHWFMEw&source=see_link. Accessed July 24, 2010.

21. Reisberg B. Functional Assessment Staging (FAST). *Psychopharmacol Bull.* 1988;24:653-659.

22. Burns A, Lliffe S. Alzheimer's disease. *BMJ.* 2009;338:467.

23. Morris JC. The Clinical Dementia Rating (CDR) current version. scores, rules. *Neurology.* 1993;43:2412.

24. Knopman D. Dementia and cerebrovascular disease. *Mayo Clin Proc.* 2006;81:223.

25. Langa K, Foster N, Larson E, et al. Mixed dementia. Emerging concepts and therapeutic implications. *JAMA.* 2004;292:2901.

26. Wright, CB. Etiology, clinical manifestations and diagnosis of vascular dementia. *Up to Date Version 17.1.* January 1, 2009:1-23.

27. Lippa CF, Duda JE, Grossman M, et al. DLB and PDD boundary issues. Diagnosis, treatment, molecular pathology, and biomarkers. *Neurology.* 2007;68:812.

28. McKeith IG, Dickenson DW, Lowe J, et al. Diagnosis and management of dementia with Lewy Bodies: Third report of the DLB Consortium. *Neurology.* 2005;65:1863.

29. Aarsland D, Perry R, Larsen JP, et al. Neuroleptic sensitivity in Parkinson's disease and Parkinsonian dementias. *J Clin Psychiatry.* 2005;66:633.

30. Tiraboschi P. What best differentiates Lewy body from Alzheimer's disease in early-stage dementia? *Brain.* 2006;129:729.

31. Yurchenko A, Lapid M, Josephs K. Frontotemporal dementia in older adults: Diagnostic and therapeutic challenge. *Clin Geriatr.* 2009;17:26-31.

32. Neary D, Snowdem J, Mann D. Frontotemporal dementia. *Lancet Neurol.* 2005;4:771.

33. Burns A, Lliffe S. Dementia. *BMJ.* 2009;14:405.

34. Ayalon L, Gum A, Filiciano L, Arean P. Effectiveness of non-pharmacological interventions for the management of neuropsychiatric symptoms in patients with dementia. A systematic review. *Arch Inten Med.* 2006;166:2182.

35. Sloane P, Hoeffer B, Mitchell M. Effect of person-centered showering and towel bath on bathing-associated aggression, agitation and discomfort in nursing home residents with dementia: A randomized control trial. *JAGS.* 2004;52:1795.

36. Sink K, Holden K, Yaffe K. Pharmacological treatment of neuropsychiatric symptoms of dementia: A review of the evidence. *JAMA.* 2005;293:596.

37. Wang P, Schneeweiss S, Avorn J, et al. Risk of death in elderly users of conventional vs. atypical antipsychotic medications. *N Engl J Med.* 2005;353:2319.

38. Birks J. Cholinesterase inhibitors for Alzheimer's disease. *Cochrane Database Syst Rev.* 2006;1:CD005593.

39. Kaduszkiewicz H, Zimmerman T, Beck-Bornholdt HP, et al. Cholinesterase inhibitors for patients with Alzheimer's disease. A systematic review of randomized clinical trials. *BMJ.* 2005; 331:321.

40. Craig D, Birks J. Galantamine for vascular cognitive impairment. *Cochrane Database Syst Rev.* 2006;1:CD004746. DOI 10.1002/14651858.

41. Reisberg B, Doody R, Stoffler A, et al. Memantine in moderate to severe Alzheimer's disease. *N Engl J Med.* 2003;348:1333.

42. Tariot PN, Farolow MR, Grossberg GT, et al. Memantine treatment in patients with moderate to severe Alzheimer's dementia already receiving donepezil: A randomized controlled trial. *JAMA.* 2004;291:317.

43. Orgogozo JM, Rigaud AS, Stoffler A. Efficacy and safety of memantine in patients with mild to moderate vascular dementia: A randomized, placebo-controlled trial. *Stroke.* 2002;33:1834.

44. McShane R, Aresoa Sastre A, Minakaran N. Memantine for dementia. *Cochrane Database Syst Rev.* 2006:CD 003154.

POST-TEST

1. The diagnosis of Alzheimer dementia does NOT include:
   A. Agnosia
   B. Aphasia
   C. Anhedonia
   D. Apraxia

2. Which of the following is more powerful for diagnosing dementia?
   A. Neuroimaging
   B. Reports of memory loss and functional decline from a caregiver
   C. A Mini-Mental State Exam score of 24
   D. Abnormal thyroid tests

3. How can patients with early dementia be distinguished from those with mild delirium?
   A. Patients with dementia have impaired social skills while those with delirium do not.
   B. Patients with dementia have word-finding difficulties while those with delirium have intact language skills.
   C. Patients with dementia have altered consciousness while those with delirium have problems with attention.
   D. Patients with dementia have a relatively stable immediate course while delirium widely fluctuates.

4. Which of the following is appropriate patient counseling for a diagnosis of mild cognitive impairment?
   A. Mild cognitive impairment has a benign course.
   B. Mild cognitive impairment is a mild form of dementia.
   C. Cholinesterase inhibitors will prevent the progression to dementia.
   D. Cognition may be normal on follow-up evaluations.

5. Which is TRUE about diagnosing vascular dementia?
   A. Patients often experience bradyphrenia more than memory impairment.
   B. Cognitive decline that begins more than 6 months after a stroke excludes the diagnosis.
   C. The diagnosis can be made based on evidence of multiple silent infarcts, which indicates a stepwise decline in cognition but no findings on neuroimaging.
   D. Abnormalities in language, object naming, and executing complex motor activities make vascular dementia unlikely as these are the features of Alzheimer dementia.

6. Which is CORRECT for patients with Lewy body dementia?
   A. There is a dose-related toxicity associated with neuroleptics, and therefore high doses should be avoided.
   B. Marked fluctuations in mental status and hallucinations are uncommon and signal the need to treat delirium.
   C. The parkinsonian features are expected to respond as robustly to levodopa as in Parkisonson disease.
   D. The onset of cognitive symptoms generally occurs within 1 year of the onset of motor symptoms.

7. Which is a correct statement about side effects of the treatments commonly used in dementia?
   A. Atypical antipsychotics have a higher risk of extrapyramidal side effects than typical antipsychotics.
   B. Acetylcholinesterase inhibitors cause constipation and gastrointestinal upset.
   C. Antipsychotics may increase mortality when used in this population.
   D. Memantine often causes orthostatic hypotension and confusion.

ANSWERS TO PRE-TEST

1. C
2. D
3. D
4. B

ANSWERS TO POST-TEST

1. C
2. B
3. D
4. D
5. A
6. D
7. C

32

Polypharmacy

Claudene J. George, MD, RPh

● **LEARNING OBJECTIVES**

1. Define polypharmacy.
2. Describe the prevalence, risks, and outcomes for polypharmacy in older adults.
3. Discuss the process of reducing polypharmacy including good prescribing habits, evaluation of patient medications, and discontinuation of medications.
4. Describe principles for reducing polypharmacy.
5. Contrast polypharmacy with undertreatment of patients.

PRE-TEST

1. **Polypharmacy is:**
   A. The use of two medications with different mechanisms of action
   B. The use of more medications than are clinically indicated
   C. Using two medications in combination that have been shown to be effective to treat a medical condition
   D. Using one medication to treat multiple conditions

2. **Risk factors for polypharmacy include all of the following EXCEPT:**
   A. Having multiple medical problems
   B. Seeing multiple subspecialists
   C. Frequent hospitalizations
   D. Obtaining multiple medications from the same pharmacy

3. **In order to reduce polypharmacy:**
   A. All medications should be stopped and restarted one by one to determine which ones are actually needed.
   B. A systematic approach should be considered to determine which medications are necessary for a patient given his or her co-morbidities.
   C. Medications that have been newly started should be stopped first.
   D. If more than one medication is being used to treat the same condition, the "extra" medication should be stopped.

INTRODUCTION

Definition

Polypharmacy is the use of more medications than are clinically indicated, or when a medication regimen contains at least one unnecessary drug.[1-3] Although alternative definitions have included the use of five or more medications, appropriate treatment of complex conditions in older adults with multiple co-morbidities may justify the use of multiple pharmacologic agents. The use of multiple medications that are clinically warranted has been termed "therapeutic polypharmacy."

Prevalence

In the United States, 45% to 55% of adults aged 65 years and older take five or more medications, and 12% take 10 or more.[4] In studies looking at inappropriate use of drugs in elderly patients, 44% to 60% of patients have no indication for use, are on unnecessary or ineffective drugs, or have duplication of therapy.[5-9]

Risk Factors

Risk factors for polypharmacy can be characterized as those that are patient-specific, prescriber (physician)-specific, or specific to the health care system. Table 32–1 lists patient-specific risk factors for polypharmacy. Patients who are predisposed to polypharmacy are more likely to be older, white, of higher education level, in poor health, have multiple chronic medical conditions, and use over nine medications.[10] The presence of knowledge deficits in the area of geriatric pharmacology, a willingness to prescribe, and reluctance to discontinue medications are prescriber (physician)-specific risk factors (Table 32–2). If physician-specific risk factors are coupled with a patient who has a high level of expectation for pharmaceutical therapy for a given condition, then polypharmacy is more likely to occur. Some risks inherent to the health care system include an increased number of health care provider visits, pharmacies, available drugs, and increased pharmaceutical company marketing (Table 32–3). A visit to the physician's office increases the likelihood that a patient will obtain a new prescription. Additionally, patients who use over-the-counter (OTC) and herbal agents may not report the use of these agents to their physicians.[11,12]

● TABLE 32–1 Patient-Specific Risk Factors for Polypharmacy
Increased age
White race
Education
Poor health
Medical conditions (depression, hypertension, anemia, asthma, angina, diverticulosis, osteoarthritis, gout, diabetes
Use of ≥ 9 medications
Data from Hajjar et al.[10]

● TABLE 32–2 Prescriber-Specific Risk Factors for Polypharmacy
Knowledge deficits in geriatric pharmacology
Willingness to prescribe new medications
Reluctance to stop medications

Polypharmacy increases the risk of adverse drug events, drug interactions, nonadherence, morbidity, mortality, and health care costs (Figure 32–1). A complication such as a fall precipitated by the use of multiple psychotropic agents can lead to hospitalization, institutionalization, and loss of independence in an older patient. Inappropriate drug use in the hospital setting can predispose patients to delirium and a prolonged hospital stay. This can be further complicated by additional diagnostic evaluations. A prescriber should be on the alert for risk factors that are modifiable so that the negative effects of polypharmacy can be averted.

REDUCING POLYPHARMACY

In order to reduce the negative outcomes attributed to polypharmacy interventions should be aimed at promoting rational prescribing. This process involves a systems approach to drug use by physicians and patients in a population (Figure 32–2). Physician prescribing is a complex behavior incorporating knowledge about drug availability, pharmacology, use, toxicity, and skills in the therapeutic use of a drug.[13] Prescribing is also influenced by health care insurance, drug formularies, and patient compliance. In older adults, prescribing should be individualized and based upon functional status and goals of care. A systematic approach to evaluating a patient's drug regimen should be considered (described in the next section).

Efforts geared toward reducing polypharmacy have included criteria or tools aimed at identifying potentially inappropriate medications, educational interventions geared toward physicians, and interventions involving medication review by physicians and/or pharmacists. Drug utilization review tools such as the Beers Criteria[14-16] and the Improved Prescribing in the Elderly Tool (IPET)[17] have been used to identify potentially inappropriate prescriptions in older adults. They list medications that have a high potential for adverse effects. A review article by Hajjar and colleagues details five studies in which the interventions used decreased

● TABLE 32–3 Health Care System–Specific Risk Factors for Polypharmacy
Increased number of health care provider visits
Availability of multiple pharmacies
Increased number of available drugs
Increased pharmaceutical company marketing
Data from Hajjar et al.[10]

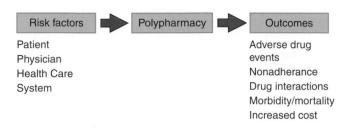

FIGURE 32–1. Complications of polypharmacy.

● TABLE 32–4 Steps to Reducing Polypharmacy
Document a complete medication list including herbal and over-the-counter agents.
Match medications to known medical problems, and question duplications or deficiencies.
Stop medications without known benefit, intolerable adverse effects, or serious drug interactions.
Avoid the prescribing cascade.
Simplify the medication regimen (decrease the number or doses or medication taken in a 24-hour period) and ensure appropriate dosing (evaluate renal and hepatic function).
Address patient-specific issues such as preferences.

Source: From the Medication Screening Questionnaire (MSQ), 2009.

polypharmacy.[10] These interventions included instructing patients at risk to bring their medications to their physician for review, mailing physicians a list of their patients who had been identified as taking inappropriate medications, the use of medication review sheets by residents in the inpatient setting to reduce the number of medications taken upon discharge, and the use of geriatric evaluation and management.

A Systematic Approach to Reducing Polypharmacy

Steps to Reducing Polypharmacy

The first step to reducing polypharmacy is to ensure that all medications have been documented (Table 32–4). This includes OTC and herbal therapies. In the outpatient setting, patients should bring all of their medications to the visit.

After documenting a complete medication list, the medications should be matched to a known medical problem. Drugs that are not indicated, have concerning drug interactions, or cause intolerable adverse events should be considered for discontinuation. If one medication is being used to treat the side effect of another, an alternative agent that has more tolerable side effects should be considered. This will help prevent a prescribing cascade. The patient's regimen should be simplified by reducing the number of medications or dosages taken within a 24-hour period. The creatinine clearance should be calculated in order to ensure that the appropriate dose is being administered. Nonpharmacologic therapy should be considered prior to initiating a new drug. Finally, patient-specific preferences such as mode of administration and tolerance of expected side effects should be discussed. These basic principles are applicable to any health care setting.

CASE PRESENTATION: MR. BENJAMIN CARLYLE

A 77-year-old man who lives alone and has a past medical history of hypertension, hyperlipidemia, osteoporosis, atrial fibrillation, and depression, Mr. Benjamin Carlyle is admitted to the hospital for progressive shortness of breath of 1-week duration. He has associated cough, fever, and chills.

On exam his blood pressure is 110/90 mm Hg, heart rate 60 bpm, and oxygen saturation 94% on room air. His weight is 76 kg. He has decreased breath sounds in the right base, an irregularly irregular heart rhythm, and bilateral lower extremity edema.

Labs reveal a white blood cell count of 15×10^3/mL (15×10^9/L) with a left shift. He is not anemic. His potassium level is 3.0 mEq/L (3.0 nmol/L). His blood urea nitrogen and creatinine are 70 mg/dL (24.9 nmol/L) and 2.0 mg/dL (176 umol/L), respectively. Digoxin level is 1.6. ng/mL (2.0 nmol/L; normal range 0.8-1.6 ng/mL [1.0-2.0 nmol/L]).

A chest x-ray is performed and reveals right lower lobe pneumonia with a small associated pleural effusion. The left lung is clear.

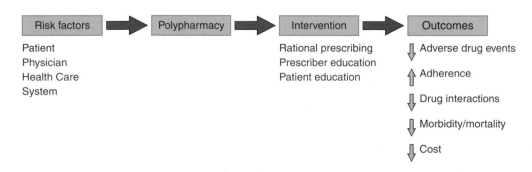

FIGURE 32–2. Decreasing negative polypharmacy outcomes.

● **TABLE 32–5** Matching Problems with Medications

Hypertension	Lisinopril 10 mg daily
	Hydrochlorothiazide 25 mg daily
	Amlodipine 5 mg daily
Atrial fibrillation No anticoagulation	Digoxin 0.125 mg daily
Osteoporosis	Fosamax 70 mg once a week
	Calcium w/vit D 500/200 tid
No documented indication	Omeprazole 40 mg daily
No documented indication	Furosemide 40 mg every AM

His EKG shows atrial fibrillation at a rate of 66 bpm. A transthoracic echocardiogram (TTE) shows a normal ejection fraction of 55%, mild mitral regurgitation, mild tricuspid regurgitation, and normal left ventricular relaxation.

Home Medications

Digoxin 0.125 mg by mouth daily
Furosemide 40 mg by mouth every morning
Alendronate 70 mg by mouth once a week
Calcium/vitamin D 500/200 one tablet by mouth tid
Omeprazole 40 mg by mouth daily
Lisinopril 10 mg by mouth daily
Hydrochlorothiazide 25 mg by mouth daily
Amlodipine 5 mg by mouth daily

Mr. Carlyle is a victim of polypharmacy. A review of his medication list suggests that he has likely been prescribed the lisinopril, hydrochlorothiazide, and amlodipine for blood pressure; the alendronate and calcium and vitamin D for osteoporosis; and digoxin for atrial fibrillation (Table 32–5). The indication for use of the omeprazole is not known. The furosemide might be used for lower-extremity edema; otherwise, he has no documented history of congestive heart failure and his TTE does not reveal significant abnormalities. There are no medications listed for hyperlipedemia or depression. He has not been anticoagulated with warfarin for atrial fibrillation.

CASE PRESENTATION (continued)

When asked about the use of herbal or over-the-counter agents he reports the use of St. John's wort to help with his mood, ginkgo to help with his memory, and aspirin to help his heart and protect him from stroke

Complete List: Home Medications

Digoxin 0.125 mg daily
Furosemide 40 mg every AM
Alendronate 70 mg once a week
Calcium/vitamin D 500/200 tid
Omeprazole 40 mg daily
Lisinopril 10 mg daily
Hydrochlorothiazide 25 mg daily
Amlodipine 5 mg daily
St. John's wort 1 or 2 tablets daily
Ginkgo biloba 1 capsule by mouth daily
Aspirin 81 mg daily

Hospital Course

B.C. is admitted to the hospital, and started on levofloxacin 500 mg for pneumonia. Furosemide and hydrochlorothiazide are held, as his creatinine is higher than his baseline of 1.1 mg/dL (97.2 μmol/L). His low potassium is repleted. He reports that furosemide was started for lower-extremity edema but that it has not been helpful. His legs are normal in the morning, but swell by the end of the day. He recalls being started on omeprazole for upper abdominal discomfort shortly after his diagnosis of osteoporosis. During his first hospital night he is provided diphenhydramine 25 mg at bedtime for sleep. This proves to be effective, so it is provided as a standing order for the remainder of his hospital stay. His herbal agents are not continued during his hospitalization.

Hospital Medications

Digoxin 0.125 mg po daily
~~Furosemide 40 mg every AM~~
Alendronate 70 mg once a week
Calcium/vitamin D 500/200 tid
Omeprazole 40 mg daily
Lisinopril 10 mg daily
~~Hydrochlorothiazide 25 mg daily~~
Amlodipine 5 mg daily
~~St. John's wort~~
~~Ginkgo biloba~~
Aspirin 81 mg daily
Levofloxacin 500 mg by mouth daily
Diphenhydramine 25 mg by mouth at bedtime

By hospital day number 3, his fever resolves and symptoms of shortness of breath and cough continue to improve. His blood pressure increases to 160/90 on lisinopril 10 mg and amlodopine 5 mg daily. On hospital day 4 he falls while trying to walk to the bathroom in the early morning. He reports feeling confused and dizzy prior to the fall. His BUN/creatinine has improved to his baseline of 20/1.1 mg/dL.

Mr. Carlyle could have been ready for discharge from the hospital on an oral antibiotic for continued treatment of pneumonia. His hospital stay has now been complicated by a fall. Review of his medication list reveals a potential cause. The most recently started agent is diphenhydramine. It has significant anticholinergic properties, and thus can cause confusion, dizziness, and lack of coordination in older adults. It is not recommended for continued use in older adults.

CASE PRESENTATION (continued)

In order to decrease his risk of oversedation, falls, and confusion, the diphenhydramine is held. His dizziness improves, but does not completely resolve. After a thorough exam and investigation for injury from his fall, he is seen by physical therapy and deemed safe for discharge to home with services (physical therapy and nurse visit for blood pressure monitoring).

How can we alter Mr. Carlyle's home regimen to decrease polypharmacy and its adverse outcomes?

1. Increase the dose of lisinopril and discontinue amlodipine. Amlodipine might be contributing to his lower-extremity edema. Monitor blood pressure.
   Principle: Simplify medications by decreasing the number of doses, or number of medications taken, in a 24-hour period.
2. Stop furosemide and consider the use of compression stockings for venous insufficiency. Advise Mr. Carlyle to elevate his lower extremities while sitting, and observe for improvement.
   Principle: Stop medications without known benefit, with intolerable adverse effects, or with serious drug interactions.
3. Ask Mr. Carlyle to describe how he administers the bisphosphonate alendronate. If not taken appropriately, potential side effects include dyspepsia and nausea. Consider discontinuing omeprazole, and observing for the presence of dyspepsia or reflux. Proton pump inhibitors can increase the risk of community-acquired *Clostridium difficile*,[18,19] pneumonia,[20] and hip fracture.[21,22] Provide instructions on the appropriate administration of the alendronate. He should take it in the morning on an empty stomach with a full glass of water. He should remain in an upright position for 30 minutes afterward.
   Principle: Stop medications without known benefit, with intolerable adverse effects, or with serious drug interactions.
4. Decrease the dose of digoxin to 0.125 mg every other day, and monitor potassium, as low potassium can predispose to digoxin toxicity. The digoxin level is 1.6, which is at the upper limits of normal. Though AV blockade and bradycardia are more serious complications, dizziness and weakness can be more subtle side effects with supra-therapeutic levels of digoxin.
   Principle: Stop medications without known benefit, with intolerable adverse effects, or with serious drug interactions.
   Principle: Simplify the medication regimen (decrease the number of doses or medications taken in a 24-hour period) and ensure appropriate dosage (evaluate renal and hepatic function).
5. In patients with low to moderate risk of stroke, and no major risk factors, warfarin has been shown to be more effective in decreasing the risk of stroke in 2 years than aspirin alone.[23] The risk versus benefits of initiation of warfarin should be discussed with Mr. B.C. and his primary care provider. One must be certain that absolute contraindications to the initiation of warfarin are not present.
6. Educate Mr. B.C. about the use of herbal and OTC agents. Though some of these agents may be effective to treat certain medical conditions, others can cause unwanted side effects, interact with conventional medications, or have unpredictable quantities of the active ingredient. He should be informed that ginkgo can increase the risk of bleeding with aspirin or warfarin (if warfarin is initiated). St. John's wort is a mild antidepressant, and can decrease the concentration of digoxin. He would benefit from an appropriate screen for depression and administration of a more effective agent if his symptoms are not significantly helped by St. John's wort. He should be told to inform his primary care provider of all medications taken including herbal and OTC agents.

CASE PRESENTATION (continued)

Current Hospital Medications

1. Digoxin 0.125 mg daily
2. ~~Furosemide 40 mg every AM~~
3. Alendronate 70 mg once a week
4. Calcium/vitamin D 500/200 tid
5. Omeprazole 40 mg daily
6. Lisinopril 10 mg daily
7. ~~Hydrochlorothiazide 25 mg daily~~
8. ~~Amlodipine 5 mg daily~~
9. Levofloxacin 500 mg daily
10. ~~St. John's wort~~
11. ~~Ginkgo biloba~~
12. Aspirin 81 mg daily
13. ~~Diphenhydramine 25 mg hs~~

Discharge Medications

1. Levofloxacin 400 mg for a total of 10 days, then stop
2. Lisinopril 20 mg daily, f/u K in 1 week

3. Alendronate 70 mg q week in early AM prior to other meds
4. Calcium/vitamin D 500/200 bid
5. Digoxin 0.125 mg every other day
6. St. John's wort
7. Ginkgo biloba (discontinue if initiation of warfarin)
8. Aspirin 81 mg daily
9. Warfarin 5 mg daily (if approved by patient and primary physician)

Medications Held upon Discharge

Furosemide 40 mg every AM
Hydrochlorothiazide 25 mg
Amlodipine 5 mg daily
Omeprazole 40 mg daily

Additional Considerations for the Outpatient Setting

Compression stockings for venous insufficiency.

Initiation of coumadin and discontinuation of ginkgo after discussion with primary care provider and confirmation of willingness to follow INR.

Disclosure of complete medication list to primary care provider.

Formal screening for depression.

Evaluation of fasting cholesterol, as hyperlipidemia is noted in his past medical history, but he is not on a medication. Explore whether dietary management has been considered.

Follow-up of digoxin level, blood pressure and heart rate, and potassium level.

Discontinuation

In addition to rational prescribing, improving the medication discontinuation process is also an important consideration.[24] A growing body of research indicates that in certain patient populations the discontinuation of medications did not worsen outcomes,[25-27] but led to deceased adverse drug reactions[28] and costs attributable to medications.[29] A systematic review of published trials of medication withdrawal reveals that withdrawal of antihypertensives, benzodiazepines, and psychotropic agents in older patients did not lead to significant harm and yielded short-term effectiveness.[30] Withdrawal of psychotropic medications was associated with a reduction in falls and improved cognition. After withdrawal of antihypertensive agents in normotensive elderly patients, 20% to 85% remained normotensive or did not require reinstatement of therapy for 6 months to 5 years. In one randomized controlled trial, patients with Alzheimer dementia who continued treatment with an antipsychotic agent had an increased risk of mortality at 12 months compared to those whose antipsychotic medication was discontinued.[31] Though abrupt discontinuation is possible with some medications, other agents can cause withdrawal or rebound effects, and should be tapered off gradually if discontinuation is appropriate. The patient should be followed for at least 4 months for evaluation for adverse outcomes or exacerbation of the underlying condition.[32] An adverse drug withdrawal event can present as an exacerbation of the underlying disease or a physiologic withdrawal reaction. In one retrospective review, beta-blockers and benzodiazepines were most implicated in the onset of a physiologic drug withdrawal reaction.[32] So despite lack of significant harm in some patients, tapering and close monitoring is the most prudent option. Generally, medications without known benefits, with intolerable adverse effects, or with serious drug interactions should be considered for discontinuation. The precise method of discontinuation depends on the pharmacology of the drug, specific patient characteristics including co-morbidities, presence or absence of a potential withdrawal syndrome, and the feasibility of appropriate monitoring for side effects or rebound effects.

Undertreatment

While we should focus on reducing polypharmacy by discontinuing unnecessary drugs or those with intolerable side effects, undertreatment is another important issue in older adults. Undertreatment has been noted with beta-blockers and ACE inhibitors in older adults with chronic heart failure, and with warfarin in patients with atrial fibrillation.[33] Other conditions such as osteoporosis, diabetes, and pain have also been undertreated with pharmacotherapy. With this in mind, clinicians must carefully consider the benefits of decreasing the number of medications with those of initiating new agents that have been shown to decrease morbidity and mortality. After a risks-versus-benefits discussion with the patient or appropriate surrogate decision-maker, a new medication should be initiated if the burden of taking additional pills is less than the benefits of treatment.

Use of Herbal and Over-the-Counter Agents

According to data from the National Health Interview Survey 2007, 58.4% of adults age 60 and over used biologically based therapies or nonvitamin, nonmineral natural products.[34] The most common reasons for use among older adults were to improve general wellness, help manage arthritis, help prevent or manage colds, and to improve memory.[35] The most common herbal agents used, in decreasing order of frequency, were fish oil (omega 3 or DHA), glucosamine, echinacea, flaxseed oil, ginseng, combination herb pills, ginkgo biloba, and co-enzyme Q10. Despite the frequency of use and good intentions, many patients do not report the use of these agents to their physicians,[11,12] and physicians often do not ask. Many patients may view these products as natural, and therefore safe and effective. Unfortunately, many natural products have the potential to cause adverse drug events and significant drug interactions with conventional medications. Questions about the use of these OTC agents should be asked during the initial patient assessment in order to document a complete medication list.

Self-Medication

Increased availability of information about disease states and drug therapy, dissatisfaction with a prescribed regimen, a desire to improve or supplement a current regimen, or increased cost of drugs might encourage self-medication and noncompliance among older adults. Physicians should explore the reasons for self-medication and educate patients about the dangers.

CONCLUSION

There are over 36 million adults over the age of 65 years in the United States, representing 12.3% of the population. This number is expected to increase to 54 million by the year 2020, when 1 in 6 Americans will be over the age of 65.[36] According to data from the National Center for Health Statistics, 71% of office visits and 91% of hospital emergency department visits involve drug therapy.[37] Given continued advances in medicine, physicians will continue to be faced with the task of medication management and the prevention of polypharmacy in even their most robust elderly patients.

There are approximately 12,900 prescription drugs approved by the FDA,[38] and a greater number of OTC and herbal agents available. Focusing on rational prescribing, or selection of the most appropriate therapeutic regimen for a specific patient, will offer more benefit in preventing the complications of polypharmacy than reducing the number of medications alone. Careful thought should be given to both the medication discontinuation process and the initiation process. Physicians should be prepared to discuss complementary and alternative therapies or cite reliable sources of information. A systematic approach should be used to combat polypharmacy, and periodic medication review and monitoring should be performed.

References

1. Carlson JE. Perils of polypharmacy: 10 steps to prudent prescribing. *Geriatrics*.1996;51:26-35.

2. Montamat SC, Cusack B. Overcoming problems with polypharmacy and drug misuse in the elderly. *Clin Geriatr Med*. 1992;8:143-158.

3. Bushardt RL, Massey EB, Simpson TW, et al. Polypharmacy: Misleading, but manageable. *Clin Interv Aging*. 2008;3:383-389.

4. Kaufman DW, Kelly JP, Rosenberg L, et al. Recent patterns of medication use in the ambulatory adult population in the United States: The Slone Survey. *JAMA*. 2002;287:337-344.

5. Schmader K, Hanlon JT, Weinberger M, et al. Appropriateness of medication prescribing in ambulatory elderly patients. *J Am Geriatr Soc*. 1994;42:1241-1247.

6. Lipton HL, Bero LA, Bird JA, McPhee SJ. The impact of clinical pharmacists' consultations on physicians' geriatric drug prescribing. A randomized controlled trial. *Med Care*. 1992;30:646-658.

7. Hajjar ER, Hanlon JT, Sloane RJ, et al. Unnecessary drug use in frail older people at hospital discharge. *J Am Geriatr Soc*. 2005;53: 1518-1523.

8. Schmader KE, Hanlon JT, Pieper CF, et al. Effects of geriatric evaluation and management on adverse drug reactions and suboptimal prescribing in the frail elderly. *Am J Med*. 2004;116:394-401.

9. Steinman MA, Landefeld CS, Rosenthal GE, et al. Polypharmacy and prescribing quality in older people. *J Am Geriatr Soc*. 2006;54: 1516-1523.

10. Hajjar ER, Cafiero AC, Hanlon JT. Polypharmacy in elderly patients. *Am J Geriatr Pharmacother*. 2007;5:345-351.

11. Kuo GM, Hawley ST, Weiss LT, et al. Factors associated with herbal use among urban multiethnic primary care patients: A cross-sectional survey. *BMC Complement Alt Med*. 2004;2:18.

12. Zeilmann CA, Dole EJ, Skipper BJ, et al. Use of herbal medicine by elderly Hispanic and non-Hispanic white patients. *Pharmacotherapy*. 2003;23:526-532.

13. Sellers EM. Defining rational prescribing of psychoactive drugs. *Br J Addict*. 1988;83:31-34.

14. Beers MH, Ouslander JG, Rollingher I, et al. Explicit criteria for determining inappropriate medication use in nursing home residents. *Arch Intern Med*. 1991;151:1825-1832.

15. Beers MH. Explicit criteria for determining potentially inappropriate medication use by the elderly. An update. *Arch Intern Med*. 1997; 157:1531-1536.

16. Fick Dm, Cooper JW, Wade W, et al. Updating the Beers criteria for potentially inappropriate medication use in older adults: Results of a US Consensus panel of experts. *Arch Intern Med*. 2003;163: 2716-2724.

17. Naugler CT, Brymer C, Stolee P, et al. Development and validation of an improved prescribing for the elderly tool. *Can J Clin Pharmacol*. 2000;7:103-107.

18. Dial S, Delaney JA, Barkun AN, Suissa S. Use of gastric acid-suppressive agents and the risk of community acquired *Clostridium difficile*-associated disease. *JAMA*. 2005;294:2989-2995.

19. Choudhry MN, Soran H, Ziglam HM. Overuse and inappropriate prescribing of proton pump inhibitors in patients with *Clostridium difficile*-associated disease. *QIM*. 2008;101:445-448.

20. Laheij RJ, Sturkenboom MC, Hassing RJ, et al. Risk of community-acquired pneumonia and use of gastric acid suppressive drugs. *JAMA*. 2004;292:1955-1960.

21. Yang YX, Lewis JD, Epstein S, Metz DC. Long-term proton pump inhibitor therapy and risk of hip fracture. *JAMA*. 2006;296: 2947-2953.

22. Targownik LE, Lix LM, Metge CJ, et al. Use of proton pump inhibitors and risk of osteoporosis-related fractures. *CMAJ*. 2008: 179:319-326.

23. Go AS, Hylek EM, Chang Y, et al. Anticoagulation therapy for stroke prevention in atrial fibrillation: How well do randomized trials translate into clinical practice? *JAMA*. 2003;290:2685-2692.

24. Bain KT, Holmes H, Beers MH. Discontinuing medications: A novel approach for revising the prescribing stage of the medication-use process. *J Am Geriatr Soc*. 2008;56:1946-1952.

25. Nelson MR, Reid CM, Krum H, et al. Predictors of normotension on withdrawal of antihypertensive drugs in elderly patients: Prospective study in second Australian National Blood Pressure Study cohort. *BMJ*. 2002;325:815.

26. McGowan MP. There is no evidence for an increase in acute coronary syndromes after short-term abrupt discontinuation of statins in stable cardiac patients. *Circulation*. 2004;110:2333-2335.

27. Black DM, Schwartz AV, Ensrud KE, et al. Effects of continuing or stopping alendronate after 5 years of treatment: The Fracture Intervention Trial Long Term Extension (FLEX): A randomized trial. *JAMA*. 2006;296:2927-2938.

28. Van der Velde N, van den Meiracker AH, Pols HA, et al. Withdrawal of fall-risk-increasing drugs in older persons: Effect on tilt-table test outcomes. *J Am Geriatr Soc*. 2007;55:734-739.

29. Zarowitz BJ, Stebelsky LA, Muma BK, et al. Reduction of high-risk polypharmacy drug combinations in patients in a managed care setting. *Pharmacotherapy*. 2005;25:1636-1645.

30. Iyer S, Naganathan V, McLachlan AJ, et al. Medication withdrawal trials in people aged 65 years and older: A systematic review. *Drugs Aging*. 2008;25:1021-1031.

31. Ballard C, Hanney ML, Theodoulou M, et al. The dementia antipsychotic withdrawal trial (DART-AD) long-term follow-up of a randomized placebo-controlled trial. *Lancet Neurol*. 2009;8:151-157.

32. Graves T, Hanlon JT, Schmader E, et al. Adverse events after discontinuing medications in elderly outpatients. *Arch Intern Med*. 1997;157:2205-2210.

33. Sloane PD, Gruber-Baldini A, Zimmerman S, et al. Medication undertreatment in assisted living settings. *Arch Intern Med*. 2004;164:2031-2037.

34. Barnes PM, Bloom B, Nahin RL. Complementary and alternative medicine use among adults and children: United States, 2007. *Natl Health Stat Report*. 2009;12:1-23.

35. Marinac JS, Buchinger CL, Godfrey LA, et al. Herbal products and dietary supplements: A survey of use, attitudes, and knowledge among older adults. *J Am Osteopath Assoc*. 2007;107:13-23.

36. US Census Bureau. *Current Population Survey, Annual Social and Economic Supplement* 2008. http://www.census.gov/population/www/socdemo/age/older_2008.html.

37. Cherry DK, Hing E, Woodwell DA, et al. National Ambulatory Medical Care Survey. US Department of Health and Human Services, Centers for Disease Control and Prevention. National Center for Health Statistics. http://www.cdc.gov/nchs/FASTATS/drugs.htm.

38. http://www.fda.gov, report as of June 1, 2009.

POST-TEST

1. **All of the following include steps to reduce polypharmacy EXCEPT:**

   A. Matching medications to known medical problems, and questioning deficiencies

   B. Stopping medications without known benefit or with intolerable adverse effects

   C. Ensuring that side effects of medications are appropriately treated with the addition of medications

   D. Simplifying medication regimens by decreasing the number of doses

2. **An 85-year-old female with hypertension and advanced dementia has developed diarrhea during the fourth day of hospitalization for aspiration pneumonia. Her discharge medications include the following:**

   Levofloxacin 500 mg daily for 6 more days

   Metronidazole 500 mg tid for 10 days

   Lisinopril 10 mg daily

   Colace 100 mg po tid

   Aricept 10 mg daily

   Namenda 5 mg bid

   Senna 87 mg at bedtime

   In order to reduce polypharmacy, which of the following medications could be discontinued?

   A. Levofloxacin and metronidazole

   B. Aricept and Namenda

   C. Colace and Senna

   D. Aricept and Colace

3. **Judie Alexis is a 78-year-old female with hypertension, osteoarthritis, and osteopenia. She lives alone and has a great functional status. She takes aspirin 81 mg daily, lisinopril 10 mg daily, and amlodipine 10 mg daily. She is interested in maintaining her good health and asks about the use of herbal and OTC agents. She does not have a history of nephrolithiasis or constipation. Which one of the following statements about the use OTC and herbal agents would be INAPPROPRIATE for Ms. Alexis?**

   A. Herbal agents are natural products, and so are therefore safe for patients taking multiple medications.

   B. 1200 mg of calcium and 800 IU of vitamin D would be good additions to her current regimen.

   C. Patients should keep an accurate account of the dosage and frequency of use of selected agents.

   D. Patients should report OTC and herbal agent use to health care providers.

ANSWERS TO PRE-TEST

1. B
2. D
3. B

ANSWERS TO POST-TEST

1. C
2. C
3. A

33

Urinary Incontinence

Camille P. Vaughan, MD, MS

Theodore M. Johnson II, MD, MPH

● LEARNING OBJECTIVES

1. Define urinary incontinence and the types.
2. Describe common symptoms and physical exam findings to direct an accurate diagnosis of the type of urinary incontinence.
3. Identify reversible causes of urinary incontinence.
4. Describe treatment options for urinary incontinence including behavioral, lifestyle, and medication interventions.
5. Discuss the possible side effects of medications used to treat urinary incontinence.
6. Delineate appropriate criteria for referral to a specialist.

PRE-TEST

1. **What type of urinary incontinence is preceded by the sudden desire to void that is difficult to defer?**
   A. Stress
   B. Mixed
   C. Urge
   D. Overflow

2. **What type of urinary incontinence is most often precipitated by coughing, sneezing, or laughing?**
   A. Stress
   B. Urge
   C. Overflow
   D. Mixed

3. **Which of the following is NOT a potentially reversible cause of urinary incontinence?**
   A. Infection
   B. Polypharmacy
   C. Polyuria
   D. Diarrhea

● INTRODUCTION

Urinary incontinence (*involuntary leakage of urine*) has physical, psychological, social, and economic consequences for older adults. Because patients may not mention the problem, it is also often undetected by primary care providers unless patients are directly questioned regarding difficulty with their bladder. Urinary incontinence (UI) is associated with an increased risk of skin breakdown, accidental falls and subsequent fractures, sleep disturbance, and recurrent urinary tract infections. The embarrassment caused by UI for some can lead to social withdrawal and isolation, and may be associated with depression and anxiety. Caregivers often cite the inability to manage UI as a factor leading to institutionalization. In the United States alone, it is estimated that the health care costs related to UI were $20 billion in the year 2000.

Anatomy and Physiology

Maintenance of continence depends on multiple factors, which include normal physiologic function of the lower urinary tract, pelvic, and neurologic systems. The urinary bladder is a low-pressure collecting system that actively relaxes during filling and is made up of transitional epithelium and smooth muscle, referred to as the detrusor muscle. The urinary bladder, urethra, and other pelvic organs are supported by pelvic floor muscles, which also serve to augment the seal between the bladder outlet and urinary sphincter. Normal voiding involves relaxation of the external sphincter, which is composed of striated skeletal muscle, followed by contraction of the detrusor muscle. This process is coordinated through the parasympathetic, sympathetic, and somatic nervous systems. The parasympathetic nervous system is primarily responsible for contraction of the detrusor muscle through the interaction of acetylcholine with M3 subtype muscarinic receptors, although other types of receptors may also play a role. The sympathetic nervous system is involved in relaxation of the external sphincter. The somatic nervous system coordinates sensory inputs between the bladder and the central nervous system, conveying information particularly regarding bladder distension to signal the need to void (Figure 33–1). Higher centers in the cerebral cortex, cerebellum, and limbic system normally send inhibitory signals through the pontine mesencephalic reticular formation located in the midbrain to prevent detrusor contraction. When signals are received indicating bladder fullness, these higher centers cease to inhibit detrusor contraction and normal voiding is facilitated.

Aging and the Lower Urinary Tract

The prevalence of UI increases with age. Approximately 15% of women and 10% of men over the age of 60 report at least weekly UI. Several factors that are associated with aging may predispose older individuals to develop UI as well as other bothersome lower urinary tract symptoms. Nocturnal urine production may increase as the normal circadian pattern of urine production changes with aging, leading to more frequent nocturia (*waking at night to void*). Changes in cortical

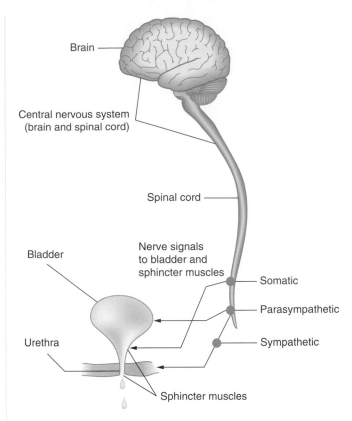

FIGURE 33–1. The bladder and central nervous system. (*Adapted from: http://kidney.niddk.nih.gov/Kudiseases/pubs/nervedisease/index.htm*)

control of the bladder can lead to involuntary detrusor contractions. Older persons may also have an increased risk for incomplete emptying secondary to both decreased detrusor pressure and diminished flow rates during micturition, leading to residual urine in the bladder. These physiologic changes may be compounded in men who often develop benign prostatic hyperplasia (BPH). While bladder capacity does not necessarily decrease with age, it can be markedly decreased particularly in individuals who experience involuntary detrusor contractions. The sensory pathways between the bladder and the central nervous system may also become dysfunctional, leading to less warning time when the bladder reaches filling capacity.

Terminology

The International Continence Society standardized terminology in reference to lower urinary tract symptoms in 2002.[1] *Stress incontinence* refers to UI associated with effort or exertion, or on sneezing or coughing. *Urge UI* is described as incontinence accompanied by or immediately preceded by urgency, which is the sudden compelling desire to pass urine that is difficult to defer. The "overactive bladder syndrome" describes urgency that is often accompanied by frequency and/or nocturia and may or may not be associated with urge UI. *Mixed incontinence* occurs when symptoms of both urgency and stress incontinence are present. *Overflow incontinence* is a nonstandardized term, but occurs in the presence of urethral obstruction, detrusor muscle weakness, or both, which can lead to accumulation of urine in the bladder.

● TABLE 33–1 Types of Urinary Incontinence

Type of Urinary Incontinence	Risk Factors	Associated Symptoms
Stress	a. Weakened pelvic floor muscles and urethral hypermobility b. Weakness of urethral sphincter c. Obesity	Usually small volume UI that occurs with activity that increases intra-abdominal pressure—typically coughing, sneezing, effort, or exertion
Urge	Detrusor hyperactivity due to: a. Lower urinary tract factors (tumor, stones, or outflow obstruction) and/or b. Central nervous system factors (spinal cord injury, parkinsonism, previous stroke)	Variable volume UI that is accompanied by or immediately preceded by urgency—sudden compelling desire to void that is difficult to defer
Mixed	Combination of factors leading to both stress and urgency UI	Variable volume UI that occurs either with increased intra-abdominal pressure or prior to a void associated with urgency
Overflow	a. Outflow obstruction b. Impaired detrusor contractility c. Detrusor-sphincter dysynergia	Usually small volume UI, urinary frequency, sensation of incomplete emptying
Functional	a. Impaired mobility b. Psychological factors c. Advanced dementia	UI secondary to limited mobility, psychomotor slowing, or dependence in activities of daily living

Functional incontinence does not describe a pathologic state of the lower urinary tract, but rather incontinence that is due to a factor such as impaired mobility, psychomotor slowing from depression, or severe cognitive impairment leading to diminished independence in activities of daily living (Table 33–1).

This chapter will explore the evaluation and management of UI in geriatric patients through two cases describing scenarios that are common in outpatient practice.

CASE PRESENTATION 1: MS. LEAKE

Ms. Leake is 78 years old and comes for a routine follow-up appointment. She has a past medical history of hypertension, diabetes diagnosed 3 years ago, hyper-cholesterolemia, osteoarthritis of both knees, and mild cognitive impairment. She had three pregnancies and all were vaginal deliveries without complications when she was in her 20s. Her current medications include atenolol 50 mg daily, lisinopril 40 mg daily, metformin 500 mg twice daily, acetaminophen 1000 mg three times a day as needed for pain, aspirin 81 mg daily, pravastatin 20 mg each evening, and trazodone 50 mg each evening as needed for insomnia. She presently lives in an assisted living facility and receives daily set-up help with her medications. She had been participating actively in recreational outings and programs, but recently stopped going on trips because of frequent severe urgency and the occasional accidental loss of urine. She denies any recent dysuria, hematuria, fever, or chills. She occasionally has accidents when she bends over or reaches to pick up something. This has occurred for several years. Within the past year, she has had increasing difficulty with the sensation of a sudden need to urinate. About once a week she will leak a small amount of urine when she hears water running or she is rushing to the bathroom to void. She would prefer not to take an additional medication if possible and asks for your recommendations.

CASE PRESENTATION 2: MR. DAMPIER

Mr. Dampier is 86 years old and reports to your clinic today for his annual follow-up. He has a past medical history of hypertension, BPH, and gastroesophageal reflux disease. He lives alone and frequently travels to Florida, where he spends the winter months. For several years he has been treated for BPH with a nonselective alpha-blocker, terazosin 10 mg, at bedtime. In addition, he is taking amlodipine 10 mg daily, enteric-coated aspirin 81 mg, and omeprazole 20 mg daily. His weak urinary stream and hesitancy had initially improved with the addition of terazosin, yet he has noted increasing frequency of urination. He awakens two or three times nightly to void, which he says is bothersome because it disrupts his sleep. He denies any snoring or difficulty breathing during sleep. He has also begun to notice it is more difficult to make it to the toilet in time during the day when he has the urge to urinate, and about once a week he will leak a small amount of urine prior to reaching the bathroom. In addition, he complains that when he leaves the car after an extended drive, he has an overwhelming sense of urinary urgency that often leads to UI. He finds occasional UI very embarrassing.

● INITIAL EVALUATION

History and Symptom Assessment

When assessing symptoms in order to characterize the type of UI, the temporality of the symptoms is important to consider. UI that is new in onset or has occurred within the last 6 months may be secondary to a reversible cause. UI that has developed insidiously over more than 6 months is generally persistent, and while reversible causes should be ruled out as contributors, long-term treatments may be necessary to improve the condition.

Reversible causes of UI can be remembered using the mnemonic DRIP, which represents some of the most common potentially reversible factors (Table 33–2). The treatment of UI secondary to one of these conditions requires treatment of the underlying cause. Delirium or restricted mobility may be a source of functional incontinence. Infections such as acute prostatitis or urinary tract infections are common causes of an acute worsening of bladder symptoms. Urinary retention could be due to an acute condition such as prostatitis or a drug side effect. Inflammation refers to irritation of tissues related to estrogen deficiency that may respond with local topical estrogen in certain patients. Fecal impaction can lead to incontinence through anatomic obstruction of urine flow. Polyuria causing potentially reversible UI may be addressed by treating a metabolic condition such as diabetes or hypercalcemia, volume overload secondary to poorly controlled co-morbid disease, or lifestyle interventions such as decreasing or eliminating caffeine-containing beverages or alcohol. Pharmaceutical agents can lead to UI secondary to medication side effects. Common culprit medications include medications with significant anticholinergic properties such as centrally acting antihistamines, antiparkinsonian agents, and tricyclic antidepressants, which can predispose to urinary retention. Acetylcholinesterase inhibitors, by increasing levels of available acetylcholine, also can worsen symptoms of urinary urgency leading to incontinence. Some psychotropic medications have been associated with an increased risk of incontinence by worsening urgency, as well as anesthetic agents, which can increase the risk of acute urinary retention. Opioid agents increase the risk of constipation, which can worsen urinary urgency. Diuretics, particularly rapidly acting loop diuretics, may lead to polyuria. Often decreasing the dose of a culprit medication, modifying the timing of a dose, or eliminating unnecessary drugs can reduce the impact that pharmaceutical agents may have on UI.

● TABLE 33–2 DRIP Mnemonic
Delirium
Restricted mobility
Retention
Infection
Inflammation
Impaction
Pharmaceuticals
Polyuria

Ms. Leake and Mr. Dampier both describe symptoms that have been present for more than 6 months and represent persistent incontinence. To further characterize the type of incontinence, assessing both patient-related and environmental factors that precipitate episodes of incontinence is helpful in directing treatment options. It is important to remember that symptoms do not always accurately predict pathophysiology, but will often lead to an appropriate initial management strategy.

Stress incontinence typically occurs with activities that increase intra-abdominal pressure such as coughing, sneezing, bending, or reaching. During the physical exam, a cough test can be utilized to assess for stress incontinence. While this test is not very sensitive, it is specific. The cough test involves having the patient hold a cloth close to the perineum while standing with a full bladder. The patient then produces several forceful coughs and the cloth is removed to assess for the presence of wetness secondary to UI.

Urge UI occurs with a strong sense of urgency that can also be brought about by sounds such as running water or activities such as hand washing. It is often also accompanied by complaints of urinary frequency and nocturia. If nocturia is present, the clinician should also inquire about symptoms of an underlying sleep disorder such as obstructive sleep apnea or sleep-related movement disorder. Among frail elderly, urge UI secondary to detrusor hyperactivity may coexist with impaired detrusor contractility, leading to concomitant urinary retention. The diagnosis of this condition is made during urodynamic investigation, and is the combination of inappropriate bladder contractility during filling and weak detrusor contractions during bladder emptying, which leaves an elevated postvoid residual. This condition is termed detrusor hyperactivity with impaired contractility (DHIC).

Symptoms associated with overflow incontinence such as dribbling, weak urinary stream, intermittency, hesitancy, frequency, and nocturia may result from bladder outlet obstruction (BPH, significant pelvic organ prolapse) or impaired detrusor contractility (DHIC, neurologic conditions, spinal cord injury). Some of these symptoms also overlap with other types of UI, which can make the diagnosis of overflow incontinence challenging. Factors that predispose to functional incontinence may be elicited by an assessment of the patient's cognitive status, mood, mobility, and conditions related to his or her living environment such as accessibility of toilets and proper signage to direct residents to bathroom facilities.

In addition to eliciting a thorough history related to the events that precipitate episodes of incontinence, the time course of symptoms, medications being used, and potentially reversible contributing causes, it is very important to assess the impact urinary symptoms are having on the individual's quality of life and what the individual's goals are for treatment. Satisfaction with care often depends upon alignment between the provider's and patient's goals in evaluating treatment effects.

Targeted Physical Examination

The physical examination should focus on determining the presence of potentially reversible conditions, clarifying the type of UI, and identifying conditions that will impact treatment choices or require referral to a consultant. Continuation of the case examples provides more information regarding the physical exams for Ms. Leake and Mr. Dampier.

CASE PRESENTATION 1 (continued)

Ms. Leake is 165 cm tall and weighs 84 kg. Her blood pressure and pulse measured in the sitting position are 137/60 mm Hg and 62. After standing for 1 minute her blood pressure and pulse are 122/56 mm Hg and 73, respectively. She is afebrile and has a respiratory rate of 14. She walks into the examination room with the assistance of a cane, but her gait appears stable. On a brief test of memory, she is able to recall 2/3 items and is able to draw the face of a clock and appropriately place the hands of the clock so that the time reads 10 minutes after 11 o'clock. Her lung fields are clear to auscultation and her heart sounds are regular in rate and rhythm with a 2/6 harsh systolic murmur at the right upper sternal border that does not radiate. Her abdomen is soft, nontender, and nondistended with regular bowel sounds. Examination of her extremities reveals 1+ pitting edema to the calves in both legs. She has bony changes of osteoarthritis of the knees, but no erythema or effusion is present bilaterally. On neurologic examination her deep tendon reflexes are 2+ and symmetric throughout. Her sensation of light touch is intact on the plantar surfaces of both feet. She has no evidence of cogwheel rigidity or bradykinesia on exam. A pelvic examination reveals thin external labia and vaginal tissues without erythema. A manual examination reveals stage one pelvic organ prolapse. Ms. Leake is able to adequately isolate her pelvic floor muscles during the manual examination and produces a moderate squeeze, which she maintains well for 2 seconds. A rectal exam reveals soft, brown stool, but no impaction. A cough test performed prior to voiding elicits a few drops of urine on a cloth towel. After voiding, a bladder ultrasound shows no significant postvoid residual urine in the bladder. A urinalysis is negative for any abnormal cells or glucose.

CASE PRESENTATION 2 (continued)

Mr. Dampier is 180 cm and weighs 100 kg. His blood pressure while sitting is 122/70 mm Hg, with a pulse of 60. After standing for 1 minute his blood pressure is 100/58 mm Hg with a pulse of 80. He is afebrile and has a respiratory rate of 16. He reports some lightheadedness with standing, but this resolves and he is able to walk to the examination room without assistance. A brief test of memory reveals recall of 3/3 items and a normal clock-drawing test. An assessment using the American Urological Association eight-question Symptom Inventory (AUA SI, Figure 33–4) reveals a score of 13 with an equal distribution among irritative and obstructive symptoms. Auscultation of the lungs and heart are unremarkable. His abdominal examination reveals normal bowel sounds and no tenderness to palpation. His neurologic examination reveals 2+ muscle stretch reflexes that are symmetric throughout. He has no evidence of cogwheel rigidity and his sensation to light touch is intact. His lower extremity examination reveals 2+ pitting edema to the calves bilaterally. On rectal examination, you note a nontender, enlarged prostate, without nodularity. He has no evidence of fecal impaction. He is able to isolate his pelvic floor muscles on examination and produces a strong squeeze which he can maintain for 3 seconds. After voiding, a bladder ultrasound reveals a postvoid residual of 25 mL. A urinalysis is negative for red blood cells or evidence of infection.

Utilizing the information gathered from the history and clinical evaluation of Ms. Leake and Mr. Dampier, the clinician is able to assess the likely etiology of incontinence and to devise a management plan. Each case will be discussed separately to highlight the unique aspects of the clinical presentation of UI in these two patients.

Mixed Incontinence

While Ms. Leake describes an insidious onset of symptoms, reversible conditions can still play a role in acute exacerbations of chronic conditions. Through the history and physical evaluation we are able to assess for potentially reversible causes of UI. She does not have evidence of delirium, significantly restricted mobility, or psychomotor slowing. While she has evidence of decreased estrogen status, the pelvic exam did not reveal inflammation from atrophic vaginitis. She has no evidence of fecal impaction or infection, and while she has minimal lower extremity edema, there are no other signs of volume overload. A review of her medication list reveals polypharmacy, but each medication is appropriately prescribed and is unlikely to have significant side effects that are worsening her urinary symptoms. While she has a diagnosis of diabetes, her urinalysis shows no evidence of glucosuria, which would precipitate polyuria. Testing of her glycosylated hemoglobin would further determine if uncontrolled diabetes is contributing significantly to her symptoms of urinary urgency.

Her symptoms are most consistent with mixed UI because she describes both stress and urge UI. The positive cough test corroborates her history of stress-related symptoms, and the absence of postvoid residual urine in the bladder rules out significant urinary obstruction or impaired detrusor contractility. She has no signs on exam of an underlying disorder such as neurologic disease or impaired mobility that should lead to functional incontinence. Further information about fluid intake or other habits that could influence her condition could be obtained by a 3-day bladder diary (Figure 33–2), which asks the patient to record voids, the number and frequency of episodes of UI, consumption of fluids, and activities associated with incontinence episodes. Examples of this type of bladder diary can be found at www.niddk.nih.gov. Her history also gives insight toward her goals of care. While it appears she was tolerating the stress symptoms, the urgency symptoms have driven her to seek care from a clinician and are the more bothersome as they have led to restriction of social activities. She would prefer to limit additional medications if possible.

Treatment options for mixed incontinence begin by targeting the symptoms that the patient finds most bothersome. For Ms. Leake, these are her urgency symptoms. Therapeutic interventions for urge UI can include behavioral and lifestyle interventions and/or medications. Since Ms. Leake would like to avoid an additional medication, the clinician might begin with behavioral and lifestyle interventions, which are virtually side-effect free. Lifestyle interventions could involve assessing fluid and caffeine intake and educating her regarding scheduled voiding techniques. Cutting back on caffeine, which is irritating to the bladder, may improve urgency symptoms. Limiting alcohol intake is often helpful. Typically, fluid restriction is not recommended unless the individual is drinking more than 64 ounces (1.9 L) of fluid per day, as insufficient fluid intake can worsen constipation. Scheduled toileting describes regular voiding to avoid involuntary bladder contractions and using techniques to delay voiding until that time. Typically, scheduled voiding involves attempting to void at an appropriate, individualized interval such as every 2 hours regardless of the sense of urgency (Figure 33–3). The appropriate voiding interval can be determined using a 3-day bladder diary completed by the patient.

Other behavioral interventions involve techniques to prevent incontinence without the addition of a medication. These include bladder training and pelvic floor muscle exercises (also called Kegel exercises) combined with urge suppression strategies, which have been shown to be as effective as drug therapy for urge UI in some studies. Patients can be

Time	Drinks	Urinated in toilet	Accidental loss of urine	Activity when leakage happened
6:35 am		✓	✓	Rushing to toilet
7:00 am	2 cups coffee			
8:10 am		✓	✓	Rushing to toilet
11:30 am		✓		
12:50 pm	1 glass water +1 glass iced tea		✓	Sneezed
2:00 pm	1 glass lemonade	✓	✓	Waited too long
3:30 pm		✓		
5:45 pm	1 glass water +1 cup coffee			
7:00 pm		✓	✓	Waited too long
9:15 pm	1 glass water	✓		
11:30 pm		✓		
2:20 am		✓		
5:00 am		✓		

FIGURE 33–2. Sample bladder diary: Day 1.

Time 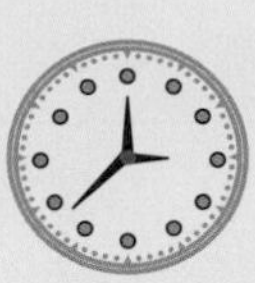	Drinks 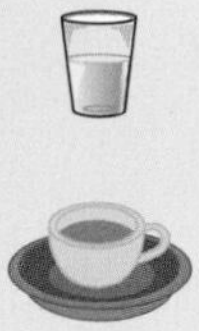	Urinated in toilet 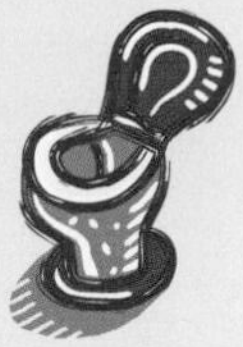	Accidental loss of urine 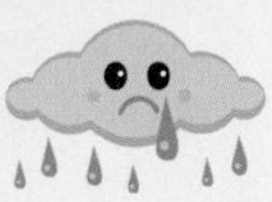	Activity when leakage happened
6:35 am		✓	✓	Rushing to toilet
7:00 am	2 cups coffee			
9:10 am		✓	✓	Rushing to toilet
12:50 pm	1 glass water +1 glass iced tea			
2:00 pm		✓	✓	Waited too long
4:30 pm		✓		
5:45 pm	1 glass water			
7:45 pm		✓	✓	Waited too long
10:00 pm	1 glass water	✓		
11:45 pm		✓		

Possible scheduled voiding routine based on the above diary

	Awakening	9 am	12 pm	3 pm	6 pm	9 pm	Bedtime
Scheduled void	✓	✓	✓	✓	✓	✓	✓

FIGURE 33–3. Sample bladder diary—leading to scheduled voiding routine.

taught pelvic floor muscle exercises during the physical exam or with a self-help booklet and then are given a home exercise routine to follow. If an individual has difficulty learning these techniques, the use of computer-assisted biofeedback or help from a specialist, such as a physical therapist, may be available in some locations to teach the techniques. Urge-suppression strategies teach patients to prevent urge incontinence by employing pelvic floor muscle exercises in situations that precipitate incontinence. Bladder training involves using these urge-suppression strategies to train the bladder to empty at less frequent time intervals, typically by gradually lengthening the time between voids. The utility of behavioral interventions may be limited by the patient's cognitive ability, as they typically require coordination and concentration to implement a pattern of exercise. Ms. Leake displays some evidence of mild cognitive impairment, as she needs assistance with her medications and her recall is mildly impaired. But if she is motivated to implement lifestyle and behavioral changes, she could avoid the need for an additional medication.[2]

Medications for urge UI are typically directed at preventing the contraction of bladder smooth muscle by blocking muscarinic receptors, which normally bind acetylcholine (Table 33–3). Several antimuscarinic drugs are available with similar efficacy to reduce urgency incontinence in clinical trials (typically 60-80%). Common side effects of these medications include dry mouth and constipation, which may be bothersome. Cognitive side effects may be possible if the medication is less selective for the bladder's muscarinic receptors or easily crosses the blood–brain barrier. Older persons taking anticholinergic drugs should be monitored carefully for worsening of cognitive function or drug-induced delirium. These medications are typically available in once-daily formulations, which are more expensive yet are typically better tolerated with fewer side effects than formulations with a shorter half-life. Medications may also enhance the effectiveness of behavioral interventions. Other medications targeting different bladder-specific receptors are also under development. Previously, there were no surgical treatments for urgency and urge UI that was refractory to medication and behavioral therapy. Now for refractory urgency-related symptoms, evaluation for treatment with botulinum toxin or a sacral nerve stimulator might be a reason to consider referral to a specialist.

For Ms. Leake's stress incontinence, behavioral interventions are typically first-line therapy. Strengthening of the pelvic floor muscles, which support the organs of the pelvis, may improve incontinence related to stretching or reaching. Ms. Leake can also be taught to squeeze her

● **TABLE 33–3** Drugs Used to Treat Symptoms of Overactive Bladder

Drugs	Usual Adult Dose	Level of Evidence/Grade of Recommendation[a]	Comments
Drugs with Predominantly Anticholinergic or Antimuscarinic effects			
Hyoscyamine	0.375 mg twice daily orally	2/D	The drug is also available in sublingual and elixir forms; it has prominent anticholinergic side effects.
Darifenacin	7.5–15.0 mg daily orally	1/A	The drug is selective for the bladder M3 muscarinic receptor and may have less cognitive side effects than other anticholinergic agents.
Fesoterodine	4–8 mg daily orally	1/A	This prodrug is easily converted to an active metabolite, which is chemically identical to the active metabolite of tolterodine.
Oxybutynin	2.5–5.0 mg 3 times daily orally (short-acting) 5–30 mg daily orally (long-acting) 3.9 mg over a 96-hr period (transdermal)	1/A	Long-acting and transdermal preparations have fewer side effects than short-acting preparations. The transdermal patch can cause local skin irritation in some patients.
Propantheline	15–30 mg 4 times daily orally	2/B	The drug has prominent anticholinergic side effects.
Propiverine	15 mg 3 times daily orally	1/A	The drug has complex pharmacokinetics with several active metabolites; it is not currently available in the United States.
Solifenacin	5–10 mg daily orally	1/A	The drug has some selectivity for the bladder M3 muscarinic receptor over other muscarinic receptors.
Tolterodine	2–4 mg daily orally	1/A	The drug has relatively low lipophilicity with limited ability to penetrate the CNS.
Trospium	20 mg twice daily orally 60 mg daily orally (long-acting)	1/A	The agent is a quaternary ammonium compound, which does not cross the blood-brain barrier and may have fewer cognitive side effects than other anticholinergic agents.
Estrogen (for Women)			
Vaginal estrogen preparations	Approximately 0.5 g cream applied topically nightly for 2 weeks, then twice per week Estradiol ring, replaced every 90 days Estradiol, 1 tablet daily for 2 weeks, then 1 tablet twice a week	4/D	Local vaginal preparations are probably more effective than oral estrogen, but definitive data on effectiveness are lacking.
Alpha-Adrenergic Antagonists (for Men)			
Alfuzosin (selective) Doxazosin (nonselective) Prazosin (nonselective) Tamsulosin (selective) Terazosin (nonselective)	10 mg daily orally 1–8 mg daily orally at bedtime 1–5 mg twice daily orally 0.4–0.8 mg daily orally 1–10 mg daily orally at bedtime	1/A	These agents are useful in men. Postural hypotension can be a serious side effect. Doses of nonselective agents must be increased gradually to facilitate tolerance.
5-Alpha Reductase Inhibitors			
Dutasteride Finasteride	0.5 mg daily orally 5 mg daily orally	4/D[b]	May be added for men with benign prostatic enlargement.

[a]Levels of evidence are based on the Oxford System: A score of 1 indicates evidence from randomized, controlled trials; a score of 2 evidence from good-quality prospective cohort studies; a score of 3 evidence from good-quality retrospective case-control studies; and a core of 4 evidence from good-quality case series. The grade of recommendations is based on the definitions used by the International Consultation on Urological Diseases.
A indicates consistent level 1 evidence; B consistent level 2 or 3 evidence or major evidence from randomized, controlled trials; C level 4 evidence or major evidence from level 2 or 3 studies, or expert opinion based on the Delphi method; and D inconclusive, inconsistent, or nonexistent evidence based on expert opinion only.
[b]This rating is for symptoms of overactive bladder, not for overall symptoms of benign prostatic hyperplasia.
Adapted from Ouslander JG.[4]

pelvic floor muscles immediately prior to activities that precipitate an accident, such as prior to sneezing or coughing. These techniques are typically most effective after several weeks of practice and can be maintained with continued exercise. For obese or overweight patients, weight loss of at least 8% can also lead to reductions in stress UI frequency.[3] If significant pelvic organ prolapse (typically greater than stage 2 or with protrusion past the vaginal introitus) is present, a referral to a gynecologist may be considered for further evaluation. A pessary may improve stress incontinence symptoms if pelvic organ prolapse is present, but must be fitted, and the patient must be willing to undertake necessary hygiene for the device. Surgical options to improve stress incontinence are also available, including periurethral injection of bulking agents, bladder suspension, or sling procedures to support the bladder and external sphincter. Ms. Leake's clinician might also consider referral for urologic or gynecologic evaluation if she did not meet her goals of care after undertaking an adequate trial of behavioral and/or drug therapy.

● LOWER URINARY TRACT SYMPTOMS AND BPH

Although Mr. Dampier describes symptoms that have slowly progressed over months to years, it is important to assess for any potentially reversible causes for his complaints. His mental status assessment and physical exam do not suggest delirium or a significant functional impairment that would predispose him to functional incontinence. Because his postvoid residual is less than 50 mL, he is considered to have adequate bladder emptying. A postvoid residual measurement > 200 mL would warrant consultation with a specialist. His physical exam and urinalysis rule out a source of infection or impaction.

In assessing his medication list, two of his current medications, terazosin and amlodipine, may warrant further evaluation. One concerning finding on exam is evidence of orthostatic hypotension. This condition places him at increased risk for falling, particularly as he is also experiencing urinary frequency and nocturia. If other sources of orthostatic hypotension such as anemia or volume depletion have been ruled out, this likely represents a common side effect of terazosin, which would warrant consideration of a selective alpha-blocker for his symptoms of BPH. In addition, he appears to have significant lower-extremity edema, which may be a side effect of a calcium channel blocker. It may be reasonable to stop this medication, particularly in light of his orthostatic hypotension, and monitor his blood pressure to assess for the need of another class of antihypertensive.

In Mr. Dampier's case, there may be potentially reversible factors that could lead to improvement in his symptoms, although the chronicity of symptoms indicates evidence of persistent incontinence as well. While his physical exam reveals evidence of BPH, his lower urinary tract symptoms of urge UI accompanied by frequency and nocturia are also typical of overactive bladder syndrome. In men, these symptoms may coexist with BPH. As in the first case, it is important to

assess Mr. Dampier's goals of care in initiating a treatment plan and to focus on the symptoms he finds most bothersome. He reports that UI is very embarrassing and he is not sleeping well because of nocturia. These are the symptoms to attempt to address first. He does not express any particular preference for therapy, but it is important for the clinician to assess this as well as his potential interest in surgical interventions if they were offered.

In order to further assess the severity of his lower urinary tract symptoms secondary to BPH, the AUA SI (also called the International Prostate Symptom Score [IPSS]; Figure 33–4) is an assessment that can be used. This brief questionnaire assesses for both obstructive (hesitancy, weak stream, incomplete emptying, intermittent stream) and irritative (frequency, nocturia, urgency) symptoms as well as the severity of symptoms. The resulting score guides the clinician in management and may serve as a follow-up measure if the questionnaire is repeated on subsequent visits. A score less than 8 reveals mild symptoms, 8 to 19 moderate symptoms, and greater than 19 severe symptoms. Mr. Dampier's AUA-SI score of 13 suggests moderate symptoms related to BPH. Society guidelines suggest that medical therapy would be most appropriate for initial management of moderate symptoms.

For Mr. Dampier's symptoms related to BPH, medical therapy usually involves an alpha-blocker as well as the possible addition of a 5-alpha-reductase inhibitor. He is already taking a nonselective alpha-blocker, terazosin, at an appropriate dose, which did initially improve his symptoms. Now, he may be experiencing side effects from terazosin and would benefit by changing to a selective alpha-blocker such as alfuzosin or tamsulosin. These medications are more selective for prostate and urethral tissue and have less frequent side effects on blood pressure. Clinicians should be aware of the increased risk of "floppy iris syndrome" with the use of tamsulosin in men who may undergo surgical removal of cataracts. This condition may be addressed in the perioperative period, but represents a potentially serious surgical complication secondary to the affinity of tamsulosin for the α-1a receptor, which is found in the smooth muscle of the bladder and prostate as well as the dilator smooth muscle of the iris. This effect is irreversible, even if the drug is discontinued prior to surgery. If cataract removal surgery is planned, it is recommended to delay the start of tamsulosin until the postoperative period. If an individual is already taking tamsulosin prior to a planned cataract surgery, the primary clinician should confirm that the patient's ophthalmologist is aware. A 5-alpha reductase inhibitor such as finasteride or dutasteride may also provide some improvement in his prostate-related symptoms over time, by preventing the conversion of testosterone to dihydrotestosterone and limiting prostate growth. These drugs are more effective for symptom relief and prevention of obstruction in men with larger prostates.

Overactive Bladder with Urge UI

Mr. Dampier also describes symptoms consistent with overactive bladder and is significantly bothered by incontinence. In men, as in women, both behavioral and medication

THE AMERICAN UROLOGICAL ASSOCIATION SYMPTOM INDEX

TAKING THE QUIZ Please circle the answer that best represents your response to each of the following questions. the questions are designed to gauge the severity of any symptoms you may be experiencing.	Not at all	Less than 1 time in 5	Less than half the time	About half the time	More than half the time	Almost always	Patient score
1. INCOMPLETE EMPTYING Over the past month, how often have you had a sensation of not emptying your bladder completely after you have finished urinating?	0	1	2	3	4	5	
2. FREQUENCY Over the past month, how often have you had to urinate again less than 2 hours after you have finished urinating?	0	1	2	3	4	5	
3. INTERMITTENCY Over the past month, how often have found you stopped and started again several times when you urinated?	0	1	2	3	4	5	
4. URGENCY Over the past month, how often have found it difficult to postpone urination?	0	1	2	3	4	5	
5. WEAK STREAM Over the past month, how often have you had a weak urinary stream?	0	1	2	3	4	5	
6. STRAINING Over the past month, how often have you had to push or strain to begin urination?	0	1	2	3	4	5	
7. NOCTURIA Over the past month, how many times did you most typically get up to urinate from the time you went to bed at night until the time you got up in the morning?	0	1	2	3	4	5+	
				Your total score			

	Delighted	Pleased	Mostly satisfied	Mixed	Mostly dissatisfied	Unhappy	Terrible
QUALITY OF LIFE DUE TO URINARY SYMPTOMS If you were to spend the rest of your life with your urinary condition the way it is now, how would you feel about that?	0	1	2	3	4	5	6

SCORING THE QUIZ
Add the numbers from your answers to questions 1 through 7. The maximum possible score is 35. The final question will help you judge how you feel about your symptoms.

PLEASE NOTE: This test is used to measure the severity of your symptoms. It is not a diagnostic test. In other words, it will not tell you whether or not you have BPH. Talk to your doctor to determine whether your symptoms are due to BPH.

Reference: 1. McConnell JD, Barry MJ, Bruskewitz RC, et al. Benign Prostatic Hyperplasta: Diagnosis and Treatment. Clinical Practice Guideline, Number 8, AHCPR Publication No. 94-0582. Rockville, Md: agency for Health Care Policy and Research, Public Health Service, U.S. Department of Health and Human Sevices, February 1994.

Remember: This information is not intended as a substitute for medical treatment.

FIGURE 33–4. AUA SI (also called International Prostrate Symptom Score [IPSS]). (*Source: Barry MJ et al. the American Urological Association symptom index for benign prostatic hyperplasia. J. Urol 1992;148:1549-1557.*)

approaches can be used to address these symptoms. Behavioral and lifestyle approaches may be informed by a 3-day bladder diary. A bladder diary that accounts for fluid intake as well as his caffeine and alcohol use would help identify lifestyle factors that might lead to improvement in symptoms. Urge-suppression strategies that involve pelvic floor muscle exercises may also be beneficial to prevent incontinence and are virtually side-effect free. Frequent or scheduled toileting may also be beneficial. Because Mr. Dampier is able to effectively empty his bladder, he is a candidate for antimuscarinic therapy if he has not achieved his goals of care through behavioral changes alone.[1] The same medications that are used in women for overactive bladder can be utilized in men and often are used in combination with alpha-blockers (Table 33–3). In men whose PVR is > 50 mL, but less than 200 mL, antimuscarinic agents can be utilized, but the patient should be monitored for urinary retention. In one recent study, urinary retention requiring catheterization typically occurred in < 1% of subjects.[5]

Nocturia

Mr. Dampier is also bothered by nocturia because it disrupts his sleep. Nocturia can have multiple causes in addition to being associated with the overactive bladder syndrome and BPH. Clinicians should also consider underlying sleep disorders and causes of nighttime polyuria. While Mr. Dampier denies a history of snoring or episodes of awakening short of breath, because he lives alone, the clinician may consider further questionnaire-based evaluations to assess the need for a formal sleep evaluation. Several studies have indicated that obstructive sleep apnea is prevalent among older persons who complain of nocturia. The Epworth Sleepiness Scale and the Berlin Questionnaire can be used to assess for the degree of hypersomnolence and probability of obstructive sleep apnea, respectively. Mr. Dampier's physical exam and history do not suggest a movement disorder or restless leg syndrome, but these conditions may also be associated with disrupted sleep that manifests as a complaint of nocturia.

Nocturia can also result from conditions that lead to excessive nighttime urine production such as poorly controlled congestive heart failure or diabetes mellitus, nocturnal polyuria, or peripheral edema. Mr. Dampier does not have a history suggestive of conditions such as heart failure or diabetes, but his physical exam does suggest lower-extremity edema. Changing his antihypertensive therapy, as discussed previously, may lead to resolution if this is the result of a medication side effect. Compression stockings during the day can also be utilized to prevent significant daytime accumulation of fluid in the lower extremities. To assess for nocturnal polyuria, a 24-hour record of voided urine volumes would also be helpful in determining the proportion of urine that is produced during the daytime hours compared with nighttime hours once the patient is asleep. Greater than 30% of urine production during sleeping hours compared with waking hours is considered abnormal and would constitute nocturnal polyuria.

Treatments for nocturia depend on the underlying factors contributing to its pathogenesis. Often multiple causes are present in a single individual, as in Mr. Dampier's case, in which he has evidence of BPH, overactive bladder syndrome, and lower-extremity edema. Treatment of these conditions may reduce his nightly nocturia frequency. Lifestyle interventions may include limiting fluid intake within 2 to 3 hours of bedtime, although adequate daily fluid intake is important to prevent constipation. Limiting afternoon and evening caffeine and alcohol may also reduce nighttime urine production and bladder irritation overnight. Behavioral interventions may involve using pelvic floor muscle exercises with urge suppression strategies that have been shown to be effective in reducing nocturia among women with urge UI who also have nocturia. Attempting to void immediately prior to bedtime may also be a useful strategy. If a 24-hour voided volume record reveals evidence of nocturnal polyuria, this condition may be amenable to pharmacologic intervention, but is often challenging to treat. Off-label drug treatment with 1-desamino-8-d-arginine vasopressin (ddAVP) may be helpful in selected patients, but has a significant risk of causing severe hyponatremia in patients over 65 years of age and is generally not recommended. An afternoon dose of a loop diuretic can lead to diuresis prior to bedtime, which may lessen overnight urine production. In persons at risk for UI, increased urinary frequency caused by a diuretic may have unacceptable side effects.

Depending on Mr. Dampier's goals of care and response to multiple possible interventions to address his urinary incontinence and other lower urinary tract symptoms, a referral to a urologist may be warranted in the future. Surgical intervention to reduce prostate size could impact his symptoms as well, but further evaluation by a specialist would determine his candidacy for a procedure. Post-prostatectomy incontinence is a condition that can affect men after either transurethral resection of the prostate or, more commonly, after a radical prostatectomy. Typically these symptoms manifest as stress incontinence from damage to the urethral sphincter during surgical manipulation. Conservative treatment options include pelvic floor muscle exercises to strengthen support tissues and improve sphincter closure. External penile clamps can also be used to prevent urine leakage, but patients must be educated regarding maintenance of the device, appropriate timing of bladder emptying, and prevention of damage to the external genitalia. Typically, post-prostatectomy incontinence will improve within 12 months following prostate resection. If the condition continues to be bothersome despite the use of conservative treatments, surgical options could include implantation of an artificial urinary sphincter or sling to support the bladder and external sphincter.

● WHEN TO REFER TO A SPECIALIST

Reasons to refer a patient to a urologist, gynecologist, or urogynecologist that have been discussed include when the patient has not achieved his or her goals for care after a sufficient trial of lifestyle, behavioral, and pharmaceutical therapies and an elevated postvoid residual (> 200 mL). Other reasons to consider a referral include persistent hematuria (> 5 red blood cells per high-power field) in the absence of infection, pelvic organ prolapse past the vaginal introitus, an abnormal prostate exam, inability to pass a 14-French straight catheter, two or more symptomatic urinary tract infections in the past 12 months, and surgery or irradiation involving the pelvic area or lower urinary tract in the past 6 months.[6]

● ABSORPTIVE INCONTINENCE PRODUCTS AND CATHETERS

While complete continence is often a goal of care, this is not practical in every patient situation and incontinence products such as pads, absorptive undergarments, and adult diapers are available to prevent skin irritation and improve hygiene. These products are usually expensive and are not covered under most insurance plans. Further information for patients and caregivers regarding continence products and education can be found through the following websites: www.medlineplus.gov (United States National Library of Medicine/National Institute of Heath), www.nafc.org (National Association for Continence), and www.simonfoundation.org (Simon Foundation). Indwelling urinary catheters are rarely needed for incontinence and should not be routinely used. Sometimes catheters are used for comfort at the end of life for those in whom bed and clothing changes are distressing. Indwelling catheters may also be utilized to prevent soiling or further irritation of sacral wounds. Clean intermittent catheterization may be necessary for certain bladder conditions such as those with bladder emptying difficulty or a high postvoid residual. While absorptive products and catheters should not be considered first-line treatments for incontinence, use of these products may be appropriate in certain situations as the clinician and patient align goals of care.

CONCLUSION

UI is a bothersome condition that affects a significant number of older adults and is often unrecognized by their care providers. While UI often represents a persistent condition that has progressed insidiously, reversible factors frequently influence the condition. Treatment of UI can improve the quality of life for older adults. Improvement in symptoms often occurs with lifestyle interventions and behavioral therapies, but pharmaceutical agents are sometimes necessary. Clinicians should always consider the goals of care of the patient when weighing different therapeutic options.

References

1. Abrams P, Cardozo L, Fall M, et al. The standardisation of terminology of lower urinary tract function: Report from the Standardisation Sub-committee of the International Continence Society *Neurourol Urodyn.* 2002;21:167-178.

2. Burgio KL, Locher JL, Goode PS, et al. Behavioral vs. drug treatment for urge urinary incontinence in older women: A randomized controlled trial. *JAMA.* 1998;280:1995-2000.

3. Subak LL, Wing R, West DS, et al. Weight loss to treat urinary incontinence in overweight and obese women. *N Engl J Med.* 2009;360:481-490.

4. Ouslander JG. Management of overactive bladder. *N Engl J Med.* 2004;350:786-799.

5. Kaplan SA, Roehrborn CG, Rovner ES, et al. Tolterodine and tamsulosin for treatment of men with lower urinary tract symptoms and overactive bladder: A randomized controlled trial. *JAMA.* 2006;296:2319-2328.

6. Gibbs CF, Johnson II TM, Ouslander JG. Office management of geriatric urinary incontinence. *Am J Med.* 2007; 120:211-220.

POST-TEST

1. **Risk factors associated with the development of overflow-type UI include all of the following EXCEPT:**

   A. Outflow obstruction

   B. Weakened pelvic floor muscles

   C. Impaired detrusor contractility

   D. Detrusor-sphincter dysynergia

2. **Which of the following is NOT a nonpharmacological treatment of stress incontinence?**

   A. Pessary

   B. Pelvic floor muscle exercises

   C. Scheduled voiding

   D. Fluid restriction

3. **Dribbling, weak urinary stream, intermittency, hesitancy, frequency, and nocturia associated with BPH are related to which type of UI?**

   A. Stress

   B. Urge

   C. Overflow

   D. Mixed

ANSWERS TO PRE-TEST

1. C
2. A
3. D

ANSWERS TO POST-TEST

1. B
2. D
3. C

34

Falls and Mobility Disorders

David A. Ganz, MD, PhD

Wessam Labib, MD, MPH

Laurence Z. Rubenstein, MD, MPH

● **LEARNING OBJECTIVES**

1. Explain why falls are an important geriatric syndrome.

2. Identify common risk factors for falls in older adults.

3. Discuss multifactorial fall assessment.

4. Describe the role of exercise in preventing falls in community-dwelling elders.

5. Describe strategies to minimize injury in patients who fall frequently.

PRE-TEST

1. Which of the following is MOST correct regarding the role of exercise in preventing falls in community-dwelling older people?

A. Exercise is effective only in older people who are at higher than average risk of falls.

B. An exercise program that challenges balance, uses a higher dose of exercise, and provides continued supervision is the most likely to be effective in preventing falls.

C. An aerobic exercise program is probably the most effective intervention for preventing falls.

D. There is no evidence that exercise helps in preventing falls in community-dwelling older people.

2. Which of the following is the LEAST helpful to assess as part of a multifactorial fall risk assessment?

A. Hearing impairment

B. Gait and balance problems

C. Visual impairment

D. Risky medications

3. Which of the following injury reduction strategies has the MOST evidence to support its use among community-dwelling elders?

A. Hip protectors

B. Pharmacologic treatment of osteoporosis

C. Low beds

D. Energy-absorbent floors

CASE PRESENTATION: A PATIENT AT RISK

A 78-year-old woman, Ms. R., comes to your office for a new patient visit. She has macular degeneration, osteoarthritis, hypertension, and mild hearing loss. Today she reports no symptoms except bilateral knee pain when she walks and a transient sense of imbalance that can occur while walking. She denies any light-headedness or vertigo, and she has not fallen in the past year. She takes lisinopril 10 mg daily, a daily multi-vitamin, calcium, vitamin D, episodic acetaminophen for her knee pain, and diphenhydramine as needed to help her sleep. She lives alone, having survived her husband of 50 years who passed away 2 years ago.

On exam, Ms. R.'s blood pressure is 138/80 mm Hg, pulse 75/min, temperature 98.2°F (36.8°C), respirations 14/min, weight 150 lb (68 kg), and height 5 ft 3 in (1.6 m). Examination is notable for crepitus on passive range of motion of both knees, symmetric gait with mildly decreased gait speed, and ability to stand with the feet close together but not in a tandem stance (heel of one foot touching toe of the other foot). The rest of the exam is within normal limits, except for decreased visual acuity in both eyes.

Other data include a normal hemoglobin checked 6 months ago as well as a normal screening colonoscopy performed 6 years ago. Papanicolaou tests were performed up until age 70 and were all normal. A bone densitometry scan checked last year demonstrated a T score of −0.9 at the femoral neck. Ms. R. is up to date in her pneumonia and influenza vaccines. At the end of the visit Ms. R. tells you that she has a friend who fell and broke his hip a month ago. She is afraid she might fall, given her problems with balance. She asks you for recommendations on how to prevent falls.

BACKGROUND

Falls are a serious concern for older adults, both those who are in generally good health and those who are frail. Although people are at risk of falls throughout the lifespan, older people tend to fall more frequently and are more likely to experience an injury from a fall (such as a hip fracture) than younger people. In addition, older people's fear of falling may induce a downward spiral through self-restriction of physical activity, decreased physical function, and increased vulnerability to falls and injuries.

Like many problems encountered by older adults, falls are caused by multiple interacting factors. Ms. R. does not report a fall, but she is nonetheless at risk for falling. Her impaired balance is the most obvious risk factor, but her decreased visual acuity may also contribute, as can the diphenhydramine

that she takes as a sleep aid. We do not know details of her home environment, but she may be at risk for falls in the home if there is poor lighting, a high level of clutter, or particular items that are easy to trip over (electrical cords, throw rugs). Outside the home, uneven pavement could be a risk.

What is the best approach to preventing falls in older people who live in their own homes? Principles similar to those that guide injury prevention in automobile drivers are applicable to fall prevention in older people. Just as the risk of an injurious automobile crash is a function of the driver's level of attention, the condition of the car, the design of the road, and the car's safety features, so also a fall is a function of both factors intrinsic to the patient (both cognitive and physical) and factors in the patient's environment. Older people may be inclined to see the solution to preventing the next fall as "being more careful the next time," but remember that such a solution is partial at best and that you, as a health care professional, have more to offer.

We define a fall as "an event whereby an individual unexpectedly comes to rest on the ground or another lower level without known loss of consciousness." About one-third of community-dwelling individuals age 65 and older fall at least once during the year,[1] and about 5% to 10% of these falls result in major injuries.[2] One of the most devastating forms of major injury resulting from a fall is a hip fracture, from which older people may never fully regain function. Other serious injuries include head trauma, internal bleeding, and other types of fractures. Another serious complication of a fall is post-fall restriction of activity, from fear of falling or injury, with its attendant further tendency toward inactivity, deconditioning, and paradoxically increasing fall risk. Because of the potential safety problems associated with recurrent falls, older people may be forced to move out of their own homes into a more structured living environment, such as a nursing home, if there are repeated falls.

GAIT AND BALANCE

Problems with gait and balance are among the strongest predictors of future falls.[1] Although gait changes predictably with normal aging, most gait problems affecting older people are not due to aging itself, but to specific diseases. Normal gait and balance involve a network of neural connections and centers. Figure 34–1 shows a diagram of the normal gait cycle, which can be divided into two phases: swing phase (when the particular limb is above the ground) and stance phase (when the limb is in contact with the ground). As either limb progresses through the gait cycle at a slow pace, about 40% of time is spent in swing phase, with the remaining 60% in stance phase. "Single support" refers to the phases of the gait cycle where only one limb is in contact with the ground, while "double support" refers to the period of time where both limbs are in contact with the ground.

Normal gait and balance depend on joints being able to move freely, muscles contracting at the appropriate time and with the appropriate intensity, and normal sensory input from the nervous system.[3,4] Aging can lead to several physical changes that affect these basic processes: (1) stiffening of

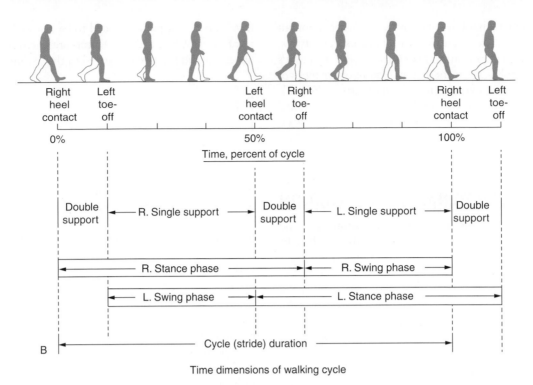

FIGURE 34–1. The gait cycle. (*Reprinted with permission, from a chapter by V. T. Inman et al., which appeared on page 26 of Human Walking, published by Williams & Wilkins, Baltimore, MD; 1981.*)

connective tissue, (2) decreased muscle strength, (3) prolonged reaction times, (4) decreased visual acuity and depth perception, (5) impaired vibratory and proprioceptive sensation, and (6) increased postural sway. In general, aging introduces a modest (20%) slowing in average walking speed. Walking speed depends on stride length (the sum of the left and right step lengths) and cadence (steps per unit time). Stride length averages 1.5 m in a normal younger person. Older adults have shorter stride lengths and compensate somewhat by increasing cadence. The decreased stride length most likely reflects instability or muscle weakness during single-limb support of the opposite leg.

In addition to changes of aging that affect gait in many, often subtle ways, many specific disease processes lead to specific gait problems. Pathologic gait, whatever the cause, generally is due to one or more of the following problems: (1) pain, (2) joint limitation, (3) muscle weakness, (4) spasticity or rigidity, (5) sensory and balance deficits, and (6) impaired central integration or processing.

● ASKING ABOUT FALLS

Older people may be reluctant to report falls to their health care providers. Older adults may connect falls with the stigma of disability, or may fear what a fall portends for their future. Or they may be concerned about their health care provider initiating a costly or time-consuming evaluation as a consequence of his or her report. Accordingly, clinical guidelines recommend that older people be asked annually about a history of falls in the previous year,[5] rather than waiting for patients to report falls. If there is no history of falls in the past year, it is also reasonable to ask a follow-up question about the presences of any walking or balance problems, since these are among the strongest risk factors for future falls.[1]

● EXERCISE AND ITS ROLE IN FALL PREVENTION

Even though Ms. R. did not report a fall to you, she is at risk for future falls because of her self-reported balance problem and specific risk factors noted on your subsequent examination. Essential components of a plan to reduce Ms. R.'s risk of future falls include exercise and reduction of risk factors found on multifactorial assessment, which includes a medical risk factor evaluation and assessment of the home for hazards.

The mainstay of fall prevention for all older adults, regardless of fall risk, should be exercise, which has been shown in a systematic review of randomized trials to reduce subsequent falls.[6] In this review, exercise reduced the fall rate by 17% on a relative basis. As an example, this means that for a person whose previous fall rate was 1 fall per year, exercise would reduce the projected number of falls for the following year to 0.83 per year. This systematic review also showed that exercises that challenge balance may be more effective at preventing falls. Such balance exercises include programs that ask older adults to practice standing on one leg or with their legs closer together, encourage them to minimize use of their hands to assist in the exercise, and practice controlled movements of their center of mass.[6] Also, a higher dose of exercise over the duration of the program (total of at least 50 hours, eg, twice weekly for 25 weeks) is likely to lead to a greater reduction in falls. These data are helpful in informing your patients about what kind of exercise to engage in for fall prevention, if they are open to a variety of exercise types. However, it is also important to take into account a patient's other medical problems, as these may require other types of exercise (eg, aerobic exercise for coronary artery disease). Most importantly, clinicians need to account for patients' preferences for different types of exercise (eg, individual vs. group), since any exercise program requires patients' willingness to participate.

● THE MULTIFACTORIAL FALL EVALUATION

In addition to exercise, patients with a demonstrated gait and balance problem, or those with a history of falls, may benefit from a multifactorial fall evaluation, with tailored interventions based on the evaluation.[1] The most recent data suggest that multifactorial interventions can reduce the number of people who fall by 10% to 20% on a relative basis,[7-9] and the rate of falls by 30% to 40% on a relative basis,[7] depending on the intensity of interventions used and the patient populations studied.

We base our recommended multifactorial fall evaluation on seven risk factors commonly addressed in a systematic review of randomized fall prevention studies (Table 34–1).[7] Different health care professionals conduct the multifactorial fall evaluation in somewhat different ways, but the principles should be the same. The evaluation starts with an understanding that falls are caused by a confluence of interacting risk

factors, and that patients need to be assessed for all of these risk factors. Whichever risk factors are uncovered in the evaluation should then be mitigated to the extent possible.

Falls History

Prior to beginning this evaluation, however, it is important to obtain a falls history and a history regarding gait or balance problems. In the case of Ms. R., we already know that she has not fallen in the past year but does have balance problems. However, if we did not know these facts already, we would want to ask her about gait, balance, and history of falls. If Ms. R. had fallen, we would want to ask her some basic questions about the fall. In addition, if Ms. R.'s fall was witnessed by someone else, we would want to obtain collateral information from the witness. Table 34–2 contains examples of questions that can be asked when taking a falls history, which can be very important in determining whether further medical evaluation is needed beyond the basic multifactorial evaluation. For example, finding out that the patient became light-headed or lost consciousness prior to the fall might suggest that workup for syncope or near-syncope is indicated. Assuming that the history does not point toward an underlying acute illness as the dominant cause for the fall, it is reasonable to proceed to the multifactorial fall evaluation.

Gait, Balance, and Strength Evaluation

The multifactorial fall evaluation begins with an assessment of gait, balance, and strength. Problems with gait, balance, and strength may be due to a variety of chronic illnesses such as osteoarthritis, Parkinson disease, peripheral neuropathy, or sequelae from a stroke. Or these problems may be due to

● TABLE 34–1	Important Risk Factors for Falls with Assessment and Treatment Options	
Risk Factor	Assessment	Treatment
Gait or balance problems	Gait and balance examination	Physical therapy Exercise program Assistive device
Medications	Medication review	Discontinue or decrease dose of relevant medications
Visual impairment	Eye exam	Cataract surgery Correction of refractive error
Orthostatic hypotension	Orthostatic vital signs	Discontinue or decrease dose of relevant medications Intervene to treat orthostatic hypotension (eg, volume expansion, compression stockings, medications)
Cognitive impairment	Mental status examination and dementia evaluation	Treat underlying disorder Supervise patient
Functional impairment	Review basic and instrumental activities of daily living	Occupational therapy Equipment to support activities of daily living
Home hazards	Home safety evaluation	Remove hazards Add safety equipment (eg, grab bars)

● TABLE 34–2	Basic Elements of a Falls History
Element	Areas to Cover in History-Taking
Circumstances	*How, where, and when did the fall occur?* *Why do you think you fell?* *What were you doing when you fell?* *Were you having any symptoms (eg, lightheadedness, dizziness) when you fell?* *Did something around you cause you to fall?* *Have there been any recent changes in your health?* *Have there been any recent changes to your medication?*
Chronic medical conditions	*Determine all of the patient's chronic medical conditions*
Medications	*Determine all of the medications that the patient is taking, whether prescribed or not*
Mobility	*Identify the patient's level of mobility* Ambulatory without assistance Ambulatory with assistive device (eg, cane, walker) Uses wheelchair Remains in bed

sarcopenia or frailty syndrome associated with advanced age (for more on frailty, see Chapter 36). The focus of the gait, balance, and strength exam is initially not on the cause of the gait, balance, or strength problem—these should be worked up in accordance with your diagnostic hypotheses. Rather, the exam focuses on simply identifying the presence of a gait, balance, or strength problem that may put a patient at risk for falls.

Gait

Gait can be examined relatively easily by watching the patient walk. This can be done in a variety of ways, using formal methods such as the Tinetti's Performance-Oriented Mobility Assessment to score a patient's gait and balance,[10] or just by making an initial judgment as to whether the gait looks normal or abnormal, something you can practice by simply watching people walk. While watching a patient walk, view him or her from the side and from the back. While viewing the side, note the type of initial contact (heel strike, foot-flat, or forefoot contact). Observe the knee during limb loading (ie, as the patient begins to bear weight on the limb during walking); for example, does the patient have excessive or absent knee flexion? Note single limb stance. The hip and knee should be neutral (neither flexed nor extended) with the ankle moving into slight dorsiflexion, as body weight progresses over the stance limb. Observe for normal heel-off during terminal stance. Normally, the heel should leave the ground before the opposite limb makes contact. In addition, watch for deviations at the trunk and pelvis, which may indicate proximal muscle weakness. Determine how the patient is propelling the limb forward during swing phase. Is the patient achieving the normal motion required during swing phase to clear the floor with the limb? From the front or rear, note lateral trunk and limb deviations. Watching for asymmetries and comparing the right and left gait will lead to the recognition of major gait deviations.

With practice, you will learn to identify specific abnormalities of gait through direct observation, such as path deviation (not walking in a straight line), width of gait (how far the feet are apart from one another as the patient walks), positioning of the feet and knees, gait asymmetry, degree to which feet clear the floor, and gait speed. If you do identify an abnormal gait and the patient's history of falls suggests that the problem was related to the abnormality you uncovered, you may want to refer the patient to a health care professional such as a physiatrist or physical therapist for further evaluation.

Balance

There are a variety of ways to examine a patient for balance problems. A simple one is the Romberg test, in which you first ask the patient to stand with feet together and eyes open, and check whether the patient can maintain balance. If the patient can maintain balance, you ask the patient to close the eyes for up to 1 minute. This test is designed to elicit whether the patient's sensory inputs to balance are intact. Making the patient close the eyes challenges balance, because it forces the patient to rely on other sensory inputs to balance besides vision, including the proprioceptive and vestibular systems.

You can also test a patient's balance using the sternal nudge, in which you ask the patient to stand (with open eyes), warning the patient that you will be pushing on his or her breastbone to test balance. When you do this, you want to push firmly, but not overwhelmingly, on the sternum. Patients should be instructed that it is all right to take a step backward if needed. Normally, in response to the sternal nudge, patients will not move, or take one step backward. However, they should not continue walking backward, nor should they lose their balance. Naturally, you should also be prepared to catch the patient when you do this test or the Romberg test. Also note that neither test is necessary in situations where the patient is obviously unsteady on direct observation of gait.

Patients with gait and balance problems may benefit from an assistive device, such as a cane or walker, to provide extra support. The simplest approach is to watch patients walk both with and without a cane (or walker, if appropriate) and see if their gait improves or their subjective sense of steadiness improves. Patients can then be referred to a health care professional with expertise in assistive devices for teaching on proper fitting and use. For more details on assistive devices, see Chapter 26.

Strength

Patients should also be examined for their strength, particularly in the lower extremities, which are critical to maintaining balance.[11] Quadriceps strength can be easily assessed by asking patients to arise from an armless chair without using their own arms. There are a range of possible responses ranging from normal (patients can arise from the chair without difficulty) to intermediate (patients require multiple attempts to arise from the chair, but ultimately succeed) to abnormal (patients cannot arise from a chair without using their arms for assistance). Patients who have weakness in the quadriceps muscles may benefit from further assessment from a qualified professional of other lower-extremity muscles, with strength training as needed.

Medication Review

Medication review is a critically important part of the multifactorial fall evaluation. Physicians and allied health care professionals who prescribe medications have a special responsibility to ensure that these medications are not harming the patient. Both the total number of medications and certain high-risk medications (typically those that are active in the central nervous system) have been implicated in falls.[12,13] As the total number of medications increases, the number of possible drug–drug interactions increases exponentially. Since most drugs have not been studied in patients on multiple other medications, the exact consequences of polypharmacy may remain unknown. Most importantly, each drug on the patient's medication list should be reviewed for its risk–benefit profile (see Chapter 13 for details). High-risk medications, particularly sedative/hypnotic drugs (eg, benzodiazepines), antidepressants (both tricyclic and newer antidepressants), and antipsychotic medications, should have a clear justification for use. These medications may affect cognitive function, cloud patients' sensorium, or cause orthostatic hypotension. Tapering high-risk medications has been shown to reduce falls in one randomized trial,[6] although many patients whose medications were tapered resumed these medications after they were discontinued.

Assessment of Vision

Visual acuity should be checked as part of a multifactorial fall evaluation, since inability to see hazards may be implicated in a fall. Alternatively, if the patient has had an eye examination in the past year by an eye care professional, it may not be necessary to check visual acuity, unless the patient has new visual complaints. Finding a visual acuity problem warrants referral to an eye care professional, since some interventions (such as first-eye cataract surgery) may reduce falls.[7] For more details on visual problems and checking visual acuity, see Chapter 8.

Orthostatic Vital Signs

Orthostatic hypotension could potentially lead patients to fall because of light-headedness or loss of consciousness.[14] Thus, orthostatic vital signs should be checked in patients with a history of falls. Orthostatic hypotension has been defined as a drop in systolic blood pressure of 20 mm Hg or diastolic blood pressure of 10 mm Hg within 3 minutes of standing.[8] Orthostatic vital signs can be performed in a variety of ways; if patients can lie supine and stand, then supine and standing measurements should be performed in preference to supine/sitting or sitting/standing. Most importantly, patients should wait at least 2 minutes supine prior to measuring supine vital signs, and wait for at least 1 minute standing prior to measuring standing vital signs,[9] to allow time for the normal physiologic adjustment to a new position. Pulse should also be measured, because if the patient has a ≥ 20 beat per minute pulse rise from supine to standing, this is suggestive of hypovolemia, in which the body is appropriately attempting to maintain blood pressure by increasing cardiac output. In contrast, in neurogenic orthostatic hypotension (eg, from diabetes or Parkinson disease), patients cannot mount an adequate response to an orthostatic challenge[14]; accordingly, the pulse is not expected to change markedly. Of note, if the patient complains of dizziness, light-headedness, or unsteadiness while standing, it is probably better for the patient's safety to abort this test; most people would consider these symptoms to be a sign of likely orthostasis and impending syncope.

If a patient is found to be orthostatic, acute causes such as hypovolemia should be ruled out first. Then, medications should be carefully reviewed. The list of medicines potentially causing orthostatic hypotension is long, and includes antihypertensives, alpha-blocker medications commonly used for benign prostatic hyperplasia, antipsychotic medications, and antidepressants. If a risky medication is identified, the risk–benefit ratio should be reviewed in the context of the degree of orthostatic hypotension. Sometimes, no obvious medication-related cause will be found for orthostasis. In this case, chronic illnesses that can cause orthostatic hypotension should be considered.[14]

Cognitive Assessment

Cognitive impairment may be a considerable risk factor for falls. Patients with cognitive impairment often have poor insight, judgment, memory of hazards, or awareness of their surroundings and may also have visuospatial disturbances.[15] Cognitive impairment can be screened for easily with the Mini-Cog (a 3-item recall test together with a clock-drawing test).[10] If cognitive impairment is detected, reversible causes should be ruled out. For more details on cognitive impairment, see Chapter 31. Barring reversible causes, the most important fall prevention intervention for cognitively impaired patients is adequate supervision. The degree of supervision will depend greatly on the patient's willingness to accept help and upon economic, social, and cultural factors.

Functional Status Assessment

The multifactorial fall evaluation also includes a functional status assessment. Knowing patients' functional limitations will determine whether there is a mismatch between their expectations of what they can do, and their actual capabilities. A fall can occur when a patient believes he or she is capable of a task, but in fact is not. Thus, collateral information on the patient's actual capabilities is key. For example, a patient may claim to be able to bathe herself, but a family member may indicate that the patient actually is not coordinated enough to do so. Functional status assessment includes basic activities of daily living, such as bathing, dressing, toileting, transferring (eg, from bed to chair), and continence. It also includes a review of instrumental activities of daily living, such as food preparation, housework, and gardening. Detection of functional impairment that is potentially remediable should prompt a referral to an occupational therapist or similarly qualified health care professional, who will evaluate the patient for the need for equipment in the home (such as grab bars in the shower or near the toilet, a shower chair, or a bedside commode). For more details on how to perform a functional status assessment, see Chapter 7.

Home Hazard Assessment

The final recommended aspect of the basic multifactorial fall evaluation is an assessment of hazards in the patient's home, since many patients who are prone to falling spend a majority of time at home, and most falls occur in the home.[16] For cognitively intact patients, a home safety checklist may be adequate (see Figure 34–2 for an example). The checklist suggests removing obstacles, improving lighting, making it easier to reach commonly used items, and modifying the home to improve safety (eg, installing grab bars in the bathroom). A complement to the home safety checklist is a home safety evaluation, which can be performed by a health care professional such as a physical therapist, occupational therapist, visiting nurse, or social worker. This individual can help the patient identify home hazards as well as devise a plan to mitigate these hazards.

Check for Safety: A Home Fall Prevention Checklist for Older Adults

FALLS AT HOME

Each year, thousands of older Americans fall at home. Many of them are seriously injured, and some are disabled. In 2002, more than 12,800 people over age 65 died and 1.6 million were treated in emergency departments because of falls.

Falls are often due to hazards that are easy to overlook but easy to fix. This checklist will help you find and fix those hazards in your home.

The checklist asks about hazards found in each room of your home. For each hazard, the checklist tells you how to fix the problem. At the end of the checklist, you'll find other tips for preventing falls.

FLOORS: Look at the floor in each room.

Q: When you walk through a room, do you have to walk around furniture?
Ask someone to move the furniture so your path is clear.

Q: Do you have throw rugs on the floor?
Remove the rugs or use double-sided tape or a non-slip backing so the rugs won't slip.

Q: Are there papers, books, towels, shoes, magazines, boxes, blankets, or other objects on the floor?
Pick up things that are on the floor. Always keep objects off the floor.

Q: Do you have to walk over or around wires or cords (like lamp, telephone, or extension cords)?
Coil or tape cords and wires next to the wall so you can't trip over them. If needed, have an electrician put in another outlet.

STAIRS AND STEPS: Look at the stairs you use both inside and outside your home.

Q: Are there papers, shoes, books, or other objects on the stairs?
Pick up things on the stairs. Always keep objects off stairs.

Q: Are some steps broken or uneven?
Fix loose or uneven steps.

Q: Are you missing a light over the stairway?
Have an electrician put in an overhead light at the top and bottom of the stairs.

Q: Do you have only one light switch for your stairs (only at the top or at the bottom of the stairs)?
Have an electrician put in a light switch at the top and bottom of the stairs. You can get light switches that glow.

Q: Has the stairway light bulb burned out?
Have a friend or family member change the light bulb.

Q: Is the carpet on the steps loose or torn?
Make sure the carpet is firmly attached to every step, or remove the carpet and attach non-slip rubber treads to the stairs.

Q: Are the handrails loose or broken? Is there a handrail on only one side of the stairs?
Fix loose handrails or put in new ones. Make sure handrails are on both sides of the stairs and are as long as the stairs.

KITCHEN: Look at your kitchen and eating area.

Q: Are the things you use often on high shelves?
Move items in your cabinets. Keep things you use often on the lower shelves (about waist level).

Q: Is your step stool unsteady?
If you must use a step stool, get one with a bar to hold onto. Never use a chair as a step stool.

BATHROOMS: Look at all your bathrooms.

Q: Is the tub or shower floor slippery?
Put a non-slip rubber mat or self-stick strips on the floor of the tub or shower.

Q: Do you need some support when you get in and out of the tub or up from the toilet?
Have a carpenter put grab bars inside the tub and next to the toilet.

BEDROOMS: Look at all your bedrooms.

Q: Is the light near the bed hard to reach?
Place a lamp close to the bed where it's easy to reach.

Q: Is the path from your bed to the bathroom dark?
Put in a night-light so you can see where you're walking. Some night-lights go on by themselves after dark.

Other Things You Can Do to Prevent Falls

Exercise regularly. Exercise makes you stronger and improves your balance and coordination.

Have your doctor or pharmacist look at all the medicines you take, even over-the-counter medicines. Some medicines can make you sleepy or dizzy.

Have your vision checked at least once a year by an eye doctor. Poor vision can increase your risk of falling.

Get up slowly after you sit or lie down.

Wear shoes both inside and outside the house. Avoid going barefoot or wearing slippers.

Improve the lighting in your home. Put in brighter light bulbs. Florescent bulbs are bright and cost less to use.

It's safest to have uniform lighting in a room. Add lighting to dark areas. Hang lightweight curtains or shades to reduce glare.

Paint a contrasting color on the top edge of all steps so you can see the stairs better. For example, use a light color paint on dark wood.

Other Safety Tips

Keep emergency numbers in large print near each phone.

Put a phone near the floor in case you fall and can't get up.

Think about wearing an alarm device that will bring help in case you fall and can't get up.

FIGURE 34–2. Home safety checklist from the US Centers for Disease Control and Prevention.

Three years later, Ms. R. developed shortness of breath and fever. She was taken to the Emergency Department where a chest film revealed pneumonia with pleural effusion. Further workup showed that the pleural effusion was loculated, and Ms. R. underwent chest tube placement to drain what was found to be an empyema. She was started on around-the-clock morphine for pain control, given the discomfort associated with the chest tube. Four days after admission, Ms. R. requested a sleeping pill to overcome her insomnia; she was treated with a benzodiazepine. Later that night, she got up from her bed alone to go to the bathroom and fell to the floor. No injuries were reported from her fall.

FALLS IN THE HOSPITALIZED PATIENT

Falls in the acute-care hospital are a serious concern, because they occur in environments where, at least in theory, falls might be preventable with adequate supervision of patients. However, hospitals are subject to resource constraints that make intense staffing unavailable except for the most critically ill patients. Even in intensely staffed environments, human factors such as fatigue and distraction make a goal of zero falls unrealistic.

The best approach to preventing falls in health care institutions is not as clear as it is in community-dwelling elders.[17] In hospitals, where patients are admitted and discharged within a matter of days, there is often inadequate time to intervene on some of the risk factors that are often targeted in the community. Thus, programs to prevent falls in hospitals target multiple areas for improvement: patient risks, the physical environment, and staff behavior. Many hospitals (as well as nursing homes) find it helpful to complete a fall risk assessment and fall prevention plan for all patients who are admitted. If a fall should occur, this assessment and plan are updated to take into account causes of the fall.

In Ms. R.'s case, some contributing risks to her fall might have been avoided. Nonpharmacologic measures focused on insomnia might have been tried prior to starting a benzodiazepine.[18] Also, the morphine Ms. R. was taking for pain control might have been administered on an as-needed, rather than around-the-clock basis, if her pain was under adequate control. More frequent nighttime nurse visits, a prompted toileting program, or a bedside commode might also have prevented Ms. R.'s fall.

If a patient does fall in the hospital (or in another setting), the question of what workup is needed arises. If the fall was witnessed, talking to the witness regarding the circumstances of the fall is appropriate (Table 34-2). If the patient is able to provide history, this can be helpful as well in guiding appropriate treatment. On examining the patient, clinicians should focus on whether the patient has any pain, and if so, where the pain is located. Also, the patient should be inspected for abrasions, lacerations, or bleeding. Pain in a particular location should lead to a more focused assessment of the area. If the patient is ambulatory, making sure the patient can walk and bear weight on both extremities is important in assessing for a potential hip fracture. Imaging should be guided by physical findings on examination. If the patient is at higher risk for bleeding due to anticoagulant medications, there should be a lower threshold for imaging studies and neurologic monitoring (if the patient might have hit her head), and for monitoring of hemoglobin/hematocrit.

After a 10-day stay in the hospital Ms. R. was discharged to her own home with physical and occupational therapy home visits set up, and her daughter agreed to stay with her until she recovered more fully. Ms. R. is now here to see you for a follow-up visit 2 weeks after hospital discharge. She arrives at your office in a wheelchair. In the exam room, Ms. R.'s daughter reports that Ms. R. was improving during the immediate post hospital period. However, yesterday she sustained a fall when she was getting out of the bathtub; her legs got caught in the edge of the bathmat on the floor. She had no obvious bruises, no head trauma, and no loss of consciousness, but she has been complaining of pain over her left hip since then and has been unable to walk without assistance.

Ms. R. has now had two falls within a several-week period. This most recent fall is concerning for hip fracture, given her inability to walk. (See Chapter 40 for more details on hip fractures.) You evaluate Ms. R. for the Heuter sign by tapping on her pubic symphysis while listening to each patella with your stethoscope, and each side produces a bright, clear tapping sound (see Chapter 6). You then send Ms. R. for an imaging study, and as it turns out there is no evidence of a fracture. You prescribe pain medication for Ms. R. and in the next few days, her ambulation improves. Besides removing the bathmat and making sure the home physical therapy and occupational therapy recommendations (eg, grab bars) are implemented, you wonder what else you can do for Ms. R. given that you've already completed a multifactorial fall assessment on her.

STRATEGIES TO MINIMIZE INJURIES

Patients like Ms. R., who are at high fall risk, may benefit from injury minimization measures in addition to fall prevention strategies. The most important injury minimization measure is to screen and treat appropriate patients for osteoporosis (see Chapter 41 for details), which can reduce the risk of subsequent fractures. Other strategies include hip protectors. Hip protectors are special undergarments that are designed to dissipate the impact of a fall on the hips. Unfortunately, recent studies suggest that hip protectors may not be effective in community-dwelling elders because many patients find hip protectors unpleasant to wear, and adherence can be low.[19] Hip protectors may be more effective in nursing home patients.[19] Also, not all marketed hip protectors provide adequate coverage of the greater trochanter area, which is important to reduce the impact of a fall on the femoral neck.[20]

Another strategy that may prevent injuries is the use of low beds, especially in institutional care, although these measures have not been definitely proven to prevent injuries. Low beds can be helpful to the extent that if a patient falls out of bed, the impact would be less severe than in a regular bed. Unlike osteoporosis medications, which are often prescribed to relatively healthy older patients (both those who are at average or higher risk of falls), hip protectors and low beds are usually reserved for patients with very frequent falling episodes.

EMERGING APPROACHES TO FALL PREVENTION

Vitamin D, which has been used to maintain or improve bone density, possibly has a role in preventing falls and fractures.[21,22] The optimal vitamin D dose for older adults for fall prevention is not clear, but recent literature suggests that the dose should be greater than 400 IU for fracture prevention[22]; amounts such as 800 or 1000 IU orally once daily are commonly prescribed. Many aspects of our understanding of the role of vitamin D in fall prevention still need to be worked out.

Older people's footwear may affect their risk of falls.[23] However, it is not clear that recommending different kinds of footwear leads to a reduced rate of falls. One randomized trial in a snowy winter climate found that a gait-stabilizing device attached to usual footwear could reduce the rate of outdoor falls during the winter.[24]

Sensor technologies are being developed to create "smart homes" that can detect if an older person is at risk for a fall and alert people at a central location.[25] Researchers are even exploring whether rapid fall detection systems could allow the deployment of an inflatable hip protector to prevent a hip fracture in the event of a fall.[26] These technologies are still in the early stages of development and data on fall-related outcomes are not yet available.

Whole-body vibration training is being explored as a means for improving physical function and may have beneficial effects on gait, balance, mobility, and bone mineral density.[27] However, whole-body vibration may also have detrimental effects on the neurologic and vascular systems, and there are no studies to date on whether whole-body vibration training reduces the rate of falls.[27]

SOCIAL AND PSYCHOLOGICAL ASPECTS OF FALL PREVENTION

Preventing falls requires a high level of motivation, both on the patient's and the health care professional's part. For example, a patient may need to change long-established behaviors, such as overcoming a sedentary lifestyle by participating in an exercise program, removing clutter from the home to make it safer, or overcoming the perceived stigma of using a cane or walker. Similarly, health care professionals need to be highly motivated to help patients, since performing a multifactorial fall evaluation is significantly more complicated than prescribing a medicine. Data show that fall prevention programs are more likely to work when the person detecting the fall risk factor is the same person who intervenes to fix it,[9] but this is not always possible in many settings. When multiple providers are involved in performing the multifactorial fall evaluation (such as a physical therapist, a pharmacist, and a physician), the patient's primary care provider needs to coordinate and track the results of each component of the assessment and make sure to communicate recommendations for all components to the patient (see Chapter 19 for details of multiprofessional team care).

Given the complexity of fall prevention and that patients may have high levels of inertia regarding behavior change, the provider must adopt a patient but proactive approach. Recommendations should be gently reinforced at visits with the patient, regardless of whether they are implemented. Sometimes communicating recommendations to family or friends involved in the patient's care (with the patient's permission) may help. Also, framing the discussion of recommendations as helping to keep the older person independent and in good physical function may be a more acceptable message than speaking about preventing falls.[28]

In cases where patients with recurrent falls suffer from early dementia and live alone, patients may be uncooperative or decline additional supervision that might be important for their own safety. Many patients with early dementia retain decision-making capacity and cannot be forced to accept supervision against their will. However, if the patient is an immediate threat to self or to others, or lacks decision-making capacity, involving a social worker may be valuable. In some jurisdictions in the United States, health care providers are mandated reporters of elder self-neglect.

COMMUNITY-BASED STRATEGIES FOR FALL PREVENTION

In an ideal world, fall prevention would be an effort undertaken at the community level. This means that health care providers, public agencies, and local media would collaborate to increase community awareness about the importance of preventing falls, as well as undertaking concrete steps for fall prevention, such as home hazard reduction and group exercise programs.[29] Proof of principle for this approach comes from several studies undertaken in different parts of the world that have demonstrated that community-based approaches can reduce falls.[30,31] Such community-based approaches would help support health care professionals in their efforts to prevent falls. In the meantime, where such comprehensive community-based supports are not available, health care providers need to become knowledgeable about local community resources, such as exercise programs, to which they can refer patients if needed. Several good references are available.[32-34]

CONCLUSION

Falls are a preventable cause of suffering in older people. Your role as a health care professional is to recommend exercise to all people who are capable of it, screen people for fall risk on a regular basis, and perform a multifactorial fall evaluation on people who are at high risk for future falls. You can then use the results of the evaluation to determine a treatment strategy that is individualized to the needs of your patient.

References

1. Ganz DA, Bao Y, Shekelle PG, Rubenstein LZ. Will my patient fall? JAMA. 2007;297:77-86.

2. Rubenstein LZ, Josephson KR. The epidemiology of falls and syncope. Clin Geriatr Med. 2002;18:141-158.

3. Woollacott MH, Shumway-Cook A, Nashner L. Postural reflexes and aging. In: Mortimer JA, Pirozzolo FJ, Maletta GJ, eds. The Aging Motor System. New York: Praeger; 1982:98-119.

4. Perry J. Gait characteristics. In: Jackson OL, ed. Therapeutic Considerations for the Elderly. New York: Churchill Livingstone; 1987:113-123.

5. American Geriatrics Society, British Geriatrics Society Clinical Practice Guideline (online). Prevention of falls in older persons. http://www.americangeriatrics.org/health_care_professionals/clinical_practice/clinical_guidelines_recommendations/prevention_of_falls_summary_of_recommendations. Accessed July 22, 2010.

6. Sherrington C, Whitney JC, Lord SR, et al. Effective exercise for the prevention of falls: A systematic review and meta-analysis. J Am Geriatr Soc. 2008;56:2234-2243.

7. Chang JT, Morton SC, Rubenstein LZ, et al. Interventions for the prevention of falls in older adults: Systematic review and meta-analysis of randomised clinical trials. BMJ. 2004;328:680.

8. Beswick AD, Rees K, Dieppe P, et al. Complex interventions to improve physical function and maintain independent living in elderly people: A systematic review and meta-analysis. Lancet. 2008;371:725-735.

9. Gates S, Fisher JD, Cooke MW, et al. Multifactorial assessment and targeted intervention for preventing falls and injuries among older people in community and emergency care settings: Systematic review and meta-analysis. BMJ. 2008;336:130-133.

10. Tinetti ME. Performance-oriented assessment of mobility problems in elderly patients. J Am Geriatr Soc. 1986;34:119-126.

11. Wolfson L, Judge J, Whipple R, King M. Strength is a major factor in balance, gait, and the occurrence of falls. J Gerontol A Biol Sci Med Sci. 1995;50:64-67.

12. Campbell AJ, Borrie MJ, Spears GF. Risk factors for falls in a community-based prospective study of people 70 years and older. J Gerontol. 1989;44:M112-M117.

13. Weiner DK, Hanlon JT, Studenski SA. Effects of central nervous system polypharmacy on falls liability in community-dwelling elderly. Gerontology. 1998;44:217-221.

14. Goldstein DS, Sharabi Y. Neurogenic orthostatic hypotension: A pathophysiological approach. Circulation. 2009;119:139-146.

15. Kaskie B, Storandt M. Visuospatial deficit in dementia of the Alzheimer type. Arch Neurol. 1995;52:422-425.

16. Norton R, Campbell AJ, Lee-Joe T, et al. Circumstances of falls resulting in hip fractures among older people. J Am Geriatr Soc. 1997;45:1108-1112.

17. Oliver D, Connelly JB, Victor CR, et al. Strategies to prevent falls and fractures in hospitals and care homes and effect of cognitive impairment: Systematic review and meta-analyses. BMJ. 2007;334:82.

18. Flaherty JH. Insomnia among hospitalized older persons. Clin Geriatr Med. 2008;24:51-67, vi.

19. Parker MJ, Gillespie WJ, Gillespie LD. Effectiveness of hip protectors for preventing hip fractures in elderly people: Systematic review. BMJ. 2006;332:571-574.

20. Minns RJ, Marsh AM, Chuck A, Todd J. Are hip protectors correctly positioned in use? Age Ageing. 2007;36:140-144.

21. Cranney A, Horsley T, O'Donnell S, et al. Effectiveness and safety of vitamin D in relation to bone health. Evid Rep Technol Assess (Full Rep). 2007;158:1-235.

22. Bischoff-Ferrari HA, Willett WC, Wong JB, et al. Prevention of nonvertebral fractures with oral vitamin D and dose dependency: A meta-analysis of randomized controlled trials. Arch Intern Med. 2009;169:551-561.

23. Koepsell TD, Wolf ME, Buchner DM, et al. Footwear style and risk of falls in older adults. J Am Geriatr Soc. 2004;52:1495-1501.

24. McKiernan FE. A simple gait-stabilizing device reduces outdoor falls and nonserious injurious falls in fall-prone older people during the winter. J Am Geriatr Soc. 2005;53:943-947.

25. Cheek P, Nikpour L, Nowlin HD. Aging well with smart technology. Nurs Adm Q. 2005;29:329-338.

26. Nyan MN, Tay FE, Murugasu E. A wearable system for pre-impact fall detection. J Biomech. 2008;41:3475-3481.

27. Brooke-Wavell K, Mansfield NJ. Risks and benefits of whole body vibration training in older people. Age Ageing. 2009;38:254-255.

28. Hughes K, van Beurden E, Eakin EG, et al. Older persons' perception of risk of falling: Implications for fall-prevention campaigns. Am J Public Health. 2008;98:351-357.

29. Ganz DA, Alkema GE, Wu S. It takes a village to prevent falls: Reconceptualizing fall prevention and management for older adults. Inj Prev. 2008;14:266-271.

30. McClure R, Turner C, Peel N, et al. Population-based interventions for the prevention of fall-related injuries in older people. Cochrane Database Syst Rev. 2005;1:CD004441.

31. Tinetti ME, Baker DI, King M, et al. Effect of dissemination of evidence in reducing injuries from falls. N Engl J Med. 2008;359:252-261.

32. Stevens JA, Sogolow ED. Preventing Falls: What Works. A CDC Compendium of Effective Community-Based Interventions from Around the World. Atlanta: Centers for Disease Control and Prevention, National Center for Injury Prevention and Control; 2008.

33. National Center for Injury Prevention and Control. Preventing Falls: How to Develop Community-Based Fall Prevention Programs for Older Adults. Atlanta: Centers for Disease Control and Prevention; 2008.

34. Fall Prevention Center of Excellence. http://www.stopfalls.org. Accessed June 25, 2009.

POST-TEST

1. **Which of the following medication classes has been most consistently associated with a risk of future falls in epidemiologic studies?**
   A. Benzodiazepines (eg, diazepam)
   B. Proton pump inhibitors (eg, omeprazole)
   C. Beta2-agonists (eg, albuterol)
   D. 5-alpha-reductase inhibitors (eg, finasteride)

2. **Which of the following is TRUE about assessing orthostatic vital signs?**
   A. Measuring supine and sitting blood pressure and pulse is equivalent to measuring supine and standing blood pressure and pulse.
   B. Standing blood pressure and pulse should be assessed within 1 minute of the patient standing.
   C. Consensus recommendations define orthostatic hypotension as a drop of 20 mm Hg in systolic blood pressure, or a drop of 10 mm Hg in diastolic blood pressure.
   D. All patients who report dizziness when asked to stand up for standing blood pressure and pulse should be asked to continue standing as long as they can so that orthostatic vital signs can be completed accurately.

3. **Which of the following is NOT true about multifactorial fall risk assessment and intervention?**
   A. Multifactorial fall risk assessment takes a standard approach to assessing a patient's risk factors for falls, but interventions for a patient's risk factors are individually tailored to that patient's needs.
   B. In community-dwelling older people, multifactorial fall risk assessment and intervention have been shown to reduce falls in randomized trials.
   C. Multifactorial fall risk assessment and intervention are currently recommended for all older adults.
   D. Assessing older adults' cognition is part of the multifactorial fall risk assessment.

ANSWERS TO PRE-TEST

1. B
2. A
3. B

ANSWERS TO POST-TEST

1. A
2. C
3. C

35

Weight Loss

Alexandra E. Leigh, MD

Christine S. Ritchie, MD, MSPH

● **LEARNING OBJECTIVES**

1. Define and describe unintentional weight loss and malnutrition.
2. Describe the causes associated with unintentional weight loss and undernutrition in the older adult.
3. Compare and contrast screening tools used for weight loss and nutritional status.
4. Discuss the processes associated with weight loss.
5. Describe management options for unintentional weight loss and undernutrition, including dietary options, environmental changes, physical activity, and appetite stimulants.
6. Discuss the issue of obesity in older adults.
7. Describe management strategies for weight reduction in older adults.
8. Discuss the special issues associated with end-of-life nutrition, including artificial nutrition.

PRE-TEST

1. Mr. V. is a 71-year-old retired schoolteacher with rheumatoid arthritis who has had a 7-pound unintentional weight loss since his last visit to your office 3 months ago. He has no new complaints today and a review of systems is negative. His body mass index (BMI) is currently 28. What type of assessment, if any, does Mr. V. need?

   A. None. As his review of systems is negative, there is no cause for concern.
   B. Administer a nutritional screening tool to further elicit the cause of weight loss.
   C. Follow-up with a repeat weight in 6 months to see if his weight loss is a trend.
   D. Congratulate Mr. V. on his weight loss, as his BMI has improved.

2. Mrs. A. is a 69-year-old homemaker with advanced non–small-cell lung cancer on chemotherapy. Despite well-controlled nausea, she has had ongoing weight loss. Calorie intake on assessment has been relatively stable. What is the MOST likely cause of her new weight loss?

   A. Poor caloric intake
   B. Chemotherapy-induced nausea
   C. Deconditioning due to limited mobility
   D. Cachexia from lung cancer

3. Mr. T. is a 90-year-old nursing home resident with congestive heart failure and hypertension. He recently has begun losing weight, and a Mini-Nutritional-Assessment shows he is at risk of malnutrition. His heart failure and hypertension remain wellcontrolled though he complains of a tooth ache. Which of the following is TRUE regarding oral health and weight loss in older adults?

A. Older patients are at low risk for oral health problems.

B. Older patients without teeth actually consume more calories than those with maintained dentition.

C. Poor oral health is a risk factor for undernutrition in older patients.

D. Dentures have been shown to reverse weight loss in older patients with oral pain.

CASE PRESENTATION 1: UNINTENTIONAL WEIGHT LOSS

Mr. P. is an 82-year-old retired piano teacher with a medical history of hypertension, atrial fibrillation, benign prostatic hypertrophy, and remote tobacco use who presents to clinic for his semiannual check-up. He has no new complaints and states he is "doing fine." On review of his vital signs you note that his weight, on your office scale, has fallen 12 lbs (5.5 kg) since his last visit 6 months ago. Medications, which have not been changed for 24 months, are warfarin, metoprolol, hydrochlorothiazide, and finasteride. Review of systems is negative for fevers, night sweats, cough, abdominal pain, or change in bowel habits. He states that he has not been trying to lose weight, nor has he noticed the weight loss.

Generally, he appears well-groomed, thin, and in no distress. His blood pressure is 138/82, heart rate is 62, and respirations are 16 and unlabored. His height is 5'11" (180.3 cm), his current weight is 165 lbs (75 kg), and his body mass index (BMI) is 23. His conversation and thought are directed though he seems preoccupied and avoids direct eye contact. His examination is remarkable for well-fitting upper dentures, poor dentition inferiorly, an irregularly irregular heartbeat, and trace pedal edema. You are troubled about Mr. P.'s weight loss but feel reassured by his still "normal" BMI.

● WEIGHT LOSS IN OLDER ADULTS

Weight loss in older persons is common. Unintentional weight loss may be a sign of a new condition, such as malignancy or depression. Yet usually, as with most geriatric syndromes, it is a multifaceted issue with health, social, and behavioral features. Even after adjustment for baseline health status, weight loss is independently associated with increased morbidity and mortality, especially in older adults. Because weight loss in older adults can have many components, consideration of weight loss etiologies and subsequent interventions must likewise be multidimensional.

Large epidemiologic studies that have followed individuals for many years show that, on average, adults tend to gain weight in their 40s and 50s and tend to lose weight from 65 onward. This weight loss in part may be due to decreased intake from early satiety in advanced age or from underlying processes that are less benign. Weight loss of as little as 5% over 3 years in community-dwelling geriatric patients is an independent predictor of mortality, regardless of patients' starting weight.[1]

Weight loss can be a component of the so-called "frailty syndrome." Frailty in older persons (see Chapter 36) is a progressive, multisystem impairment and decreased physiologic reserve resulting in a state of increased vulnerability. Frailty is due in part to the physiologic changes of normal aging as well as chronic disease processes and social and emotional factors. The frailty cycle begins with the accumulation of multiple factors associated with aging, which can include poor nutrition, weight loss, and little physical exercise. It leads to a loss of functional abilities, independence, and increased mortality. However, frailty is not inevitable. The ability to stop the trend toward frailty, by intervening in these processes, may allow us to avoid frailty. This is one of the goals in avoiding and reversing weight loss in older persons.[2]

Malnutrition is a general term that can include any state with improper diet or nutrition including undernutrition, overnutrition, or micronutrient deficiencies. For the purposes of this chapter, malnutrition will be considered as undernutrition, a nutritional deficiency of calories or an inability to properly utilize those calories. The prevalence of undernutrition in community-dwelling elders is 2% with those at risk compromising nearly one-quarter of this population. In hospitalized and institutionalized older adults the prevalence is much greater, at 23% in hospitals and 21% in institutions such as nursing homes. Forty-six percent of older adults who are hospitalized are at risk for undernutrition, and 51% are at risk among those in nursing homes.[3] Though weight loss does not always accompany undernutrition, an assessment of weight loss nearly always considers the risk of undernutrition.

● SCREENING FOR WEIGHT LOSS

Nutritional assessment and screening for weight loss and malnutrition should be a component of health care maintenance for all geriatric patients. For the community-dwelling elder, measurement of weight should be done at every clinic visit. Long-term care facilities in the United States are required by law to conduct periodic weight assessments of all patients. What measure of loss constitutes clinically important weight loss in the elder is not entirely clear. A loss of as little as 4% of one's previous weight in 1 year increases subsequent 2-year mortality. The annual incidence of this amount of weight loss in outpatient veterans is 13%.[4] The federally mandated Minimum Data Set (MDS) for patients in long-term care facilities defines significant weight loss as ≥ 5% in 30 days or ≥ 10% in 180 days. Certainly, as weight loss is a marker of frailty and a predictor of mortality, even minimal weight loss should prompt concern for the provider, even if the patient is obese or overweight to start.

A number of screening and assessment tools designed to identify older patients at risk for weight loss and malnutrition are available and easy to use in clinical settings. These are valuable both before weight loss has occurred and to recognize those patients at risk. The choice of which tool to use hinges on the clinical setting, the ability to take measurements of the patient, and the ability of the patient to answer questions. Currently there is no single "gold-standard" reference to assess nutritional status.

The Mini Nutritional Assessment (MNA) is a two-part nutrition screening and assessment tool designed for patients age 65 and above to identify those who are malnourished or those at risk of malnourishment (Figure 35–1). The MNA-short form (MNA-SF) is a six-item screening component to ascertain if the entire MNA needs to be completed. The full MNA assesses nutritional status based on anthropomorphic measurements, diet, functional status, lifestyle, and a subjective assessment of health. The MNA has been validated in numerous studies.[3,5,6] Moreover, using the MNA score as a basis for intervention can stop weight loss in those at risk or in those who are already malnourished. The sensitivity and specificity of the MNA are 96% and 98%, respectively, with a positive predictive value of 97%.

The Malnutrition Universal Screening Tool (MUST) is designed to recognize those with or at risk of malnutrition in all settings, even if height and weight cannot be measured. Unlike the MNA it was developed for all adults, not just older adults. Its ease and simplicity allow it to be applied quickly to groups of hospitalized or institutionalized patients; there is no subjective component as with the MNA so the patient does not have to be able to answer questions. In British hospitalized patients over 65 (with malnutrition rates near 40%), MUST scores have shown correlations with outcomes and mortality.[7]

The Simplified Nutrition Assessment Questionnaire (SNAQ) is a screening tool for prediction of anorexia-related weight loss developed for community-dwelling adults and long-term care residents. Like the MNA-SF, it is short and requires patient cooperation to answer questions. Unlike the MNA-SF, the focus is mainly on appetite. The SNAQ has sensitivities and specificities for 5% and 10% weight losses of 81% and 76% and 88% and 84%, respectively.[8]

Of note, there is also a Dutch screening tool for malnutrition also termed SNAQ (the Short Nutrition Assessment Questionnaire). It is a three-item questionnaire that has been applied to both outpatient and hospitalized patients with good results.[9]

Subjective Global Assessment (SGA) is a clinical technique for bedside nutritional assessment in adults. It assesses nutritional status based on the history and physical exam as well as the examiner's clinical judgment. The SGA is widely used in hospital settings and has been well validated in numerous populations of adult patients, both medical and surgical. Of importance, the SGA does not allow for the classification of mild malnutrition and does not detect acute declines in nutritional status.[10] Use of the SGA in long-term care patients and hospitalized patients has been shown to be highly indicative of mortality and nutrition-related hospital readmission.[11] The SGA is not recommended for the detection of malnutrition in obese persons.

SCREEN II (Seniors in the Community: Risk Evaluation for Eating and Nutrition Version II) is designed to identify community-dwelling older adults at risk for poor nutrition. It is a 17-item questionnaire intended for broad use in the community, or even over a phone. The sensitivity of SCREEN II is 84% and specificity is 62%, with a positive predictive value of 85% and a negative predictive value of 61%.[12]

● PROCESSES OF WEIGHT LOSS

Sarcopenia

There are numerous processes by which older persons lose weight. Ubiquitous to all persons is the process of sarcopenia, an age-associated loss of skeletal muscle mass and strength. Though sarcopenia refers to the process of muscle loss, the term sarcopenia is often used to refer to persons with a skeletal muscle mass deemed to be in an unhealthy range or occurring to the extent that it places a person at a disability risk. Sarcopenic obesity is a term used to describe persons with sarcopenia who also have a body mass index ≥ 30 kg/m². Numerous studies have found an association between sarcopenia and functional impairment, physical disability, infection risk, and even mortality.[13] However, most older persons who become sarcopenic do not lose weight, due to increased fat mass seen with aging.

Cachexia

In contrast to sarcopenia, cachexia occurs due to the inflammatory effects of acute or chronic disease. It is defined as a complex metabolic syndrome associated with underlying illness, typified by loss of muscle with or without loss of fat mass. Primary depression, hyperthyroidism, malabsorption, starvation, and sarcopenia must be ruled out before the diagnosis can be made. Cachexia increases mortality. Inflammation, insulin resistance, and increased muscle protein breakdown are frequently associated.[14] Anorexia is nearly always seen in cachectic states. The anorexia-cachexia syndrome, the coupling of cachexia with poor dietary intake, is likely due to ineffective appetite stimulation despite an ongoing

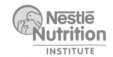

Mini Nutritional Assessment
MNA®

Last name:		First name:	
Sex:	Age:	Weight, kg:	Height, cm:	Date:

Complete the screen by filling in the boxes with the appropriate numbers. Total the numbers for the final screening score.

Screening

A Has food intake declined over the past 3 months due to loss of appetite, digestive problems, chewing or swallowing difficulties?
0 = severe decrease in food intake
1 = moderate decrease in food intake
2 = no decrease in food intake ☐

B Weight loss during the last 3 months
0 = weight loss greater than 3 kg (6.6 lbs)
1 = does not know
2 = weight loss between 1 and 3 kg (2.2 and 6.6 lbs)
3 = no weight loss ☐

C Mobility
0 = bed or chair bound
1 = able to get out of bed/chair but does not go out
2 = goes out ☐

D Has suffered psychological stress or acute disease in the past 3 months?
0 = yes   2 = no ☐

E Neuropsychological problems
0 = severe dementia or depression
1 = mild dementia
2 = no psychological problems ☐

F1 Body Mass Index (BMI) (weight in kg)/(height in m²)
0 = BMI less than 19
1 = BMI 19 to less than 21
2 = BMI 21 to less than 23
3 = BMI 23 or greater ☐

IF BMI IS NOT AVAILABLE, REPLACE QUESTION F1 WITH QUESTION F2.
DO NOT ANSWER QUESTION F2 IF QUESTION F1 IS ALREADY COMPLETED.

F2 Calf circumference (CC) in cm
0 = CC less than 31
3 = CC 31 or greater ☐

Screening score
(max. 14 points) ☐☐

12-14 points: Normal nutritional status
8-11 points: At risk of malnutrition
0-7 points: Malnourished

For a more in-depth assessment, complete the full MNA® which is available at www.mna-elderly.com

Ref.   Vellas B, Villars H, Abellan G, et al. *Overview of the MNA® - Its History and Challenges.* J Nutr Health Aging 2006;10:456–465.
Rubenstein LZ, Harker JO, Salva A, Guigoz Y, Vellas B. *Screening for Undernutrition in Geriatric Practice: Developing the Short-Form Mini Nutritional Assessment (MNA-SF).* J, Geront 2001;56A: M366–377.
Guigoz Y. *The Mini-Nutritional Assessment (MNA®) Review of the Literature - What does it tell us?* J Nutr Health Aging 2006; 10:466–487.
® Société des Produits Nestlé, S.A., Vevey, Switzerland, Trademark Owners
© Nestlé, 1994, Revision 2009. N67200 12/99 10M
For more information: www.mna-elderly.com

FIGURE 35–1. The mini-nutritional assessment. (*Source: Vellas B, Villars H, Abellan G, et al. Overview of the MNA®—Its History and Challenges.* J Nutr Health Aging. *2006;10: 456-465.*)

energy deficit. Though cachexia is classically considered a disease-related process, age > 70 alone may induce similar cytokine changes to that seen in disease states. However, cytokine elevations seen with aging are minimal and difficult to teaseout from unknown subclinical illnesses that may be present. If age has an effect on cytokines and cachexia, the contribution is likely small.[15]

Undernutrition

Inadequate intake as a cause of weight loss, termed undernutrition, is the final major process of weight loss in the older person.[16] Normally, energy intake remains the same or declines with aging. This decline in intake occurs in a setting where total energy expenditure is also falling, due in part to the decreasing physical activity, decreasing resting metabolic rate, and hormonal changes that accompany aging.[17] In older persons who maintain weight, the decline in intake is coupled with a decline in energy expenditure that, together, maintain equilibrium. In undernutrition, the physiologic decline in intake is exacerbated by other conditions. Disability, oral health issues, and social isolation are just a few reasons an older person might lose weight due to undernutrition. Loss of appetite, or anorexia, is also common and, independent of other disease processes, likely related to myriad hormonal changes and gastrointestinal slowing that occur with aging. In nursing home residents, inadequate oral intake has been observed to be major component of weight loss due to the individual's lack of control over access to food.[18]

● CAUSES OF UNDERNUTRITION

Access to Food

Access to food can be hindered in many ways. For the community-dwelling elders, lack of transportation or physical disability can hinder their ability to prepare food or travel to the grocery store. Older persons typically live on fixed incomes, often near the poverty line, which may limit the food they purchase. They may find they have to choose between paying for medications or utilities versus paying for nutrient-dense foods. An individual's social support system often thins as he or she ages, so friends or family who assisted with shopping or meal preparation may be unavailable. Institutionalized patients rely on others to prepare and, often, assist them with feeding. Inadequate feeding assistance in nursing homes has been identified as the major component of weight variation in residents across nursing homes.[18]

Oral Issues

Oral issues are an important cause of decreased intake in the older person. They include dry mouth, oral pain, oral lesions, the inability to chew properly, and poor occlusion. According to the United States National Health and Nutrition Examination Survey (NHANES) from 1999 to 2004, 18% of those 65 and older had untreated tooth decay.

According to the National Health Interview Survey (NHIS) of 2005 to 2007, an additional 26% of these older patients were edentulous. Poor oral health has been shown to be associated with undernutrition in patients in long-term care facilities. Edentate patients are more likely to have chewing pain and poor appetite.[19] Edentulousness, regardless of denture status, has been shown to be an important independent risk factor for significant weight loss of > 4% in a year in community-dwelling older adults.[20] Difficulty in chewing food has been shown to correlate highly with malnutrition and risk of malnutrition in older hospitalized patients.[21]

Dysphagia

The risk of dysphagia increases with age. Among community-dwelling older persons, between 7% and 10% complain of difficulty swallowing. For individuals residing in long-term care facilities, these numbers may approach 30% to 40%.[22] There may be age-related reasons for some component of dysphagia. Esophageal motility may become depressed after the eighth decade; and with aging, peristalsis throughout the gut declines. However, dysphagia among older persons is more likely due to medical conditions. Stroke, Parkinson disease, neuromuscular disease, and head and neck cancer are common causes of oropharyngeal dysphagia. Strictures, achlasia, medication-induced injury, and esophageal cancer are some causes of esophageal dysphagia. Dysphagia can cause food avoidance and significant weight loss.[23]

Eating Alone

Recently widowed persons, such as Mr. P., are at a special risk of developing weight loss.[24] This is thought to be due to eating alone, consuming more commercial meals, and eating fewer snacks. Widowed persons, and likely many older adults accustomed to eating with others, find less enjoyment in eating when eating alone. An examination of more than 200 older persons at risk of or with malnutrition found that over 60% were widowers and 40% were living alone.[25]

● ASSESSMENT OF WEIGHT LOSS

For Mr. P., determining the presence of weight loss is relatively straightforward, as he has had serial weight measurements and was able to use a standing scale. For other patients, this may be difficult or impossible. When persons are unable to stand on a scale, bed or chair scales can be used. In situations where the provider has never seen a patient before and has no prior records, patient or family concern about weight loss alone should prompt further investigation. Physical examination may yield additional clues such as loose-fitting clothing or a belt that shows evidence of recently being adjusted tighter. Despite the ease of detecting weight loss and the risk for malnutrition, providers more often than not fail to recognize or act on it.[21]

After determination of weight loss, a focused investigation into the cause of the loss should follow. A screening test, such as the Simplified Nutrition Assessment Questionnaire (SNAQ) or Mini-Nutritional Assessment (MNA), can help determine if the loss is due to poor appetite or if another process of weight loss, such as cachexia, may be ongoing. A complete history and physical exam can help direct efforts. The provider should remember that both new and chronic processes can be at fault. Laboratory evaluations to consider include a fasting glucose, complete blood count (CBC), basic metabolic profile, and thyroid stimulating hormone (TSH). Additional studies, such as imaging studies or further laboratory workup, should be ordered as the history and physical examination dictate. Currently, there are no established guidelines for the evaluation of involuntary weight loss.

● UNINTENTIONAL WEIGHT LOSS

The medical reasons for unintentional weight loss are numerous. Fear of an occult malignancy is often foremost in both the patient's and provider's mind. Chronic diseases such as heart failure, end-stage renal disease, Parkinson disease, and chronic obstructive pulmonary disease can cause weight loss through anorexia, early satiety, increased energy expenditure, and impaired functional status. New medication side effects, depression, thyroid disease, diabetes mellitus, autoimmune disease, and infections are additional causes of weight loss in an older adult, as in younger individuals. By no means are these lists exhaustive. Drug or alcohol dependence should be considered, as they are often not obvious to providers.

Psychiatric disorders including obsessive-compulsive disorder and anorexia nervosa persist in older persons and can contribute to weight loss as well.[26,27]

Studies that have examined unintentional weight loss in older persons have found that the cause of weight loss—or at least an important contributor—can usually be identified. In one chart review of 46 community-dwelling elders, depression ranked as the most common recognizable cause of weight loss in 30%. Poorly controlled diabetes and malignancy ranked equally after depression at 9% each. Therapeutic diets, oropharyngeal disease, and dementia are other important recognized causes of weight loss in these patients. Only 7% of patients had entirely unexplained weight loss.[27] In a similar examination of nursing home patients, depression was likewise found to be the primary cause of weight loss, present in 36%.[26] Such data offer reassurance to providers and patients that causes for weight loss are detectable in the majority of patients. However, providers should keep in mind that occasionally more than one cause may be present. Furthermore, the interplay of medical issues with the complex physiologic, behavioral, and social issues of aging may further complicate matters.

● DEPRESSION

Depression among older adults is common and under-recognized. It is an important cause of weight loss due to undernutrition in older persons both in the community and in long-term facilities. Estimates on the prevalence of depression among older patients are concerning. A review of diagnoses among over 76,000 nursing home residents in the state of Ohio revealed that 48% of patients carried a diagnosis of active depression.[28] In a study from the Netherlands, nearly 27% of newly admitted patients to nursing homes had depressive symptoms.[29] The presence of depression also correlates independently with low Mini-Nutritional Assessment (MNA) scores.[30]

Mr. P.'s score on the Geriatric Depression Scale raises concern for depression as the primary cause for his weight loss. His recent widowhood, increased social isolation, and dentate status are likely also contributing. A full assessment with MNA could delineate if he has fallen into the category of malnourished, if he is at risk solely, or if he is well nourished. Certainly, directed additional tests are also needed to assure no other ongoing medical problem is present.

MNA, including the aforementioned measurements, Mr. P. scores a 22, placing him in the category "at risk for malnutrition."

At a repeat visit a week later, you discuss your findings with Mr. P. His laboratory values were within normal limits. His chest x-ray showed no sign of disease. Given his poor appetite, his GDS score, and his depressed behavior in your office, you feel confident that depression is the primary source of Mr. P.'s weight loss. You share your concern with Mr. P. that his grief for the loss of his wife may have become something more. You also point out that he has become at risk for malnutrition due to depression and perhaps other factors. After discussing depression and potential steps toward treatment, Mr. P. asks what he may do "to stop losing weight."

● REVERSING WEIGHT LOSS

Reversal of weight loss in older adults can be more challenging than in younger adults. Older persons are less able to adapt to periods of low food intake during times of illness. Weight loss that would be quickly regained in a younger patient may persist in an older patient. In long-term care populations, younger age is the strongest correlate over 6 months for appetite improvement.[31] Physiologic loss of smell, impairments in taste, and decreased appetite seen with aging may contribute. Yet, though challenging, there are proven ways in which weight loss can be halted and reversed in older individuals. Multidimensional solutions are often the most effective.

First, if a primary medical problem has been found, it is crucial to treat the problem. For Mr. P., this will involve treatment of his depression. For the cachectic patient, treating the cause is especially crucial, as weight is usually unmoved by increased calorie intake. The "MEALS ON WHEELS" mnemonic includes common, often reversible causes of weight loss to consider in all patients (Figure 35–2).

Medication (digoxin, theophylline, psychotropics)
Emotional (depression)
Anorexia/alcoholism
Late-life paranoia
Swallowing disorders

Oral and dental disease
No money (absolute or relative poverty)

Wandering (dementia/behavioral disorders)
Hyperthyroidism/hyperparathyroidism
Entry problems
Eating problems
Low salt or restricted diets
Shopping and food preparation problems

FIGURE 35–2. MEALS ON WHEELS acronym for common causes of under-nutrition in older persons. (*Source: Morley JE. Anorexia of aging: Physiologic and pathologic. Am J Clin Nutr. 1997;66:760-763.*)

The Council for Nutritional Clinical Strategies in Long-Term Care and the American Academy of Home Care Physicians offer guidelines for recognizing and managing weight loss and malnutrition in long-term care and home care patients, respectively.[30,32] At times, the cause of poor nutrition may be irreversible or unable to be addressed due to a patient's wishes. At this point, it should be decided which interventions are consistent with the individual's goals of care.

Nutritional Modifications

Diet modifications are often the first focus in efforts to stop or reverse weight loss. Early involvement of a nutrition specialist to assess a patient's current diet and decide on appropriate interventions is recommended for both community-dwelling and long-term patients. Dietary histories or calorie-counting are needed to establish a baseline. However, how further diets should be structured is still a matter of some debate. The average protein intake in older adults is often below that of younger adults. Thus, aiming for the RDA of protein intake, something many older persons may not be hitting, may improve both weight and sarcopenia.[13] For patients in long-term care, the American Dietetic Association recommends removing restrictive, therapeutic diets as a way of improving intake, weight gain, and quality of life.[33] In addition, therapeutic diets are an important contributor to weight loss in 7% of older outpatients,[27] so removing such restrictions for community-dwelling patients may also be of benefit.

Increasing the nutrient density of food through food choices or preparation can drastically increase caloric and nutrient intake. For older individuals with slower gastric emptying times and increased satiety, moving from the standard three meals a day to five smaller meals may be of benefit. Likewise, frequent snacking with healthful options should be encouraged.

Oral nutritional supplements such as Boost, Ensure, and Carnation are heavily marketed and often prescribed for elderly patients with weight loss or at risk of malnutrition. A recent large meta-analysis of the benefits of protein-energy supplementation for older people had mixed conclusions. The mean weight gain for patients on supplements was only 2.2%. If patients were undernourished at the start of the study, a small mortality benefit was present compared to control groups. This mortality benefit was not seen for those who were not undernourished. No benefit in hospital length of stay for supplemented patients or improvement in functionality was found.[34] Protein supplements alone have been found to increase protein consumption in elderly persons, but no data at this time have shown if this intervention alone can slow or reverse loss of muscle strength or disability due to sarcopenia.[13,35] However, resistance training with or without protein supplementation has been shown to be of benefit to strength and functional status in elderly adults.[36] Given these results, providers should target therapies with such supplements for persons who are undernourished to begin with as a means of effecting weight gain and improving mortality.

Environment and Food Aesthetics

Improvements in dining environment and food aesthetics can have a significant impact on calorie consumption in older persons. Comfortable seating, warm lighting, ambient music, and even use of china plates have been shown to promote increased intake.[37] Nursing residents receiving family-style meals or cafeteria-style meals with waitress service consume more calories than those given fixed-portion trays.[38,39] Interestingly, this effect may be more pronounced in patients with low BMIs and cognitive impairment.[40] When other persons are present at meals, intake can increase to over 100 kcal more per meal than when eating in isolation.[41] Aside from benefits to weight and malnutrition risk, improved dining environment, food-choice autonomy, and improved ratio of staff to residents have been shown to improve quality of life indicators in nursing home residents.[42]

Physical Activity

Physical activity such as strength training has shown the most promise in preventing and reversing sarcopenia as defined by muscle mass. Resistance training has been shown to increase skeletal muscle strength and mass in older women and men.[36,43] Such training needs to be regimented and of at least moderate intensity, occurring at least two or three times weekly, according to the American College of Sports Medicine. Six weeks of resistance training, which increases muscle mass by approximately 1% each week, may reverse the muscle lost in a decade.[13]

Appetite Stimulants

Appetite stimulants, or orexigenic agents, hold a place for select patients with weight loss or malnutrition. First, insufficient appetite must be one of the causes of poor nutrition in order for them to be of any utility. Currently there are no drugs approved by the FDA for treatment of age-related anorexia.[16] As appetite stimulants, most drugs are approved for those with cancer or HIV/AIDS. The side-effect profiles of these agents need to be considered and many are expensive. Consideration for use should be taken on an individual basis.

Megestrol acetate is synthetic progesterone that has been well studied in cancer patients. A recent meta-analysis and systematic review in patients with anorexia-cachexia syndrome showed an improvement in appetite and weight gain for patients on megestrol acetate. However, there was no improvement in survival for patients on megestrol acetate and benefit on quality of life was not confirmed.[44] A trial of megestrol acetate in elderly nursing home patients with anorexia-cachexia syndrome showed improved weight gain in those receiving 800 mg a day though there were no effects on survival. Appetite and well-being appeared to be improved in those on megestrol, though these were secondary outcomes.[45] The most significant side effect is edema; thromboembolism, adrenal suppression, and decreased muscle strength have also been noted. Megestrol acetate should not be given for more than 8 to 12 weeks.

Dronabinol, a cannabis derivative, is approved by the FDA for anorexia in HIV/AIDs and for nausea and vomiting associated with chemotherapy. It is not as effective in appetite improvement and weight gain as megestrol acetate is for advanced cancer patients.[46] For older patients, the side-effect profile of sedation and euphoria warrant extreme caution, especially for those individuals who cannot be closely monitored. A small study evaluating dronabinol in long-term care patients with anorexia and significant weight loss found that a small majority gained weight on the drug and that therapy was well tolerated.[47]

Testosterone levels decline with aging and it has been suggested that replacement could improve cognition, energy levels, functional status, and lean body mass in older men. Certainly such improvements would be beneficial to Mr. P. A recent randomized control trial comparing 6 months of testosterone supplementation to placebo found that lean body mass, relative to fat mass, increases in older men on testosterone therapy. However, these changes did not correlate with improved functional ability or muscle strength. Weight, as measured by BMI, remained stable.[48]

CASE PRESENTATION 2: WEIGHT LOSS IS DESIRED

Ms. G. is a 68-year-old bus driver with a medical history of type 2 diabetes, hypertension, and osteoarthritis of her knees who is concerned about her weight. Recently she took part in a health fair at her local health department and found that her BMI was 31, classifying her as obese. She wonders what health benefits she might gain from losing weight and asks you to recommend a weight loss program.

On review of her records you see that she is 5'4" (63 cm) and for the past 5 years her weight has been relatively stable at 180 lbs (82 kg). Her calculated BMI today in the office is 30.9. Her diabetes has been relatively well controlled since diagnosis 4 years ago. Her prescribed medications include hydrochlorothiazide, enalapril, metformin, glucophage, aspirin, simvastatin, and a multivitamin. She takes an over-the-counter acetaminophen tablet up to twice daily for knee pain.

Examination today is relatively unchanged from prior exams. She is afebrile, blood pressure is 132/68, heart rate is 78, and respirations are 16. She is well dressed, pleasant, and appears obese. Abdominal exam shows no striae; waist circumference is 36 inches (91.4 cm). She has bilateral crepitus of her knees and mild tenderness along her femoral–tibial junction medially. She rises somewhat guardedly from her chair but her gait appears normal. Laboratory tests sent 3 months prior show a normal thyroid stimulating hormone (TSH) level and total cholesterol. Glycosylated hemoglobin A[1c] was 7.4% (0.074 proportion of total hemoglobin)

Further questioning reveals that Ms. G.'s major concern about her health is her knees. She wishes she were not so troubled by her arthritis, which makes it difficult to climb in and out of her bus due to stiffness and pain. She worries if her arthritis progresses that she will be unable to work.

● OVERWEIGHT AND OBESITY IN OLDER ADULTS

The last 25 years have seen a rise in older persons who are overweight or obese (Figure 35–3).[24] For young and middle-aged adults, obesity and overweight are associated with large decreases in life expectancy and increases in early mortality.[49] However, for older persons, longitudinal studies have shown that as persons age, the mortality risk associated with being overweight or obese declines.[50,51] Such data have been interpreted as suggesting that overweight and obesity are less harmful in older persons than in young or middle-aged adults. For the practitioner, this elicits the question, what are our goals for weight loss in the overweight or obese older patient?

Body Mass Index

BMI is a widely used measurement used to define underweight, overweight, and obese adults. It is defined as the weight in kilograms divided by the square of the height in meters (kg/m^2). The World Health Organization (WHO) defines underweight adults as those with a BMI < 18.5, overweight adults as having a BMI of 25 to 29.99, and obese adults as having a BMI >30 (Figure 35–4). In the United States, the prevalence of obesity in persons over 60 years of age is approximately 30% in men and 35% in women.[52]

As we age, changes in body composition occur. The percentage of fat-free mass, peaking at 20 to 30 years, declines with aging, while fat mass rises until 60 to 70 years. After age 70, both fat-free mass and fat mass decline. Fat also redistributes with aging. Subcutaneous fat thins relative to visceral, intramuscular, and intrahepatic fat. Though easy to calculate and apply, BMI does not take into account fat, fat-free mass, or muscle mass. At any given BMI, fat deposits in older persons may be different than in younger persons. Declines in height with aging may further alter the reliability of BMI. It has been recommended that, if available, the height prior to age 50 should be used when calculating BMI to compensate for the effects of kyphosis or spinal compression fractures.[16] For those patients for whom a prior height is not available or able to be recalled, as in a nursing home, arm span may be substituted for height.[53] Yet, despite its shortcomings, BMI remains the most commonly used measure of weight status.

An Ideal Weight for Older Persons?

Optimum weight in the older person may fall above the "normal" BMI range. Moreover, it appears that a larger and higher BMI range may be well-tolerated in older persons. Though some large studies have shown minimum mortality at normal-weight BMIs of 20.5 to 25[51] for older adults, most

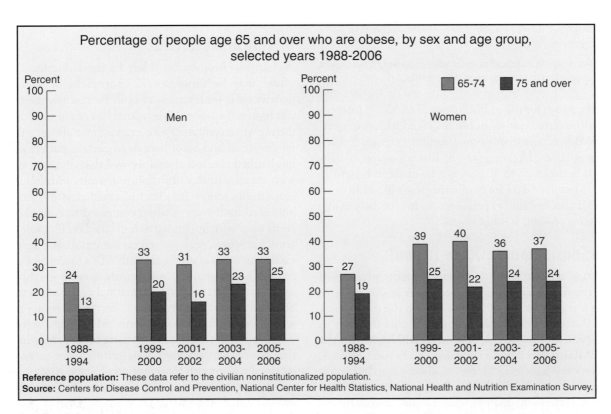

Reference population: These data refer to the civilian noninstitutionalized population.
Source: Centers for Disease Control and Prevention, National Center for Health Statistics, National Health and Nutrition Examination Survey.

FIGURE 35–3. International classification of adult underweight, overweight, and obesity according to the body mass index (BMI).

Classification	BMI (kg/m²)	
	Principal Cut-Off Points	Additional Cut-Off Points
Underweight	**<18.50**	**<18.50**
Severe thinness	<16.00	<16.00
Moderate thinness	16.00–16.99	16.00–16.99
Mild thinness	17.00–18.49	17.00–18.49
Normal range	**18.50–24.99**	**18.50–22.99**
		23.00–24.99
Overweight	**≥25.00**	**≥25.00**
Pre-obese	25.00–29.99	25.00–27.49
		27.50–29.99
Obese	**≥30.00**	**≥30.00**
Obese class I	30.00–34.99	30.00–32.49
		32.50–34.99
Obese class II	35.00–39.99	35.00–37.49
		37.50–39.99
Obese class III	≥40.00	≥40.00

Source: Adapted from WHO, 1995, WHO, 2000, and WHO, 2004. WHO. Physical status: The use and interpretation of anthropometry. Report of a WHO Expert Committee. WHO Technical Report Series 854. Geneva: World Health Organization, 1995. http://whqlibdoc.who.int/trs/WHO_TRS_854.pdf. WHO. Obesity: Preventing and managing the global epidemic. Report of a WHO Consultation. WHO Technical Report Series 894. Geneva: World Health Organization, 2000. http://whqlibdoc.who.int/trs/WHO_TRS_894.pdf. WHO expert consultation. Appropriate body-mass index for Asian populations and its implications for policy and intervention strategies. The Lancet, 2004; 157-163. http://www.ncbi.nlm.nih.gov/entrez/query.fcgi?cmd=Retrieve&db=pubmed&dopt=Abstract&list_uids=14726171.

FIGURE 35–4. International classification of adult underweight, overweight, and obesity according to the body mass index (BMI).

have shown nadirs for risk at BMIs from 27 to 30.[50,54] Interestingly, health-related quality of life is ranked higher in overweight BMI veterans than normal-weight veterans.[55] Such data suggest that addressing weight loss for older patients with BMIs between 25 to 30 may not be of much benefit to mortality. Moreover, data are conflicting regarding if an overweight BMI affects ability to perform activities of daily living; if the effect is present, it is likely small.[56]

Special Consideration: Obese Patients

The question remains what to do with patients whose BMI falls within the category of "obese," such as our patient, Ms. G. It is important to realize that though the relative risk of death due to an elevated body-mass index declines as persons age, the absolute risk of death is still higher for the highest BMIs in older persons until age 75. (Beyond 75 years, the association is less clear.) Moreover, obesity is an important contributor to many medical conditions among older adults including hypertension, dyslipidemia, arthritis, urinary incontinence, and perhaps certain cancers. Obesity can adversely affect quality of life in older persons. The loss of muscle mass that occurs with aging, in the setting of large amounts of adiposity, may cause obese older adults to be particularly vulnerable to declines in physical functioning. As with older persons experiencing unintentional weight loss, those with BMIs > 30 have very high frailty rates and decreased quality of life.[57,58] Obesity is an independent predictor of disability in the ability to perform activities of daily living (ADLs).[56] Epidemiologic data from the United States suggest that as obese persons are living longer, due likely to improvements in cardiovascular mortality, disability is becoming more common.[59]

A recent examination of approximately 2000 elderly individuals found that in those with a self-reported normal weight at age 50, classified as a BMI of 20 to 25, weight gain of as little as 5% (as well as weight loss of at least 10%) was associated with increased disability in activities of daily living after age 65, even with adjustment for chronic diseases. In those persons who were already obese at age 50, subsequent weight gain was even more associated with increased disability. Interestingly, for these already obese persons, weight loss was not associated with greater odds of disability—though in normal-weight persons, as has been wellestablished in prior epidemiologic studies, there is an association.[56]

● APPROACHING WEIGHT LOSS

The means of approaching weight loss is of particular importance in the obese elderly patient. Weight loss should be considered on an individual basis, taking into consideration ongoing medical illnesses, current functional capacity, and the likelihood that a patient can comply with an exercise program. Weight loss for the purpose of weight loss alone is likely not indicated. However, weight loss should be considered if it is a means to improving physical functioning or quality of life.

Dieting and Exercise

Weight loss brought on solely by the reduction of caloric intake may be dangerous in overweight or obese elderly patients as it leads to loss of both fat and fat-free mass that can hasten the normal age-related loss of muscle.[60] However, dieting when combined with exercise may alleviate the loss of fat-free mass and be of benefit in certain patients. A small randomized controlled trial showed that diet in conjunction with exercise in sedentary, obese persons with mild to moderate frailty scores does lead to significant weight loss and improved frailty scores when compared to controls. Participants were initially defined as frail based on Physical Performance Test scores, peak oxygen consumption, and self-reported need for assistance or difficulty with ADLs (using the Functional Status Questionnaire). Importantly, despite weight loss, the study group's fat-free mass remained relatively unchanged. Scores in physical performance, oxygen consumption, and self-reported ability to perform ADLs were significantly improved with treatment.[61] A more recent study has shown that overweight or obese long-term cancer survivors who received a 12-month intervention of home-based counseling that promoted exercise, improved diet, and modest weight loss did reduce the rate of self-reported functional decline.[62] At this point it is impossible to say if these improvements in quality of life and functional status correlate with survival, as no randomized controlled trials have evaluated that question. In total, these results suggest that exercise in some form (preferably through resistance training) is a necessary component to healthy weight loss in older persons.

Weight Cycling

Weight cycling, or the repeated intentional loss and then regaining of weight, has been thought to be associated with increased mortality. However, a recent prospective study of older women did not find an association with all-cause or cardiovascular mortality.[63] Thus concerns over weight cycling as a deterrent for weight loss in select obese, older patients is likely not warranted.

The Metabolic Syndrome

Ms. G. qualifies as obese, as her BMI is > 30. Interventional trials examining specific disease processes have shown some benefit to weight reduction in obese persons older than 65; these disease processes include both arthritis and the metabolic syndrome.[64] The metabolic syndrome is characterized by insulin resistance, central adiposity, abnormal lipid profiles, and elevated blood pressure. Ms. G., given her diabetes, hypertension, and waist circumference, has metabolic syndrome by Adult Treatment Panel III (ATP III) criteria. It is most prevalent in older, obese adults. A small, randomized trial with 24 patients showed that older patients were able to improve all indices of the metabolic syndrome, including their weight, with exercise alone or exercise and mild caloric restriction.[65]

Knee Osteoarthritis

In overweight and obese older adults with knee osteoarthritis, moderate exercise and dietary weight loss have been shown in randomized trials to improve health-related quality of life, knee pain, and physical function compared with diet or exercise alone.[66,67] However, if an older patient is not able to lose or sustain weight loss, exercise alone can provide some benefit to physical ability.[67] One of the risks of weight loss in the elderly is adverse effects on bone mineral density and increased risks of fracture. Weight loss induced by dieting alone seems to be particularly harmful.[61] The addition of exercise, both weight-bearing and resistive, has been shown to prevent and perhaps reverse bone loss in the femoral neck and trochanter, but not the spine, in older persons.[68,69]

Ms. G. is obese. Her disability from her knee arthritis affects her life on a daily basis and she may benefit from weight loss. In addition, weight loss might bring about improvement of her metabolic syndrome parameters such as her insulin resistance and hypertension. As her practitioner, suggesting a plan of weight loss in conjunction with supervised exercise likely could improve her quality of life. If weight loss proved impossible for Ms. G, exercise alone could provide an improvement in her physical ability. As with any older person, assessment of bone density is crucial, especially when considering a weight loss program. Ms G. should also be advised that dieting or calorie restriction for the purposes of weight loss alone, without the addition of exercise, should be avoided.

CASE PRESENTATION 3: NURSING HOME RESIDENT APPROACHING END OF LIFE

Mrs. B. is an 83-year-old nursing home resident with a medical history of progressive vascular dementia, coronary artery disease, congestive heart failure, and hypertension. Over the past 3 years, Mrs. B. has gone from being partially independent with activities of daily living such as feeding and dressing to requiring full assistance with all aspects of her care. For 8 months she has been bed-bound and without intelligible speech. Over the past year, Mrs. B. has had frequent admissions to her local hospital for repeated aspiration pneumonias and exacerbations of her heart failure. A bedside swallowing evaluation performed 1 month ago showed pharyngeal dysphasia. As a result her diet was changed to puree with nectar-thickened liquids.

Following her last hospital discharge, Mrs. B.'s daughter, as her next of kin, decided that resuscitation and intubation were no longer in line with Mrs. B.'s goals of care. Mrs. B. returned to the nursing home with a "do not attempt resuscitation or intubation" order. At each mealtime, a staff member continued to sit by Mrs. B.'s bedside and offer her a "cardiac-prudent" pureed diet by mouth. According to her chart, she usually finished about 25% of her meal before refusing further bites or sips or spitting them out.

Two days ago, Mrs. B.'s son arrived from out of town and was very upset to find his mother looking very thin and, in his words, "starving to death." He asks what may be done to improve her weight and mentions a feeding tube.

On examination, Mrs. B. is lying in bed. She is afebrile, blood pressure is 104/52, heart rate is 88, and respirations are 18 and unlabored. Her weight, by bed scale, is 104 lbs (47.3 kg). (Prior height, according to her chart was 5'5" or 165 cm.) She appears very thin with temporal wasting. Her clothes are clean and dry. She is awake and appears to smile when spoken to. She occasionally makes moaning sounds but is not conversational. She has slightly dry mucous membranes. She is edentulous and does not wear dentures. Her lips are cracked and peeling. Abdomen is thin, without palpable masses, and nontender. Skin is without rashes and is free from breakdown. Extremities are slightly cool. During the examination, Mrs. B shows no grimacing or movements suggestive of pain or discomfort. Review of Mrs. B.'s chart shows that she is on stool softeners and has a bowel movement every 2 days.

WEIGHT LOSS IN THE END-OF-LIFE PATIENT

Weight loss and anorexia in the end-of-life patient can be distressing for patients and their families. Weight loss and a wasted appearance are visible harbingers of a nearing death. As patients take in less food and drink, families may worry that starvation may hasten the end. When a terminal patient takes in little, family members may fear he or she is suffering. Decreased intake in the last weeks to days of life is nearly universal and should be considered part of the dying process. As providers, giving patients and families accurate expectations about what to anticipate may help prepare them for the decreased intake and weight loss nearing death. Providing information about what is and is not helpful in this time is crucial and should be framed within the goals of care for the patient.

Family Expectations

Families and loved ones, such as Mrs. B.'s son, are often more concerned than the patient about weight loss or indifference to food or drink. Though weight loss is often an expected step toward death, the erroneous notion that "if they would just eat, they would get better" is commonplace. Preparing food and feeding a patient are often comforting measures that allow family members to feel they are contributing to the care of their loved one. Loss of this role may lead to feelings of inadequacy or guilt. Again, providers can educate families that decreased intake is not the cause of the patient's decline; rather, it is a part of the process. Data suggest that many dying patients are not hungry or thirsty, despite poor intake. In a study of comfort-care patients who were mentally aware and competent, 62% of patients never experienced hunger or thirst. In those patients who did have hunger or thirst, all patients received relief with small amounts of oral food or fluids.[70]

Causes of Weight Loss at the End of Life

As with any geriatric patient, weight loss at the end of life is usually multifaceted. For cancer patients, cachexia and anorexia may be a part of their ongoing disease process. For those with terminal dementia, swallowing can become difficult or a patient may essentially "forget" how to eat or what food is. The satisfaction received from eating may wane. Depression, delirium, and pain can further influence hunger and the desire to eat or drink. Oral thrush, mucositis, and dry mouth may make eating uncomfortable or outright painful. The social, emotional, and behavioral features discussed earlier in the chapter also need to be considered.

ADDRESSING NUTRITION AT THE END OF LIFE

A systematic approach to addressing nutritional support in the older patient with advanced or terminal disease can assist both the provider and the caregiver in minimizing the distress often experienced with poor intake. The first question to consider is if decreased intake or weight loss is affecting the patient's quality of life. Interestingly, patients in palliative care units that find appetite loss distressing may not disclose it unless formally asked.[71] Sometimes, family expectations alone are the concern. When weight loss is deemed a problem, the provider should look for easily reversible causes of poor intake. The trajectory of the patient's weight loss or poor appetite can provide clues to the nature of the weight loss. Is this an acute process, or is this a subacute or chronic process? Acute medical problems like infection, new constipation, or urinary retention may contribute to altered intake and with treatment intake may improve.

Symptom Burden

Pain is a common symptom at the end of life. A patient in pain may be so focused on pain that hunger goes unnoticed or eating is intolerable. Medications may also be a source of decreased intake. Opioids commonly lead to nausea, anorexia, or constipation. Selective serotonin reuptake inhibitors (SSRIs), anti-epileptics, stimulants, and even nonsteroidal anti-inflammatory drugs can diminish appetite (though long-term use of SSRIs may lead to weight gain). Anticholinergics and diuretics may cause dry mouth; the former have also been associated with swallowing dysfunction and urinary retention.

Rethinking Dietary Restrictions

Lifting dietary restrictions in patients nearing death is appropriate and may improve intake, or at least make eating more enjoyable for the patient. Diabetics, if blood sugars are not reaching dangerously elevated levels, may feel liberated if offered a favorite food, regardless of carbohydrate or fat content. If the patient is able, involve him or her in meal planning. Consider offering smaller meals more frequently and increasing personal assistance with meals. Other, less well-studied maneuvers include offering hot or cold foods instead of lukewarm foods and adding gravy or juices to foods.[72]

On exam, Mrs. B. did not appear to be in any discomfort nor does her exam indicate acute infection or constipation. Weight loss in Mrs. B. is likely due primarily to her advanced terminal dementia. Though she still takes food with assistance, after consuming a small portion of her meals she signals to the nursing home staff by spitting out food that she is finished. Though it is impossible to directly ask Mrs. B. if she is suffering or is hungry, together the evidence suggests that she is, for the most part, comfortable. Certainly, a first step for the provider would be to share this information with Mrs. B.'s family, especially her son. Ascertaining more about the son's concerns for his mother is also necessary. Remorse, guilt, and fear about his mother's death may be more of a worry than the actual weight loss itself. Sometimes, especially for a family member who has been far away, time alone may be necessary to come to terms with the nearing death.

Oral Care

Improved oral hygiene for Mrs. B. would be appropriate at this time. Her exam shows dry oral mucosa and peeling lips. Addressing this with frequent mouth moistening and use of lip emollients might improve Mrs. B.'s comfort. Involving her family members in oral care may alleviate their focus on her intake and help them contribute to her well-being. If the focus on food for the family persists, offering more frequent small meals by hand may alleviate some concern. Lifting Mrs. B.'s cardiac-prudent diet restriction at this time is recommended and may also allow family to bring in favorite foods from home. The provider should warn the family that her intake, despite these measures, may not appreciably change. However, the symbolism of such acts may be a relief for the family.

● CONSIDERATION OF ARTIFICIAL FEEDING

Enteral feeding is often intended or prescribed to prevent aspiration, prolong life, improve nutrition, and provide comfort. In select populations, such as head and neck cancer patients and dysphasic stroke patients, placement of nasogastric or percutaneous gastrostomy tubes has proven benefit during the patient's early recovery. However, such prescriptions for terminally ill patients are not upheld by the existing medical literature. A recent meta-analysis of feeding tubes in patients with advanced dementia found no conclusive evidence that enteral tube feedings prolonged survival, improved quality of life, or improved nourishment.[73] Moreover, placement of percutaneous gastrostomy tubes comes with risks. A large meta-analysis reported an all-comer procedure-related morbidity of 9% and mortality of 0.5%.[74] Smaller studies that have included larger proportions of dementia patients reported 30-day all-cause mortality rates as high as 22% to 54%.[75]

It is important to remember the logistics and burdens of a feeding tube. Care of the tube may involve dressing changes and common leakage problems, potentially requiring repeat visits to the Emergency Room or physician's office. Stool and urine output may increase with tube feedings, causing need for increased diaper or bed changes and raising the risk for pressure ulcers. Both nasogastric tubes and percutaneous gastrostomy tubes can be uncomfortable or unfamiliar to patients. For the delirious, demented, or dying patients, restraints are often needed as patients try to pull or remove their tubes. Such restraints can be very distressing for many patients and families. Often, patients on feeding tubes no longer receive oral intake, taking away pleasure the patient may have gotten from eating or drinking or removing the daily contact the patient may have had during mealtimes with families or nursing home staff.[76,77] Informing the patient and family of these risks is essential.

Despite the clinical evidence on the lack of benefit of feeding tubes in patients at the end of life, some families and patients may persist with desire for placement. The provider should support informed decisions, even if current scientific literature does not demonstrate clear benefit. Recognize that many patients and families rely on emotional, cultural, or religious principles when making the decision about artificial hydration and nutrition. In the United States, terminally ill patients on tube feedings are still eligible for hospice benefits.

CONCLUSION

Weight loss at the end of life need not be an unforeseen, feared occurrence. Education about what to expect is necessary for both patients and families. Though decreased appetite may not be a concern for most patients, ascertaining the importance of appetite cannot be done unless a patient is asked. Family concerns may not be the same as those of the patients and, though forcing intake is possible, feeding is an emotive issue. The patient's goals of care should be the framework upon which any interventions are built.

References

1. Newman AB, Yanez D, Harris T, et al. Weight change in old age and its association with mortality. *J Am Geriatr Soc.* 2001;49: 1309-1318.

2. Lang PO, Michel JP, Zekry D. Frailty syndrome: A transitional state in a dynamic process. *Gerontology.* 2009. DOI: 10.1159/000211949.

3. Guigoz Y. The Mini Nutritional Assessment (MNA) review of the literature—What does it tell us? *J Nutr Health Aging.* 2006; 10:466-485.

4. Wallace JI, Schwartz RS, LaCroix AZ, et al. Involuntary weight loss in older outpatients: Incidence and clinical significance. *J Am Geriatr Soc.* 1995;43:329-337.

5. Guigoz Y, Lauque S, Vellas BJ. Identifying the elderly at risk of malnutrition. The Mini Nutritional Assessment. *Clin Geriatr Med.* 2002;10:737-757.

6. Sieber CC. Nutritional screening tools: How does the MNA compare? Proceedings of the session held in Chicago May 2-3, 2006 (15 years of Mini Nutritional Assessment). *J Nutr Health Aging.* 2006;10:488-492.

7. Stratton RJ, King CL, Stroud MA, et al. "Malnutrition Universal Screening Tool" predicts mortality and length of hospital stay in acutely ill elderly. *Br J Nutr.* 2006;95:325-330.

8. Wilson MM, Thomas DR, Rubenstein LZ, et al. Appetite assessment: Simple appetite questionnaire predicts weight loss in community-dwelling adults and nursing home residents. *Am J Clin Nutr.* 2005; 82:1074-1081.

9. Neelemaat F, Kruizenga HM, de Vet HC, et al. Screening malnutrition in hospital outpatients. Can the SNAQ malnutrition screening tool also be applied to this population? *Clin Nutr.* 2008; 27:439-446.

10. Covinsky KE, Covinsky MH, Palmer RM, et al. Serum albumin concentration and clinical assessments of nutrional status in hospitalized older people: Different sides of different coins? *J Am Geriatr Soc.* 2002;50:631-637.

11. Sacks GS, Dearman K, Replogle WH, et al. Use of subjective global assessment to identify nutrition-associated complications and death in geriatric long-term care facility residents. *J Am Coll Nutr.* 2000;19:570-577.

12. Keller HH, Goy R, Kane SL. Validity and reliability of SCREEN II (Seniors in the Community: Risk Evaluation for Eating and Nutrition, version II). *Eur J Clin Nutr.* 2005;59:1149-1157.

13. Janssen I. Sarcopenia. In: Bales CW, Ritchie CS, eds. *Nutrition and Health: Handbook of Clinical Nutrition and Aging.* 2nd ed. Totowa, NJ: Humana Press; 2009:183-205.

14. Evans WJ, Morley JE, Argiles J, et al. Cachexia: A new definition. *Clin Nutr.* 2008;27:793-799.

15. Thomas DR. Cachexia: Diagnosis and treatment. In: Bales CW, Ritchie CS, eds. *Nutrition and Health: Handbook of Clinical Nutrition and Aging.* 2nd ed. Totowa, NJ: Humana Press; 2009:207-217.

16. Bales CW, Ritchie CS. Redefining nutritional frailty: Interventions for weight loss due to undernutrition. In: Bales CW, Ritchie CS, eds. *Nutrition and Health: Handbook of Clinical Nutrition and Aging.* 2nd ed. Totowa, NJ: Humana Press; 2009:157-182.

17. Villareal DT, Apovian CM, Kushner RF, et al. Obesity in older adults: Technical review and position statement of the American Society for Nutrition and NAASO, the Obesity Society. *Obes Res.* 2005;13:1849-1863.

18. Simmons SF, Garcia ET, Cadogan MP, et al. The minimum data set weight-loss quality indicator: Does it reflect differences in care processes related to weight loss? *J Am Geriatr Soc.* 2003;51: 1410-1418.

19. Lee JS, Weyant RJ, Corby P, et al. Edentulism and nutritional status in a biracial sample of well-functioning, community-dwelling elderly: The health, aging, and body composition study. *Am J Clin Nutr.* 2004;79:295-302.

20. Ritchie CS, Joshipura K, Silliman RA, et al. Oral health problems and significant weight loss among community-dwelling older adults. *J Gerontol A Biol Sci Med Sci.* 2000;55:M366-M371.

21. Wilson MM. Undernutrition in medical outpatients. *Clin Geriatr Med.* 2002;18:759-771.

22. Achem SR, Devault KR. Dysphagia in aging. *J Clin Gastroenterol.* 2005;39:357-371.

23. Lorefalt B, Granerus AK, Unosson M. Avoidance of solid food in weight losing older patients with Parkinson's disease. *J Clin Nurs.* 2006;15:1404-1412.

24. Shahar DR, Schultz R, Shahar A, et al. The effect of widowhood on weight change, dietary intake, and eating behavior in the elderly population. *J Aging Health.* 2001;13:189-199.

25. Feldblum I, German L, Castel H, et al. Characteristics of undernourished older medical patients and the identification of predictors for undernutrition status. *Nutr J.* 2007;6:37. doi:10.1186/1475-2891-6-37

26. Morley JE, Kraenzle D: Causes of weight loss in a community nursing home. *J Am Geriatr Soc.* 1994;42:583-585.

27. Wilson MM. Prevalence and causes of undernutrition in medical outpatients. *Am J Med.*1998;104:56-63.

28. Levin CA, Wei W, Akincigil A, et al. Prevalence and treatment of diagnosed depression among elderly nursing home residents in Ohio. *J Am Med Dir Assoc.* 2007;8:585-594.

29. Achterberg W, Pot AM, Kerkstra A, et al. Depressive symptoms in newly admitted nursing home residents. *Int J Geriatr Psychiatry.* 2006;21:1156-1162.

30. Thomas DR, Ashmen W, Morley JE, et al. Nutritional management in long-term care: Development of a clinical guideline. Council for Nutritional Strategies in Long-Term Care. *J Gerontol A Biol Sci Med Sci.* 2000;55:725-734.

31. Sullivan DH, Morley JE, Johnson LE, et al. The GAIN (Geriatric Anorexia Nutrition) registry: The impact of appetite and weight on mortality in long-term care population. *J Nutr Health Aging.* 2002; 6:275-281.

32. Milne AC, Avenell A, Potter J. Meta-analysis: Protein-energy supplementation in older people. *Ann Intern Med.* 2006;144: 37-48.

33. Niedert KC. Position of the American Dietetic Association: Liberalization of the diet prescription improves quality of life for older adults in long-term care. *J Am Diet Assoc.* 2005;105: 1955-1965.

34. Milne AC, Potter J, Vivanti A, et al. Protein and energy supplementation in elderly people at risk from malnutrition. *Cochrane Database Syst Rev.* 2009;2:CD003288.

35. Lauque S, Arnaud-Battandier R, Mansourian R. Protein-energy oral supplementation in malnourished nursing-home residents. A controlled trial. *Age Ageing.* 2000;29:51-56.

36. Fiatarone M, O'Neill E, Ryan ND, et al. Exercise training and nutritional supplementation for physical frailty in very elderly people. *N Engl J Med.* 1994;330:1769-1775.

37. Stroebele N, De Castro JM. Effect of ambience on food intake and food choice. *Nutrition.* 2004;20:821-838.

38. Nijs KA, de Graaf C, Kof FJ, et al. Effect of family style mealtimes on quality of life, physical performance, and body weight of nursing home residents: Cluster randomised controlled trial. *BMJ.* 2006; 332:1180-1184.

39. Nijs KA, de Graaf C, Siebelink K, et al. Effect of family-style meals on energy intake and risk of malnutrition in Dutch nursing home residents: A randomized controlled trial. *J Gerontol A Biol Sci Med Sci.* 2006;61:935-942.

40. Desai J, Winter A, Young KW, et al. Changes in type of food service and dining room environment preferentially benefit institutionalized seniors with low body mass indexes. *J Am Diet Assoc.* 2007;107: 808-814.

41. Locher JL, Robinson CO, Roth DL, et al. The effect of the presence of others on caloric intake in homebound older adults. *J Gerontol A Biol Sci Med Sci.* 2005;60:1475-1478.

42. Carrier N, West GE, Ouellet D. Dining experience, food services and staffing are associated with quality of life in elderly nursing home residents. *J Nutr Health Aging.* 2009;13:565-570.

43. Roth SM, Ivey FM, Martel GF. Muscle size responses to strength training in young and older men and women. *J Am Geriatr Soc.* 2001;49:1428-1433.

44. Lesniak W, Bala M, Jaeschke R, et al. Effects of megestrol acetate in patients with cancer-anorexia syndrome—A systematic review and meta-analysis. *Pol Arch Med Wewn.* 2008;118: 636-622.

45. Yeh SS, Lovitt S, Schuster MW. Usage of megestrol acetate in the treatment of anorexia-cachexia syndrome in the elderly. *J Nutr Health Aging.* 2009;13:448-454.

46. Jatoi A, Windschitl HE, Loprinzi CL, et al. Dronabinol versus megestrol acetate versus combination therapy for cancer-associated anorexia: A North Central Cancer Treatment Group study. *J Clin Oncol.* 2002;20:567-573.

47. Wilson MM, Philpot C, Morley JE. Anorexia of aging in long term care: Is dronabinol an effective appetite stimulant? A pilot study. *J Nutr Health Aging.* 2007;11:195-198.

48. Emmelot-Vonk MH, Verhaar HJ, Nakhai Pour HR, et al. Effect of testosterone supplementation on functional mobility, cognition, and other parameters in older men: A randomized controlled trial. JAMA. 2008;299:39-52.

49. Peeters A, Barendregt JJ, Willekens F, et al. Obesity in adulthood and its consequences for life expectancy: A life-table analysis. Ann Intern Med. 2003;138:24-32.

50. Allison DB, Gallagher D, Heo M, et al. Body mass index and all-cause mortality among people 70 and over: The Longitudinal Study of Aging. Int J Obes Relat Metab Disord. 1997;21:424-431.

51. Calle EE, Thun MJ, Petrelli JM, et al. Body-mass index and mortality in a prospective cohort of US adults. N Engl J Med. 1999;341:1097-1105.

52. Hedley AA, Ogden CL, Johnson CL, et al. Prevalence of over-weight and obesity among US children, adolescents, and adults, 1999-2002. JAMA. 2004;291:2847-2850.

53. Nygaard HA. Measuring body mass index (BMI) in nursing home residents: The usefulness of measurement of arm span. Scand J Prim Health Care. 2008;26:46-49.

54. Heiat A, Vaccarino V, Krumholz HM. An evidence-based assessment of federal guidelines for overweight and obesity as they apply to elderly persons. Arch Intern Med. 2001;161:1194-1203.

55. Arterburn DE, McDonnell MB, Hendrick SC, et al. Association of body weight with condition-specific quality of life in male veterans. Am J Med. 2004;117:738-746.

56. Busetto L, Romanato G, Zambon S, et al. The effects of weight changes after middle age on the rate of disability in an elderly population sample. J Am Geriatr Soc. 2009;57:1015-1021.

57. Villareal DT, Banks M, Siener C, et al. Physical frailty and body composition in obese elderly men and women. Obes Res. 2004;12:913-920.

58. Villareal DT, Apovian CM, Kushner RF, et al. Obesity in older adults: Technical review and position statement of the American Society for Nutrition and NAASO, the Obesity Society. Obes Res. 2005;13:1849-1863.

59. Alley DE, Chang VW. The changing relationship of obesity and disability 1988–2004. JAMA. 2007;298:2020-2027.

60. Roubenoff R. Sarcopenia: Effects on body composition and function. J Gerontol A Biol Sci Med Sci. 2003;58:1012-1017.

61. Villareal DT, Banks M, Sinacore DR, et al. Effect of weight loss and exercise on frailty in obese older adults. Arch Intern Med. 2006:166:860-866.

62. Morey MC, Snyder DC, Sloane R, et al. Effects of home-based diet and exercise on functional outcomes among older, overweight long-term cancer survivors: RENEW: A randomized controlled trial. JAMA. 2009;301:1883-1891.

63. Field AE, Malspeis SM, Willett WC. Weight cycling and mortality among middle-aged or older women. Arch Intern Med. 2009;169:881-886.

64. Bales CW, Buhr G. Is obesity bad for older persons? A systematic review of the pros and cons of weight reduction in later life. J Am Med Dir Assoc. 2008;9:302-312.

65. Yassine HN, Marchetti CM, Krishnan RK, et al. Effects of exercise and caloric restriction on insulin resistance and cardiometabolic risk factors in older obese adults: A randomized clinical control trial. J Gerontol A Biol Sci Med Sci. 2009;64:90-95.

66. Rejeski WJ, Focht BC, Messier SP, et al. Obese, older adults with knee osteoarthritis: Weight loss, exercise, and quality of life. Health Psychol. 2002;21:419-426.

67. Messier SP, Loeser RF, Miller GD, et al. Exercise and dietary weight loss in overweight and obese older adults with knee osteoarthritis: The Arthritis, Diet, and Activity Promotion Trial. Arthritis Rheum. 2005;50:1501-1510.

68. Ryan AS. Nicklas BJ, Dennis KE. Aerobic exercise maintains regional bone mineral density during weight loss in postmenopausal women. J Appl Physiol. 1998:84:1305-1310.

69. Ryan AS, Ivey FM, Hullbut DE, et al. Regional bone mineral density after resistive training in young and older men and women. Scand J Med Sci Sports. 2004;14:16-23.

70. McCann RM, Hall WJ, Groth-Juncker A. Comfort care for termi-nally ill patients. The appropriate use of nutrition and hydration. JAMA. 1994;272:1263-1266.

71. White C, McMullan D, Doyle J. "Now that you mention it doctor...": Symptom reporting and the need for systematic ques-tioning in a specialist palliative care unit. J Palliat Med. 2009;12:447-450.

72. Finucane T, Christmas C, Travis K. Tube feeding in patients with advanced dementia. A review of the evidence. JAMA. 1999;282:1365-1370.

73. Sampson EL, Candy B, Jones L. Enteral tube feeding for older people with advanced dementia. Cochrane Database Syst Rev. 2009;2:CD007209.

74. Wollman B, D'Agostino HB, Walus-Wigle JR, et al. Radiologic, endoscopic and surgical gastrostomy; an institutional evaluation and meta-analysis of the literature. Radiology. 1995;197:699-704.

75. Potack JZ, Chokhavatia S. Complications of and controversies asso-ciated with percutaneous endoscopic gastrostomy: Report of a case and literature review. Medscape J Med. 2008;10:142.

76. Scott AG, Austin HE. Nasogastric feeding in the management of severe dysphagia in motor neuron disease. Palliat Med. 1994;8:45-49.

77. Gillick MR. Rethinking the role of tube feeding in patients with advanced dementia. N Engl J Med. 2000;342:206-210.

POST-TEST

1. Mr. R. is a 73-year-old retired banker with metastatic colon cancer currently undergoing systemic chemotherapy. He is concerned about his poor appetite and asks about appetite stimulants. Which of the following statements is TRUE?

   A. Megestrol acetate has been shown to increase weight in cancer patients with anorexia-cachexia syndrome.

   B. Dronabinol improves quality of life in elderly patients with weight loss.

   C. The side effects of appetite stimulants are minimal.

   D. Megestrol acetate improves survival in elderly patients with weight loss.

2. Mrs. N. is an 80-year-old nursing home resident with advanced Alzheimer disease. She is bed-bound and only able to say three words. Her family asks if a feeding tube would improve her ability to function or her prognosis. Which of the following information is TRUE?

   A. Feeding tubes help prevent bed sores in patients with dementia.

   B. Feeding tubes increase the interaction between patients and nursing home staff.

   C. Feeding tubes have not been shown to improve survival in patients with advanced dementia.

   D. Quality of life indicators in demented patients improve once a feeding tube is placed.

3. Mr. V. is a 67-year-old grocer with type II diabetes, hypertension, and a recent wrist fracture. He is obese with a BMI of 33 and is interested in dieting to lose weight. Which of the following weight loss regimes is recommended for this patient?

   A. No weight loss regime is recommended for persons over 65.

   B. A combined diet and resistive or weight-bearing exercise program.

   C. A low-carbohydrate diet with a goal caloric intake of less than 1200 kcal a day.

   D. Replacement of one meal with a meal supplement, such as Boost.

ANSWERS TO PRE-TEST

1. B
2. D
3. C

ANSWERS TO POST-TEST

1. A
2. C
3. B

36

The Frailty Syndrome

Peter Khang, MD, MPH, FAAFP

Kuo-Wei Lee, MD

● **LEARNING OBJECTIVES**

1. Define frailty, and describe the aspects of this syndrome.
2. Discuss the conditions that contribute to the development of frailty.
3. Describe the role of diminished physiologic reserve and other classic geriatric syndromes to frailty.
4. Delineate clinical signs, symptoms, and assessment tools that clinicians may use to identify frail and "pre-frail" patients.
5. Discuss interventions to prevent frailty.

PRE-TEST

1. **How would you define frailty?**

   A. A medical term for the common observation of the changes in an individual as they age

   B. A syndrome characterized by impairments across multiple systems that leads to a state of increased vulnerability

   C. A normal process of chronologic aging that makes those 65 years and older susceptible to medical complications

   D. A state of weakness that results solely from the synergistic effects of multiple chronic medical conditions

2. **All of the following have been identified as criteria that define frailty EXCEPT:**

   A. Gradual weight gain

   B. Low grip strength

   C. Slow gait speed

   D. Lower levels of activity

3. **Which of the following statements is FALSE?**

   A. Interventions involving physical reconditioning yield the most benefit in the pre-frail population as compared to the severely frail population.

   B. Because of some commonality between geriatric syndromes and frailty, interventions that address geriatric syndromes may have a benefit in decreasing disability associated with frailty.

   C. Results of frailty intervention trials vary depending on the population type, namely community-dwelling versus nursing home residents.

   D. Studies on frailty interventions have all showed a mortality benefit in the frailest group.

CASE PRESENTATION: A CHANGE IN WALKING

Mr. Devereaux is an 82-year-old retired accountant living with his wife in Los Angeles. He has a past medical history of hypertension, dyslipidemia, and osteoporosis. He is physically active, taking daily 30-minute walks in his neighborhood and he volunteers at the community hospital twice a week. He is independent in all basic and instrumental activities of daily living, but he reports it just takes him a little longer to do anything. He is still driving and his wife accompanies him for the visit to your office. She reports that he is doing pretty well, but she has noticed that he is walking more slowly. On further questioning, Mr. Devereaux admits to a 3- to 4-month history of decreased energy levels and being less physically active. He does not endorse any symptoms of depression or anhedonia. Review of systems is negative for fevers, night sweats, cough, dyspnea, abdominal pain, nausea, vomiting, diarrhea, or constipation.

INTRODUCTION

Geriatricians view frailty as a core geriatric syndrome, and provide skillful care to this highly vulnerable population. For years, clinicians have intuitively characterized some of their older patients as frail, based on their subjective impression. In the past two decades, working definitions of frailty have evolved—definitions that may lend themselves to research and clinical practice. Frailty is a serious public health issue. The frail elderly utilize health care and hospitals at a higher rate, and have the highest rates of disability. The main adverse outcomes associated with frailty include disability, hospitalization, and death. Estimates from studies suggest that approximately 7% of all adults over 65 years old are frail,[1] and that between 20% and 40% of those over 80 years old are frail. This will gain greater importance as the fastest-growing segment of the population—those who are 85 years and older—will have the highest proportion of frail elderly. This chapter introduces the reader to the important aspects of frailty, including the underlying biological and physiologic science, and the clinical approach to managing frailty.

THE FRAILTY SYNDROME DEFINED

Frailty is defined as a progressive, multisystem impairment and decreased physiologic reserve resulting in a state of increased vulnerability to stressors. The progressive impairment in multiple systems includes physiologic, inflammatory, immune, and biochemical systems. This intersystem dysregulation lowers physiologic reserves that are called upon to maintain homeostasis, thereby rendering the patient less able to withstand stressors such as infection or medication side effects. This state of increased vulnerability contributes to the high rate of adverse outcomes in the frail elderly.

As in other classical "syndromes," the pathogenesis, pathophysiology, and clinical manifestations of frailty are not fully understood or agreed upon.[2] Researchers have begun to define more precisely criteria for a variety of geriatric syndromes,[3] including frailty, and to relate these syndromes to emerging understandings of "multiple morbidity" that include system impairments, as opposed to cumulative effects of diagnosed diseases.[4] In fact, about 7% of patients who are clinically frail may have no accompanying illness, and one-quarter only one co-morbid disease.[5] Yet frailty may also occur after acute illness or with an end-stage chronic condition such as atherosclerosis, cancer, infection, and depression. These diseases, and conditions such as cognitive or balance impairment, anorexia, sarcopenia, and decreased physical activity, appear to play a large role in development of frailty.[6] Frailty should not be confused with its concomitant or resultant disabilities,[7] nor should old-age disability be confused with frailty. A minority of older people with IADL or ADL disabilities are frail, as their disabilities are not the result of multiple organ system failures but chronic disease processes such as dementia.[5]

The first study that successfully tackled the challenge of operationally defining frailty and linking it to outcomes was done by Linda Fried and colleagues in 2001.[1] Using the Cardiovascular Health Study, a prospective study of over 5000 adults over the age of 65, five criteria defined frailty:

- Weakness (low grip strength)
- Self-reported exhaustion
- Poor mobility (slow gait speed)
- Unintentional weight loss (10 lbs in the last year)
- Low levels of physical activity

Three or more of the criteria indicated frailty; intermediate frailty was having one or two of these. The primary outcomes were falls, institutionalization, decline in BADL/IADL function, and death. The incidence of frailty increased with age, from just 3.2% of the 65 to 70 age range to 25.7% of the 85 to 89 age group.[1] Frailty is more common in women, and in people with chronic illnesses, depression, disability, and lower income and education levels.[5] In the study by Fried and associates, frailty, as compared to the non-frail population, was independently associated with a higher rate of falls, hospitalization, worsening ADL disability and worsening mobility disability, and mortality.[1] People meeting the frailty criteria were shown to be at risk for these outcomes even when they were relatively functional. Thus, determining whether a patient is frail or at risk should be of considerable value in the clinical setting both for prognosis and possible interventions.

In an alternative approach, Rockwood and Minitski define frailty as a multifactorial and dynamic health state affected by an accumulation of a variety of deficits. Their Frailty Index measures these deficits, which include co-morbid illnesses, poor health attitudes, signs of disease, and self-reported disabilities. This measure combines items into a single index, which recognizes that frailty is multifactorial and dynamic. The conceptual basis of the "accumulation of deficit model" is the simple underlying probabilistic consideration: The more things individuals have that are wrong with them, the greater the likelihood they will be frail.[8] In a 2005 paper, Rockwood and colleagues introduced the Clinical Frailty Scale (CFS),[9]

● **TABLE 36–1** Canadian Study of Health and Aging Clinical Frailty Scale
1 *Very fit*—robust, active, energetic, well motivated, and fit; these people commonly exercise regularly and are in the most fit group for their age
2 *Well*—without active disease, but less fit than people in category 1
3 *Well, with treated comorbid disease*—disease symptoms are well controlled compared with those in category 4
4 *Apparently vulnerable*—although not frankly dependent, these people commonly complain of being "slowed up" or have disease symptoms
5 *Mildly frail*—with limited dependence on others for instrumental activities of daily living
6 *Moderately frail*—help is needed with both instrumental and non-instrumental activities of daily living
7 *Severely frail*—completely dependent on others for the activities of daily living, or terminally ill

Source: Rockwood K, Song X, MacKnight C, et al. CMAJ. 2005;173. doi:10.1503/cmaj.050051.

Based on the Canadian Study of Health and Aging Study, a 5-year prospective cohort study of 10,263 persons over the age of 65 years. The CFS is a seven-level scale (Table 36–1), which was used by practicing physicians and then correlated with previously established tools.

The authors found that each one-category increment on the CFS significantly increased the medium-term risk of death (21.2%) and becoming institutionalized (23.9%) in multivariate models. The CFS was judged an effective measure of frailty; it provided predictive information, similar to that of the established tools, about death or the need for institutionalization. Notably, the CFS mixes items such as co-morbidity, cognitive impairment, and disability that some other groups separate in focusing on physical frailty. A unique feature of the CFS is that it incorporates practitioners' judgment, and as such can be readily employed in the office setting. This judgment-based system seems to be a reasonable way to measure relative fitness and frailty and is widely accessible without the need for extensive data collection.[8]

CONDITIONS CONTRIBUTING TO DEVELOPMENT OF FRAILTY

Information around the underlying physiology and biochemistry of frailty has many implications in terms of early identification. The current state of knowledge of the relationship between frailty and underlying biochemical and physiologic processes is still evolving. A commonly accepted concept is that multisystem dysregulation narrows the breadth of complexity of responses that the body has available to maintain homeostasis.

Reduction of caloric intake and loss of appetite are to some extent part of normal aging. However, certain diseases, decreased physical activity, dysphoria, and poor oral health can result in chronic undernutrition and resulting weakness, wasting and micronutrient deficiencies (see Chapter 35). Anorexia can thus contribute to sarcopenia, decreased activity, and worsening of chronic diseases such as atherosclerosis.

Chronic inflammation is thought to play a role. Several studies have identified significant positive correlations between frailty and the inflammatory cytokine interleukin 6 (IL-6), C-reactive protein, and clotting factor VIII. Higher levels of these markers were associated with disability and mortality.[10,11] The correlation with frailty persists even after excluding persons with cardiovascular disease or diabetes.[12] Research demonstrates a biological link between elevated IL-6 and bone and muscle loss, anemia, insulin resistance, and altered immune system modulation.[12] The impact of these inflammatory markers is that they precede the features of frailty, such as weakness, exhaustion, low levels of activity, weight loss, and slow gait speed.

Age-related hormonal changes may also contribute. Age-related declines of growth hormone, insulin-like growth factor 1 (IGF-1), and the adrenal androgen, dehydroepiandrosterone sulfate (DHEA-S), are associated with loss of muscle mass and bone mass—both key components of physical frailty. DHEA-S has been shown to have a role in suppressing inflammatory signal transduction; declines in this hormone are likely to contribute to chronic inflammation.[11] Further, these hormonal problems can contribute to anorexia. Replacement with DHEA-S may reverse these changes in muscle when accompanied by exercise and in bone when taken alone.[13,14]

Sarcopenia—excessive loss of muscle mass associated with aging—can be viewed as the clinical hallmark of frailty and a central component. Currently, we think of older adults as being sarcopenic when the lean body mass is less than two standard deviations of the sex-specific mean in a young, healthy sample.[15] Muscle mass declines 15% from the third to eighth decades of life, and other studies suggest a more rapid rate of loss in the later decades, up to 15% per decade.[16] With sarcopenia, strength declines, leading to poor endurance, mobility, balance, and slowed gait. There is an accumulating body of knowledge of some of the potential contributing factors to sarcopenia. With aging, normal muscle tissue may be replaced by fat (myosteatosis) or fibrotic tissue, which results in a decline in muscle function.[15] Vitamin D deficiency can lead to poor muscle function. While sarcopenia is thought to be genetically determined to some extent, decreased physical activity, testosterone, and growth hormone deficiencies may aggravate sarcopenia, and present targets for intervention.[17]

In line with the concept of intercommunication of systems, the maintenance of a robust musculoskeletal system involves neurologic, hormonal, inflammatory, nutritional, and activity components. Thus, sarcopenia can be the result of the dysregulation of multiple systems, as well as disease and lack of physical activity. Musculoskeletal weakness may be the strongest, most unifying manifestation of the frailty phenotype, with its manifold implications for functional decline.

THE CONCEPT OF PHYSIOLOGIC RESERVE

Frailty involves a diminished physiologic reserve resulting in increased vulnerability to stressors to the system. What exactly does diminished physiologic reserve entail? All organisms

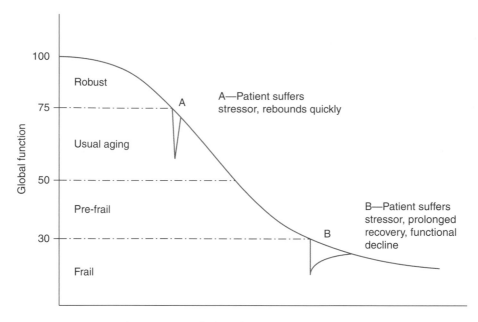

FIGURE 36-1. Impact of stressor on non-frail and frail patients.

exhibit redundant structure and function, called physiologic reserve. This reserve is called upon when a person experiences a stressor, such as a common cold or a hip fracture. Most body systems, when examined individually, need 30% of normal organ function as the threshold for adequate function.[7] In general, this means that there is a 70% margin of loss before the systems' impairment becomes evident. As a quantitative example, Bassey and colleagues have identified that young persons have 5 W/kg of strength in their legs. In order to walk, one needs 1.2 W/kg, or 24% of baseline. Below 0.5 W/kg, walking is no longer possible.[18]

It is not just the physiology of each organ, but perhaps more importantly, the intercommunication of organ systems that is central to frailty. It has been hypothesized that complex physiologic pathways allow for a wide range of adaptive responses, both quantitatively and qualitatively, in vital non-frail organisms.[10] Accordingly, frailty may result from one or more organs systems reaching a threshold of decline, which may trigger dysregulation in related systems, leading to a generalized decline in multiple clinical domains, including worsening of function and exacerbation of existing co-morbidities.[10]

Figure 36–1 illustrates the consequences of the resultant decline in functional reserve as well as the trajectory of persons who have the frailty syndrome. It is important to note that frailty is not a static condition, and as one travels down the "slippery path" of continual functional decline the reserve to handle stressors such in trauma, infection, stroke, and similar insults continues to be more and more limited. The end result of this is death. Patients have a life expectancy of 2 to 5 years at the time the diagnosis of frailty is made.[1]

● CLINICAL ASSESSMENT OF FRAILTY

While our understanding of the frailty syndrome evolves, research has established a set of clinical signs, symptoms, and assessment tools that clinicians may use to identify frail and

● TABLE 36–2 Clinical Indicators of Frailty	
Indicators/Criteria	Possible Measures
Mobility	Gait speed, Timed-Up-and-Go (TUG)
Strength	Grip (upper extremity) strength, chair-rise, knee extensor (lower extremity) strength
Endurance	Lack of energy, tiredness, oxygen consumption
Nutrition	Undernutrition/poor food intake, weight loss, body mass index, obesity
Physical inactivity	Under-use syndrome; frequency and duration of walking and bicycling in the previous week; average amount of time spent monthly on hobbies, gardening, odd jobs, and sports
Balance	Items from Berg Balance Scale (sit to stand, stand to sit, standing unsupported)
Motor processing	Coordination, movement planning, movement speed

Adapted from Daniels et al.[27]

"pre-frail" patients who have increased susceptibility to functional decline and to study interventions that may reverse or prevent further disability. Following Fried, mobility, strength, balance, motor processing, nutrition, endurance, and physical activity are the criteria for the syndrome.[19] Table 36–2 lists these criteria together with various measures that have been used in research and may be used in the clinical setting.

CASE PRESENTATION (continued)

When Mr. Devereaux enters the exam room, you notice that he is slightly stooped over and his gait is definitely slower than what you previously remember. However, his vital signs including his weight and exam are unchanged from previous visits, and clinically he looks about the same. There do not appear to be any new problems or diagnoses, such as knee arthritis, recent medical illness, Parkinson disease, or a recent stroke to explain why he has "slowed down." Since you have the proper arrangement of furniture you do a Timed Up and Go test as well as a measured gait speed test. Upon starting the Timed Up and Go test, you notice just a slight hesitation getting out of the chair and the first few steps are sluggish, but then he perks up and completes the activity in just under 13 seconds. Similarly, when you do the timed gait speed test, over 10 meters his gait velocity works out to 1.1 m/s. You are a bit puzzled as to what might explain his situation, but you are concerned that Mr. Devereaux might be "pre-frail" and worry about what further declines might bring. You suggest that he consider tai-chi classes offered at the community senior center to improve his balance and endurance.

INTERVENTIONS TO PREVENT FRAILTY

In their attempts to prevent and treat frailty, researchers have explored a broad array of interventions, including supplementation of vitamin D, vitamin E, carotenoids, creatine, or DHEA[20]; lower-extremity resistance training; walking programs; gait speed training; and balance training through computer feedback systems or traditional tai-chi quan forms.

The most promising interventions to date involve physical reconditioning, although the exact mode (strength, aerobic, balance, functional) and setting (individualized, group) have yet to be refined. The interpretation of studies reported as "positive" is tricky because of the heterogeneity of the elderly population, especially as it applies to the oldest old. For this reason, researchers often study a multicomponent regimen that incorporates nutritional supplementation and socialization in addition to a set of physical training components. A comprehensive review of interventions is beyond the scope of this chapter. Instead, we will focus on a few representative studies aimed at treating frailty.

Tai chi is an ancient form of Chinese martial arts. Tai chi has been employed by elderly Chinese as a daily exercise routine for centuries. The literature has shown positive benefits of tai chi on various health markers, including the reduction of falls in recurrent fallers.[21] Building on previous work, Wolf and associates found that in pre-frail elderly with a history of a previous fall, a 48-week intervention with tai chi was able to improve functionality. Specifically, participants of the tai chi intervention group reduced their time needed to complete three chair-rises, an outcome measure that correlates with the physical frailty indicator of muscle strength. By increasing lower-extremity strength, the tai chi intervention reduced the rate of falls and thus potential disability.[22]

Another group examined the effects of preventative moderate-intensity group exercise programs on physically pre-frail (one or two of Fried's five criteria) and frail (three or more criteria) elderly living in long-term care (LTC) facilities.[23] The three-armed study compared control subjects to those receiving a functional walking (FW) or an in-balance (IB) intervention. The FW intervention involved exercises that consisted of standing up from a chair, reaching while stepping forward and sideways, heel and toe standing, walking and turning, stepping on and over an obstacle, stair climbing, tandem foot standing, and single-limb standing. The IB intervention comprised seven therapeutic elements of tai chi that have been found to be the most beneficial in elderly persons, with emphasis placed on slow and continuous movements, trunk rotations, and weight shifting. Statistically significant fall reduction was achieved in the pre-frail group only after the interventions lasted for 11 or more weeks. The findings suggest that interventions aimed at preventing falls should be challenging (push the limits of balance) but safe, targeted to pre-frail individuals, and need to be of sufficient duration to see a benefit. The study also revealed that frail (not pre-frail) participants had a higher rate of falling after being randomized to either FW or IB, and no benefits were gained from these interventions. This is consistent with the notion that as a person progresses toward frailty with worsening physiologic reserve and progressive sarcopenia, there is a point at which interventions cannot reverse the downward decline toward disability and death.[15,24]

Chin and colleagues studied 157 frail community-dwelling elderly participating in a multidimensional trial consisting of five arms: control, exercise, nutritional supplementation, exercise, and nutrition. The trained participants showed statistically significant improvements in their functional performance and physical fitness scores, but not in their disability scores.[25] The successful component from this study was a twice-weekly group exercise routine that lasted for 17 weeks. Micronutrient supplementation was not associated with any functional benefits, consistent with other studies.[26] Results from this study show that community-dwelling frail individuals can improve in functional and physical fitness measures after intervention.

Daniels and colleagues recently reviewed clinical trials involving the prevention of disability in frail community-dwelling individuals.[27] There was again no evidence for nutritional interventions as a means of impacting disability outcomes. The trials that showed statistically significant improvements on disability outcomes were relatively long lasting (10-18 months) high-intensity multicomponent programs focused on strength, flexibility, balance, and endurance. One study found that the majority of disability outcomes were seen in participants with moderate but not severe frailty.[27]

GERIATRIC SYNDROMES AND FRAILTY

There is an intimate link between frailty and other classic geriatric syndromes, such as falls, depression, and incontinence. Tinetti and colleagues identified factors common to both.[28] For incontinence, falls, and functional dependence (the end result of frailty), four independent predisposing risk factors were identified: lower-extremity impairment (slowed chair-rise time), upper-extremity impairment (decreased arm strength), sensory impairment (decreased vision and hearing), and affective impairments (high anxiety or depression scores). The proportion of functional dependence doubled (from 7-14% to 28-60%) as the number of risk factors increased, and similar increases were observed for the other syndromes. Independent of these four risk factors, incontinence and falling were also associated with more functional dependence.[28] These results have important implications. First, the results confirm the importance of sarcopenia and its detrimental effect on upper- and lower-extremity strength as a manifestation of frailty. Second, the risk factors for frailty and for geriatric syndromes are themselves a mix of physical frailty indicators (upper- and lower-extremity weakness) and other geriatric syndromes (decreased sensorium, anxiety/depression). Just as interventions that address physical decline can reduce the adverse outcomes associated with frailty, interventions that treat geriatric syndromes may also impact adverse outcomes associated with frailty. In other words, addressing geriatric syndromes may provide a pathway for management of the frail elderly patient.

One proven and available method of addressing geriatric syndromes is comprehensive geriatric assessment (CGA) and management. CGA is a multidimensional interdisciplinary diagnostic process focused on determining a frail elderly person's medical, psychological, and functional capabilities in order to develop a coordinated and integrated plan for treatment and long-term follow-up.[29] While CGA programs are diverse, systematic reviews show that programs staffed by interdisciplinary teams providing long-term management and targeting older patients with features of geriatrics syndromes and frailty are likely to improve care outcomes.[30] Accordingly, the American Geriatrics Society states that CGA is most effective when targeted toward older adults who are at risk for functional decline (physical or mental), hospitalization, or nursing home placement, and that elements of CGA should be incorporated into the care provided to these at-risk elderly individuals. Unfortunately, in the United States these programs are not widely available. However, older patients having features of frailty and the geriatric syndromes might best be referred where these services exist (eg, in the VA health care system).[31]

CASE PRESENTATION (continued)

Seven months and several missed clinic appointments later you see Mr. Devereaux in the office again. This time he is accompanied by both his wife and daughter, who report that "we are concerned he is starting to really go downhill." In the intervening period, his wife and daughter report that he has really slowed down. He stopped his afternoon walks and quit his volunteering job at the hospital because he was "just too tired." He tends to spend much of the day now resting on the couch or doing only minimal activity. He is no longer able to open jars for his wife that she has trouble opening. After taking your history of Mr. Devereaux, you perform a careful review of his medication list, active medical problems, co-morbidities, and self-reported function. You look for any medications considered inappropriate to use in the elderly and find none. He has had no localizing symptoms, no pain, no shortness of breath, no changes in his condition other than he feels like he doesn't have the stamina he used to have. He admits to eating less, but says this is because his appetite is poor and not due to lack of access to food. His health screening is up to date, his last colonoscopy was 2 years ago, he had a PSA that was normal done within the last 8 months as well.

On exam, his blood pressure is 138/50 mm Hg, pulse 68, respirations/minute 18, temperature 98.8°F (37.1°C). His height is 70 in (1.78 m), weight has decreased from 170 to 157 lbs (77.3 to 71.4 kg), about 13 lbs (5.9 kg) lighter than the last visit. BMI = 22.5 (down from 24.4). On your exam, you note that he leans forward and pushes with his arms on the armrests of the chair getting up to go to the exam table. The musculoskeletal exam reveals mild bitemporal, interosseous, and quadriceps atrophy. Neurologic exam is unremarkable except for a generalized weakness, and the remainder of his exam provides no additional information other than he looks a bit deconditioned and thin. You perform a Timed Up and Go test. He has difficulty getting out of the chair, as you noted earlier, and his time to cover 10 feet (3.05 m) and sit down again is 24 seconds. You then have him walk a timed 10 meters (32.8 feet), which takes him 16.7 seconds, generating a gait speed of 0.6 m/s. These are both significant changes from your exam just a few months ago. You also have a hand dynamometer in the office, which shows a grip strength of 15 lbs (6.8 kg) in his dominant hand, which is significantly less than the mean of 65.8 lbs (29.9 kg) for men his age.

Laboratory studies show normal hemoglobin, white count, and platelets. Minerals and kidney function are normal, as is his thyroid stimulating hormone (TSH). A urinalysis shows no proteinuria or ketones and no signs of infection. His liver function tests were normal with the exception of albumin, which was low at 2.7 g/dL (27 g/L).

You believe that you have ruled out malignancy and exacerbation of any co-morbid condition. Based on his weight loss, slow gait speed, weakness, and symptom of exhaustion, you make the diagnosis of frailty. Based on your understanding of this syndrome, you discuss with Mr. Devereaux and his wife and daughter what to expect in terms of his condition and prognosis and ask that they begin to think about advanced care planning. The daughter states that she is concerned and she will need to think about the information but will probably have more questions in the next few days.

CASE DISCUSSION

Mr. Devereaux is an example of the clinical presentation of a pre-frail developing into frail older adult. Based on your knowledge of pre-frail states and the frailty syndrome, you took seriously his declines, ruled out other causes, and then made the correct diagnosis of frailty syndrome. You recognized that decreased levels of energy, slower gait speed, lower levels of physical activity, and weight loss were all components of the Fried frailty model. You evaluated Mr. Devereaux for major medical problems, but upon making the diagnosis of frailty informed him and his family that he would be vulnerable to stressors as well as a continued decline in function and health. In addition to your typical physical exam, you also measured gait speed as well as Timed Up and Go, knowing that it might provide information concerning the mobility component of frailty.

After suspecting that the patient might be pre-frail, you prescribed a community-based tai chi exercise regimen. You chose tai chi because it was a physical reconditioning intervention that would improve strength and dynamic balance. Ideally, you would have wanted Mr. Devereaux also to participate in a more multifaceted program that incorporated endurance and flexibility.

At this point in his care, it would be reasonable to refer Mr. Devereaux to a CGA clinic for further management. CGA clinic assessment of his medications to ensure that there were no medications contributing to his symptoms and condition, as well as administering screening tests for commonly seen geriatric syndromes such as depression, cognitive impairment, and falls, as well as care planning for his future dependency, would be in order. Unfortunately, as outlined in this chapter, the treatments available for frailty are very limited and generally have not been shown to have an effect. However, there does appear to be some benefit to identifying and treating pre-frail conditions. Nonetheless, good interdisciplinary team care can make Mr. Devereaux's transition to a more dependent person with declining health much easier and less distressing for his family.

CONCLUSION

Frailty is a common condition that increases in prevalence with age. It is also important to remember that it is a condition distinct from co-morbidity or multi-morbidity and functional decline. Clinicians should take every opportunity to recognize and intervene in those patients who appear to entering a pre-frail condition, as once the criteria for frailty are met the possibility for successful interventions diminishes greatly. Recognition of this condition should involve a team approach as well as health care planning involving both the patient and his or her family.

An exercise in assessing frailty is included at the end of the chapter (Table 36–3).

References

1. Fried LP, Tangen CM, Walston J, et al. Frailty in older adults: Evidence for a phenotype. *J Gerontol.* 2001;56A:M146-M156.

2. Bergman H, Ferrucci L, Guralnik J, et al. Frailty: An emerging research and clinical paradigm. Issues and controversies. *JGMS.* 2007;63:731-737.

3. Inouye SK, Studenski S, Tinetti ME, Kuchel GA. Geriatric syndromes: Clinical, research, and policy implications of a core geriatric concept. *J Am Geriatr Soc.* 2007;55:780-791.

4. Boyd CM, Ritchie CS, Tipton EF, et al. From bedside to bench: Summary from the American Geriatrics Society/National Institute on Aging Research Conference on Comorbidity and Multiple Morbidity in Older Adults. *Aging Clin Exp Res.* 2008;20: 181-188.

5. Ahmed N, Mandel R, Fain MJ. Frailty: An emerging geriatric syndrome. *Am J Med.* 2007;120:748-753.

6. Gillick M. Pinning down frailty. *J Geronol Med Sci.* 2001;56: M146-M156. Also RW Kressig, SL Wolf, RW Sattin. et al. Associations of demographic, functional, and behavioral characteristics with activity-related fear of falling among older adults transitioning to frailty. *J Am Geriatr Soc.* 2001;49:1456-1462.

7. Bortz W. A conceptual framework of frailty: A review. *J Gerontol A Biol Sci Med Sci.* 2002:57:M283-M288.

8. Rockwood K, Minitski A. Frailty in relation to the accumulation of deficits. *J Gerontol.* 2007;62A:722-727.

9. Rockwood K, Song X, MacKnight C, et al. A global clinical measure of fitness and frailty in elderly people. *CMAJ.* 2005:173:489-495.

10. Walston J, McBurnie MA, Newmann A, et al. Frailty and activation of inflammation and coagulation systems with and without clinical comorbidities. *Arch Intern Med.* 2002;162:2333-2341.

11. Leng SX, Cappola AR, Andersen RE, et al. Serum levels of insulin-like growth factor-1 and dehydro-epandrosterone sulfate (DHEA-S), and their relationships with serum interleukin-6, in the geriatric syndrome of frailty. *Aging Clin Exp Res.* 2004;16:153-157.

12. Walston J, Hadley EC, Ferrucci L, et al. Research agenda for frailty in older adults: Toward a better understanding the physiology and etiology: Summary from the American Geriatrics Society/National Institute on Aging Research Conference on Frailty in Older Adults. 2006;54:991-1001.

13. Jankowski CM, Gozansky WS, Schwartz RS, et al. Effects of dehydroepiandrosterone replacement therapy on bone mineral density in older adults: A randomized, controlled trial. *J Clin Endocrinol Metab.* 2006;91: 2986-2993.

14. Villareal DT, Holloszy JO. DHEA enhances effects of weight training on muscle mass and strength in elderly women and men. *Am J Physiol Endocrinol Metab.* 2006;291:E1003-E1008.

15. Morley JE, Haren MT, Rolland Y, et al. Frailty. *Med Clin North Am.* 2006;90:837-847.

16. Fried LP, Walston J. Frailty and failure to thrive. *Geriatric Medicine and Gerontology.* 5th ed. New York: McGraw-Hill; 2003.

17. Morley JR, Baumgartner RN, Roubenoff R, et al. Sarcopenia. *J Lab Clin Med.* 2001;137:231-243.

18. Bendall MJ, Bassey EJ, Pearson EJ. Factors affecting walking speed of elderly people. *Age Aging.* 1989;18:327-332.

19. Ferrucci L, Guralnik JM, Studenski S, et al. Designing randomized, controlled trials aimed at preventing or delaying functional decline and disability in frail, older persons: A consensus report. *J Am Geriatr Soc.* 2004;52:625-634.

20. Cherniak EP, Florez HJ, Troen BR. Emerging therapies to treat frailty syndrome in the elderly. *Altern Med Rev.* 2007;12:246-258.

21. Wolf SL, Barnhart HX, Kutner NG, et al. Reducing frailty and falls in older persons: An investigation of tai chi and computerized balance training. *J Am Geriatr Soc.* 2003;51:1794-1803.

22. Wolf SL, O'Grady M, Easley KA, et al. The influence of intense tai chi training on physical performance and hemodynamic outcomes in transitionally frail, older adults. *J Gerontol A Biol Sci Med Sci.* 2006;61:184-189.

23. Faber MJ, Bosscher RJ, Chin A, et al. Effects of exercise programs on falls and mobility in frail and pre-frail older adults: A multicenter randomized controlled trial. *Arch Phys Med Rehabili.* 2006; 87:885-896.

24. Fried LP, Xue Q-L, Cappola AR, et al. Nonlinear multisystem physiological dysregulation associated with frailty in older women: Implications for etiology and treatment. JGMS. 2009; 64A:1049-1057.

25. Chin A, Paw MJ, de Jong N, EG, et al. Physical exercise and/or enriched foods for functional improvement in frail, independently living elderly: A randomized controlled trial. *Arch Phys Med Rehabil.* 2001;82:811-817.

26. Fiatarone MA, O'Neill EF, Ryan ND, et al. Exercise training and nutritional supplementation for physical frailty in very elderly people. *N Engl J Med.* 1994;330:1769-1775.

27. Daniels R, van Rossum E, de Witte L, et al. Interventions to prevent disability in frail community-dwelling elderly: A systematic review. *BMC Health Serv Res.* 2008;8:278.

28. Tinetti ME, Inouye SK, Gill TM, Doucette JT. Shared risk factors for falls, incontinence, and functional dependence. Unifying the approach to geriatric syndromes. JAMA. 1995;273:1381-1383.

29. Rubenstein LZ. An overview of comprehensive geriatric assessment: Rationale, history, program models, basic components. In: Rubenstein LZ, Wieland D, Bernabei R, eds. *Geriatric Assessment Technology.* Milan: Kurtis; 1995.

30. Wieland D. The effectiveness and cost of comprehensive geriatric assessment. *Crit Rev Oncol Hematol.* 2003;48:227-237.

31. American Geriatrics Society. Comprehensive Geriatric Assessment Position Statement Last Updated August 26, 2005. http://www .americangeriatrics.org/products/positionpapers/cga.shtml.

POST-TEST

1. **The MOST promising frailty prevention/ intervention to date has been:**
   A. Social support
   B. Walking programs
   C. Nutritional interventions
   D. Physical reconditioning

2. **The strongest, most unifying manifestation of the frailty phenotype is:**
   A. Age-related hormone changes
   B. Musculoskeletal weakness
   C. Chronic inflammation
   D. Undernutrition

3. **Models of physical frailty include the following characteristics EXCEPT:**
   A. Weakness
   B. Slow walking speed
   C. Fatigue/exhaustion
   D. Morbid obesity (BMI > 50)

ANSWERS TO PRE-TEST

1. B
2. A
3. D

ANSWERS TO POST-TEST

1. D
2. B
3. D

● TABLE 36–3 Clinical Assessment of Frailty

As an exercise in assessing frailty, please rate the following cases on a scale of 0 to 100 in terms of frailty. Zero signifies a robust, non-frail person. One hundred signifies the frailest frail. Write your score in the adjacent box.

Conditions and Impairments	Score (0-100)
Unintended weight loss (20 lbs) + fear of falling	
Hypertension only	
HTN + arthritis + DM-well controlled on oral agents, fatigues on performance of ADLs + mild dementia (MMSE = 25), unsteady gait + in bed or chair most of day	
HTN + arthritis + DM-well controlled on oral agents	
Occasional urinary incontinence + unsteady gait + undernourished + difficulty with BADL due to weakness	
Dementia (MMSE = 20), dependent in IADL, independent for BADL	
Arthritis + depression + anxiety about gait stability (no falls) + poor stamina, goes outdoors infrequently + 2 falls in past 4 months	
Arthritis, independent in IADL and BADL	
Dementia (MMSE = 20), dependent in IADL, independent for BADL + generalized weakness, goes outdoors infrequently + unintended weight loss (20 lbs)	
Osteoporosis + h/o single compression fracture + generalized weakness	

Exercise 1: Results for Clinical Assessment of Frailty

While the operationalization of the definition of frailty and the research models continue to evolve, there is one certainty: there are many frail patients in our health care system. In a very illustrative study, experienced geriatricians were given several different patient descriptions and were asked to rate them on an arbitrary "frailty" scale of 0 to 100. The results of their collective appraisals are listed in the next part of the table. How did you compare to the geriatricians?

Some important findings came from that study. Ninety-eight percent of the respondents said that frailty and disability were separate clinical entities, but they thought that they were causally related. Importantly, individual diseases were not sufficient for identification of those who were frail. Nor were any two diseases or two disabilities alone. These findings from expert geriatricians suggest that it is the accumulation, or critical mass, of impairments or geriatric conditions that comprise the frailty phenotype.[2]

Geriatricians' Appraisal of What Is Clinically Identifiable Frailty

Conditions and Impairments	Score (± SD)	Comment
Hypertension only	5.8(13)	This was the lowest score.
Arthritis, independent in IADL and BADL	13.6(20)	
HTN + arthritis + DM-well controlled on oral agents	15.3(16)	
Dementia (MMSE = 20), dependent in IADL, independent for BADL	30.2(22)	So cognition has some role in frailty.
Osteoporosis + h/o single compression fracture + generalized weakness	37.3(23)	
Unintended weight loss (20 lbs) + fear of falling	42.6(22)	
Arthritis + depression + anxiety about gait stability (no falls) + poor stamina, goes outdoors infrequently + 2 falls in past 4 months	52.3(23)	The fear of falling can propagate a cycle of deconditioning.
HTN + arthritis + DM-well controlled on oral agents, fatigues on performance of ADLs + mild dementia (MMSE = 25), unsteady gait + in bed or chair most of day	64.6(24)	
Dementia (MMSE = 20), dependent in IADL, independent for BADL + generalized weakness, goes outdoors infrequently + unintended weight loss (20 lbs)	74.3(20)	
Occasional urinary incontinence + unsteady gait + undernourished + difficulty with BADL due to weakness	76(18)	Notice how the addition of functional deficits renders the patient more frail (even in absence of true diagnosis). This was the highest score.

Source: Fried LP, Ferruci L, Darer J, et al. Untangling the concepts of disability, frailty, and comorbidity: Implications for improved targeting and care. Journal of Gerontology: Medical Sciences (A). *2004;59:258.*

37

Evaluating and Treating Depression in Older Adults

Stephen Thielke, MD, MSPH, MA

Steven Vannoy, PhD, MPH

● **LEARNING OBJECTIVES**

1. Define depression in older adults, and describe how it presents in older adults.
2. Discuss the experience of older patients with depression.
3. Discuss diagnostic challenges in identifying and treating patients with depression.
4. Describe assessment of outcomes and treatment response during depression treatment.
5. Identify practical strategies for treating depression in clinical settings.

PRE-TEST

1. **What time frame is correct as a minimum requirement for diagnosis of major depression?**

   A. Two days, if they are severe enough

   B. One week

   C. Two weeks

   D. One month

2. **Which of the following is NOT one of the nine main symptoms of major depression?**

   A. Weight change

   B. Pessimism

   C. Thoughts of death or suicide

   D. Hearing voices or paranoia

3. **Which of the following is TRUE about minor depression?**

   A. Antidepressant treatments have little benefit for minor depression compared to placebo.

   B. Minor depression progresses into major depression.

   C. Minor depression is the same as adjustment disorder.

   D. In deciding a treatment, it does not matter what type of depression a patient has.

4. **Which of the following is TRUE about the origins of depression?**

   A. The causes of depression are easy to identify.

   B. Genetics are a main factor in determining who becomes depressed.

   C. Risk factors can explain almost all of the cases of depression.

   D. Older women are more likely than older men to be depressed.

CASE PRESENTATION: GETTING MY LIFE BACK

Mrs. Watson is a 76-year-old woman whose family told her she needed to return to her doctor because she kept crying and could not fall asleep. It took her over a year to do so. Eight years ago, her daughter died of breast cancer. Three years ago, her husband died after a short illness. She continued with all of her former activities, but became upset when her friends at her pottery class would talk about their husbands and children. Listening to them made her feel cheated, and she thought that it was unfair that she now was alone. She felt that her health was declining, although her only chronic medical condition was hypertension. She had occasional bouts of gastrointestinal distress and heart palpitations, which were worked up, but no cause identified. She stopped going to pottery class and spent more time at home. She noticed problems with her memory, losing her keys and misplacing her glasses. She had trouble falling asleep, and lost 5 lbs over the period of a year. She had thought about dying as a way to be with her husband, but did not have suicidal thoughts. When asked, she denied being depressed, saying, "It's been hard, but I get through. I need to keep going on. I think it's normal to feel like this after what I've been through." She had bouts of crying every few days, but said this was normal for someone in her situation. Two years ago her son and daughter encouraged her to seek help, and her primary physician, after hearing her symptoms, prescribed citalopram (Celexa) 10 mg per day, which she has taken since. During follow-up appointments, when asked about her mood, she replied, "Fine," and always denied suicidal ideation. Over the last year, she had been less active, and largely stayed at home. Her primary care provider continued to prescribe citalopram, but did not ask her how often she took it.

As part of a new program in her primary care clinic, Mrs. Watson received a screening test for depression, which suggested that she had major depression. She was enrolled in a collaborative care treatment program, in which a depression care manager met with her and reviewed her history and her preferences for treatment, then discussed the case with a consulting psychiatrist. The consulting psychiatrist recommended increasing the citalopram to 20 mg per day; her primary care provider prescribed this. Mrs. Watson's care manager found that she had not been taking the medication every day, since she was worried about the side effects. The care manager contacted her every 2 weeks by phone to ask how she was doing, to encourage taking the citalopram every day, and to administer a depression assessment tool, the PHQ-9, which was tracked in a database. There was no improvement in her symptoms after 3 months. The psychiatrist recommended increasing the citalopram to 30 mg per day, and Mrs. Watson began coming in to see the care manager to work on problem-solving treatment, identifying actionable steps she could take in her life. Her main goal was to start going to pottery class again. After 2 more months, her scores on the PHQ-9 suggested that her depression had remitted, and she was no longer having problems concentrating, with sleep, or with thoughts of death. "I feel like I have my life back," she told the care manager. The care manager continued to contact her every 2 months for the next year, and there were no further signs of depression.

● DEPRESSION AS A DIAGNOSIS

Almost everyone has experienced feeling down or sad at times. Particularly in response to stressful events, people describe themselves as blue, unhappy, or not well. Such low mood states are often accompanied by trouble sleeping, poor appetite, problems concentrating, lack of interest, distraction, and low energy. As Arateus, a Greek physician, described in AD 150, people with low mood appear "dull or stern, dejected or unreasonably torpid . . . They also become peevish, dispirited and start up from a disturbed sleep." Yet these sorts of experiences almost always abate, and human beings show a remarkable resilience and adaptation, even to extreme circumstances. People generally explain these sorts of reactions as natural, expect them to resolve, and almost never seek treatment for anticipated transitory states (thinking, "this will get better").

Yet in many cases, symptoms of low mood persist at an intense level, for weeks, months, or years. Mrs. Watson, for instance, continued to experience serious, daily symptoms for more than a year. At the outset, no one, probably not even a specialized mental health provider, could have predicted how long her symptoms would linger. This persistent state of low mood represents more than just a "bad day," "trouble coping," or "feeling stressed." It constitutes a specific clinical entity and diagnosis, called "major depression." The criteria used to define major depression entail:

- Low mood or loss of interest or pleasure
- Weight loss or weight gain
- Sleeping too much or too little
- Agitated or slowed down physical state
- Loss of energy
- Feelings of worthlessness or guilt
- Trouble concentrating
- Psychotic experiences (like hearing voices or paranoia)
- Thoughts of death or suicide

● **TABLE 37–1** Criteria for Major Depression

A. Five (or more) of the following symptoms have been present during the same 2-week period and represent a change from previous functioning; at least one of the symptoms is either (1) depressed mood or (2) loss of interest or pleasure. **Note:** Do not include symptoms that are clearly due to a general medical condition, or mood-incongruent delusions or hallucinations.

   (1) Depressed mood most of the day, nearly every day, as indicated by either subjective report (eg, feels sad or empty) or observation made by others (eg, appears tearful).

   (2) Markedly diminished interest or pleasure in all, or almost all, activities most of the day, nearly every day (as indicated by either subjective account or observation made by others).

   (3) Significant weight loss when not dieting or weight gain (eg, a change of more than 5% of body weight in a month), or decrease or increase in appetite nearly every day.

   (4) Insomnia or hypersomnia nearly every day.

   (5) Psychomotor agitation or retardation nearly every day (observable by others, not merely subjective feelings of restlessness or being slowed down).

   (6) Fatigue or loss of energy nearly every day.

   (7) Feelings of worthlessness or excessive or inappropriate guilt (which may be delusional) nearly every day (not merely self-reproach or guilt about being sick).

   (8) Diminished ability to think or concentrate, or indecisiveness, nearly every day (either by subjective account or as observed by others).

   (9) Recurrent thoughts of death (not just fear of dying), recurrent suicidal ideation without a specific plan, or a suicide attempt or a specific plan for committing suicide.

B. The symptoms do not meet criteria for a Mixed Episode (of bipolar disorder).

C. The symptoms cause clinically significant distress or impairment in social, occupational, or other important areas of functioning.

D. The symptoms are not due to the direct physiologic effects of a substance (eg, a drug of abuse, a medication) or a general medical condition (eg, hypothyroidism).

E. The symptoms are not better accounted for by bereavement (eg, after the loss of a loved one), and the symptoms persist for longer than 2 months or are characterized by marked functional impairment, morbid preoccupation with worthlessness, suicidal ideation, psychotic symptoms, or psychomotor retardation.

Source: Based upon the Diagnostic and Statistical Manual of Mental Disorders *(DSM-IV) of the American Psychiatric Association.*

For a formal diagnosis, 5 of these 9 symptoms must occur every day for 2 weeks or more. If these symptoms do not occur every day, but do occur more than half the days for 2 years or more, the diagnosis "dysthymia" applies. "Mild depression" defines those cases in which symptoms interfere with functioning or engagement in life, but either not enough of them (not 5 of 9) are present or their current duration is less than 2 weeks. Table 37–1 summarizes these criteria for major depression published in the *Diagnostic and Statistical Manual of Mental Disorders* (DSM-IV) of the American Psychiatric Association.

● DSM-IV DEPRESSION CRITERIA

Older adults with low mood often expect that their concerns do not merit attention or that they will spontaneously resolve, and that they thus ought to "tough it out" and avoid seeking or applying treatments. Many older adults hesitate to report mood symptoms, and instead present with physical symptoms such as insomnia, pain, fatigue, heart palpitations, headache, or gastrointestinal distress.[1] Patients may describe feeling anxious, worried, or distressed rather than depressed. Mrs. Watson, for instance, believed that her difficulties resulted from her life stressors, had physical symptoms, and only reluctantly admitted to low mood. Her provider never sought more information besides screening questions about mood and suicidality, both of which received negative responses.

Differentiating major depression from other mood problems among older adults may seem of only academic importance, but it has great relevance for diagnosis, prognosis, and treatment. Minor depression includes some of the symptoms listed earlier, but not 5 present for at least 2 weeks. Minor depression sometimes progresses into major depression, but often remits spontaneously. Current research suggests that some treatments for minor depression among older adults may have no more benefit than placebo.[2,3] Dysthymia, the presence of some depressive symptoms (but not enough for a diagnosis of major depression) for 2 years or more, often proves resistant to standard treatments for depression. Adjustment disorder, a response to a specific serious stressor, typically resolves on its own, and merits observation rather than aggressive treatment. As will be discussed later in the chapter, these differences between types of depression deserve attention in treatment planning. In the case of Mrs. Watson, the characteristics of her case that are consistent with major depression—presence of daily symptoms, no symptom-free periods, and a longer duration—all decrease the likelihood that her mood disorder will remit spontaneously, but also increase the likelihood that treatments for major depression could improve her condition. The clinician's assessment of a patient's type and degree of mood symptoms thus will modify treatment choice and affect treatment response.

Once present, major depression frequently persists, and about three-quarters of older adults with significant depressive symptoms continue to have them 1 year later.[4,5] Older adults with major depression often become "stuck" in this state. At the same time, most patients do not seek treatment for symptoms of low mood. As in the case of Mrs. Watson, patients often present to clinic only at the urging of their family members, and after prolonged periods of suffering. Despite strides to reduce the stigma surrounding mental health problems, patients find it difficult to admit feeling depressed, and sometimes perceive their symptoms (such as guilt, low energy, and trouble concentrating) as signs of moral weakness. Patients frequently present complaining of physical symptoms such as pain, insomnia, or fatigue,[6] when they primarily suffer from depression.

● DEPRESSION AS AN EXPERIENCE

Identifying the constellation of symptoms that occur in major depression does little to capture the experience of those who suffer from depression. Patients use a number of metaphors to describe how they feel, such as "swimming through concrete," "all out of gas with nowhere to go," or "stuck in park," as well as terms like "blue," "down," "in the dumps," "dark," "bleak," "a pit," or "an abyss." Psychologist Aaron Beck found that depressed patients hold negative views of themselves, the world, and the future—the so-called "cognitive triad of depression."[7] Depressed patients often cannot say exactly how they feel, and even those gifted in language have difficulty communicating about their internal depressed state. The author William Styron explored this core dilemma in his memoir, *Darkness Visible*: "Depression is a disorder of mood, so mysteriously painful and elusive in the way it becomes known to the self—to the mediating intellect—as to be very close to being beyond description."[8] He also found fault with the term *depression*: "For over seventy-five years the word has slithered innocuously through the language like a slug, leaving little trace of its intrinsic malevolence and preventing, by its very insipidity, a general awareness of the horrible intensity of the disease when out of control."

The theme of pain occurs frequently in accounts of depression, and depressed patients frequently report that their minds and bodies hurt. As Styron observed, "The gray drizzle of horrors induced by depression takes on the quality of physical pain." Often patients experience depression as even more painful, intense, and disabling that any sort of physical pain. As one patient noted, "I have suffered from severe, recurrent depression for 40 years. The psychological pain that I felt during my depressed periods was horrible and more severe than my current physical pain associated with metastases in my bones from cancer."[9] Research about suicide has identified psychological pain (also called "psychache") as a central theme in suicide notes, especially in the phrase "I can't stand the pain any longer."[10] Research has shown that physical pain and depression interact strongly, and that patients with pain respond poorly to many structured treatments for depression.[11,12] People with depression often, but not always, have thoughts of death or suicide. Some patients report that the state of death seems preferable to that of depression: "I would be better off dead."

Anxiety frequently co-occurs with depression. Although anxiety constitutes a separate diagnostic category from depression, in practice depression and anxiety generally represent two sides of the same coin, and the two occur, worsen, and improve simultaneously. Anxiety, in essence, is a state that arises when a person recognizes a mismatch or gap between how things are and how they should be—"something is not right." A small amount of anxiety is a normal, and in fact healthy, experience, and can motivate positive health behaviors (for instance, recognizing that one has not learned enough material before a test creates anxiety, which in turn prompts studying). But it can also become maladaptive, and occur with intense distress (as during panic attacks) and create worry around itself (called anticipatory anxiety—worry about being worried). Depression, in the same framework, is a state in which people are unable to move from where they are to where they want to be. The patients' descriptions given earlier about being "stuck" or "swimming in concrete" well encapsulate this dilemma. Depression has been also termed "learned helplessness," signifying the inability to accomplish aims or to direct energy toward improving one's situation.

The treatments for depression also generally improve anxiety, and psychotherapies geared at anxiety often focus both on the perceived mismatch between desired state and real state, as well as ways of becoming activated enough to move from one to the other.

● AGING, DISEASE, AND DEPRESSION

Patients and providers may perceive depression as a natural part of getting older, brought on by role changes, medical illness, declines in functioning, and deaths of friends or family. Some research, however, has found that the prevalence of major depression decreases with advancing age.[13] Recent longitudinal research suggests that the incidence of depression (how often it appears) does not vary with advancing age, but that the probability of depression resolving (how often it goes away) decreases, which results in an overall increase in the prevalence of depressive symptoms in older adults.[4] The existing evidence provides no evidence for the belief that depression occurs naturally as people age, or that it is an expected part of getting older. Research has repeatedly confirmed the association of depression with chronic medical conditions, such as diabetes, lung disease, heart disease, cancer, and chronic pain. Having a chronic condition increases a patient's likelihood of experiencing depression, and having depression compromises how patients maintain healthy behaviors and manage chronic diseases. The association is, in other words, bidirectional. Yet notwithstanding the strong association between chronic disease and depression, the majority of patients with even multiple co-morbidities do not become depressed,[14] so depression should not be seen as an inevitable consequence of medical illness.

Clinicians and researchers have sought to identify what causes depression in older adults, and if certain genetic, biological, or social factors predispose to its development as patients age. Such efforts have, in general, failed to identify highly specific predictive factors. Original typologies, such as "reactive" (in response to a situation or stressor) versus "endogenous" (genetic or without cause) depression, have lost favor because they correspond poorly to how real patients present, or to treatment response.[15] Genetic differences between people, despite initially promising results, appear not to predict depression,[16] and inheritance patterns have less relevance for the onset of depression in older compared with younger adults.[17] Older women become depressed more often than older men, although the rates of persistence or recurrence of depression do not differ significantly between the sexes.[5,18] Married older adults experience less depression than the widowed or divorced.[19] In general, risk factors account for only a small amount of the variance in the cause or persistence of depression in older adults,[20] and attempting to uncover exactly *why* someone becomes depressed mainly has little advantage for clinicians.[21]

While the same DSM-IV diagnostic criteria apply regardless of an adult patient's age, depression manifests differently in older compared with younger adults. Older adults less often endorse having a depressed mood, and show more frequent insomnia, anxiety, somatization (physical symptoms of distress), and hypochondriasis (concerns about and symptoms of medical illnesses that do not exist).[22] Research has found higher prevalence of cognitive problems, psychotic symptoms (such as auditory or visual hallucinations, or paranoia) in older compared with younger adults.[17] The death of a spouse, far more common in older than younger adults, frequently precedes depression,[20] and caring for a spouse with dementia also greatly increases the risk of depression.[17] Speculative work suggests that perceptions of relative disadvantage (comparing oneself negatively to one's social peers, as a consequence of social, physical, economic, or psychological changes during aging) may constitute the core of the experience of depression in older adults.[23] Mrs. Watson's depression started after her husband died, and she became caught up in feelings of relative disadvantage compared to her peers—she felt cheated that they still had their husbands.

Older adults often worry about having or getting Alzheimer dementia, and depression can, as noted, interfere with clarity of thought. As a depressed patient said, "I feel like I couldn't think my way out of a paper bag." Depressed patients have trouble concentrating, and often present with the concern that they are losing their minds or memories. The term "pseudodementia" applies to a state of serious cognitive impairment secondary to depression: when the depression lifts, normal memory and thinking return. While this concept seems plausible, extensive research has found that "pseudodementia" does not accurately describe patients' symptoms or prognosis. While patients with severe depression have troubles with concentration and attention, they do not manifest problems with memory or thinking similar to those of dementia.[2] Patients who present with both serious cognitive problems and depression often have, in fact, early dementia, and their cognitive symptoms do not improve if or when the depression remits. Depression may mark people at greater risk for cognitive problems, but does not in itself cause dementia.[24] Older adults who present with concerns about their memory thus merit a thorough medical evaluation and screening for memory problems, but most of those who have concerns about memory do not have dementia. For instance, the problems that Mrs. Watson reported (losing keys, misplacing glasses) stem from trouble with concentration rather than from memory loss, and do not raise red flags for early dementia, although she felt great distress about them.

• CHALLENGES IN TREATMENT OF DEPRESSION

This background about depression in older adults suggests some of the challenges in treating depression in clinical settings. Prior research has identified other key barriers that hinder older adults from receiving adequate care for depression, including knowledge deficits, social isolation, multiple medical problems, and lack of financial resources.[25,26] In discussing treatment, we will focus on issues most relevant for clinicians in their daily practice, and will then discuss how systems of care can improve management of depression. As we shall see, effectively treating depression depends not on picking the "one best treatment" at the outset, but on recognizing how patients present with and experience depression, applying and persistently reapplying

objective measures of treatment response, and making changes until the patient improves. It takes more than just one individual to accomplish these ends, and research has identified that "collaborative care" approaches for depression have significantly better outcomes than usual clinical care. Principles from collaborative care, discussed in more detail later, undergird this clinical approach to depressed older adults presented here.

Engaging Depressed Patients

Patients with depression often cannot explain in words how they feel despite self-awareness of suffering. The patient's low mood can darken a clinical encounter, and bring the interviewer down, too. The symptoms of depression directly impair engagement with others: few people enjoy talking with those who harbor negative thoughts, act sluggishly, feel guilty, cannot concentrate, do not care, have little energy, and have not slept well; nor does discussing these topics often make for stimulating dialogue. Providers sometimes report "having to do all the work" to elicit symptoms from depressed patients, or that clinical interviews with them feel "like pulling teeth." Patients may keep presenting with multiple nonspecific physical complaints such as pain or fatigue, none of which shows an objective cause, yet which require time-consuming medical workup, which would naturally frustrate providers. Patients may also, despite showing overt signs of depression, minimize their symptoms, or may give answers that discourage further questioning. Mrs. Watson, for instance, continued to report being "fine" despite little improvement in her condition. Providers, in turn, may experience relief when patients talk about another topic besides low mood. Research has confirmed these observations: primary care physicians, even when under observation, often fail to assess older adults for depression, and if they do, they spend an average of about 2 minutes on the entire process.[27,28]

Providers may find it especially hard to talk with people who have suicidal thoughts, not only because the subject requires time and care to address, but also because the patient's wish to die may seem illogical, outside the domain of normal shared human experience, or morally wrong—seeing the world from the patient's perspective would require the provider to connect with, acknowledge, or share in the patient's deep despair. In fact, research suggests that physicians with personal or vicarious experience with depression (through a family member or close friend) spent more time talking with depressed patients than those without this experience.[29] Yet for all providers, establishing rapport with, empathizing with, and working to help depressed patients can prove challenging.

Providers can deal with this barrier to treatment by recognizing their own emotional reactions while talking with patients. Automatic thoughts may sometimes suggest, even to mental health providers, that a patient is overreacting to stressors, is intentionally remaining sad, is not trying hard enough, or should just "pull herself up." Recognizing that depression constitutes a clinical condition, that it frequently lingers for years, and that patients cannot simply will themselves out of it, can help reframe one's perspective on depressed patients who receive care in clinical settings.

Identifying Causes

As described earlier in the chapter, differentiating major depression from adjustment disorder and minor depression has relevance for treatment selection and prognosis. Patients only rarely present with the complaint, "I am depressed," and busy clinical visits allow little time for extensive questioning about mood status, coping, and mental health symptoms. Patients often present with physical symptoms (pain, gastrointestinal distress, palpitations, insomnia) rather than complaints of low mood, and endorse physical (also called somatic) symptoms rather than psychological ones. Even when time allows, and when the clinician has expertise in mental health, the differences between major depression, minor depression, and adjustment disorder with depressed mood remain subtle. The contexts in which patients provide information may also determine how they present their symptoms; often patients have a harder time expressing despair in face-to-face interviews than on paper. A very experienced family physician reported (in personal communication to the author) a case of a patient, whom he had treated for over 30 years, and whom he had never identified with a mental health problem, who endorsed all the symptoms of depression, including a long-standing plan to shoot himself, when given a computer-directed screening instrument in the waiting room.

Research has found that instruments to screen for and track depression reliably identify and quantify depression in older adults, and determine when improvements occur. Current clinical guidelines strongly recommend using such instruments. Examples include the Patient Health Questionnaire (PHQ-2 and PHQ-9), the Geriatric Depression Scale (GDS-15), the Center for Epidemiological Studies-Depression Scale (CES-D), and the Zung Depression Rating Scale Inventory.[30] None of these appears superior to the others, and the patient-level benefit likely arises out of the act of measuring and monitoring, and not from specific organization or content of these screening or tracking tools.

A shorter version, the PHQ-2, includes two questions about symptoms during the last 2 weeks. Clinical work demands efficiency, and for identifying cases initially the PHQ-2 has shown "the best mix of brevity, sensitivity, and ease of administration,"[31] and has been tested in older adult populations.[32]

PHQ-2

Over the past two weeks, how often have you been bothered by any of the following problems?

1. Little interest or pleasure in doing things.
   0 = Not at all
   1 = Several days
   2 = More than half the days
   3 = Nearly every day
2. Feeling down, depressed, or hopeless.
   0 = Not at all
   1 = Several days
   2 = More than half the days
   3 = Nearly every day

Total point score: _____

A score of 3 or greater on the PHQ-2 is associated with a 75% probability of a depressive disorder,[33] and justifies further evaluation, such as completion of the full PHQ-9 or another instrument. Other instruments to screen for and track depression in community practice include the Center for Epidemiological Studies Depression Scale (CES-D), the Geriatric Depression Scale (GDS), and the Zung Self-Rating Depression Scale (ZSDS). Few substantial differences have been found between these instruments,[34] and it is more important routinely and consistently to apply a systematic tool for quantifying depression than to focus on finding the one best tool. Mrs. Watson's depression, for instance, went unidentified for a long period because her provider asked her only general questions and applied a subjective sense of her mood state. We recommend that clinicians try a number of different screening and tracking instruments to determine which fits best with their particular clinical environments.

Evaluating Suicidal Risk

Anyone who has experienced the suicide of a family member, friend, colleague, or acquaintance, or has even only heard second-hand about a suicide, has felt some of the hurt, loss, sadness, and tragedy of the event. Most people find it very unpleasant and aversive to talk with those who say they want to die, and human impulse may discourage us from bringing up the topic. Yet suicide happens—not commonly but not uncommonly—in depressed patients, and remains a significant cause of death in older adults. As such, it demands treatment. Every evaluation of a depressed patient should include some assessment of suicidal risk.

Suicides are the eighth leading cause of death for males and the seventeenth for females.[35] Older adults have the highest suicide rates, and among adults 65 years and older, suicide attempts are more lethal: for every four suicide attempts one results in death. Older men have higher rates of completed suicide than older women. Non-Hispanic white men and women have higher rates than other ethnic groups. Older men with alcohol dependence and mood disorders have especially high rates of completed suicide, about ten times that of the general population. The most common means of suicide, in older men, remains firearms, and in older women, poisoning. Access to firearms greatly increases the risk of completed suicide.[36]

Clinical encounters provide an opportunity for assessing suicide and taking steps to prevent it. Patients often seek medical treatment in the period before they attempt or complete suicide, more commonly from general medical providers than from mental health specialists.[37] All providers can thus intervene to reduce the risk of completed suicide. Yet several misconceptions impede the evaluation of suicide in primary care settings. First, providers may worry that bringing up suicide will "put thoughts in the patient's head" and encourage action. In fact, asking about suicide-related topics, such as thoughts of death, wish to die, access to lethal means, or prior attempts, does not increase the chance that patients will take action to hurt or kill themselves.[38] Providers should thus ask patients about suicidal thoughts whenever assessing depression. Second, providers may expect that patients will not admit to having suicidal thoughts, that "If I asked, they wouldn't tell me the truth anyway." But extensive clinical experience and research suggest that patients will—if asked—share honestly how they feel and think about suicide, as well as their wishes or plans around it. Providers should thus ask, and accept what patients say at face value. Patients will generally also share this information on paper-based or electronic screening forms.[39,40]

Third, providers may worry that if a patient completes suicide after being asked, the provider will be at fault and open to a lawsuit, and that they can thus protect themselves by not asking at all. This expectation, in addition to showing a disregard for the patient, also confuses malpractice with an error in judgment. While every provider who cares for patients could find himself or herself the target of a lawsuit, cases in which the provider asked the patient about suicidality, documented the answer, and deemed risk level as low almost never have resulted in malpractice suits or in judgments against the provider. Cases, however, where the provider did not assess suicidality in very depressed patients, documented high suicidality without any other information or plan, or took no steps to limit risks create the most medicolegal exposure. Providers should thus not worry that talking about suicide increases their liability.

How, then should providers screen for and assess suicidality in older adults? The tracking instruments for depression described above each contain questions about suicide. Providers should become familiar asking a question such as "Have you had thoughts of hurting or killing yourself?" and should ask this as part of every depression evaluation. No single approach can dictate how to respond when a patient expresses suicidal thoughts or reports self-harm, but some general principles apply to the type of information to obtain. First, providers should ask for details about the plan, for instance time, place, means, and other details (eg, "Do you have an actual plan of how you would kill yourself?"). If yes, assess for the accessibility of means (eg, "Do you have a gun? Do you have ammunition? How strong is your wish to die? What would it take to make you act on these thoughts?") Second, providers should assess the lethality and availability of the means (such as guns, medications, or poisons). Third, they should examine protective factors, such as religious or cultural beliefs, family ties, or concerns about the afterlife.[41,42] Fourth, providers should make an assessment of the degree of risk of suicide, and document this in the medical record. Fairly broad qualitative categories suffice, such as "very low," "low to moderate," "moderate," and "high."

Fifth, if a provider believes that a patient poses an imminent risk, he or she must take steps to secure the patient's immediate safety, as by arranging for psychiatric hospital admission, consulting immediately with a mental health specialist, or contacting legal agencies. Even without imminent risk, providers can give patients contact information for suicide hotlines and other local resources. Sixth, it is important to validate the patient's thoughts and feelings and level of distress. This can be done with simple reflections, "You are feeling like life just isn't worth it anymore" and then following up with "I'm sorry that you are feeling so distressed, your life is important to me and I'd like to discuss this further." With good rapport established on this topic, providers should feel free to suggest that patients not attempt suicide, pointing out

that it is a "bad problem-solving approach," "a decision that cannot be reversed," or "a really bad way to try to solve your problems." This approach attempts to instill a "reasonable doubt" in the minds of patients, to discourage them from making a dramatic and irreversible mistake. Providers can also educate patients that, while no person can know exactly what happens after we die, we know the tragedy of suicide for survivors, and also know that the surviving family members of those who completed suicide, and especially their children, suffer enormously and have a higher probability of completing suicide themselves.[43]

Finally, providers must continue to reassess depressed patients for suicidal thoughts. The absence of suicidality at one time point does not ensure its absence later, and research has found that suicidal thoughts often appear during the course of depression.[44] All of these steps in evaluation of suicidal intent may appear intimidating, but do not take much time during a clinical interview, and function directly to sustain the life and well-being of the patient. Consider how hard a provider would strive, with medications, treatments, and advice, to improve some health-related parameter like blood sugars, to save a limb, or to extend a patient's lifespan. Addressing and dealing with suicide has just as much, or probably even more, overall benefit for patients and the population as do more objective medical approaches to improving health.

We recommend that providers develop their own brief protocol for identifying people at risk, assessing their level of risk, making clinical decisions about how to manage that risk, executing the clinical management plan, and conducting follow-up. Such a protocol should include any standard assessment items that the provider wants to collect, some guidelines for assigning level of risk, a list of mental health professionals that the provider can contact and refer suicidal patients to, and some mechanism to ensure follow-up with this patient in a short time frame as well as over time.

Practical Suggestions for Treating Depression in Older Adults

Health care providers have several options for treating depression, some of which they can provide themselves, and some of which require referral to other providers. At first glance, the best treatment approach might seem obvious: use medications designed and marketed to treat depression (antidepressants), or refer to providers specializing in mental health (psychiatrists or psychologists). Unfortunately, most such "single-prong" approaches to depression treatment fail to achieve significant improvements. For example, in the largest depression intervention among older adults to date, patients in the "usual care" arm of the study, in which primary care physicians managed depression, had a very high likelihood of remaining depressed: only 19% of them had a significant reduction in their symptoms of depression at one year.[45] Other studies have confirmed this theme of limited response, and have also found that efforts to improve practice in primary care settings through better screening, guidelines, or referral to specialists generally fail.[46]

Given this theme of limited response to standard methods of treating depression, what can providers do? We propose that paying more attention to nuanced differences in treatments (for instance, one antidepressant medication versus another, or one type of therapy versus another, or a medication versus a medication with therapy), will help providers very little. Published research often suggests to clinicians that attending to novel, "statistically significantly better," or "evidence-based" approaches will result in better patient outcomes, but doing so often diverts attention from the real-world issues faced by providers, and has little evidence of benefit. Instead of presenting a comprehensive algorithm for treating depression in older adults, or offering a canonical framework for describing and incorporating the complex interplay of medical, psychological, and social issues into treatment planning, we offer several practical recommendations about treating depression in older adults, which may apply differently to different clinical settings.

Ask about Alcohol Abuse

Depression and problem drinking often co-occur.[47] While adults 65 years and older have fewer problems with substance abuse than do younger adults, and only rarely with drugs,[48] roughly 2% report heavy alcohol use, and roughly 6% report binge drinking. Screening for alcohol abuse or dependence takes only a few minutes, and should happen as part of all clinical encounters about mental health. Various tools can be used for screening, such as CAGE, AUDIT-C, and RAPS4. For instance, the CAGE questionnaire asks four questions about alcohol use: Have you ever felt you should cut down on your drinking? Have people annoyed you by criticizing your drinking? Have you ever felt bad or guilty about your drinking? Have you ever had a drink first thing in the morning to steady your nerves or get rid of a hangover (eye-opener)? Two or more positive responses is considered clinically significant. As with depression screening, it is more important that screening be performed than that providers pick the one best test. Recognizing and treating problem drinking can greatly improve depression, as well as providing benefit in itself.

When Using Medications, Avoid Undertreatment

Antidepressant medications have become the mainstay of therapy for mood disorders. Antidepressants have demonstrated efficacy over placebo, but must be used appropriately to have benefit. For some treatments, a direct relationship exists between dose and response; for instance, a half dose of a medication would produce half of the outcome. For others, no response happens until the patient takes a threshold dose of the medication. While the mechanism of antidepressant effect remains somewhat nebulous, some evidence suggests that antidepressants given at low doses or to treat mild symptoms may have no clinical benefit over placebo.[49] Providers, however, in an attempt to minimize risks, sometimes offer treatments at doses lower than the "full" doses, or may assume that older adults require less medication than their younger counterparts. Medication doses in primary care tend to fall short of recommended doses.[50] Mrs. Watson, for instance,

took 10 mg of citalopram (about half of a full dose) for several years. Using the "right" dose of treatment does not guarantee success, but using an inadequate dose will ensure lack of drug benefit.

Even with an appropriate dose, many patients do not take antidepressants as prescribed: in one study, almost one-third (28%) of older adults with depression did not adhere to the prescribed antidepressant treatment, and non-adherence was associated with worse depression outcomes. Perhaps the biggest factor in undertreatment is the assumption on the part of the provider that if the patient is not improving, the patient will seek a change in treatment. While this may hold true for acute conditions like rashes and sore throats, depressed patients are often already demoralized, and a failure to respond to treatment is likely to instill a hopeless attitude; hence providers must be vigilant in tracking progress, proactively adjusting treatment appropriately, and encouraging adherence. Mrs. Watson, for instance, never told her provider that she was not taking the antidepressant medication every day, nor did the provider ask about this.

Antidepressant side effects can also interfere with adherence and successful outcomes. The newer antidepressants (such as mirtazapine, fluoxetine, sertraline, citalopram, escitalopram, paroxetine, venlafaxine, duloxetine, and bupropion) cause fewer serious side effects than older medications, but still have important side effects which patients dislike. These include stomach upset, a feeling of being "revved up," weight loss, and sexual dysfunction (difficulty with erections in men, or interest in sex, arousal, or orgasm in both men and women). Most of these side effects (except sexual dysfunction) resolve spontaneously over the first few weeks of medication use. The choice between various antidepressant medications can be complicated, but several practical principles can help with older adults. Mirtazapine tends to increase appetite and cause sedation, which often are advantageous side effects in older adults who have insomnia and weight loss. Drug interactions with antidepressants are common, especially in older patients who are taking a large number of medications, and citalopram or escitalopram is often used because both have fewer interactions. Bupropion does not cause sexual dysfunction, although it can worsen anxiety. We recommend that prescribing providers review side effect profiles carefully with their patients.

The key to effective medication use therefore lies not in picking the one and only best treatment initially, but in monitoring outcomes and making changes if treatment response does not occur. Recent psychiatric research has stressed that while many patients do not achieve adequate responses from the first antidepressant regimen they take, with ongoing medication monitoring and modification most cases of depression can either remit or improve considerably.[51]

Measure and Track Outcomes

When treating a patient for high blood pressure, a provider would measure blood pressure at every visit. While we lack a tool like a blood pressure cuff to measure depressive symptoms, numerous scales (like the PHQ-9 and GDS-15, described earlier) can quantify degree of depression over time. Treating depression as a "laboratory value" can help remind providers of the primary importance of outcomes.[52] Asking a patient, "How are you?" and taking an answer of "Fine" to signify absence of depression (as in the case of Mrs. Watson) does not suffice. Commonly, the clinician will identify a patient as depressed, prescribe a medication, and see the patient back for multiple follow-up visits, but never measure how the depressive symptoms change over time. Although well intentioned, and probably better than doing nothing, this unmeasured approach does little to make patients better. Successful interventions for improving depression, such as collaborative care programs described later in this chapter, use systematic tracking systems to monitor symptoms of depression over time. Some rely on sophisticated Internet-based tracking tools.[53] These approaches affirm that "If you're not measuring something, you can't assume it's getting better." Large-scale analyses have suggested that patient outcomes greatly improve when patients receive systematic tracking and follow-up.[54] Depressive episodes frequently recur, and even after patients improve providers should continue to monitor symptoms for at least a year.[50]

Change Treatments If They Have No Positive Effect after About 2 Months

No treatment for depression will guarantee success, and the most effective interventions for geriatric depression produce clinically relevant remission of depressive symptoms in roughly 50% of patients.[55] As mentioned earlier, usual care shows remission rates of roughly 20% at one year.[45] Given these low rates of response, providers must monitor symptoms and consider switching to another treatment (different dose of medication, different medication, different modality of therapy) if the patient has not improved. As a rule of thumb, if the scores on depression tracking tools remain high and unchanged after 2 months of "full-dose" treatment, then the provider should change the treatment. This principle urges providers to define and to provide full-dose treatment to depressed patients. More commonly, as in the case of Mrs. Watson, patients begin and remain on an ineffective treatment for months or years, and continue to have the same limited response: "If you always do what you've always done, you'll always get what you've always got." Providers, who work hard to help their patients, can be lulled into believing that the sincerity of their efforts will suffice to combat depression, and that providing treatments, advice, or referrals must be enough. Such an approach relies on the "fallacy of good reasons" and the "fallacy of good intentions"—that if someone tries earnestly enough, successful outcomes are guaranteed. In fact, systematic reviews of depression treatments have underlined the importance of adapting treatments around objective measures of response, and not relying on the provider's intentions or goals.

Consider Nonphamacologic Treatments

Of the available treatments for depression, medications fit most naturally into medical settings—providers feel comfortable prescribing drugs, and patients often ask directly for them. Marketing on television and in magazines encourages patients to ask for specific medications. Physicians may thus perceive antidepressant medications as their primary tool for

treating depressed patients. But this should not imply either that most patients want medications, or that medications most effectively treat depression. In fact, many patients seek to avoid taking medications,[56,57] and want instead to talk about their current stressors and to build skills at dealing with their mood problems. Psychotherapy can produce lasting benefits, confers few or no side effects, and may be cost-effective.[58,59] Researchers have found no substantial or general differences between antidepressant treatments and psychotherapy in patient outcomes.[57] These perspectives encourage providers to offer psychotherapy or counseling to depressed patients, either in addition to or instead of medications. There are common misconceptions that older adults are not amenable to psychotherapy interventions, but the literature is clear: psychotherapy for older adults is a viable treatment option. Undertreatment is a problem for therapies as well as for medications. Even brief psychotherapies for depression require more than just one or two visits,[58] and advice ("Get over it," "Cheer yourself up," "Try to get active") or bibliotherapy (recommending books to read), if not supplemented, are inadequate to address the main issues.

Refer to Specialty Care As Needed, But Do Not Assume It Will Occur

Ideally, busy providers could refer patients to specialists in mental health care, who would conduct a thorough assessment, develop a treatment plan with the patient, follow up on depressive symptoms over time, and more generally, assume responsibility for the patient's mental health. In reality, most patients referred for specialty mental health care either never have an initial appointment, or quit coming after one or two appointments with a psychiatrist, psychologist, or other mental health professional. For instance, even mental health specialists provide inadequate (as defined by HEDIS measures) follow-up for depression in roughly half of cases.[60] Patients "fall through the cracks" when referred for specialty care, either because they experience stigma about having a mental health diagnosis, because of cost, because they prefer to receive treatment in their primary care setting, because they believe the risks outweigh the benefits, or for other reasons.

An indication of patients' general preference against receiving treatments for depression appears in the high rates of discontinuing treatments: in primary care practices, about half of patients with depression had no follow-up visit for depression at 6 weeks, and over one-third did not refill their prescription for an antidepressant medication.[50] These problems occurred as much in specialty care as in primary care.[61] Providers should thus not assume that a referral to a psychologist, psychiatrist, counseling, or therapist will suffice to cure or even apply novel treatments for depression, and providers in general medical settings remain the primary agents for monitoring symptoms and changing treatments. The likelihood of follow-up with specialty providers should inform the decision about when to refer out of primary care. There is no single right answer about when to refer a depressed older adult to specialty mental health treatment, but as with other specialty services, referrals work best when some dialogue is sustained between the primary care provider and the specialist.

Specialty mental health providers conduct thorough evaluations to determine if other psychiatric or medical conditions may be responsible for the patient's symptoms. Occasionally, patients are found to suffer from bipolar disorder rather than depression. Specialty clinics can apply some treatments not commonly available in primary care. They may initiate psychotherapy. They may augment treatment with other medications such as antipsychotics. For patients who do not respond to initial treatments, electroconvulsive therapy (ECT) can be tried. ECT is considered a safe treatment in older adults, and is the single most effective short-term treatment for severe depression.[62] Because it is a significant medical procedure and carries some significant side effects, in particular short-term memory loss, it is undertaken only with care and with the informed consent of the patient.

It May Be Clinically Acceptable to Watch and Wait

This discussion of the importance of treatment should not pressure providers to treat depression frenetically or desperately. The principles discussed here encourage careful monitoring and follow-up, but do not identify one best treatment, or require the use of any treatment for all patients with depression. The low rates of remission in most treatments for depression (about 20% in usual care) argue against a pressured urgency in applying treatments. This situation contrasts with other conditions, such as infections, where treatments have a very high likelihood of producing benefit, or where failure to treat guarantees a bad outcome. Treating depression with a medication or therapy may, in many cases, show no difference from no formal treatment. Many patients, even those under observation in research studies, express preference for this form of "watchful waiting" over active treatment.[63, 64] The lack of clinically significant differences between treatment and placebo occurs especially among patients with less severe symptoms.[49] Adjustment disorder, the low mood that results in response to a specific stressor, typically resolves spontaneously. In other words, in cases where the provider cannot exactly differentiate major depression from minor depression, or major depression from adjustment disorder, the effects of active treatment may produce the least benefit. In these cases, frequent monitoring of symptoms and frequent reconsideration of treatments may produce as much benefit for patients as a medication or psychotherapy, and may fit better with the patient's desires. This approach is not the same as ignoring symptoms or telling a patient that "nothing can help you"; rather, it entails discussing with the patient the risks and benefits of treatments, agreeing on observation as a treatment plan, and continuing to monitor symptoms over time. Patients in "watchful waiting" may feel more empowered to work through their own methods for dealing with depression; so while they are not using "medical" treatments, they are not doing nothing.

Understand That Depression Impacts How Patients Make Decisions

For most medical conditions, we may rightly assume that patients' decisions about treatment derive from their knowledge, values, and preferences, and that if appropriately informed patients will make decisions which others should respect and accept. Severely depressed patients, however, often neglect themselves and make poor medical decisions. They may not take important medications to control diabetes or blood pressure, or may have severe weight loss. These patients may at the same time refuse treatment either for depression or for their other medical problems. Providers may feel at a loss for how to help these patients either to combat depression or to address pressing medical problems. Mrs. Watson did not suffer from any life-threatening illnesses requiring treatment, but often older patients with severe depression will refuse to have conditions treated, for which the treatment would be expected to effect a cure. For instance, depressed patients may be unwilling to accept treatment for tumors that can be removed surgically, metabolic abnormalities that can be corrected, or chronic conditions like severe hypertension that put patients at great risk. In some cases, providers will refer patients to mental health courts, who decide if a patient has the decisional capacity to refuse treatment for existing conditions, and if treatment can be mandated. Although such referral requires careful consideration, and may result in treatment that is formally against the will of the patient, addressing the patient's depression through forced treatment can in some cases save the patient's life.

Collaborative Care for Depression

Extensive research has demonstrated that improving treatments of depression for older adults necessitates more than simply better screening, treatment selection, more referrals, or better follow-up. In fact, most carefully studied interventions have found that single-prong quality improvement interventions geared at provider behavior do not produce patient-level improvements.[26,46] Put simply, effective treatment for depression in general clinical settings requires more than a single provider who "does it all alone." Rather, it requires a team approach, involving the patient, the provider, a mental health consultant, and a designated agent, called a depression care manager or depression care coordinator. This approach, called collaborative care, developed and tested over the last decade, has demonstrated superiority to usual care across diverse clinical settings in the treatment of depression among older adults. Rather than describing how collaborative care has better outcomes than usual care,[55,65,66] we will give an example and outline its key components. As we shall see, collaborative care addresses many of the patient-level, provider-level, and systemic barriers already discussed.

Mrs. Watson benefited from collaborative care, with a process that worked as follows. Her primary care provider gave her a screening tool, which identified significant depressive symptoms, and as a result she was referred to the depression care manager (CM). The CM met with her at her primary care clinic, reviewed her history and symptoms, discussed treatment options, and agreed on an approach. The CM reviewed the case with a consulting psychiatrist, who recommended increasing the citalopram to 20 mg. The CM informed the primary care provider, who prescribed the higher dose of medication. Mrs. Watson continued to have symptoms, and the consulting psychiatrist recommended increasing the dose to 30 mg. Mrs. Watson met with the CM, and related her recent stressors and problems coping with life changes. She and the CM decided to conduct problem-solving treatment (a structured, brief form of psychotherapy[67]), which they continued once per week for 6 weeks. After that, the CM made contact with Mrs. Watson every week or so, either in person or on the phone. At each encounter the CM completed a PHQ-9 form to measure depressive symptoms, and entered the data into an electronic database. The consulting psychiatrist and the CM reviewed Mrs. Watson's case once a month, by looking at a graph of her symptoms over time, talking about her treatment, and determining if they should make changes. Mrs. Watson's scores on the PHQ-9 fell after about 2 additional months. The CM and consulting psychiatrist developed a relapse prevention plan, which involved taking the medication for 9 months and then reassessing. The CM continued to contact Mrs. Watson once a month to measure her degree of symptoms.

The essential elements of collaborative care, as seen in this example, involve the roles and functions described in the next sections.

Care Manager

Based in a primary care clinic, the care manager gets to know the patient, and formulates current symptoms, stressors, coping mechanisms, and treatment preferences. Based on familiarity with the patient, the CM provides tailored patient education about depression and treatment and collaborates with the patient to develop a treatment plan. The CM measures and tracks symptoms over time using a database, and checks with the patient about treatment use—for instance, medication adherence and side effects. He or she consults with the consulting psychiatrist to determine treatment plans, making changes if no improvement has occurred after about 2 months. The CM provides education about the role of behavioral activation in combating depression and reinforces the patient for engaging in regular pleasant activities. The CM often, but not always, offers brief structured therapy, such as problem-solving therapy. The CM recommends treatment changes to the primary care provider, who prescribes them to the patient. After the depression has improved, the CM develops a relapse prevention plan, and continues to contact the patient and to measure degree of depression.

Consulting Psychiatrist

The consulting psychiatrist reviews the case and provides suggestions for treatment changes. These activities happen in scheduled meetings with the CM, usually once per week, at which time they look over all of the cases, usually using the summaries from the tracking tool. In cases where the patient does not improve, or shows other psychiatric symptoms, the consulting psychiatrist may schedule a visit with the patient, and then discuss the case further with the CM.

Primary Care Provider

The primary care provider identifies patients with depression and refers them to the CM. The primary care provider receives feedback from the CM about suggested treatment changes, and prescribes any medications.

Although this brief account only sketches out how collaborative care works, it suggests how including a structured treatment plan and a responsible agent, the care manager, overcomes some of the barriers to treating depression in older adults. The CM has responsibility and dedicated time for addressing depression, ensuring that patients do not "fall through the cracks" or that other medical issues do not push depression down the list of immediate concerns. By using a structured tracking tool, the CM continues to measure outcomes and recommend treatment changes if no improvement occurs after several months, ensuring that ineffective treatments do not continue unchanged. The CM serves as a connection between a mental health expert and a primary care provider, allowing specialty care to happen efficiently within a primary care setting. The CM discusses treatment preferences with the patient, and tries to provide matching treatments, which increases patient engagement.[56] The CM does not drop patients after their depression improves, but develops a relapse prevention plan, continues to track their symptoms, and provides more intense care if depressive symptoms recur.

Collaborative care interventions are the most effective treatments known for depression in older adults, but many clinical settings do not have access to them at present. Providers can learn about these models of care, and attempt to incorporate their principles, such as by using structured screening and tracking tools, discussing patient preferences, monitoring symptoms over time, changing ineffective treatments, and planning for relapse prevention after depression improves. Practically, however, providers will have trouble managing all these tasks within busy clinical settings, and experience has shown the importance of a dedicated, responsible agent (the care manager) in organizing and following through on the details. Systems of care will likely increasingly adopt collaborative care approaches in the future, especially as they show economic advantages over usual care.[68]

SUMMARY

Depression can bring more suffering to patients than many other medical problems, yet patients often do not tell their providers about feeling depressed. Older patients especially become "stuck" in a depressed state, and may consider it to be normal. Many treatments for depression can succeed, and providers can greatly improve their patients' lives, or even give them a sense of a new life, by treating their depression. At the center of this process, as we have seen, lie process-related issues: consistently tracking and monitoring depression and not letting patients fall through the cracks or linger in depression. There is no one "right" way to treat depression, but the maxim "Never do nothing" applies well, encouraging us to talk with patients about how to approach their treatment, to assess risk frequently, to try and change treatments until improvements happen, to use structured treatment programs like collaborative care when available, and to persist in these aims.

References

1. Weinberger MI, Raue PJ, Meyers BS, Bruce ML. Predictors of new onset depression in medically ill, disabled older adults at 1 year follow-up. *Am J Geriatr Psychiatry.* 2009;17:802-809.

2. Alexopoulos GS. Clinical and biological interactions in affective and cognitive geriatric syndromes. *Am J Psychiatry.* 2003;160:811-814.

3. Ackermann RT, Williams JW Jr. Rational treatment choices for non-major depressions in primary care: an evidence-based review. *J Gen Intern Med.* 2002;17:293-301.

4. Thielke S, Diehr P, Unützer J. Prevalence, incidence, and persistence of major depressive symptoms in the Cardiovascular Health Study. *Aging Mental Health.* In press.

5. Harris T, Cook DG, Victor C, et al. Onset and persistence of depression in older people—Results from a 2-year community follow-up study. *Age Ageing.* 2006;35:25-32.

6. Simon GE, VonKorff M, Piccinelli M, et al. An international study of the relation between somatic symptoms and depression. *N Engl J Med.* 1999;341:1329-1335.

7. Brown GP, Hammen CL, Craske MG, Wickens TD. Dimensions of dysfunctional attitudes as vulnerabilities to depressive symptoms. *J Abnorm Psychol.* 1995;104:431-435.

8. Styron W. *Darkness Visible: A Memoir of Madness.* London: Jonathon Cape; 1991.

9. Mee S, Bunney BG, Reist C, et al. Psychological pain: A review of evidence. *J Psychiatr Res.* 2006;40:680-690.

10. Shneidman ES. Perspectives on suicidology. Further reflections on suicide and psychache. *Suicide Life Threat Behav.* 1998;28:245-250.

11. Thielke SM, Fan MY, Sullivan M, Unutzer J. Pain limits the effectiveness of collaborative care for depression. *Am J Geriatr Psychiatry.* 2007;15:699-707.

12. Kroenke K, Shen J, Oxman TE, et al. Impact of pain on the outcomes of depression treatment: Results from the RESPECT trial. *Pain.* 2008; 134:209-215.

13. McDougall FA, Kvaal K, Matthews FE, et al. Prevalence of depression in older people in England and Wales: The MRC CFA Study. *Psychol Med.* 2007;37:1787-1795.

14. Katon W, Lin EH, Kroenke K. The association of depression and anxiety with medical symptom burden in patients with chronic medical illness. *Gen Hosp Psychiatry.* 2007;29:147-155.

15. Paykel ES. Basic concepts of depression. *Dialogues Clin Neurosci.* 2008;10:279-289.

16. Risch N, Herrell R, Lehner T, et al. Interaction between the serotonin transporter gene (5-HTTLPR), stressful life events, and risk of depression: A meta-analysis. *JAMA.* 2009;301:2462-2471.

17. Gottfries CG. Is there a difference between elderly and younger patients with regard to the symptomatology and etiology of depression? *Int Clin Psychopharmacol.* 1998;13(suppl):S13-S18.

18. Luijendijk HJ, van den Berg JF, Dekker MJ, et al. Incidence and recurrence of late-life depression. *Arch Gen Psychiatry.* 2008;65: 1394-1401.

19. Mancini AD, Bonanno GA. Marital closeness, functional disability, and adjustment in late life. *Psychol Aging.* Sep 2006;21(3):600-610.

20. Schoevers RA, Smit F, Deeg DJ, et al. Prevention of late-life depression in primary care: Do we know where to begin? *Am J Psychiatry.* 2006;163:1611-1621.

21. Monroe SM, Reid MW. Gene-environment interactions in depression research: Genetic polymorphisms and life-stress polyprocedures. *Psychol Sci.* 2008;19:947-956.

22. Shahpesandy H. Different manifestation of depressive disorder in the elderly. *Neurol Endocrinol Lett.* 2005;26:691-695.

23. Blazer DG. How do you feel about...? Health outcomes in late life and self-perceptions of health and well-being. *Gerontologist.* 2008;48:415-422.

24. Modrego PJ, Ferrandez J. Depression in patients with mild cognitive impairment increases the risk of developing dementia of Alzheimer type: A prospective cohort study. *Arch Neurol.* 2004;61:1290-1293.

25. Unutzer J, Katon W, Sullivan M, Miranda J. Treating depressed older adults in primary care: Narrowing the gap between efficacy and effectiveness. *Milbank Q.* 1999;77:225-256.

26. Thielke S, Vannoy S, Unutzer J. Integrating mental health and primary care. *Prim Care.* 2007;34:571-592, vii.

27. Tai-Seale M, Bramson R, Drukker D, et al. Understanding primary care physicians' propensity to assess elderly patients for depression using interaction and survey data. *Med Care.* 2005;43:1217-1224.

28. Tai-Seale M, McGuire T, Colenda C, et al. Two-minute mental health care for elderly patients: Inside primary care visits. *J Am Geriatr Soc.* 2007;55:1903-1911.

29. Geraghty EM, Franks P, Kravitz RL. Primary care visit length, quality, and satisfaction for standardized patients with depression. *J Gen Intern Med.* 2007;22:1641-1647.

30. Sharp LK, Lipsky MS. Screening for depression across the lifespan: A review of measures for use in primary care settings. *Am Fam Physician.* 2002;66:1001-1008.

31. Watson LC, Zimmerman S, Cohen LW, Dominik R. Practical depression screening in residential care/assisted living: Five methods compared with gold standard diagnoses. *Am J Geriatr Psychiatry.* 2009;17:556-564.

32. Li C, Friedman B, Conwell Y, Fiscella K. Validity of the Patient Health Questionnaire 2 (PHQ-2) in identifying major depression in older people. *J Am Geriatr Soc.* 2007;55:596-602.

33. Kroenke K, Spitzer RL, Williams JB. The Patient Health Questionnaire-2: Validity of a two-item depression screener. *Med Care.* 2003;41:1284-1292.

34. Snowden M, Steinman L, Frederick J, Wilson N. Screening for depression in older adults: Recommended instruments and considerations for community-based practice. *Clin Geriatr.* 2009;17:26-32.

35. National Center for Injury Prevention and Control WISQARS (Web-based Injury Statistics Query and Reporting System). http://www.cdc.gov/injury/wisqars/. Accessed Jan. 15, 2010.

36. Miller M, Lippmann SJ, Azrael D, Hemenway D. Household firearm ownership and rates of suicide across the 50 United States. *J Trauma.* 2007;62:1029-1034; discussion 1034-1025.

37. Luoma JB, Martin CE, Pearson JL. Contact with mental health and primary care providers before suicide: A review of the evidence. *Am J Psychiatry.* 2002;159:909-916.

38. Hall K. Suicide prevention topic 7: Does asking about suicidal ideation increase the likelihood of suicide attempts? *NZHTA Report,* 2002.

39. Mann JJ, Apter A, Bertolote J, et al. Suicide prevention strategies: A systematic review. *JAMA.* 2005;294:2064-2074.

40. Fliege H, Becker J, Walter OB, et al. Evaluation of a computer-adaptive test for the assessment of depression (D-CAT) in clinical application. *Int J Methods Psychiatr Res.* 2009;18:23-36.

41. SLAP Scale. http://www.ssw.umich.edu/simulation/rube-assessmentScales pdf. Accessed Jan 15, 2010.

42. Mitty E, Flores S. Suicide in late life. *Geriatr Nurs.* 2008;29: 160-165.

43. Barrero SA. Preventing suicide: A resource for the family. *Ann Gen Psychiatry.* 2008;7:1.

44. Vannoy SD, Duberstein P, Cukrowicz K, et al. The relationship between suicide ideation and late-life depression. *Am J Geriatr Psychiatry.* 2007;15:1024-1033.

45. Unutzer J, Katon W, Callahan CM, et al. Collaborative care management of late-life depression in the primary care setting: A randomized controlled trial. *JAMA.* 2002;288:2836-2845.

46. Simon GE, Fleck M, Lucas R, Bushnell DM. Prevalence and predictors of depression treatment in an international primary care study. *Am J Psychiatry.* 2004;161:1626-1634.

47. Kirchner JE, Zubritsky C, Cody M, et al. Alcohol consumption among older adults in primary care. *J Gen Intern Med.* 2007;22:92-97.

48. Substance use among older adults. *National Household Survey on Drug Abuse* http://www.oas.samhsa.gov/2k1/olderadults/olderadults.htm. Accessed Jan. 15, 2010.

49. Kirsch I. Challenging received wisdom: Antidepressants and the placebo effect. *Mcgill J Med.* 2008;11:219-222.

50. Lin EH, Katon WJ, Simon GE, et al. Low-intensity treatment of depression in primary care: Is it problematic? *Gen Hosp Psychiatry.* 2000;22:78-83.

51. Rush AJ, Warden D, Wisniewski SR, et al. STAR*D: Revising conventional wisdom. *CNS Drugs.* 2009;23:627-647.

52. Oslin DW, Ross J, Sayers S, et al. Screening, assessment, and management of depression in VA primary care clinics. The Behavioral Health Laboratory. *J Gen Intern Med.* 2006;21:46-50.

53. Unutzer J, Choi Y, Cook IA, Oishi S. A web-based data management system to improve care for depression in a multicenter clinical trial. *Psychiatr Serv.* 2002;53:671-673, 678.

54. Solberg LI, Trangle MA, Wineman AP. Follow-up and follow-through of depressed patients in primary care: The critical missing components of quality care. *J Am Board Fam Pract.* 2005;18:520-527.

55. Williams JW Jr, Gerrity M, Holsinger T, et al. Systematic review of multifaceted interventions to improve depression care. *Gen Hosp Psychiatry.* 2007;29:91-116.

56. Gum AM, Arean PA, Hunkeler E, et al. Depression treatment preferences in older primary care patients. *Gerontologist.* 2006; 46:14-22.

57. Chilvers C, Dewey M, Fielding K, et al. Antidepressant drugs and generic counselling for treatment of major depression in primary care: Randomised trial with patient preference arms. *BMJ.* 2001; 322:772-775.

58. Churchill R, Hunot V, Corney R, et al. A systematic review of controlled trials of the effectiveness and cost-effectiveness of brief psychological treatments for depression. *Health Technol Assess.* 2001;5:1-173.

59. Bosmans JE, van Schaik DJ, de Bruijne MC, et al. Are psychological treatments for depression in primary care cost-effective? *J Ment Health Policy Econ.* 2008;11:3-15.

60. National Committee for Quality Assurance (NCQA). The State of Health Care Quality: Industry trends and analysis. Quality Compass. Washington, DC; 2007

61. Simon GE, Von Korff M, Rutter CM, Peterson DA. Treatment process and outcomes for managed care patients receiving new antidepressant prescriptions from psychiatrists and primary care physicians. *Arch Gen Psychiatry.* 2001;58:395-401.

62. Little A. Treatment-resistant depression. *Am Fam Physician.* 2009; 80:167-172.

63. Johnson MD, Meredith LS, Hickey SC, Wells KB. Influence of patient preference and primary care clinician proclivity for watchful waiting on receipt of depression treatment. *Gen Hosp Psychiatry.* 2006;28:379-386.

64. Dobscha SK, Corson K, Gerrity MS. Depression treatment preferences of VA primary care patients. *Psychosomatics.* 2007;48: 482-488.

65. Hunkeler EM, Katon W, Tang L, et al. Long term outcomes from the IMPACT randomised trial for depressed elderly patients in primary care. *BMJ.* 2006;332:259-263.

66. Gilbody S. Depression in older adults: Collaborative care model seems effective. *Evid Based Mental Health.* 2008;11:44.

67. Haverkamp R, Arean P, Hegel MT, Unutzer J. Problem-solving treatment for complicated depression in late life: A case study in primary care. *Perspect Psychiatr Care.* 2004;40:45-52.

68. Unutzer J, Katon WJ, Fan MY, et al. Long-term cost effects of collaborative care for late-life depression. *Am J Manag Care.* 2008;14:95-100.

POST-TEST

1. **Which of the following is useful as a SCREENING instrument for depression, but NOT a tracking instrument?**
   A. The Geriatric Depression Scale (GDS)
   B. The Center for Epidemiological Studies-Depression Scale (CES-D)
   C. The Zung Depression Rating Scale
   D. The Two-Item Patient Health Questionnaire (PHQ-2)

2. **Which group has the highest rate of completed suicide?**
   A. Older (> 65 years old) women
   B. Younger (< 50 years old) women
   C. Older (> 65 years old) men
   D. Younger (< 50 years old) men

3. **Which of the following is FALSE about assessing suicide?**
   A. No suicidal thoughts on initial assessment does not mean they will not surface later.
   B. Asking about suicidal thoughts increases a patient's likelihood of attempting suicide.
   C. Providers who find that a patient is at imminent risk for suicide are obligated to make a plan for immediate safety.
   D. Providers can express sincere concern about a patient's distress, and suggest that the patient not attempt suicide.

4. **Which statement is TRUE about nonpharmacologic treatments (such as therapy or counseling) for depression?**

   A. Nonpharmacologic treatments do not work as well as medications.

   B. Most patients prefer medications to other forms of treatment.

   C. Psychotherapy is often cost-effective.

   D. Advice (such as "cheer yourself up") is an effective treatment.

ANSWERS TO PRE-TEST

1. C
2. B
3. A
4. D

ANSWERS TO POST-TEST

1. D
2. C
3. B
4. C

38

Pressure Ulcers

David R. Thomas, MD

● **LEARNING OBJECTIVES**

1. Describe the pathophysiology for development and changes present in pressure ulcers.
2. Discuss the intrinsic and extrinsic risk factors for pressure ulcers.
3. Explain strategies for reducing pressure, shear, and friction.
4. Delineate the general principles of pressure ulcer therapy.
5. Compare and contrast local wound treatment for pressure ulcers.
6. Describe the process for wound debridement.
7. Discuss complications associated with pressure ulcers.

PRE-TEST

1. **The single most important strategy in the prevention of pressure ulcers is to:**
   A. Operationalize a risk-assessment tool.
   B. Relieve pressure.
   C. Massage the skin.
   D. Use a skin lubricant.

2. **The single most important strategy in the treatment of pressure ulcers is to:**
   A. Change the dressing daily.
   B. Culture the wound.
   C. Use a topical antimicrobial.
   D. Maintain a moist wound environment.

3. **The single most important strategy in nutritional support of pressure ulcers is to:**
   A. Provide 1.2 to 1.5 g of protein/kg body weight per day.
   B. Provide 4000 kilocalories per day or 30% over recommended intake.
   C. Provide arginine supplements three times a day.
   D. Provide 2000-mg supplements of vitamin C daily.

CASE PRESENTATION: A CONCERNING DEVELOPMENT

Mrs. Jones is a 76-year-old African American widow who has long-standing type 2 diabetes mellitus with complications of peripheral neuropathy, retino-proliferative eye disease without blindness, and chronic kidney disease stage 3. Her other medical conditions include hypertension, peripheral vascular disease with an ankle arm index of 0.75 on the left leg and 0.60 on the right leg, diastolic dysfunction congestive heart failure with normal left ventricular function, and degenerative arthritis of most of her large joints with total joint replacement of her left knee, 3 years ago. She is on 15 different medications for her medical conditions, many of which she doesn't know what they are for.

She lives in her own home but has a part-time aide who helps with her with medications, preparing meals, shopping, and bathing. While getting up to go to the toilet last night, she slipped on the bathroom rug and fractured her right hip. A total hip replacement was performed in the hospital. By the third post-operative day she developed a stage 3 pressure ulcer on her coccyx. She also reports that her right leg was painful and her aide notices an oval red ulcer on the right lateral malleolus of her ankle measuring approximately 2 cm by 1 cm.

• INTRODUCTION

Pressure ulcers are rare, affecting only about 0.5% of the total population. The distribution is clustered into two groups, peaking once in younger, mostly neurologically impaired persons and again in older persons. The cluster in the geriatric population accounts for about 70% of all pressure ulcers.[1]

Pressure ulcers are a frequent complication of hospitalization, but only about 1% of hospitalized patients develop a pressure ulcer. The frequency is particularly common in patients with hip fracture, in those who require treatment in the intensive care unit, or those who undergo neurologic or cardiovascular surgical procedures. Up to 36% of patients with a hip fracture develop a postoperative pressure ulcer.[2]

About 95% of pressure ulcers occur in the lower part of the body. The sacral and coccygeal areas, ischial tuberosities, and greater trochanteric areas account for the majority of pressure ulcer sites.[3] The sacrum is the most frequent site (36% of ulcers). The heel is the next most common site (30%), with other body areas each accounting for about 6% of pressure ulcers.[4,5] In hospital settings, pressure ulcers often develop within 72 hours of a surgical procedure.

• PATHOPHYSIOLOGY

A pressure ulcer is the visible evidence of a pathologic interruption in blood flow to dermal and intradermal tissues.[6] The chief cause has historically been attributed solely to pressure, or force per unit area, applied to susceptible tissues. Pressure is concentrated wherever weight-bearing points come in contact with surfaces. These weight-bearing points usually occur over a bony prominence.[7]

Although the cause of pressure ulcers is sometimes naively attributed solely to external pressure, factors intrinsic to the patient also contribute to the development of a pressure ulcer.[8] The high incidence in hospitalized patients may result from unavoidable immobilization after surgery, the need for support of blood pressure with pressors, low cardiac output, or tissue hypoxia. In the case of Mrs. J., the presence of peripheral arterial disease increases the risk of developing a pressure ulcer and may result in delayed healing. The presence of diabetes and its associated complications (microvascular circulatory changes and altered pain perception) also contribute to the development of a pressure ulcer.

Provocative research into skin blood flow may shed some light on the development of pressure ulcers. In patients selected for lengthy abdominal or spine surgery, skin blood flow was monitored before and during surgery. Pressure ulcers developed in 36% of subjects. Contrary to the hypothesis that prolonged pressure reduces skin blood flow, an increase in skin blood flow was observed in most subjects during surgery. However, skin blood flow decreased to half of the preoperative level in persons who developed pressure ulcers, while skin blood flow increased to 500% of maximum baseline value in persons who did not develop pressure ulcers.[9] In other studies, the skin's neural response to cold stimulation produces differences in skin blood flow among older subjects who do or do not develop pressure ulcers. A positive correlation exists between the blood flow response time over the greater trochanter and the development of pressure ulcers.[10]

• RECOGNIZING RISK

A primary risk factor for development of a pressure ulcer is immobility. Immobility may result from casting, or abduction pillows in hip fracture patients, but other reasons include the inability to position patients due to treatments in the intensive care unit, immobility due to cerebrovascular disease, paralysis, or immobility due to other conditions.

Considerable effort has been directed to predicting patients who have a high risk of developing a pressure ulcer, thus directing increased efforts towards prevention (Table 38–1). A commonly used risk assessment instrument in the United States is the Braden Scale. This instrument assesses six items: sensory perception, moisture exposure, physical activity, mobility, nutrition, and friction/shear force. Each item is ranked from 1 (least favorable) to 3 or 4 (most favorable) for a maximal total score of 23. A score of 16 or less indicates a high risk.

The Braden Scale has good sensitivity (83-100%) and specificity (61-77%) but has a poor positive predictive value (around 37% when the pressure ulcer incidence is 20%).

Variable	Norton	Braden	Waterlow
Mobility	X	X	X
Moisture exposure	X	X	X
Physical activity	X	X	
General condition	X		X
Nutrition		X	
Appetite			X
Friction/shear force		X	
Sensory perception		X	
Mental status	X		
Skin type			X
Medication			X
Weight			X
Age			X
Gender			X
Other (e.g., disease)			X

● TABLE 38–1 Comparison of Risk Assessment Instruments for Pressure Ulcers

X = present in risk assessment scale.

In populations with an incidence of pressure ulcers less than 20%, such as nursing homes, the same sensitivity and specificity would produce a positive predictive value of 2%.[11] A systematic review of 33 clinical trials of risk assessment found no decrease in pressure ulcer incidence that could be attributed to use of a risk assessment scale.[12]

PREVENTION

In patients similar to Mrs. J. who are undergoing a surgical procedure, relief of extrinsic pressure should begin in the operating room. Orthopedic and cardiac surgical procedures performed in the supine position on the operating room table are associated with pressure ulcers.[13] A number of devices have been used to lessen pressure ulcer development during the intraoperative period, including pillows, blankets, gel pads, and foam pads, but their effectiveness has not been demonstrated. Several studies suggest that the use of warming devices and standard operating room table mattresses increases the risk of pressure ulcer development.[14,15] When two or more anesthetic agents (categories) were used in orthopedic procedures, 63% of patients developed a pressure ulcer.[16] These data suggest that intraoperative factors play an important role in the development of a pressure ulcer.

CASE PRESENTATION (continued)

Evaluation

The wound care team is consulted to evaluate Mrs. Jones. They examine the ulcers and report the coccyx ulcer is 3 × 4 cm, oval with a depth of 0.5 cm with a red beefy base. No odor, purulence, or abnormal drainage is noted.

A hydrocolloid dressing is applied to the coccyx and a low air-loss mattress overlay is ordered as well as every 4 hour repositioning with the limitations of her recent hip fracture repair noted. The orthopedics doctor approves the repositioning order.

REDUCING PRESSURE, SHEAR, AND FRICTION

In the case of Mrs. J., a stage 3 pressure ulcer developed on her coccyx. Pressure ulcers are characterized by a clinical staging system (Table 38–2). This system was developed empirically and characterizes the pressure ulcer by depth of penetration into the skin and subcutaneous tissues. It should be emphasized that this system pertains only to pressure ulcers and should not be used for wounds of other etiologies.

In addition to intrinsic risk factors, pressure applied to the tissues compromises blood flow. Therefore, the first treatment principle is to relieve pressure. Postoperatively, the goal should be early mobilization. In those patients who cannot be mobilized out of bed, the most commonly recommended method for reducing pressure is frequent turning and positioning. A 2-hour turning schedule for spinal-injury patients was deducted empirically in 1946.[17] However, an exact interval for optimal turning to prevent pressure ulcers is unknown. The interval may be shortened or lengthened by intrinsic factors. In healthy older volunteers, intervals of 1 to 1½ hours rather than the traditional 2-hour schedule were required to prevent skin erythema on a standard mattress.[18]

● TABLE 38–2 Pressure Ulcer Staging System

Suspected Deep Tissue Injury	Purple or maroon localized area of discolored intact skin or blood-filled blister due to damage of underlying soft tissue from pressure and/or shear. The area may be preceded by tissue that is painful, firm, mushy, boggy, warmer, or cooler as compared to adjacent tissue.
Stage 1	Intact skin with non-blanchable redness of a localized area usually over a bony prominence. Darkly pigmented skin may not have visible blanching; its color may differ from the surrounding area.
Stage 2	Partial-thickness loss of dermis presenting as a shallow open ulcer with a red pink wound bed, without slough. May also present as an intact or open/ruptured serum-filled blister.
Stage 3	Full-thickness tissue loss. Subcutaneous fat may be visible but bone, tendon, or muscle are not exposed. Slough may be present but does not obscure the depth of tissue loss. May include undermining and tunneling.
Stage 4	Full-thickness tissue loss with exposed bone, tendon, or muscle. Slough or eschar may be present on some parts of the wound bed. Often includes undermining and tunneling.
Unstageable	Full-thickness tissue loss in which the base of the ulcer is covered by slough (yellow, tan, gray, green, or brown) and/or eschar (tan, brown, or black) in the wound bed.

Adapted from the National Pressure Ulcer Advisory Panel. http://www.npuap.org/resources.htm.

A systematic review of published strategies for prevention of pressure ulcers through June 2006 found only 59 randomized controlled trials: 51 addressing impaired mobility, 5 addressing nutrition, and 3 addressing impaired skin condition.[19] The data confirm that pressure-reducing devices appear to have an advantage over standard beds, but little difference has been shown between devices. No trial of measures for addressing impaired skin met criteria for study design, and only one trial of turning and positioning suggested a reduction in pressure ulcer incidence.

Turning and positioning may be difficult to achieve because of a patient's self-positioning or medical treatments that interfere with the ability to position the patient. Because of this difficulty, a number of medical devices have been designed in an attempt to relieve pressure. These devices can be classified as static or dynamic. Static devices include air-, gel-, or water-filled containers that reduce the tissue-surface interface. Dynamic devices use a power source to fill compartments with air that supports the patient's weight or alternates the pressure on different areas of the body. Static devices are acceptable when the patient has good bed mobility. A dynamic device is useful when the patient cannot self-position in bed.

Results of reported clinical trials do not favor one device over another. The choice should be based on durability, ease of use, and patient comfort. A simple check for so-called "bottoming out" should be done for all devices. Your hand should be inserted palm upward under the patient's sacrum between the device and the bed surface. If there is not an air column between the patient and the bed surface, the device is ineffective and should be changed.

When compared to a standard hospital mattress, most pressure-reducing devices lower the incidence of pressure ulcers by about 60%.[20] No device is effective in reducing heel pressure, the second most common site for development of a pressure ulcer.

When a pressure-reducing device is combined with turning and positioning, the effective interval for turning may be increased. In a randomized, controlled trial in high-risk nursing home residents, four different turning schedules were used. Subjects were turned every 2 hours on a standard institutional mattress, every 3 hours on a standard institutional mattress, every 4 hours on a viscoelastic foam mattress, or every 6 hours on a viscoelastic foam mattress. The incidence of non-blanchable erythema (a stage 1 pressure ulcer) was not different between the groups (35-38%). However, the incidence of stage 2 and higher pressure ulcers was 3% in the 4-hour turning interval group, compared with incidence figures in the other groups varying between 14% and 24%. Turning every 4 hours on a viscoelastic foam mattress resulted in a significant reduction in the number of higher-stage pressure ulcer lesions and suggests that less frequent turning in combination with a pressure-reducing mattress is effective and feasible.[21,22]

Studies in turning and positioning suggest an optimum interval of 4 hours while on a pressure-reducing device. More frequent turning schedules, including the often-suggested 2-hour interval, have not been demonstrated to prevent pressure ulcers.

● LOCAL WOUND TREATMENT

Pressure ulcers are chronic wounds. Acute wounds proceed to healing through a well-researched sequential progression. Pressure ulcers, like other chronic wounds (diabetic ulcers, venous stasis ulcers, and arterial ulcers), fail to proceed through an orderly and timely process to produce anatomic or functional integrity. This results in rather long healing times for these chronic wounds. Although improvement in a standardized healing score occurred in 71% of stage 3 or 4 pressure ulcers in a nursing home setting, the median days to healing was 140 days.[23] The considerable length of time to healing increases the morbidity and cost of treating pressure ulcers and is often frustrating to the patient and caregivers.

Local wound treatment is directed to providing an optimum wound environment and improving intrinsic factors. The first principle of pressure ulcer management is to maintain a moist wound environment. Maintaining a moist wound environment is associated with more rapid healing rates compared to dressings that are allowed to dry. A moist wound base can be maintained by saline-soaked gauze, a hydrogel, or an occlusive type dressing. Newer wound dressings provide a low moisture vapor transmission rate (MVTR), a measure of how quickly the dressing allows drying. An MVTR of less than 35 g of water vapor per square meter per hour is required to maintain a moist wound environment. Woven gauze has an MVTR of 68 g/m^2 per hour, and impregnated gauze has an MVTR of 57 g/m^2 per hour. By comparison, hydrocolloid dressings have an MVTR of 8 g/m^2 per hour. Dressings with low MVTR provide a moist wound environment that encourages granulation tissue formation and epithelialization. A meta-analysis of five clinical trials comparing a hydrocolloid dressing with a dry dressing demonstrated that treatment with a hydrocolloid dressing resulted in a statistically significant improvement in the rate of pressure ulcer healing, with a positive odds ratio of 2.6.[24]

Moisture-retentive or occlusive dressings can be divided into broad categories of polymer films, polymer foams, hydrogels, hydrocolloids, alginates, and biomembranes (Table 38–3). Each has advantages and disadvantages. No single agent is perfect. The choice of a particular agent depends on the clinical circumstances. Nonpermeable polymers can be macerating to normal skin. Polymer films are not absorptive and may leak, particularly when the wound is highly exudative. Most films have an adhesive backing that may remove epithelial cells when the dressing is changed.

Hydrogels are hydrophilic polymers that are insoluble in water but absorb aqueous solutions and are available in amorphous gels or sheet dressings. They are poor bacterial barriers and are non-adherent to the wound. Because of their high specific heat, these dressings are cooling to the skin, aiding in pain control and reducing inflammation. Most of these dressings require a secondary dressing to secure them to the wound.

Hydrocolloid dressings are complex dressings similar to ostomy barrier products. They are impermeable to moisture and bacteria and highly adherent to the skin. Hydrocolloid dressings have an accelerated healing of 40% compared to

● **TABLE 38–3** Available Types of Occlusive Dressings for Pressure Ulcers

Agent	Mechanism of Action	Dressing Changes	Benefits	Side Effects	Notes
Hydrocolloid	Maintains moist environment	Change 3 to 7 days, depending on when seal is open around wound	Accelerates rate of healing compared to dry dressing	None	Five trials have shown improved rate of healing compared to dry dressings; no difference among types of hydrocolloids has been found.
Hydrogel	Maintains moist environment	Daily to four times per day, depending on drying	Accelerates rate of healing compared to dry dressing	None	Most trials have not shown inferiority compared to hydrocolloid dressings.
Film dressing	Protects wound	Daily or less frequently	Use in superficial ulcers may protect undamaged skin	None	Most trials have not shown inferiority compared to hydrocolloid dressings.
Alginates	Absorbent; maintains moist environment when sufficient wound fluid is present	Daily to less frequently, depending on exudate	Absorbs exudate	None	May be useful in overly moist wounds; may be used under other dressings or sequentially with other dressings.
Moist saline gauze	Maintains moist environment	Three times daily or more frequently	Maintains moist environment	May macerate healthy tissue	Most trials show superiority of hydrocolloid dressings.
Petroleum gauze dressings	Maintains moist environment	Daily to four times daily	Maintains moist environment	None	May require more frequent dressing changes.
Hypertonic saline wet gauze dressings	Maintains moist environment	Twice daily to more frequently	Has antimicrobial activity	Hypertonicity may damage healthy tissue	
Iodine-solution wet gauze dressing	Broad-spectrum antiseptic	Daily to four times daily	Has antimicrobial activity	May damage healthy tissue	Specifically not recommended by some experts due to potential toxicity to fibroblasts.

moist gauze dressings. Hydrocolloid dressings are particularly suited for areas subject to urinary and fecal incontinence. Their adhesiveness to surrounding skin is higher than some surgical tapes, but they are non-adherent to wound tissue and do not damage epithelial tissue in the wound. The adhesive barrier is frequently overcome in highly exudative wounds. Hydrocolloid dressings should be used with caution over tendons or on wounds with eschar formation.

Alginates are complex polysaccharide dressings that are highly absorbent in exudative wounds. This high absorbency is particularly suited to exudative wounds. Alginates are non-adherent to the wound, but if the wound is allowed to dry, damage to the epithelial tissue may occur with removal. Alginates may be used under other dressings to absorb exudates. The biomembranes are very expensive and not readily available (Table 38–4).

● **TABLE 38–4** Comparison of Occlusive Wound Dressings

	Moist Saline Gauze	Polymer Films	Polymer Foams	Hydrogels	Hydrocolloids	Alginates, Granules	Biomembranes
Pain relief	+	+	+	+	+	±	+
Maceration of surrounding skin	±	±	–	–	–	–	–
O₂ permeable	+	+	+	+	–	+	+
H₂O permeable	+	+	+	+	–	+	+
Absorbent	+	–	+	+	±	+	–
Damage to epithelial cells	±	+	–	–	–	–	–
Transparent	–	+	–	–	–	–	–
Resistant to bacteria	–	–	–	–	+	–	+
Ease of application	+	–	+	+	+	+	–

Source: Data from Helfman T, Ovington L, Falanga V. Occlusive dressings and wound healing. Clin Dermatol. 1994;12:121-127; and Witkowski JA, Parish LC. Cutaneous ulcer therapy. Int J Dermatol. 1986;25:420-426.

Stage 1 and 2 pressure ulcers can be managed with a polymer film or hydrocolloid dressing. Stage 3 and 4 pressure ulcers may be treated with a film or hydrocolloid dressing. In addition, some stage 3 and 4 wounds with dead space or tunneling may require wound filler, such as a calcium alginate or an amorphous hydrogel, to obliterate dead space and decrease potential for anaerobic colonization.

Because the theory of augmenting ulcer healing under the newer dressings suggests that wound fluid contains favorable healing factors, it is important not to change the dressings too frequently. Unless the wound fluid seeps from under the dressing, it should not be changed more often than every 3 to 7 days. The use of occlusive-type dressings is more cost-effective than gauze dressings primarily because of a decrease in nursing time for dressing changes.

A systematic review of published trials on topical wound dressings for pressure ulcers through 2003 found only 21 published randomized, controlled trials.[25] Hydrocolloid wound dressings were superior to saline dressings in 6 trials, while comparisons in 5 trials using other treatment modalities (dextranomer beads, paraffin gauze, polyurethane dressing, amorphous hydrogel) showed no differences compared to saline gauze. In 9 trials comparing hydrocolloid dressings with various other advanced dressings, no difference was observed between the intervention and comparison group. A trial comparing two different polyurethane dressings showed no difference.

Vacuum-assisted closure is used in both acute and chronic wounds. Only two randomized, controlled trials in pressure ulcers have been reported. A total of 22 patients with 35 pressure ulcers were randomized to the vacuum-assisted closure device or a system of wound gel products for 6 weeks. Two patients in the vacuum-assisted closure group and two patients in the wound gel group healed completely. There was no difference in reduction in ulcer volume between groups.[26] Vacuum-assisted closure was compared to gauze moistened with Ringer's solution in a small trial of pressure ulcer treatment. Time to reach 50% of the initial wound volume was 27 days in the vacuum-assisted group and 28 days in the moist gauze–treated group.[27]

In both trials, vacuum-assisted closure was not superior to treatment with a hydrogel or moistened gauze, at a higher cost. Five other trials in various other chronic wounds (surgical, diabetic, and venous stasis ulcers) have been published. No benefit in wound healing was observed for VAC therapy.[28] Topical agents such as zinc, phenytoin, aluminum hydroxide, sugar, yeast, aloe vera gel, or gold were not effective in clinical trials.

Encouraging granulation tissue formation and promoting re-epithelialization are goals of therapy. Growth factors have shown promising early results, but the data do not suggest accelerated healing of pressure ulcers.[29] It is important not to affect granulation and epithelial tissue negatively. A number of wound cleaners and antiseptics are toxic to fibroblasts and epithelial tissues, including benzalkonium chloride, povidone-iodine solution (Betadine), Dakin's solution, hydrogen peroxide, Granulex, Hibiclens, and pHisoHex. The use of these agents in a pressure ulcer should be limited to use in infected ulcers and strictly limited in duration.

CASE PRESENTATION (continued)

Postop

On postoperative day 5 the wound care team happens to run into the orthopedic doctor for Mrs. Jones while on rounds. He explains, "We need to discharge this patient as soon as possible, we need these beds, so I think we need to be more aggressive with her treatment to heal this pressure ulcer." He suggests nasogastric feedings to increase her caloric intake, adding a zinc supplement to her medications and a wound culture to "make sure it's not infected."

● SUPPORTIVE TREATMENT

Nutritional status has been thought to influence the incidence, progression, and severity of pressure sores.[30] Experimental studies in animal models suggest a biologically plausible relationship between undernutrition and development of pressure ulcers.[31] These data suggest that pressure damage occurs independent of nutritional status, but malnourished animals may have impaired healing after a pressure injury.

The primary link between pressure ulcers and nutritional status derives from epidemiologic observational studies. For example, at hospital admission, patients who are defined as undernourished are twice as likely to develop pressure ulcers as patients who are not undernourished.[32] In a long-term-care setting, 59% of residents were diagnosed as undernourished on admission. Among these residents, 7.3% were classified as severely undernourished. Pressure ulcers occurred in 65% of these severely undernourished residents. No pressure ulcer developed in the mild-to-moderately undernourished or well-nourished groups.[33]

The association of undernutrition with pressure ulcers is problematic, because there is no accepted gold standard for the diagnosis of undernutrition.[34] The markers used for the diagnosis of nutritional status may reflect underlying disease rather than undernutrition in older ill persons. Cachexia and wasting diseases also produce weight loss and decreases in acute phase reactants such as albumin and prealbumin.[35]

This critical distinction between undernutrition and the effect of wasting diseases is important because undernutrition due to starvation can be reversed by provision of adequate nutrients, while cachexia and wasting diseases are remarkably resistant to hypercaloric feeding.[36] This overlap between undernutrition and cachexia may account for the disappointing results of nutritional interventions in the prevention of pressure ulcers. A systematic review of nutritional intervention for prevention of pressure ulcers found only one of four trials suggesting that nutritional supplements may reduce the incidence of pressure ulcers in critically ill older persons.[37] In the single positive trial, two drinks of a mixed nutritional supplement produced a modest-sized effect at 15 days. The cumulative incidence of pressure ulcers was 40% in the nutritional supplemented group compared to 48% in the control group.[38]

The deficiency of several vitamins has significant effects on wound healing. However, supplementation of vitamins to accelerate wound healing is controversial. High doses of vitamin C have not been shown to accelerate wound healing.[39] In a 12-week study of 88 patients who received either 10 mg or 500 mg of ascorbic acid twice daily, the healing rates and the healing velocity of their pressure ulcers was not different in the higher-dosed group.[40] Zinc supplementation has not been shown to accelerate healing except in zinc-deficient patients.[41] High serum zinc levels interfere with healing and supplementation above 150 mg/day may interfere with copper metabolism.[42]

The use of enteral feeding has been disappointing. In a study of enteral tube feedings in long-term care, 49 patients were followed for 3 months.[43] Patients received 1.6 times basal energy expenditure daily, 1.4 g of protein per kilogram per day, and 85% or more of their total recommended daily allowance. At the end of 3 months, there was no difference in number or healing of pressure ulcers. In a study of survival among residents in long-term care with severe cognitive impairment, 135 residents were followed for 24 months.[44] The reasons for the placement of a feeding tube included the presence of a pressure ulcer. Having a feeding tube was not associated with increased survival; in fact, the risk was slightly increased. These data suggest that the effectiveness of enteral feeding in pressure ulcers is not established.

In addition to nutrition, reduction in tissue pressure should be provided. This can be achieved by manual turning and positioning or the use of pressure-reducing devices. The same principles for these modalities apply as discussed under "Prevention" earlier in the chapter. Greater rates of healing have been demonstrated for pressure-reducing devices compared to standard hospital mattresses.

An important part of supportive treatment is to assess and treat pain. Pressure ulcers do not always result in pain, particularly in insensate patients. However, some pressure ulcers do result in pain and should be aggressively treated. Oral or parenteral pain medications should be used to control symptoms.

● WOUND DEBRIDEMENT

Necrotic debris increases the possibility of bacterial infection and delays wound healing in animal models.[45] This delay in healing results from slow removal of debris required by phagocytosis. Although widely recommended, it remains unclear whether wound debridement is a beneficial process that results in a greater frequency of complete wound healing.[46] There are no studies that compared debridement with no debridement as the control in wound healing.[47] The use of debridement can result in a shorter time to a clean wound bed in anticipation of surgical therapy.

Options for debridement include sharp surgical debridement, mechanical debridement with dry gauze dressings, autolytic debridement with occlusive dressings, or application of exogenous enzymes. Surgical sharp debridement produces the most rapid removal of necrotic debris and is indicated in the presence of infection. Surgical or mechanical debridement can damage healthy tissue or fail to completely clean the wound. Mechanical debridement can be easily accomplished

by letting saline gauze dry before removal, but may produce pain with removal. Re-moistening of gauze dressings in an attempt to reduce pain can defeat the debridement effect.

Thin portions of eschar can be removed by occlusion under a semi-permeable dressing. Enzymatic debridement can dissolve necrotic debris but possible harm to healthy tissue is debated. Penetration of enzymatic agents is limited in eschar and requires either softening by autolysis or cross-hatching by sharp incision prior to application. Both autolytic and enzymatic debridement require periods of several days to several weeks to achieve results.

Collagenase is the only enzyme available in the United States for topical debridement. A trial in 21 patients with pressure ulcers found a greater reduction in necrotic tissue using papain/urea (95.4%) compared to collagenase (35.8%) at 4 weeks, but the rate of complete healing was not different between groups.[48]

A total of five trials have not shown that enzymatic agents increased the rate of complete healing in chronic wounds compared to control treatment.[49] One trial showed an increase in wound size with both collagenase and the control treatment, but the increase was significantly less in the enzyme-treated group. Only one trial out of four that compared a hydrogel with a control treatment found a statistically significant difference between treatments. The single favorable trial suggested a small benefit from treatment with a hydrogel compared with a hydrocolloid dressing. In a single trial comparing different hydrogels, no statistically significant difference was seen between the two hydrogels.

Trials of other debridement agents have shown mixed results. Three trials of dextranomer polysaccharide found a statistically significant difference compared to control, while two trials found the control treatment more effective. A hydrogel significantly reduced necrotic wound area compared with dextranomer polysaccharide paste in one trial, but not in another. Dextranomer polysaccharide was not better than an enzymatic agent in two trials. There are no randomized, controlled trials using the papain/urea/chlorophyll combination.

● COMPLICATIONS

Pressure ulcers should be assessed for the presence of infection. Quantitative microbiology alone is a poor predictor of clinical infection in chronic wounds. All pressure ulcers are colonized with bacteria, usually from skin or fecal flora. The presence of microorganisms alone (colonization) does not indicate an infection in pressure ulcers. The diagnosis of infection in chronic wounds must be based on clinical signs: erythema, warmth, pain, edema, odor, fever, or purulent exudates. In the presence of clinical signs of infection, enteral or parenteral antibiotics should be used. In ulcers that are not progressing toward healing, an empirical trial of topical antimicrobials may be considered, although the data are inconclusive.

A number of heavy metal-impregnated dressings or solutions have been evaluated for chronic wounds, based on the hypothesis that an antimicrobial effect would enhance wound healing. Topical silver and silver-impregnated dressings have been evaluated in three trials of mixed-type wounds suspected of being infected. Only one trial included pressure ulcers as a wound type. In that trial, there was no difference in complete healing or absolute or relative wound size, but a small effect was calculated for healing rate per day.[50]

● DIFFERENTIAL DIAGNOSIS

While pressure ulcers generally occur in soft tissues over a bony prominence, Mrs. J. also has a wound on her lateral malleolus, rather than the more common site of the heel. This should immediately suggest an alternate pathophysiology for this wound. A careful examination of peripheral pulses is mandatory. A search for sources of pressure to this area should also be undertaken.

Chronic ulcers of the skin include arterial ulcers, venous stasis ulcers, diabetic ulcers, and pressure ulcers. The treatment of wounds due to these various etiologies differs considerably.

Arterial ulcers frequently occur in the distal digits or over a bony prominence in the context of diminished pulses, cool skin temperature, and atropic changes of the lower leg. In diabetic wounds, the usual clinical course is repetitive trauma and callous formation at the site of the diabetic ulcer, usually occurring from footwear or other repetitive pressure. Diabetic ulcers occur in regions of callus formation, and venous stasis ulcers occur on the mid-tibial aspect of the lower leg. The most likely diagnosis of Mrs. J.'s lateral malleolus wound is peripheral arterial disease. However, atypical presentations may occasionally obscure the etiology.

The presence of two different wounds on the same patient illustrates the difference in chronic wound treatment. The treatment of an arterial ulcer differs from treatment of a pressure ulcer. The primary objective is to improve circulation. The ankle-brachial index should be repeated. Worsening of arterial supply to the extremity may have occurred as a complication of surgery. There is no standard of therapy for the topical treatment of arterial ulcers. The principle is to maintain a dry wound base. Moisture in an arterial ulcer, so-called wet gangrene, may increase the likelihood of infection. Topical Betadine is often used achieve a dry wound base. Addressing medical issues including good control of diabetes, cessation of smoking, assessing lipid status, and consideration of antiplatelet drugs is appropriate.

CASE PRESENTATION (continued)

Case Conclusion

Mrs. Jones is discharged to a rehabilitation facility on postoperative day 9. Her sacral ulcer is now 2 × 2 cm with a depth of 2.5 mm, without signs of infection, and appears to be healing well. Likewise her lateral malleolus ulcer is healing as well. Five weeks later both ulcers have closed and Mrs. Jones is now walking independently with the aid of a cane.

SUMMARY

The accumulating data for the prevention and management of pressure ulcers permit an outline of clinical strategies (Table 38–5). Risk assessment remains problematic because of poor predictive validity and an apparent floor effect in preventing all pressure ulcers, but can highlight patient-specific risk factors for development of a pressure ulcer. Pressure-reducing devices are clearly superior to a standard hospital mattress in preventing pressure ulcers. However, it is difficult to distinguish superiority among various devices. The impact of nutrition on the prevention of pressure ulcers remains controversial. Limited data suggest that nutritional supplementation may have an effect on reducing incidence. Nutritional status should be evaluated in all clinical settings as a process of good care.

Limited evidence and clinical intuition support pressure-reducing devices in improving the healing rate of pressure ulcers. The amount of dietary protein intake seems linked to improved rates of healing, but the results of enteral feeding to achieve this result are disappointing. Other nutritional interventions including specific amino acids and vitamin or mineral supplements have not shown an effect on healing rate.

Local wound treatment should aim at maintaining a moist wound environment. Options include hydrocolloid dressings and other occlusive moist dressings. The choice of a particular dressing depends on wound characteristics such as the amount of exudate, dead space, or wound location. Debridement by any of several methods may improve time to a clean wound bed, but the effect of debridement on time to healing remains to be demonstrated. The use of topical growth factors in improving healing rates is in its infancy but has not been remarkably effective thus far. A thorough evaluation of pain is a component of good wound management.

● TABLE 38–5 General Principles of Pressure Ulcer Management	
Principle	Management
Assess pain	Treat systemic pain with systemic drugs. Consider systemic pre-treatment for painful dressing changes. Consider topical pain medications during dressing changes.
Relieve pressure	Try overlays or low-air-loss devices for prevention. Use dynamic support devices (eg, alternating-air mattresses) for patients who cannot self-position. Consider air-fluidized beds for patients who do not otherwise respond to treatment or who have more severe ulcers. Heel devices should completely eliminate pressure on the heels (eg, L'Nard or Multi-podus Splints).
Maintain moist wound environment	Choose a specific dressing based on wound characteristics. See Table 38–4.
Assess nutrition	Provide adequate calories. Consider optimum protein range from 1.2 to 1.5 g/kg body weight/day unless contraindicated.
Control infection	Monitor for clinical signs of infection. Avoid superficial wound cultures. Consider empiric topical antibiotics for non-healing wounds. Use systemic antibiotics for systemic infection.
Debridement	Consider surgical debridement for clinically infected wounds. Use autolytic or mechanical debridement for non-infected wounds.
Monitor healing status	Consider a change in treatment regimen if wound is not progressing toward healing week by week.

References

1. Whittington K, Patrick M, Roberts JL. A national study of pressure ulcer prevalence and incidence in acute care hospitals. *J Wound Ostomy Continence Nurs.* 2000;27:209-215.

2. Baumgarter M, Margolis DJ, Orwig DL, et al. Pressure ulcers in elderly patients with hip fracture across the contnuum of care. *J Am Geriatr Soc.* 2009;57:863-870.

3. Vasconez LO, Schneider WJ, Jurkiewicz MJ. Pressure sores. *Curr Probl Surg.* 1977;62:83-89.

4. Meehan M. National pressure ulcer prevalence survey. *Adv Wound Care.* 1994;7:27-37.

5. Barbenel J. The prevalence of pressure sores. National symposium on the care, treatment, and prevention of decubitus ulcers. Conference proceedings. 1984:1-9.

6. Thomas DR. Management of pressure ulcers. *J Am Med Dir Assoc.* 2006;7:46-59.

7. Thomas DR. Issues and dilemmas in managing pressure ulcers. *J Gerontol Med Sci.* 2001;56:M238-M340.

8. Thomas DR. Prevention and management of pressure ulcers. *Clin Rev Gerontol.* 2008;17:1-17.

9. Sanada H, Nagakawa T, Yamamoto M, et al. The role of skin blood flow in pressure ulcer development during surgery. *Adv Wound Care.* 1997;10:29-34.

10. Van Marum RJ, Meijer JH, Ribbe MW. The relationship between pressure ulcers and skin blood flow response after a local cold provocation. *Arch Phys Med Rehabil.* 2002;83:40-43.

11. Thomas DR. Prevention and management of pressure ulcers. *Rev Clin Gerontol.* 2001;11:115-130.

12. Pancorbo-Hidalgo PL, Garcia-Fernandez FP, Lopez-Medine IM, Alvariex-Nieto C. Risk assessment scales for pressure ulcer prevention: A systematic review. *J Adv Nurs.* 2006;54:94-110.

13. Aronovitch SA. Intraoperatively acquired pressure ulcer prevalence. *J WOCN.* 1999;26:130-136.

14. Bliss M, Simini B. When are the seeds of pressure sores sown? *BJM.* 1999;319:864.

15. Marchette L, Arnell I, Redick E. Skin ulcers of elderly surgical patients in critical care units. *Appl Res.* 1991;10:321-329.

16. Aronovitch SA. Intraoperatively acquired pressure ulcers: Are there common risk factors? *Ostomy Wound Manage.* 2007;53:57-69.

17. Kenedi RM, Cowden JM, Scales JT, eds. *Bedsore Biomechanics.* Baltimore: University Park Press; 1976.

18. Knox DM, Anderson TM, Anderson PS. Effects of different turn intervals on skin of healthy older adults. *Adv Wound Care.* 1994;7:48-56.

19. Reddy M, Gill SS, Bouchon PA. Preventing pressure ulcers: A systematic review. *JAMA.* 2006;296:974-984.

20. Cullum N, McInnes E, Bell-Syer SEM, Legood R. Support surfaces for pressure ulcer prevention. *Cochrane Database Syst Rev.* 2004;3.

21. Defloor T, Bacquer DD, Grypdonck MHF. The effect of various combinations of turning and pressure reducing devices on the incidence of pressure ulcers. *Int J Nurs Stud.* 2005;42:37-46.

22. Defloor T. Less frequent turning intervals and yet less pressure ulcers. *Tijdschr Gerontol Geriatr.* 2001;32:174-177.

23. Lynn J, West J, Hausmann S, et al. Collaborative clinical quality improvement for pressure ulcers in nursing homes. *J Am Geriatr Soc.* 2007;55:1663-1669.

24. Bradley M, Cullum N, Nelson EA, et al. Systematic reviews of wound care management: Dressings and topical agents used in the healing of chronic wounds. *Health Techn Assess.* 1999;3: 1-135.

25. Bouza C, Saz Z, Munoz A, Amate J. Efficacy of advanced dressings in the treatment of pressure ulcers: A systematic review. *J Wound Care.* 2005;14:193.

26. Ford CN, Reinhard ER, Yeh D, et al. Interim analysis of a prospective, randomized trial of vacuum-assisted closure versus the Healthpoint system in the management of pressure ulcers. *Ann Plast Surg.* 2002;49:55-61.

27. Wanner MB, Schwarzl F, Strub B, et al. Vacuum-assisted wound closure for cheaper and more comfortable healing of pressure sores: A prospective study. *Scand J Plast Reconstruct Surg Hand Surg.* 2003;37:28-33.

28. Ubbink DT, Westerbos SJ, Evans D, et al. Topical negative pressure for treating chronic wounds. *Cochrane Lib.* 2009;1.

29. Thomas DR. The promise of topical nerve growth factors in the healing of pressure ulcers. *Ann Intern Med.* 2003;139: 694-695.

30. Thomas DR. The role of nutrition in prevention and healing of pressure ulcers. *Geriatr Clin North Am.* 1997:13:497-512.

31. Takeda T, Koyama T, Izawa Y, et al. Effects of malnutrition on development of experimental pressure sores. *J Dermatol.* 1992;19: 602-609.

32. Thomas DR, Goode PS, Tarquine PH, Allman R. Hospital acquired pressure ulcers and risk of death. *J Am Geriatr Soc.* 1996;44: 1435-1440.

33. Pinchcofsky-Devin GD, Kaminski MV Jr. Correlation of pressure sores and nutritional status. *J Am Geriatr Soc.* 1986;34:435-440.

34. Thomas DR. Improving the outcome of pressure ulcers with nutritional intervention: A review of the evidence. *Nutrition.* 2001;17: 121-125.

35. Thomas DR. Distinguishing starvation from cachexia. *Geriatr Clin North Am.* 2002;18:883-892.

36. Thomas DR. Loss of skeletal muscle mass in aging: Examining the relationship of starvation, sarcopenia and cachexia. *Clin Nutr.* 2007;26:389-399.

37. Langer G, Schloemer G, Knerr A, et al. Nutritional interventions for preventing and treating pressure ulcers. *Cochrane Database Syst Rev.* 2007;1.

38. Bourdel-Marchasson I, Barateau M, Rondeau V, et al. A multi-center trial of the effects of oral nutritional supplementation in critically ill older inpatients. GAGE Group. Groupe Aquitain Geriatrique d'Evaluation. *Nutrition.* 2000;16:1-5.

39. Vilter RW Nutritional aspects of ascorbic acid: Uses and abuses. *West J Med.* 1980;133:485.

40. ter Riet G, Kessels AG, Knipschild PG. Randomized clinical trial of ascorbic acid in the treatment of pressure ulcers. *J Clin Epidemiol.* 1995;48:1453-1460.

41. Sandstead HH, Henriksen LK, Greger JL, et al Zinc nutriture in the elderly in relation to taste acuity, immune response, and wound healing. *Am J Clin Nutr.* 1982;36(suppl):1046-1059.

42. Thomas DR. The role of nutrition in prevention and healing of pressure ulcers. *Geriatr Clin North Am.* 1997:13:497-512.

43. Henderson CT, Trumbore LS, Mobarhan S, et al. Prolonged tube feeding in long-term care: Nutritional status and clinical outcomes. *J Am Coll Clin Nutr.* 1992;11:309.

44. Mitchell SL, Kiely DK, Lipsitz LA. The risk factors and impact on survival of feeding tube placement in nursing home residents with severe cognitive impairment. *Arch Intern Med.* 1997;157:327-332

45. Constantine BE, Bolton LL. A wound model for ischemic ulcers in the guinea pig. *Arch Dermatol Res.* 1986;278:429-431.

46. Thomas DR. Managing pressure ulcers: Learning to give up cherished dogma. *J Am Med Dir Assn.* 2007;8:347-348.

47. Bradley M, Cullum N, Sheldon T. The debridement of chronic wounds: A systematic review. *Health Technol Assess.* 1999;3:1-78.

48. Alvarez OM, Fenandez-Obregon A, Rogers RS, et al. Chemical debridement of pressure ulcers: A prospective, randomized, comparative trial of collagenase and papain/urea formulations. *Wounds.* 2000;12:15-25.

49. Bradley M, Cullum N, Sheldon T. The debridement of chronic wounds: A systematic review. *Health Technol Assess.* 1999;3:1-78.

50. Meaume S, Vallet D, Morere MN, Teot L. Evaluation of a silver-releasing hydroalginate dressing in chronic wounds with signs of local infection. *J Wound Care.* 2005;14:411-419.

POST-TEST

1. **A pressure ulcer that has partial-thickness loss of dermis presenting as a shallow open ulcer with a red pink wound bed, without slough is classified as:**
   A. Stage 1
   B. Stage 2
   C. Stage 3
   D. Unstageable

2. **A risk assessment tool for pressure ulcers that has very poor positive predictive value in nursing home patients is the:**
   A. Braden scale
   B. Norton scale
   C. Waterlow scale
   D. Derm scale

3. **The most frequent site for pressure ulcers is:**
   A. Malleolus
   B. Greater trochanteric
   C. Sacrum
   D. Heel

ANSWERS TO PRE-TEST
1. B
2. D
3. A

ANSWERS TO POST-TEST
1. B
2. A
3. C

● **TABLE 39–1** Dysphagia: Diagnostic/Management Pearls

1. Distinguish between oropharyngeal or esophageal dysphagia, by history, before starting the workup.
2. The differential diagnosis of esophageal dysphagia should be based on the consistency of the inciting food(s) (solids only vs. solids and liquids) and progression of symptoms (slow vs. rapid).
3. Treatments should be targeted toward the specific cause.
4. Patients with esophageal dysphagia should be referred to a gastroenterologist.

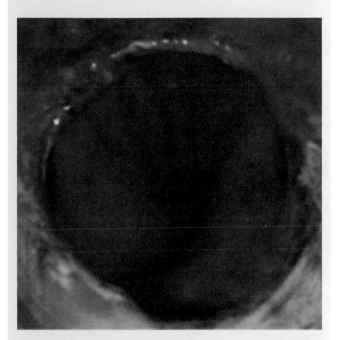

FIGURE 39–1. Peptic (reflux-induced) esophageal stricture at the level of the distal esophagus.

● NSAID GASTROPATHY

CASE PRESENTATION 2: "I HAVE NO ENERGY"

Mrs. K. is a 75-year-old retired school teacher who comes to you for follow-up, after you referred her to an orthopedic surgeon for severe degenerative arthritis pain of the right knee, which was limiting her ability to take her usual daily walks. She has underlying type 2 diabetes mellitus, with no known complications, and hypertension for which she takes amlodipine. The surgeon recommended starting celecoxib but she did not want to due to the cost; she decided to start ibuprofen instead, which was much cheaper and also easily available over the counter. She got good relief from it and has been taking 400 mg three times a day for the past 6 weeks. When you walk into the exam room Mrs. K. does not look her usual self. When you ask her, she responds, "Doctor, for the past few days, I have had no energy. It's a struggle just to do simple things around the house. I get short of breath with minimal activity and I need to rest several times during the day. This morning when I got up I was dizzy and light-headed and also had a black and tarry bowel movement." You review her vital signs and note that the nurse obtained orthostatic vitals. Supine, her pulse was 72 with a blood pressure of 124/78 and standing, after 2 minutes, her pulse was 96 with a blood pressure of 98/64. The nurse notes that she complained of light-headedness particularly just after she stood up.

Forty percent of the 30 million people worldwide who take NSAIDs on a daily basis are older than 60 years. NSAIDs block the cyclo-oxygenase type-1 (COX-1)-mediated generation of cytoprotective prostanoids, such as prostaglandin E2 and prostacyclin, leading to gastroduodenal mucosal vulnerability to gastric acid. There is poor correlation between epigastric or upper abdominal discomfort (dyspepsia) and ulcer development and asymptomatic, endoscopically demonstrable ulcers have been found in up to 40% of long-term NSAID users. Fortunately, serious complications such as bleeding, perforation, or obstruction are rare, with an annual incidence of around 1.5%. However, given the scale at which these medications are used, even this low incidence translates into a significant impact at the population level. Serious gastrointestinal complications are three- to fivefold higher in NSAID users compared to nonusers.[7] Low-dose aspirin (LDA; defined as ≤ 300 mg daily) has been shown to increase the risk of upper gastrointestinal bleeding in a dose-dependent manner, with fourfold odds at a dose of 300 mg/day, when compared to both hospital and community controls.[8] Even more importantly, concomitant NSAID and LDA usage doubles the risk of ulcer bleeding, compared to taking either alone.[8] A meta-analysis of 22 randomized placebo-controlled trials that included over 57,000 patients found that the pooled incidence of major gastrointestinal bleeding in the placebo group was 0.12% per year, with LDA doubling that risk (RR 2.07, 95% CI 1.61-2.66).[9]

Risk stratification of patients before instituting NSAID therapy is essential. Variables that increase the risk of gastrointestinal complications from NSAID use are history of gastroduodenal ulcer or hemorrhage (most important risk factor, increases risk 13-fold), age 65 years or above, long-term use of high-dose NSAIDs, usage of more than one NSAID at the same time, concomitant use of corticosteroids, antiplatelet agents or anticoagulants, and serious co-morbidities such as cardiovascular disease or renal or hepatic impairment (Table 39–2). Corticosteroids alone do not increase the risk of ulceration; however, the risk is increased fourfold when steroids are taken together with NSAIDs.[10]

The gastrointestinal complications of NSAID or aspirin use can be prevented with the use of mucosal protective agents such as proton pump inhibitors (PPIs) or misoprostol, a prostaglandin agonist, or by the substitution for the NSAID with a selective cyclo-oxygenase 2 (COX-2) inhibitor. Concomitant PPI use was shown to be useful for the primary

● TABLE 39–2 Risk Factors for NSAID-Related Gastrointestinal Complications
Prior history of gastroduodenal ulcer or hemorrhage related to the use of NSAIDs
Age greater than 65 years
Long-term use of high-dose NSAIDs
Concomitant usage of aspirin or other NSAIDs
Concomitant usage of anticoagulants, anti-platelet agents, or corticosteroids
Serious co-morbidities (cardiovascular, renal, hepatic, etc.)

prevention of NSAID-induced injury by a meta-analysis that pooled the results of five randomized controlled trials; the use of PPIs was associated with a much lower risk of endoscopically identified gastric ulcers (RR 0.40, 95% CI 0.32-0.51) and duodenal ulcers (RR 0.19, 95% CI 0.09-0.37) as compared to placebo.[11] Overall, endoscopic ulcers were identified in 14.5% using PPIs versus 35.6% in the placebo group. Even though the current literature provides strong evidence indicating the usefulness of PPIs in preventing NSAID-induced endoscopic lesions, the impact on reduction in the risk of clinically significant events, such as gastrointestinal hemorrhage or perforation, is not fully known. A small trial (150 patients) compared 1 week of *Helicobacter pylori* eradication therapy with 6 months of PPI (omeprazole) use in high-risk users of NSAIDs who were *H. pylori*-positive patients and had a history of NSAID-related ulcer bleeding.[12] The PPI group was found to have significantly lower probability of recurrent ulcer bleeding (18.8% vs. 4.4%, $p = 0.005$). A case-control study involving 2777 patients with endoscopically confirmed peptic ulcer bleeding (PUB) who were matched to 5532 control subjects found that PPIs decreased the risk of both NSAID-related PUB (adjusted relative risk 0.33, CI 0.27-0.39) and aspirin (all doses)-related PUB (adjusted RR 0.30, CI 0.20-0.44).[13]

Misoprostol offers efficacy equivalent to PPIs in reducing the risk of NSAID-induced GI complications, albeit with a lower effectiveness due to its high frequency (20%) of adverse effects of diarrhea, abdominal cramps, and nausea, which limit patient compliance. A meta-analysis demonstrated that patients receiving misoprostol with NSAIDs when compared to those receiving placebo and NSAIDs, had a decrease in the incidence of gastric ulcers by 74% and in duodenal ulcers by 53%.[11] COX-2 inhibitors alone for pain control offer an efficacy equivalent to that of an NSAID and PPI combination, in terms of risk reduction for GI complications. A trial that randomized 287 NSAID users with a recent episode of ulcer bleeding to either the COX-2 inhibitor celecoxib alone (400 mg daily), or the nonselective NSAID diclofenac (75 mg daily) plus omeprazole (20 mg daily), for 6 months[14] showed no difference in the incidence of recurrent endoscopic gastroduodenal ulcer between the two groups (18.7% vs. 25.6%, $p = 0.21$). Another study demonstrated a benefit of combining a COX-2 inhibitor with a PPI compared to COX-2 alone in patients with recent NSAID-induced upper GI bleeding: the former group had a 0% incidence of recurrent ulcer bleeding after 12 months compared to 8.9% ($p < 0.001$) in the latter.[15] The risk for

cardiovascular adverse effects with COX-2 inhibitors, such as coronary or cerebrovascular events, should be weighed against the gastrointestinal risks of NSAIDs before making management decisions.

CASE PRESENTATION 2 (continued)

You decide to admit Mrs. K. for further evaluation. She is started on intravenous fluids and is found to be anemic with hemoglobin of 7.8 g/dL (78 g/L). She undergoes an upper endoscopy and is found to have a large NSAID-induced, antral ulcer containing a visible vessel (Figure 39–2). Urease testing for *H. pylori* is negative. Endoscopic hemostasis, using epinephrine injection in combination with heater probe application, is applied, a blood transfusion is given, and intravenous PPI infusion is initiated. She recovers uneventfully from the current episode and is discharged on an oral PPI (once daily for 2 months to heal the ulcer) and a COX-2 inhibitor (for control of arthritis pain and inflammation) and is told to discontinue the ibuprofen. This decision is based on her requirements for continued pain control, low cardiovascular risk (no significant risk factors except her age), and high gastrointestinal risk (prior history of ulcer bleeding). This episode of gastrointestinal bleeding could have been prevented had she been on a mucosal protective agent (Table 39–3).

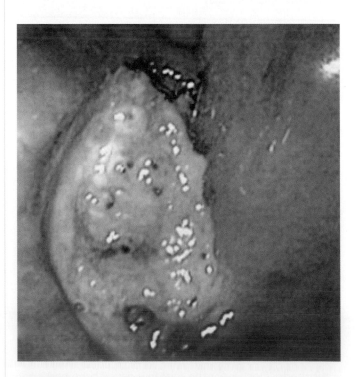

FIGURE 39–2. Large NSAID-induced antral ulcer with a visible vessel at its lower surface.

TABLE 39–3 NSAID Gastropathy: Diagnostic/Management Pearls

1. Prior history of gastroduodenal ulcer or hemorrhage as a result of NSAID use is the biggest risk factor.
2. Concomitant aspirin, other NSAIDs, warfarin, or prednisone use increases the risk.
3. Co-therapy with a PPI or misoprostol is effective for prevention.
4. COX-2 inhibitor alone can be considered to lower GI risk in those at low risk for cardiovascular toxicity.

BACTERIAL OVERGROWTH IN THE SMALL BOWEL

CASE PRESENTATION 3: AN EMBARRASSING PROBLEM

Mr. H., a 76-year-old Caucasian retired engineer, has long-standing poorly controlled diabetes, the latter secondary to noncompliance with medications. He tried metformin and pioglitazone initially but had to be started on lantus insulin when his Hb_{A1c} hit a plateau around 9, after having decreased gradually from 11.5 at baseline. He does not follow with you on a regular basis, as instructed. On a recent visit, he was diagnosed with early cirrhosis felt to be from nonalcoholic steatohepatitis. During his office visit today, he sheepishly tells you about his "excessive gas problem" that started a month ago. He tells you, "Doc, I feel embarrassed eating out in the restaurants." On further questioning, he also admits to occasional watery diarrhea, unexplained 10-lb weight loss, and upper abdominal bloating. His physical examination is significant for palpable nodular left liver lobe and decreased sensation to touch in both the upper and lower extremities. Diarrhea, weight loss, and peripheral neuropathy make you wonder if he has a malabsorptive condition. A complete blood count reveals hemoglobin of 10.2 g/dL (102 g/L) with MCV of 104. You send off for vitamin B_{12} as well as folate levels; the former comes back as low, and he is started on supplementation therapy. After your initial workup, you re-evaluate his presentation and decide to rule out small intestinal bacterial overgrowth, given the risk factors—advanced age, diabetes mellitus, as well as cirrhosis.

Small intestinal bacterial overgrowth (SIBO) is a condition caused by the overgrowth of bacteria in the small intestine resulting in malabsorption. The classical description of SIBO was vitamin B_{12} deficiency and steatorrhea, typically in the setting of bowel surgery leading to short bowel syndrome. However, it is now recognized that it most often presents with

symptoms of diarrhea, abdominal bloating, and flatulence. Additionally, it may cause dyspepsia and weight loss. The two most common predisposing factors for SIBO include structural and functional disorders of the small bowel. Structural abnormalities include the presence of a blind loop (after Billroth partial gastrectomy), small intestinal diverticulosis, and strictures (such as with Crohn disease). Disorders affecting the function (peristalsis) of the small bowel leading to SIBO include diabetes mellitus, scleroderma, and chronic radiation enteritis. Other causes include hypochlorhydria (including that induced by proton pump inhibitor therapy), cirrhosis, chronic pancreatitis, celiac disease, and atrophic gastritis. SIBO is likely underdiagnosed in the elderly,[16] and in fact advancing age may be an independent risk factor[16,17]; SIBO was reported in 15% of unselected asymptomatic nursing home residents.[18] It may be an under-recognized cause of malnutrition in the elderly.[19]

Other clinical manifestations of SIBO may include symptoms related to anemia, peripheral neuropathy, night blindness, or osteoporosis, resulting from vitamin deficiencies. Physical examination may show evidence of past abdominal surgeries or a succussion splash. Laboratory testing can indicate a macrocytic anemia; vitamin B_{12} levels may be low but folate levels are normal or high (the latter is produced by the intestinal bacteria). A small bowel series to evaluate for diverticulosis, strictures, or abnormal transit would be appropriate in the right clinical setting. The gold standard for diagnosis is a jejunal aspirate culture demonstrating the presence of more than 100,000 colony-forming units of bacteria (normal range 100-1000). Aspirate can be collected during an upper endoscopy; small-bowel biopsy can be obtained at the same time to rule out the presence of celiac sprue. The other commonly used diagnostic modality is breath testing. It utilizes the fact that the intestinal bacteria produce hydrogen or carbon (radiolabeled) when metabolizing glucose, xylose, or lactulose, ingested by the patient. These gases or associated radioactivity are measured in the exhaled breath to diagnose SIBO. Even though these breath tests are simple and noninvasive, their accuracy has varied in different clinical studies and several patient-related factors such as diet, exercise, or smoking may affect their performance. A 2-week trial of antibiotics may be used as a diagnostic modality; significant improvement in symptoms strongly suggests the diagnosis of SIBO.

The treatment of SIBO is with oral antibiotics: ciprofloxacin, metronidazole, tetracycline, cotrimoxazole, amoxicillin, and rifaximin have all been found to be effective. After a 2-week course of treatment, clinical response should be assessed. Many patients, especially those with underlying anatomic or motility problems, will require long-term treatment; it is prudent to rotate treatment with another antibiotic or cycle therapy with off-and-on periods to prevent development of resistance and occurrence of adverse effects. Rifaximin is an attractive choice given its extremely low systemic absorption. Management of patients with SIBO should also include a search for and treatment of associated nutritional deficiencies. A lactose-free diet and discontinuation of medications that lower stomach acidity, such as PPIs, should be considered. Lastly, if possible, the predisposing factors for SIBO (such as blind loops) should be surgically corrected, if possible.

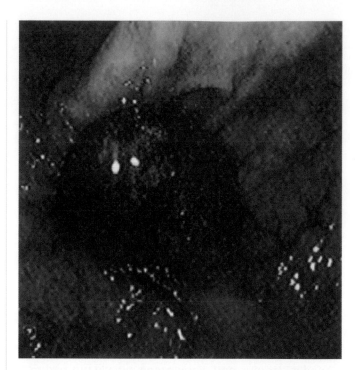

FIGURE 39–3. Large pedunculated colon polyp.

CASE PRESENTATION 3 (continued)

You refer Mr. H. to your gastroenterology colleague with a request to perform an upper endoscopy with jejunal aspirate. The aspirate culture grows more than 100,000 colony-forming units of bacteria and the small bowel biopsies are negative for celiac sprue. You start him on ciprofloxacin and he experiences rapid resolution of his symptoms. Unfortunately, symptoms recur at a 3-month follow-up visit and he needed to be retreated (Table 39–4).

● **TABLE 39–4** Small Intestinal Bacterial Overgrowth: Diagnostic/Management Pearls

1. Nonspecific symptoms of diarrhea and abdominal bloating, in a patient with risk factors, may indicate SIBO.
2. Breath tests, jejunal aspirate, or trial of antibiotics can be used to diagnose SIBO.
3. SIBO should be considered in the differential diagnoses when encountering an elderly, malnourished patient.
4. Patients frequently require prolonged therapy.

● COLON POLYPS

CASE PRESENTATION 4: AM I OK?

Mr. S., a 72-year-old African American retired military man, presents to your office with a request for a referral for a screening colonoscopy. He suffers from hypercholesterolemia, hypertension, chronic kidney disease, and obesity. He does not have a family history of colon cancer or polyps. He denied any hematochezia or involuntary weight loss. You determine that he is at average risk for colorectal cancer and refer him for a colonoscopy. At a follow-up visit 1 month later, you inform him of the results of his colonoscopic examination, which was significant for one 10-mm polyp in his sigmoid colon (Figure 39–3). The endoscopy report mentioned excellent quality of the bowel preparation. The polyp was removed completely using a snare and it was found to be a tubular adenoma on pathologic examination, without any features of high-grade dysplasia or of villous histology. He asks, "What does that mean and do I need to do anything different?"

Polyps are ingrowths of the colonic mucosa into the lumen. They may be pedunculated (with a stalk), sessile (no stalk), or flat/depressed. Broadly, polyps are classified as neoplastic (adenomas) or non-neoplastic (hyperplastic). They are usually asymptomatic but occasionally may cause overt or occult bleeding (latter manifesting as anemia and positive fecal occult blood test). Only about 5% or fewer of adenomas will progress to colonic adenocarcinoma. However, such cancer progression can be halted if they are detected and completely resected; herein lies the rationale for colon cancer screening using colonoscopy. The prevalence of adenomas increases with age: 25% of population at age 50 and 50% of those at age 75 will have adenomas; thus, age is a significant predictor.[20] Another predictor is gender, since men are more likely to have adenomas. Based on their glandular architecture on histologic examination, adenomas are classified as tubular, villous, or tubulo-villous. Overall, advanced age, size, and villous architecture of an adenoma are independent predictors of malignancy.

In the United States, colorectal cancer is the third most common cancer and the second leading cause of cancer death. Approximately 60% of the adenomas are distal and 40% proximal to the splenic flexure; the former are within reach of a sigmoidoscopic examination. Women, the elderly, and likely African Americans are more likely to harbor right-colonic adenomas. Therefore, a colonoscopy would be an ideal test to detect as well as remove adenomas from the entire colon. It is currently recommended that screening examination should start at age 50 (45 for African Americans). If no adenomas are detected after a meticulous exam, repeat colonoscopy should be performed after 10 years. After age 80, screening programs lose their cost-effectiveness and are not recommended. Furthermore, if the life expectancy of an individual is less than 10 years, screening is unlikely to prolong

● TABLE 39–5	Suggested Guidelines for the Interval before a Repeat Colonoscopy
Surveillance Interval	Findings on Screening Colonoscopy
10 years	No polyps or small hyperplastic polyps
5 years	1 or 2 tubular adenomas, ≤ 1 cm in size, without any high-grade dysplasia
3 years	3-10 tubular adenomas (≤ 1 cm in size, no high-grade dysplasia) or any adenoma ≥ 1 cm in size, or any adenoma with predominantly villous histology, or any adenoma with high-grade dysplasia
1-3 years	> 10 adenomas (consider workup for familial syndromes)

Adapted from Winawer et al.[37]

survival. After the index colonoscopy, the optimal interval before the repeat colonoscopy is guided by the malignant potential of the polyp. This is based on the number, size, and histologic type of the polyp/s, and also by the presence or absence of high-grade dysplasia (Table 39–2). A large prospective study[21] from the Veteran Affairs hospitals evaluated the incidence of advanced neoplasia (defined as tubular adenoma ≥ 10 mm, adenoma with villous histology, adenoma with high-grade dysplasia, or invasive cancer) at 5.5 years after a screening colonoscopy and found that the relative risk varied based on the findings on the screening colonoscopy:

- 1.92 (95% CI 0.83-4.42) with 1 or 2 tubular adenomas < 10 mm
- 5.01 (95% CI 2.10-11.96) with 3 or more tubular adenomas < 10 mm
- 6.40 (95% CI 2.74-14.94) with tubular adenoma ≥ 10 mm
- 6.05 (95% CI 2.48-14.71) for villous adenoma
- 6.87 (95% CI 2.61-18.07) for adenoma with high-grade dysplasia

The recommendations for the interval before a repeat colonoscopy assume that the bowel preparation was adequate, the colonoscopy was complete (to the cecum), the mucosa was carefully examined, and the removal of any polyps, if detected, was complete. If any of these conditions is not met, a repeat exam is warranted in 3 to 6 months (Table 39–5).

CASE PRESENTATION 4 (continued)

You inform Mr. S. of the malignant potential of the tubular adenoma and reassure him that it was completely removed. Importantly, you tell him that based on the current guidelines, he needs a repeat colonoscopy in 3 years (Table 39–6).

● TABLE 39–6	Colon Polyps: Diagnostic/Management Pearls

1. Advanced patient age, and size and villous architecture of a polyp, are independent predictors of malignancy.
2. Recommendations for the duration before the next colonoscopy are only valid if the colon preparation was good and the exam was complete.

● ISCHEMIC COLITIS

CASE PRESENTATION 5: MILD DIFFUSE ABDOMINAL PAIN

A 76-year-old Asian American retired nurse comes to your office complaining of mild diffuse abdominal pain that started yesterday, soon after she finished hemodialysis. This morning, she also noticed a few bloody, loose stools. Her renal failure has been the result of long-standing diabetic nephropathy. She recalls suffering from a similar pain, occasionally in the past, especially after a long session of hemodialysis. She does not have any nausea or vomiting. She denies eating any unusual foods, especially any raw shellfish. There is no family history of inflammatory bowel disease. She also denies any new medications or use of any illicit drugs; her medication list includes metoprolol, lisinopril, aspirin 81 mg daily, sevelamer, lantus insulin at night, and human lispro insulin pre-meals. She had had a cholecystectomy, appendectomy, and two cesarean sections in the distant past. Her physical examination reveals some dryness of her mucous membranes as well as slightly decreased skin turgor. She has left lower quadrant tenderness with mild guarding but no rebound tenderness. Bowel sounds are normal. You decide to admit her to the hospital and order complete blood count, metabolic panel, serum lactic acid, stool culture, stool for fecal leucocytes, as well as a CT scan of her abdomen, and seek consultation with gastroenterology.

Ischemic colitis (IC) is the most common presentation of mesenteric ischemia, the latter caused by a reduction in the blood flow to the intestines. It can be occlusive (rare) or non-occlusive (common). It can also be defined as gangrenous (15% of all IC cases) or non-gangrenous (85%). Elderly individuals (over age 60) account for more than 90% of cases.[22] The two common areas of involvement in the colon are the so-called "watershed areas": rectosigmoid junction and splenic flexure, owing to their greater susceptibility to decreased blood flow; over 75% of IC occurs in the left colon and the rectum is usually spared.

The various causes of IC include (1) states of decreased perfusion such as congestive heart failure, perioperative period, hemodialysis, cardiopulmonary bypass, and shock; (2) vascular occlusion caused by aortic reconstructive surgery (2-3% incidence), aortic dissection, and mesenteric artery thrombosis; (3) drugs such as alosetron, diuretics, tegaserod, digitalis, cocaine, NSAIDs, statins, chemotherapeutic agents (taxanes and vinca alkaloids), and hormones (estrogens); (4) mesenteric venous thrombosis caused by hypercoagulable states (eg, anti-phospholipid syndrome, factor V Leiden); and (5) miscellaneous causes such as marathon running, infections (*E. coli* 0157:H7), colon cancer, adhesions, and fecal impaction.

The clinical presentation of IC varies with its severity. Typically, there is rapid onset of abdominal pain (usually mild), urgent desire to defecate, and diarrhea. Mild to moderate amounts of hematochezia are seen within 24 hours of the onset of pain. On examination, tenderness can be appreciated over the affected area of colon. Peritoneal signs indicate transmural infarction from the ischemia and require urgent surgical evaluation. Laboratory testing may reveal leucocytosis and elevated serum amylase, creatine phosphokinase, and lactate. Abdominal x-ray usually is unrevealing; however, one-third of patients may have signs such as "thumb-printing." Barium enema can be helpful; however, it should be avoided when suspecting severe ischemia or when a colonoscopy is contemplated since barium may coat the colonic mucosa and make endoscopic interpretation difficult. A CT scan with intravenous contrast can reveal segmental colonic wall thickening or may be entirely normal. Colonoscopy (or sigmoidoscopy) is probably the best test to diagnose IC. The findings encompass pale-appearing mucosa, petechial hemorrhages, hemorrhagic nodules, cyanotic mucosa, mucosal edema, pseudomembranes (occasionally), and black areas (gangrenous), depending on the underlying severity. Typically, segmental distribution, rectal sparing, and abrupt transition of normal and abnormal mucosa are seen. Histology of the biopsies taken from the involved areas shows edema, capillary thrombosis, crypt distortion, granulation tissue, and inflammatory infiltrate in the lamina propria.

The treatment of IC varies from supportive care only to surgery, depending upon the severity. Medications that may cause mesenteric ischemia should be discontinued. Intravenous fluids, oxygen supplementation, and broad-spectrum antibiotics to cover the gut flora should be initiated. Bowel rest is advisable. Exploratory laparotomy should be considered when a patient deteriorates despite optimal supportive care or peritoneal signs emerge. Segmental colonic resection may be needed in cases of severe disease. If colonic infarction develops, the mortality, despite surgery, can rise up to 75%.[23]

The prognosis for the majority of the patients with IC is good and patients typically improve within 24 to 48 hours. Yet up to 20% may end up requiring surgery.[24] IC without evidence of gangrene carries low risk of mortality (~6%).[24] Right-sided IC fares worse than left-sided, with a twofold mortality and fivefold need for surgical intervention.[25] In about 20% of the patients, the IC will become chronic, resulting from persistent ischemia, and may result in colonic strictures, bloody diarrhea, abdominal pain, and repeated episodes of sepsis.[26]

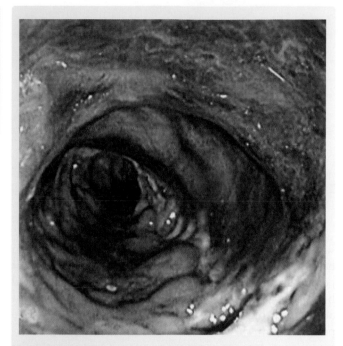

FIGURE 39–4. Endoscopic appearance of ischemic colitis.

colonoscopy that reveals bluish-black–appearing mucosa with friability, edema, and nodularity involving the sigmoid and descending colon (Figure 39–4). The rest of the colon appears unremarkable. Her symptoms improve rapidly in the next 24 hours and she is discharged home on the third hospital day (Table 39–7).

● **TABLE 39–7** Ischemic Colitis: Diagnostic/Management Pearls

1. The presentation can vary from mild to life threatening.
2. Endoscopy is likely the single best test for diagnosis.
3. Consider exploratory laparotomy if patient deteriorates despite optimal care.
4. Twenty percent of the patients may develop chronic ischemic colitis.

● C. DIFFICILE DIARRHEA

CASE PRESENTATION 6: "I THINK THE PIZZA WAS BAD!"

You receive a call from Mrs. J., a 69-year-old Hispanic housewife whom you treated with a 3-day course of oral ciprofloxacin for an uncomplicated urinary tract infection 1 week ago. She reports frequent watery, nonbloody bowel movements that started yesterday and are associated with diffuse abdominal cramping. No fever, nausea, or vomiting have accompanied these episodes. Her husband does not have any of these symptoms. Her grandchildren do visit her occasionally. You recall that she is sexually active and has had two previous episodes of UTI over the past year, but never

CASE PRESENTATION 5 (continued)

The patient receives gentle intravenous hydration, oxygen supplementation, and bowel rest. CBC shows slight leucocytosis (WBC 10.6) and mild anemia (Hb 11.2g/dL, 112 g/L). Stool studies and serum lactate level come back as normal. Her pain persists initially and the CT scan reveals colonic thickening in the left lower quadrant. She is started on IV ceftriaxone and undergoes a had any gastrointestinal symptoms accompany those episodes. She thinks that the pizza that she ate at the local shopping mall the day before might have been "bad." When you examine her at your office, she has mild tenderness in the left lower quadrant. She asks "Doctor, do you think that I should cancel our air tickets for tomorrow, to Hawaii? I and my husband had this vacation planned for a while!" You suspect viral gastro-enteritis but decide to check stool for *Clostridium difficile* toxin given her recent history of antibiotic use.

Clostridium difficile is a spore-forming bacterium, transmitted through a fecal–oral route, and can cause a variety of disease states in humans as a result of its toxin production (collectively termed C. *difficile*-associated disease, or CDAD). The spectrum varies from mild diarrhea to severe colitis (including formation of pseudomembranes), megacolon, bowel perforation, and death. CDAD is mostly seen in hospitalized patients receiving antibiotics, although intestinal surgery and chemotherapy also increase the risk. The number of patients diagnosed with CDAD during a hospitalization is increasing in the United States and was reported at 546 cases per 100,000 patients in 2003.[27] Hospitalized elderly patients are particularly affected and are prone to more severe disease.[28] Furthermore, those living in a nursing home or rehabilitation facility are also at risk,[29] and in fact, 50% of them may be infected, without any associated symptoms.[30] During an outbreak of C. *difficile* infection, patients older than 65 years are 10-fold more likely to contract the infection.[31] Recently, a highly virulent strain of C. *difficile* termed BI/NAP1/027 has been identified and is associated with a threefold higher risk of death than the other strains.[32]

C. *difficile* persists in the environment in its spore form and undergoes transformation to vegetative form inside the human host, where it produces toxins (A, B, and binary) that act as cytotoxins and cause disease, most commonly clinical watery diarrhea. The most notable inciting antibiotics include clindamycin, cephalosporins, fluoroquinolones, and penicillin. On physical examination, mild abdominal tenderness may be present: laboratory studies typically reveal leucocytosis, sometimes quite profound. The gold standard diagnostic test is a stool cytotoxicity assay; however, direct detection of the toxin in stool with enzyme immunoassay is a more commonly used test. The latter has good sensitivity (60-95%) and excellent specificity (99%). Endoscopic examination may be a useful adjunct, especially if clinical suspicion is high but stool tests are negative, or if the patient does not respond to therapy and an alternate diagnosis (such as ischemic colitis) cannot be ruled out.

Management of CDAD consists of stopping the inciting antibiotic, if possible. Definitive treatment of mild-to-moderate disease consists of oral (or intravenous) metronidazole, 500 mg thrice daily. For severe disease, oral vancomycin, 125 mg every 6 hours, is superior to metronidazole.[33] Importantly, intravenous vancomycin has no effect in CDAD. Therapy is usually given for 10 to 14 days. Relapses of CDAD can also be treated with metronidazole or vancomycin (especially if there is severe disease). Rifaximin has also been used in the management of CDAD, though it is not a front-line therapy. Severe CDAD, unresponsive to standard therapy, may require intracolonic fecal infusion using feces from a blood relative, to replenish the natural colonic flora; it has been shown to be effective in some studies. Surgery (partial or total colectomy) may be required when other options fail in severe CDAD.

CASE PRESENTATION 6 (continued)

You advise Mrs. J. to defer her trip and start taking frequent liquids as well as electrolyte solutions. However, she continues to have frequent diarrhea and develops mild to moderate dehydration, necessitating hospitalization and intravenous fluids. Her abdominal tenderness worsens slightly and she also develops a low-grade fever. Stool assays come back positive for *C. difficile* toxin. Colonoscopy reveals pseudomembranous colitis (Figure 39–5). She is started on intravenous metronidazole with subsequent symptomatic improvement. She is discharged 2 days later on oral metronidazole. She leaves for her vacation 2 weeks later, by which time her symptoms have completely resolved (Table 39–8).

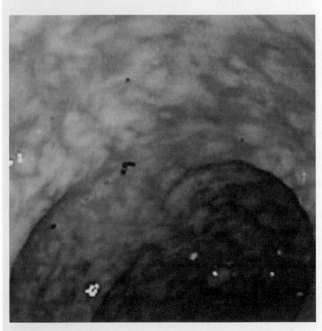

FIGURE 39–5. Endoscopic appearance of *C. difficile* colitis.

● **TABLE 39–8** *Clostridium difficile* Colitis: Diagnostic/ Management Pearls

1. Presentation varies from mild diarrhea to severe colitis.
2. Hospitalized elderly patients are particularly at risk.
3. Endoscopic examination may be considered if clinical suspicion is high but stool toxin assays are negative.
4. Oral vancomycin is preferred to metronidazole for severe disease.

● CHOLELITHIASIS

CASE PRESENTATION 7: INTERMITTENT PAIN NOW MORE ACUTE

Mrs. T., a 70-year-old short and stocky Hispanic woman, a retired judge, seeks your expertise regarding a pain in her right upper side of abdomen that has been bothering her intermittently for the past 3 years but now is more acute and severe for the past 2 days. She did note feeling warm with an occasional chill. The pain comes on only occasionally and especially after eating fried food. She has tried over-the-counter antacids as well as acetaminophen to no avail. She is widowed and lives by herself. Active and with no other significant medical problems, she loves to visit the families of her four grown-up children. Her surgical history consists of an appendectomy at age 12 and a hysterectomy for large fibroids at age 54. She has a remote history of social alcohol intake socially but has not had a drink in over 20 years. She denies any diarrhea or weight loss. On examination she is quite tender upon palpation of the right upper quadrant of her abdomen. Her oral temperature is 100.3°F (37.9°C) with normal BP but slight tachycardia (HR 98). Laboratory tests reveal white blood cell count of 15,700 but with normal AST, ALT, alkaline phosphatase, and total bilirubin. What is the next step in the management of this patient?

Gallstone disease, one of the most common gastrointestinal diseases in the United States, afflicting 6 million men and 14 million women between the ages of 20 and 74.[34] The major risk factors include age, gender (more in women), ethnicity (more in Hispanics), pregnancy, obesity, and cirrhosis. Other risk factors include rapid weight loss (eg, after bariatric surgery), total parenteral nutrition, and family history of gallstones. The majority (~85%) of gallstones are cholesterol stones.

Most of the gallstones are asymptomatic. Typical symptoms, when present, include sharp pain in the epigastric or right upper quadrant (RUQ) area, accompanied by nausea and vomiting. The pain increases in intensity to a peak level and then remains constant for a few hours. Examination may be normal or may reveal RUQ tenderness. Laboratory data may be unremarkable or show hyperbilirubinemia or elevated liver enzymes, particularly alkaline phosphatase. Ultrasound is an excellent test to detect the presence of gallstones; it has a sensitivity of 84% and specificity of 99%. Cholescintigraphy (HIDA scan) is not indicated for the diagnosis of cholelithiasis unless acute cholecystitis is suspected. Complications of gallstone disease include acute cholecystitis, cholangitis, choledocholithiasis, obstructive jaundice, pancreatitis, chronic cholecystitis, Mirizzi syndrome, and rarely, gallbladder cancer. In patients with symptomatic cholelithiasis, there is a 70% chance of recurrent symptoms and complications within 2 years of initial presentation.[35]

Management of gallstone disease depends on whether it is symptomatic or not and the presence or absence of any associated complications. Asymptomatic cholelithiasis, discovered incidentally, does not need to be treated. Symptomatic cholelithiasis requires adequate pain control with oral diclofenac or intravenous ketorolac, depending on its severity. Definitive treatment is surgical removal of the gallbladder, either laparoscopically or via an open incision. Oral chenodeoxycholic acid or ursodeoxycholic acid may be helpful in dissolving small stones in a minority of patients and are suitable options for patients who are not surgical candidates. If jaundice or cholangitis are present, an endoscopic retrograde cholangiography should be considered in order to identify and remove common bile duct stones through a sphincterotomy and stone extraction using a balloon or basket. Such stone clearance facilitates the resolution of cholangitis and the subsequent performance of a laparoscopic cholecystectomy.

CASE PRESENTATION 7 (continued)

Based on her history as well as associated risk factors, you suspect Mrs. T. of having cholelithiasis with possible acute cholecystitis, and the next step in her management is obtaining a RUQ ultrasound. It confirms the diagnosis of acute cholecystitis (Figure 39–6) and she undergoes a laparoscopic cholecystectomy with subsequent resolution of her symptoms (Table 39–9).

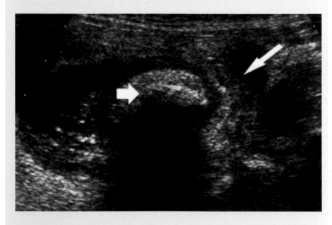

FIGURE 39–6. Right upper quadrant ultrasound in acute cholecystitis.

● **TABLE 39–9** Cholelithiasis: Diagnostic/Management Pearls

1. Most gallstones are asymptomatic and require no treatment.
2. Ultrasound is an excellent test for detection.
3. Management depends upon the presence or absence of symptoms and of complications.
4. Cholecystectomy is the only definitive treatment.

• PANCREATIC CANCER

CASE PRESENTATION 8: RECENT WEIGHT LOSS

Mr. G., a 77-year-old Caucasian retired minister, comes to visit you at the insistence of his wife, who is worried about his recent weight loss. As you shake his hand, you notice that he has temporal wasting and icteric sclerae. On further questioning, he admits to recent change in the color of his urine and stools. He also describes a dull ache in his upper abdomen. His appetite has decreased somewhat. He denies any family history of gastrointestinal cancers though his father died at age 67 of lung cancer. Mr. G. started smoking cigarettes in his early teenage years but quit once he became a minister in his mid-20s. He denies any alcohol history. While listening to his story, the word "malignancy" pops up in your head, as you mentally visualize the anatomic relations of the various abdominal organs. His wife, seeing the worried look on your face, inquires further about your concerns and you tell her that you are worried about the possibility of pancreatic cancer.

Pancreatic cancer is the fifth leading cause of cancer death in men and women and is the second most common gastrointestinal cancer. Its age-adjusted incidence is 12.9 per 100,000 men and 10 per 100,000 women; 32,000 new cases were diagnosed during 2004 in the United States. Because of the high associated mortality, the number of deaths per year from pancreatic cancer closely matches the number of new cases per year. More than 90% of pancreatic cancer is ductal adenocarcinoma. The majority (60%) of pancreatic cancers arise in the head of the pancreas. Risk factors include age (> 45 years), gender (males more commonly affected), race (more common in blacks), hereditary pancreatitis, chronic pancreatitis, smoking, diabetes mellitus, obesity, and possibly heavy alcohol use.

The clinical presentation varies depending on the location of cancer within the pancreas. Tumors in the head of the pancreas manifest with jaundice, weight loss or, in a minority of cases, with vague epigastric pain. Those in the body or tail present with weight loss and possibly epigastric pain. Other associated symptoms may include anorexia, nausea, steatorrhea, malaise, and migratory thrombophlebitis. However, by the time any symptoms appear, the cancer is already in an advanced stage and only 20% are resectable.[36] An abdominal mass may be felt in 20% of the patients. Laboratory tests may reveal elevated serum bilirubin and alkaline phosphatase. Serum levels of CA 19-9 and CA 125 can help establish a diagnosis of cancer in pancreatic tumors. The best imaging study is a thin-slice, helical CT scan of the pancreas, which is 97% accurate; it is also used for staging as well as for obtaining a biopsy to establish tissue diagnosis. Endoscopic ultrasound with fine-needle aspiration can be helpful to establish a diagnosis in cases of small tumors.

Surgery offers the best chance of a cure; unfortunately, by the time a patient presents to the clinician, only about 10% to 15% of pancreatic cancers are resectable. The Whipple procedure and pylorus-preserving pancreaticoduodenectomy have similar outcomes. Chemotherapy (neoadjuvant or adjuvant) with 5-fluoruracil and/or gemcitabine improves survival, but the overall 5-year survival remains dismal at less than 5%. Even with "curative" surgery, median survival ranges from 10 to 20 months only. The predictors of improved outcome include a tumor less than 3 cm in size, no lymph node involvement, negative margins after surgery, and well-differentiated tumors. Palliation of inoperable tumors involves chemotherapy, radiotherapy, endoscopic biliary stent placement to relieve obstructive jaundice, celiac plexus block to relieve pain, and gastric decompression (for intractable nausea and vomiting secondary to duodenal obstruction from the tumor) using a gastrostomy tube. Hospice care should be considered for those with advanced disease.

CASE PRESENTATION 8 (continued)

You further explain to Mr. G and his wife that your suspicion of pancreatic cancer is based on his presenting symptoms of epigastric pain, significant weight loss, and features of obstructive jaundice—icterus, acholic stools, and dark urine. You arrange for appropriate laboratory tests and a pancreatic protocol CT scan. It reveals a pancreatic head low-attenuation mass causing obstruction of both the bile and pancreatic ducts (Figure 39–7). You make an urgent referral for an oncologist for treatment options and also schedule a follow-up visit to see him in 2 weeks (Table 39–10).

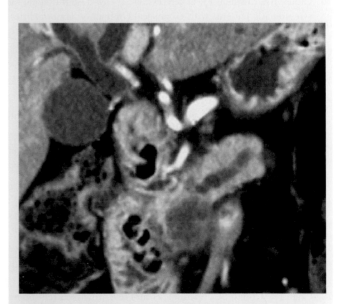

FIGURE 39–7. Coronal CT images of a pancreatic head mass which obstructs the pancreatic duct.

● **TABLE 39–10** Pancreatic Cancer: Diagnostic/Management Pearls

1. Associated with high mortality.
2. Majority arise in the head of the pancreas.
3. Thin-slice, helical pancreatic CT scan is a highly accurate test for diagnosis.
4. Endoscopy ultrasound with fine-needle aspiration can be helpful for small tumors.

CONCLUSION

Clinicians involved in the care of elderly patients need to be well cognizant of the conditions discussed in this chapter and should include them in the differential diagnoses of gastrointestinal complaints. An understanding of these should help in working closely with a gastroenterologist and in taking better care of these patients. Issues unique to the geriatric population, such as presence of multiple co-morbid illnesses as well as atypical presentation of various disorders, need to be considered.

References

1. Everhart JE, Ruhl CE. Burden of digestive diseases in the United States part I: Overall and upper gastrointestinal diseases. *Gastroenterology.* 2009;136:376-386.

2. Bloem BR, Lagaay AM, van Beek W, et al. Prevalence of subjective dysphagia in community residents aged over 87. *BMJ.* 1990;300: 721-722.

3. Barczi SR, Sullivan PA, Robbins J. How should dysphagia care of older adults differ? Establishing optimal practice patterns. *Semin Speech Lang.* 2000;21:347-361.

4. Shamburek RD, Farrar JT. Disorders of the digestive system in the elderly. *N Engl J Med.* 1990;322:438-443.

5. Cattau EL Jr., Castell DO, Johnson DA, et al. Diltiazem therapy for symptoms associated with nutcracker esophagus. *Am J Gastroenterol.* 1991;86:272-276.

6. Clouse RE, Lustman PJ, Eckert TC, et al. Low-dose trazodone for symptomatic patients with esophageal contraction abnormalities. A double-blind, placebo-controlled trial. *Gastroenterology.* 1987; 92:1027-1036.

7. Chan FK. NSAID-induced peptic ulcers and *Helicobacter pylori* infection: Implications for patient management. *Drug Saf.* 2005; 28:287-300.

8. Weil J, Colin-Jones D, Langman M, et al. Prophylactic aspirin and risk of peptic ulcer bleeding. *BMJ.* 1995;310:827-830.

9. McQuaid KR, Laine L. Systematic review and meta-analysis of adverse events of low-dose aspirin and clopidogrel in randomized controlled trials. *Am J Med.* 2006;119:624-638.

10. Piper JM, Ray WA, Daugherty JR, Griffin MR. Corticosteroid use and peptic ulcer disease: Role of nonsteroidal anti-inflammatory drugs. *Ann Intern Med.* 1991;114:735-740.

11. Rostom A, Dube C, Wells G, et al. Prevention of NSAID-induced gastroduodenal ulcers. *Cochrane Database Syst Rev.* 2002;4: CD002296.

12. Chan FK, Chung SC, Suen BY, et al. Preventing recurrent upper gastrointestinal bleeding in patients with *Helicobacter pylori* infection who are taking low-dose aspirin or naproxen. *N Engl J Med.* 2001; 344:967-973.

13. Lanas A, Garcia-Rodriguez LA, Arroyo MT, et al. Effect of antisecretory drugs and nitrates on the risk of ulcer bleeding associated with nonsteroidal anti-inflammatory drugs, antiplatelet agents, and anticoagulants. *Am J Gastroenterol.* 2007;102:507-515.

14. Chan FKL, Hung LCT, Suen BY, et al. Celecoxib versus diclofenac plus omeprazole in high-risk arthritis patients: Results of a randomized double-blind trial. *Gastroenterology.* 2004;127:1038-1043.

15. Chan FK, Wong VW, Suen BY, et al. Combination of a cyclooxygenase-2 inhibitor and a proton-pump inhibitor for prevention of recurrent ulcer bleeding in patients at very high risk: A double-blind, randomised trial. *Lancet.* 2007;369:1621-1626.

16. Roberts SH, James O, Jarvis EH. Bacterial overgrowth syndrome without "blind loop": A cause for malnutrition in the elderly. *Lancet.* 1977;2:1193-1195.

17. McEvoy A, Dutton J, James OF. Bacterial contamination of the small intestine is an important cause of occult malabsorption in the elderly. *Br Med J (Clin Res Ed).* 1983;287:789-793.

18. Lewis SJ, Potts LF, Malhotra R, Mountford R. Small bowel bacterial overgrowth in subjects living in residential care homes. *Age Ageing.* 1999;28:181-185.

19. Montgomery RD, Haboubi NY, Mike NH, et al. Causes of malabsorption in the elderly. *Age Ageing.* 1986;15:235-240.

20. Williams AR, Balasooriya BA, Day DW. Polyps and cancer of the large bowel: A necropsy study in Liverpool. *Gut.* 1982;23:835-842.

21. Lieberman DA, Weiss DG, Harford WV, et al. Five-year colon surveillance after screening colonoscopy. *Gastroenterology.* 2007;133: 1077-1085.

22. Binns JC, Isaacson P. Age-related changes in the colonic blood supply: their relevance to ischaemic colitis. *Gut.* 1978;19:384-390.

23. Longo WE, Ward D, Vernava AM III, Kaminski DL. Outcome of patients with total colonic ischemia. *Dis Colon Rectum.* 1997;40: 1448-1454.

24. Longo WE, Ballantyne GH, Gusberg RJ. Ischemic colitis: Patterns and prognosis. *Dis Colon Rectum.* 1992;35:726-730.

25. Sotiriadis J, Brandt LJ, Behin DS, Southern WN. Ischemic colitis has a worse prognosis when isolated to the right side of the colon. *Am J Gastroenterol.* 2007;102:2247-2252.

26. Cappell MS. Intestinal (mesenteric) vasculopathy. II. Ischemic colitis and chronic mesenteric ischemia. *Gastroenterol Clin North Am.* 1998;27:827-860, vi.

27. Ricciardi R, Rothenberger DA, Madoff RD, Baxter NN. Increasing prevalence and severity of *Clostridium difficile* colitis in hospitalized patients in the United States. *Arch Surg.* 2007;142:624-631; discussion, 631.

28. Carignan A, Allard C, Pepin J, et al. Risk of *Clostridium difficile* infection after perioperative antibacterial prophylaxis before and during an outbreak of infection due to a hypervirulent strain. *Clin Infect Dis.* 2008;46:1838-1843.

29. Pepin J, Saheb N, Coulombe MA, et al. Emergence of fluoroquinolones as the predominant risk factor for *Clostridium difficile*-associated diarrhea: A cohort study during an epidemic in Quebec. *Clin Infect Dis.* 2005;41:1254-1260.

30. Riggs MM, Sethi AK, Zabarsky TF, et al. Asymptomatic carriers are a potential source for transmission of epidemic and nonepidemic *Clostridium difficile* strains among long-term care facility residents. *Clin Infect Dis.* 2007;45:992-998.

31. Pepin J, Valiquette L, Cossette B. Mortality attributable to nosocomial *Clostridium difficile*-associated disease during an epidemic caused by a hypervirulent strain in Quebec. *CMAJ.* 2005;173:1037-1042.

32. Warny M, Pepin J, Fang A, et al. Toxin production by an emerging strain of *Clostridium difficile* associated with outbreaks of severe disease in North America and Europe. *Lancet*. 2005;366:1079-1084.

33. Zar FA, Bakkanagari SR, Moorthi KM, Davis MB. A comparison of vancomycin and metronidazole for the treatment of *Clostridium difficile*-associated diarrhea, stratified by disease severity. *Clin Infect Dis*. 2007;45:302-307.

34. Everhart JE, Khare M, Hill M, Maurer KR. Prevalence and ethnic differences in gallbladder disease in the United States. *Gastroenterology*. 1999;117:632-639.

35. Thistle JL, Cleary PA, Lachin JM, et al. The natural history of cholelithiasis: The National Cooperative Gallstone Study. *Ann Intern Med*. 1984;101:171-175.

36. Warshaw AL, Fernandez-del Castillo C. Pancreatic carcinoma. *N Engl J Med*. 1992;326:455-465.

37. Winawer SJ, Zauber AG, Fletcher RH, et al. Guidelines for colonoscopy surveillance after polypectomy: A consensus update by the US Multi-Society Task Force on Colorectal Cancer and the American Cancer Society. *Gastroenterology*. 2006;130: 1872-1885.

POST-TEST

1. Which of the following is NOT an effective treatment for *Clostridium difficile*–associated disease?

A. Oral metronidazole

B. Intravenous metronidazole

C. Oral vancomycin

D. Intravenous vancomycin

2. Which of the statements is FALSE regarding gallstone disease?

A. Hispanic ethnicity is a risk factor.

B. Most older adults are symptomatic.

C. The definitive treatment is cholecystectomy.

D. It is more common with increasing age.

3. Which of the following patients has a higher comparative risk of developing pancreatic cancer?

A. A 34-year-old Caucasian man with diabetes mellitus of 5 years duration

B. A 53-year-old Caucasian woman with a history of ingesting 2 or 3 alcoholic drinks per day for the past 10 years

C. A 67-year-old African American man with a 20 pack-year smoking history

D. A 42-year-old Hispanic man with a BMI of 36

ANSWERS TO PRE-TEST

1. D
2. C
3. B
4. C

ANSWERS TO POST-TEST

1. D
2. B
3. C

40

Hip Fractures

Susan M. Friedman, MD, MPH

Daniel A. Mendelson, MS, MD

Stephen L. Kates, MD

● **LEARNING OBJECTIVES**

1. Identify common consequences of hip fractures.
2. Describe the evaluation of a patient with an acute hip fracture.
3. List the common co-morbidities of patients who have hip fractures.
4. Explain the importance of getting patients with hip fractures to surgery in a timely fashion.
5. Discuss the different types of hip fracture and implications for repair.
6. Identify common complications following hip fracture repair, and how to reduce their incidence.
7. Describe systematic ways to optimize hip fracture care.

PRE-TEST

1. **The most common postoperative complication for hip fracture patients is:**
   A. Arrhythmia
   B. Delirium
   C. Pressure sore
   D. Urinary tract infection

2. **Which of the following is NOT true regarding perioperative management of hip fracture patients?**

   A. Communication with patients and family members promotes care planning, reduces anxiety, and prevents information from "slipping through the cracks."
   B. Hydration status can be monitored via assessing blood pressure, mucous membranes, urine output, and renal function.
   C. "Tethers," such as Foley catheters, restraints, and intravenous fluids, should be limited to whatever extent possible.
   D. Surgical delay to investigate every chronic, stable co-morbidity is likely to improve outcomes.

3. **Which of the following is TRUE about the surgical management of hip fractures?**

A. Approximately 60% of patients who fracture their hips will undergo surgical repair of the fracture.

B. Indications for surgical repair include restoration of function and mobility, and reduction of pain.

C. Patients who are bed-bound should not receive surgical repair, since surgery will not change their ambulatory status.

D. Patients with unstable fractures have minimal care needs, and surgical intervention is therefore usually not indicated.

CASE PRESENTATION 1: UNINTENDED CONSEQUENCES OF DELAYS

F.P. is a 90-year-old Caucasian woman who lives independently but must descend and climb one flight of stairs every time she leaves and returns to her apartment. She lives alone, but has a daughter who lives nearby, whom she visits at least twice a week. She has been in good health with only well-controlled hypertension and mild cataracts not needing surgery, but otherwise no significant past medical history. She doesn't smoke or drink alcohol. Her mother fractured her hip in her 80s after a fall. Her only medication is a diuretic. She is 5 feet tall (152 cm) and weighs 110 pounds (50 kg).

• INTRODUCTION

Hip fractures are a common and serious problem, associated with substantial morbidity and mortality. Because of the aging of the population worldwide, the incidence of hip fractures is increasing across the globe (Figure 40–1).[1] A 50-year-old white woman has a 15.6% lifetime risk of hip fracture, a 15% risk of Colles fracture, and a 32% risk of at least one atraumatic vertebral fracture.[1a] Each year 350,000 hip fractures occur in the United States,[2] and this number may grow to 500,000 by 2040.[3]

At least 20% of patients die within a year of hip fracture surgery.[4] One-fourth of those who lived in the community will need long-term nursing home care.[5] A year after a hip fracture, 40% are still unable to walk independently, 60% have difficulty with at least one activity of daily living, and 80% need assistance with an instrumental activity of daily living,

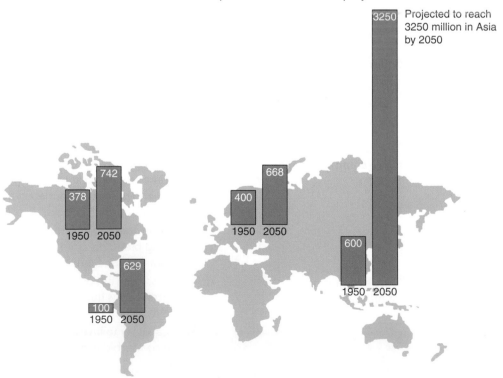

Dimension of the problem—worldwide projection

Estimated number of hip fractures (1000s)

FIGURE 40–1. World incidence of hip fractures historical and projected. (*Adapted from Cooper C, Campion G, Melton U. Hip fractures in the elderly. A world-wide projection. Osteoporosis Intl. 1992;3:285-289.*)

such as shopping or house cleaning.[6] Individuals who have sustained a hip fracture may experience increased fear of falling,[7] and may have difficulties with gait and balance,[5] which may in turn limit mobility and functioning.

Hip fractures occur predominantly in older adults, particularly those with frailty in whom homeostatic systems are impaired. They often have multiple co-morbidities and may function well until they have a serious acute event.[8] At that point, they are at high risk of developing complications and are likely to have difficulty recovering or will be at risk for further complications, which can set off a vicious downward spiral. The road to recovery of function can be slow, with frequent setbacks. Management of co-morbidities and anticipation of common complications affords an opportunity to dramatically improve the quality of care and outcomes for patients who suffer hip fragility fractures.

It is estimated that 90% of hip fractures result from a fall (for more on gait and falls see Chapter 34).[9] For this reason, some argue that the focus of hip fracture prevention should be fall prevention.[10,11] Most hip fractures in older adults occur in the setting of low-energy falls in patients with osteoporosis or osteopenia. Patients who have osteoporosis can sustain hip fractures after falling from a standing or even sitting height. Metabolic bone disease, such as osteomalacia and Paget disease, can lead to stress fractures. Less commonly, primary or metastatic cancer can result in hip fractures.

● RISK FACTORS FOR SUSTAINING A HIP FRACTURE

The FRAX score is a WHO-developed tool to help determine the 10-year risk of hip fracture and other fragility fractures.[12] This tool is free, available online (http://www.shef.ac.uk/FRAX/), and was developed based on population-based cohort studies in Europe, North America, Asia, and Australia. By entering age, gender, height, weight, previous history of fracture, parental history of hip fracture, smoking history, use of glucocorticoids, history of rheumatoid arthritis, a chronic condition associated with secondary osteoporosis, alcohol history, and bone mineral density if available, a 10-year risk of subsequent fracture can be determined. According to this tool, without having all the information about whether she has osteoporosis, our patient, Mrs. F. P., has a 33% risk of sustaining a hip fracture over the next 10 years

CASE PRESENTATION 1 (continued)

F.P. feels well prior to going to bed one evening. However, she sustains a fall onto her right side after tripping over a slipper on the way to the bathroom at 3:00 in the morning, without her glasses. She has no dizziness, loss of consciousness, or light-headedness surrounding the fall. She notes immediate, severe right hip pain and is unable get up off the floor. She is eventually able to crawl to her bedside nightstand and call for an ambulance. On presentation to the emergency room she is examined, is noted to have a leg length discrepancy by the ER physician as well as tremendous pain with any attempt to move the right leg. X-rays of the right hip and pelvis show a moderately displaced right intertrochanteric hip fracture, but no other fractures. Labs are normal except for a BUN-to-creatinine ratio of 24. She is evaluated by the orthopedic surgery team and a surgical repair of her fracture is recommended. Her admission orders are written by the orthopedic team, but her admission to the ward is delayed by a full hospital census as well as cardiac testing that has been ordered. An echocardiogram, obtained 48 hours after admission, shows an ejection fraction of 58%, mild mitral regurgitation, normal chambers sizes, and no other significant abnormalities.

● ACUTE EVALUATION OF PATIENTS WITH HIP FRACTURE

Acute evaluation of the hip fracture patient should include questioning about the circumstances of the fall. If the patient is unable to give a reliable history, it is helpful to question any family, caregivers, or witnesses (see Chapter 34). For our patient, as is seen in many patients, the fall was probably multifactorial, resulting from an environmental hazard in a patient who has some visual impairment and was not wearing her glasses. In addition, her labs suggest that she may have some dehydration, which also could have contributed to the fall.

In addition to the circumstances surrounding the fall, it is prudent to assess what other injuries or problems the patient may have. Did the patient fall directly on his or her hip? Did the patient hit his or her head? Are there other injuries? How long did the patient lie on the floor before help arrived?

Falls are a common nonspecific outcome of acute illness, such as acute infection, dehydration, or cardiac disease. It is therefore important to take a thorough history in addition to the specific falls history. In Mrs. P.'s case, it does not appear that she was feeling ill prior to her fall, and she does not describe any symptoms consistent with a urinary tract infection, though this can be misleading (see Chapter 9). However, it may be worthwhile to ask her about how much fluid she drinks and whether she has reduced her intake for any reason.

Physical exam involves evaluation of the acute injury, assessment for evidence of other injuries, investigation of possible causes of the fall, assessment of evidence of osteoporosis such as severe kyphosis or low body weight, determination of the presence of other acute illness that might delay surgery, and identification of significant co-morbidities that may result in postoperative complications or require additional attention before or after surgery. Essential elements include vital signs, evaluation for head trauma, a thorough cardiorespiratory evaluation, abdominal exam, evaluation of the injured extremity, and other targeted exam as directed by history.

Orthopedic examination starts with an evaluation of the affected extremity. Check for osteophony (bone sound), by placing the diaphragm of your stethoscope on the pubic symphysis. Gently percuss each kneecap with your forefinger. An intact bone will produce a clear, bright tapping sound. A hip fracture will give a muffled, distant sound. Other approaches include using a tuning fork on the patella or listening over each iliac crest rather than the pubic symphysis. Observe for shortening or rotational deformity at the level of the feet. This is best assessed from the foot of the bed. Because movement of a fractured hip is frequently painful, "log-rolling" of the affected extremity is useful to diagnose a fracture (see Chapter 6 for more on the geriatric physical exam). Once the fracture has been noted, however, movement should be minimized to reduce bleeding and pain experienced by the patient.

The orthopedic exam should include an examination of all four extremities as well as the pelvis and spine. Presence of ecchymosis, crepitus, hematoma, pain, and deformity should all be noted in the medical record. The pelvis should be palpated as well to exclude the presence of injury. It is not uncommon to have knee pain with hip fracture and the ipsilateral knee should be assessed for tenderness, crepitus, or effusion that could represent injury. An examination looking for other injuries is completed for Mrs. P., with no other injuries noted.

Neurologic examination should include evaluation of the active motion and sensory examination of both feet, and findings should be recorded. Vascular examination should include palpation of pedal pulses and observation of lower leg skin for presence of chronic venous congestion changes. Capillary refill in the extremities should also be assessed.

Examination of the skin should include evaluation for the presence of ecchymosis, wounds, or ulceration. The presence of a pressure ulcer in the setting of a hip fracture usually indicates a much worse than average prognosis.

Patients who sustain hip fractures are at high risk for having another hip fracture,[15] in part because of the presence of osteoporosis, and in part because persons who fall are at high risk for falling again. For this reason, it is important to assess for other fall risk factors. Is this a person who has had multiple falls in the past? If so, is there a pattern to the falls? How is the patient's vision? Were there any environmental issues related to the fall? Did the patient have problems with gait and balance prior to this fall? Is there any evidence of alcoholism (commonly under-recognized in older adults)? Review medications—is the patient on medications that put him or her at high risk of falls,[16] such as psychotropics, sedatives, or antidepressants? Are there any new medications or dose changes?

REASONS FOR SURGICAL REPAIR OF HIP FRACTURES

The majority of patients who experience a hip fracture will require and benefit from surgical repair.[13] Indications for hip fracture surgery include:

- Preservation of function and mobility
- Pain control
- Promote fracture healing
- Improve the ability to care for the patient

For most, the primary reason is restoration of function and mobility. However, pain control is also an important reason for surgery. Particularly for unstable fractures, patients generally will have substantial pain related to turning, moving, or other functions related to being cared for. Turning patients regularly for bathing and hygiene-related care, and prevention of pressure sores, may be painful for the patient, requiring potent systemic opioids to preserve comfort. For that reason, even patients who have severely restricted mobility may benefit from surgical fracture repair.[14] Non-operative treatment is indicated in patients who have extremely short life expectancy (days to weeks) in whom the risks outweigh the benefits; patients who present late and show signs of healing; patients who are immobile with a stable fracture that is not associated with significant pain; and patients who do not want to have surgery after understanding the risks and benefits.

COMMON CO-MORBIDITIES IN PATIENTS WITH HIP FRACTURE

Because hip fracture incidence increases with age, and because patients over age 85 have the highest incidence of hip fracture, they commonly present with multiple co-morbidities. A list of common co-morbidities can be found in Table 40–1. Assessment of co-morbidities preoperatively helps determine medical stability, individualize treatment, anticipate potential complications, and plan both acute and follow-up care. Some common co-morbidities in a hip fracture population include osteoporosis, dementia, coronary artery disease and congestive heart failure, chronic obstructive pulmonary disease, hypertension, and diabetes. We will discuss some clinical implications of each of these co-morbidities next.

Osteoporosis is present in most patients who are admitted with acute hip fractures, and many have osteomalacia as well. Unfortunately, only about 20% of patients who undergo hip fracture surgery receive secondary prevention,[17] and the result is that they are at high risk of sustaining a second fracture. *Osteomalacia* is also commonly seen, particularly in frail and nursing home or homebound patients, who may spend minimal time outdoors. At a minimum, patients should have a calcium and 25-OH vitamin D level drawn, and have a follow-up assessment with their primary care physician for evaluation and treatment of osteoporosis.

TABLE 40–1 Common Co-Morbidities in Patients with Hip Fracture

1. Osteoporosis
2. Osteomalacia
3. Dementia
4. Coronary artery disease
5. Congestive heart failure
6. Chronic obstructive pulmonary disease
7. Hypertension
8. Diabetes

Dementia increases with age, and is most common in those over the age of 85 (see Chapter 31). Dementia increases the risk of postoperative delirium.[18] Anticholinergic stress during the perioperative period, whether from medications, anesthesia, the stress of surgery, sudden changes in blood pressure, or infection, adds to the risk of delirium. Responses to previous surgery will help assess the added level of risk of delirium (see Chapter 30). The perioperative period may also be a time of "unmasking" of a dementia that was previously unrecognized by family members or caregivers. Changes in cognition that have progressed slowly over time may be identified, thus leading to opportunities for further evaluation, treatment, and care planning. For patients with advanced dementia, the return to full weight-bearing status following surgery is critical, because they will be unlikely to be able to follow instructions for partial weight-bearing.

Coronary artery disease is also seen frequently in older adults. The presence of stable coronary artery disease should not delay surgery.[19] A history determining whether there has been a recent escalation of ischemic symptoms should be obtained, as well as symptoms at the time of the fall, to determine whether it is likely that the patient has had an acute coronary event. A history of usual activity level and absence of cardiac symptoms is helpful to estimate exercise tolerance and risk of acute coronary events in the perioperative period.

The presence of *congestive heart failure* is important to determine so as to anticipate issues related to perioperative fluid management. As a result of bleeding and third-space losses into the fracture site, patients are often dehydrated on admission (as we see in our F.P.'s case). This will need to be treated with intravenous hydration initially, with clinical monitoring of volume status. The presence of congestive heart failure at baseline is a risk factor for developing multiple complications, including cardiac complications, delirium, and renal insufficiency postoperatively. Previous echocardiogram results can provide useful information as to the mechanism of congestive heart failure, but it is rare that surgery should be delayed in order to obtain an echocardiogram.

Evaluation of *chronic obstructive pulmonary disease* is important in determining surgical and anesthetic risks. Some patients will not tolerate intubation and general anesthesia or may be particularly sensitive to sedation used with regional anesthesia. Patients with significant pulmonary disease require careful care coordination with the medical, surgical, and anesthesia teams. Often patient with chronic obstructive pulmonary disease have coronary and other vascular disease as well as renal disease.

Orthostatic hypotension and hypertension are relatively common chronic conditions in older adults. Orthostatic hypotension should be a consideration in the etiology of any fall, and evidence of this should be elicited from the history. Mrs. P. doesn't give a history to suggest orthostatic hypotension, but her lab values suggest that she may have some dehydration. Well-controlled hypertension should not be a contraindication to surgery but the medications related to blood pressure control should be monitored because of the significant fluid shifts that occur perioperatively. Patients often have significantly lower blood pressures than normal after surgery. Sudden shifts in blood pressure put patients at risk for developing delirium, as well as other end-organ damage. For this reason, it may be useful to discontinue some blood pressure medications immediately postoperatively and restart them when the blood pressure increases. For most patients with fragility fractures, low blood pressure is much more of an issue than high blood pressure and it is important not to overtreat elevated blood pressure. When fracture patients have dramatically elevated blood pressure, consider inadequately managed pain and carefully assess volume status.

Patients with *diabetes mellitus* may have pre-existing end-organ damage, such as renal impairment and coronary artery disease that may lead to postoperative complications. Renal, coronary, and other vascular disease due to diabetes may be subclinical, but still impact risk and prognosis. Additionally, because of the stresses of surgery and decreased oral intake initially, glucose control may be variable. It is therefore useful initially to hold long-acting medications (both insulins and oral agents), provide short-acting insulin until oral intake improves, and then resume the previous regimen when the patient is stable. There is growing evidence that poor glycemic control increases morbidity and mortality.[20] In frail older adults, particularly those with dementia and/or delirium, who may not be able to report symptoms, this must be weighed against the risks of hypoglycemia.

● TIMELY SURGICAL INTERVENTION

There is considerable observational evidence that delays in surgery for patients who are otherwise stable lead to worse outcomes, including increased complication rates, longer lengths of stay, lower likelihood of returning to independent living, and higher mortality.[21-23] Longer times to surgery increase the risks of immobility, including venous thromboembolism, skin breakdown, deconditioning, pulmonary decompensation, and infection. Delays lead to longer durations of acute preoperative pain, anxiety, and associated complications. A delay in surgery also delays weight-bearing and post-fracture rehabilitation. For these reasons, surgery should be completed as soon as medically appropriate and as facilities allow. In other words, hip fracture surgery should be considered urgent but not emergent. Patients who sustain a hip fracture as a result of a fall caused by an acute illness may require additional medical optimization prior to surgery; patients who have multiple co-morbidities that are stable, on the other hand, should not need to have surgery delayed.

Although it is possible to optimize the patient's condition, it should be understood and communicated to patients and their families that surgery remains a substantial risk. A careful discussion of risks and benefits of surgery, within the context of the patient's preoperative status and goals of care, should be completed prior to the surgery. It is helpful to establish advance directives prior to surgical intervention.

Preoperative evaluation should be targeted to workup that will likely change management and outcome (see Chapter 21). It is important to ensure that chronic co-morbidities are stable, and to identify and treat acute, unstable conditions. It is reasonable to include in the initial evaluation the following items:

- History and physical exam
- CBC with differential
- Electrolytes and renal function
- Coagulation studies
- Urinalysis
- Bone radiographs
- EKG

Radiographic examination should include films of the pelvis and entire ipsilateral femur. Any other painful body site or positive findings on examination should be followed up with detailed radiographs of that area. Routine cardiac evaluation including echocardiogram, cardiac markers, and chest radiograph should be *avoided* without focal findings, symptoms, or a history that suggests the presence of active cardiovascular disease. In this case, since Mrs. P. did not have any symptoms to suggest active cardiac disease, an echocardiogram was not necessary to include preoperatively and contributed to a delay in her surgery.

There are several clinical conditions that may potentially delay surgery. Many elderly hip fracture patients are being treated with warfarin prior to their injury. They may need warfarin for a variety of different reasons, including atrial fibrillation, mechanical heart valves, cardiac thrombus, stroke, or history of thromboembolism. Many centers use a target INR of < 1.5 before taking a patient to surgery. It is useful to understand the type of fracture, and type of procedure planned in determining the aggressiveness of reducing the INR. The type of anesthesia may also affect the target INR based on whether regional, spinal, or general anesthesia is utilized. Methods for treating an elevated INR include delay (with the considerations as listed), use of vitamin K, or administration of fresh frozen plasma. Studies evaluating effectiveness of oral versus intravenous vitamin K have shown similar efficacy at 24 hours[24]; subcutaneous and intramuscular vitamin K should be avoided as absorption is less predictable and may lead to warfarin resistance when anticoagulation is reinitiated. There exists a small risk of anaphylaxis when vitamin K is administered as an intravenous preparation. Oral or intravenous vitamin K usually takes at least 6 hours to begin to be effective. If fresh frozen plasma is chosen, it must be timed correctly with the start of surgery, since its effectiveness only lasts for about 6 hours; it is sometimes useful to consider infusing additional fresh frozen plasma during surgery based on clinical need.

Clopidogrel is an irreversible platelet inhibitor that is used frequently in acute coronary syndromes and stroke. Because of the risk of bleeding, clopidogrel should be discontinued 7 days prior to *elective surgery*. However, hip fracture surgery is considered an urgent procedure. One recent survey of orthopedic surgery residency programs found that about 74% of those surveyed felt it was acceptable to wait 3 days or fewer, and 25% felt that no delay was necessary.[25] Some centers routinely transfuse platelets for patients who were previously on clopidogrel, although there is currently no good evidence assessing this practice. Careful assessment of the type of procedure, expected duration of surgery, and expected blood loss is useful

in optimizing care and in determining the risks and benefits of delayed surgery.

Several cardiac conditions may lead to a delay in surgery according to the 2007 ACC/AHA perioperative guidelines.[19] These include acute coronary syndromes, decompensated congestive heart failure, severe valvular heart disease, and significant arrhythmias. Full evaluation of these conditions and discussions with the anesthesiologist and cardiologist will help in optimizing surgical and postoperative management. A history of compensated, stable congestive heart failure alone should not result in a delay to surgery for further cardiac evaluation.

Severe infection, such as pneumonia or sepsis, will also lead to surgical delay. Issues that will require treatment prior to surgery include respiratory status, blood pressure, and clearing of septicemia. It is imperative to avoid placing an implant when a patient is potentially bacteremic.

● OPERATIVE CONSIDERATIONS

Hip fracture surgery in older adults presents several challenges. The combination of requiring urgent surgery in a patient with multiple co-morbidities and poor bone quality results in the need for a high level of expertise in surgical management of the patient.

Certain surgical principles are important to follow in order to optimize care. First, prophylactic antibiotics that provide anti-staphylococcal coverage should be administered, with the first dose given within 60 minutes of skin incision, and lasting for less than 24 hours.[26] This practice has been shown to reduce deep and superficial infections by 60%. Local resistance patterns and medication allergies may dictate antibiotic choice.

Second, patients who are medically stable should have surgery within 48 hours of admission (and ideally within 24 hours), preferably during normal working hours. It is best to avoid having fresh postoperative patients with significant co-morbidities and frailty returning to the hospital unit when nurse and medical staffing levels are lowest overnight.[27]

Third, maintaining hydration before, during, and after surgery will help reduce complications such as hypotension, renal failure, and delirium. Urine output, renal function, blood pressure, and heart rate are usually the best indicators of volume status. Skin tenting is often unreliable due to natural aging of the skin and loss of elastin. Many elderly patients who are supine in bed will develop crackles on exam.

Fourth, rehabilitation allowing weight-bearing as tolerated status shortly after surgery is preferred. Restoring mobility decreases the risk of skin breakdown, delirium, pneumonia, and urinary tract infection. Many fragility fracture patients cannot reliably follow directions for partial weight-bearing due to cognitive dysfunction and/or alterations in proprioception or musculoskeletal function.

Although somewhat controversial at this point,[28] low-dose beta blockers may reduce risk in the perioperative period for those with known or suspected coronary artery disease.[29] There is suggestion that patients with the highest cardiac risk have the most benefit from beta-blockers.[30] The largest randomized controlled trial to date, POISE, comprising 8351 patients, showed a reduction in myocardial infarction at 30 days, but an increase in strokes and mortality.[31] However, this study used very high doses of metoprolol, and treatment for 30 days, with a high frequency of hypotension, suggesting that lower doses might be better tolerated. Most postoperative myocardial infarctions occur within 5 days of surgery, and it is unclear that continuing the beta-blocker for more than a week confers significant benefit. The combination of beta-blockers, maintenance of blood volume, and excellent pain control may reduce the risk of postoperative atrial fibrillation.

An understanding of the type of fracture sustained and the type of repair planned helps to plan effectively for the patient's best management.

● TYPES OF HIP FRACTURES

Fractures are classified according to the main location of the fracture line. Many classification schemes exist for hip fractures. For simplicity, fractures are divided into those within the hip joint capsule (intracapsular) and those external to the hip joint capsule (extracapsular). Furthermore, each of these fractures may be displaced or non-displaced and may be simple or multifragmentary (comminuted). Each of these fracture types has different treatment considerations from a surgical standpoint, so it is important to understand the various patterns. The different types of fracture are depicted on the picture of the femur in Figure 40–2, and the common types of repair for each type are given in Table 40–2.

Intracapsular Hip Fractures

Most intracapsular hip fractures in the elderly occur at the lower edge of the femoral head but occasionally extend to the base of the femoral neck. These commonly are termed

TABLE 40–2 Common Types of Repair for Hip Fracture	
Fracture Type	Surgical Treatment
Intertrochanteric—simple	Dynamic hip screw
Intertrochanteric—complex	Intramedullary nail
Subtrochanteric	Intramedullary nail
Displaced femoral neck fracture, debilitated	Partial hip replacement
Displaced femoral neck fracture, healthy	Total hip replacement
Undisplaced femoral neck fracture	Screw fixation

subcapital fractures. Treatment is based upon displacement of the fracture and bone quality. Undisplaced femoral neck fractures are most frequently treated with in-situ cannulated screw fixation (Figure 40–3). This procedure can be accomplished through a very small incision. Displaced femoral neck fractures are typically treated with prosthetic replacement. Because much of the blood supply to the femoral head enters the femoral neck within the capsule, fractures in this area may damage the blood supply to the femoral head and reduce the chances of healing. Partial hip replacement is the most commonly performed procedure in the elderly patient (Figures 40–4 and 40–5). Total hip replacement is becoming more common in the healthy active elderly patient. Total hip replacement is a somewhat larger procedure and carries with it a higher risk of hip dislocation. Numerous recent studies show that total hip replacement is associated with better function and better hip scores.[32] Hip scores measure pain relief, function, and range of movement following hip surgery.

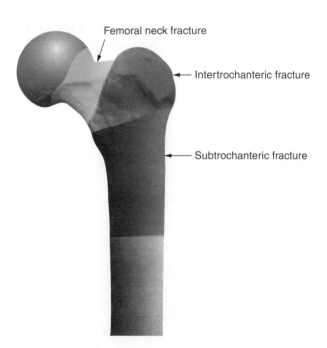

FIGURE 40–2. Location of different fracture types.

Femoral neck fracture

Intertrochanteric fracture

Subtrochanteric fracture

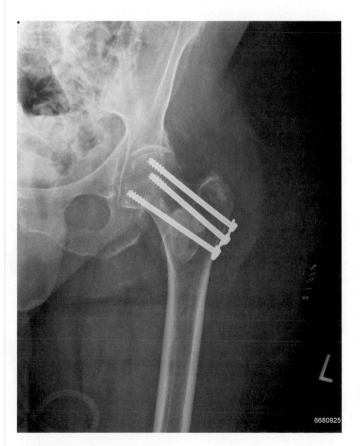

FIGURE 40–3. Cannulated screws.

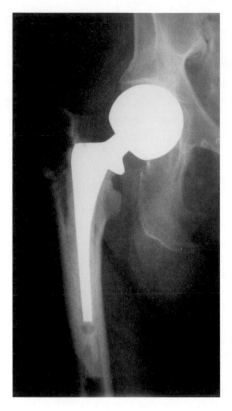

FIGURE 40–4. Partial hip replacement.

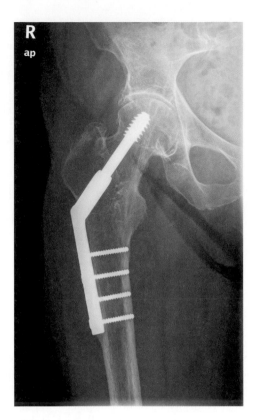

FIGURE 40–6. Dynamic hip screw.

Extracapsular Hip Fractures

Extracapsular fractures can be divided into intertrochanteric and subtrochanteric locations and are subclassified into stable and unstable patterns. The location and pattern of the fracture lines determine the choice of treatment. Stable fracture patterns are typically treated with a compression screw-plate device (sliding hip screw or dynamic hip screw; Figure 40–6). Unstable fracture patterns are best treated with a trochanteric entry intramedullary nail (Figure 40–7). Use of the intramedullary nail is becoming a common treatment with some

surgeons for all extracapsular fractures. This procedure is usually performed on a fracture table (Figure 40–8) under spinal or general anesthesia. The subtrochanteric fracture patterns are typically more difficult surgeries and are associated with higher blood losses and longer operative times. Patients with a subtrochanteric fracture usually have displaced fractures and deformity on presentation. They may lose a great deal of blood prior to surgery, and this should be considered when examining and optimizing these patients for surgery.

From an anesthesia standpoint, the patient with a hip fracture presents a challenge in many cases. It is essential to

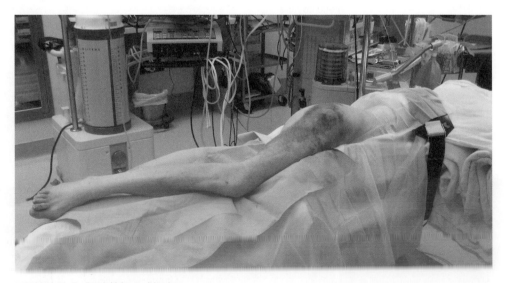

FIGURE 40–5. Partial hip positioning.

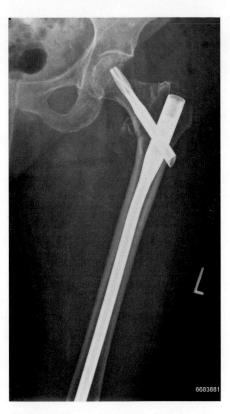

FIGURE 40-7. Intramedullary nail.

CASE PRESENTATION 1 (continued)

F.P. is taken to the OR after being given the okay by the internal medicine consultant. She undergoes an uneventful right intramedullary nail placement and is transferred to the recovery room. Later that evening, while back on the orthopedics ward, she develops an agitated delirium, unrecognized by her orthopedists. She is placed in arm restraints to prevent her from pulling out the urinary catheter and intravenous catheter. She is given haloperidol, 2 mg every 6 hours and subsequently becomes somnolent. On postoperative day 2 she develops a fever and is found to have a pneumonia, which is presumed due to aspiration; she is made "NPO" (nothing by mouth) by the internal medicine team that is now following her medical care. She later becomes hypoxic and hypotensive; she develops atrial fibrillation with a rapid ventricular rate, which is treated with oxygen, IV fluids, and IV esmolol. She undergoes a head CT, which shows atrophy but no acute bleed or stroke. She is slowly stabilized and over the next 8 days she makes significant improvement. On postoperative day 12 she is transferred to skilled rehabilitation for gait training and leg strengthening.

consider the patient's fluid balance, coagulation status, and overall medical status. Spinal anesthesia and general anesthesia are commonly used anesthetic choices. Peripheral nerve blocks can be used to augment anesthesia as well as for pre- and postoperative pain management. Collaboration and coordination with the anesthesiologist can facilitate timely surgery and improve pain management while minimizing the risk of systemic medications.

● MINIMIZING POSTOPERATIVE COMPLICATIONS

General Principles

As F.P.'s case illustrates, postoperative complications are common among hip fracture patients, and can often set off a "chain reaction" of further complications. For this reason, it is

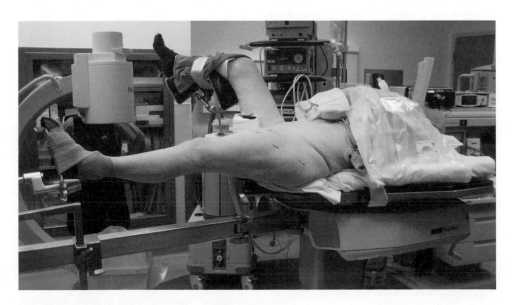

FIGURE 40-8. Patient positioning for an intramedullary nail.

important to anticipate potential complications and to use some common principles to reduce postoperative risk.

First, limit "tethers." This includes avoiding restraints altogether, but also includes removal of indwelling urinary catheters as soon as possible, discontinuing use of intravenous fluids when the patient is eating and drinking well, and discontinuing supplemental oxygen as soon as it is no longer needed. Knee immobilizers should be avoided. Telemetry boxes or cardiac monitors should not be used unless they are likely to change management. For F.P., who was already agitated, restraining her probably contributed to worsening her agitation. She would have been better served by removing her Foley catheter and bringing her into the hallway to provide redirection and reorientation. Although low-dose antipsychotics (eg, haloperidol, 0.5 mg every 6 hours as needed) may be useful when patients remain severely agitated despite comprehensive treatment for delirium, high doses may result in oversedation, risking the development of aspiration pneumonia, pressure sores, malnutrition, and other problems.

Second, as with preoperative management, maintain hydration. Monitor blood pressure, heart rate, mucous membranes, urine output, and renal function. In this patient, it would have been appropriate to hold her diuretic postoperatively until it is clear that she is euvolemic.

Third, mobilize the patient on the first postoperative day. A stable surgical repair that enables weight-bearing helps this process, as does discontinuing IVs, cardiac monitors, and any other items that hold the patient to his or her bed as well, and providing satisfactory pain control; all will facilitate a more rapid recovery. Because F.P. was restrained, delirious, and in pain, she was not able to be mobilized effectively in the postoperative period.

Fourth, regularly assess and treat pain. Uncontrolled pain increases the risk of delirium,[18] atelectasis and subsequent pneumonia, poor nutrition, depression, and delay to return of function. In this case, it is clear that F.P.'s poorly controlled pain led to her delirium and decline.

Fifth, optimize nutrition. Patients often have a diminished appetite after surgery. They must be monitored for development of a postoperative ileus. Elderly patients often feel overwhelmed by large trays of food and usually benefit from smaller portions with high caloric content snacks between meals. Family members should be encouraged to bring in favorite foods if the patient is able to eat but suffering from poor appetite.

Communication between care team members and patients and their families is critical throughout the hospitalization. Communication helps to establish goals of care early and to prevent these important issues from "slipping through the cracks." This reduces patient and family anxiety, and facilitates planning for care needs. Making the family a part of the care team may increase their satisfaction in the overall management of their loved one.

Specific Common Postoperative Complications

Common postoperative complications are summarized in Table 40–3. Here these complications are explored separately.

● TABLE 40–3 Common Postoperative Complications Following Hip Fracture Repair
Delirium
Infection
Pain
Renal insufficiency
Venous thromboembolism
Acute blood loss anemia
Arrhythmia
Pressure sores

Delirium

Delirium is extremely common following hip surgery, in part because of the patient population that is involved, and in part because of the processes involved in the surgery. The incidence of delirium is approximately 10% to 30% in hospitalized medical patients, but can be as high as 60% in postoperative hip fracture patients.[33] Delirium is characterized by an acute change in cognition with fluctuating course, and involves inattention, disorganized thinking, and changes in level of consciousness. It is important to identify because it can contribute to many adverse outcomes.[34] These include increased length of stay, lower likelihood of returning to previous level of function, and higher risk of nursing home admission and death. A delirious patient cannot participate in rehabilitation and has a much greater chance of developing a pressure sore.

There are many risk factors for postoperative delirium in hip fracture patients, and these are listed in Table 40–4. There is sometimes hesitation to treat pain due to fear that it may induce delirium. However, a recent study found that individuals with severe pain were nine times more likely to develop delirium, and those who were treated with less than 10 mg of parenteral morphine equivalent were five times as likely to develop delirium.[18] Avoidance of anticholinergic medications such as diphenhydramine and promethazine can help reduce risk of developing delirium. Use of appropriate assistive devices such as glasses and hearing aids can optimize communication and reduce risk the risk of delirium. Finally, if delirium does develop, reassuring both patient and family that this is a common, acute, and reversible condition, and enlisting family for emotional support of the patient, will help reduce the anxiety associated with this condition.

● TABLE 40–4 Risk Factors for Postoperative Delirium in Hip Fracture Patients	
Delayed surgery	Previous delirium
Medications	Dementia
Constipation	Dehydration
Severe pain	Sleep interruption
Infection	Sensory impairment
Hypoxia	Hypotension during surgery
Alcohol withdrawal	Congestive heart failure
"Tethers" (catheters, oxygen, IVs, telemetry)	

Infection

Infection is common after hip fracture surgery, with the most common infections being urinary tract infections, pneumonia, *Clostridium difficile*–induced colitis, and wound infections.[35-37] Urinary tract infections (UTIs) can be minimized by keeping the patient well hydrated and removing the urinary catheter promptly after surgery.[38] Documenting absence of an infection on admission helps determine whether the UTI was acquired during hospitalization or prior to admission. Early postoperative mobilization, elevation of the head of the bed, and optimal pain control can help minimize development of atelectasis and reduce risk of subsequent pneumonia. Prophylactic antibiotics (as mentioned earlier) at the time of surgery will reduce the incidence of wound infection.

Pain

Pain is common following a hip fracture. Although it is substantially reduced by surgical repair, pain is usually experienced postoperatively, and untreated pain can lead to other complications. Scheduled assessment and treatment of pain, with short-acting opioids in addition to round-the-clock acetaminophen, and additional as-needed medicine, is useful initially. Meperidine should be avoided, as its long-acting metabolite, normeperidine, can accumulate and lead to delirium, dysphoria, and seizures.

Renal Insufficiency

Worsening renal function is commonly seen in the first few days postoperatively, due to dehydration, intraoperative bleeding, and blood loss into the hematoma that occur with the hip fracture. It may be prudent to discontinue diuretics prior to surgery and restart them once the patient is fully rehydrated and taking oral fluids well. It is usually easier to manage modest fluid overload than to manage acute tubular necrosis that can result from renal hypoperfusion.

Venous Thromboembolism

Deep venous thrombosis (DVT) and pulmonary embolism are very common in the perioperative period, and the process starts early. The rate of DVT without prophylaxis is 46% to 75% by venography and of pulmonary embolism is 15% to 20%, although most of these are asymptomatic. Hip fracture patients are considered by the American College of Chest Physicians (ACCP) to be in the highest risk category for thromboembolism.[39] Prophylaxis has been shown in many studies to reduce the risk of venous thromboembolism and is considered a quality measure. It is unclear at this point which medication is the most effective, and so choice of prophylaxis should take into account the patient's clinical co-morbidities. The ACCP recommends treating with fondaparinux, low-molecular-weight heparin, warfarin, or low-dose unfractionated heparin. The ACCP recommends against using aspirin alone as a prophylactic therapy.[39] Anticoagulation should be continued for a minimum of 10 days, up to 45 days postoperatively; optimal duration of prophylaxis is not clear and individual clinical factors should be considered.[40]

Acute Blood Loss Anemia

Because the proximal femur has a rich blood supply from the profunda femoris artery, substantial blood loss in the perioperative period is common. The threshold for transfusion is controversial at this point, and should take into account symptoms, vital signs, co-morbidities, and rate of drop of the hematocrit.

Arrhythmias

Patients undergoing hip fracture surgery are at risk for developing arrhythmias due to dehydration, acute blood loss, pain, electrolyte shifts, as well as stress of surgery. A history of previous arrhythmia helps to identify risk, and a baseline EKG can provide a point of reference for patients who do develop arrhythmias postoperatively. Atrial fibrillation is the most common postoperative cardiac arrhythmia and often resolves with conservative medical management.

Pressure Sores

Because of the immobility that accompanies the perioperative period, as well as poor nutrition, patients are at risk of developing skin breakdown. Keeping heels off the bed, frequent turning and positioning, early mobilization, early surgery to promote early return to eating and mobility, and attentive nursing can reduce risk. It is also important to maintain attention to personal care and to keep the skin clean and dry. Adequate hydration may help improve tissue turgor and perfusion and thus reduce the risk of pressure breakdown (see Chapter 38).

CASE PRESENTATION 2: OPTIMIZING THE APPROACH

Better Process, Better Outcome

You are rounding at the local nursing home and are called urgently to the bedside of B.B., an 81-year-old man with a history of hypertension, depression, mild dementia, and atrial fibrillation, and a distant history of lymphoma. The nurse reports that an aide heard a thump from the hallway and when she went to the room there was Mr. B.B. lying on the floor moaning in pain. Evidently he was on his way to the bathroom at his nursing home when he slipped and fell. On your exam he is unable to bear weight and had an obvious hip deformity. An ambulance is called and on the way to the hospital, he is given 4 mg of intravenous morphine with good pain relief. At the hospital, x-rays reveal a left intertrochanteric fracture, but no other injury. He is seen, shortly after arrival, by the orthopedic surgeon and the consulting geriatrician. His medical records are reviewed. There does not appear to be any acute illness or change in his condition other than the noted left hip fracture. An echocardiogram from 4 months ago shows an LVEF of 48% and his labs including CBC, UA, electrolyte panel, coagulation studies, and EKG are all found to be at his usual baseline. The consulting geriatrician writes his admission orders including referral for the hospital discharge planner to work on rehabilitation placement if his facility is not able to conduct his postoperative rehabilitation. He is evaluated by the anesthesiologist and goes to surgery 16 hours after admission for a dynamic hip screw. He receives prophylactic antibiotics, and postoperatively receives low-molecular-weight heparin for thromboprophylaxis. Following the surgery he is weight-bearing as tolerated, and is evaluated by the physical therapist on postop day 1. In addition, family members, who live in the area, are asked to take turns spending the night with him as well as bring in foods that he likes. Pain is controlled via a standardized pain protocol that includes frequent assessments of pain, initially with intravenous morphine until he is able to take medications by mouth, and the nursing team routinely assesses him for pain. He is started on a bowel program to prevent narcotic-associated constipation and his family is also asked to bring some familiar items from his nursing home room to be placed in his hospital room. He is well hydrated throughout his hospitalization, with minimal change in his renal function acutely. The urinary catheter that had been placed upon admission is removed on postop day 1. He is seen daily by the orthopedics and geriatrics team, who communicate regularly about his course and inform the family about his progress as well.

COORDINATED CARE: THE GERIATRIC FRACTURE CENTER APPROACH

This case illustrates some of the medical and surgical optimization that was discussed earlier in the chapter. This case also addresses a systems approach to improve hip fracture care. The Geriatric Fracture Center (GFC) model is a total quality management program that has been shown to improve both processes and outcomes of care.[41,42] These include lower-than-expected in-hospital mortality and readmission, and a reduction in time to surgery, length of stay, and complications.

Principles of the GFC model are presented in Table 40–5, and include expert surgical stabilization of the fracture in

a timely fashion, co-management by an orthopedic surgeon and geriatrician with frequent communication, standardized protocols addressing common clinical issues, and early discharge planning. Co-management has been shown in many health care systems around the world to effectively improve outcomes, but has been routine only in a few centers in the United States until recently. In a co-managed approach, patients are seen daily by each team, with "co-ownership" of the patient. In other words, orders are written by both teams, and communication is frequent between the orthopedic and geriatric care providers, and also between care providers, patient, and family. Protocols for common issues, such as pain management and delirium prevention, apply evidence-based best practices, while leaving the final decision to the clinician based on the patient's specific clinical circumstances. In this manner, patient care is individualized, but with avoidance of unwarranted variability. The social worker meets with the patient and family soon after admission, to review the patient's prior living situation and goals, and to plan for rehabilitation. The social worker has frequent communication with both the surgical and medical teams to determine readiness for discharge. The rehabilitation staff meets and evaluates the patient on the first postoperative day, to begin the rehabilitation process.

CASE PRESENTATION 2 (continued)

Mr. B.'s vitamin D level is found to be low, at 15 ng/mL (37.4 nmol/L), and he is started on ergocalciferol 50,000 units three times per week. The hospital team calls the admitting physician at the rehabilitation nursing home to update him on the condition of the patient as well as items that will require further follow-up. A stat discharge summary is dictated for inclusion in the transfer papers, which also notes, in addition to the usual items, his dietary likes and dislikes, his code status, and important follow-up items. Changes in his previous medication regimen, including the addition of warfarin and ergocalciferol, are highlighted in the discharge summary as well. The team also adds to the medication list that the nursing home consider an oral or IV bisphosphonate for osteoporosis. On postoperative day 3 he is transferred to the nursing home with appointments, already made, for the orthopedist and his regular geriatric physician.

FOLLOWING HOSPITALIZATION

The determination of post-hospital rehabilitation plans depends on several factors, including patient characteristics, social support systems, financial resources, community resources, and hospital "culture." In some centers, most patients transition to skilled nursing facility rehabilitation,

---

● TABLE 40–5 Principles of the Geriatric Fracture Center

1. Most patients benefit from surgical stabilization of their fracture.
2. The sooner patients have surgery, the less time they have to develop iatrogenic illness.
3. Co-management with frequent communication avoids iatrogenic issues.
4. Standardized protocols decrease unwarranted variability.
5. Discharge planning begins at admission.

Source. Friedman et al.[11]

whereas others use a combination of inpatient, SNF, and community rehabilitation.

Secondary Prevention of Hip Fractures

Patients who sustain hip fractures are at high risk for developing future fractures, in part because of their osteoporosis, and in part because of their risk of falls. In one study following patients for a year after a hip fracture, 12% sustained another fracture, and 5% sustained another hip fracture.[15] Unfortunately, secondary prevention efforts remain suboptimal, leading to recurrent fracture and functional decline.

Currently, the rate of treatment for osteoporosis among patients who have had hip fractures is in the range of 20%.[17] The reasons for this are multiple. Traditionally, there has been reluctance on the part of most orthopedic surgeons to initiate evaluation and treatment in the hospital. Often, surgeons prefer to leave treatment of osteoporosis to the primary care physician. Because patients are frequently discharged to rehabilitation prior to returning to the community, recommendations for follow-up may get lost, or may be considered less important than addressing other more acute issues. Primary care physicians may not feel comfortable evaluating and managing osteoporosis. Finally, evaluation and definitive treatment can be expensive, so that hospitals do not want to include these costs in the acute care DRG (diagnosis related group) reimbursement.

The evaluation and treatment of osteoporosis is discussed in Chapter 41, so we will not discuss this in detail here. However, it is clearly important with respect to secondary prevention, both for reduction of morbidity and preservation of function, that osteoporosis be addressed following a hip fracture.

Falls are also extremely common after a hip fracture. Patients who sustain hip fractures were at high risk of falls prior to the fracture, and afterward they are at even higher risk. In the study mentioned earlier, 42% of patients with a hip fracture had another fall in the year prior to their fracture, and in the year following, 56% had another fall.[15] The increased risk of falls can be thought of in terms of six "D's" following hip fracture surgery, as outlined in Table 40–6. One risk factor that is particularly relevant in this setting, however, is vitamin D deficiency, and a level of 25 hydroxy vitamin D ≤ 25 ng/mL (62.4 nmol/L) was associated with an almost fourfold increase in risk of falls in the subsequent year.[15]

● TABLE 40–6	The 6 D's: Why Are Hip Fracture Patients at Increased Risk for Falls?
Deconditioning	
Dehydration	
Delirium	
Drugs	
Leg length discrepancy	
Vitamin D deficiency	

SUMMARY

Hip fractures are a common and serious condition in older adults, and the incidence is on the rise. Consideration of patients' multiple co-morbidities, anticipation of potential complications, and attentive, well-organized interdisciplinary care can improve outcomes for these patients. Because patients are at increased risk of sustaining other fractures after their presentation, attention to secondary prevention is essential.

References

1. Kates SL, Kates OS, Mendelson DA. Advances in the medical management of osteoporosis. *Injury*. 2007;38(suppl):S17-S23.

1a. Cummings SR, Black DM, Rubin SM. Lifetime risks of hip, Colles', or vertebral fracture and coronary heart disease among white postmenopausal women. *Arch Int Med*. 1989;149: 2445-2448

2. Morris AH, Zuckerman JD. National Consensus Conference on Improving the Continuum of Care for Patients with Hip Fracture. *J Bone Joint Surg Am*. 2002;84A:670-674.

3. Cummings SR, Rubin SM, Black D. The future of hip fractures in the United States. Numbers, costs, and potential effects of postmenopausal estrogen. *Clin Orthop Relat Res*. 1990:163-166.

4. Braithwaite RS, Col NF, Wong JB. Estimating hip fracture morbidity, mortality and costs. *J Am Geriatr Soc*. 2003;51:364-70.

5. Magaziner J, Hawkes W, Hebel JR, et al. Recovery from hip fracture in eight areas of function. *J Gerontol A Biol Sci Med Sci*. 2000;55:M498-M507.

6. Cooper C. The crippling consequences of fractures and their impact on quality of life. *Am J Med*. 1997;103(2A):12S-17S; discussion 17S-19S.

7. McKee KJ, Orbell S, Austin CA, et al. Fear of falling, falls efficacy, and health outcomes in older people following hip fracture. *Disabil Rehabil*. 2002;24:327-333.

8. Greenfield S, Apolone G, McNeil BJ, Cleary PD. The importance of co-existent disease in the occurrence of postoperative complications and one-year recovery in patients undergoing total hip replacement. Comorbidity and outcomes after hip replacement. *Med Care*. 1993;31:141-154.

9. Youm T, Koval KJ, Kummer FJ, Zuckerman JD. Do all hip fractures result from a fall? *Am J Orthop*. 1999;28:190-194.

10. Jarvinen TL, Sievanen H, Khan KM, et al. Shifting the focus in fracture prevention from osteoporosis to falls. *BMJ*. 2008;336:124-126.

11. Grisso JA, Kelsey JL, Strom BL, et al. Risk factors for falls as a cause of hip fracture in women. The Northeast Hip Fracture Study Group. *N Engl J Med*. 1991;324:1326-1331.

12. Kanis J. FRAX: *WHO Fracture Risk Assessment Tool*. Sheffield, UK: World Health Organization Collaborating Centre for Metabolic Bone Diseases, University of Sheffield; 2009.

13. Zuckerman JD. Hip fracture. *N Engl J Med*. 1996;334:1519-1525.

14. Hay D, Parker MJ. Hip fracture in the immobile patient. *J Bone Joint Surg Br*. 2003;85:1037-1039.

15. Lloyd BD, Williamson DA, Singh NA, et al. Recurrent and injurious falls in the year following hip fracture: A prospective study of incidence and risk factors from the Sarcopenia and Hip Fracture study. *J Gerontol A Biol Sci Med Sci*. 2009;64:599-609.

16. Tinetti ME, Speechley M, Ginter SF. Risk factors for falls among elderly persons living in the community. *N Engl J Med*. 1988; 319:1701-1707.

17. Elliot-Gibson V, Bogoch ER, Jamal SA, Beaton DE. Practice patterns in the diagnosis and treatment of osteoporosis after a fragility fracture: A systematic review. *Osteoporos Int.* 2004;15:767-778.

18. Morrison RS, Magaziner J, Gilbert M, et al. Relationship between pain and opioid analgesics on the development of delirium following hip fracture. *J Gerontol A Biol Sci Med Sci.* 2003;58:76-81.

19. Fleisher LA, Beckman JA, Brown KA, et al. ACC/AHA 2007 guidelines on perioperative cardiovascular evaluation and care for noncardiac surgery: A report of the American College of Cardiology/American Heart Association Task Force on Practice Guidelines (Writing Committee to Revise the 2002 Guidelines on Perioperative Cardiovascular Evaluation for Noncardiac Surgery) developed in collaboration with the American Society of Echocardiography, American Society of Nuclear Cardiology, Heart Rhythm Society, Society of Cardiovascular Anesthesiologists, Society for Cardiovascular Angiography and Interventions, Society for Vascular Medicine and Biology, and Society for Vascular Surgery. *J Am Coll Cardiol.* 2007;50:e159-e241.

20. Gale SC, Sicoutris C, Reilly PM, et al. Poor glycemic control is associated with increased mortality in critically ill trauma patients. *Am Surg.* 2007;73:454-460.

21. Rogers FB, Shackford SR, Keller MS. Early fixation reduces morbidity and mortality in elderly patients with hip fractures from low-impact falls. *J Trauma.* 1995;39:261-265.

22. Orosz GM, Magaziner J, Hannan EL, et al. Association of timing of surgery for hip fracture and patient outcomes. *JAMA.* 2004;291: 1738-1743.

23. Gdalevich M, Cohen D, Yosef D, Tauber C. Morbidity and mortality after hip fracture: The impact of operative delay. *Arch Orthop Trauma Surg.* 2004;124:334-340.

24. Lubetsky A, Yonath H, Olchovsky D, et al. Comparison of oral vs intravenous phytonadione (vitamin K1) in patients with excessive anticoagulation: A prospective randomized controlled study. *Arch Intern Med.* 2003;163:2469-2473.

25. Lavelle WF, Demers Lavelle EA, Uhl R. Operative delay for orthopedic patients on clopidogrel (plavix): A complete lack of consensus. *J Trauma.* 2008;64:996-1000.

26. Fletcher N, Sofianos D, Berkes MB, Obremskey WT. Prevention of perioperative infection. *J Bone Joint Surg Am.* 2007;89:1605-1618.

27. Marsh D, Currie C, Brown P, et al. *The Care of Patients with Fragility Fracture.* Bexhill-on-Sea: Chandlers Printers; 2007.

28. Devereaux PJ, Beattie WS, Choi PT, et al. How strong is the evidence for the use of perioperative beta blockers in non-cardiac surgery? Systematic review and meta-analysis of randomised controlled trials. *BMJ.* 2005;331:313-321.

29. Wiesbauer F, Schlager O, Domanovits H, et al. Perioperative beta-blockers for preventing surgery-related mortality and morbidity: A systematic review and meta-analysis. *Anesth Analg.* 2007;104:27-41.

30. Lindenauer PK, Pekow P, Wang K, et al. Perioperative beta-blocker therapy and mortality after major noncardiac surgery. *N Engl J Med.* 2005;353:349-361.

31. Devereaux PJ, Yang H, Yusuf S, et al. Effects of extended-release metoprolol succinate in patients undergoing non-cardiac surgery (POISE trial): A randomised controlled trial. *Lancet.* 2008;371: 1839-1847.

32. Blomfeldt R, Tornkvist H, Eriksson K, et al. A randomised controlled trial comparing bipolar hemiarthroplasty with total hip replacement for displaced intracapsular fractures of the femoral neck in elderly patients. *J Bone Joint Surg Br.* 2007;89: 160-165.

33. Robertson BD, Robertson TJ. Postoperative delirium after hip fracture. *J Bone Joint Surg Am.* 2006;88:2060-2068.

34. Marcantonio ER, Flacker JM, Michaels M, Resnick NM. Delirium is independently associated with poor functional recovery after hip fracture. *J Am Geriatr Soc.* 2000;48:618-624.

35. Khasraghi FA, Christmas C, Lee EJ, et al. Effectiveness of a multidisciplinary team approach to hip fracture management. *J Surg Orthop Adv.* 2005;14:27-31.

36. Zuckerman JD, Sakales SR, Fabian DR, Frankel VH. Hip fractures in geriatric patients. Results of an interdisciplinary hospital care program. *Clin Orthop Relat Res.* 1992;274:213-225.

37. Phy MP, Vanness DJ, Melton LJ III, et al. Effects of a hospitalist model on elderly patients with hip fracture. *Arch Intern Med.* 2005;165:796-801.

38. Wald HL, Ma A, Bratzler DW, Kramer AM. Indwelling urinary catheter use in the postoperative period: analysis of the national surgical infection prevention project data. *Arch Surg.* 2008;143: 551-557.

39. Geerts WH, Bergqvist D, Pineo GF, et al. Prevention of venous thromboembolism: American College of Chest Physicians Evidence-Based Clinical Practice Guidelines (8th edition). *Chest.* 2008;133(suppl):381S-453S.

40. Eriksson BI, Lassen MR. Duration of prophylaxis against venous thromboembolism with fondaparinux after hip fracture surgery: A multicenter, randomized, placebo-controlled, double-blind study. *Arch Intern Med.* 2003;163:1337-1342.

41. Friedman SM, Mendelson DA, Kates SL, McCann RM. Geriatric co-management of proximal femur fractures: Total quality management and protocol-driven care result in better outcomes for a frail patient population. *J Am Geriatr Soc.* 2008; 56:1349-1356.

42. Friedman SM, Mendelson DA., Bingham KW, Kates SL. Impact of a comanaged geriatric fracture center on short-term hip fracture outcomes. *Arch Intern Med.* 2009;169:1712-1717.

POST-TEST

1. **Which of the following is TRUE about the evaluation and treatment of F.P.?**

   A. An echocardiogram should be a standard, routine preoperative screening test for patients.

   B. A head CT is a "high-yield" procedure in the evaluation of patients with postoperative delirium, and should be performed on all delirious patients.

   C. Pain medication should be avoided or given minimally in order to prevent postoperative delirium.

   D. F.P. was probably dehydrated on admission to the hospital, and this may have put her at risk for multiple postoperative complications such as hypotension, delirium, and rapid atrial fibrillation.

2. **Which of the following is TRUE of postoperative delirium in patients with hip fractures?**

   A. Delirium can lead to increased length of stay, higher risk of other complications, and higher risk of functional decline.

   B. It is best to exclude families from participating in the care of patients with delirium, as it will be upsetting to them.

   C. High-dose haldol (2-5 mg every 3 hours) should be a first-line treatment of delirium.

   D. Delirium is unusual, occurring in about 5% of patients postoperatively.

3. **Which of the following is TRUE with respect to the surgical management of patients with hip fractures?**

   A. Anti-pseudomonal antibiotics should be administered for 3 days perioperatively, to reduce the risk of wound infection.

   B. Most patients should maintain partial weight-bearing status for 6 weeks following surgery, to allow the fracture time to heal.

   C. Subtrochanteric fracture repair is often a more difficult surgery, associated with more blood loss and longer operative times than fractures in other locations.

   D. Undisplaced femoral neck fractures are most commonly treated with total hip replacement.

ANSWERS TO PRE-TEST

1. B
2. D
3. B

ANSWERS TO POST-TEST

1. D
2. A
3. C

41

Osteoporosis

Susan Ott, MD

● **LEARNING OBJECTIVES**

1. Identify risk factors for osteoporosis and potential fractures as a result of osteoporosis.
2. Discuss secondary causes of osteoporosis and describe the pathology that leads to this disorder.
3. Discuss routine laboratory testing for osteoporosis and explain the process of bone density screening.
4. Discuss prevention and treatment strategies for osteoporosis.
5. Describe the most appropriate medications for patients with osteoporosis, their dosage recommendations, side effects, and monitoring requirements.
6. Differentiate osteoporosis in males from that in females.

PRE-TEST

1. **All of the following are risk factors for osteoporosis EXCEPT:**
   A. Early menopause
   B. Smoking
   C. Maternal history of osteoporosis
   D. Obesity

2. **A subtle first manifestation of osteoporosis is:**
   A. Height loss
   B. Fracture
   C. Rising calcium level
   D. Weakness

3. **Which of the following factors is most important in predicting osteoporotic fractures?**
   A. Calcium intake
   B. Alcohol consumption
   C. Race
   D. Rheumatoid arthritis

● INTRODUCTION

Osteoporosis is a bone disorder that is distinguished by lower bone density and a weakening of bone structure that ultimately results in greater bone fragility and increased risk of fracture.[1] The most typical of the fractures associated with osteoporosis are at the spine, hip, shoulder, and forearm. The lifetime risk of a fracture of the hip, spine, or forearm is 40% in white women and 13% in white men. African Americans have fewer fractures than people of other races.[1] Fracture rates also vary among countries, races, ethnic backgrounds, and between urban and rural areas. The incidence of hip fractures rises exponentially with age in women after the age of 60 and in men after the age of 70. Vertebral fractures also increase with aging, and the prevalence of these fractures reaches about 20% in men and 30% to 40% in women (Figure 41–1).[2]

Osteoporosis is a common disease but it is not simple. Bone cells respond to a large variety of hormonal messages and use many of the same signaling pathways as the immune system. The major bone cells are osteoclasts, which resorb bone; osteoblasts, which form new bone; and osteocytes, which form a network inside the bone. The osteocytes detect minor changes in force applied to the bone and direct bone formation to the most appropriate place. In adults, bone is continuously remodeling. This allows repair of micro-cracks that occur with ordinary acts of daily living. When an area of bone has been damaged, it is resorbed by osteoclasts, and then osteoblasts form new bone to fill in the cavities. Osteoporosis develops if the resorption exceeds the formation; this happens with either too much resorption or too little formation.

Pathology of Osteoporosis

With estrogen deficiency, resorption is increased; this is the most common kind of osteoporosis. Osteoblasts respond by increasing bone formation but they are unable to completely restore the bone that was lost; therefore, bone mass decreases inexorably. The micro-architecture of the bone is destroyed as the hyperactive osteoclasts perforate the bone structures; this further weakens the bone. This kind of osteoporosis can be termed "high-turnover-osteoporosis."

Another type of osteoporosis is seen when the osteoblasts fail to form new bone; this is "low-turnover-osteoporosis." This physiology is analogous to anemia, which can be caused by hemolysis, blood loss, or hypoproliferative marrow. Although iron deficiency is the most common cause of anemia, physicians do not treat every case with iron! In the future, as better drugs become available, osteoporosis may be treated more specifically with anti-resorptive drugs for the high-turnover disease and anabolic drugs for those with low-turnover disease.

Bone Density Loss with Aging

During childhood growth, the density of the bones does not change very much but the bones become larger. After adolescents attain their adult height, the bone density increases and reaches a peak in the third decade. In men the bone density then decreases gradually and is about 20% lower at age 85 than at age 25. In premenopausal women, the skeleton loses and then regains 5% to 10% during each reproductive cycle of pregnancy and lactation. During the menopausal transition bone is lost rapidly, and postmenopausal women continue to lose bone. The average bone density at age 85 ("the age of fracture") is 30% lower than it was at age 25.

At any age, there is a wide range of bone density values; the standard deviation is 13%. It is important to remember that risk of fracture depends on age as well as bone density. For example, at age 25 a woman with a bone density of 832 mg/cm^2 (total hip, standardized) would be one standard deviation *below* the mean (T-score = −1). This same bone density would be one standard deviation *above* the mean for an 80-year-old woman. But the older woman would have almost 10% risk of a hip fracture in the next decade, whereas the younger one would have less than 0.1% risk of a hip fracture.

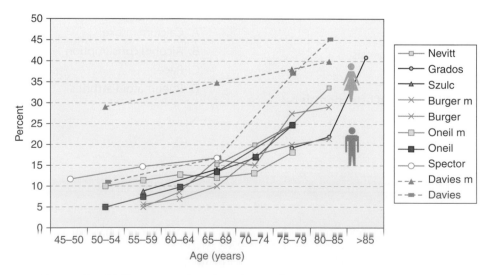

FIGURE 41–1. Vertebral fracture prevalence by various studies.

● RISK FACTORS FOR OSTEOPOROSIS

Many factors are involved in the development of osteoporosis. Risk factors for the development of osteoporosis can be classified as non-modifiable and modifiable/lifestyle-related factors.

Non-modifiable risk factors include gender, age, race/ethnicity, and family history. By far, women are more likely to develop osteoporosis by almost a 4:1 ratio. This is related to the generally lighter skeletal framework of women in comparison to men, and the bone impact associated with the dramatic decrease in estrogen that occurs with menopause. Estrogen has a protective effect on bone health and the rapid drop in levels with menopause are associated with loss of bone density. Loss of estrogen promotes osteoclast maturation, leading to increased bone resorption compared with bone formation.[2] Age is another risk factor for osteoporosis, since with time come the previously described changes in bone density. Osteoporosis affects all races and ethnicities, but certain groups are more likely to develop the disorder. Asian and non-Hispanic Caucasian women have a greater risk for osteoporosis than African American and Hispanic groups. This may be related to ethnic variations in body size, genetics, diet, activity level, and starting bone density levels. Finally, family history and genetics are likely to play a role in osteoporosis through the influence of a number of genes that affect hormone levels and control bone formation, bone loss, calcium management, and even protein formation. So those who have a parent or first-degree relative with osteoporosis are at greater risk for osteoporosis development.

Age, race, and gender are the most important risk factors for osteoporotic fractures. Men and women with the same age and bone density will have about the same risk of a fracture, but overall women have more fractures because they have lower bone density and they live longer. Persons of African ancestry have better bone density than other races; furthermore, at the same bone density they have about 30% fewer fractures. Asians have fewer fractures than Caucasians, despite similar bone density values.

Modifiable risk factors for osteoporosis include nutritional and dietary factors, inactivity, alcohol excess, and cigarette smoking.

Nutritional and Dietary Factors

Calcium Intake

Calcium is a major component of bone. Many people have an inadequate amount in their diet. With limited calcium intake there is not enough mineral to provide for the optimal strength of the bone. The parathyroid glands sense a low calcium intake and respond by secreting parathyroid hormone, which enhances bone resorption. There is individual variation in the amount of calcium necessary to maintain bone health, but an intake of 1200 mg/day is usually adequate. Most of the epidemiologic studies do not find that low calcium intake is the major risk factor for osteoporosis, but it is a contributing factor. Calcium is further discussed in "Treatment for Osteoporosis" later in the chapter.

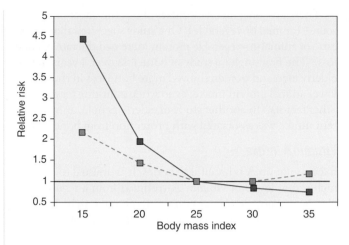

FIGURE 41–2. Body mass index (BMI) and risk of osteoporosis and hip fracture. (*Source: De Laet et al.*[3])

Calories and Weight

Weight and bone are very closely linked. Meta-analyses of 60,000 men and women throughout the world documented that low body mass index (BMI) is an important risk factor for osteoporosis and hip fractures (Figure 41–2).[3] Notice that the risk of a hip fracture is twice as high in somebody with a BMI of 20 compared to somebody with a BMI of 25; partly this is explained by low bone density, but even after adjustment, the BMI is a significant risk factor for hip fractures. The total caloric intake is more closely related to bone density than any of the specific nutrients. Even when overweight persons voluntarily lose weight, the bone density decreases. In the Women's Healthy Lifestyle Project, women were randomized into an intervention that encouraged lower dietary fat and exercise. After 18 months the active group lost 3.2 kg and the control group gained 0.4 kg. The bone density decreased twice as fast in the active group.[4] The prospective Study of Osteoporotic Fractures found that elderly women who lost more than 5% of their weight over 4 years had twice as many hip fractures as those who did not lose weight. This was true even if they were initially overweight.[5]

Protein Intake

Approximately half of the weight of bone is from protein, and adequate protein nutrition is essential for bone health. Proteins contain sulfur and phosphate, which are fixed acids that must be renally excreted. In elderly persons with impaired ability to excrete acid, a slight metabolic acidosis will develop. This is buffered by the bone, but at the expense of some bone loss. High-protein diets also cause slight increases in urine calcium, but this is because there is more calcium absorbed from the intestines. Also, amino acids can increase the glomerular filtration rate, which can increase urine calcium.

These potential negative effects of protein appear to be balanced by positive effects. A placebo-controlled trial of protein supplement (dairy-based) in patients with recent hip fracture showed attenuated bone loss in the femur.[6] The calcium resorbed from the bones is actually decreased with high protein intake.[7] One of the beneficial effects of protein is an increase in insulin-like growth factor, which stimulates bone formation rates.

There are some inconsistencies about the effect of protein source (animal or vegetable). One study suggested that a high ratio of animal-to-vegetable protein increased the rate of bone loss.[8] The Framingham study of bone loss over 4 years in 614 elderly men and women showed more bone loss in those with lower animal protein intake, even when adjusting for multiple other factors.[9] In another study of elderly people, animal protein intake was associated with protection from bone loss.[10]

Vitamin A Intake

Excess vitamin A is harmful to bones. It is unusual to develop high serum levels of vitamin A (retinol) from a regular diet. However, many supplements and fish oils contain high levels. The Institute of Medicine recommends an intake of 2330 IU = 700 µg for women, and 3000 IU = 900 µg for men, which is less than the current recommended daily intake for labeling (5000 IU).

Other Modifiable Factors

Inactivity

Active women who walk for exercise have a lower risk of osteoporosis and hip fracture than sedentary women. This may be due to positive effects of exercise on the skeleton or to decreasing the risk of high impact with a fall. It also may be a reflection of the fact that healthier people are more likely to be active.

Excess Alcohol

Excess alcohol intake inhibits osteoblast activity and proliferation and chronic use may have an adverse effect on PTH as well. It also interferes with vitamin D absorption, a necessary factor for bone tissue replacement.[11]

Cigarette Smoking

Smoking interferes with the body's use of calcium, and in women decreases the level of estrogen. Women smokers have actually been found to experience menopause earlier, which compounds a person's risk for osteoporosis. Smokers may have associated duplicate risk factors in that they may also be thinner than nonsmokers, drink more alcohol, be less physically active, and have poorer diets. All of these factors serve to increase osteoporosis risk.[12]

CASE PRESENTATION 1: FIRST SIGNS OF OSTEOPOROSIS

Mrs. W., an artist, recently exhibited her newest paintings featuring multicultural aspects of landscaping. At the opening of her exhibit she was honored for 50 years of service and education at the art academy. Now she comes to your office for follow-up of a bladder infection. While she is showing you the photos of her exhibit she mentions that her granddaughter, who had not seen her for several years, came to see the show, and noticed that she was getting shorter. She is a delightful 76-year-old woman, who is generally active and in good health.

She takes eye drops for mild glaucoma, one multiple vitamin on most days, and Tylenol on occasion for headaches.

Her past history includes menopause at age 42 without hormone replacement. Prior to that she had irregular periods, and as a young woman she was infertile. She has had a breast biopsy that was negative, and otherwise her past history is unremarkable.

Her family history is positive for breast cancer in her sister and grandmother. Her parents did not have hip fractures. She does not smoke cigarettes. She consumes about one glass of wine at dinner. She does not take calcium supplements and she regularly eats two servings/day of dairy products. She has not lost any weight over the last 5 years.

On physical examination she does not have scoliosis or noticeable kyphosis. Her height is 5'2" (157 cm) and weight is 110 lbs (50 kg). She is nontender and has a good range of motion. You review her chart and see that her height was measured 5 years ago at 5'4" (163 cm), and has not been checked since then.

● CLINICAL MANIFESTATIONS OF OSTEOPOROSIS

The first sign of osteoporosis for many is a fracture. However, before that event there may be a subtle manifestation as seen with Mrs. W., height loss. This is frequently asymptomatic and usually gradual. Height loss can be caused by disc narrowing, kyphosis (forward curvature of the spine,) and worsening of scoliosis (sideways curvature of the spine). Loss of over 2.6 cm is seen in the majority of older women.[13,14]

Compression fractures from osteoporosis also are a factor in height loss. Loss of greater than 4 cm is seen in 27% of women without vertebral fractures and 41% of women with fractures. Almost all persons who have lost greater than 6 cm have vertebral fractures.[15] Lateral radiographs of the thoracic and lumbar spine should be obtained in any elderly men or women who have lost over 4 cm of height, especially if they have kyphosis or tenderness. On physical exam the patients with a fracture may have point tenderness over one vertebra, but this does not occur unless the fractures are recent. Fixed kyphosis and a "Dowager's hump" are seen in serious cases (Figure 41–3). Patients should be examined for scoliosis, which worsens after menopause.

CASE PRESENTATION 1 (continued)

Upon conclusion of your exam you reflect on the fact that Mrs. W. had an early menopause and was infertile with a long history of irregular periods. You suspect a life long mild estrogen deficiency. This would be a

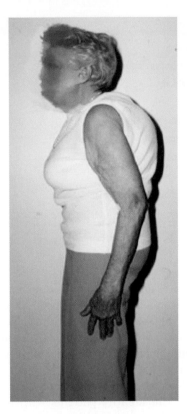

FIGURE 41–3. Dowager's hump.

secondary cause of bone loss. She does not have any major chronic diseases, but at 76 years of age Mrs. W. is already at risk for osteoporosis. Her body mass index is 20, which is at the low end of the normal range for a young adult and thus an additional risk factor. She has height loss that suggests she might already have vertebral compression fractures. Therefore, you decide that the next step is to order a CBC, calcium and phosphate level, metabolic profile, thyroid stimulating hormone level, as well as a 25-OH vitamin D level. In addition, you order radiographs of her spine.

● DIAGNOSIS OF OSTEOPOROSIS

The goals of testing in osteoporosis are to determine whether the patient has risk for the disease, low bone density, or osteoporosis itself. As a primary risk factor for osteoporosis, hormone deficiency also needs to be ascertained, as does any underlying condition that may be causing or exacerbating bone loss.

Laboratory Testing

For baseline testing, the *complete blood count* (CBC) is done to check for anemia and bone marrow diseases that could lead to osteoporosis. Anemia also is a clue that a patient could

have asymptomatic celiac sprue, or a chronic immunologic or rheumatologic disease causing bone loss. The *calcium level* should be checked because a high value may be seen with hyperparathyroidism, sarcoidosis, malignancy, or vitamin D intoxication, all of which are associated with bone loss. Low calcium is seen in some cases of malabsorption, vitamin D deficiency, or patients with conditions that cause low serum albumin. Hypogonadism is the most common contributing cause of osteoporosis. In men, the *testosterone* levels should be measured, because levels that are low enough to cause osteoporosis may not cause more overt signs of hypogonadism. Elderly women do not need *estrogen* level measurements because they all are postmenopausal and will have low levels. Women who are not known to be postmenopausal should have *follicle-stimulating hormone (FSH)* levels obtained to determine if menopause has occurred.

A chronically low *phosphate* will result in osteomalacia, which may mimic osteoporosis in older patients. The *creatinine* is measured to determine the stage of kidney disease, which is an important contributing cause of osteoporosis in elderly patients. Also the renal function can influence the dosages of some of the medications. The creatinine should be entered into an equation that will estimate the glomerular filtration rate. A "normal" creatinine is very misleading in a thin, elderly person. The *bicarbonate* is a check for renal tubular acidosis, which causes osteoporosis and/or osteomalacia. *Thyroid stimulating hormone* (TSH) should be checked because early hyperthyroidism or overzealous thyroid replacement are common causes of bone loss (Table 41–1).

The *alkaline phosphatase* test is a screen for liver abnormalities, particularly primary biliary cirrhosis, although this is usually known by the time a patient is elderly. Alkaline phosphatase is also secreted by osteoblasts and increases with osteomalacia, Paget disease, vitamin D deficiency, metastatic bone disease, and acute fractures.

Based upon the calcium level, *vitamin D* and parathyroid hormone (PTH) levels should be obtained. Vitamin D deficiencies can lead to decreased calcium absorption. Baseline vitamin D values and subsequent correction for lower levels are important in appropriate treatment. Vitamin D should be measured in elderly patients who have osteoporosis, as it is frequently low, and these frail patients show reduction in hip fractures when treated with vitamin D. The 25-hydroxyvitamin D levels should be greater than 20 ng/dL (52 nmol/L in international units); there is some controversy

● TABLE 41–1 Routine Tests
Complete blood count
Calcium
Phosphate
Creatinine
Bicarbonate
Thyroid stimulating hormone
25-OH-vitamin D
Alkaline phosphatase
Testosterone (in men)

about whether levels between 20 and 30 ng/dL (52-75 nmol/L) are adequate. The highest level of vitamin D seen in healthy young people exposed to sunlight is 60 ng/dL (150 nmol/L).[16] It is important to measure the 25-hydroxyvitamin D, not the 1,25-dihydroxyvitamin D. The latter is not as stable, more expensive, and may be misleading because people with moderate vitamin D deficiency actually have elevated levels of 1,25-dihydroxyvitamin D.

Parathyroid hormone (PTH) should be checked if the calcium is increased or if the patient has stage 3 or 4 chronic kidney disease. If a patient has primary hyperparathyroidism, then surgical removal of the parathyroid adenoma results in improvement of bone density, particularly in the spine.

Most testing for osteoporosis is done to rule out the many different secondary diseases and conditions that may cause osteoporosis. Some of these conditions are listed in Table 41–2.

Other Laboratory Testing

Routine tests for patients with newly diagnosed compression fractures are shown in Table 41–3. In a patient with a new, painful vertebral compression fracture, multiple myeloma is in

● TABLE 41–3 Specialized Tests

Parathyroid hormone
Serum AND urine protein electrophoresis
24-hour urine calcium
Urine cortisol
Antibodies for celiac sprue (TTG)
Bone turnover markers:
N-telopeptide (resorption)
C-telopeptide (resorption)
Bone alkaline phosphatase (formation)
P1NP (formation)

● TABLE 41–2 Secondary Causes of Osteoporosis/Fractures

Medications	Corticosteroids, dilantin and other anticonvulsants, gonadotropin-releasing hormone agonists, loop diuretics, methotrexate, excess thyroid, heparin, depo-medroxyprogesterone acetate, anti-neoplastic agents, cyclosporin, proton-pump inhibitors, selective serotonin reuptake inhibitors, aromatase inhibitors
Hereditary skeletal/connective tissue diseases	Osteogenesis imperfecta, rickets, hypophosphatasia, Marfan syndrome, pseudoglioma
Endocrine and metabolic	Hypogonadism, prolactinoma, hypopituitarism, hyperparathyroidism, hyperthyroidism, Cushing syndrome, acidosis, diabetes type I and type II, androgen insensitivity, Gaucher disease, hemochromatosis
Gastro-intestinal	Celiac sprue, malabsorption, malnutrition, inflammatory bowel disease, chronic hepatic disease
Rheumatologic diseases	Systemic lupus, ankylosing spondylitis, rheumatoid arthritis
Marrow diseases	Myeloma, mastocytosis, thalassemia, leukemia
Renal disease	Chronic kidney disease, renal tubular acidosis, hypercalciuria
Neurologic diseases	Spinal cord injury, stroke, Parkinson disease, history of polio
Psychiatric diseases	Alcoholism, depression, anorexia nervosa
Pulmonary diseases	Chronic obstructive pulmonary disease, cystic fibrosis
Other	Organ transplantation, lactation, AIDS, transient regional osteoporosis, any disease that causes serious weight loss or prolonged bed rest
Fractures not caused by osteoporosis	Severe trauma, cancer metastatic to the bone, Paget disease, tuberculosis (Pott disease), avascular necrosis, fibrous dysplasia, osteomalacia, repetitive injury (march fractures)

the differential diagnosis, and both serum and urine protein electrophoresis should be tested. About 20% of cases have normal serum values but abnormal urine values.

In unexplained osteoporosis, the *24-hour urine calcium* is helpful because it identifies patients with hypercalciuria, who can be treated with thiazides. On a diet of 1000 mg of calcium, the 24-hour urine calcium should be less than 300 mg. This test also can identify patients with malabsorption, because they will usually have low urine calcium (less than 50 mg/day). If there are any signs of Cushing syndrome then a cortisol measurement can be done on the urine collection. Osteoporosis may be the first clinical sign of an adrenal tumor.

Biochemical Markers of Bone Turnover. It is possible to distinguish between high-turnover osteoporosis and low-turnover bone disease, but currently the markers are not recommended to make decisions about initiating therapy. Almost all of the medications work by inhibiting bone resorption. In the future, as anabolic medications become available and affordable, it may become more important to decide whether a patient has high or low bone formation. For example, a post-hoc analysis of women in the alendronate fracture intervention trial examined the relationship between bone formation and the reduction in fractures with alendronate. Those in the lowest tertile of bone formation did not have any decrease in fracture rates when comparing alendronate to placebo, whereas those in the highest tertile had significant reduction in fractures with alendronate.[17]

The markers for bone resorption are based on cross-linking of collagen (serum or urine N-telopeptide or C-telopeptide). Bone formation can be assessed by the bone specific alkaline phosphatase (BAP) or by the procollagen type I N-propeptide (P1NP). These markers are sensitive and are suppressed by 50% to 90% with effective anti-resorbing medications. In epidemiologic studies the markers predict the risk of an osteoporotic fracture, but there is enough variation that they are not currently recommended for routine use in patients with osteoporosis. They are helpful for other diseases of bone, such as Paget disease, and in unusual cases. The markers increase after a fracture, because there is increased activity due to repair of the fracture, so they may not reflect the underlying bone turnover rate.

The markers can help decide if an anti-resorbing medication is being absorbed from the intestinal tract. Some suggest that they should be used to test for compliance, but for most cases it is sufficient and preferable to ask the patient. In patients who appear to have unexpectedly lost bone density, the N-telopeptide or C-telopeptide markers can be useful. High levels suggest that the bone loss was real, whereas low levels suggest there could have been technical problems with the bone density measurements. In patients who have taken bisphosphonates for an extended time, these markers are very low, and if a bisphosphonate is discontinued the markers can stay decreased for up to 5 years. Patients can be followed with markers to help determine when it is time to restart an anti-resorbing medicine. More research is necessary to determine the best ways to use these markers.

CASE PRESENTATION 1 (continued)

Two weeks later, Mrs. W. returns to the clinic to review her lab tests and x-rays. Her calcium level is 9.4 mg/dL (2.35 mmol/L). She had a normal blood count and chemistry panel. Her TSH was also normal, but her vitamin D was 18 ng/dL (45 nmol/L). You tell her that this level is low and will need to be corrected with oral vitamin D supplementation as part of the treatment. Radiographs of Mrs. W. reveal two mild compression fractures at T10 and T12, and you tell her that she has already suffered two osteoporosis-related fractures.

Bone Density Testing. Bone density screening is used to decide about initiating drug therapy. Many organizations recommend screening bone density tests for all women older than 65 and men older than 70, and also for those older than 50 with a clinical risk factor. The most reliable method of measuring bone density is with dual energy x-ray absorptiometry (DEXA). This radiographic method is widely used, has very low radiation exposure, and has well-established normative data ranges. Three manufacturers produce these densitometers, and unfortunately the results are about 8% different from one another. Therefore, the results are typically expressed as "T-scores," which are standard deviations from a reference base of young persons. Bone is invariably lost with age, so the average T-score of an 82-year-old woman is −2.1.

Discordant Results. Spine measurements are frequently inaccurate due to scoliosis, osteoarthritis, vascular calcifications, and narrowing of the disk space, all of which increase the DEXA readings. These factors are common in elderly persons, so the spine bone density should not be considered unless it is lower than the hip bone density. Some hormonal and nutritional factors affect the spine more than the hip. For example, glucocorticosteroids show more severe effects on spine bone density, whereas primary or secondary hyperparathyroidism decreases hip density more than spine.

If there is a discrepancy between these measurements that is not explained by anatomic reasons, then the fracture risk is site specific. Women with osteoporosis at the hip but not at the spine show higher risk of hip fractures than of spine fractures.[18]

However, it is not clear if screening is necessary in an older woman who already has vertebral compression fractures, because she already meets a well-accepted criterion for initiating treatment. One approach is to estimate the fracture risk using clinical risk factors, and then measure bone density in those whose fracture risk is near a treatment threshold. Those who clearly have low risk and those who clearly need treatment may not require bone density. This approach is used in the United Kingdom and the assessment threshold is on the UK FRAX chart.

Bone Density Testing and Fracture Risk. The World Health Organization has analyzed 1.2 million person-years of data from around the world to formulate and validate a fracture risk assessment model called FRAX.[19] The risk factors were chosen because they were included in the primary cohorts, could be easily checked by questionnaire, were significantly related to fractures, and were common. The model predicts fracture risks based on clinical risk factors as shown in Table 41–4. Bone density can be added if it has been measured. This approach is currently the best way to estimate fracture risk, but it does have some limitations: it cannot accommodate all known risk factors and it lacks detail on some risk factors. It depends on adequacy of epidemiologic information. Data from poor countries are not available. FRAX estimations are relevant only for untreated patients.

Two large studies in the United States (SOF[20] in women and MrO[21] in men) have examined risk factors that were statistically independent of bone density, as shown in Tables 41–5 and 41–6. Some of these were not in the FRAX risk-factor list because the other studies did not provide enough detailed information.

Chronic abnormalities of nearly every system result in bone loss (Table 41–2) and secondary osteoporosis.

● TABLE 41–4 Clinical Risk Factors for Fracture: FRAX Model	
FACTOR	Risk Ratio
Age	
Gender	
Race	
BMI (20 vs. 25)	1.95
Parenteral hip fracture	2.27
Glucocorticoids	2.31
Prior adult fracture	1.85
Current smoking	1.84
High alcohol intake	1.68
Rheumatoid arthritis	1.95
From Kanis et al.[19]	

● TABLE 41–5	Clinical Risk Factors for Fracture: SOF Model
FACTOR[a]	Risk Ratio
Anticonvulsants	2.0
Hyperthyroid history	1.7
On feet < 4 hr/day	1.7
Inability to rise from chair	1.7
Resting pulse > 80	1.7
Benzodiazepines	1.6
Poor general health	1.6
Depth perception	1.4
Weight loss	

[a]Adjusted for age and bone density.
From Cummings and Black.[20]

The presence of these diseases may not increase the fracture risk above that estimated from the FRAX model, if the disease merely caused low bone density. On the other hand, if a disease also increases the risk of falling or the quality of the bone, then the FRAX model will not be accurate. For example, patients with epilepsy have low bone density, but they also have poor bone quality due to effects of anti-epileptic medications, and during seizures they experience more falls, so their fracture risk is worse than expected from FRAX.

CASE PRESENTATION 1 (continued)

You try using FRAX to estimate the risk of fracture using the clinical risk factors. With a BMI of 20 and a previous fracture as an adult, Mrs. W.'s risk of a major fracture is 26% in the next decade. For a woman her age, the assessment threshold is about 30% (ie, treat if the risk is higher than 30% and get BMD if it is lower than 30%). You then include "secondary osteoporosis" because she had an early menopause; this increases the risk to 37%. FRAX treats all adult fractures the same, and you know that a vertebral compression fracture is a particularly strong risk factor, especially

● TABLE 41–6	Clinical Risk Factors for Fracture: MrOS Model
FACTOR[a]	Risk Ratio
Tricyclic	2.39
Unable to do narrow walk	1.98
Depressed mood	1.8
Fall during past year	1.56

[a]Unadjusted, independent factors.
From Lewis et al.[21]

for vertebral osteoporosis. You tell her that you don't think she requires bone density screening, but it would be a reasonable consideration if she is interested. The patient says she wants to know her bone density results, as this is what her friends talk about. Because bone density screening is widely promoted, patients expect their doctors to check it. Given her situation and the possibility of using the bone density test to follow her response to therapy, you order a bone density test.

Bone Density Testing and Treatment. Why should a bone density test be done if a physician has already decided to treat the patient? In the future it may be helpful to decide which drug to use depending on the severity of bone loss, but currently the therapeutic choices are limited. There is not enough evidence that the treatment response depends on the baseline bone density in patients who already have an osteoporotic fracture. Bone density could potentially be used to monitoring drug therapy, but recent studies have questioned this approach. The bone density reproducibility is so close to the expected change with treatment that the results can be misleading and do not usually alter therapy.[22]

If a bone density test is done, there remains some controversy about what the treatment thresholds should be. This depends on the cost, safety, and efficacy of the medications. Several expert groups have made recommendations based on the currently available medicines, including the National Osteoporosis Guideline Group in the United Kingdom and the National Osteoporosis Foundation (NOF) in the United States.[23] The UK recommendations are based on an age-specific threshold for fracture risk, from about 2% hip fracture risk over the next decade in a 50-year old person to 70% in a 90-year-old person. The NOF guidelines recommend treatment above a 10-year hip fracture risk of 3% or a major fracture risk of 20%.

If the NOF guidelines were used, then almost everybody over the age of 75 would be treated, as shown in papers using data from the Study of Osteoporotic Fractures,[24] or the NHANES data[23] shown in Figure 41–4. More studies on the effectiveness and safety of the medications should be done before such widespread use is advocated.

Alternatives to Bone Density Testing. Peripheral measurements such as ultrasound of the calcaneus or single photon absorptiometry of the arm or ankle are also able to predict hip fractures, but they have not been used as often as DEXA. Quantitated computed tomography (CT) can measure the bone density in three dimensions and can separate cortical from trabecular bone. This test requires very specific techniques and calibrations that are not usually possible in a clinical setting, and in elderly persons the T-scores are two or three standard deviations lower than those with DEXA.

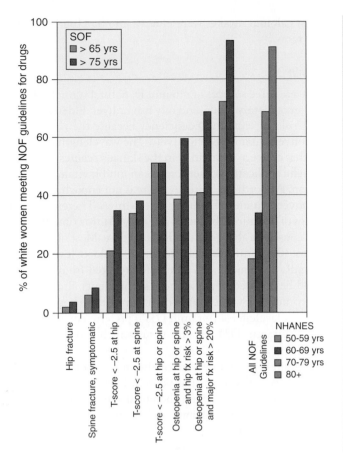

FIGURE 41–4. National Osteoporosis Foundation (NOF) recommendations on medication use for osteoporosis. (*Source: Dawson-Hughes et al.*[23])

CASE PRESENTATION 1 (continued)

The results of the bone density DEXA scan show a spine T-score of −2.3 and the hip of −1.8. The bone density report returned with fracture risk calculations using the T-score for the hip. Without consideration of clinical risks, there was 12% chance of a major osteoporotic fracture and 2.9% chance of a hip fracture (below the treatment threshold). Including the previous fracture, these risks increased to 18% and 4%, respectively. You were not surprised that the hip bone density was not in the osteoporotic range (T-score less than −2.5), because you realize that most fractures happen in women with only moderate bone loss. The risk of a fracture is highest in those with bone density lower than −2.5, but the majority of fractures occur in women with T-score between −1 and −2.5 because there are so many more women in that range. You also know that your patient's problem is with her vertebral fractures, and the FRAX calculator does not include that level of detail. Her bone density at the spine is close to osteoporosis, and she has had a fracture. Based upon this and the other diagnostics, you conclude she needs treatment.

● TREATMENT FOR OSTEOPOROSIS
Prevention and Supportive Treatment

General Nutrition

Some older women strive to maintain a low weight to look fashionably thin. Many underweight patients do not realize that this "healthy" diet is not optimal for them. Better sources of calories such as oils, carrot cake, chocolate, yogurt, and nuts should be emphasized. Weight loss due to change in a living situation, depression, or illness may be difficult to treat but increased calories and more frequent meals should also be encouraged. Protein intake should be adequate and balanced.

Exercise

Controlled studies show a benefit from ongoing exercise, particularly weight-bearing exercise, which promotes muscle development and bone health. Walking is a weight-bearing activity that a woman can do her entire life, and it does not require any expensive equipment. Back extension exercises and tai chi have also been found to be beneficial. Exercise of some type, particularly weight bearing, should be encouraged for all older adults, as even frail skeletons can respond to exercise with lowered risk of future fractures.

Smoking

Cigarette smoking contributes to osteoporosis as well as a host of other medical conditions.[25] The increased risk of hip fractures in cigarette smokers is shown in Figure 41–5. Quitting smoking has been found to reduce the risk of both osteoporosis and fractures, but generally requires years being smoke-free before the risk begins to approach that of a non-smoker (Figure 41–5).

Alcohol

Hip fractures more frequent in persons who drink more than 24 g of ethanol a day, which is approximately two "standard drinks" in the United States. Modest alcohol intake increases

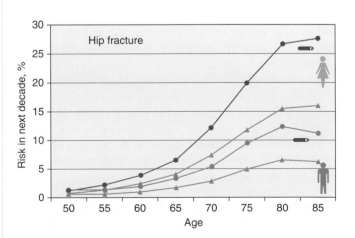

FIGURE 41–5. Hip fracture risk in cigarette smokers. (*Source: Kanis et al.*[25])

the bone density, probably because it enhances aromatase and thus raises estrogen levels, but nevertheless the risk of fracture is increased. Alcohol should be limited and taken in moderation.

Calcium

For adult men and women the current evidence suggests a total elemental calcium intake of 1000 to 1500 mg/day. This includes both dietary calcium and calcium supplements. The average total daily intake should not exceed 2000 mg. Calcium alone cannot prevent or treat osteoporosis, but an adequate calcium intake is needed for any other treatment to work.

Calcium carbonate is the most cost-effective source of calcium. Contrary to some advertisements, the intestinal absorption of calcium citrate and calcium carbonate is the same except when there is no acid in the stomach.[26] Side effects from a reasonable dose of calcium (1000 mg/day) are very low.

Constipation is associated with higher doses of calcium supplements (1200 mg/day in addition to 900 mg/day from dietary sources) and in one study caused constipation in 13% of subjects compared to a 9.1% rate of constipation in the control group.[27] To help prevent constipation, a patient should not take more calcium than necessary, increase intake of fruit juices and water, try getting calcium from food sources instead of tablets, take calcium with magnesium, or try calcium citrate or calcium chews. Gastritis is occasionally seen, which might be caused by taking calcium carbonate between meals, thus stimulating rebound acid production.

Calcium supplements may increase the risk of kidney stones if the dose is too high (over 2000 mg/day). On the other hand, inadequate dietary calcium can also cause kidney stones. This is because most kidney stones are caused by oxalate, and calcium inhibits the intestinal oxalate absorption. Patients with kidney stones should collect a 24-hour urine sample for calcium and oxalate measurements. If hypercalciuria with normal oxalate is found, it is reasonable to slightly limit calcium intake (between 800 and 1000 mg/day). Patients with hypercalciuria and low bone density can be treated with low doses (12.5-25 mg/day) of thiazide, using potassium bicarbonate as necessary to keep serum potassium normal. If oxalate is the culprit, then old-fashioned advice about avoiding calcium increases the risk of both osteoporosis and another kidney stone! Decreasing salt and protein may also help decrease the incidence of calcium-oxalate kidney stones.

The Women's Health Initiative studied 36,000 women for 7 years in a randomized clinical trial, and the calcium group had as many fractures as the placebo group. However, the baseline intake was 1100 mg/day, and a post-hoc analysis of those whose intake was lower than 800 mg/day did show a benefit.[28] Therefore, it is most likely that an intake of 1200 mg/day is adequate.

A meta-analysis of 29 randomized trials of calcium with or without vitamin D suggested that there was an overall 12% reduction in the risk of osteoporotic fractures with calcium. Addition of vitamin D did not make very much difference. The benefit was greatest in the people who had lowest calcium intake, were elderly, and had high compliance rates.[29]

Vitamin D

There are three sources of vitamin D: natural sunlight, fortification of dietary foods, and oily fish or liver. Elderly people are at risk for vitamin D deficiency because their skin does not convert vitamin D effectively. The wavelength of radiation that converts vitamin D in the skin also causes sunburn, so careful application of sunscreen can inhibit vitamin D production. At northern latitudes, there is not enough radiation to convert vitamin D during the winter. Therefore, oral sources of vitamin D become necessary. At this time there is not a consensus about the optimal oral dose. Most of the time 800 to 1000 units/day will result in a blood level above 20 ng/dL (50 nmol/L). Vitamin D prepared from fish oils should be avoided because these supplements also contain high contents of vitamin A, which can increase bone resorption. Cholecalciferol (vitamin D3) is preferred over ergocalciferol (vitamin D2) because it sustains blood levels for a longer time.[30-32]

Vitamin D is actually a steroid hormone, with pleiotropic effects. It is well known that vitamin D increases the intestinal absorption of calcium, thereby decreasing parathyroid hormone and making calcium available to bones. Other more recently described effects include strengthening of muscle and inhibition of cell proliferation and promotion of differentiation, which might suppress cancer growth. Intracellular conversion of 25-OH-vitamin D in T-cells results in expression of cathelicidin, an enzyme that is necessary to kill mycobacteria. This explains results described by Niels Finsen, the 1903 Nobel Prize winner, who observed that sunlight exposure treated lupus vulgaris (cutaneous tuberculosis).

Like other steroids, adverse effects are seen with either high or low levels of vitamin D. Prospective and observational studies have shown that levels of vitamin D lower than 20 ng/dL (50 nmol/L) are associated with higher fracture rates[33] and higher mortality.[34] However, excess vitamin D may cause complications such as nephrolithiasis and hypercalcemia. Early reports of a protective effect on prostate cancer have not been substantiated in large studies. In the prospective Prostate, Lung, Colorectal and Ovarian Cancer Screening Trial of 38,350 men, high vitamin D levels were associated with higher incidence of aggressive prostate cancer.[35] Some studies have suggested that vitamin D could reduce the risk of breast cancer, but this has not been seen in recent larger prospective studies.[32,36,37] The majority of recent, large clinical trials of vitamin D have not found significant reduction in fracture rates in community-dwelling persons. Meta-analyses of clinical trials of vitamin D produce mixed results. The most consistent beneficial finding is that vitamin D combined with calcium reduces hip fractures in elderly subjects living in nursing homes, particularly if their food sources are not fortified with vitamin D.[38]

Fall Prevention and Protection

Fall prevention is very important to older patients with osteoporosis, and this is covered in detail in Chapter 34.

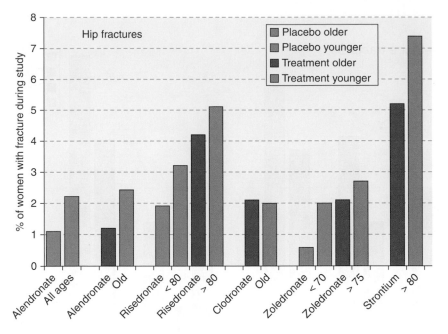

FIGURE 41–6. Osteoporosis medications, treatment, age, and hip fractures.

CASE PRESENTATION 1 (continued)

You discuss the possible treatments with Mrs. W. First, you estimate that her calcium intake from food sources is 600 mg/day. You then suggest calcium tablets containing 300 mg each, to take one with breakfast and one with dinner. You also explain the importance of vitamin D. She does not really need the other vitamins in her multiple vitamin tablet, which contained 400 units of ergocalciferol. Instead you tell her to take a brand of cholecalciferol that provides 1000 international units per day.

Medications to Treat Osteoporosis

Several medications are approved for treatment of osteoporosis. Recent reviews have commented on the irony that the majority of hip fractures occur in patients older than 80, but they are scarcely represented in clinical trials of medications to treat osteoporosis.[39-43] Results from studies of women in their 60s and 70s should not automatically be applied to older patients, who frequently have more complex risk factors. A database study from Quebec included all patients with a hip fracture from 1996 to 2002 who returned home after the fracture (N = 20,644). Anti-resorptive medications were prescribed to 6779 patients. Those younger than 80 who had taken medications had 47% fewer recurrent hip fractures. In those older than 80, however, there was only an 8% reduction. This age effect was significant.[44] Geriatric patients may have more diseases that contribute to bone weakness. For example, many have moderate chronic kidney disease, which has been an exclusion criterion for all of the major clinical trials. Weight loss and frailty are common, and falls are more frequent than in younger people. Bone loss accelerates in women older than 80, and once the bone mass becomes very low, treatment can cause a significant improvement in bone mass that may nevertheless not be enough to prevent a fracture.

Figure 41–6 shows the results from randomized clinical trials in elderly women with osteoporosis. Several of these studies compared the efficacy in older than 75 or 80 years old to younger women. In general, these medications are effective in otherwise healthy elderly women, although sometimes the effect is better in the younger groups (Figure 41–7).

Bisphosphonates

Bisphosphonates are analogs of pyrophosphate, a natural inhibitor of mineralization. They bind tightly to mineral and inhibit osteoclasts, thus reducing bone resorption and preventing bone loss. Cavities in the bone that were recently resorbed will fill with new bone during the first 6 months of treatment; after that the bone volume stabilizes and no further resorption will occur. This prevents the microarchitectural deterioration that occurs in patients with high bone turnover. When bone resorption is inhibited, there is no stimulus for bone formation, which decreases by 75% to 90% after several months of bisphosphonates. In women or men with an osteoporotic bone density (T-score of the hip lower than −2.5), bisphosphonates reduce the incidence of fractures and improve the quality of life. Bisphosphonates are less effective in preventing fractures in people with osteopenia.

Several different bisphosphonates have been approved for treatment of osteoporosis. To date there is no convincing evidence that any one is better than the others. There are now choices between oral and intravenous preparations. The intravenous forms are more expensive, but they can be advantageous in patients with dementia or inability to remember their medications, or those with esophagitis.

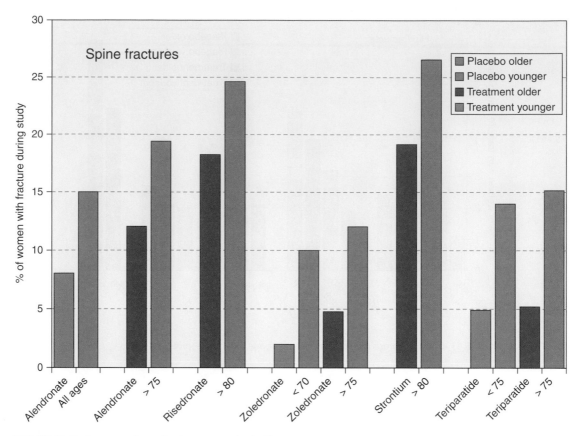

FIGURE 41–7. Osteoporosis medications, age, and spinal fractures.

Dosage adjustments have not been recommended for elderly patients, but in a large study of risedronate, 5445 women between 70 and 79 years old were randomized to placebo, 2.5 mg/day, or 5 mg/day. There was a significant reduction in hip fracture risk with a dose of 2.5 mg/day; the results with 5 mg/day were not quite statistically significant.[45] When given orally, it is imperative that the medicine is taken on an empty stomach without food or beverages except plain water, because the bisphosphonates are absorbed very poorly and food reduces the absorption further. In addition, to avoid esophageal irritation, the pill should be taken with about 4 oz of water and the patient should avoid lying down or bending over. Excess water is not optimal because it can cause reflux.

Bisphosphonates are excreted by the kidneys and are not recommended for persons with stage 4 or 5 chronic kidney disease. Often elderly, thin women with low muscle mass have a deceptively normal creatinine. This should be taken into account when prescribing bisphosphonates. Also, it is especially important to insure adequate vitamin D levels before starting bisphosphonates, because serious hypocalcemia can develop after bisphosphonates in people with vitamin D deficiency.

Gastrointestinal irritation is a common adverse effect, and when taken improperly esophageal ulceration may occur. There have been some findings of atrial fibrillation, but a review by the FDA concluded that these were not related to the medications. Uncommon adverse events include severe generalized bone pain, nephrotic syndrome, eye inflammation, or allergic rash. Hypocalcemia was not noted in the clinical trials, but subjects were not enrolled unless they had normal vitamin D and PTH; in practice, hypocalcemia occurs in patients who are deficient in vitamin D or who have malabsorption. The incidence of jaw osteonecrosis is less than 1/10,000 when used in osteoporosis doses, but the risk is higher in patients who have malignancies and are treated with higher doses. Intravenous forms cause fever, transient leukopenia, and an acute-phase reaction. Unusual diaphyseal femur fractures have been associated with prolonged alendronate use; the incidence rate is uncertain.

Information about long-term use of bisphosphonates is limited. Subjects who participated in clinical trials have been observed for up to 10 years, with stable bone density and without increase in fracture rates, which would otherwise be expected as they aged. One randomized placebo-controlled trial enrolled women who had already taken alendronate for an average of 5 years. They were then treated with either placebo or alendronate for 5 years. The bone density gradually decreased in the placebo group but not in the alendronate group. In the placebo group, P1NP (formation marker) increased moderately but was still 24% below baseline after 5 years; the bone alkaline phosphatase gradually increased toward baseline, and the bone resorption markers remained suppressed. In the alendronate group all markers remained suppressed for 10 years. The overall clinical fractures and vertebral fractures documented by radiographs were similar in those who took alendronate compared with those who were on placebo.[46] The bisphosphonates remain deposited in the bone with a half-life greater than 10 years, so it appears safe to discontinue alendronate after 5 years. However, there are no practice guidelines about this issue and experts disagree about when to stop bisphosphonates.

These medications are effective in women aged 75 to 80. Limited data on women older than 80 show that bone density improves, and hip fracture rates are decreased but the statistical significance is variable (Figure 41–6). In the Alendronate Fracture Intervention Trial the women between 75 and 80 who had established osteoporosis showed improvement in bone density and fracture reduction that was similar to the women aged 55 to 75.[47] Risedronate did not reduce hip fracture rates in women older than 80, even among the 941 women who had osteoporosis by bone densitometry. This poor result could have been due to low power.[45] In the recent report of zoledronic acid the average age was 73 and women up to age 89 were enrolled. These women with established osteoporosis had a significant reduction in fractures, including hip fractures. A post-hoc analysis showed that women younger than 70 had a better response than women older than 75.[48] In another zoledronic acid study in patients who had experienced a recent hip fracture, the average age was 74 and 292 subjects (14%) were older than 85. Those who received zoledronic acid had an absolute risk reduction of 5.3% for clinical fracture. The hip fracture rate was decreased but did not reach statistical significance.[49]

Raloxifene

Raloxifene is a selective estrogen receptor modulator that has estrogenic actions on skeletal tissue but anti-estrogenic actions on reproductive tissues. Thus, it improves bone strength and reduces risk of breast cancer. Clinical trials consistently show reductions in the rates of vertebral fractures and of breast cancer. The skeletal effects are not as strong as native estrogen, and the rates of non-vertebral fractures are not significantly reduced with raloxifene as they are with estrogen.

The dose of raloxifene is 60 mg/day. It can be taken at any time with or without food. It has been studied in placebo-controlled trials with durations up to 8 years.

The most serious adverse effect is an increase in coagulopathy similar to that seen with estrogen. The risk of thrombophlebitis is increased. In women who had confirmed coronary artery disease, raloxifene did not affect the rate of myocardial infarction or overall strokes, but did increase the risk of fatal strokes. In women with osteoporosis or a high risk of breast cancer there was no difference in the rate of fatal strokes. Raloxifene may cause hot flashes and leg cramps.

The clinical trials have not included many women older than 80. In the RUTH (Raloxifene Use for The Heart) study, 39% of subjects were older than 70. The clinical vertebral fracture rate was slightly better in the older women, where the incidence was 3.2% in those on placebo and 1.8% in those taking raloxifene. In the younger group, these rates were 1.1% and 0.9%, respectively.[50]

Calcitonin

Calcitonin, a hormone produced by cells in the thyroid gland, acts directly on osteoclasts (via specific receptors on the cell surface). The osteoclasts shrink and stop bone resorption.

Bone biopsies from patients treated with the drug show no effects on mineralization. It has a short half-life. This is a milder medication that modulates bone resorption but does not totally inhibit it.

The clinical trials of calcitonin have not enrolled as many subjects as trials of other approved osteoporosis medications. A significant reduction in vertebral fractures was seen with a dose of 200 units/day, but not with higher or lower doses. Non-vertebral fracture rates were not reduced. Some measurements of bone quality as determined by high-resolution magnetic resonance have shown improvements on the microstructure of the bone with calcitonin.[51]

This medication was previously given as a subcutaneous injection, with several side effects. The current recommended dose is the nasal spray formulation, which delivers 200 units per metered dose. This should be sprayed daily in alternate nostrils.

Calcitonin is a very safe medication with no serious side effects. Nasal irritation or allergic reactions may occur.

Teriparatide

Parathyroid hormone is naturally an 84-amino-acid polypeptide. In 2002 the FDA approved recombinant PTH 1-34, chemical name teriparatide. Teriparatide is currently the only approved *anabolic* medication that reduces the incidence of osteoporotic fractures. Anabolic drugs work by increasing formation of new bone, whereas other drugs block the resorption of bone.

This medication is expensive and there are no long-term data, so currently it is indicated for patients with severe osteoporosis and vertebral compression fractures, patients who have fractures despite prolonged bisphosphonate use, those with a very high risk of fractures and low bone formation (for example, T-score less than −3.5 and low markers of bone turnover), and osteoporotic patients with prolonged use of high-dose glucocorticosteroids.

In animal studies and some early clinical observations, teriparatide can help with fracture healing, so it could be considered in patients with pelvic insufficiency fracture or delayed fracture healing.

In clinical trials, the bone density increases, particularly in the trabecular bone, where the average increase is 18%. Fracture rates of the vertebrae and all clinical fractures are significantly decreased.

Currently only one dose is available, 20 μg/day given by subcutaneous injection. The anabolic effects of teriparatide begin to wane after about a year, so therapy should not be continued for longer than 2 years. Thereafter, it is important to follow with an anti-resorbing medication, or the gains in bone will be rapidly lost.

In the largest trial, nausea was seen in 8% (similar to placebo), headache in 8%, dizziness in 9%, leg cramps in 3%, hypercalcemia in 11% (usually mild), and the uric acid increased by an average of 13%.

In laboratory rats, an increased risk of osteosarcoma was observed with moderate to large doses of teriparatide. This has not been observed in other species or in humans. However, the drug should be avoided in persons with a high risk of osteosarcoma, including those with history of cancer, radiation to the bone, Paget disease, or other diseases with high turnover. It also should not be used in patients with hyperparathyroidism, hypercalcemia, or gout.

This medicine has not been studied in patients with liver disease, and since liver enzymes can break down PTH, it is not known if the anabolic effects of PTH will work. The drug has not been studied in those with later stages of chronic kidney disease, or in those with kidney stones. In persons between 75 and 86 years old, there was a beneficial effect on fracture rates that was similar to the reduction in fractures seen in the younger patients (Figure 41–7).[52]

CASE PRESENTATION 1 (continued)

In weighing the various treatment options for Mrs. W., you consider that you want to use a medication that has been shown to reduce the risk of vertebral fractures and is safe over time. You do not use estrogen because she is more than 10 years past menopause and the risks of cardiovascular complications make that a poor choice given the Women's Health Initiative study. It would have been a good choice for a woman within 5 years of menopause, particularly if she also had hot flashes. You also do not prefer calcitonin in this case because it has a weaker effect and the other medications are more potent. You might use this in somebody who seems to have a reaction to everything and won't take a medicine unless it is very safe. Your first choices are a bisphosphonate or raloxifene. The study that directly compared these drugs failed to enroll enough women to definitely determine which was superior, but in that study they had similar effects on vertebral fractures. You therefore tell your patient that either of these medications would be helpful. She is interested in the raloxifene because her sister had breast cancer. This is an important consideration because women who do not take raloxifene develop breast cancer twice as often as women who take it. She also is reluctant to take alendronate because her neighbor had heartburn with that medication. The main contraindication to raloxifene is a history of thromboembolism. Your patient has never had that problem, so you prescribe raloxifene. You also make a referral to the physical therapist for instruction in back care and gentle back extension exercises.

● FRACTURES AND OSTEOPOROSIS

Incidence and Prevalence

The lifetime risk of a fracture of the hip, spine, or forearm is 40% in white women and 13% in white men. African Americans have fewer fractures than people of other races.[53] Fracture rates also vary among countries, races, ethnic backgrounds, and between urban and rural areas.

The incidence of hip fractures rises exponentially with age in women after the age of 60 and in men after the age of 70. Vertebral fractures also increase with aging, and the prevalence of these fractures reaches about 20% in men and 30% to 40% in women.[54]

Low bone density is not the only cause of fractures. The strength of the bone also depends on the micro-architecture and shape of the bone, as well as factors called "bone quality," which include the flexibility of the bone material, the crystal size, and the ability to repair micro-damage. For example, a new branch of a willow tree will sway with the wind, but an old, brittle branch with the same amount of wood will snap and break.

The stress applied to the bone also determines whether the bone will fracture. Trauma, falls, lifting heavy objects, twisting, and forceful muscle contractions can all precipitate a fracture. Falls are especially important causes in geriatric populations, and the direction of the fall makes a difference. Falls to the side, which result in direct hit to the hip, are six times more likely to cause a fracture than forward falls.[55]

Compression Fractures

Compression fractures vary in severity, and mild fractures may be difficult to distinguish from natural variation in the shape of the vertebrae. Several methods have been proposed for ascertaining whether a "deformity" is a fracture in clinical trials, but they all result in some overlap between "normal" and compressed vertebrae. For practical purposes in the clinic, a vertebra can be considered compressed if the anterior height is less than 80% of the posterior height, or if the height of one vertebra is less than 80% of the adjacent one (Figure 41–8). A new fracture should show a loss of at least 4 mm from a previous radiograph.

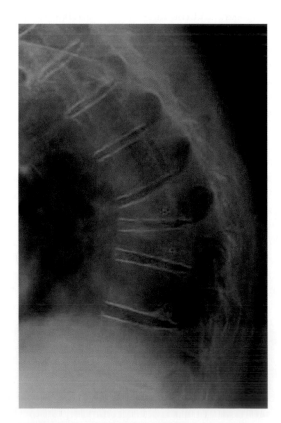

FIGURE 41–8. Compression fractures.

Asymptomatic Vertebral Fractures

When looking at a pair of vertebral radiographs showing a new compression fracture, it is difficult to imagine that it did not cause a great deal of pain. However, an observational study of 7223 women, with radiographs taken at baseline and at 3.7 years, found that only 43% of the women with new vertebral fractures reported increasing back pain.[8] Virtually all of the clinical trials of osteoporosis medications have found that "morphometric fractures" (those measured by standard radiographs) occur three to four times as often as "clinical fractures" (those which came to their primary physician's attention, usually due to symptoms). On the other hand, fractures can cause severe pain, which is typically located at the site of the fracture, and which lasts about a month. The pain then gradually improves and usually resolves by 3 months. The most likely explanation for the differences between clinical and morphometric fractures is that the former occur suddenly, and are caused by a high stress such as lifting a heavy weight, whereas the silent fractures are gradual compressions due to fragile bone structure.

Vertebral Fractures Strongly Predict Future Fractures, But ...

Radiologists do not mention vertebral fractures in about half of the radiology reports from standard chest x-rays. Even when the fractures are included on the report, they are often not treated by the physicians. This is undesirable, because even a mild or an asymptomatic vertebral fracture predicts future fractures. After adjusting for the age and bone density, a person with a fracture is four times more likely to have another fracture as a person without one. The more severe the prevalent vertebral fractures, the higher the risk of a new fracture. In the first year after a vertebral fracture, the average risk of a new fracture is 20%. Hip fractures are also seen more often in patients with a previous vertebral fracture. These new fractures can be prevented with treatment and should not be ignored.[54]

Hip Fractures

Hip fractures are a devastating manifestation of osteoporosis and they frequently result in loss of independence in elderly men and women. These are discussed in Chapter 40.

● MALE OSTEOPOROSIS

CASE PRESENTATION 2: NEW VERTEBRAL FRACTURE IN A MALE

A retired mechanical engineer who is now 83 years old comes to your office complaining of lower back pain for the last week. It is severe and began when he was lifting some rocks while he was working in his garden. His medical problems include history of TURP for early-stage prostate cancer, moderate hearing loss,

and hypertension. Current medications are HCTZ 25 mg/day, aspirin 81 mg/day, and vitamin D 4000 units/day. He does not have any of the clinical risk factors for osteoporosis. On most days he eats one bowl of cereal that contains 1000 mg of calcium.

On physical exam he has point tenderness over the midspine in the lower lumbar region. Otherwise his exam is unchanged from his previous visits. You decide he needs further evaluation and order an x-ray of his spine and bone density test. You also request labs tests, including a complete blood count, prostate specific antigen, and testosterone level. Because you suspect this is a new fracture, you check serum and urine protein electrophoresis to rule out myeloma.

Osteoporosis in men is under-recognized and understudied.[56] In men, the increase in hip fracture rates shows the same exponential increase as in women, but this begins when they are a decade older. The longer lifespan of women also increases the proportion of hip fractures experienced by women. When men fracture a hip, their age-adjusted mortality is about twice that of women. Vertebral fractures and kyphosis are also serious problems in men. Studies that assess the prevalence of vertebral fractures by taking radiographs of community populations show overall similar rates in men and in women, but in men there are more vertebral fractures when they are in their 50s and the incidence in older life is lower (Figure 41–1). This suggests that some of the prevalent fractures were caused by work-related injuries.

The diagnostic workup is similar in both men and women, but should include measurement of testosterone for men. Low levels of testosterone can be seen even when there are no overt symptoms of hypogonadism.

CASE PRESENTATION 2 (continued)

His x-ray shows a compression fracture at L2. Bone density of the spine showed a T-score of −2.8 and hip (femoral neck) of −2.9. His 10-year risk of a hip fracture is 11%. Labs show mild hypokalemia (3.4 mg/dL), low testosterone, and a prostate-specific antigen (PSA) at 3 ng/mL (considered normal by this lab). His vitamin D level was 80 ng/dL (200 nmol/L). Otherwise the laboratory tests are unremarkable, including a normal serum and urine protein electrophoresis. You decide to order a bone scan because he has a previous history of prostate cancer.

Treatment in Men

Gonadal hormones largely explain the differences in bone biology between men and women. During growth, the androgens are responsible for more periosteal expansion, so the bones in men are larger, and the cortical thickness is greater. Men do not experience menopause. Although gradual decreases in testosterone are common in elderly men, this is not a universal finding. In the bones of men, testosterone is converted to estrogens that maintain the bone turnover rate at a healthy level. Patients with aromatase deficiency have osteoporosis despite abundant testosterone, and this reverses with estrogen. Thus, estrogen is a requirement for bone health in both men and women.

Testosterone

In hypogonadal men, testosterone increases the bone density.[57] This has been a consistent finding, but the clinical trials have not been large enough to document the reduction in fracture rates that would be expected with the improved bone density. Micro-magnetic resonance imaging has shown improved micro-architecture in men after 2 years of testosterone treatment.[58]

Testosterone may be administered by intramuscular injection or transdermally, and both routes will improve bone density. Adverse effects include increased cholesterol, hematocrit, and liver function tests. Hypogonadism results in smaller size of the prostate, and replacement with testosterone increases the prostate to the size that would be expected if there had not been hypogonadism. In some cases this will cause symptoms of urinary obstruction.

Testosterone has not been shown to cause prostate cancer, but it can exacerbate existing cancer and should be avoided in men with a history of prostate cancer or an elevated PSA.

CASE PRESENTATION 2 (continued)

Your patient returns to clinic. His bone scan showed increased uptake at L2, the same location as the fracture, and this is suggestive of a relatively new fracture, as was seen on the plain films. There is no other uptake to suggest a malignancy. His pain is slightly better. You ordered a testosterone test to see if this was the cause of his osteoporosis, and this now seems the most likely explanation. However, you are reluctant to prescribe this because he had a history of prostate cancer. Instead, you suggest a bisphosphonate, because he is at an elevated risk of both another vertebral fracture and a hip fracture. Alendronate is the most cost-effective choice, and he is a motivated and intelligent man who follows instructions. You also tell him the most recent studies do not show a benefit of vitamin D for prostate cancer, even though early studies had suggested this. He will discontinue the vitamin D, and you suggest he return to clinic in 4 months.

At the return visit he is feeling much better. His pain is now present only on occasion and is mild. He is taking the alendronate as prescribed without any side effects. You check his vitamin D again and it is now 40 ng/mL

(99.8 nmol/L), so you recommend that he take a supplement of 400 units a day until next year. You plan to check this again and would increase the dose if his level decreased below 20 ng/mL (50 nmol/L). This also is a good time to send him to the physical therapist for some gentle back extension exercises and instructions in back care and encourage him to remain active.

CONCLUSION

Osteoporosis and osteoporosis-related fractures are a significant problem for older adults. With the growing population of older adults, rates of osteoporosis will continue to climb. Despite the availability of techniques to diagnose osteoporosis as well as the increasing number of treatment options, osteoporosis is still widely under-diagnosed and undertreated. Only with vigilant care by providers who recognize both the risk factors as well as silent indicators of disease will sufficient numbers of older adults be appropriately diagnosed and treated for this disabling disease.

References

1. US Department of Health and Human Services. Bone health and osteoporosis: A report of the surgeon general. Rockville, MD: US Department of Health and Human Services, Office of the Surgeon General; 2004.

2. Hothauer LC, Schoppet M. Clinical implications of the osteoprotegerin /RANKL/RANK system for bone and vascular diseases. JAMA. 2004; 292:490-495.

3. De Laet C, Kanis JA, Oden A, et al. Body mass index as a predictor of fracture risk: A meta-analysis. *Osteoporos Int*. 2005;16:1330-1338.

4. Salamone LM, Cauley JA, Black DM, et al. Effect of a lifestyle intervention on bone mineral density in premenopausal women: A randomized trial. *Am J Clin Nutr*. 1999;70:97-103.

5. Ensrud KE, Ewing SK, Stone KL, et al. Intentional and unintentional weight loss increase bone loss and hip fracture risk in older women. *J Am Geriatr Soc*. 2003;51:1740-1747.

6. Schurch MA, Rizzoli R, Slosman D, et al. Protein supplements increase serum insulin-like growth factor-I levels and attenuate proximal femur bone loss in patients with recent hip fracture. A randomized, double-blind, placebo-controlled trial. *Ann Intern Med*. 1998;128:801-809.

7. Kerstetter JE, O'Brien KO, Caseria DM, et al. The impact of dietary protein on calcium absorption and kinetic measures of bone turnover in women. *J Clin Endocrinol Metab*. 2005;90:26-31.

8. Sellmeyer DE, Stone KL, Sebastian A, Cummings SR. A high ratio of dietary animal to vegetable protein increases the rate of bone loss and the risk of fracture in postmenopausal women. Study of Osteoporotic Fractures Research Group. *Am J Clin Nutr*. 2001;73:118-122.

9. Hannan MT, Tucker KL, Dawson-Hughes B, et al. Effect of dietary protein on bone loss in elderly men and women: The Framingham Osteoporosis Study. *J Bone Miner Res*. 2000;15;2504-2512.

10. Promislow JH, Goodman-Gruen D, Slymen DJ, Barrett-Connor E. Protein consumption and bone mineral density in the elderly: The Rancho Bernardo Study. *Am J Epidemiol*. 2002;155:636-611.

11. Sampson HW. Alcohol's harmful effect on bone. *Alcohol Health Res World*. 1998;22:190-194.

12. NIH Osteoporosis and Related Bone Diseases, National Resource Center. Smoking and Bone Health. 2009. Accessed at www.niams.nih.gov/bone.

13. Nevitt MC, Ettinger B, Black DM, et al. The association of radiographically detected vertebral fractures with back pain and function: A prospective study. *Ann Intern Med*. 1998;128:793-800.

14. Kaptoge S, Armbrecht G, Felsenberg D, et al. When should the doctor order a spine X-ray? Identifying vertebral fractures for osteoporosis care: Results from the European Prospective Osteoporosis Study (EPOS). *J Bone Miner Res*. 2004;19:1982-1993.

15. Siminoski K, Warshawski RS, Jen H, Lee K. The accuracy of historical height loss for the detection of vertebral fractures in postmenopausal women. *Osteoporos Int*. 2006;17:290-296.

16. Binkley N, Novotny R, Krueger D, et al. Low vitamin D status despite abundant sun exposure. *J Clin Endocrinol Metab*. 2007;92: 2130-2135.

17. Bauer DC, Garnero P, Hochberg MC, et al. Pretreatment levels of bone turnover and the antifracture efficacy of alendronate: The fracture intervention trial. *J Bone Miner Res*. 2006;21:292-299.

18. Fink HA, Harrison SL, Taylor BC, et al. Differences in site-specific fracture risk among older women with discordant results for osteoporosis at hip and spine: Study of osteoporotic fractures. *J Clin Densitom*. 2008;11:250-259.

19. Kanis JA, Oden A, Johnell O, et al. The use of clinical risk factors enhances the performance of BMD in the prediction of hip and osteoporotic fractures in men and women. *Osteoporos Int*. 2007; 18:1033-1046.

20. Cummings SR, Black D. Bone mass measurements and risk of fracture in Caucasian women: A review of findings from prospective studies. *Am J Med*. 1995;98:24S-28S.

21. Lewis CE, Ewing SK, Taylor BC, et al. Predictors of non-spine fracture in elderly men: The MrOS study. *J Bone Miner Res*. 2007;22:211-219.

22. Bell KJ, Hayen A, Macaskill P, et al. Value of routine monitoring of bone mineral density after starting bisphosphonate treatment: Secondary analysis of trial data. *BMJ*. 2009;338:B2266.

23. Dawson-Hughes B, Looker AC, Tosteson AN, et al. The potential impact of new National Osteoporosis Foundation guidance on treatment patterns. *Osteoporos Int*. 2009;21:41-52.

24. Donaldson MG, Cawthon PM, Lui LY, et al. Estimates of the proportion of older white women who would be recommended for pharmacologic treatment by the new U.S. National Osteoporosis Foundation Guidelines. *J Bone Miner Res*. 2009;24:675-680.

25. Kanis JA, Johnell O, Oden A, et al. Smoking and fracture risk: A meta-analysis. *Osteoporos Int*. 2005;16:155-162.

26. Heaney RP, Dowell MS, Barger-Lux MJ. Absorption of calcium as the carbonate and citrate salts, with some observations on method. *Osteoporos Int*. 1999;9:19-23.

27. Prince RL, Devine A, Dhaliwal SS, Dick IM. Effects of calcium supplementation on clinical fracture and bone structure: Results of a 5-year, double-blind, placebo-controlled trial in elderly women. *Arch Intern Med*. 2006;166:869-875.

28. Jackson RD, LaCroix AZ, Gass M, et al. Calcium plus vitamin D supplementation and the risk of fractures. *N Engl J Med*. 2006;354: 669-683.

29. Tang BM, Eslick GD, Nowson C, et al. Use of calcium or calcium in combination with vitamin D supplementation to prevent fractures and bone loss in people aged 50 years and older: A meta-analysis. *Lancet*. 2007;370:657-666.

30. Glendenning P, Chew GT, Seymour HM, et al. Serum 25-hydroxyvitamin D levels in vitamin D-insufficient hip fracture patients after supplementation with ergocalciferol and cholecalciferol. *Bone*. 2009;45:870-875.

31. Armas LA, Hollis BW, Heaney RP. Vitamin D2 is much less effective than vitamin D3 in humans. *J Clin Endocrinol Metab*. 2004;89: 5387-5391.

32. McCullough ML, Stevens VL, Patel R, et al. Serum 25-hydroxyvitamin D concentrations and postmenopausal breast cancer risk: A nested case control study in the Cancer Prevention Study-II Nutrition Cohort. *Breast Cancer Res*. 2009;11:R64.

33. Cauley JA, Lacroix AZ, Wu L, et al. Serum 25-hydroxyvitamin D concentrations and risk for hip fractures. *Ann Intern Med*. 2008; 149:242-250.

34. Melamed ML, Michos ED, Post W, Astor B. 25-hydroxyvitamin D levels and the risk of mortality in the general population. *Arch Intern Med*. 2008;168:1629-1637.

35. Ahn J, Peters U, Albanes D, et al. Serum vitamin D concentration and prostate cancer risk: A nested case-control study. *J Natl Cancer Inst*. 2008;100:796-804.

36. Chlebowski RT, Johnson KC, Kooperberg C, et al. Calcium plus vitamin D supplementation and the risk of breast cancer. *J Natl Cancer Inst*. 2008;100:1581-1591.

37. Freedman DM, Chang SC, Falk RT, et al. Serum levels of vitamin D metabolites and breast cancer risk in the prostate, lung, colorectal, and ovarian cancer screening trial. *Cancer Epidemiol Biomarkers Prev*. 2008;17:889-894.

38. Cranney A, Weiler HA, O'Donnell S, Puil L. Summary of evidence-based review on vitamin D efficacy and safety in relation to bone health. *Am J Clin Nutr*. 2008;88:513S-519S.

39. Boonen S, McClung MR, Eastell R, et al. Safety and efficacy of risedronate in reducing fracture risk in osteoporotic women aged 80 and older: Implications for the use of antiresorptive agents in the old and oldest old. *J Am Geriatr Soc*. 2004;52:1832-1839.

40. Parikh S, Avorn J, Solomon DH. Pharmacological management of osteoporosis in nursing home populations: A systematic review. *J Am Geriatr Soc*. 2009;57:327-334.

41. Inderjeeth CA, Foo AC, Lai MM, Glendenning P. Efficacy and safety of pharmacological agents in managing osteoporosis in the old old: Review of the evidence. *Bone*. 2009;44:744-751.

42. Schneider DL. Management of osteoporosis in geriatric populations. *Curr Osteoporos Rep*. 2008;6:100-107.

43. Wilkins CH, Birge SJ. Prevention of osteoporotic fractures in the elderly. *Am J Med*. 2005;118:1190-1195.

44. Morin S, Rahme E, Behlouli H, et al. Effectiveness of antiresorptive agents in the prevention of recurrent hip fractures. *Osteoporos Int*. 2007;18:1625-1632.

45. McClung MR, Geusens P, Miller PD, et al. Effect of risedronate on the risk of hip fracture in elderly women. Hip Intervention Program Study Group. *N Engl J Med*. 2001;344:333-340.

46. Black DM, Schwartz AV, Ensrud KE, et al. Effects of continuing or stopping alendronate after 5 years of treatment: The Fracture Intervention Trial Long-term Extension (FLEX): A randomized trial. *JAMA*. 2006;296:2927.

47. Ensrud KE, Black DM, Palermo L, et al. Treatment with alendronate prevents fractures in women at highest risk: Results from the Fracture Intervention Trial. *Arch Intern Med*. 1997;157: 2617-2624.

48. Eastell R, Black DM, Boonen S, et al. Effect of once-yearly zoledronic acid five milligrams on fracture risk and change in femoral neck bone mineral density. *J Clin Endocrinol Metab.* 2009;94: 3215-3225.

49. Lyles KW, Colon-Emeric CS, Magaziner JS, et al. Zoledronic acid in reducing clinical fracture and mortality after hip fracture. *N Engl J Med.* 2007;357:nihpa40967.

50. Ensrud KE, Stock JL, Barrett-Connor E, et al. Effects of raloxifene on fracture risk in postmenopausal women: The Raloxifene Use for the Heart Trial. *J Bone Miner Res.* 2008;23:112-120.

51. Chesnut CH III, Azria M, Silverman S, et al. Salmon calcitonin: A review of current and future therapeutic indications. *Osteoporos Int.* 2008;19:479-491.

52. Boonen S, Marin F, Mellstrom D, et al. Safety and efficacy of teriparatide in elderly women with established osteoporosis: Bone anabolic therapy from a geriatric perspective. *J Am Geriatr Soc.* 2006;54:782-789.

53. US Department of Health and Human Services. Bone Health and Osteoporosis: A Report of the Surgeon General. Rockville, MD: US Department of Health and Human Services, Office of the Surgeon General; 2004.

54. Ott SM. Osteoporosis and Bone Physiology. http://courses.washington.edu/bonephys 2009.

55. Greenspan SL, Myers ER, Kiel DP, et al. Fall direction, bone mineral density, and function: Risk factors for hip fracture in frail nursing home elderly. *Am J Med.* 1998;104:539-545.

56. Ebeling PR. Clinical practice. Osteoporosis in men. *N Engl J Med.* 2008;358:1474-1482.

57. Amory JK, Watts NB, Easley KA, et al. Exogenous testosterone or testosterone with finasteride increases bone mineral density in older men with low serum testosterone. *J Clin Endocrinol Metab.* 2004;89: 503-510.

58. Benito M, Vasilic B, Wehrli FW, et al. Effect of testosterone replacement on trabecular architecture in hypogonadal men. *J Bone Miner Res.* 2005;20:1785-1791.

POST-TEST

1. **Which one of these medications improves osteoporosis by stimulating osteoblasts to make more bone?**
   A. Teriparatide
   B. Alendronate
   C. Raloxifene
   D. Calcitonin

2. **Which of these is NOT an important effect of vitamin D?**
   A. Increases intestinal calcium absorption
   B. Decreases level of parathyroid hormone
   C. Enables white blood cells to kill mycobacteria
   D. Decreases bone cell production of fibroblast growth factor 23

3. **In a 65-year-old woman with osteopenia, which of these risk factors would suggest treatment with an approved osteoporosis medication?**
   A. Her father suffered a hip fracture.
   B. She had a mild, asymptomatic vertebral compression fracture noted on a chest x-ray.
   C. She is of African heritage.
   D. She smokes cigarettes.

ANSWERS TO PRE-TEST

1. D
2. A
3. C

ANSWERS TO POST-TEST

1. A
2. D
3. D

42

Approach to Common Infections in Older Adults

Stephen G. Weber, MD, MS

● LEARNING OBJECTIVES

1. Discuss the biological and epidemiologic factors that influence the incidence and severity of infection among older individuals.
2. Describe and illustrate a practical and consistent approach to the selection of empirical antimicrobial therapy for older patients with known or suspected infection across the spectrum of clinical care.
3. Identify clinical and biological features that help predict the most likely causative pathogen in older patients with known or suspected infection.
4. Discuss factors that help determine the most appropriate breadth of empirical antimicrobial therapy for older patients with known or suspected infection, with a focus on the severity of infection and the likelihood of antimicrobial resistance.
5. Identify pharmacologic considerations that shape the final selection of appropriate antimicrobial therapy for older patients with known or suspected infection.

PRE-TEST

1. A 71-year-old woman who lives with her daughter and four grandchildren presents to the office describing a low-grade fever after the onset of a painful "spider-bite" on her left ankle. Her vital signs are stable and she generally looks well. Which antibiotic choice is MOST appropriate?
   A. Oral dicloxacillin
   B. Oral cephalexin
   C. Oral clindamycin
   D. Intravenous vancomycin

2. Each of the following pathogens are common etiologic agents of lower respiratory infection among community-dwelling older individuals EXCEPT:

   A. Influenza
   B. *Pseudomonas aeruginosa*
   C. *Streptococcus pneumoniae*
   D. *Mycoplasma* spp.

3. The single most significant physiologic change affecting the level and distribution of antimicrobial agents among older individuals is:
   A. Reduced creatinine clearance
   B. Reduced GI absorption
   C. Impaired liver metabolism
   D. Changes in volume of distribution

● GENERAL APPROACH TO INFECTION

Older individuals disproportionately endure both the risk and consequences of infection. For older patients in all care settings, the incidence of serious infection exceeds that observed in younger adult populations.[1] Moreover, for older patients, the consequences of infection are also more severe. The frequency of fatal infection is greater than that observed for other patient groups.[2] Furthermore, infections in older patients are associated with prolonged length of hospital stay, more frequent complications, and significant impairment of functional status.[3]

A number of well-studied changes in the host immune response predispose older patients to the likelihood of infection. Among many older individuals, both qualitative and quantitative impairments of both the cellular and humoral immune response have been described.[4] These innate changes that come about with aging (collectively termed "immunosenescence") are further compounded by the impact of co-morbid conditions that themselves can result in considerable impairment of the host response to bacterial, viral, and fungal pathogens. Examples of these often common conditions are diabetes mellitus, congestive heart failure, and neoplastic disease.

Given these challenges, the diagnosis and management of infection in older patients must be approached in a systematic manner so as to ensure that a rational and consistent strategy is applied to every case. In this manner, even in the face of misleading signs and symptoms of infection in this vulnerable population, the clinician will not only pursue the most appropriate diagnostic workup but also initiate timely and rational empirical antimicrobial therapy when indicated. In this chapter, a specific algorithm for approaching the older patient with known or suspected infection is described that is both practical and evidence-based. Particular focus is placed on the selection of empirical antimicrobial therapy, arguably the most challenging aspect of managing these patients. To encourage the reader to become more proficient in employing this algorithm, the strategy is applied to a pair of clinical scenarios describing cases of infection among older patients in varied care settings. In each case, the practicality and adaptability of this approach are illustrated in conjunction with up-to-date information about new evidence-based practices, therapeutic options, and epidemiologic trends. Before addressing the cases, it is worthwhile to first introduce the overall approach to the challenge of managing older patients with known or suspected infection.

In essence, the clinician tasked with the diagnosis and treatment of a patient with possible infection (whether older or younger) must consider three critical factors in determining the most appropriate empirical antimicrobial therapy: (1) the anticipated microbiology or likely identity of the causative pathogen, (2) the breadth of coverage necessary to safely treat infection, and (3) pharmacologic considerations. Each of these factors is outlined in Figure 42–1 and discussed in detail in the sections that follow.

Anticipated Microbiology

In order to ensure that systemic or localized infection is effectively treated, the prescribing clinician must ensure that the antimicrobial regimen chosen possesses specific activity in killing or at least inhibiting the growth of the most likely causative pathogen. The failure to administer appropriate therapy in a timely fashion has been associated with worsened clinical outcomes for a number of infections commonly seen among older patients.[5] For a clinician faced with an older patient with known or suspected infection, the challenge is to make use of available data to formulate the most appropriate antimicrobial regimen that can be administered until the results of definitive cultures are available or other conclusive microbiological testing is completed. Obviously, important information about the likely pathogen is derived from an understanding of the suspected site of infection. Specific clinical syndromes, such as pneumonia or urinary tract infection, are linked through experience and the available literature with specific pathogens. These associations are discussed in greater detail in the context of the specific clinical scenarios described later in this chapter. In addition, pathogens commonly associated with a range of clinical syndromes in older patients are summarized in Table 42–1.

While awaiting the results of confirmatory testing from the clinical microbiology laboratory, a more informed estimate of the most likely causative pathogen can be inferred based on other available data. Epidemiologic information can be especially valuable. These clues may be more precisely classified as (1) those related to the individual patient or the specific signs and symptoms of infection and (2) those inferred from the population or environmental context in which the patient is evaluated. Included in the first group are specific clinical features that are associated with infection caused by particular microbial pathogens. For example, a

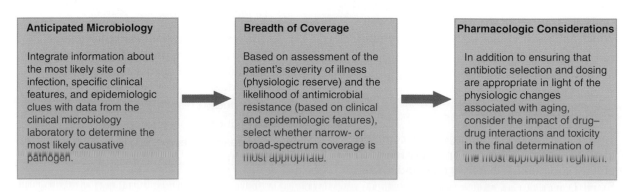

FIGURE 42–1. General approach to selection of antimicrobial therapy for older patients.

● TABLE 42–1	Common Pathogens Associated with Infection at Specific Sites in Older Patients
Site of Infection	Common Pathogens
Lung (pneumonia)	Varies between community (*S. pneumoniae*, atypical bacteria and viral pathogens), long-term care (*S. pneumoniae*, influenza, Enterobacteriaceae, *P. aeruginosa*), and hospital (*P. aeruginosa* and Enterobacteriaceae)
Urinary tract	Enterobacteriaceae (*E. coli*), Enterococcal spp, *Candida* spp. (in patients with urinary catheters)
Skin and soft tissue	*S. aureus* (including MRSA), streptococci, rare Gram-negative bacteria (especially in patients with diabetes mellitus)
Bone and joint	*S. aureus* (including MRSA), streptococci, coagulase negative staphylococci (prosthetic joints), rare Gram-negative bacteria (especially in patients with diabetes mellitus)
Central nervous system	*S. pneumoniae*, *Listeria moncytogenes*, herpes simplex virus (HSV)

hospitalized patient with profuse diarrhea who recently was administered a broad-spectrum antimicrobial regimen is more likely than not to be infected with *Clostridium difficile*. Of course, one must be careful in relying too heavily on these associations; some generally-accepted clinical "pearls" are in fact spurious. For example, a patient presenting with pneumonia and gastrointestinal symptoms is probably only slightly more likely to be infected with *Legionella pneumophila* (with which these symptoms are commonly linked in the minds of many clinicians) than a patient with pulmonary symptoms and no such associated complaints.

Apart from these patient-specific characteristics, additional epidemiologic clues drawn from an understanding of the overall context in which the patient is seeking care should also influence the selection of empirical antimicrobial therapy. For example, an older patient presenting with high fever and cough in the middle of January is more likely to be suffering from influenza infection than a similar patient presenting in July (at least in the Northern hemisphere). In this circumstance, local data and experience are most valuable. In the setting of an outbreak of methicillin-resistant *Staphylococcus aureus* (MRSA) skin and soft-tissue infections in a long-term care facility, a clinician evaluating a resident with a boil would be compelled to include MRSA among the pathogens he or she targets with initial antimicrobial therapy.

While such trends and epidemiologic clues are indeed valuable, there remains no substitute for the timely collection of definitive microbiological samples from older patients with known or suspected infection. When pursuing such sampling, the yield of testing must be weighed against the risk or discomfort of the procedure required to obtain the specimen and other possible complications. The decision to pursue invasive sampling for definitive culture is especially challenging and important for older patients. Too often, the clinician may overestimate the risk and discomfort associated with a specific procedure or diagnostic test and simultaneously underestimate the potential value of achieving a confirmed diagnosis. In such cases, disagreement over whether an older patient can "tolerate" a test may impede the rational selection and

optimization of antimicrobial treatment. Specific examples are provided in association with the clinical cases discussed later in this chapter.

Breadth of Coverage

Having determined the most likely causative pathogen, the clinician evaluating the older patient with known or suspected infection must next make a decision about the most appropriate breadth of initial antimicrobial coverage (generally before the results of confirmatory microbiological testing are available). Is a single narrow-spectrum agent, active against just a few select pathogens, the best choice, or should the clinician opt for a combination of powerful (but sometimes toxic) antibiotics that treat a range of microbes? To a great extent, this decision is a reflection of the confidence that the prescribing clinician has in his or her ability to predict the most likely causative agent. Put another way, after a clinician has determined the most likely causative pathogen, he or she must ask: "How certain am I of this and can I afford to be wrong?" If the consequence of inappropriately narrow coverage could be a worsened clinical outcome for the patient (and even death), then the clinician is obliged to prescribe a regimen with a broader spectrum of activity. However, that is not to say that all older patients should be prescribed broad-spectrum coverage. To do so is not only to increase risk of toxicity and drug interactions but also to contribute to the emergence and dissemination of antibiotic resistant pathogens in this population.

Two main factors may be used to guide the most appropriate breadth of coverage for an older patient with infection. First is the severity of patient's illness. An older patient with less physiologic reserve is more likely to have a poor clinical outcome if treated with inadequate antimicrobial therapy. These patients cannot tolerate an inaccurate determination of the most likely causative pathogen. Unfortunately, the actual severity of illness for an infected older patient may be difficult to quantify, especially given the sometimes protean signs of infection in this group.[6] In the absence of well-validated bedside tools for quantifying severity of illness across all care settings, close monitoring of vital signs and organ function (eg, urine output and mental status) is especially important. The clinician must simultaneously be certain not to inappropriately equate co-morbidity with severity. While the presence of one or more underlying medical conditions (such as diabetes or congestive heart failure) can certainly contribute to more severe illness, many older patients with even multiple co-morbid conditions can present with less severe manifestations of infection.

The other major factor that contributes to the determination of the appropriate breadth of antimicrobial coverage is the likelihood of drug resistance. Many clinicians inappropriately conclude that older age independently confers a specific risk of colonization and infection with multidrug-resistant organisms (MDRO). Based on this faulty assumption, these providers may needlessly extend the breadth of coverage for all older patients with signs or symptoms of infection (sometimes even after confirmatory microbiological testing has been completed) under the mistaken impression that antimicrobial resistance is necessarily likely. In truth, older age is not an independent risk for all MDRO, but rather a surrogate for other known risk factors for resistance, including more frequent hospitalization and the presence of certain co-morbid conditions. Therefore, not every older patient is at increased risk for resistance. An extremely valuable resource when assessing the likelihood of resistance for an infected hospital patient is the institutional annual susceptibility report ("antibiogram"). This tool, generally available to clinicians at most US hospitals, quantifies the risk of resistance for a wide range of pathogens commonly encountered at the facility. The potential value of these reports may be enhanced for the management of older patients if separate data can be provided for bacterial isolates recovered from this higher-risk group.[7]

Pharmacologic Considerations

A comprehensive discussion of the complexity of pharmacokinetics and pharmacodynamics among older patients is well beyond the scope of this chapter. However, a number of essential points on this subject must be addressed in determining the most appropriate antimicrobial regimen for the older patient with known or suspected infection. This practical approach not only ensures that the selection and breadth of coverage is optimized for these patients, but also that needless toxicity and expense are averted.

A number of factors related to the absorption, metabolism, and excretion of antimicrobial agents are considerably altered among older patients (Table 42–2).[8] In almost all cases, these changes come about both as the result of the direct physiologic effects of aging and the impact of other co-morbid conditions. Considering the extent and complexity of these changes, it is understandable that appropriate selection and dosing of antimicrobial drugs can be exceptionally challenging. That said, both experimental testing and clinical experience have consistently demonstrated that the single factor contributing to the altered metabolism of antimicrobial agents in older patients relates to the compromise in kidney function resulting in impaired urinary excretion of antibiotics and associated metabolites.[9] As the glomerular filtration rate becomes progressively impaired among older adults, serum drug levels (and therefore delivery to the primary site of infection) become less predictable. Compounding matters, as renal function worsens, drug toxicity related to inappropriately high serum levels may further complicate the overall clinical picture.

While arguably less well studied and often less appreciated than the metabolic changes already discussed, there are other more practical pharmacologic issues that clinicians must consider when managing the older patient with known or suspected infection. Principal among these factors are the issues of drug toxicity and drug–drug interactions. Older patients, in part because of physiologic compromise as a result

of both underlying co-morbid conditions and the direct consequences of aging, are more susceptible to end-organ toxicity including renal dysfunction, hepatotoxicity, and hematologic dyscrasias.[10] As has already been noted, the impaired renal excretion of many antibiotics observed among older patients may itself increase the risk of subsequent toxicity, compounding this problem. Specific examples of the potential consequences of drug toxicity among older patients with infection are described in the case discussions later in the chapter.

The other practical consideration that must be addressed when managing the infected older patient is the increased likelihood of drug–drug interactions and non-adherence in this population.[11] Both phenomena arise as the result of the often complicated medical regimens prescribed for older patients. Interactions are commonly encountered between specific antimicrobial classes and a wide range of pharmaceutical agents commonly prescribed for older patients, including oral anticoagulants, digoxin, and certain diuretic agents. In all cases, it is vitally important when making the final decision on an antimicrobial regimen for an older patient that a careful history of other concurrent medical therapy is obtained. This list should include not only prescription agents but also over-the-counter medications and even alternative medicines and herbal supplements.

● PNEUMONIA IN A LONG-TERM CARE FACILITY RESIDENT

CASE PRESENTATION 1: "SHE'S SWEATING REALLY BAD"

Mrs. Miller is a 77-year-old resident at the long-term care facility where you are rounding. According to her caregiver, this morning Mrs. Miller did not eat her breakfast and told her friend, also a resident of the facility, that she "could not get her breath." When Mrs. Miller's son Ronald visited later this morning, he insisted that you be called. When you enter the room, he looks concerned, noting, "I've never seen her look this way before. She's sweating really bad and her breathing looks awful."

You begin to evaluate the patient. She states that she first started feeling sick yesterday afternoon when she noted some difficulty breathing when coming upstairs after watching a movie. She denies any coughing whatsoever. You pull her chart and are reminded that she has diabetes (well-controlled), hypothyroidism, and hypertension. Her current medications include metformin, levothyroxine sodium, and an ACE inhibitor. She also takes a baby aspirin every day. In her chart, it is noted that she is allergic to "-micins." She smoked in the distant past and does not drink alcohol.

You carefully assist Mrs. Miller back to her bed, noting that her top is soaked with perspiration, and conduct a

● **TABLE 42–2** Factors Affecting the Absorption, Metabolism, and Excretion of Antimicrobial Agents in Older Patients

Physiologic Changes of Aging Affecting Antimicrobial Selection and Dosing
Decreased GI blood flow, absorptive surface area, and motility
Decreased hepatic drug delivery and impairment of metabolic pathways
Malnutrition and decreased lean body mass and total body water
Impaired renal excretion as a result of decreased glomerular filtration rate

thorough physical examination. Overall, she appears to be quite fatigued. Her vital signs reveal a temperature of 38.8°C, a heart rate of 110 beats per minute, and a respiratory rate of 18 breaths per minute. She is mildly orthostatic. Her breathing, while not labored, permits her to complete only a short sentence without interruption. Her skin is dry and there are other signs of volume depletion. Her cardiac exam reveals tachycardia without any extra heart sounds. Auscultation of her lungs demonstrates decreased breath sounds in the bilateral mid-lung zones. There are accompanying crackles.

Overview of Pneumonia in Older Patients

Infection of the respiratory tract, including the lungs, represents one of the most common infections responsible for hospital admission among older patients. In part due to the aging of the population, the absolute number of older patients hospitalized for pneumonia is still rising, even in the face of more intensive efforts at prevention.[12]

Despite advances in supportive care (including increasingly sophisticated ventilatory and hemodynamic support), the incidence of mortality among older patients hospitalized with lung infection remains high. While there remains considerable variability in the risk of death depending on the pathogen causing infection and the underlying physiologic reserve of the host, pneumonia remains a serious and potentially lethal illness for all patients. Given the ease and rapidity with which pulmonary infection can claim a patient, it is for good reason that Sir William Osler famously described pneumonia as "the old man's friend."[13]

The clinical syndrome of pneumonia may be particularly difficult to detect in older individuals, as is the case for a number of common infections (see Chapter 9). Many older patients with pneumonia do not demonstrate the classic signs and symptoms of the infection. Specifically, fever may be absent and respiratory symptoms may be subtle, if not altogether unapparent. Many older patients with pneumonia will not even report a cough, as is true for Mrs. Miller. Older pneumonia patients may only describe fatigue, malaise, decreased appetite, or alteration in mental status. Pneumonia is common enough in this population that even nonspecific signs of physiologic decline should prompt an evaluation for pulmonary infection, including consideration of pulse oximetry and chest radiography.

In general, older patients with pneumonia can be classified into one of three etiologic groups: (1) community-acquired infection, (2) hospital-acquired disease, and (3) pneumonia contracted in nursing homes or other long-term care facility. Of course, the distinction between each category can be somewhat blurred, especially considering the frequency with which some older patients move between both acute and chronic care (or residential) facilities. Given Mrs. Miller's current residential arrangement, it is this last category of disease upon which this part of the chapter will focus. Nonetheless, both community- and hospital-acquired pneumonia will

be discussed in comparison throughout the sections that follow. Fortunately, the same algorithm for guiding the approach to all infected patients (discussed in the introduction to this chapter) applies across the spectrum of pneumonia, no matter where infection was acquired.

Anticipated Microbiology

As has already been noted, determination of the most likely etiologic agent is a crucial first step in guiding the approach to empirical therapy for patients. What is the most likely pathogen to be causing Mrs. Miller's symptoms? While the points discussed next provide the clinician with the means by which to use clinical clues to anticipate the causative organism, it is imperative in most cases to initiate the steps to actually confirm the microbiological diagnosis as soon as possible after first evaluating the older patient with pneumonia. Of course, the most reliable and time-tested manner to achieve a microbiological diagnosis is through recovery of the pathogen from a clinical culture specimen. As such, many experts encourage that older patients with pneumonia also have both sputum (or other available respiratory secretions) and blood assessed by culture to evaluate for determination of microbial etiology. However, controversy surrounds both methods. The utility of sputum Gram stain and culture has been a point of disagreement between clinical experts, investigators, and professional societies. Critics observe that the actual sensitivity of the test even in experienced hands does not justify the resources required to ensure timely specimen collection in analysis. This perspective is compounded by the decreased availability of materials and expertise in processing and interpreting culture and Gram stain, particularly at the bedside. Nonetheless, the sputum Gram stain and culture, when interpreted with caution, could point to the involvement of a number of specific common pathogens, including *Streptococcus pneumoniae* and, less commonly, *Staphylococcus aureus*.[14] The outlook on the utility of blood cultures is similarly muddled. Most experienced clinicians will observe that the relative infrequency with which blood cultures from pneumonia patients are positive, especially among those with community-acquired disease, does not warrant the performance of the testing in all such patients. In contrast, blood culture proponents will argue that in as much as the mortality of pneumonia (specifically infection with *S. pneumoniae*) increases dramatically among patients with bloodstream involvement, the information remains useful. This debate has been compounded by the inclusion of timely blood culture collection among the so-called pay-for-performance measures applied to the management of pneumonia patients in the emergency departments of US hospitals.[15]

In terms of non-culture methods, many clinical laboratories offer more sophisticated techniques including urinary antigen testing for both common pathogens such as *S. pneumoniae* and even more esoteric causes of pneumonia (eg, *Histoplasma capsulatum*). Also available is a noninvasive test for *Legionella pneumophila*. The results of these studies offer considerable positive predictive value but will not reliably assist the clinician in excluding these diagnoses when confronted with the patient with known or suspected pulmonary infection. It is also important to note that these particular non-culture measures have not been exceptionally well studied in older patients and therefore unpredictable variation in test performance could occur.

While discussing the multitude of confirmatory tests widely available in the acute care setting, it seems appropriate to also address the question of whether patients such as Mrs. Miller, who develop the signs and symptoms of pneumonia while in long-term care or other settings, are best managed in the hospital as opposed to remaining at their primary residence. This is an important and controversial subject that has considerable implications regarding resource utilization and patient satisfaction. While a definitive answer to this question is beyond the scope of this review, it is worth noting that some of the testing described thus far is unlikely to be available at even well-resourced long-term care facilities and nursing homes.

Unfortunately, it will take some time for the results of Mrs. Miller's confirmatory testing to become available, and you still think that she likely requires empirical antibiotic therapy. How might you go about trying to formulate a rational regimen while awaiting these critical results? Based on what is known about the various settings in which pneumonia is encountered, some general assumptions can be made regarding the most likely etiologic agent for each. In this case, the focus is on pneumonia arising in a patient who resides in a long-term care facility, as opposed to community- or hospital-acquired infection. The most common pathogens encountered among older patients with pneumonia in each of these three distinct settings were introduced in Table 42–1. In general, for patients in the community, the most frequently encountered organism (at least among those patients for whom a microbiological diagnosis is attained) is *S. pneumoniae*.[14] Also common are the so-called atypical organisms, including *Mycoplasma pneumoniae* and *Chlamydia pneumoniae*. Less frequently, but particularly in cases of severe disease, is *Legionella pneumophila* encountered. For patients in the hospital, a wider array of microbial pathogens is associated with pneumonia. In these cases, probably the most significant additional pathogen for consideration is *Pseudomonas aeruginosa*, which may exhibit resistance to a broad range of antibacterial agents. Also more frequently encountered in this group are members of the family *Enterobacteriaceae*. Of course, in both the hospital and the community, patients at risk for aspiration are more apt to be infected with anaerobic pathogens and other oral flora.[16]

For Mrs. Miller and other residents of long-term care facilities, the usual suspects associated with pneumonia occupy an intermediate portion of the microbiologic spectrum between those pathogens affecting patients in the community and those in the hospital. Put more specifically, LTCF residents remain susceptible to all of the common pathogens encountered in the community (including *S. pneumonia* and atypical pathogens). At the same time, more frequent exposure to antibiotic therapy and contact with the health care system (such as repeated hospital admissions for other co-morbid conditions) place these same patients at risk for *P. aeruginosa* and other more aggressive hospital pathogens. Furthermore, the importance of viral pathogens, and particularly influenza, cannot be overstated in this group. Outbreaks of viral infections

in LTCFs are well-described in the literature and have been associated with considerable morbidity and even mortality.[17]

Apart from these more general observations about patterns of microbiological involvement in older patients with pneumonia, are there data that might be informative in directing our initial management of Mrs. Miller? In the introduction to this chapter, it was observed that many so-called pearls that link specific clinical findings to particular pulmonary pathogens often lack reliable predictive value to inform clinical management. While in some cases these findings might be helpful in tracking the overall course of disease (and eventual recovery), they offer little meaningful guidance to even the most experienced clinician. In Mrs. Miller's case, the absence of cough or sputum production offers no guidance in detecting the likely pathogen. Similarly, the absence of classic signs and symptoms of viral infection (myalgias, headache) does not exclude the diagnosis of influenza.

CASE PRESENTATION 1 (continued)

In reviewing Mrs. Miller's medical chart, you note that she has not recently been admitted to the hospital and there is no recent prescription for antibiotic therapy documented in the record. She has no other recent microbiological testing results to provide information about colonizing strains of bacteria. Based on your experience with such patients, and after a quick consultation with a pocket guide to antibiotic therapy, you conclude that the most likely pathogens responsible for Mrs. Miller's symptoms include *S. pneumoniae*, atypical pathogens, *Enterobacteriaceae* such as *E. coli* or *K. pneumoniae*, and influenza virus. You request that a sputum Gram stain and culture be collected if possible and that phlebotomy be performed to check a complete blood count, a metabolic panel, and two sets of peripheral blood cultures. In addition, you ask that a chest radiograph be performed in the morning when the technician returns to duty.

Breadth of Coverage

When determining the most appropriate breadth of antimicrobial coverage for Mrs. Miller (or any older patient with pneumonia), the treating clinician is challenged to answer two related questions: (1) how certain am I that the antibiotic selected is adequate to cover the most likely pathogen and (2) what are the consequences of being wrong? Recalling the general approach introduced at the beginning of this chapter (Figure 42–1), these questions can be approached in light of two factors that together inform the determination of the most appropriate breadth of antimicrobial therapy: the likelihood of antimicrobial resistance in the causative pathogen and the physiologic reserve or severity of illness of the affected patient. To illustrate the usefulness of this approach, each factor is discussed as it applies to the case of Mrs. Miller.

When estimating the likelihood of antimicrobial resistance, the thoughtful clinician applies an approach similar to that employed in determining the most likely causative pathogen. Information is integrated first about the general population and then supplemented with available data concerning the individual patient and the local environment in which he or she is evaluated. Among patients with pneumonia, in general it can be assumed that the likelihood of antimicrobial resistance is greater among pneumonia patients residing in long-term care facilities when compared with patients with community-acquired pneumonia. For the most part, this increased risk is generally believed to be mediated through the more frequent exposure of these individuals to systemic antimicrobial therapy. To individualize the risk for resistance for a single patient such as Mrs. Miller, the medical history can be evaluated to determine if she has had substantial prior exposure to systemic antibiotic therapy.

Among older pneumonia patients from long-term care facilities, the heightened risk for antimicrobial resistance is further potentiated by the increased likelihood of transmission of resistant pathogens between residents. In this setting, the risk for horizontal spread is magnified by the sometimes inconsistent application of infection prevention best practices in some LTCFs. While the increased risk for resistance associated with this phenomenon is difficult or even impossible to quantify for an individual patient or facility, it further supports the conclusion that an older patient with pneumonia at a long-term care facility generally is more likely to be infected with an antibiotic-resistant pathogen.

Sometimes additional data may be available to more precisely quantify the likelihood of infection with antibiotic resistant pathogens among LTCF residents. Some facilities now make available to clinicians a periodic antibiotic susceptibility report ("antibiogram") such as is commonly distributed at acute care hospitals. These helpful tools provide prescribers with comprehensive information about the proportion of a range of common pathogens that are resistant to a wide array of available antimicrobial agents. With such a report in hand, a clinician who has already deduced that a given infection is likely caused by a particular pathogen has immediate access to a tool that quantifies the likelihood that a specific regimen will provide adequate coverage. Of course, the best and most reliable means by which to determine the appropriate breadth of coverage for an older patient with pneumonia is to obtain microbiological confirmation of the causative organism itself. Both culture and non-culture testing methods can be helpful in securing this critical information.

If the likelihood of resistance highlights the confidence with which a clinician views his or her antibiotic choice, the potential consequence of being wrong is integrated by estimating the physiologic reserve of the patient with pneumonia. As was noted in the chapter introduction, the severity of illness must be carefully distinguished from other factors, such as co-morbid conditions, when evaluating an older patient with pneumonia. Unfortunately, semi-quantitative tools that have been widely disseminated as a prognostic aids for patients with community-acquired pneumonia are of limited value in treating patients like Mrs. Miller. Moreover,

the performance of these instruments has not been examined for pneumonia patients admitted from long-term care facilities.[2] Without the availability of more comprehensive severity metrics, important information can be gleaned by careful and quantitative assessment of the patient's ventilatory and hemodynamic status. While bedside pulse oxymetry can be helpful in this regard, more precise and comprehensive information is available through performance of an arterial blood gas assessment and close monitoring of blood pressure.

For the older patient with pneumonia exhibiting a pronounced degree of physiologic compromise or end-organ involvement, most clinicians will favor a broader approach to empirical therapy. In this setting it is prudent to begin the broadest justifiable antimicrobial coverage with the understanding that as more information becomes available (including the results of definitive microbiologic confirmation), the therapeutic regimen can be narrowed in a rational manner. To a degree, the risk/benefit analysis of selecting broad versus narrow coverage can be quantified. For example, a clinician equipped with an up-to-date antibiogram may know that the selection of monotherapy with drug A will cover 85% of the pathogens likely affecting the patient. The clinician can then decide whether the likely clinical consequences associated with the 15% risk of treatment failure warrant the addition of a second agent or an altogether different regimen.

CASE PRESENTATION 1 (continued)

As you carefully consider the most appropriate breadth of coverage to treat Mrs. Miller's pneumonia, the results of preliminary lab testing become available. Her white blood cell count is found to be $14.5 \times 10^3/\mu L$ ($14.5 \times 10^9/L$) and there is a dramatic left shift (to more immature forms). Serum chemistry reveals a creatinine of 1.6 mg/dL (141.4 μmol/L). You are very concerned for the possible involvement of highly resistant Gram-negative organisms based on the fact that three other residents of the same wing of the facility in which Mrs. Miller lives have been recently diagnosed with infection with such pathogens. While this recent outbreak has convinced the medical director to compile an antibiogram for the facility, the susceptibility report has not yet been made available to all providers.

Your concern for Mrs. Miller is heightened when you note that her respiratory rate has increased since you initiated your evaluation. Her oxygen saturation based on bedside pulse oxymetry has decreased to 87% on room air and you request that supplemental oxygen be brought to her room. She remains tachycardic but the nursing assistant notes that she is maintaining her blood pressure and continues to generate good urine output.

Pharmacologic Considerations

In terms of pharmacodynamic and pharmacokinetic considerations, there are few if any specific complicating factors when it comes to treating lung infection, even for older patients with poor functional status. As was pointed out in the introduction to this chapter, the single most important pharmacologic issue influencing antibiotic selection and administration in this population is decreased renal function and impaired urinary clearance. Renal insufficiency is exceedingly common among older patients, whether or not they have been formally diagnosed with a primary or secondary disease of the kidneys. With this in mind, the prescribing clinician needs to exercise great care when managing these patients in terms of both the dose and selection of antimicrobial agents.

Even with these concerns in mind, most of the antimicrobial agents recommended for the management of patients with community-acquired pneumonia are generally safe even in the face of impaired creatinine clearance. For community-based patients who do not require hospital admission, the use of either fluoroquinolone antibiotics or macrolides (such as azithromycin) facilitates ease of dosing and lessens concern for renal toxicity. These agents are generally exceptionally well tolerated and dose adjustment for renal dysfunction is generally not needed. However, when it comes to the management of pulmonary infection among hospitalized older patients or those residing in long-term care facilities, the situation becomes quite a bit more complex. Specifically, given the need to cover for enteric Gram-negative pathogens (as has been discussed), clinicians will likely be confronted with the need to use agents associated with an increased risk of complications and toxicity. For example, if the clinician elects for broad coverage to treat both anaerobic pathogens and *Pseudomonas aeruginosa*, he or she may choose the combination agent piperacillin/tazobactam. In this case, the prescriber needs to both ensure that sufficient drug be administered to maintain efficacy against this potentially lethal pathogen (which often requires especially high dosing when *P. aeruginosa* is suspected) while simultaneously adjusting the dose to avoid the accumulation of toxic drug levels in the face of impaired renal clearance.

Of course, other more practical issues are apt to have a greater influence on antimicrobial selection and dosing when treating the older patient with pneumonia. The issues of toxicity and drug–drug interactions are especially critical. Drug toxicities that might otherwise be unimportant and even trivial in a young and healthy population can lead to life-threatening complications for a patient like Mrs. Miller. For example, it should never be underestimated that the fluoroquinolone antibiotics nearly as a class are all associated with the possibility of inducing prolonged QT interval on the patient's electrocardiogram.[18] For an older patient who may have underlying cardiac dysrhythmia or who may be on other medications that themselves can prolong the QT interval, the consequences could be serious.

CASE PRESENTATION 1 (continued)

Given your concerns for the involvement of more resistant pathogens and Mrs. Miller's declining physiologic state, you have decided to order broad-spectrum intravenous antibiotic therapy. While your concern for *P. aeruginosa* is relatively low (given the lack of recent hospitalization or structural lung disease), you still want to be certain to cover for more resistant strains of *E. coli* and *K. pneumoniae*. Her worsening renal function also has you concerned about complicated dosing regimens. You consult a table outlining specific antimicrobial regimens for patients with pneumonia (Table 42–3). Ultimately, you decide to select cefepime plus levofloxacin. The former offers excellent activity against most resistant Gram-negative pathogens while still retaining excellent anti-pneumococcal activity. The latter not only extends the coverage to include atypical pathogens but may complement the cefepime in terms of the extent of enteric organisms covered.

Because of Mrs. Miller's poor physiologic reserve and her overall declining status, you elect to have her transferred to the acute care hospital located close to the long-term care facility. There, she ultimately requires admission to the intensive care unit after demonstrating

---

● **TABLE 42–3** Typical Antimicrobial Regimens Selected for Older Patients with Pneumonia

Setting	Anticipated Microbiology	Typical Empirical Regimen
Community-acquired	*S. pneumoniae*, atypical bacteria (*M. pneumoniae, C. pneumoniae*)	Respiratory fluoroquinolone (levofloxacin or moxifloxacin)
Community-acquired, admitted to hospital	*S. pneumoniae*, atypical bacteria (*M. pneumoniae, C. pneumoniae*)	Third-generation cephalosporin (eg, ceftriaxone) plus azithromycin, or respiratory fluoroquinolone
Community-acquired, admitted to intensive care unit	*S. pneumoniae*, *Legionella* spp.	Third-generation cephalosporin PLUS respiratory fluoroquinolone
Long-term care facility resident	*S. pneumoniae*, Enterobacteriaceae, *P. aeruginosa*, *S. aureus* (including MRSA)	Third-generation cephalosporin PLUS respiratory fluoroquinolone PLUS vancomycin (if MRSA suspected) PLUS anti-pseudomonal agent (if *P. aeruginosa* suspected)
Hospital-acquired	*P. aeruginosa*, Enterobacteriaceae, *S. aureus* (including MRSA)	Cefepime, imipenem or piperacillin/tazobactam PLUS respiratory fluoroquinolone PLUS vancomycin or linezolid (MRSA suspected)

evidence of evolving sepsis in the emergency room. Sputum and blood cultures (collected at the LTCF) ultimately turn positive for *K. pneumoniae* that is susceptible to both cefepime and fluoroquinolone. The treating physician continues to treat with cefepime during her time in the hospital, but ultimately switches to PO levofloxacin at the time of hospital discharge. She returns to your facility demonstrating clear signs of improvement and expressing considerable gratitude for your thoughtful and expert care.

SKIN AND SOFT-TISSUE INFECTION IN AN ACTIVE OLDER PATIENT

CASE PRESENTATION 2: A LITTLE RED SPOT

Elliot Wingate, a 71-year-old former accountant, is a very active member of the local tennis club. In addition to serving as treasurer, he is among the top-ranked players in the club's masters division. Three days ago, while in the locker room after a long match, he noticed some redness on his right ankle. The area was somewhat warm and tender to the touch. He observed a central area that was particularly inflamed, which he later described as a "nasty bug bite or pimple." Mr. Wingate, a busy man, did not think much of the lesion and returned home to finish some gardening. When he awoke the next morning, he noted that the ankle was even more tender. In addition, he observed to his wife that he felt "cold as hell," despite the intense heat of the day. She also noted that he seemed a bit "sluggish" and did not even walk to the end of the driveway to get the newspaper. By that afternoon, Mr. Wingate was feeling progressively worse and even cancelled his standing Tuesday match for the first time in his wife's memory. At her urging, he called your office and was scheduled for an appointment the next day.

In the office, you note that Mr. Wingate is febrile (39.1°C) and tachycardic (112 beats per minute). His blood pressure is 108/55 mm Hg and he is breathing at 14 breaths per minute. In general he looks exhausted, quite uncharacteristic in comparison to your findings at his regular checkup 6 weeks ago.

Overview of Skin and Soft Tissue Infection in Older Patients

Skin and soft-tissue infection, while among the most frequently encountered bacterial diseases in patients of all ages, is frequently underappreciated by even experienced clinicians

in terms of the potential for progressive disease and complications. The wide range of clinical manifestations, from impetigo and other superficial infections to furunculosis, cellulites, and even deeper and more serious infections such as necrotizing fasciitis, presents an array of diagnostic and therapeutic challenges. Recognizing the signs and symptoms distinguishing more benign syndromes from potentially life-threatening complications is especially difficult when confronted with the older patient with skin and soft-tissue infection. As has been the case for the other infectious syndromes described in this chapter, classic findings of infection in this vulnerable population may be blunted, modified, or even absent.

Recently observed changes in the epidemiology and microbiology of skin and soft-tissue infections, and the as-yet-undetermined manner and degree to which these phenomena affect older patients, warrant particular attention to this subject. While these changes are discussed in detail in the remainder of this section, it is important to note that in general both the incidence and severity of skin and soft-tissue infections appear to be on the rise.[19]

Before examining these epidemiologic trends, it is worth considering the factors that predispose older patients to these potentially life-threatening infections. As has already been noted, a number of changes in both cellular and humoral immunity predispose older patients to the likelihood of infection. However, it is not such complex elements of immunosenescence that are likely the main contributing factor to the high frequency of skin and soft-tissue infection in this group. Rather, it is the physical and mechanical breakdown of the integument that accompanies even normal aging that most likely predisposes older patients to these infections.[20] The skin of the older individual tends to become drier and less elastic with aging, factors that serve to predispose to skin breaks even in the absence of significant trauma. When other complications of aging are considered, including co-morbid conditions such as diabetes mellitus (and the possibility of neuropathic injury, especially to the feet and lower extremities), and impairments of functional status (which might lead to increased falls and other trauma), the high incidence of skin and soft-tissue infections in this group is perhaps not surprising.

While this chapter will focus on illustrating a rational approach to the initial management of one particular manifestation of disease, the diversity and severity of skin and soft-tissue infections among older adults mirrors that seen in younger patients. An older patient may present to his or her primary clinician or a walk-in clinic with a boil or furuncle requiring nothing more than an incision and drainage procedure. Alternatively, older patients with poorly controlled diabetes mellitus may present with complicated foot infection in part exacerbated by neuropathic changes that predispose to local trauma. Most worrisome may be the onset of rapidly progressive deep tissue infection such as necrotizing fasciitis. These infections, often mediated by toxin-producing strains of bacteria, may precipitate a rapid and catastrophic clinical decline requiring ICU admission and even emergent surgical debridement.

Anticipated Microbiology

While the general rule can be applied to infection at almost any body site, the dictum that patients generally become infected with the same microbes with which they are colonized is never more applicable than in the case of skin and soft-tissue infection. Even while acknowledging the infrequent involvement of more unusual pathogens such as Gram-negative bacteria and even anaerobes in some cases, most skin and soft-tissue infections among both older and younger adult patients are caused by streptococci and staphylococci. Taken together, these pathogens are ubiquitous as colonizers of the skin and other superficial sites among even healthy older adults. As a result, it should come as no surprise that any compromise of the integument can permit the introduction of streptococci and staphylococci as a precipitant to skin and soft-tissue infection in all patients.

The relatively predictable involvement of streptococci and staphylococci in skin and soft-tissue infections would seem to offer little incentive to busy clinicians to devote the time or resources to confirm the microbiological diagnosis when confronted with a patient with classical signs and symptoms of infection. In many clinical settings, the prevalent practice centers on the administration of empirical antimicrobial regimens with exceedingly limited breadth of activity (exclusively targeting Gram-positive pathogens). With this mindset, specimens from these patients may never be sent to the clinical microbiology lab. Unfortunately, as is suggested later in this section, this rather presumptuous approach is rapidly becoming outmoded and even obsolete in an era of emerging pathogens and antimicrobial resistance.

Of course, in the case of many skin and soft-tissue infections, even the most meticulous clinician may be limited in his or her ability to confirm the causative pathogen. Among older patients with skin and soft-tissue infection, microbiological sampling can be challenging to obtain, especially for more superficial infections. Blood cultures are very infrequently positive, even in the case of severe disease.[21] There are protocols available to guide clinicians in microbiological sampling from patients with cellulitis (such as aspiration and culture of fluid injected into the so-called "leading edge" of the inflamed tissue).[22] However, these methods have proven to be cumbersome and insufficiently sensitive to be accepted into routine clinical practice. Perhaps even more confusing is the microbiological diagnosis of deeper infections, especially those involving wounds or other skin defect. In these cases, the treating clinician must be cautious about interpreting the results of cultures of superficial material and skin surfaces. These samples, frequently collected with cotton or synthetic swabs, lack reliable predictive value in distinguishing primary pathogens from superficial colonizing strains. As a result, the findings can be not only imprecise but even misleading.

In the case of more discrete and superficial skin and soft-tissue infections, there is considerably more opportunity to confirm the causative pathogen through additional testing. Where there is a collection of inflamed material, such as a boil, furuncle, or skin abscess, incision and drainage at the bedside or in the clinic offers both diagnostic and therapeutic value. The potential yield of incision and drainage of superficial skin lesions is so great that any clinician with a busy primary care practice would be well-served to attain proficiency in the performance of this relatively straightforward procedure. For complicated skin and soft-tissue infections that do not lend themselves to simple bedside drainage, timely referral to an experienced surgeon offers the opportunity to confirm the microbiological diagnosis through culture of deep samples of fluid or even tissue.

In cases where microbiological confirmation is not feasible, or when the results of such testing are pending, what information is available to the clinician to guide the rational selection of empirical antimicrobial therapy? Stated in a more practical manner in the case of skin and soft-tissue infections, when should the clinician be concerned for pathogens apart from streptococci and staphylococci? Epidemiologic clues may be helpful to the clinician who takes the time to carefully review the patient's history. For example, the nature of the inciting or precipitating event leading up to skin and soft-tissue infection may be helpful. For example, a patient with new onset of erythema, pain, and drainage at a surgical wound during the first several days after an operation is likely at higher risk for involvement by health care–associated pathogens such as methicillin-resistant *S. aureus* (MRSA) and even Gram-negative pathogens. Other information from the patient's medical history may also be of use. Some co-morbid conditions are associated with increased risk for skin and soft-tissue infection with specific pathogens. A history of eczema should raise specific concern for *S. aureus* and even MRSA. A diabetic patient with complicated skin and soft-tissue infection may be at risk for infection with gram negative pathogens, including *P. aeruginosa* (although it is worth mentioning that streptococci and staphylococci still predominate in this population). These and other associations are outlined in Table 42–4.

Specific findings on the physical examination and appearance of the abnormal skin surface itself may also be informative to the savvy clinician formulating a rational differential diagnosis for an older patient with skin and soft-tissue infection. For example, the honey-colored crusting of impetigo is highly suggestive of streptococcal or staphylococcal disease. The well-demarcated plaque-like erythema of erysipelas is more specifically associated with group A streptococci and is especially common in older patients. In contrast, more diffuse erythema and scaling, especially when confined to the intertriginous zones, may be more consistent with skin infection due to *Candida* species.

● TABLE 42–4 Epidemiological Clues for the Involvement of Specific Pathogens in Skin and Soft Tissue Infections in Older Patients

Epidemiological/Clinical Factor	Associated Pathogen(s)
Recent hospitalization or antibiotics	Healthcare-associated MRSA
Described by patient as a "spider bite"	Community-associated MRSA
Diabetes mellitus, hepatic cirrhosis	Gram-negative pathogens
Salt water swimming or immersion	*Vibrio vulnificus*
Infected animal bite	*Capnocytophaga canimorsus* (dog), *Pasteurella multocida* (cat)
Deep puncture wound	*Clostridium* spp.

CASE PRESENTATION 2 (continued)

Mr. Wingate adamantly denies any antecedent trauma at the site of the new skin lesion. While acknowledging the initial appearance of the rash, he reaffirms that he can recall no specific insect bite at the site in the hours or days leading up to the onset of infection. He also denies recent travel and generally does no swimming, remarking that he avoids the club's pool and hot tub because "we cut some of the regular servicing and cleaning out of the budget." During your meeting, he is reminded that one of his playing partners at the club recently was treated for "boils." As a result, signs had been posted in the locker room advising members not to share towels.

On examination, the central area of inflammation on Mr. Wingate's ankle remains especially tender. While you cannot detect a discrete fluid collection, the overall appearance suggests a degree of fluctuance. After obtaining Mr. Wingate's informed consent, you perform an incision and drainage of the central aspect of the affected area. 2.5 mL of frank pus are recovered and sent to the lab for culture. You duck into the small lab in your office and quickly and carefully perform a Gram stain on some retained material. Under the scope, you see sheets of Gram-positive cocci in clusters.

Breadth of Coverage

As has already been introduced, the principal factors that should help guide the breadth of coverage when selecting empirical antimicrobial therapy for an older patient are the severity of illness (physiologic reserve) and the likelihood of antimicrobial resistance. Both factors weigh heavily in the evaluation of Mr. Wingate and all older patients with suspected skin and soft-tissue infection.

The severity of illness is especially critical to delineate in the case of skin and soft-tissue infection in an older patient. The consequences of failing to detect more severe and aggressive types of superficial infection could be catastrophic. Unlike the other infectious processes already discussed, in the case of skin and soft-tissue infection, systemic signs and symptoms alone may not be sufficiently predictive to reliably identify the patient at risk for complications related to superficial infection. Instead, the evidence that should raise concern for more severe disease includes local findings demonstrating progressive involvement at the original site of infection, such as progressive expansion of the area of involved skin. Among the more severe manifestations of skin and soft-tissue infection most familiar to many clinicians is necrotizing fasciitis (NF), in which infection and inflammation disseminate rapidly and broadly via the fascial planes underlying the skin and more superficial soft-tissue structures. In cases of NF, compromise of the vascular communications across the fascial plane can result in widespread devitalization of superficial tissue. This aggressive clinical course is mimicked by infection with bacterial strains elaborating extracellular toxins (which may or may not be consistently associated with true NF). These pathogens, most commonly strains of streptococci and (less commonly) staphylococci, have attained notoriety in the lay press and in the popular consciousness as "flesh-eating bacteria."

With this in mind, one of the most important responsibilities of any clinician evaluating an older patient with skin and soft-tissue infection is to ensure that there is no evidence for rapidly progressive disease. One effective strategy employed by many experienced clinicians is to use a pen or marker to draw a line that circumscribes the extent of the visible inflammation on the skin. Next, the site is re-evaluated within an hour or two to document the extent of spread of infection beyond the original margin. Depending on the amount of time that has passed, the area of involvement should not exceed the drawn margin by more than a centimeter. Other signs associated with rapidly progressive infection include crepitations, analgesia over the involved site, and hemodynamic changes consistent with evolving sepsis.

As is true for most other infectious syndromes, the clinician selecting the initial breadth of coverage must also tailor his or her decision based on the likelihood of antimicrobial resistance. Obviously, the final determination of the susceptibility of the infecting pathogen will be revealed by the findings of confirmatory cultures, which lends added value to the timely collection of appropriate samples for analysis. Nevertheless, in cases in which specimens were not or could not be sent to the clinical microbiology lab or even when culture and susceptibility data are still pending, additional clues are available from the patient's history to help predict the likelihood of antimicrobial resistance. While many patient-level risk factors for resistance are unique to one multidrug-resistant organism or another, certain clinical findings are almost universally associated with resistance across the microbiological spectrum. For example, prior contact with the health care system, and specifically recent exposure to systemic antimicrobial therapy, has been established as an important risk factor for a wide spectrum of resistant pathogens including MRSA, vancomycin-resistant enterococci (VRE), and highly resistant Gram-negative bacteria.[23] Specific co-morbid conditions, which are frequently more prevalent among older patients, have also been independently associated with the risk of colonization or infection with antimicrobial-resistant pathogens. For example, diabetes mellitus has been associated with colonization and infection with a multitude of multidrug-resistant organisms.[24,25]

Sometimes more individualized data are available from the patient's record to help stratify him or her according to the risk of skin and soft-tissue infection with antimicrobial-resistant bacteria. Particularly for an older patient, documentation of previous colonization or infection with an MDRO can be especially useful in predicting the likelihood of resistance when subsequent infections arise (even if at a different body site, including the skin). At least one study demonstrated that colonization with MRSA can persist for years, even among younger and relatively healthy individuals.[26] The extent to which the physiologic changes of aging influence this phenomenon has not yet been completely determined. Knowing that the patient has previously been affected by an MDRO should automatically trigger the concern of a clinician contemplating subsequent antimicrobial therapy for that individual, even if the time span between episodes is prolonged.

CASE PRESENTATION 2 (continued)

In considering the case of Mr. Wingate, you do not find him to be severely ill in appearance. While clearly exhausted, his overall demeanor and outlook are not all that far from his baseline. You look again more closely at the inflamed area on his ankle. While he acknowledges that the degree of inflammation appears worse than when he first noticed the lesion at the club yesterday, he is not convinced that the actual area of involvement has progressed. There appears to be no tracking of infection proximally or distally. You smile when you note that your nurse took a moment to draw a line around the rash with her pen when she put Mr. Wingate in the exam room more than 45 minutes ago (a time span about which he reminded you when you first entered to the exam room). The rash has not extended beyond this margin.

As is suggested by his active lifestyle, Mr. Wingate does not routinely have frequent contact with the health care system. He only sees any doctor "when my wife makes me go." He says he last got an antibiotic in the army as a young man, when he was given a single shot of penicillin for reasons he fails to recall or recount. Accessing his electronic medical record, you note that the field for microbiology reports is completely unfilled.

What other information is available to the clinician selecting empirical therapy for a patient like Mr. Wingate, where nothing in his personal medical history suggests an increased likelihood of antimicrobial resistance? Can the prescriber simply conclude that any infecting organism is apt to be susceptible to most antibiotics and go ahead and prescribe exceptionally narrow coverage? We are reminded that the treatment of infection is not simply a matter of considering the individual patient but in fact relies on appreciation and integration of data about the overall context in which the infection occurs. The very nature of contagious disease demands that information about trends of disease in the community and other individuals with whom the patient has had contact must impact our outlook on both the likelihood of

infection and specifically the risk of resistance. It is in this context that Mr. Wingate's case takes on a considerably different perspective.

Perhaps the single most important change in the epidemiology of antimicrobial resistance (and arguably all of clinical bacteriology) during the past quarter century has been the emergence of community-associated MRSA (CA-MRSA) as a significant pathogen. These strains were first detected among pediatric patients with no other contact with the health care system or other specific identifiable risk factor for MRSA carriage or infection. Because these infections frequently arose outside of the hospital, the causative staphylococcal strains came to be designated as "community-acquired" or "community-associated," even where no specific source of acquisition could be identified. In these early reports, CA-MRSA strains were most commonly associated with episodes of severe and sometimes recurrent skin and soft-tissue infection. Common presentations included boils, furuncles, and episodes of folliculitis.[27] Curiously, many affected patients spontaneously reported to clinicians that at the onset of infection, the skin lesion took on the appearance of an insect or spider bite, and this observation in the clinical history has come to be regarded by many experienced clinicians as a specific indicator for infection with CA-MRSA. Of further note, despite their characteristic resistance to beta-lactam agents, CA-MRSA isolates are frequently found to remain susceptible to multiple other drugs and drug classes (including clindamycin, sulfa agents, and doxycycline)—a phenomenon that distinguishes these isolates from conventional health care–associated MRSA strains.[28]

Early recognition of the signs and symptoms of skin and soft-tissue infection with CA-MRSA is essential to the timely initiation of appropriate antimicrobial therapy. Beta-lactam and cephalosporin agents such as dicloxacillin and cephalexin, long-standing mainstays of antibiotic therapy for this type of infection, will not be effective in treating CA-MRSA. In this context, the unique susceptibility profile of the CA-MRSA presents an opportunity to call into service a number of older antimicrobial agents previously not favored as first-line agents in the treatment of staphylococcal disease. These antibiotics are discussed in greater detail in the next section.

What are the implications of the proliferation of CA-MRSA for older patients? The question, at the time of this writing, has not been definitively resolved. As yet, there have not been sufficient studies to determine whether the incidence of skin and soft-tissue infections caused by community-associated MRSA is any greater among older versus younger patients. Moreover, there has been no systematic study or even consensus among experienced and expert clinicians regarding the unique consequences of infection with this pathogen among these patients. Nonetheless, the remarkable degree to which CA-MRSA infections have been observed to spread in the community and, increasingly, in health care settings, suggests that familiarity with the key concepts of diagnosis and management of these patients is essential for any clinician responsible for the care of older patients.

Pharmacologic Considerations

CASE PRESENTATION 2 (continued)

Based on his history, physical exam findings, and your own awareness of recent epidemiologic trends, you conclude that Mr. Wingate's infection is most likely caused by CA-MRSA. You inform him of your findings and offer a brochure distributed by the local health department that provides detailed information about the CA-MRSA epidemic and advice for preventing the spread of infection to household contacts. Relieved and impressed, Mr. Wingate affirms his trust in your clinical acumen and suggests that you immediately prescribe for him "the latest and greatest antibiotic" in order to hasten his recovery so that he can participate in the club tournament next week. He reminds you that his insurance coverage is "the best" and even offers to sponsor you for membership at the club once his infection has completely resolved.

In general, when considering the selection of specific antimicrobial therapy for patients with skin and soft-tissue infection, there are relatively few potential complications related to pharmacokinetic or pharmacodynamic factors. After carefully considering both the most likely causative pathogens and having determined the most appropriate breadth of antimicrobial coverage, clinicians will generally find that the range of appropriate antibiotic choices is rarely limited by such issues as bioavailability, tissue penetration, or volume of distribution. Instead, concerns related to drug toxicity, hypersensitivity reactions, drug–drug interactions, and adherence must be a priority, especially for clinicians working with older patients.

For older patients for whom the risk of antimicrobial resistance is low but streptococci and staphylococci remain the most likely causative pathogens, a number of very effective therapeutic options are available to treat skin and soft-tissue infection. Assuming the affected patient is not allergic to beta-lactam agents or related drug classes (including the cephalosporins and carbapenems), excellent choices might include an oral first-generation cephalosporin (such as cephalexin) or a semisynthetic penicillin which retains good anti-staphylococcal activity (eg, dicloxacillin). Both agents are well tolerated although the more frequent dosing schedule required for cephalexin (four times daily) may present a challenge to some older patients, especially those already taking multiple other medications to manage co-morbid conditions. Assuming no microbiological data are returned that warrant a change in the regimen, such patients generally can be successfully treated with 2 weeks of oral therapy. In cases in which poor physiologic reserve, the severity of infection, or other factors require inpatient hospitalization, similar breadth of coverage can be assured with the intravenous agents cefazolin and oxacillin (or nafcillin).

Historically, patients infected with health care–associated MRSA strains, which are generally more resistant to non-beta-lactam agents than CA-MRSA, required administration of parenteral therapy, typically in an inpatient setting. The usual choice for these patients was vancomycin. Vancomycin has the advantage of retaining a broad spectrum of activity against a wide range of Gram-positive pathogens including nearly all strains of staphylococci and streptococci. Serum vancomycin levels can be followed by the treating clinician to ensure that sufficient drug was being administered to be effective for the specific infection, whether in the skin and soft tissue or at some deeper body site. Generally, periodic assessment of the trough drug level is sufficient for this purpose in as much as peak vancomycin levels do not reliably correspond to episodes of drug toxicity.[29]

Unfortunately, the complexity and expense of intravenous administration is a major barrier to the dependence on vancomycin as the major pharmacologic weapon for treating infections caused by HA-MRSA. Moreover, the challenge of maintaining drug levels within an appropriate therapeutic range may be especially challenging when managing an older infected patient. As has already been noted, nephrotoxicity is the single most important pharmacodynamic change experienced by such patients and demands close monitoring especially when vancomycin is prescribed. Vancomycin, particularly when administered in conjunction with other pharmacologic agents with renal toxicity, may be associated with an increased risk of acute renal failure.[29]

Given these challenges associated with vancomycin, especially in the context of managing infection potentially caused by HA-MRSA strains, the widespread availability of two newer agents with specific activity against methicillin-resistant isolates has been welcomed by clinicians. Both daptomycin and linezolid have approval from the US Food and Drug Administration for the treatment of skin and soft-tissue infection. Daptomycin, which is only available as an intravenous preparation, has excellent activity against even the most drug-resistant strains of S. aureus. The drug is generally well tolerated, even by older patients. However, because of the risk of elevation of the creatinine phosphokinase level, especially during prolonged treatment courses, periodic blood testing is advised.[30]

Linezolid, which has the advantage of being available and approved for skin and soft-tissue infection as both an oral and intravenous formulation, has been demonstrated to be very effective in treating these infections in both younger and older patients. Because of the drug's excellent oral bioavailability, linezolid is a popular choice for clinicians who wish to manage cases of known or suspected infection with MRSA without admitting the patient to the hospital or placing an intravenous line. The widespread use of linezolid has been somewhat limited, however, owing to the risk of drug–drug interactions and toxicity. Furthermore, the relatively high price of even the oral formulation of linezolid can serve as an additional barrier to use for many patients. Linezolid administration is relatively contraindicated for patients who are concurrently receiving selective serotonin reuptake inhibitors and a wide range of related drugs.[31]

So what is the best choice for Mr. Wingate? As was previously noted, the unique antibiotic susceptibility profile of CA-MRSA isolates offers the relatively uncommon opportunity to manage an emerging and potentially aggressive infection without calling upon some of the newer or more complicated regimens previously described. Specifically, in most point prevalence and observational studies of antimicrobial resistance examining CA-MRSA isolates, both clindamycin and trimethoprim/sulfamethoxazole retain very good if not excellent activity (to a lesser extent, some clinicians have also found doxycycline to be useful in this setting). Again, this stands in stark contrast to the experience with health care–associated MRSA strains, which are almost universally resistant to these agents. In the case of clindamycin, more refined microbiological testing algorithms can be used to identify even the possibility of inducible resistance to the drug, which has been associated with an increased risk of clinical failure.[32] Such confirmatory testing should be performed in any lab where these isolates are routinely received and analyzed. Because of considerable heterogeneity in the relative proportion of CA-MRSA strains adequately covered by clindamycin or trimethoprim/sulfamethoxazole in a given geographic range, consultation with an institutional or local antibiotic susceptibility report (as discussed earlier in the chapter) is especially valuable in selecting the preferred regimen.

Even considering the extensive experience of using both clindamycin and trimethoprim/sulfamethoxazole to treat infection in older patients, and despite their relatively favorable safety profile, these agents are not without risk. Among commonly used antibiotics, clindamycin is among the drugs most closely associated with *Clostridium difficile*-associated diarrhea (CDAD). The incidence of CDAD has increased dramatically over the past decade, and many of the most severe and sometimes even fatal cases are now seen among older patients. Trimethoprim/sulfamethoxazole is associated with an increased risk of hypersensitivity reactions, owing to the drug's sulfa moiety.

CASE PRESENTATION 2 (continued)

Despite Mr. Wingate's protestation that you prescribe one of the new antibiotics he saw advertised in a magazine, you prescribe a 2-week course of high-dose trimethroprim/sulfamethoxazole. Consultation with recent guidelines published by the local department of health suggests that the incidence of resistance to clindamycin among CA-MRSA isolates is on the rise. The original culture specimen eventually grows *S. aureus* that is resistant to methicillin and clindamycin but not trimethoprim/sulfamethoxazole. Although you are never invited to the club to play tennis with Mr. Wingate and no offer of sponsorship for membership is proffered, you gain great satisfaction in knowing that you contributed in a small way to Mr. Wingate's third consecutive master's trophy.

CONCLUSION

The management of infection among older patients is a topic sufficiently broad and complex as to limit the extent to which it can be meaningfully addressed in a single chapter in even the most comprehensive text. Moreover, the constantly changing landscape of emerging pathogens, evolving epidemiology, and cutting-edge therapeutic agents can render even well-thought-out and practical references obsolete within a short time after publication. In this context, an encyclopedic recitation of common presentations and pathogens, "bug-drug" pairings, and other conventional tools for introducing the subject of antimicrobial therapy for older patients to an informed readership is all but impracticable.

To address these challenges, this chapter has introduced a straightforward and intuitive algorithm for the selection of empirical antimicrobial therapy for older patients with known or suspected infection. In applying this approach to the management of two very different cases of infection in older patients, it is intended that the clinician reader can become not only proficient but ultimately master this strategy. Using this approach for their older patients, clinicians can be assured of providing care that is always rational, equitable, and evidence based.

References

1. Yoshikawa TT. Epidemiology and unique aspects of aging and infectious diseases. *Clin Infect Dis*. 2000;30:931-933.

2. Ochoa-Gondar O, Vila-Corcoles A, de Diego C, et al. The burden of community-acquired pneumonia in the elderly: The Spanish EVAN-65 Study. *BMC Public Health*. 2008;8:222.

3. High K, Bradley S, Loeb M, et al. A new paradigm for clinical investigation of infectious syndromes in older adults: Assessing functional status as a risk factor and outcome measure. *J Am Geriatr Soc*. 2005;53:528-535.

4. Castle SC, Uyemura K, Fulop T, et al. Host resistance and immune responses in advanced age. *Clin Geriatr Med*. 2007;23:463-479.

5. Frei CR, Restrepo MI, Mortensen EM, et al. Impact of guideline-concordant empiric antibiotic therapy in community-acquired pneumonia. *Am J Med*. 2006;119:865-871.

6. Juthani-Mehta M, Quagliarello VJ. Prognostic scoring systems for infectious diseases: Their applicability to the care of older adults. *Clin Infect Dis*. 2004;38:692-696.

7. Weber SG, Miller RR, Perencevich EN. The prevalence of antimicrobial-resistant bacteria isolated from older versus younger hospitalized adults: Results of a two-center study. *J Antimicrobial Chemother*. 2009;64:1291-1298.

8. Faulkner CM, Cox HL, Williamson JC. Unique aspects of antimicrobial use in older adults. *Clin Infect Dis*. 2005;40:997-1004.

9. Turnheim K. Drug dosage in the elderly. Is it rational? *Drugs Aging*. 1998;13:357-379.

10. Noreddin AM, Haynes V. Use of pharmacodynamic principles to optimise dosage regimens for antibacterial agents in the elderly. *Drugs Aging*. 2007;24:275-292.

11. George J, Elliott RA, Stewart DC. A systematic review of interventions to improve medication taking in elderly patients prescribed multiple medications. *Drugs Aging*. 2008;25:307-324.

12. Jackson ML, Neuzil KM, Thompson WW, et al. The burden of community-acquired pneumonia in seniors: Results of a population-based study. *Clin Infect Dis.* 2004;39:1642-1650.

13. Kaplan V, Clermont G, Griffin MF, et al. Pneumonia: Still the old man's friend? *Arch Intern Med.* 2003;163:317-323.

14. Mandell LA, Wunderink RG, Anzueto A. Infectious Diseases Society of America/American Thoracic Society Consensus Guidelines on the Management of Community-Associated Pneumonia in Adults. *Clin Infect Dis.* 2007;44:S27-S72.

15. Bratzler DW, Nsa W, Houck PM. Performance measures for pneumonia: Are they valuable, and are process measures adequate? *Curr Opin Infect Dis.* 2007;20:182-189.

16. American Thoracic Society, Infectious Diseases Society of America. Guidelines for the Management of Adults with Hospital-Acquired, Ventilator-Associated, and Healthcare-Associated Pneumonia. *Am J Respir Crit Care Med.* 2005;171:388-416.

17. Hui DS, Woo J, Hui E, et al. Influenza-like illness in residential care homes: A study of the incidence, aetiological agents, natural history and health resource utilisation. *Thorax.* 2008;63:690-697.

18. Stahlmann R, Lode H. Fluoroquinolones in the elderly: Safety considerations. *Drugs Aging.* 2003;20:289-302.

19. Pallin DJ, Egan DJ, Pelletier AJ, et al. Increased US emergency department visits for skin and soft tissue infections, and changes in antibiotic choices, during the emergence of community associated methicillin-resistant *Staphylococcus aureus. Ann Emerg Med.* 2008; 51:291-298.

20. Sunderkotter C, Kalden H, Luger TA. Aging and the skin immune system. *Arch Dermatol.* 1997;133:1256-1262.

21. Stevenson A, Hider P, Than M. The utility of blood cultures in the management of non facial cellulitis appears to be low. *NZ Med J.* 2005;118:U1351.

22. Sachs MK. The optimum use of needle aspiration in the bacteriologic diagnosis of cellulitis in adults. *Arch Intern Med.* 1990;150: 1907-1912.

23. Tacconelli E, De Angelis G, Cataldo MA, et al. Antibiotic usage and risk of colonization and infection with antibiotic-resistant bacteria: A hospital population-based study. *Antimicrob Agents Chemother.* 2009;53:4264-4269.

24. Zaas AK, Song X, Tucker P, et al. Risk factors for development of vancomycin-resistant enterococcal bloodstream infection in patients with cancer who are colonized with vancomycin-resistant enterococci. *Clin Infect Dis.* 2002;35:1139-1146.

25. Tentolouris N, Petrikkos G, Vallianou N, et al. Prevalence of methicillin-resistant *Staphylococcus aureus* in infected and uninfected diabetic foot ulcers. *Clin Microbiol Infect.* 2006;12: 186-189.

26. Sanford MD, Widmer AF, Bale MJ, et al. Efficient detection and long-term persistence of the carriage of methicillin-resistant *Staphylococcus aureus. Clin Infect Dis.* 1994;19:1123-1128.

27. Herold BC, Immergluck LC, Maranan MC, et al. Community-acquired methicillin-resistant *Staphylococcus aureus* in children with no identified predisposing risk. *JAMA.* 1998;279:593-598.

28. Daum RS. Clinical practice. Skin and soft-tissue infections caused by methicillin-resistant *Staphylococcus aureus. N Engl J Med.* 2007; 357:380-390.

29. Elting LS, Rubenstein EB, Kurtin D, et al. Mississippi mud in the 1990s: Risks and outcomes of vancomycin-associated toxicity in general oncology practice. *Cancer.* 1998;83:2597-2607.

30. Carpenter CF, Chambers HF. Daptomycin: Another novel agent for treating infections due to drug-resistant Gram-positive pathogens. *Clin Infect Dis.* 2004;38:994-1000.

31. Hau T. Efficacy and safety of linezolid in the treatment of skin and soft tissue infections. *Eur J Clin Microbiol Infect Dis.* 2002;21: 491-498.

32. Fiebelkorn KR, Crawford SA, McElmeel ML, et al. Practical disk diffusion method for detection of inducible clindamycin resistance in *Staphylococcus aureus* and coagulase-negative staphylococci. *J Clin Microbiol.* 2003;41:4740-4744.

POST-TEST

1. **The most common associated pathogen for a deep puncture wound is:**
   A. Community-associated MRSA
   B. Gram-negative pathogens
   C. *Clostridium*
   D. *Pasturella multocida*

2. **For a long-term care resident with pneumonia, a typical treatment regime without suspected MRSA would be:**
   A. A fluoroquinolone such as levofloxacin
   B. A third-generation cephalosporin plus fluoroquinolone plus antipseudomondal agent
   C. Fluoroquinolone alone
   D. Cefepime or piperacillin plus fluoroquinolone plus vancomycin

3. **The most common pathogen for an older adult in the community with a urinary tract infection is:**
   A. *E. coli*
   B. *S. aureus*
   C. *Candida*
   D. *Listeria monocytogenes*

ANSWERS TO PRE-TEST

1. C
2. B
3. A

ANSWERS TO POST-TEST

1. C
2. B
3. A

43

Congestive Heart Failure

Mara Slawsky, MD

Greg Valania, MD

Fadi Saab, MD

Sandra Bellantonio, MD

● **LEARNING OBJECTIVES**

1. Define heart failure (HF) with preserved left ventricular (LV) ejection fraction (HFPEF).
2. Identify risk factors for development of heart failure.
3. Determine treatment modalities in elderly patients with HFPEF including pharmacologic and nonpharmacologic interventions.

PRE-TEST

1. **What is the prognosis of patients with preserved left ventricular (LV) ejection fraction heart failure (HFPEF) compared to patients with reduced ejection fraction heart failure (HFREF)?**

   A. Patients have normal LV ejection fraction, therefore prognosis is excellent.

   B. Risk of rehospitalization is minimal.

   C. Mortality and morbidity are similar for patients with HFPEF and HFREF.

   D. HFREF patients usually die within 3 months of diagnosis

2. **Which of the following is FALSE regarding signs and symptoms of heart failure with preserved EF?**

   A. Patients will have evidence of volume overload with distended JVD and lower extremity edema.

   B. Patients who don't have rales on exam are not volume overloaded and cannot be in heart failure.

   C. The chest x-ray can look normal.

   D. Impaired exercise tolerance is a common complaint among patients with HFPEF.

3. **Which one of the following statements is TRUE regarding co-morbidities in patients with HFPEF?**

   A. HFPEF patients are less likely to suffer from arrhythmias than patients with reduced EF.

   B. Obesity does not appear to increase the risk of developing HFPEF.

   C. Hypertension is common in elderly patients and contributes to ventricular and vascular stiffness.

   D. Diabetes increases the risk of coronary artery disease in HFPEF patients but does not contribute to increased ventricular stiffness.

HEART FAILURE IN THE GERIATRIC POPULATION

Epidemiology

The prevalence of heart failure (HF) increases with increasing age. One in 100 people over the age of 65 carries this diagnosis, and heart failure is the number one cause of hospitalization in the Medicare population. Approximately 2 per 100 men and 3 per 100 women above 75 will develop heart failure, an incidence significantly greater than any other age group.[1] Over 80% of patients with a hospital discharge diagnosis of heart failure are ≥ 65 years old, and more than 50% are ≥ 75 years old.[1] In one large community study of HF patients, the mean age was 76 years.[2] Community studies and hospital registries have documented a 50% to 55% prevalence of preserved EF heart failure (HFPEF) in the geriatric population.[3] The presence of HFPEF is associated with female gender and with hypertension.[4] In patients with reduced ejection fraction heart failure (HFREF), coronary artery disease is the underlying cause in two-thirds of cases.[3] The morbidity and mortality in patients with HFPEF and HFREF are similar.[5]

A recent analysis of Medicare patients hospitalized for HF in the United States has highlighted the importance of co-morbid conditions in determining short-term (30-day) and long-term (5-year) mortality in geriatric HF patients. The mean age of patients was 80 years, 10% had dementia, and 39% had "mobility disability," defined as requiring assistance with ambulation or inability to walk. Both co-morbidities were identified as strong independent predictors of increased short- and long-term mortality.[6]

Definition and Clinical Manifestations

Current heart failure guidelines identify four stages of heart failure (A, B, C, and D). Stages A and B identify patients at risk for developing symptomatic heart failure. Stage A defines risk factors predisposing the patient to heart failure such as hypertension, diabetes, or coronary artery disease. Stage B includes patients with LV hypertrophy or impaired LV systolic function but no symptoms of heart failure. Stage C describes patients with current or past symptoms of heart failure. Stage D describes patients at an advanced state of heart failure with refractory symptoms requiring advanced treatment modalities such as device therapy, chemical support of heart function (inotropic agents), or cardiac transplantation. These treatment modalities are generally reserved for patients with advanced reduced ejection fraction heart failure (HFREF).

Heart failure patients are also classified on the basis of their functional status according to New York Heart Association (NYHA) functional classification. Depending on the degree of symptoms caused by exertion, the patient is assigned a degree between I and IV. Class I patients are essentially asymptomatic with normal activities. Class II patients develop symptoms with exertion that otherwise would not limit a person in good health. Class III refers to patients with symptoms on low-level exertion (eg, climbing less than one flight of stairs). Class IV patients have symptoms of heart failure at rest or with minimal activity. There are limitations

NYHA Class	Symptoms
I	No symptoms and no limitation in ordinary physical activity, eg, shortness of breath when walking, climbing stairs etc.
II	Mild symptoms (mild shortness of breath and/or angina) and slight limitation during ordinary activity.
III	Marked limitation in activity due to symptoms, even during less-than-ordinary activity, eg, walking short distances (20-100 m). Comfortable only at rest.
IV	Severe limitations. Experiences symptoms even while at rest. Mostly bed-bound patients.

● TABLE 43–1 New York Heart Association Health Failure Functional Classification

to these classification schemes. Determination of poor functional status due to heart failure symptoms may be particularly difficult in the elderly who often have limited functional capacity due to co-morbidities. Nonetheless, these HF classification schemes remain useful in guiding therapy and addressing prognosis (Table 43–1).

Symptoms of HF such as fatigue, decreased exercise tolerance, dyspnea, and edema are frequently attributed to aging. This results in under-recognition and undertreatment of heart failure in the elderly. Insufficient treatment of risk factors such as hypertension, diabetes mellitus, and dyslipidemia contributes to the increased prevalence of this disease in the elderly. Prevalent co-morbid conditions such as renal insufficiency, pulmonary disease, thyroid disease, atrial fibrillation, and anemia often precipitate worsening HF.[7-9] In addition, elderly patients are often prescribed medications, like nonsteroidal anti-inflammatory drugs, that can result in decompensated HF.[10]

Typical HF symptoms include gradual onset of dyspnea on exertion, orthopnea, and paroxysmal nocturnal dyspnea. Gradually worsening leg edema and increasing abdominal girth may also be present. Symptoms are often atypical in older adults who may present with fatigue, lethargy, or delirium.

Physical findings include the presence of low or elevated systolic blood pressure, rapid heart rate, displaced apical cardiac impulse, abnormal heart sounds (S3 or S4), jugular venous distension, lower extremity edema, and rales on lung exam. The best predictor of congestion is jugular venous distention.[11] Hepatojugular or abdominojugular reflux (a sustained increase in jugular venous pressure on abdominal compression) alone or in addition to jugular venous distention is a marker of elevation in left ventricular filling pressure.[12] Rales, when present on lung exam, are a strong indicator of volume overload. However, in patients with chronic heart failure, they are often not present.[13]

Changes in body weight (2 lbs [1 kg] or more) over a short time period (≤ 1 week) are an easily assessed and useful marker for heart failure decompensation. Weight gain usually precedes admission for heart failure by approximately 1 week.[14]

Markers of a low cardiac output state with poor systemic perfusion include narrowed pulse pressure, cool extremities, altered mental status, resting tachycardia, and abnormal breathing patterns such as Cheyne Stokes respiration. These are more ominous signs in heart failure patients.

In patients presenting with dyspnea, in whom the diagnosis remains unclear from history, physical examination, and chest x-ray, brain natriuretic peptide assay (BNP or NT-proBNP) is recommended to aid in the diagnosis of heart failure.

HEART FAILURE WITH REDUCED EF (HFREF)

CASE PRESENTATION 1: MR. C

You are asked to evaluate a 72-year-old African American man, Mr. C., prior to his discharge following a myocardial infarction 1 week ago. He has hypertension, dyslipidemia, and tobacco dependence.

He had initially presented to the emergency room 24 hours after a prolonged episode of left-sided chest pain associated with dyspnea and palpitations. On examination, he has a blood pressure of 104/88 mm Hg, a pulse of 102/min, a respiratory rate of 28/min, cold extremities, rales extending into the mid lung fields, and a summation gallop. EKG shows sinus tachycardia with Q-waves and associated 3-mm ST elevations in the anterior precordial leads. Emergent cardiac catheterization had revealed a proximal total occlusion of the left anterior descending (LAD) artery with no collateral flow to the vessel and a very elevated left ventricular end-diastolic pressure (LVEDP) of 35 mm Hg. Ventriculography documented severely reduced left ventricular systolic function with estimated ejection fraction of 20% (normal range 55-70%), anterior/apical akinesis, and moderate mitral regurgitation. A coronary stent was placed in the LAD. Post-procedure he required temporary mechanical ventilation for respiratory failure as well as 24 hours of inotropic support with an intra-aortic balloon pump and intravenous dopamine infusion to maintain adequate blood pressure. He received an intravenous loop diuretic infusion for treatment of pulmonary edema. Following extubation and withdrawal of inotropic/pressor support he was transitioned to the telemetry unit on an oral loop diuretic, an HMG Co-A reductase inhibitor (statin), aspirin, and clopidogrel. His subsequent hospital course has been notable for borderline low blood pressures (102/78 mm Hg), persistent anterior ST elevations and anterior Q-waves, frequent ventricular ectopy, as well as periodic nonsustained ventricular tachycardia.

Today, he reports that he is feeling better without rest chest pain, palpitations, or rest dyspnea. He is able to ambulate to the end of the hallway, at which point he stops for fatigue and dyspnea. He has no postural dizziness or light-headedness. His appetite is fair and he has had only mild difficulty with sleep secondary to the noisy hospital environment.

On examination, he has a blood pressure of 100/82 mm Hg, pulse of 92/min, respirations of 12/minute, normal jugular venous pressure, normal carotid upstrokes, clear lungs, an apical S3 and S4 sound, a 2/6 holosystolic apical murmur radiating to the axilla, and warm extremities with good distal pulses.

His primary care team had been hesitant to initiate guideline-indicated post myocardial infarction therapy with beta-blockers and angiotensin-converting enzyme inhibitors (ACEIs) due to borderline blood pressures. Mr. C. is an educated consumer and has read about benefits of beta-blockers and ACEIs after heart attacks, but he is concerned about his borderline blood pressure. He has had family members who have had heart attacks and heart failure. He asks you to make appropriate recommendations about his medical therapy prior to hospital discharge.

Evidence-Based Pharmacotherapy

The pathophysiology of HFREF begins after injury to the myocardium and leads to the characteristic hemodynamic abnormalities of reduced cardiac output and elevated cardiac filling pressures. There is an associated compensatory neurohormonal activation involving both the sympathetic nervous system (SNS) and the renin-angiotensin-aldosterone system (RAAS). This results in deleterious hemodynamic alterations, peripheral vasoconstriction, and negative myocardial remodeling with worsening of left ventricular function.[15] Multiple clinical trials have demonstrated efficacy of SNS and RAAS blocker therapy in preventing adverse cardiac remodeling and improving clinical outcomes in post-MI and heart failure patients.[16-26] Elderly patients may have variable pharmacologic responses to medications and may be susceptible to adverse events and drug–drug interactions due to concurrent treatments for co-morbidities. Close monitoring of elderly patients undergoing HF treatment is essential to ensure safety and optimal outcomes.

Beta-Blockers

Beta-blockers (BBs) exert their beneficial effect by blocking the sympathetic nervous system. Beta-blockers such as metoprolol and bisoprolol are specific for the beta-1 adrenergic receptors; carvedilol blocks the beta-1 and beta-2 receptors and, to some degree, alpha receptors as well.

Mortality reduction with BB therapy (22-65%) is observed in patients with both ischemic and non-ischemic cardiomyopathy and in patients with mild, moderate, and advanced heart failure.[20,22-25] In addition, BB therapy is associated with a 33% to 36% reduction in heart failure hospitalizations.[22-24]

There is significant reduction in the risk of reinfarction or death when BBs are begun soon after a myocardial infarction in combination with an ACE inhibitor.[14-21,26]

There were few geriatric patients included in the earlier HFREF trials. Recently, however, the SENIORS trial examined the safety and efficacy of BB therapy with nebivolol in heart failure patients ranging from 70 to 95 years in age. The majority of these patients had HFrEF (LVEF < 35%). This study demonstrated a 15% relative reduction (NNT 23.8 for 21 months) in the combined end-point of all-cause mortality and heart failure hospitalizations.[27]

Despite the evidence that BB therapy has consistently reduced morbidity and mortality in HFREF patients, these therapies are still underutilized in patients with EF < 40%).[28] In a large registry of HFREF patients, 90% of all patients were eligible for BB therapy.[29] The safety and tolerability of BB therapy (carvedilol) was highlighted in a study initiating BBs in patients with severe heart failure who were first rendered free of congestion. The BB arm of the trial demonstrated a 35% mortality reduction (NNT 14 for 10.4 months) and a 24% reduction in the combined end-point of hospitalizations and death. In the high-risk subgroup of patients in which the placebo group mortality at 1 year was 24%, the survival benefit of BB therapy was more striking, with a 39% mortality reduction.[25] The SENIORS trial[21] demonstrated a less robust reduction in mortality than had been demonstrated in the other major BB trials, but this may be attributable to the competing risk of death from co-morbid conditions that are more prevalent in older patients.[27] The tolerability of BB therapy in the SENIORS study population was better than expected, with 70% of patients reaching the target dose. There was no difference in medication discontinuation rate in patients on placebo versus study drug (Table 43–2).[27]

● TABLE 43–2 Use of Beta-Blockers with Heart Failure

Take Home Points

Indications

1. Use of evidence-based BB (carvedilol, metoprolol succinate, bisoprolol) for all stable patients with current of prior HF and reduced EF
2. Post MI patients with HF
3. Post MI patients with reduced EF and no prior HF

Contraindications

1. Cardiogenic shock
2. Severe reactive airway disease
3. High-degree AV block (2nd- or 3rd-degree block)

Use only BB with clinical trial evidence of mortality reduction such as carvedilol, metoprolol succinate (XL), or bisoprolol.

Up-titrate by doubling to target or maximally tolerated dose at 2-week intervals in stable, euvolemic patients.

	Initial Dose	Target Dose
Carvedilol	3.125 mg BID	25 mg BID (50 mg BID > 85 kg)
Metoprolol XL	12.5 or 25 mg daily	200 mg daily
Bisoprolol	1.25 mg daily	10 mg daily

From Hunt[3]

● TABLE 43–3 Use of Ace-Inhibitors with Heart Failure

Take Home Points

Indications

1. Use ACE Inhibitors for all stable patients with current or prior HF and reduced EF
2. Post MI patients with reduced EF and HF
3. Post MI patients with reduced EF and no prior HF

Contraindications

1. Pregnancy
2. Hyperkalemia (caution with K+ > 5.5 mEq/L)
3. Angioedema
4. Cardiogenic shock
5. Bilateral renal artery stenosis (only with cautious use and for clear benefits)

Cautious use in patients with creatinine > 3 mg/dL.

Up-titrate by doubling to target dose or maximally tolerated dose.

Monitor serum potassium and renal function routinely and 1-2 weeks after first dose and subsequent dosage increases.

	Initial Dose	Target Dose
Enalapril	2.5 mg BID	10-20 mg BID
Captopril	6.25 mg TID	50 mg TID
Lisinopril	2.5-5 mg daily	40 mg daily

From Hunt.[3]

Angiotensin-Converting Enzyme Inhibitors

Angiotensin-converting enzyme inhibitors (ACEIs) block the conversion of angiotensin I to angiotension II in the renin angiotensin pathway, which, like the sympathetic nervous system, is up-regulated in heart failure.

Along with BBs, ACEIs are considered first-line treatment in all patients with HFREF, and in post-MI patients with LVEF < 40% unless contraindicated[13]. A meta-analysis of large, randomized, placebo-controlled trials on angiotensin-converting enzyme inhibitors totaling 7105 patients demonstrated a 33% relative reduction in mortality and heart failure hospitalizations compared to placebo.[30] In hospitals with an 88% utilization rate for ACEIs there was a 2.1-day decrease in length of stay for heart failure patients and a 77% mortality reduction compared to hospitals with a 58% utilization rate[28]. There is trial-based evidence to support up-titration of ACEIs to target doses. In the ATLAS study there was a 12% reduction in mortality and all-cause hospitalizations when higher versus lower doses of ACEIs were used.[31] The benefit seen from individual ACEIs is believed to be a "class" effect. Even though ACEIs have documented clinical benefit, in a recent large hospital registry of systolic heart failure patients, only 44% of eligible patients were receiving ACEIs (13% were receiving alternative therapy with an angiotensin receptor blocker, described later) (Table 43–3).[28]

CASE PRESENTATION 1 (continued)

Mr. C. comes to your office for a scheduled visit. It has been several weeks after his hospitalization for a large anterior myocardial infarction complicated by heart failure. He has tolerated the initiation of carvedilol

3.125 mg BID. He has started taking an ACEI (enalapril 2.5 mg BID) and continues on furosemide 40 mg daily. He has been feeling generally well with moderate exertional dyspnea, but no orthopnea or edema. He has noted an increasingly frequent dry cough that can occur at any time during the day or night. He has not noticed a clear precipitant for the coughing episodes. On examination, his blood pressure is 98/60 mm Hg and pulse 68/min. Examination again reveals a left S3 and displaced apical impulse, clear lungs, no edema, and no jugular venous distension. His medications have not changed from what was prescribed in the hospital except for the addition of nicotine gum for smoking cessation.

On examination, he is not fatigued or short of breath at rest. His blood pressure is 100/68 mm Hg and his pulse is 62/min. His apical impulse remains laterally displaced with an apical S3 and 2/6 mitral regurgitant murmur heard at the apex. There is no JVD or peripheral edema, and his lungs are clear. His renal function parameters have remained within normal limits and his serum potassium is 3.9 mEq/L (3.9 mmol/L). After reviewing his medications and clinical condition you discuss with him the addition of an aldosterone blocker, in addition to watching his sodium intake, which may reduce his risk of rehospitalization. He is agreeable and goes home with a new prescription. Over the next 6 months he does well with no further hospitalizations or heart failure exacerbations.

Angiotensin-Receptor Blockers

Angiotensin-receptor blockers (ARBs) block the binding of angiotensin II to the AT1 receptor, which mediates the deleterious effects of this neurohormone in heart failure. ARBs reduce morbidity and mortality in patients with symptomatic HFREF and in patients with reduced LVEF post-MI to a similar extent as the ACEIs.[30-38] At present, candesartan and valsartan are FDA-approved for treatment of HFREF and are considered appropriate therapy for patients who develop a cough on ACEIs.[13] Otherwise, the contraindications and adverse effects noted for ARB are similar to those with ACEIs, with the exception of angioedema, which appears to be less frequent for ARBs. Older adults may be more vulnerable to the side effects of ACEIs and ARBs, such as worsening renal function, hyperkalemia, and hypotension, due to age-related changes in the heart and kidneys. Thus, lower doses of these drugs should be used initially with careful titration and monitoring of electrolytes and renal function.

CASE PRESENTATION 1 (continued)

Mr C. comes for a scheduled visit 3 months later, after switching his ACEI to an ARB with resolution of his cough. His interval history is notable for an admission with heart failure decompensation 2 weeks prior to this visit, for which he received intravenous diuretic therapy. This admission occurred shortly after the Christmas holiday during which time he had consumed a diet higher in sodium. He is on target doses of candesartan and carvedilol, and had a recent increase in his furosemide dose, which he is now taking twice daily. He has no orthopnea or dyspnea at rest, but he reports fatigue and shortness of breath with activities such as climbing the front stairs to his house and walking to the mailbox. He can still do his own grocery shopping if he does not have to hurry.

Aldosterone Blockers

Aldosterone production by the RAAS is increased in heart failure and causes multiple deleterious effects to the cardiovascular system that lead to worsening of cardiac function and exacerbation of systolic heart failure.[39-43] Although aldosterone production is inhibited temporarily by use of ACEIs or ARBs, this does not appear to be sustainable over time.[44] Aldosterone blockers have been shown to reduce morbidity and mortality in severely symptomatic patients with NYHA class III and IV systolic heart failure. In the RALES trial, which was undertaken prior to completion of the HF BB trials, background medications included digoxin, diuretics and ACEIs, with fewer 20% of patients on BBs. The addition of spironolactone resulted in a sizeable absolute mortality reduction of 11% (NNT of 9) and a 35% reduction in heart failure hospitalizations over 2 years.[45] More recently, in a large trial of post-MI patients with LVEF < 40% and either HF or diabetes mellitus, the addition of the aldosterone blocker eplerenone to background ACEI and BB therapy resulted in a significant early post-MI reduction in mortality, sudden cardiac death, and heart failure hospitalizations.[46] Aldosterone blockers, when used with an ACEI, can cause hyperkalemia in older adults, especially if there is coexisting diabetes or renal insufficiency. Smaller doses, not exceeding 25 mg/day, are suggested for older adults (Table 43–4).

Diuretics

Diuretics are the mainstay of therapy in the majority of patients with HFREF. They are indicated in patients with systolic heart failure for symptomatic treatment of congestive symptoms and for achieving euvolemia, which allows for safe initiation and up-titration of ACEIs and BBs.[13] Two main classes of diuretics (loop and thiazide) are used individually or in combination for increased diuretic efficacy. Diuretics are available in both IV and oral formulations. Loop diuretics have become the preferred therapy due to their sustained potency in patients with moderate renal impairment. Thiazide diuretics, with the exception of metolazone (zaroxolyn), lose

● **TABLE 43–4** Aldosterone Blockers

Take Home Points

Indications

1. Use aldosterone inhibitors in patients with moderate or severe HF with reduced EF with close monitoring of renal function and potassium levels after therapy initiation.

Contraindications

1. Creatinine > 2.5 mg/dL in men and > 2.0 mg/dL in women.
2. Serum potassium level > 5.0 mEq/L.

	Initial Dose	Target Dose
Spironolactone	12.5 mg daily	25 mg daily
Eplerenone	25 mg daily	50 mg daily

From Hunt.[3]

efficacy in patients with moderate renal impairment (creatinine clearance (CrCl) < 40 mL/min).

Diuretics have demonstrated efficacy in relief of congestive symptoms but no known positive impact on mortality in HFREF. Adverse effects of chronic diuretic use include diuretic resistance, electrolyte imbalance (hypokalemia, hypomagnesemia), and renal hypoperfusion.[13] Aggressive use of diuretics can cause dehydration, prerenal azotemia, and hyponatremia, which can precipitate delirium in the geriatric population. Diuretics may also precipitate or worsen urinary incontinence and nocturia, which are often responsible for falls in older adults. When possible, dosing diuretics early in the day helps avoid nocturia. A rational approach to the use of diuretics in older adults is to use the smallest effective dose with frequent monitoring of renal function and electrolytes. Reassessment of volume status is important to identify opportunities to taper the dose of diuretics.

Digoxin

Digoxin is a useful therapy for patients with persistent symptomatic heart failure despite optimized therapy with ACEIs, BBs, and diuretics.[13] While digoxin has a neutral effect on mortality in patients with HFREF, it does improve symptoms and quality of life and reduces hospitalizations.[47] In patients with atrial fibrillation and HFREF, digoxin is preferred for ventricular rate control.[13] Older adults are particularly vulnerable to the side effects of digoxin due to age-related decrease in renal clearance and increased volume of distribution. Thus, digoxin initiation should be gradual and the total daily dose should not exceed 0.125 mg daily in elderly patients (> 70 years old), patients with low body weight, or patients with renal impairment.[48] Target therapeutic range is 0.5 to < 1.0 ng/mL (0.64 to < 1.28 nmol/L). Markers of toxicity include cardiac arrhythmias, GI side effects (nausea, vomiting, and loss of appetite), visual disturbances, and confusion. Care should be taken in patients with hypothyroidism, hypokalemia, or hypomagnesemia as these conditions can precipitate digoxin toxicity at lower serum concentrations.[49]

Implantable Cardioverter-Defibrillators

Implantable cardioverter-defibrillators (ICDs) recognize VT and VF and deliver either a pacing technique (for VT) or intracardiac electrical shock (for refractory VT or VT), to restore normal rhythm. The implantation procedure is relatively simple and lasts 1 to 2 hours. Driving is temporarily restricted after implantation. There is debate about the clinical role of ICDs in older adults who often have co-morbidities and reduced life expectancy. Older patients were under-represented in the pivotal large randomized trials demonstrating survival benefit of ICDs in patients with HFREF. More recently, a retrospective cohort study focusing on older patients (mean age 74-75 years) with HFREF (LVEF < 35%) showed similar survival benefit from ICD implantation (29% 3-year improved survival).[50] Older adults may choose not to receive an ICD based on personal preferences or religious or cultural reasons. For others who are frail or who have other co-morbidities that would shorten their survival or diminish their quality of life, it is reasonable to defer discussion regarding ICD implantation. In advanced heart failure patients with ICDs, disabling the device should be considered as part of end-of-life care.

● HEART FAILURE WITH PRESERVED EJECTION FRACTION

CASE PRESENTATION 2: MRS. T.

Mrs. T. is a 78-year-old woman who presented to your hospital with shortness of breath. The patient reported that she found it more difficult to move around her house in the 2 weeks leading up to her presentation. She has been waking up in the middle of the night with shortness of breath that is relieved by sitting up. The patient also states that her feet have been more swollen recently. Her past medical history is notable for stage 2 systolic hypertension, moderate renal insufficiency (GFR 55 mL/min/1.73m^2), and normocytic anemia. She is fairly independent in her activities of daily living and recently enjoyed a 7-day cruise. She quit smoking 40 years ago when she decided to adopt a healthier lifestyle. She is a retired office manager. Her medications include hydrochlorothiazide 25 mg daily, losartan 25 mg daily, atenolol 25 mg daily, and a multivitamin. In the ER the patient appears slightly anxious. She has a blood pressure of 165/85 mm Hg, heart rate of 105/min, respiratory rate of 24/minute, and a normal temperature. She weighs 169 lbs (76.8 kg), which she says is 9 lbs (4.1 kg) more than her usual home weight. Lung exam reveals decreased breath sounds at both bases. There are no rales or wheezes. Her apical cardiac impulse is present in the fifth intercostal space; S1 and

S2 are present. An S3 and an S4 are appreciated. There is no pericardial rub. Examination of the neck reveals jugular venous distension with a positive hepatojugular reflux. The abdominal exam is benign. Lower extremities are warm with good distal pulses and moderate (2+) pitting edema. Laboratory evaluation shows hemoglobin of 11.5 g/dL (115 g/L), Na of 132 mEq/L (132 mmol/L), K of 4.9 mEq/L (4.9 mmol/L), BUN of 42 mg/dL (15 mmol/L), creatinine of 1.4 mg/dL (124 μmol/L), and proBNP of 600 pg/mL (normal 12-150 pg/mL). You discuss with her that you think that she has congestive heart failure, but that this should be readily treatable. To prevent further progression you encourage her to more vigorously monitor her blood pressure and take her medicines. You also tell her you would like to order an echocardiogram to evaluate her heart pump function.

Patients with heart failure with preserved ejection fraction (HFPEF) have a similar clinical presentation to patients with HFREF.[51,52] These patients often present with dyspnea on exertion and reduced exercise tolerance. Although they can present acutely with elevated blood pressure and pulmonary edema, they may also present without evidence of pulmonary congestion on exam or chest x-ray. There is an increased incidence of atrial fibrillation in the HFPEF patients. In HFPEF patients, like patients with HFREF, there is neurohormonal activation promoting sodium and water retention and vasoconstriction. However, ventricular remodeling produces concentric rather than eccentric hypertrophy resulting in increased LV mass-volume ratio contributing to LV stiffness and impaired relaxation.[7]

Pathophysiology of HFPEF

Contributing factors to the development of HFPEF include increased afterload from hypertension, cardiac myocyte hypertrophy, increased arterial stiffness, increased ventricular stiffness due to alterations in the extracellular matrix such as increased collagen deposition, and impaired calcium uptake by the cardiac myocytes.[8]

Abnormal diastolic function also contributes to HFPEF. Normal diastolic function allows the ventricle to fill adequately during rest and exercise, without an abnormal increase in diastolic pressures. The filling phase is divided into early rapid filling, diastasis, and late filling (atrial systole). Atrial systole plays an important role in patients with diastolic dysfunction. Atrial contraction is responsible for 20% of the stroke volume in a young healthy subject; however, in elderly patients with stiffer ventricles, atrial contraction can be a major contributor to stroke volume and therefore to cardiac output. This is one reason why patients with HFPEF may not tolerate atrial fibrillation in which organized atrial contraction is lost.

Co-Morbidities

Patients with HFPEF often have co-morbidities of hypertension and diabetes. Hypertension is considered one of the most common co-morbidities in patients with HFPEF. Hypertensive heart disease results in LV hypertrophy and increased ventricular and vascular stiffness. Diabetes is also common in patients with HFPEF, as it is in patients with HFREF. Hyperglycemia-associated cellular and metabolic abnormalities result in myocyte hypertrophy, increased extracellular collagen deposition, and advanced glycation end products (AGE) that contribute to increased extracellular matrix stiffness. This in turn results in increased LV mass and impaired LV relaxation.[53]

The reason for the female predominance in HFPEF is not entirely clear, but women tend to have higher LV systolic and diastolic stiffness than men.[9] Obesity is common in patients with HFPEF and appears to increase the risk of developing HF. The relationship of obesity to development of HFPEF is complex and may involve mechanisms related to insulin resistance, hypertension, dyslipidemia, and obstructive sleep apnea.[53] Finally, patients with HFPEF seem to be at a higher risk for atrial fibrillation. Atrial fibrillation can cause decompensated HF in patients with diastolic dysfunction. Conversely, diastolic dysfunction (in the absence of HF) is a risk factor for atrial fibrillation.[54]

Diagnostic Modalities

Originally HFPEF was described as diastolic heart failure. HF with preserved (or normal) ejection fraction was proposed when it became clear that other mechanisms were also involved in this disease process. In addition, it is evident that diastolic dysfunction is also present in HF with reduced ejection fraction. Diagnosing patients with HFPEF can be difficult. Numerous studies comparing clinical features between patients with reduced EF and normal EF have shown minimal differences. Therefore it is essential to rely on diagnostic modalities, mainly cardiac imaging, to establish the diagnosis and determine the illness stage.

The European Society of Cardiology, ACCF/AHA, and the Heart Failure Society of America have all published guidelines for diagnosis and treatment of HFPEF. All published guidelines to date require the presence of signs/symptoms of heart failure, evidence of normal heart function, and evidence of diastolic LV dysfunction[55] for the diagnosis of HFPEF. Because of the impracticality of invasively measuring diastolic properties in most patients, noninvasive methods for evaluating LV diastolic function have been developed. Echocardiography is the main tool utilized in defining diastolic parameters. Echo-Doppler technique is currently the method used to assess LV filling and, indirectly, diastolic function. Doppler echocardiography utilizes assessment of mitral inflow into the left ventricle during diastole to assess diastolic function (Figure 43–1). The mitral inflow pattern is composed of two components. The first component is the rapid filling portion (E), which reflects the passive filling of the left ventricle during early diastole. The second portion is the late filling (A), which reflects the flow generated by the atrial contraction during late diastole. The relationship between the early phase (E) and late phase (A)

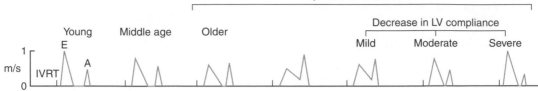

FIGURE 43–1. Mitral inflow and the relationship between early (E) and late (A) filling patterns.

inflow patterns determines the degree of diastolic dysfunction. There are other Doppler parameters that are used to define the degree of diastolic dysfunction but discussion of these is beyond the scope of this chapter.

With aging, the late-filling portion (A wave) from atrial systole, or "atrial kick," becomes a major contributor to stroke volume. As the ventricle becomes stiffer and diastolic dysfunction becomes more severe, the contribution from atrial systole is much less prominent.

Studies have shown that brain natriuretic peptide (BNP) and N-terminal (NT) proBNP assay results are elevated in patients with HFPEF; however, when compared with HFREF, BNP and NT–proBNP values are, on average, lower in patients with HFPEF.[56] BNP levels tend to increase with age and are higher in females; therefore, these values should be interpreted with caution.

CASE PRESENTATION 2 (continued)

Mrs. T. was admitted to the hospital and treated with intravenous furosemide, low-sodium diet, and fluid restriction. Her weight was monitored daily. No Foley catheter was inserted to decrease the risk of urinary tract infection. On intravenous diuretic therapy, she lost 4 lbs (1.8 kg) over the next 24 hours. She felt much better and was able to walk to the bathroom with minimal dyspnea. The next day the patient was walking back from the bathroom when she suddenly became dyspneic and complained of palpitations. On exam her heart rate was increased at 140 beats per minute and irregular, and she was tachypneic with a respiratory rate of 24/min and a blood pressure of 110/70 mm Hg. Her lung exam did not reveal any rales or wheezes. On cardiac exam, heart rate was irregular. There were no murmurs or extra heart sounds. EKG showed atrial fibrillation with rapid ventricular response at 140/min. She was given a calcium-channel blocker, and her heart rate slowed to the 100 to 110 bpm range. Although the patient felt more comfortable, she still noted palpitations and shortness of breath on ambulation down the hallway. Since her symptoms were felt to be due to loss of atrial contraction due to atrial fibrillation, a transesophageal echo (TEE) guided cardioversion was recommended and IV heparin was initiated

for anticoagulation. The TEE showed no thrombus in the left atrium or left atrial appendage, and the patient was cardioverted uneventfully into normal sinus rhythm. Over the next 2 days, the patient lost another 5 lbs (2.3 kg) on diuretic therapy with resolution of symptoms and signs of heart failure decompensation. She was discharged on warfarin anticoagulant therapy without other changes in her home medications. She was also referred to the outpatient cardiac rehabilitation program. She was instructed on a low-sodium diet, and a 1.5L-per-day fluid restriction was recommended. She also received education on the risks of warfarin therapy. An appointment was scheduled with her regular doctor. Her questions were answered and she appeared to have a good understanding of her condition as well as her treatment.

Treatment

Medical therapy with BBs and RAAS blockers (ACEIs, ARBs, aldosterone blockers) in patients with HFREF has documented efficacy in reducing both morbidity and mortality. Currently, none of these agents has proven mortality benefit in the HFPEF population, although a reduction in heart failure morbidity has been identified.

The SENIORS trial (Study of Effects of Nebivolol Interventions on Outcomes and Rehospitalization in Seniors with Heart Failure) is the only BB HF trial so far that has included patients with relatively preserved LVEF. This study examined the efficacy of a vasodilating BB, nebivolol, in heart failure patients older than 70 years. Prespecified study groups included patients with LVEF ≤ 35% and LVEF > 35%. Approximately 20% of the study population had relatively preserved LV systolic dysfunction with LVEF ≥ 45%. This study demonstrated benefit of BB therapy in reducing morbidity and mortality independent of LVEF.[27]

The PEP-CHF trial evaluated the use of an ACEI, perindopril versus placebo in elderly patients (> 70 years)[57] with HFPEF (defined as LVEF > 40%). Mean LVEF was 65% versus 64% in perindopril and placebo groups, respectively. Inclusion criteria for this study also required documentation of diastolic dysfunction by echocardiogram. Because of a significant crossover of patients to open-label ACEIs, the study did not have enough power to identify any benefit of ACEI therapy at the study end point of 2 years. However, an analysis of 1-year data, when most patients were on the study drug, did show significant benefit of ACEI therapy in reducing the combined end point of mortality and HF hospitalization.[15]

The CHARM (Candesartan in Heart Failure Assessment of Mortality and Morbidity) trial randomized 3000 patients with preserved LV function to an ARB (candesartan) versus placebo. There was no benefit of ARB therapy on cardiovascular mortality, but there were fewer hospitalizations in the candesartan group.[58] In the more recent I-PRESERVE study (Irbesartan in Heart Failure with Preserved Systolic Function), however, there was no morbidity/mortality benefit with the ARB, irbesartan, compared to placebo.[59]

Digoxin is one of the oldest medications in use for treatment of patients with HFREF. The digitalis investigation group trial included a subset of patients with HPPEF. In the HFPEF group, treatment with digoxin reduced the hospitalization rate, but had no effect on mortality.[60]

Aldosterone has been implicated in myocardial fibrosis and hypertrophy, which are important pathologic processes underlying HFPEF. The effect of aldosterone antagonism on HFPEF is being investigated in two large outcome trials: ALDO-DHF (Aldosterone Receptor Blockade in Diastolic Heart Failure) and TOPCAT (Treatment of Preserved Cardiac Function Heart Failure with an Aldosterone Antagonist) trials.

As discussed, randomized controlled trials to date have failed to show a clear advantage of treatments in HFPEF that have proven benefit in patients with HFREF. As a result, the current guideline recommendations for management of HF with preserved LV ejection fraction target control of factors that precipitate or exacerbate HF decompensation.[3] Class I recommendations include treatment of hypertension, control of ventricular rate in patients with atrial fibrillation, and treatment of pulmonary congestion or peripheral edema with a diuretic. Coronary revascularization has been recommended for selected patients. Current guidelines also suggest consideration of ACE inhibitors, beta-blockers, or digitalis to relieve HF symptoms, and restoration of sinus rhythm in patients with atrial fibrillation.

• CARDIAC REHABILITATION

Older adults with HF benefit from cardiac rehabilitation, a customized, medically supervised 12-week program designed to improve quality of life and reduce symptoms related to heart disease. An interdisciplinary team of health professionals, often a cardiologist, a nurse specialist, a dietitian, an exercise therapist, and a physical therapist, collaborate to design, implement, and oversee an individualized rehabilitation plan. Cardiac rehabilitation includes education about self-management of hypertension and hyperlipidemia, and information on a heart-healthy diet, smoking cessation, and stress reduction. Exercise is a large component of cardiac rehabilitation; the cardiac rehabilitation team is very involved initially and provides close monitoring of heart rate and symptoms during exercise. Eventually patients are able to exercise independently and monitor their own heart rate. The goal of the 12-week program is to teach patients how to independently carry out the program at home or a local gym. The British Heart Foundation, American Heart Association,

and American College of Cardiology all recommend cardiac rehabilitation programs. Cardiac rehabilitation programs may begin during an acute hospitalization and can continue in nursing facilities, at home, in outpatient clinics, or in rehabilitation hospitals.

• AVOIDING REHOSPITALIZATIONS

Readmissions in older adults with HF are commonly due to medication non-adherence, poor access to care, co-morbid conditions, and polypharmacy. Rehospitalizations can have a negative impact on the patient's quality of life and functional status, and contribute to excess health care expenditures. Both outpatient clinic visits and home visits by an interdisciplinary health care team who assess, monitor, and manage heart failure have been shown to decrease rehospitalization and costs related to HF. The key components of these programs include patient and caregiver education around lifestyle such as daily physical activity, avoiding excessive salt, the importance of daily weights, and flexible diuretic dosing based on changes in weight. In older adults with cognitive impairment, involvement of family to enhance understanding and compliance is essential. Typical members of the interdisciplinary team include a nurse coordinator, dietician, social worker, pharmacist, primary care physician, and a cardiologist.

CASE PRESENTATION 2 (continued)

Mrs. T. comes for her fourth follow-up visit. She has now completed her outpatient cardiac rehabilitation. With medications, a reduced sodium diet, and exercise, Mrs. T. is pleased to tell you her systolic blood pressures are now consistently running in the 115 to 125 mm Hg range and that she is walking almost 1 mile (1.6 km) per day. She feels well, and has had no further palpitations or shortness of breath. She understands that she has to remain vigilant about her diet and exercise to maintain her health. You are encouraged by her report and tell her you are most pleased with her progress.

CONCLUSION

Heart failure is an increasingly common condition in older adults, and is responsible for excess morbidity and mortality as well as hospitalizations. Treatment for both HFREF and HFPEF should be targeted at reducing risk factors as well as treating symptoms. While good data on treatment modalities exist for HFREF, unfortunately the evidence base for HFPEF is significantly smaller. Nonetheless, with good team care, close follow-up, and risk factor reduction interventions, the risks of both progression and hospitalization can be reduced.

References

1. Lloyd-Jones D, Adams RJ, Brown TM, et al. Heart disease and stroke statistics—2010 update: A report from the American Heart Association. *Circulation*. 2010;121:e46-e215.

588

2. Bursi F, Weston SA, Redfield MM, et al. Systolic and diastolic heart failure in the community. JAMA. 2006;296:2209-2216.

3. Hunt SA. ACC/AHA 2005 guideline update for the diagnosis and management of chronic heart failure in the adult: A report of the American College of Cardiology/American Heart Association Task Force on Practice Guidelines (Writing Committee to Update the 2001 Guidelines for the Evaluation and Management of Heart Failure). J Am Coll Cardiol. 2005;46:e1-e82.

4. Ceia F, Fonseca C, Mota T, et al. Prevalence of chronic heart failure in Southwestern Europe: The EPICA study. Eur J Heart Fail. 2002;4:531-539.

5. Bhatia RS, Tu JV, Lee DS, et al. Outcome of heart failure with preserved ejection fraction in a population-based study. N Engl J Med. 2006;355:260-269.

6. Chaudhry SI, Wang Y, Gill TM, Krumholz HM. Geriatric conditions and subsequent mortality in older patients with heart failure. J Am Coll Cardiol. 2010;55:309-316.

7. Kitzman DW, Little WC, Brubaker PH, et al. Pathophysiological characterization of isolated diastolic heart failure in comparison to systolic heart failure. JAMA. 2002;288:2144-2150.

8. Katz AM, Zile MR. New molecular mechanism in diastolic heart failure. Circulation. 2006;113:1922-1925.

9. Redfield MM, Jacobsen SJ, Borlaug BA, et al. Age- and gender-related ventricular-vascular stiffening: A community-based study. Circulation. 2005;112:2254-2262.

10. Heerdink ER, Leufkens HG, Herings RM, et al. NSAIDs associated with increased risk of congestive heart failure in elderly patients taking diuretics. Arch Intern Med. 1998;158:1108-1112.

11. Cesario D, Clark J, Maisel A. Beneficial effects of intermittent home administration of the inotrope/vasodilator milrinone in patients with end-stage congestive heart failure: A preliminary study. Am Heart J. 1998;135:121-129.

12. Drazner MH, Hamilton MA, Fonarow G, et al. Relationship between right and left-sided filling pressures in 1000 patients with advanced heart failure. J Heart Lung Transplant. 1999;18:1126-1132.

13. Hunt SA, Abraham WT, Chin MH, et al. 2009 Focused update incorporated into the ACC/AHA 2005 Guidelines for the Diagnosis and Management of Heart Failure in Adults. A Report of the American College of Cardiology Foundation/American Heart Association Task Force on Practice Guidelines Developed in Collaboration with the International Society for Heart and Lung Transplantation. J Am Coll Cardiol. 2009;53:e1-e90.

14. Chaudhry SI, Wang Y, Concato J, et al. Patterns of weight change preceding hospitalization for heart failure. Circulation. 2007;116:1549-1554.

15. Fonarow GC. Vasopeptidase inhibition in patients with heart failure. Rev Cardiovasc Med. 2001;2:104.

16. A randomized trial of propranolol in patients with acute myocardial infarction. I. Mortality results. JAMA. 1982;247:1707-1714.

17. Chadda K, Goldstein S, Byington R, Curb JD. Effect of propranolol after acute myocardial infarction in patients with congestive heart failure. Circulation. 1986;73:503-510.

18. Pfeffer MA, Braunwald E, Moye LA, et al. Effect of captopril on mortality and morbidity in patients with left ventricular dysfunction after myocardial infarction. Results of the survival and ventricular enlargement trial. The SAVE Investigators. N Engl J Med. 1992; 327:669-677.

19. The Acute Infarction Ramipril Efficacy (AIRE) Study Investigators. Effect of ramipril on mortality and morbidity of survivors of acute myocardial infarction with clinical evidence of heart failure. Lancet. 1993;342:821-828.

20. Waagstein F, Bristow MR, Swedberg K, et al. Beneficial effects of metoprolol in idiopathic dilated cardiomyopathy. Metoprolol in Dilated Cardiomyopathy (MDC) Trial Study Group. Lancet. 1993; 342:1441-1446.

21. ISIS-4 (Fourth International Study of Infarct Survival) Collaborative Group. ISIS-4: A randomised factorial trial assessing early oral captopril, oral mononitrate, and intravenous magnesium sulphate in 58,050 patients with suspected acute myocardial infarction. Lancet. 1995;345:669-685.

22. Packer M, Bristow MR, Cohn JN, et al. The effect of carvedilol on morbidity and mortality in patients with chronic heart failure. U.S. Carvedilol Heart Failure Study Group. N Engl J Med. 1996;334: 1349-1355.

23. The Cardiac Insufficiency Bisoprolol Study II (CIBIS-II): A randomised trial. Lancet. 1999;353:9-13.

24. Effect of metoprolol CR/XL in chronic heart failure: Metoprolol CR/XL Randomised Intervention Trial in Congestive Heart Failure (MERIT-HF). Lancet. 1999;353:2001-2007.

25. Packer M, Coats AJ, Fowler MB, et al. Effect of carvedilol on survival in severe chronic heart failure. N Engl J Med. 2001;344: 1651-1658.

26. Pfeffer MA, McMurray JJ, Velazquez EJ, et al. Valsartan, captopril, or both in myocardial infarction complicated by heart failure, left ventricular dysfunction, or both. N Engl J Med. 2003;349: 1893-1906.

27. Flather MD, Shibata MC, Coats AJ, et al. Randomized trial to determine the effect of nebivolol on mortality and cardiovascular hospital admission in elderly patients with heart failure (SENIORS). Eur Heart J. 2005;26:215-225.

28. Fonarow GC, Yancy CW, Heywood JT. Adherence to heart failure quality-of-care indicators in US hospitals: Analysis of the ADHERE Registry. Arch Intern Med. 2005;165:1469-1477.

29. Gheorghiade M, Abraham WT, Albert NM, et al. Systolic blood pressure at admission, clinical characteristics, and outcomes in patients hospitalized with acute heart failure. JAMA. 2006;296: 2217-2226.

30. Garg R, Yusuf S. Overview of randomized trials of angiotensin-converting enzyme inhibitors on mortality and morbidity in patients with heart failure. Collaborative Group on ACE Inhibitor Trials. JAMA. 1995;273:1450-1456.

31. Massie BM, Armstrong PW, Cleland JG, et al. Toleration of high doses of angiotensin-converting enzyme inhibitors in patients with chronic heart failure: Results from the ATLAS trial. The Assessment of Treatment with Lisinopril and Survival. Arch Intern Med. 2001; 161:165-171.

32. Cohn JN, Tognoni G. A randomized trial of the angiotensin-receptor blocker valsartan in chronic heart failure. N Engl J Med. 2001;345:1667-1675.

33. Crozier I, Ikram H, Awan N, et al. Losartan in heart failure. Hemodynamic effects and tolerability. Losartan Hemodynamic Study Group. Circulation. 1995;91:691-697.

34. Gottlieb SS, Dickstein K, Fleck E, et al. Hemodynamic and neurohormonal effects of the angiotensin II antagonist losartan in patients with congestive heart failure. Circulation. 1993;88:1602-1609.

35. Mazayev VP, Fomina IG, Kazakov EN, et al. Valsartan in heart failure patients previously untreated with an ACE inhibitor. *Int J Cardiol.* 1998;65:239-246.

36. McKelvie RS, Yusuf S, Pericak D, et al. Comparison of candesartan, enalapril, and their combination in congestive heart failure: Randomized evaluation of strategies for left ventricular dysfunction (RESOLVD) pilot study. The RESOLVD Pilot Study Investigators. *Circulation.* 1999;100:1056-1064.

37. Riegger GA, Bouzo H, Petr P, et al. Improvement in exercise tolerance and symptoms of congestive heart failure during treatment with candesartan cilexetil. Symptom, Tolerability, Response to Exercise Trial of Candesartan Cilexetil in Heart Failure (STRETCH) Investigators. *Circulation.* 1999;100:2224-2230.

38. Sharma D, Buyse M, Pitt B, Rucinska EJ. Meta-analysis of observed mortality data from all-controlled, double-blind, multiple-dose studies of losartan in heart failure. Losartan Heart Failure Mortality Meta-analysis Study Group. *Am J Cardiol.* 2000;85:187-192.

39. Barr CS, Lang CC, Hanson J, et al. Effects of adding spironolactone to an angiotensin-converting enzyme inhibitor in chronic congestive heart failure secondary to coronary artery disease. *Am J Cardiol.* 1995;76:1259-1265.

40. Duprez DA, De Buyzere ML, Rietzschel ER, et al. Inverse relationship between aldosterone and large artery compliance in chronically treated heart failure patients. *Eur Heart J.* 1998;19:1371-1376.

41. Hensen J, Abraham WT, Durr JA, Schrier RW. Aldosterone in congestive heart failure: Analysis of determinants and role in sodium retention. *Am J Nephrol.* 1991;11:441-446.

42. MacFadyen RJ, Barr CS, Struthers AD. Aldosterone blockade reduces vascular collagen turnover, improves heart rate variability and reduces early morning rise in heart rate in heart failure patients. *Cardiovasc Res.* 1997;35:30-34.

43. Rocha R, Chander PN, Khanna K, et al. Mineralocorticoid blockade reduces vascular injury in stroke-prone hypertensive rats. *Hypertension.* 1998;31:451-458.

44. Struthers AD. Aldosterone escape during angiotensin-converting enzyme inhibitor therapy in chronic heart failure. *J Card Fail.* 1996;2:47-54.

45. Pitt B, Zannad F, Remme WJ, et al. The effect of spironolactone on morbidity and mortality in patients with severe heart failure. Randomized Aldactone Evaluation Study Investigators. *N Engl J Med.* 1999;341:709-717.

46. Pitt B, Williams G, Remme W, et al. The EPHESUS trial: Eplerenone in patients with heart failure due to systolic dysfunction complicating acute myocardial infarction. Eplerenone Post-AMI Heart Failure Efficacy and Survival Study. *Cardiovasc Drugs Ther.* 2001;15:79-87.

47. The Digitalis Investigation Group. The effect of digoxin on mortality and morbidity in patients with heart failure. *N Engl J Med.* 1997;336:525-533.

48. Jelliffe RW, Brooker G. A nomogram for digoxin therapy. *Am J Med.* 1974;57:63-68.

49. Fogelman AM, La Mont JT, Finkelstein S, et al. Fallibility of plasma-digoxin in differentiating toxic from non-toxic patients. *Lancet.* 1971;2:727-729.

50. Hernandez AF, Fonarow GC, Hammill BG, et al. Clinical effectiveness of implantable cardioverter-defibrillators among medicare beneficiaries with heart failure. *Circ Heart Fail.*3:7-13.

51. Yancy CW, Lopatin M, Stevenson LW, et al. Clinical presentation, management, and in-hospital outcomes of patients admitted with acute decompensated heart failure with preserved systolic function: A report from the Acute Decompensated Heart Failure National Registry (ADHERE) Database. *J Am Coll Cardiol.* 2006;47:76-84.

52. Fonarow GC, Abraham WT, Albert NM, et al. Factors identified as precipitating hospital admissions for heart failure and clinical outcomes: Findings from OPTIMIZE-HF. *Arch Intern Med.* 2008; 168:847-854.

53. Desai A, Fang JC. Heart failure with preserved ejection fraction: Hypertension, diabetes, obesity/sleep apnea, and hypertrophic and infiltrative cardiomyopathy. *Heart Fail Clin.* 2008;4:87-97.

54. Tsang TS, Gersh BJ, Appleton CP, et al. Left ventricular diastolic dysfunction as a predictor of the first diagnosed nonvalvular atrial fibrillation in 840 elderly men and women. *J Am Coll Cardiol.* 2002;40:1636-1644.

55. Paulus WJ, van Ballegooij JJ. Treatment of heart failure with normal ejection fraction: An inconvenient truth! *J Am Coll Cardiol.* 2010; 55:526-537.

56. Munagala VK, Burnett JC Jr, Redfield MM. The natriuretic peptides in cardiovascular medicine. *Curr Probl Cardiol.* 2004;29:707-769.

57. Cleland JG, Tendera M, Adamus J, et al. The perindopril in elderly people with chronic heart failure (PEP-CHF) study. *Eur Heart J.* 2006;27:2338-2345.

58. Yusuf S, Pfeffer MA, Swedberg K, et al. Effects of candesartan in patients with chronic heart failure and preserved left-ventricular ejection fraction: The CHARM-Preserved Trial. *Lancet.* 2003;362: 777-781.

59. Massie BM, Carson PE, McMurray JJ, et al. Irbesartan in patients with heart failure and preserved ejection fraction. *N Engl J Med.* 2008;359:2456-2467.

60. Ahmed A, Rich MW, Fleg JL, et al. Effects of digoxin on morbidity and mortality in diastolic heart failure: The ancillary digitalis investigation group trial. *Circulation.* 2006;114:397-403.

POST-TEST

1. **Which of the following statements is TRUE concerning initiation of BB and/or ACEI therapy after myocardial infarction?**

   A. It is appropriate to start ACEI and BB therapy in the outpatient setting when the patient is more stable.

   B. The risk of adverse drug effects of ACEIs or BBs, particularly in elderly patients with borderline or low blood pressure, outweighs their long-term clinical benefit.

   C. In patients with heart failure during myocardial infarction, there is no benefit to adding BBs once they are stable and euvolemic due to the possible precipitation of heart failure.

   D. Initiation of a low-dose BB after the patient has demonstrated tolerance to ACEI therapy reduces morbidity and mortality in patients with myocardial infarction complicated by heart failure.

2. **What is the appropriate next step in the management in a patient with stage 3, class D CHF on a low-dose ACEI and BB as well as a statin and diuretic who complains of an intermittent dry cough that can occur any time day or night?**

   A. Continue up-titration of the BB and ACEI, since these are both at low doses, and schedule a follow-up visit in 2 weeks.

   B. Check renal function parameters and potassium level, and if they are good, increase the ACEI dose at the next visit.

   C. Stop the ACEI and substitute an angiotensin receptor blocker (ARB).

   D. Add Robitussin prn.

3. **Mr. Jones is a 74-year-old patient with reduced EF heart failure who has been well managed on an ACEI, BB, statin, and medium-dose diuretic with a potassium level of 3.9 mEq/L (3.9 mmol/L). He was recently hospitalized for decompensated heart failure after perhaps increasing his sodium intake at a few holiday parties. What do you recommend now?**

   A. Increase the furosemide, as he appears to be volume overloaded.

   B. Add digoxin for inotropic support.

   C. Add an aldosterone inhibitor at low dose.

   D. Decrease the carvedilol dose, as this may be the cause of his fatigue.

Bonus: Is Mr. C. in Case Presentation 1 a candidate for implantation of an ICD? (Yes or No)

ANSWERS TO PRE-TEST

1. C
2. B
3. C

ANSWERS TO POST-TEST

1. D
2. C
3. C; Yes

44

Stroke

Mel L. Anderson III, MD

Jeffrey I. Wallace, MD, MPH

● **LEARNING OBJECTIVES**

1. Describe an appropriate initial evaluation and risk stratification for a patient presenting with a transient ischemic attack (TIA).
2. Describe time-course requirements for evaluation and interventions for a new TIA or small stroke.
3. Discuss the determination for appropriate thrombolytic therapy.
4. Compare and contrast choices for antiplatelet therapy after TIA or stroke.
5. Explain options for symptomatic carotid stenosis and the counsel of patients regarding revascularization.

PRE-TEST

1. **Which of the following statements about strokes is TRUE?**
   A. Stroke is most common cause of disability in the United States and Europe.
   B. Most strokes originate from cardiac sources.
   C. Anterior circulation strokes usually affect cranial nerves.
   D. The majority of strokes are hemorrhagic in nature.

2. **Which of the following statements BEST describes intravenous thrombolytic therapy for acute stroke?**
   A. Lytics reduce stroke mortality.
   B. Lytics can improve neurologic outcomes.
   C. Intracranial hemorrhage is a relative contraindication to lytics.
   D. Elderly patients are well represented in lytic trials.

3. **Which of the following has the GREATEST impact on reducing stroke risk?**
   A. Statin therapy
   B. Antiplatelet therapy
   C. Treatment of hypertension
   D. Increased physical activity

4. **Which of the following statements about carotid artery stenosis and carotid endarterectomy (CEA) is TRUE?**
   A. CEA is indicated only for patients with greater than 70% stenosis in the presence of stroke or TIA symptoms.
   B. CEA is less effective in elderly patients.
   C. CEA should be completed within 2 weeks of the TIA incident.
   D. CEA should be delayed until a second TIA occurs.

CASE PRESENTATION: MR. W.F.

W.F. is an 81-year-old male patient with a history of peripheral vascular disease with stable claudication, hyperlipidemia, hypertension, mild cognitive impairment, and gout. His medications include daily aspirin 81 mg, lisinopril 10 mg, atorvastatin 20 mg, and allopurinol 300 mg. He has never had neurologic symptoms until this morning, when his spouse called your clinic relating that her husband had acute onset of difficulty expressing himself and some right arm weakness. You directed her to call 911, and the patient arrived at the emergency department within 45 minutes of the onset of his symptoms. In the emergency room his blood pressure is 172/98 and pulse is 88 and regular. His neurologic exam is notable for expressive aphasia and mild weakness of the right side of the face and right arm. On cardiovascular exam he has an S4 gallop and dorsalis pedis pulses are diminished bilaterally. Electrocardiogram shows normal sinus rhythm. A complete blood count and metabolic panel including serum glucose are normal. His spouse anxiously inquires about further tests and what can be done to help resolve his symptoms.

BACKGROUND

Stroke is the number one cause of disability and the third most frequent cause of death in the United States. In the United States, there are over 750,000 new strokes a year, 250,000 to 350,000 transient ischemic attacks (TIAs, defined as a brief episode of neurologic dysfunction resulting from focal temporary cerebral ischemia not associated with cerebral infarction), and 4 million stroke survivors. About 15% of strokes are hemorrhagic and 85% are ischemic in etiology. Atherosclerotic vascular disease is the leading cause of ischemic stroke, especially among those over age 65.[1] Ischemic strokes may be thrombotic or embolic in origin, and the latter may emanate from cardiac, aortic, or carotid artery sources. Embolic strokes usually have abrupt onset with maximal deficits at the start whereas the course of thrombotic strokes may be more stuttering in nature. In terms of distribution, the middle cerebral artery (MCA) is the most commonly affected by TIAs and strokes. Strokes in the MCA *distribution* lead to neurologic deficits affecting the face and arm more than the leg. Aphasia may also be present when the dominant side is affected and neglect is a characteristic feature when the non-dominant MCA is affected. Clues to strokes in the *anterior cerebral artery distribution* include leg/foot being affected more than arm or face as well as personality change and/or frontal release signs (grasp, sucking reflexes). Cranial nerve deficits, diplopia, dysarthria, vertigo, ataxia, and/or decreased level of consciousness are suggestive of *vertebrobasilar pathology*. Small artery (lacunar) infarcts involve penetrating vessels and often result in pure motor or pure sensory deficits. Most patients with lacunar infarcts have risk factors for penetrating artery disease (eg, hypertension and/or diabetes).

This patient's difficulty with speech along with arm and facial weakness indicate a dominant MCA distribution event. As is often the case, initial medical contact was made by a family member and the call went to the physician's office rather than to emergency medical service providers.[2] Pre-hospital time accounts for the majority of delay before stroke treatment, and the interval from symptom onset to first call for medical help is the predominant part of pre-hospital delay. Efforts to improve public awareness include the "time is brain" and "brain attack" concepts to highlight that stroke should be considered a medical emergency. Also of note, this patient had multiple risk factors for stroke and evidence suggests that assessment of stroke risk using predictive models derived from Framingham stroke risk factors may increase awareness and impact provider and patient behavior to more effectively lower stroke risk.[3,4]

INITIAL EVALUATION/CONSIDERATIONS FOR THROMBOLYTICS

The initial evaluation of the patient with suspected acute stroke should focus on three items:

- Ruling out other conditions that mimic acute stroke
- Determining the onset of symptoms and whether the patient might be a candidate for thrombolysis
- Performing brain imaging to exclude intracranial hemorrhage or alternate diagnoses, and to assess for early signs of infarction

The history and physical examination should confirm the presence of focal neurologic signs and symptoms. The National Institutes of Health Stroke Scale (NIHSS) or another standardized assessment tool should be readily available and completed on all patients with acute stroke to assist with diagnosis and to objectively assess stroke severity (http://www.ninds.nih.gov/doctors/NIH_Stroke_Scale.pdf). Measurable deficits on NIHSS scores were used as inclusion criteria among clinical trials, with high scores (> 20) predicting poorer clinical outcomes and higher rates of intracranial bleeding. Three items on this scale provide the greatest positive predictive value for the presence of acute stroke: acute facial paresis, arm drift, and abnormal speech.[5] Several conditions can mimic acute stroke: brain tumors, subdural hematomas, unrecognized seizures, and toxic and metabolic confusional states—especially hypoglycemia.[6] These conditions are typically readily detected with routine laboratory testing (Table 44–1).

In one series of 336 patients presenting with suspected acute stroke, 31% were found to have stroke mimics.[7] The presence of cognitive impairment and abnormal signs in a non-neurologic system suggested a stroke mimic. Several items suggested the presence of acute stroke:

- Having an exact time of symptom(s) onset
- Presence of focal neurologic symptoms and/or signs
- Patient's symptoms lateralize to the left or right side of the brain

TABLE 44–1 Initial Diagnostic Studies of Patients with Suspected Acute Ischemic Stroke

All Patients

Neuroimaging with non-enhanced CT or MRI

12-lead EKG

Blood glucose

Serum electrolytes and creatinine

CBC including platelet count

Prothrombin time/international normalized ratio

Partial thromboplastin time

Selected Patients

Hepatic function tests

Toxicology screening including blood alcohol

Pregnancy testing

Pulse oximetry or arterial blood gas testing if hypoxia suspected

Chest radiography if lung disease suspected

Lumbar puncture if subarachnoid hemorrhage suspected and CT negative

Electroencephalography if seizures suspected

From Adams et al.[19]

- Being able to subclassify the type of stroke
- Having abnormal vascular findings on brain imaging

This same group studied the reliability of stroke history and physical examination findings between paired observers. They found that, while most items had moderate to good interobserver reliability, there was only 45% agreement for the hour and minute of symptom onset. Knowledge of these data should inform clinicians about the potential fallibility of their exams, the importance of considering multiple aspects of the history and physical exam in arriving at a correct diagnosis, and even the importance of further neurologic training for physicians treating acute stroke patients.[8]

Determining the onset of acute ischemic stroke symptoms is a crucial step in determining whether thrombolytic therapy is indicated. By convention, the last time at which neurologic function was clearly normal is the time from which onset is measured, although newer observational data suggest that "wake-up stroke" may be safely treated with thrombolytics.[9] Until wake-up stroke treatment is studied in prospective trials, clinicians should use the last time of normal neurologic function prior to going to sleep to calculate the duration of symptoms. Thrombolytics are FDA approved for use within 3 hours of the onset of symptoms, with even greater benefit among patients treated within the first 90 minutes of symptoms.[10] As in the case of acute myocardial infarction, time is of the essence: during each minute of ischemic stroke, 1.9 million neurons—7.5 miles of myelinated fibers—are destroyed.[11] The acute ischemic brain ages 3.6 years for every hour without treatment, compared with usual age-related neuronal loss. Recently, the ECASS 3 trial confirmed the benefit of lytic therapy for acute ischemic stroke up to 4.5 hours.[12] The American Heart Association and American Stroke Association published a joint Scientific Advisory recommending that the FDA extend the approved lytic time window to 4.5 hours.[13]

Emergent performance of brain imaging, usually with noncontrast computed tomography or magnetic resonance imaging, is the final necessary step of the initial evaluation. The scan should be reviewed for evidence of intracranial hemorrhage and for signs of alternate diagnoses, such as a neoplasm. The scan should be interpreted by a clinician skilled in neuroimaging assessment and formally evaluated for the presence of high-risk features, especially acute ischemic changes involving greater than one-third of the middle cerebral artery (MCA) territory.[14]

Thrombolytic trials all excluded patients with intracranial hemorrhage. The ATLANTIS study also excluded those patients with CT involvement of more than one-third of the MCA territory, loss of gray-white matter distinction and/or sulcal effacement, and patients with evidence of midline shift/mass effect.[15] The NINDS study only excluded those patients with evidence of hemorrhage. The ECASS studies excluded patients with hemorrhage and/or involvement (either hypodensity or swelling) of more than one-third of the MCA territory.[12,16] Newer trials have used magnetic resonance imaging (MRI) to select patients who may benefit from thrombolytic therapy up to 6[17] or even 9 hours[18] from the onset of symptoms. Until the MRI imaging techniques used in these trials have been further validated, the 3-hour time window is still the most universally recommended.[19]

Whether to Provide Thrombolysis

Benefits

Pooled analysis of the major recombinant tissue plasminogen activator (rt-PA) trials (NINDS, ATLANTIS, and ECASS II) showed an improvement in 3-month favorable outcome, defined as alive and with minimal disability.[10] Improvements in formal stroke scale scores provided the main measure of thrombolytic effect. As the ECASS II trial included treatment up to 6 hours from the onset of symptoms, the pooled results in this analysis are reported from 0 to 360 minutes from the onset of symptoms. Looking only at patients treated within 180 minutes across these three trials, mortality rates at 90 days were the same between treatment and placebo. There was an overall increase in favorable outcome at 3 months from 12.7% with placebo to 18% with rt-PA, an absolute increase of 5.3% (number needed to treat [NNT] was 19 for 1 favorable outcome at 90 days). Intracranial hemorrhage occurred in 0.65% of placebo-treated patients and in 4.75% of treatment patients (number needed to harm was 24 for 1 intracranial hemorrhage). More than half of the patients suffering significant intracranial hemorrhage died. In short, the current evidence shows that intravenous thrombolysis with rt-PA significantly improves the level of function at 3 months but does not offer a net mortality benefit.

Risks

Intracranial hemorrhage is the primary risk and is well documented in the prospective literature. The risk of treatment related intracranial hemorrhage increases with the time from symptom onset, patient age, the presence of significant hypertension, the extent of infarction on CT, the degree of neurologic impairment as measured by the NIHSS score, and the type and route of thrombolytic agent used. While the USFDA approved the use of rt-PA for acute ischemic stroke in 1996, its use was not approved in Canada until 1999, in Germany until 2000, and in member states of the European Agency for the Evaluation of Medicinal Products (EMEA) until 2002. The EMEA stipulates that rt-PA treatment is limited to patients treated within 3 hours of the onset of symptoms, age < 80 years old, no prior stroke or history of diabetes, no signs of extensive infarction on CT, NIHSS score < 25, documented informed consent, and entrance of presenting data and outcomes into a safety registry—the Safe Implementation of Thrombolysis in Stroke: A Multinational, Multicenter Monitoring Study of Safety and Efficacy of Thrombolysis in Stroke (SITS-MOST).[20] These constraints illustrate the caution that is proper with the use of thrombolytics.

Decision-Making

Rapid, thoughtful assessment of the risks and benefits of thrombolytic therapy is essential. Intravenous thrombolytic therapy is indicated for acute ischemic stroke in patients presenting up to 4.5 hours of the onset of symptoms, having a measurable deficit on an objective stroke scale and whose symptoms are not spontaneously clearing. Major neurologic deficits, suppression in the level of consciousness, and high scores on the NIHSS scale (eg, > 20) should caution against the use of thrombolytics. Advancing age has been associated with increased risk of in-hospital death, in particular with patients ≥ 75 years old.[21] A careful systematic review of patients over age 80 in thrombolytic studies concluded that, while absolute rates of intracranial hemorrhage were higher, there was still benefit in treating patients of this age.[22] The margins of risk and benefit are narrower, and informed consent of even greater importance for this reason. Thrombolytics should not be used in patients with marked hypertension (SBP ≥ 185 mm Hg, DBP ≥ 110 mm Hg), hypoglycemia (< 50 mg/dL), hyperglycemia (> 400 mg/dL), or other standard contraindications (Table 44–2).

Hypertension should be treated cautiously and according to a defined protocol. If the patient is not felt to be a candidate for thrombolytic therapy during the acute phase of an ischemic stroke, antihypertensives are generally not instituted for elevated blood pressure unless systolic blood pressure exceeds 220 mm Hg or diastolic pressure exceeds 120, or end-organ effects are present (eg, aortic dissection, myocardial infarction). The presence of extensive infarction by neuroimaging should caution against the use of thrombolytics, as the risk of hemorrhagic transformation is greater.[14,19] Intravenous rt-PA should be administered only after clinical, radiographic, and laboratory assessment has been completed. Patients taking oral anticoagulants or with liver disease can be treated if the International Normalized Ratio is ≤ 1.7; it is acceptable to begin thrombolytics prior to the results of coagulation testing in those patients who are not taking anticoagulants and in whom there is not a clinical suspicion of coagulopathy. Written informed consent is not required by the FDA; clearly, though, the patient and/or family should understand the risks and benefits of treatment.

● **TABLE 44–2** Features of Patients with Ischemic Stroke Who Could Be Candidates for Thrombolytics

Diagnosis of ischemic stroke causing measurable neurologic deficit on stroke scale

Neurologic deficits should not be clearing spontaneously

Neurologic deficits should not be minor and isolated

Caution should be exercised in treating patients with major deficits (eg, NIHSS score > 20)

Stroke symptoms not suggestive of subarachnoid hemorrhage (thunderclap headache)

Onset of symptoms < 3 hours before beginning treatment (with data supporting 4.5 hours)

In the previous 3 months, no head trauma, prior stroke, or myocardial infarction

In the previous 21 days, no gastrointestinal or urologic hemorrhage

In the previous 14 days, no major surgery

In the previous 7 days, no arterial puncture in a noncompressible site

No prior history of intracranial hemorrhage

Systolic blood pressure < 185 mm Hg and diastolic blood pressure < 110 mm Hg

No other signs of active bleeding or acute trauma (eg, fracture) on examination

Not taking oral anticoagulants, or if taking oral anticoagulants, INR < 1.7

If receiving heparin in the previous 48 hours, aPTT must be in the normal range

Platelet count > 100,000 mm[3]

Blood glucose ≥ 50 mg/dL

No seizure with post-ictal residual neurologic impairment

CT does not show multilobar infarction (hypodensity > 1/3 cerebral hemisphere)

Patient and family understand potential risks and benefits

From Adams et al.[19]

CASE PRESENTATION (continued)

A stroke alert is called and the patient is sent for a stat head CT scan, which shows no acute lesions and no evidence of hemorrhage. The stroke team discusses the possibility of thrombolytic therapy with the patient and his spouse. However, between 90 and 120 minutes after onset of symptoms your patient's weakness seems to be improving although he is still having trouble expressing himself. He and his wife are concerned about potential bleeding risk with thrombolytic therapy and the stroke team is encouraged by the slight clinical improvement, and the decision is made to observe without thrombolytic therapy. Over the next few hours he continues to improve. He is now able to express himself more clearly and asks what the next steps should be.

● INITIAL EVALUATION

Patients with suspected TIA or minor stroke require urgent evaluation due to a high initial stroke risk associated with TIA. Meta-analyses have suggested stroke rates of 4% to 10% in the first 48 hours after a TIA, 8% to 13% at 30 days, and 9% to 17% at 90 days.[23] TIAs associated with evidence of infarction by neuroimaging or that have large artery atherosclerosis etiologies appear to be at particularly higher risk for subsequent stroke. Further evaluation of the patient presenting with a transient ischemic attack (TIA) should focus on a few key areas:

- Observing for recurrent stroke symptoms and the need for acute thrombolytic therapy
- Identifying treatable causes of TIA and stroke
- Achieving carotid revascularization, when indicated, within 2 weeks of presentation
- Initiating evidence-based secondary prevention measures

The ABCD scoring system (Age, Blood pressure, Clinical features, Duration of symptoms) was derived and validated as part of the Oxford Vascular Study, and has served as the basis for TIA risk stratification since that time, with modifications since the initial publication.[24] This 6-point score was highly predictive of subsequent stroke (Age [> 60 years = 1], Blood pressure [systolic $\geq$ 140 mm Hg and/or diastolic blood pressure $\geq$ 90 mm Hg = 1], Clinical features [unilateral weakness = 2, speech disturbance without weakness = 1, other = 0], and Duration of symptoms in minutes [$\geq$ 60 = 2, 10-59 = 1, < 10 = 0]).

Since initial publication, the ABCD scoring system has been validated in several other patient cohorts.[25] More recently, a direct comparison of the California and ABCD scoring systems has led to a modification to ABCD, known as ABCD-2 (or ABCD^2; Table 44–3).[26] The new 7-point scoring system adds diabetes mellitus as an additional risk factor (Age, Blood pressure, Clinical features, Duration of symptoms, Diabetes). Recent guidelines recommend inpatient evaluation if a patient presents within 72 hours after onset of symptoms and the ABCD^2 score is 3 or higher, or if the ABCD^2 score is 0 to 2 but there is uncertainty about the ability to complete the diagnostic workup as an outpatient within 48 hours.[27]

● ADDITIONAL TESTING

Diagnostic recommendations include noninvasive imaging of the cervical vessels in patients who have had TIAs and indicate that noninvasive imaging of intracranial vessels is reasonable to detect atherosclerotic stenosis of the major intracranial arteries (middle cerebral artery, vertebral artery, and basilar artery), especially in blacks, Asians, and Hispanics, who have a higher prevalence of such lesions. The 2009 AHA/ASA guidelines suggest that echocardiography is reasonable when embolic stroke is suspected or no cause has been identified by other aspects of the workup and recommend cardiac monitoring with inpatient telemetry or Holter monitor to exclude atrial fibrillation in the setting of embolic TIA or stroke or for patients without a clear etiology after initial evaluation.[27] Arguments that favor hospitalization include that inpatient status allows earlier use of thrombolytics or other interventions if symptoms recur, expedited evaluation, and earlier institution of secondary prevention measures. Regardless of whether the patient is hospitalized or not, urgent assessment and management is vital as a growing body of evidence suggests that prompt evaluation and intervention can help prevent a significant number of strokes among high-risk patients.

The benefits of rapid assessment and intervention after TIA have been studied virtually and then in patient cohorts. A computer modeling study performed in 2002 concluded that an 80% to 90% reduction in stroke risk might be achieved if all these measures were undertaken rapidly and simultaneously.[28] Based upon these data, a prospective trial was conducted within the Oxford Vascular Study to determine the effect of rapid stroke risk assessment and intervention in TIA patients (EXPRESS study).[29] The intervention was deceptively simple: the investigators changed the scheduling for their local daily TIA referral clinic from appointment-based to same-day walk-in. Primary physicians received no other instruction than to send their patients (those who they were not admitting to a hospital) directly to the referral clinic rather than calling or faxing to arrange an appointment. The average time to being seen in the TIA clinic decreased from an average of 3 days to 1 day, with a significant decrease in the average time to prescriptions being filled. The results of this intervention were profound: at 1 month follow-up, the rates of clopidogrel and statin use, blood pressure control, and rates of carotid endarterectomy were all significantly improved Table 44–4). After the intervention, two-thirds of patients who needed carotid endarterectomy had it performed within 30 days, compared to only 12% prior to the intervention. The 90-day risk of recurrent stroke was 10.3% prior to the intervention, decreasing to 2.1% after the intervention (Odds ratio for stroke 0.20, 95% C.I. 0.08-0.49, p = 0.0001). Follow-up investigation shows that this intervention reduced subsequent hospital bed-days, acute costs, and 6-month disability.[30]

● **TABLE 44–3** ABCD Scoring

Factor	Points
Age	
$\geq$ 60 years	1
< 60 years	0
Blood pressure when first assessed after TIA	
Systolic $\geq$ 140 mm Hg or diastolic $\geq$ 90 mm Hg	1
Systolic < 140 mm Hg and diastolic < 90 mm Hg	0
Clinical Features	
Unilateral weakness	2
Isolated speech disturbance	1
Other	0
Duration of TIA symptoms	
$\geq$ 60 minutes	2
10-59 minutes	1
< 10 minutes	0
Diabetes	
Present	1
Absent	0
48-hour stroke risk estimate based on score	
Score 6 to 7: High 2-day risk (8.1%)	
Score 4 to 5: Moderate 2-day risk (4.1%)	
Score 0 to 3: Low 2-day stroke risk (1.0 %)	

From Johnston et al.[26]

● **TABLE 44-4** 30-Day Process of Care Endpoints in the EXPRESS Study

	Pre-Intervention	Post-Intervention	*p* Value
On antiplatelet or anticoagulant agent	292(97%)	269(97%)	1.00
On aspirin and 30-day course clopidogrel	26(10%)	137(49%)	<0.0001
On a statin	187(62%)	233(84%)	<0.0001
On one or more BP-lowering drugs	187(62%)	231(83%)	<0.0001
On two or more BP-lowering drugs	103(34%)	168(60%)	<0.0001
Average systolic blood pressure	142 mm Hg	136 mm Hg	<0.0019
Average diastolic blood pressure	80 mm Hg	76 mm Hg	<0.0001
Time to carotid surgery	n = 17	n = 15	
<7 days	0 (0%)	6(40%)	0.006
<30 days	2(12%)	10(67%)	0.001

From Rothwell et al.[29]

CASE PRESENTATION (continued)

The patient had an ABCD[2] score of 5 (age, blood pressure, unilateral weakness, and duration 10-59 minutes) and was admitted to the hospital for further evaluation. The patient's aphasia and right arm weakness completely resolved by mid-afternoon. By the next afternoon all diagnostic studies had been completed. Blood work remained unremarkable. The patient's LDL and HDL cholesterol were 86 mg/dl (2.23 mmol/L) and 38 mg/dl (0.98 mmol/L), respectively. An echocardiogram with bubble study found mild LVH, normal systolic function without any wall motion abnormalities, and no evidence of a right-to-left shunt. A carotid ultrasound study found 80% to 90% stenosis at the left carotid bifurcation and 50% to 60% stenosis of the right carotid artery. Subsequently a CT angiogram confirmed these findings. A care conference was arranged with the vascular surgeon, neurologist, and the patient's primary care provider to review intervention options with the patient and his family. At this point he was no longer a candidate for rt-PA, but there were a number of options including increasing his aspirin dosage to 325 mg per day, adding an antiplatelet agent such as clopidogrel, improving his blood pressure control, and consideration for a carotid endarterectomy. His primary care doctor thought that improvement in his medical management would substantially reduce his risk of recurrent stroke without subjecting him to the risks of surgery. The vascular surgeon of course argued for rapid intervention with a carotid endarterectomy. The neurologist thought both options were viable and suggested that either course would be reasonable.

● MEDICAL MANAGEMENT

Atherosclerotic vascular disease is the leading cause of ischemic stroke, especially among those over age 65.[1] Prevention of recurrent stroke involves controlling the factors that promote atherosclerosis, including diabetes, high blood pressure, hyperlipidemia, and smoking. Hypertension is the most important modifiable factor and is addressed briefly here and in Chapter 45. The remainder of this section then focuses primarily on antiplatelet therapy to prevent recurrent stroke (secondary prevention), with brief mention of the role of anticoagulation and of statin therapy to reduce stroke risk.

Hypertension

A large number of randomized trials have conclusively demonstrated the importance and efficacy of antihypertensive therapy for both the primary and secondary prevention of stroke. A meta-analysis of over 40 randomized controlled trials found that a 10 mm Hg reduction in systolic BP reduces stroke risk by about one-third, and cohort studies in persons age 60 to 79 suggest that this decrement in stroke risk is continuous for each 10 mm Hg reduction in systolic blood pressure down to levels of at least 115/75 mm Hg.[31] While the proportional association noted in this meta-analysis is age dependent, many other studies have demonstrated that the benefit of treating hypertension on stroke reduction persists and is strong in persons age 80 and over. These findings have been consistent across gender, regions, and for all stroke subtypes. Although clinical trials have tested and compared many antihypertensive agents, both singly and in combination, the optimal medical regimen for managing hypertension after stroke has not yet been established. While recent guidelines suggest that a thiazide diuretic or the combination of a diuretic and an ACE inhibitor may be the most appropriate initial antihypertensive choices for prevention of recurrent stroke, clinicians must also take concomitant disease into account (eg, renal or heart disease, diabetes mellitus) when selecting therapeutic antihypertensive regimens.[1] At this time current evidence indicates that effective lowering of blood pressure is more important than which agents are used to achieve that goal.

Antiplatelet Agents

Antiplatelet medications are the preferred choice for preventing ischemic events among persons who have symptomatic atherosclerotic disease at any vascular site, including TIAs or strokes. Aspirin, the combination of aspirin with extended release dipyridamole (ASA-ERDP), and clopidogrel have been shown to provide effective secondary prevention for patients after ischemic stroke.

Aspirin

Aspirin, in dosages from 30 to 1300 mg/day, has been shown to protect patients from secondary ischemic events with estimates of risk reductions in major vascular events by 13% and decreased risk of ischemic stroke by up to 22% relative to placebo.[32] In ESPS2, aspirin 50 mg/d reduced stroke rates by 18% with an ARR of 2.9%.[33] Most studies have found that 50 to 325 mg/day of aspirin is as effective as higher doses. The Antithrombotic Trialists' Collaboration found that aspirin doses of 75 to 150 mg/day produced the same risk reduction in major vascular events as 150 to 325 mg/day doses, and did not find differences in efficacy between doses ≥ 75 mg/day or < 75 mg/day, although lower doses have not been as well studied. Because efficacy of reducing ischemic events appears similar within these dose ranges and because data support that lower doses of aspirin are associated with reduced rates of gastrointestinal side-effects and bleeding, recent expert panel guidelines suggest aspirin doses of 50 to 100 mg/day for the prevention of cerebrovascular events.[34]

Aspirin Combined with Extended-Release Dipyridamole (ASA-ERDP)

Dipyridamole impairs platelet function by inhibiting the activity of adenosine deaminase and phosphodiesterase. Dipyridamole may also cause vasodilation. Dipyridamole is currently available in an immediate-release form (given in doses of 50 to 100 mg three times per day) and a patent-protected formulation containing extended-release dipyridamole (ERDP) 200 mg and 25 mg aspirin, given two times per day. Two pivotal clinical trials, the European Stroke Prevention Study 2 (ESPS-2) and the European/Australasian Stroke Prevention in Reversible Ischemia Trial (ESPRIT), have established that a combination of aspirin and extended-release dipyridamole significantly reduces the risk of recurrent stroke relative to aspirin (in variable dose of 30-325 mg/day) alone.[35,36] The risk of bleeding was not increased with combination therapy relative to aspirin monotherapy in either the ESPS-2 or ESPRIT trials. Although concerns had been expressed that dipyridamole may unfavorably impact cardioprotection due to potential coronary artery vasodilating effects, no significant differences were seen in time to first cardiac event in these two trials. However, the combination

● **TABLE 44–5** American Heart Association/American Stroke Association Guidelines for Antithrombotic Therapy in Patients with Ischemic Stroke of Noncardioembolic Origin

Guideline	Recommendation, Level of Evidence[a]
Class I Recommendations	
Antiplatelet agents recommended over oral anticoagulants	I, A
For initial treatment, aspirin (50-325 mg/d), combination of aspirin and extended-release dipyridamole, or clopidogrel are acceptable options	I, A
Combination of aspirin and extended-release dipyridamole recommended over aspirin alone	I, B
Class II Recommendations	
Clopidogrel may be considered instead of aspirin alone	IIb, B
For patients hypersensitive to aspirin, clopidogrel is a reasonable choice	IIa, B
Class III Recommendations	
Addition of aspirin to clopidogrel increases risk of bleeding. Combination not recommended unless specific indication (ie, coronary stent)	III, A

[a]*Recommendation: I = treatment is useful and effective; IIa = conflicting evidence or divergence of opinion regarding treatment usefulness and effectiveness; IIb = usefulness/efficacy of treatment is less well established; III = treatment is not useful or effective. Level of evidence: A = data from randomized clinical trials; B = data from a single randomized clinical trial or nonrandomized studies. Data from European Stroke Organisation.*[2]

requires twice-daily dosing, is less well tolerated (34% discontinuation rates for combined therapy vs. 13% for aspirin alone, most often due to headache), and is markedly more expensive than aspirin. Further, the additional beneficial effects noted, although statistically significant, are modest: in the ESPRIT trial the RR reduction was 20%, ARR was 1%, and NNT 100. AHA/ASA and Chest guidelines indicate that ASA-ERDP combination therapy is a more effective first-line treatment after TIA or stroke (Table 44–5), but in practice many providers reserve this combination of drugs for patients who have had a TIA or stroke events while on aspirin (so-called "aspirin failures"). While the short-acting dipyridamole preparation is appealing from a cost perspective (generics are available), there is currently insufficient evidence to support its use.

Clopidogrel

Clopidogrel acts by inhibiting ADP-dependent platelet aggregation. Prior to the PRoFESS study, the main trial supporting the efficacy of clopidogrel 75 mg for secondary prevention of strokes was derived from the Clopidogrel Versus Aspirin in Patients at Risk of Ischemic Events (CAPRIE).[37] In this trial of 19,000 subjects clopidogrel significantly reduced the risk of major vascular events in patients with atherosclerotic vascular disease by 8.7% relative to aspirin, an ARR of 0.51% (NNT 196). However, when the analysis was restricted to the 6000 enrollees with prior ischemic stroke, the risk reduction was not statistically significant. No increased risk of bleeding was observed. In contrast, trials that combined clopidogrel with aspirin have found no increase in efficacy of preventing major vascular events but significant increases in bleeding risk.[38,39] For example, the effect of clopidogrel 75 mg with or without aspirin 75 mg on vascular end-points was evaluated in the Management of Atherothrombosis with Clopidogrel in High-Risk Patients with Recent TIA or Ischemic Stroke (MATCH) trial.[39] This study found clopidogrel plus aspirin was not more efficacious than clopidogrel monotherapy in lowering rates of recurrent ischemic events, and that combination therapy was associated with higher rates of bleeding. Although the MATCH trial had limitations (eg, over 50% of subjects had lacunar strokes, a stroke subtype associated with a low recurrence rate), recent guidelines generally recommend against long-term use of combination aspirin and clopidogrel.[34]

Clopidogrel versus ASA-ERDP versus ASA Monotherapy

Based on indirect comparisons, ASA-ERDP appeared to have greater efficacy than clopidogrel in reducing rates of vascular events in patients with TIAs or strokes, roughly 18% to 7% added benefit relative to aspirin alone. In an effort to clarify the relative efficacy of these two antiplatelet agents, the landmark PRoFESS trial compared ASA-ERDP 25 to 200 mg BID to clopidogrel 75 mg once daily in over 20,000 patients with recent noncardioembolic ischemic stroke.[40] Recurrent stroke rates were roughly 9% in each group and there were no major differences in other efficacy end-points (eg, MI or vascular death). Rather than rely solely on this direct comparison, the accompanying editorial added PRoFESS data to prior indirect comparison data and calculated RRRs of 0.83 for ASA-ERDP and 0.87 for clopidogrel relative to aspirin alone. However, whether compared to aspirin or to each other, none of these differences was statistically significant. Using an average annual vascular event rate of 6.5% (the average of the event rates of the CAPRIE, ESPS2, ESPRIT, and PRoFESS trials) these RR reductions would translate to ARR and NNTs of 1.1% and 91 for ASA-ERDP, and 0.85% and 118 for clopidogrel. In contrast, several other editorials opined that clopidogrel might reasonably be considered the preferred agent because when compared head to head to ASA-ERDP efficacy rates were similar, bleeding rates and discontinuation rates due to side-effects (mostly headache) were higher in the ASA-ERDP group, clopidogrel is a once a day drug, and although costs are currently similar clopidogrel will become a generic agent in 2011 while ASA-ERDP will not be generic until 2015.

Choosing Initial Therapy and Recurrent Events

When deciding between the three currently available antiplatelet options, clinicians and patients may consider these factors:

1. Predisposition to adverse effects such as bleeding. In the PRoFESS trial, ASA-ERDP was associated with higher bleed rates than clopidogrel (4.1 vs. 3.6%), although the net risk-benefit as measured by recurrent stroke or major hemorrhagic event was not significantly different between the two treatments.
2. Side effects. In clinical trials discontinuation rates of ASA-ERDP have been roughly 5% higher than for clopidogrel, mostly due to headaches.
3. Cost. Aspirin costs pennies a day, while both clopidogrel and ASA-ERDP cost around $160/month in the United States.
4. Compliance. Clopidogrel and aspirin are taken once daily while ASA-ERDP is taken twice daily. Current expert panel guidelines do not prioritize between initial choice of antiplatelet agents but have not yet been revised in light of the PRoFESS trial data.

The treatment of patients who have a recurrent vascular event on antiplatelet therapy remains unclear. Alternative causes of stroke should be sought and efforts to optimize risk-factor management are essential. Reasonable treatment strategies include no change in therapy, change to another antiplatelet agent, adding another antiplatelet agent, or using oral anticoagulation.[2]

Oral Anticoagulants

Oral anticoagulants are indicated when TIA or stroke events are attributable to cardioembolic sources (eg, atrial fibrillation, patent foramen ovale, other cardiac disorders). Oral anticoagulants may also have a role for patients with prothrombotic disorders. Several clinical trials have demonstrated that oral anticoagulants are not superior to antiplatelet agents in preventing recurrent ischemic stroke, and therefore there is currently no indication for use of oral anticoagulant therapy in patients with stroke secondary to atherosclerotic disease.[1]

Statin Therapy

A review of over 20 primary prevention statin trials found these agents reduced stroke incidence from 3.4% to 2.7%.[2] Several clinical trials have demonstrated the beneficial effects of statins on reducing the risk of recurrent cardiovascular events in patients who have had an ischemic stroke. Newer data suggest that this class of drugs is also likely indicated for recurrent stroke prevention. The Stroke Prevention by Aggressive Reduction in Cholesterol Levels (SPARCL) trial enrolled nearly 5000 subjects with a history of TIA or stroke and an LDL cholesterol level of 100 mg/dL (2.6 mmol/L) to 190 mg/dL (4.9 mmol/L).[41] The study found that relative to placebo, high-dose (80 mg) atorvastatin reduced the risk of recurrent stroke (ARR 2.2%, NNT 45.5) and major cardiovascular events (ARR 3.5%, NNT 28.6) over 5 years. Although the treatment groups did not differ in the incidence of serious adverse events, the atorvastatin treatment group experienced 55 hemorrhagic strokes compared to 33 in the placebo treatment group. While concerns have been raised that statins might increase the risk of hemorrhagic stroke, to date observed increases in studies have been minimal and it appears that the benefits of statins in preventing ischemic events far outweigh this potential risk. Recent guidelines from the AHA/ASA regarding secondary stroke prevention recommend the use of statins in all patients with atherosclerotic stroke or TIA to reduce the risk of recurrent stroke as well as other cardiovascular events.[38] Further, in patients with diabetes mellitus and recent stroke, the recommended target LDL-C level in these patients is less than 70 mg/dL (1.81 mmol/L). The patient in this case had an LDL-C of 86 (2.23 mmol/L) on atorvastatin 20 mg, and based on the data given and recommendations it would be reasonable to increase his atorvastatin dose.

● CAROTID STENOSIS

Carotid Endarterectomy

Carotid endarterectomy (CEA) is one of the best-studied surgical procedures, with multiple well-conducted prospective randomized trials demonstrating efficacy treating carotid stenosis. The North American Symptomatic Carotid Endarterectomy Trial (NASCET) was the major landmark study demonstrating the efficacy of intervention.[42] This trial of patients with symptomatic carotid stenosis across a broad range of severity was stopped early for those patients with "severe" stenosis, defined as 70% to 99% narrowing by conventional angiography. At 2 years, the rate of ipsilateral stroke or postoperative death in patients with severe stenosis decreased from 26% in the medical arm to 9% in the CEA arm (NNT 5.9). Patients with "moderate" stenosis (50-69% stenosis) were followed out to 5 years, at which point they had benefit over medical therapy alone.[43] Patients with less than 50% stenosis had no benefit from CEA. Of particular interest, patients aged 75 years or older actually had a greater absolute benefit with CEA compared to patients under age 75.[44]

The VA Cooperative Trial 309[45] and the European Carotid Stenosis Trial (ECST)[46] were combined with NASCET in a pooled analysis of over 6000 patients and about 35,000 patient-years of follow-up.[47] Among patients with 70% or greater stenosis, CEA reduced the absolute 5-year risk of ipsilateral ischemic stroke and any operative stroke or death by 16% (NNT 6.3). The benefit was less pronounced among patients with 50% to 69% stenosis, in whom CEA conferred a 4.6% absolute 5-year risk reduction (NNT 21.7; Table 44–6). The medical arms of these trials required only the use of aspirin. The current practices of intensive lipid control and tight glycemic and blood pressure control would probably reduce the rate of events in both medical and surgical arms. The 30-day postoperative stroke risk was between 6% and 7% across these trials. Referring clinicians should know the operative event rates of the surgeons to whom they are referring in order to intelligently balance risk and benefit. Patients operated on by surgeons with higher perioperative surgical risk outcomes may have risk in excess of benefit with CEA. Clinicians should also only refer those patients whose anticipated life expectancy is at least 2 years for those with 70% to 99% stenosis and at least 5 years for those with 50% to 69% stenosis.

● **TABLE 44–6** Number Needed to Treat to Prevent One Stroke per Year in Patients Who Undergo Surgery for Internal Carotid Artery Stenosis

Disease	NNT
Asymptomatic (6-99%)	85
Symptomatic (70-99%)	27
Symptomatic (50-69%)	75
Symptomatic (> 50%) in men	45
Symptomatic (> 50%) in women	180
Symptomatic (> 50%) > 75 years	25
Symptomatic (> 50%) < 65 years	90
Symptomatic (> 50%) < 2 weeks after the event	25
Symptomatic (> 50%) >12 weeks after the event	625
Symptomatic (≤ 50%)	No benefit

All percentages reflect the NASCET method of measuring stenosis severity.

Data from European Stroke Organisation.[2]

Carotid Angioplasty and Stenting

Carotid angioplasty and stenting (CAS) is increasingly used as an alternative to CEA among selected patients. Two procedural developments have improved the safety of percutaneous carotid revascularization. First, distal embolic protection filters deployed prior to angioplasty collect debris associated with the mechanical intervention and limit the risk of peri-procedural stroke. Second, the use of self-expanding stents has improved long-term patency over balloon-expanding stents, which can be damaged by neck movement and external pressure. The SAPPHIRE trial was a non-inferiority trial of Stenting and Angioplasty with distal embolic Protection in Patients at High Risk for Endarterectomy.[48] Inclusion criteria were symptomatic carotid stenosis of greater than 50% or asymptomatic stenosis greater than 80%. Patients had to have one of several high-risk features to be included (Table 44–7). The cumulative incidence of postoperative stroke, myocardial infarction, death, and ipsilateral stroke within 1 year after the procedure was 20.1% in the CEA arm and 12.2% in the CAS arm, $p = 0.004$ for non-inferiority and $p = 0.053$ for superiority. The rate of post-procedural cranial nerve injury was substantially lower (zero) in the CAS arm. However, among those

● **TABLE 44–7** High-Risk Criteria from the SAPPHIRE Trial

At least one factor required:

Age > 80 yr

Clinically significant cardiac disease (congestive heart failure, abnormal stress test, or need for open-heart surgery)

Severe pulmonary disease

Contralateral carotid occlusion

Contralateral laryngeal nerve palsy

Previous radical neck surgery or radiation therapy to the neck

Recurrent stenosis after prior endarterectomy

From Yadav et al.[48]

patients with *symptomatic* carotid stenosis, the cumulative incidence of the primary end-point was 16.8% in the CAS arm and 16.5% in the CEA arm. Based upon this trial, CAS has equivalent 1-year outcomes versus CEA in a high-risk population, primarily in asymptomatic individuals. These results remained consistent out to 3 years of follow-up.[49]

However, two newer trials of CAS versus CEA in lower-risk populations cast doubt on the overall safety of CAS among symptomatic patients. The SPACE trial (Stent-Protected Angioplasty versus Carotid Endarterectomy) randomized 1200 average-risk patients with symptomatic carotid stenosis of 50% or greater by angiography or 70% or greater by ultrasound to either CAS or CEA.[50] The trial design stipulated that both surgeons and percutaneous interventionalists perform at least 25 procedures prior to inclusion in the study, and that independent quality committees review these procedures. The use of distal embolic protection devices was left to the discretion of the operators. The 30-day rate of death or ipsilateral ischemic stroke was 6.34% in the CEA arm and 6.84% in the CAS arm, $p = 0.09$ for non-inferiority. The investigators concluded that CAS is not non-inferior to CEA—that is, that CAS is inferior. The EVA-3S trial (Endarterectomy Versus Angioplasty in Patients with Symptomatic Severe Carotid Stenosis) randomized 527 patients with symptomatic carotid stenosis of 70% or greater by angiography or Magnetic Resonance Angiography (MRA) to either CAS or CEA within 2 weeks of the index event.[51] This trial design also stipulated that surgeons had performed at least 25 CEAs in the prior year. Percutaneous interventionalists did not have similar numeric procedure requirements, although the investigators provided tutoring for less experienced operators. The trial was stopped prematurely due to futility (in terms of non-inferiority) and harm within the CAS arm. The 30-day cumulative incidence of death or any stroke was 3.9% in the CEA arm and 9.6% in the CAS arm, $p = 0.01$ for superiority of CEA. The trial was powered to detect only large differences among low- and high-volume operators. Importantly, nearly 10% of patients did not have distal embolic protection devices used during their CAS procedures. The CREST trial (Carotid Revascularization Endarterectomy vs. Stenting Trial) and ICSS trial (International Carotid Stenting Study) are major studies currently under way and should provide clearer guidance on the relative roles for CEA and CAS for symptomatic carotid stenosis. Until then, clinicians should consider CEA as the primary interventional treatment for symptomatic carotid stenosis, with CAS for those patients who are high-risk and in the hands of experienced operators.[52]

Accurate Diagnosis

Different trials used different criteria for defining the percent stenosis of the diseased carotid arterial segment. These differences were based primarily on the mode of testing—conventional angiography versus ultrasound, and on what portion of the carotid artery was used as the reference or baseline segment to calculate the percent stenosis. A meta-analysis of various noninvasive modes of testing for carotid stenosis concluded that duplex ultrasound had a pooled sensitivity and specificity of 86% and 87%, respectively, to distinguish 70% to 99% stenosis from less than 70% stenosis.[53] Ultrasound screening should be followed by more definitive testing with CT or MRI angiography to more specifically detail the degree of stenosis and guide procedural decisions about revascularization. Conventional digital subtraction angiography is generally considered the gold standard test. With the need to complete revascularization within 2 weeks from incident TIA, it is pivotal that potential delays in obtaining more accurate noninvasive testing are minimized.[54]

CASE PRESENTATION (continued)

After consultation among the patient, family, attending physician, and vascular surgical consultant, W.F. decided to have a carotid endarterectomy. He underwent an uncomplicated left carotid endarterectomy 3 days later and had an uneventful postsurgical course. His medical regimen was adjusted to include more aggressive blood pressure management, a change from aspirin to clopidogrel, and increase in atorvastatin dose from 20 to 40 mg. One year later he remains without recurrent stroke symptoms and is feeling well.

CONCLUSION

Stroke is a common and potentially devastating disease. With the aging of society, the frequency of stroke will continue to increase. Patients need to be educated as to what stroke symptoms are and that they represent an emergency in which rapid response is imperative. In addition, clinicians need to be ready to recognize and diagnose stroke and TIA, provide treatment in the most efficient and timely manner, and then recognize and treat risk factors for recurrent stroke. Stroke management, like many types of geriatric care, is best provided by an interdisciplinary team in whom effective communication and evidence-based protocol-driven care is engendered as routine.

References

1. Adams HP. Secondary prevention of atherothrombotic events after ischemic stroke. *Mayo Clin Proc.* 2009;84:43-51.

2. The European Stroke Organisation (ESO) Executive Committee and the ESO Writing Committee. Guidelines for Management of Ischemic Stroke and Transient Ischemic Attack 2008. *Cerebrovasc Dis.* 2008;25:457-507.

3. Volpe M, Rosei E, Ambrosioni E, et al. Reduction in estimated stroke risk associated with practice-based stroke-risk assessment and awareness in a large, representative population of hypertensive patients. *J Hypertens.* 2007;25:2390-2397.

4. Stroke Education LtD Website. http://www.stroke-education.com/RiskCalculator.do.

5. Goldstein LB, Simel DL. Is this patient having a stroke? *JAMA.* 2005;293:2391-2402.

6. Norris JW, Hachinski VC. Misdiagnosis of stroke. *Lancet.* 1982;1: 328-331.

7. Hand PJ, Kwan J, Lindley RI, et al. Distinguishing between stroke and mimic at the bedside. The Brain Attack Study. *Stroke.* 2006;37:769-775.

8. Goldstein LB. Improving the clinical diagnosis of stroke. *Stroke.* 2006;37:754-755.

9. Barreto AD, Martin-Schild S, Hallevi H, et al. Thrombolytic therapy for patients who wake-up with stroke. *Stroke.* 2009;40: 827-832.

10. Hacke W, Donnan G, Fieschi C, et al.; ATLANTIS Trials Investigators; ECASS Trials Investigators; NINDS rt-PA Study Group Investigators. Association of outcome with early stroke treatment: Pooled analysis of ATLANTIS, ECASS, and NINDS rt-PA stroke trials. *Lancet.* 2004;363:768-774.

11. Savers JL. Time is brain—quantified. *Stroke.* 2006;37:263-266.

12. Hacke W, Kaste M, Bluhmki E, et al. Thrombolysis with alteplase 3 to 4.5 hours after acute ischemic stroke. *N Engl J Med.* 2008;359: 1317-1329.

13. del Zoppo GJ, Saver JL, Jauch EC, Adams HP on behalf of the American Heart Association Stroke Council. Expansion of the time window for treatment of acute ischemic stroke with intravenous tissue plasminogen activator. *Stroke.* 2009;40:2945-2948.

14. Latchaw RE, Alberts MJ, Lev, MH, et al. Recommendations for imaging of acute ischemic stroke: A scientific statement from the American Heart Association. *Stroke.* 2009;40:3646-3678.

15. Clark WM, Wissman S, Albers GW, et al. Recombinant tissue-type plasminogen activator (alteplase) for ischemic stroke 3 to 5 hours after symptom onset. The ATLANTIS study: A randomized controlled trial. *JAMA.* 1999;282:2019-2026.

16. Hacke W, Kaste M, Fieschi C, et al. Randomised double-blind placebo-controlled trial of thrombolytic therapy with intravenous alteplase in acute ischemic stroke (ECASS II). *Lancet.* 1998;352: 1245-1251.

17. Thomalla G, Schwark C, Sobesky J, et al. Outcome and symptomatic bleeding complications of intravenous thrombolysis within 6 hours in MRI-selected stroke patients. *Stroke.* 2006;27:852-858.

18. Hacke W, Albers G, Al-Rawi Y, et al. The Desmoteplase in Acute Ischemic Stroke Trial (DIAS): A phase II MRI-based 9-hour window acute stroke thrombolysis trial with intravenous desmoteplase. *Stroke.* 2005;36:66-73.

19. Adams HP, del Zoppo G, Alberts MJ, et al. Guidelines for the Early Management of Adults with Acute Ischemic Stroke: A Guideline From the American Heart Association/American Stroke Association Stroke Council, Clinical Cardiology Council, Cardiovascular Radiology and Intervention Council, and the Atherosclerotic Peripheral Vascular Disease and Quality of Care Outcomes in Research Interdisciplinary Working Groups; the American Academy of Neurology affirms the value of this guideline as an educational tool for neurologists. *Stroke.* 2007;38:1655-1711.

20. Accessible at http://www.acutestroke.org/.

21. Heuschmann PU, Kolominsky-Rabas PL, Roether J, et al. Predictors of in-hospital mortality in patients with acute ischemic stroke treated with thrombolytic therapy. *JAMA.* 2004;292: 1831-1838.

22. Engelter ST, Bonati LH, Lyrer PA. Intravenous thrombolysis in stroke patients of ≥ 80 versus < 80 years of age—A systematic review across cohort studies. *Age Ageing.* 2006;35:572-580.

23. Wu CM, McLaughlin K, Lorenzetti DL, et al. Early risk of stroke after transient ischemic attack: A systematic review and meta-analysis. *Arch Intern Med.* 2007;167:2417-2422.

24. Rothwell PM, Giles MF, Lovelock CE, et al. A simple score (ABCD) to identify individuals at high early risk of stroke after transient ischemic attack. *Lancet.* 2005;366:26-36.

25. Sciolla R, Melis F, for the SINPAC Group. Rapid identification of high-risk transient ischemic attacks: Prospective validation of the ABCD score. *Stroke.* 2008;39:297-302.

26. Johnston SC, Rothwell PM, Nguyen-Huynh MN, et al. Validation and refinement of scores to predict very early stroke risk after transient ischemic attack. *Lancet.* 2007;369:283-292.

27. Easton JD, Saver JL, Albers GW, et al. Definition and evaluation of transient ischemic attack: A scientific statement for healthcare professionals from the American Heart Association/ American Stroke Association Stroke Council. *Stroke.* 2009;40: 2276-2293.

28. Hackman DG, Spence JD. Combining multiple approaches for the secondary prevention of vascular events after stroke: A quantitative modeling study. *Stroke.* 2007;38:1881-1885.

29. Rothwell PM, Giles MF, Chandratheva A, et al. Effect of urgent treatment of transient ischemic attack and minor stroke on recurrent stroke (EXPRESS study): A prospective population-based sequential comparison. *Lancet.* 2007;370:1432-1442.

30. Luengo-Fernandez R, Gray AM, Rothwell PM. Effect of urgent treatment for transient ischemic attack and minor stroke on disability and hospital costs (EXPRESS study): A prospective population-based sequential comparison. *Lancet.* 2009;8:235-243.

31. Lawes CM, Bennett DA, Feigin VL, et al. Blood pressure and stroke: An overview of published reviews. *Stroke.* 2004;35: 776-785.

32. Baigent, C, Blackwell, L, Collins, R, et al. Aspirin in the primary and secondary prevention of vascular disease: Collaborative meta-analysis of individual participant data from randomised trials. *Lancet.* 2009;373:1849.

33. ESPS -2. Diener HC, Cunha L, Forbes C, et al. European Stroke Prevention Study 2: Dipyridamole and acetylsalicylic acid in the secondary prevention of stroke. *J Neurol Sci.* 1996;143:1-13.

34. Albers GW, Amarenco P, Easton JD, et al. Antithrombotic and thrombolytic therapy for ischemic stroke. *Chest.* 2008;133; 630S-669S.

35. Diener HC, Cunha L, Forbes C, et al. European Stroke Prevention Study 2: Dipyridamole and acetylsalicylic acid in the secondary prevention of stroke. *J Neurol Sci.* 1996;143:1-13.

36. ESPRIT Study Group. Aspirin plus dipyridamole versus aspirin alone after cerebral ischemia of arterial origin (ESPRIT): Randomised controlled trial. *Lancet.* 2006;367:1665-1673.

37. CAPRIE Steering Committee. A randomised, blinded, trial of clopidogrel versus aspirin in patients at risk of ischemic events (CAPRIE). *Lancet.* 1996;348:1329-1339.

38. Adams RJ, Albers G, Alberts MJ, et al. Update to the AHA/ASA recommendations for the prevention of stroke in patients with stroke and transient ischemic attack. *Stroke.* 2008;39: 1647-1652.

39. Diener H-C, Bogousslavsky J, Brass LM, et al; MATCH Investigators. Aspirin and clopidogrel compared with clopidogrel alone after recent ischemic stroke or transient ischemic attack in high-risk patients (MATCH): Randomised, double-blind, placebo-controlled trial. *Lancet.* 2004;364:331-337.

40. Sacco RL, Diener HC, Yusuf S, et al; PRoFESS Study Group. Aspirin and extended-release dipyridamole versus clopidogrel for recurrent stroke. *N Engl J Med.* 2008;359:1238-1251.

41. The Stroke Prevention by Aggressive Reduction in Cholesterol Levels (SPARCL) Investigators. High-dose atorvastatin after stroke or transient ischemic attack. *N Engl J Med.* 2006;355:549-559.

42. North American Symptomatic Carotid Endarterectomy Trial Collaborators. Beneficial effect of carotid endarterectomy in symptomatic patients with high-grade carotid stenosis. *N Engl J Med.* 1991;325:445-453.

43. North American Symptomatic Carotid Endarterectomy Trialists' Collaborative Group. The final results of the NASCET trial. *N Engl J Med.* 1998;339:1415-1425.

44. Almowitch S, Eliasziw E, Algra A, et al. for the NASCET Group. Risk, causes, and prevention of ischemic stroke in elderly patients with symptomatic internal-carotid-artery stenosis. *Lancet.* 2001; 357:1154-1160.

45. Mayberg MR, Wilson E, Yatsu F, et al. for the Veteran Affairs Cooperative Studies Program 309 Trialist Group. Carotid endarterectomy and prevention of cerebral ischemia in symptomatic carotid stenosis. *JAMA.* 1991;266:3289-3294.

46. European Carotid Surgery Trialists' Collaborative Group. Randomised trial of endarterectomy for recently symptomatic carotid stenosis: Final results of the MRC European Carotid Surgery Trial (ECST). *Lancet.* 1998;351:1379-1387.

47. Rothwell P, Eliasziw M, Gutnikov A, et al. Analysis of pooled data from the randomised controlled trials of endarterectomy for symptomatic carotid stenosis. *Lancet.* 2003;361:107-116.

48. Yadav JS, Wholey MH, Kuntz, et al., Stenting and Angioplasty with Protection in Patients at High Risk for Endarterectomy Investigators. Protected carotid-artery stenting versus endarterectomy in high-risk patients. *N Engl J Med.* 2004;351: 1493-1501.

49. Gurm HS, Yadav JS, Fayad P, et al. for the SAPPHIRE Investigators. Long-term results of carotid stenting versus endarterectomy in high-risk patients. *N Engl J Med.* 2008;358:1572-1579.

50. SPACE Collaborative Group. 30-day results from the SPACE trial of stent-protected angioplasty versus carotid endarterectomy in symptomatic patients: A randomised non-inferiority trial. *Lancet.* 2006;368:1239-1247.

51. Mas J, Chatellier G, Beyssen B, et al., EVA-3S Investigators. Endarterectomy versus stenting in patients with symptomatic severe carotid stenosis. *N Engl J Med.* 2006;355:1660-1671.

52. Levy EI, Mocco J, Samuelson RM, et al. Optimal treatment of carotid artery disease. *J Am Coll Cardiol.* 2008;51:979-985.

53. Nederkoorn PJ, van der Graaf Y, Hunink MG. Duplex ultrasound and magnetic resonance angiography compared with digital subtraction angiography in carotid artery stenosis: A systematic review. *Stroke.* 2003;34:1324-1332.

54. Wardlaw JM, Stevenson MD, Chappell F, et al. Carotid artery imaging for secondary stroke prevention: Both imaging modality and rapid access to imaging are important. *Stroke.* 2009;40: 3511-3517.

POST-TEST

1. Which statement regarding a patient presenting 2 days after a TIA event is TRUE?

A. Urgent hospitalization is always required.

B. Neuroimaging and diagnostic evaluation should be completed within 48 hours.

C. rt-PA may still be considered as a therapeutic option.

D. Elevated systolic blood over 180 mm Hg should be normalized quickly.

2. Which of the following statements about intravenous thrombolytic therapy for acute stroke is FALSE?

A. Patients with high NIHSS scores (> 20) have higher rates of intracranial hemorrhage with lytics.

B. Lytic therapy can be considered out to 4.5 hours from onset of symptoms based upon new trial data.

C. Age is not a risk factor for intracranial hemorrhage.

D. Elderly patients may still benefit from lytic therapy for acute stroke.

3. Which of the following is MOST accurate regarding the use of aspirin (ASA) for non-cardioembolic stroke?

A. ASA 325 mg/day is more effective than ASA 81 mg/day.

B. There is no difference in the gastrointestinal toxicity of low-dose (≤ 81 mg/day) versus high-dose (≥ 325 mg/day) aspirin.

C. ASA 50 to 100 mg is a reasonable initial antiplatelet treatment choice following a transient ischemic event.

D. ASA combined with short-acting dipyridamole has been well studied as a less costly and effective treatment alternative to ASA combined with extended-release dipyridamole.

4. Which of the following statements about carotid artery stenosis is FALSE?

A. Carotid stenting (CAS) is the preferred modality for the treatment of symptomatic carotid stenosis in younger patients.

B. Carotid endarterectomy (CEA) for moderate (> 50%) stenosis is safe and effective.

C. CAS is an option for high-risk patients with carotid stenosis.

D. The benefits of CEA may be offset by high perioperative surgical risk.

ANSWERS TO PRE-TEST

1. A
2. B
3. C
4. C

ANSWERS TO POST-TEST

1. B
2. B
3. C
4. A

45

Management of Hypertension in the Elderly

Ihab Hajjar, MD, MS

Dae Hyun Kim, MD, MPH

● **LEARNING OBJECTIVES**

1. Describe the epidemiology and functional consequences of hypertension in older adults.
2. Identify the challenges in the management of hypertension in a heterogeneous geriatric population.
3. Discuss the available evidence and controversies in treating hypertension in the very old.
4. Explain the general principles of selecting nonpharmacologic and pharmacologic therapy based on an individualized approach to the elderly patient.

PRE-TEST

1. **Which one of the following statements is TRUE in evaluating an 83-year-old hypertensive patient?**

   A. Hypertension is an age-related physiologic response.

   B. Current evidence does not support that treating hypertension in this age group is beneficial.

   C. Hypertension can affect both cognitive and physical function in older adults.

   D. Information on functional status and social support does not affect treatment decision-making.

2. **Which one of the following statements on hypertension awareness and control rates is TRUE?**

   A. Hypertension awareness has improved during the past two decades.

   B. Hypertension control rate is higher in older adults than in younger adults.

   C. Hypertension control rate is, in general, lower in nursing home residents than in community dwellers.

   D. Overall prevalence of hypertension has remained stable.

3. **Which one of the following statements on orthostatic hypotension is FALSE?**

   A. Orthostatic hypotension is more common in nursing home residents than in community dwellers.

   B. Uncontrolled systolic hypertension is strongly associated with orthostatic hypotension.

   C. Antihypertensive therapy should be discontinued in case of orthostatic hypotension.

   D. Orthostatic hypotension is associated with postprandial hypotension in older adults.

CASE PRESENTATION 1: MR. H.

Mr. H. is an 80-year-old male with newly diagnosed hypertension.

History

Mr. H. is an 80-year-old, healthy Caucasian man who has recently relocated to Florida after his retirement. He has not seen a primary care physician for years due to his busy work schedule. He is fully independent and does not report falls, heart disease, stroke, or diabetes mellitus. He takes no medications.

Evaluation

At the initial office visit 2 weeks ago, you discovered that he had blood pressure of 180/76 mm Hg and heart rate of 74 per minute while sitting. After 3-minute standing, blood pressure was 172/72 mm Hg and heart rate was 80 per minute. Today, blood pressure is unchanged from the previous visit and physical examination was unremarkable, including normal Mini-Mental State Examination and clock-drawing test. His balance and gait evaluation was normal. There was no evidence of kidney dysfunction on laboratory tests and left ventricular hypertrophy on electrocardiogram. You have asked Mr. H. to measure his blood pressure at home. He brings in his blood pressure records for the past 2 weeks and they are consistently in the range of 160-180/60-78 mm Hg.

CASE PRESENTATION 2: MR. A

Mr. A. is an 83-year-old male with uncontrolled hypertension and multiple co-morbid conditions.

History

Mr. A. is an 83-year-old African-American man who is transferring his care to you because his primary care physician has just retired. Other than hypertension, he has multiple co-morbid conditions, including coronary artery disease, congestive heart failure, and diabetes mellitus. He has been recently hospitalized for congestive heart failure exacerbation. He takes aspirin, lisinopril, metoprolol, furosemide, atorvastatin, and insulin. He resides alone in an assisted living facility because he has mild cognitive impairment and requires some assistance in his activities of daily living.

Evaluation

At today's visit, you found that his blood pressure was 182/54 mm Hg and heart rate was 56 per minute while sitting. After 3-minute standing, his blood pressure dropped to 164/50 mm Hg with heart rate response to 62 per minute. He did not have any light-headedness with standing. Physical examination was remarkable for grade 3/6 systolic ejection murmur with preserved S2, no volume overload, and Mini-Mental State Examination score of 24 out of 30 with abnormal clock-drawing test. He has not fallen, but ambulates slowly without using any assistive device.

CASE PRESENTATION 3: MRS. N.

Mrs. N. is an 84-year-old nursing home resident with severe dementia and hypertension.

History

Mrs. N. is an 84-year-old Caucasian woman who was recently admitted to the nursing home because of her severe dementia and need for assistance in activities of daily living. Two years ago, she had a major stroke, which caused residual right-sided weakness and aphasia. She also has hypertension, osteoporosis, and osteoarthritis. She takes donepezil, atenolol, hydrochlorothiazide, simvastatin, calcium and vitamin D supplement, and acetaminophen. She has fallen several times during the past year and ambulates with a walker. She has poor oral intake and has lost 15 lbs in 6 months.

Evaluation

Two weeks ago, her blood pressure was 166/52 mm Hg and heart rate was 60 per minute. After 3 minutes of standing, her blood pressure and heart rate were 138/48 mm Hg and 64 per minute, respectively. She reported a brief period of light-headedness with standing. On examination, she was only oriented to herself and has bilateral carotid bruits and right-sided weakness. Her Mini-Mental State Examination score was 10 and clock-drawing test was abnormal. Today, you are reviewing her blood pressure records for the past 2 weeks, which are in the range of 148-182/46-60 mm Hg.

● BACKGROUND

Although many randomized controlled trials have demonstrated the benefit of blood pressure reduction in the elderly patient with hypertension, undertreatment and under control of hypertension is common in the geriatric population.[1] Physicians' reluctance to adequately lower blood pressure and achieve control is a major contributing factor to the lower control rates in the elderly patient.[2] A national survey indicated that a significant proportion of geriatricians had a biased understanding of hypertension and different opinions about how hypertension should be treated in this population.[3] The complexities of the management of hypertension in the elderly are illustrated in the three case examples.

These cases represent the heterogeneity of the geriatric patient population, which makes it difficult to apply the same treatment guidelines on all three patients. The role of age in managing the elderly patient with hypertension is overemphasized in many current guidelines, clinical trials, and physicians' practice habits. This is most evident in managing the "very-old" hypertensive patient. The majority of randomized controlled trials of antihypertensive therapy were conducted in relatively younger elderly adults. Further, evidence from observational studies of older adults suggests that lower blood pressure is associated with a worse outcome.[4,5] Recently, the Hypertension in the Very Elderly Trial (HYVET) demonstrated, in subjects whose average age was 83.5 years, that on average a decrease of systolic blood pressure of 15 mm Hg led to a 28% lower mortality (number needed to treat for 2 years was 40), 34% reduction in stroke (number needed to treat for 2 years was 94), and 72% lower risk of congestive heart failure.[6]

In the elderly patient management goals depend on the patient's functional status and remaining life expectancy rather than age alone. Although all three cases are of similar age and have systolic hypertension, their management plans and goals will differ significantly. Mr. H. is a community-dwelling healthy elderly man. He is robust functionally and is likely to have greater life expectancy than Mrs. N. She is frail and has multiple co-morbidities, which may lead to a limited life expectancy. On the other hand, Mr. A. has mild functional and cognitive impairment and his life expectancy is probably intermediate between the other two. In addition to cognitive function, mobility and fall risk should play a role in designing hypertension management in the elderly. For example, the effect of antihypertensives on cognitive decline is relevant to Mr. A's therapy goals and the effect of blood pressure lowering on falls and orthostatic hypotension is extremely critical for Mrs. N.

Taken together, managing hypertension in the geriatric population is unique because of the heterogeneity of the population, presence of multiple co-morbid conditions and geriatric syndromes, and limited amount of evidence to guide antihypertensive therapy, especially in the very old. Management decisions in the cases presented should address the following three questions:

1. What are the risks and benefits of treating hypertension?
2. How should the blood pressure be lowered and how fast?
3. What should be the optimal target blood pressure?

The answers to these questions are not always straightforward. Therefore, it is essential that physicians understand the available evidence and the principles of management of hypertension in older adults.

The Burden of Hypertension in the Elderly Population

According to the National Health and Nutrition Examination Survey (NHANES) from 1999 to 2004, 67% of the non-institutionalized adults aged 60 and older had hypertension, which was significantly higher than 58% in NHANES III (1988-1994).[1] The prevalence increased in all age groups, in both sexes, and in non-Hispanic whites and non-Hispanic blacks. In the 1999 to 2004 survey, 74% of hypertensive old adults were aware of their diagnosis, 67% were treated, and 43% of the treated were controlled. Although these rates improved significantly over time, the rates were still lower in older adults than in younger adults. Hypertension is also common in the nursing home population. The prevalence of hypertension in the nursing home setting was 51% to 71% and its control rate was higher than that in the community setting, ranging from 60% to 85%.[7] Among 202 residents aged 50 to 98 years in an academic nursing home, 71% had hypertension and all hypertensive adults were treated, of whom 85% were controlled.[8] Hypertension is one of the most common clinical diagnoses that providers address in their elderly patients. The three cases provided are typical scenarios in geriatric primary care and provide a challenging decision-making process to the treating health care provider.

Blood Pressure and Aging

Systolic blood pressure progressively increases with age, whereas diastolic blood pressure increases until age 50 and tends to decline afterward. As a result, systolic hypertension is the predominant type of hypertension in the elderly and has several important clinical implications. In all three cases provided, systolic hypertension was characteristic. It is important to note that systolic blood pressure is a better predictor of cardiovascular events than diastolic blood pressure in hypertensive elderly adults.[9,10] However, diastolic blood pressure has been historically emphasized as a more important predictor of cardiovascular events, and physicians are more likely to react to high diastolic blood pressures than high systolic blood pressures and therefore use diastolic blood pressure to determine treatment efficacy, when this assumption has proven to be false in older adults. As a result, undertreatment of systolic hypertension makes up the majority of uncontrolled hypertension in the elderly.[11]

In addition to elevated blood pressure, hypertensive elderly individuals are more likely to have orthostatic hypotension. This is defined as a reduction in blood pressure upon standing by at least 20 mm Hg in systolic or 10 mm Hg in diastolic blood pressure, and is common in the elderly population. It is estimated that 20% to 34% of community-dwelling older adults and up to 50% of nursing home residents have orthostatic hypotension. For example, in our case three of Mrs. N., the fact that she has uncontrolled hypertension plays an important role in her also having orthostatic hypotension. To date, studies have failed to document an association between antihypertensive therapy and incident orthostatic hypotension. A small randomized trial has shown that controlled hypertension with antihypertensive therapy reduced orthostatic hypotension.[12] In addition to orthostatic hypotension, the elderly hypertensive patient is more likely to have postprandial hypotension, white-coat hypertension, and lack of nocturnal drop in blood pressure (non-dipping). All are important characteristics of geriatric hypertension that need to be considered when making decisions about management.

Significance of Hypertension in the Elderly Population

Numerous prospective epidemiologic studies have confirmed that high blood pressure is associated with cardiovascular events including coronary heart disease, stroke, congestive heart failure, and cardiomyopathy in a continuous and incremental fashion even in the very old. A meta-analysis of individual data from 61 prospective studies involving 1 million adults showed that systolic and diastolic blood pressure are associated with ischemic heart disease and stroke mortality without any indication of a threshold down to 115/75 mm Hg.[13] This relationship was observed even in adults aged 80 to 89 years, although the relative risk was attenuated in the advanced age group.

Hypertension in the elderly patient not only contributes to worse vascular outcomes but also may lead to cognitive and physical impairment. An emerging body of evidence suggests that hypertension is also a risk factor for cognitive impairment and dementia including Alzheimer disease.[5,14,15] Midlife blood pressure elevation is associated with cognitive impairment and dementia, whereas late-life blood pressure is often not. Moreover, increased midlife and late-life systolic blood pressure elevation was associated with greater functional decline and incident disability in the Charleston Heart Study.[16]

● CLINICAL EVALUATION

Every hypertensive patient needs to have the following three evaluation principles met:

1. Assessment of other cardiovascular risk factors and comorbid conditions that may affect prognosis and treatment decision
2. Examination for identifiable or secondary causes of hypertension
3. Assessment of target organ damage and cardiovascular disease[17]

In the elderly patient, evaluation should also include a risk-benefit assessment for lowering blood pressure and preferably an assessment of cognitive and physical performance for prognosis, therapeutic, and monitoring reasons (Table 45–1).

History

Although most patients with hypertension do not have any symptoms, older adults are more likely to experience symptoms. Case 1 provides a typical example of a patient with asymptomatic elevation in blood pressure. Although Cases 2 and 3 are also not necessarily symptomatic, the fact that the patients demonstrated evidence of physical and cognitive

● **TABLE 45–1** Essential Elements in Evaluating a Hypertensive Elderly Patient

History
Symptoms related to hypertension and atherosclerotic cardiovascular disease
Symptoms of orthostatic hypotension[a]
Memory loss[a]
History of falls or balance problem[a]
Basic and instrumental activities of daily living—especially medication management[a]
Living situation and social support system[a]
Medication review, adverse effects, and compliance[a]
Physical Examination
Blood pressure measurement in both arms
Orthostatic and standing blood pressure measurement[a]
Body weight and body mass index
Signs of end-organ damage
Neurologic deficits
Cognitive screening[a]
Gait and balance assessment[a]
Diagnostic Evaluation
Kidney function, electrolytes, glucose, hemoglobin, lipid panel
12-lead electrocardiogram
Further evaluation for secondary hypertension if indicated

[a]*Important in evaluating geriatric patients.*

decline may be exacerbated by their elevation in blood pressure. Headaches are reported in 20% to 30% of older adults with hypertension. They are more common in women, those with severe hypertension, and those who are aware of their blood pressure. Other symptoms are subtle and may include nocturia, cognitive impairment, and sluggishness. Case 2 is a good example for such presentation. It is important to inquire about symptoms of orthostatic hypotension and history of falling, because older adults often do not volunteer such information. Medication history should include prior blood pressure medication use, over-the-counter medication use, and allergic reactions or adverse events from medication. Family history of hypertension and other cardiovascular diseases, social history including the assessment of financial status and social support system, and functional history such as the need for assistance in medication management should be considered in formulating a treatment plan.

Blood Pressure Measurement and Physical Examination

Accurate blood pressure measurement is critical in the elderly patient to avoid under- or overtreatment, both of which can adversely affect patients' health outcomes and health care expenses. Patients should avoid caffeine, exercise, and smoking at least 30 minutes and be seated quietly for at least 5 minutes in a chair with feet, back, and arms supported before blood pressure measurement. Blood pressure should be measured in both arms, at least twice, using an appropriately sized cuff (the inflatable bladder of the cuff encircling at least 80% of the arm), and the arm with higher blood pressure should be used for follow-up measurements. Newly diagnosed hypertension in elderly patients should also undergo an out-of-the-office blood pressure measurement to rule out white-coat hypertension. This can be obtained by self blood pressure monitoring at home or ambulatory blood pressure monitoring (ABPM). Elevated office blood pressure despite self-measured blood pressure consistently less than 130/80 mm Hg, and no evidence of target organ damage, indicates white-coat hypertension. ABPM has a better predictive ability to assess cardiovascular events, and the lack of night-time reduction in blood pressure has been associated with an increased cardiovascular risk. The wide use of ABPM in clinical settings is limited by lack of insurance reimbursement in the United States. In Case 1, the home readings confirmed the office readings and hence provided further support for the clinical diagnosis of hypertension.

Pseudohypertension which results in falsely elevated blood pressure readings due to a noncompressible, thickened, calcified brachial artery; white-coat hypertension, defined as isolated high blood pressure readings in the office setting; and an auscultatory gap, defined as the interval of blood pressure in which Korotkoff sounds indicating true systolic blood pressure disappear and reappear at a lower blood pressure level, secondary to arterial stiffness; are common in the elderly population. Multiple measurements, including out-of-the-office measurements, are recommended prior to confirmation of the diagnosis. Treatment should not be initiated on the basis of a single measurement. The suspicion of pseudohypertension should be considered based on certain clinical clues:

- Severe hypertension without target organ damage
- Hypertension not responding to antihypertensive therapy
- Significant postural hypotension from low doses of antihypertensive agents
- A very wide pulse pressure

Blood pressure should also be measured in standing position, especially in patients who report symptoms consistent with orthostatic hypotension. Standing blood pressure measurement is essential in frail, elderly patients in long-term care facilities such as in our Case 3, because the risks of overtreatment can be serious.

Physical examination is performed to look for the evidence of secondary causes of hypertension and target organ damage. It should include a funduscopic examination to screen for hypertensive retinopathy, such as arteriovenous nicking, retinal hemorrhage, cotton wool spots, and papilledema; neck examination to examine jugular venous distension, carotid pulse and bruit, and thyroid enlargement; cardiopulmonary examination to look for the third and fourth heart sounds, murmurs, and displacement of point of maximal impulse; abdominal examination to detect enlarged kidneys, masses, pulsating aorta, and bruits of renal artery stenosis or abdominal aortic aneurysm; extremity examination to check peripheral pulses and edema, as well as signs of peripheral arterial disease; and neurologic examination to evaluate for any focal deficits. Measurements of body weight and height to calculate body mass index and waist circumference to determine central adiposity are also useful.

● **TABLE 45–2** Hypertension Stages

Category	Systolic		Diastolic
Normal	<120	*and*	< 80
Pre-hypertension	120-39	*or*	80-89
Hypertension			
Stage 1	140-159	*or*	90-99
Stage 2	≥160	*or*	≥100

Adapted from the JNC-7 Guidelines contained in Chobanian et al.[17]

The elevation of blood pressure is commonly reported by stage of blood pressure elevation. Hypertension stages should be based on the average of two or more readings taken after two or more visits after the initial examination (Table 45–2).

Laboratory Tests and Other Diagnostic Procedures

Initial laboratory evaluation should include the assessment of kidney function (with estimated glomerular filtration rate [GFR]), electrolytes including calcium level, glucose, hematocrit, lipid profile, and urinalysis. Screening for microalbuminuria or albumin/creatinine ratio are useful and should be performed annually in high-risk patients with diabetes or chronic kidney disease, because they are associated with an increased risk of cardiovascular events, even in the absence of reduction in GFR.[18] A 12-lead electrocardiogram can be used to detect left ventricular hypertrophy or an old myocardial infarction.

Secondary hypertension, although very rare, is more prevalent with increasing age. Additional investigation for a secondary cause is indicated if one of these factors applies:

- Hypertension is newly diagnosed after age 70
- Blood pressure control is not achieved despite adequate treatment with three antihypertensive agents including a diuretic
- Previously controlled blood pressure becomes uncontrolled for unknown reasons
- The initial evaluation suggests secondary hypertension

Causes of secondary hypertension in the elderly include renovascular hypertension, hyperaldosteronism, chronic kidney disease, hyperparathyroidism, hyperthyroidism, chronic alcohol use, obstructive sleep apnea, and drug-induced hypertension (such as from nonsteroidal anti-inflammatory agents). Pheochromocytoma and abuse of substances such as cocaine as causes of blood pressure elevation are rare in older hypertensive patients.

CASE PRESENTATION 1 (continued)

Evaluation

Mr. H., the 80-year-old male with newly diagnosed hypertension, has uncontrolled stage 2 isolated systolic hypertension but does not have any evidence of adverse clinical and functional consequences of hypertension. Since he has good life expectancy and uncontrolled hypertension significantly increases the risk of cardiovascular events, especially stroke, the risk-to-benefit ratio of antihypertensive therapy is favorable. Antihypertensive therapy has been shown to prolong survival and reduce major cardiovascular events. It may also prevent disability and cognitive decline.

CASE PRESENTATION 2 (continued)
Evaluation

Recall that Mr. A. is the 83-year-old male with uncontrolled hypertension and multiple co-morbid conditions. His mild cognitive impairment, especially executive dysfunction, and slow gait probably have resulted from uncontrolled hypertension. His life expectancy is likely over 2 years, and he remains at high risk for cardiovascular events and further functional and cognitive decline. Adequate control of hypertension and cholesterol, along with evidence-based treatment for congestive heart failure, is likely to reduce cardiac morbidity and mortality as well as hospitalization for congestive heart failure. Therefore, intensifying his antihypertensive regimen should be considered.

CASE PRESENTATION 3 (continued)
Evaluation

Mrs. N., the 84-year-old nursing home resident, has severe dementia and hypertension. She has cerebrovascular disease and dementia, both of which are well-known consequences of uncontrolled hypertension. Her orthostatic hypotension is likely multifactorial in origin, from uncontrolled hypertension, autonomic dysfunction, dehydration from inadequate fluid intake, and antihypertensive medications. It is an important contributor to her recurrent falls. The combination of atenolol and donepezil may cause significant bradycardia, which may lead to syncope. Despite the persistent risk of recurrent stroke, it is unclear whether antihypertensive therapy will provide any meaningful survival benefit or improvement in her quality of life.

• MANAGEMENT

The decision regarding whom and how we should treat should be individualized after consideration of the following factors: the severity of hypertension, presence of other co-morbid

conditions and cardiovascular risk factors, potential risk of polypharmacy, financial burden, functional status, life expectancy, and geriatric-specific syndromes. In general, blood pressure should be targeted to 140/90 mm Hg or less, because this has been associated with a lower risk of cardiovascular events.[19] In the very old, the target may be 150/90 mm Hg based on the HYVET. The goal may be lower in patients with diabetes mellitus or kidney disease. Whether or not treating uncomplicated stage 1 hypertension in the elderly is beneficial has not been tested. There is no evidence to suggest that those with preserved function and cognition would not fare as well as younger patients. For example, in Case 1, Mr. H. does not have any cognitive or functional impairment and has minimal co-morbidities; he is likely to tolerate, comply with, and benefit from the treatment. In Case 2, due to his diabetes, congestive heart failure, and other risk factors, it will be prudent to improve vascular risk factors. Due to his cognitive impairment, a simple regimen is recommended. In contrast, Mrs. N. has short life expectancy and is at increased risk of potential drug-induced complications. There is limited evidence to suggest an improved outcome in these cases with further lowering of blood pressure. Discussions with the patient's proxy should include clarifications of goals of care and describing the lack of evidence to support lowering blood pressure in high-risk frail older adults. In addition, polypharmacy is a particular concern in older adults with multiple co-morbid conditions, because most elderly adults need two or more antihypertensive agents to achieve effective blood pressure control. Underprescribing beneficial medications has been linked to higher morbidity, mortality, and reduced quality of life.[20] Thus, it is important to achieve the balance between the risk of polypharmacy and the benefit of a rational antihypertensive therapy.

The general prescribing principle in geriatrics, "start low and go slow," should be applied in treating the frail, elderly population who may not tolerate aggressive blood pressure lowering and are at high risk for complications from treatment. It is better to prescribe one medication at a time and at the lowest effective dose. The frequency and timing of dosing can be modified to avoid abrupt blood pressure reduction, which may exacerbate orthostatic hypotension and postprandial hypotension. Another important consideration is to assess the patient's financial condition and insurance coverage to afford the medication you are prescribing. Prescription of generic medications should be considered for cost reasons as well as often the presence of a larger evidence base. Judicious use of fixed-dose combination pills can reduce the number of medications, patients' copay, and may reduce side effects from the use of higher dose of individual medications. The quality of life should also be assessed periodically by asking the patient's satisfaction and ability to perform instrumental and basic activities of daily living as well as any medication-related side effects.

Nonpharmacologic Treatment

Most evidence for lifestyle modification comes from young adults with high-normal blood pressure and stage 1 hypertension. Dietary sodium reduction to no more than 100 mmol per day (2.4 g of sodium) and weight loss of 10 lbs (4.5 kg) have been shown to prevent hypertension.[21,22] A diet rich in vegetables, fruits, and low-fat dairy products that contain low cholesterol and saturated fat and high calcium and potassium reduced systolic blood pressure by 8 to 14 mm Hg.[23] Alcohol intake restricted to two drinks per day (30 mL or 1 oz) in men and one drink per day (15 mL or 0.5 oz) in women reduced systolic blood pressure by 2 to 4 mm Hg.[24] Progressive resistance exercise and regular aerobic exercise at least 30 minutes per day, most days of the week, lowered systolic blood pressure by 1 to 4 mm Hg and 3 to 5 mm Hg, respectively.[25,26] Implementation of a combination of lifestyle changes lowers blood pressure, delays the onset of hypertension, and has a favorable effect on other cardiovascular risk factors.[27] Smoking cessation should be offered to current smokers for overall cardiovascular benefit.

In contrast to younger adults, there are only limited data on lifestyle modification in older adults. The Trial of Non-Pharmacological Interventions in the Elderly (TONE) was a multicenter randomized controlled trial that evaluated the effect of sodium reduction and weight loss (for obese adults) on blood pressure in hypertensive adults between ages 60 and 80.[28] After a median of 29-month follow-up, sodium reduction reduced the need for antihypertensive medications by 31% and weight loss reduced the need by 36%. Their combination reduced the need for antihypertensive medications by 53%. This study proved that lifestyle modification should be an essential part of antihypertensive treatment even in the elderly population. Therefore, lifestyle modification should be the first step in treating stage 1 hypertension and an essential part in treating stage 2 hypertension whenever patients can comply with these interventions. In elderly patients who are starting lifestyle modifications, it is important to evaluate their cardiovascular status and balance safety before exercise and monitor for excessive weight loss beyond their ideal body weight. Of the three cases, Cases 1 and 2 are ideal for starting a lifestyle-changing program.

Selection of Antihypertensive Agents

As a first-line agent, thiazide diuretics are usually preferred, but other classes, such as angiotensin-converting enzyme inhibitors, angiotensin receptor blockers, or calcium-channel blockers are also appropriate. In the Antihypertensive and Lipid-Lowering Treatment to Prevent Heart Attack Trial (ALLHAT), there was no difference in fatal or nonfatal myocardial infarction and mortality among chlorthalidone, lisinopril, and amlodipine, but chlorthalidone was superior in preventing heart failure (to amlodipine and lisinopril) and stroke (to lisinopril).[29] Side effects include metabolic disturbance such as hypokalemia, hyperuricemia, and diabetes mellitus. But low-dose thiazide diuretics are generally well-tolerated, safe with appropriate laboratory monitoring, and less expensive. Therefore, thiazide diuretics are recommended as the initial agent or as the first add-on therapy.

Similar to treating hypertension in younger adults with co-morbid conditions, there are compelling indications for the use of specific antihypertensive classes: heart failure (angiotensin converting enzyme inhibitor [ACEI], angiotensin receptor blocker [ARB], beta-blocker, diuretic, and aldosterone antagonist); myocardial infarction (ACEI, beta-blocker, and aldosterone antagonist); diabetes (ACEI, ARB, beta-blocker, calcium-channel blocker [CCB], and diuretic); chronic kidney disease (ACEI and ARB); stroke (ACEI and diuretic); and high coronary disease risk (ACEI, beta-blocker, CCB, and diuretic). In older adults with osteoporosis, a thiazide can be considered to maintain positive calcium balance and improve bone density.[30] In the absence of heart failure with a low ejection fraction, a combination of ACEI and ARB should be avoided due to high risk of adverse events, including hypotension, syncope, and renal dysfunction as compared to either agent alone.[31]

Recently, several meta-analyses have questioned the efficacy of beta-blockers in treating uncomplicated hypertension.[32] Compared to placebo, beta-blockers, especially atenolol, provide no reduction in all-cause mortality and myocardial infarction, and only modest reduction in stroke, which is smaller than the risk reduction seen with ACEIs, ARBs, and CCBs.[33] Several explanations have been proposed: suboptimal central aortic pressure lowering effect, lower efficacy on reversing left ventricular hypertrophy and endothelial dysfunction, increased risk of diabetes, decreased exercise tolerance, and poor tolerability. Based on available evidence, beta-blockers are not preferred as a first-line agent, unless there is a strong indication, such as heart failure, prior myocardial infarction, acute coronary syndrome, stable angina, prevention of perioperative cardiac complications, or hypertrophic obstructive cardiomyopathy.[32]

A frequently raised concern is the possibility of increased mortality with excessive reduction of diastolic blood pressure in older adults with isolated systolic hypertension, or the so-called "J-curve phenomenon." This concern often contributes to suboptimal control of hypertension in the elderly by providers. The following hypotheses have been proposed to explain this relationship: (1) low diastolic blood pressure increases mortality by compromising the perfusion to target organs, (2) it merely reflects the arterial stiffness from advanced cardiovascular disease, or (3) it relates to underlying poor health conditions. To explain the underlying mechanism, secondary analyses of data from randomized controlled trials have been performed. Pooled analysis of individual data from seven randomized controlled trials revealed that increased mortality from low blood pressure was observed for both cardiovascular and noncardiovascular mortality and for both treated and untreated patients.[34] This suggests that low blood pressure may be related to poor health-related conditions. In addition, randomized placebo-controlled trials conducted in isolated systolic hypertension demonstrated significant reduction in cardiovascular events. In the Systolic Hypertension in Europe trial, cardiovascular events were not increased with treated diastolic blood pressure as low as 55 mm Hg.[35] However, in patients with coronary heart disease, cardiovascular events tended to increase with treated diastolic blood pressure below 70 mm Hg.[35] Based on this evidence, antihypertensive therapy should be intensified in patients with uncontrolled systolic hypertension and close monitoring for ischemic symptoms is required for those with known coronary heart disease.

Very Old Population

There is an ongoing debate that lowering blood pressure with antihypertensive therapy might be harmful in the very old, because low blood pressure has been associated with poor outcomes in observational studies conducted in this population. In a cohort study of adults aged 85 and older, systolic blood pressure lower than 120 mm Hg was associated with increased mortality, whereas systolic blood pressure of 164 mm Hg was associated with the lowest mortality.[4] In another study of older adults, however, the inverse relationship between blood pressure and mortality disappeared after adjustment of health status.[36]

It was not until the results from HYVET became available that the direct evidence for antihypertensive therapy in this population emerged. HYVET was a randomized placebo-controlled trial of indapamide with or without perindopril in adults over age 80 with stage 2 hypertension.[6] Participants were generally healthy and only 12% had cardiovascular disease at baseline. Those with accelerated or secondary hypertension, hemorrhagic stroke in the previous 6 months, heart failure requiring treatment with antihypertensives, a serum creatinine greater than 1.7 mg/dL (129.6 μmol/L), gout, dementia, and requiring nursing care were excluded. Blood pressure was lowered from 173/91 mm Hg to 144/78 mm Hg in the treatment group. The trial was terminated early because of significant reduction in all-cause mortality by 21% (relative risk reduction; 81 patients need to be treated for 1 year to prevent 1 death) and heart failure by 64% (relative risk reduction; 105 patients need to be treated for 1 year to prevent 1 case of heart failure) and trends toward decreased stroke by 30% and CV mortality by 23%. Some benefits became apparent within the first year. Although there are unanswered questions regarding target blood pressure in this population and its generalizability to frail, elderly adults, these findings strongly suggest that robust, very old adults should be treated.

Long-Term Care Residents

Many frail older adults in long-term care facilities pose a special challenge due to a greater risk of adverse events including orthostatic hypotension, postprandial hypotension, and falls, which can significantly compromise the quality of remaining life. Such patients remain at high risk for cardiovascular events, especially stroke, which can further worsen their physical and cognitive function. However, the evidence to guide antihypertensive treatment is lacking, because they were not included (often specifically excluded) in randomized controlled trials. Therefore, antihypertensive therapy should be carefully contemplated after considering the patient's functional status and competing co-morbid conditions that may limit his or her life expectancy. Given that antihypertensive therapy reduced the risk of cardiovascular events as soon as within the first year of treatment,[6] it seems reasonable to treat stage 2 hypertension in relatively well-functioning, nursing home residents who have a life expectancy of at least 2 years and can tolerate blood pressure reduction. Once the treatment is initiated, close monitoring for orthostatic hypotension, postural hypotension, and falls is

recommended. Conversely, antihypertensive therapy is less likely to offer a meaningful improvement in the quality of life or a survival benefit to the residents who are progressively declining from an end-stage condition, such as advanced dementia or cancer.

Orthostatic Hypotension

Initiation or up-titration of any antihypertensive agents and the associated risk of developing orthostatic hypotension is not clear but should always be considered. It is important to remember that uncontrolled hypertension is strongly associated with orthostatic hypotension, and treatment of uncontrolled hypertension may ameliorate the orthostatic drop in blood pressure. Nonpharmacologic and pharmacologic management of orthostatic hypotension and postprandial hypotension have been described elsewhere.[37,38] It is reasonable to avoid using peripheral vasodilators such as CCBs or drugs that may decrease intravascular volume in those with orthostatic hypotension. ACEIs or ARBs may be appropriate in these scenarios. Withdrawing unnecessary medications, maintaining adequate intravascular volume, slow rising from supine position, avoiding straining and prolonged standing, raising the head of the bed to 10 to 20 degrees, small meals, elastic waist-high stockings, and regular exercise can improve orthostatic hypotension. Administration of antihypertensive medications between meals rather than before or during meals can reduce exaggerated meal-induced blood pressure change. If nonpharmacologic interventions fail, fludrocortisone and midodrine, with close monitoring, can be tried to ameliorate symptoms and improve the patient's functional status.

CASE PRESENTATION 1 (continued)
Management
Mr. H. should be treated with a thiazide diuretic as well as nonpharmacologic lifestyle changes to lower blood pressure, at least to the target level of 150/90 mm Hg in HYVET. Since the risk of cardiovascular events increases continuously with blood pressure, it would be reasonable to attempt to lower blood pressure to 140/90 mm Hg as long as he can tolerate the treatment without undue side effects.

CASE PRESENTATION 2 (continued)
Management
Although there have not been any randomized controlled trials including high-risk, very old patients, Mr. A. will probably benefit from blood pressure lowering by both nonpharmacologic and pharmacologic management. Ideally, his blood pressure target should

be 130/80 mm Hg. But sometimes such a degree of blood pressure reduction is not well-tolerated by the patient. Therefore, a careful attempt to intensify antihypertensive therapy can be made by increasing the dose of lisinopril or metoprolol or by adding a third agent (such as amlodipine) to the lowest effective dose. If he develops treatment-related side effects, including orthostatic hypotension and falls, aggressive antihypertensive therapy should be discontinued and a more moderate regimen instituted.

CASE PRESENTATION 3 (continued)
Management

In Mrs. N., a frail, elderly woman, antihypertensive therapy could be attempted very carefully, but it may not be possible to achieve the acceptable blood pressure control without causing further harm or side effects. When the treatment cannot be intensified due to unfavorable risk-to-benefit ratio or her intolerance to the drugs, this should be clearly documented and communicated to her health care proxy.

CONCLUSIONS

Effective control of hypertension is an important goal in older adults, because uncontrolled hypertension increases the risk of cognitive and physical impairment as well as that of cardiovascular events. In evaluating an elderly hypertensive adult, physicians should focus on accurate measurements of blood pressure, evidence of end-organ damage, functional and cognitive assessment, fall and balance assessment, financial and social support, and goals of care. Such information is essential to understand the heterogeneity of geriatric patients and formulate an individualized treatment plan based on the risk and benefit assessment. Current evidence suggests that treating stage 2 hypertension is beneficial and blood pressure below 140/90 mm Hg (or 130/80 mm Hg for diabetic patients) is associated with lower cardiovascular morbidity and mortality. However, there is little evidence to guide antihypertensive therapy in the very old and nursing home residents. Pharmacologic treatment of stage 1 hypertension has not been studied among elderly adults. Based on the results from HYVET, generally healthy older adults over age 80 should be offered antihypertensive therapy for stage 2 hypertension, with the target blood pressure of 150/90 mm Hg or lower. However, frail, elderly patients with multiple co-morbid conditions, or nursing home residents with end-stage conditions such as severe dementia, may not tolerate aggressive blood pressure lowering and are at high risk for complications from treatment. The general prescribing principle in geriatrics, "start low and go slow," should be applied and antihypertensive

therapy needs to be adjusted to the maximal tolerable level to avoid treatment-related adverse effects. If the risk of blood pressure lowering exceeds the benefit due to patients' co-morbid conditions and limited life expectancy, this should be documented in the records and communicated with health care proxy.

References

1. Ostchega Y, Dillon CF, Hughes JP, et al. Trends in hypertension prevalence, awareness, treatment, and control in older U.S. adults: Data from the National Health and Nutrition Examination Survey 1988 to 2004. J Am Geriatr Soc. 2007;55:1056-1065.

2. Hyman DJ, Pavlik VN, Vallbona C. Physician role in lack of awareness and control of hypertension. J Clin Hypertens (Greenwich). 2000;2:324-330.

3. Hajjar I, Miller K, Hirth V. Age-related bias in the management of hypertension: A national survey of physicians' opinions on hypertension in elderly adults. J Gerontol A Biol Sci Med Sci. 2002; 57:M487-M491.

4. Molander L, Lovheim H, Norman T, et al. Lower systolic blood pressure is associated with greater mortality in people aged 85 and older. J Am Geriatr Soc. 2008;56:1853-1859.

5. Verghese J, Lipton RB, Hall CB, et al. Low blood pressure and the risk of dementia in very old individuals. Neurology. 2003;61: 1667-1672.

6. Beckett NS, Peters R, Fletcher AE, et al. Treatment of hypertension in patients 80 years of age or older. N Engl J Med. 2008;358: 1887-1898.

7. Aronow WS. Hypertension in the nursing home. J Am Med Dir Assoc. 2008;9:486-490.

8. Koka M, Joseph J, Aronow WS. Adequacy of control of hypertension in an academic nursing home. J Am Med Dir Assoc. 2007,8.538-540.

9. Benetos A, Thomas F, Bean K, et al. Prognostic value of systolic and diastolic blood pressure in treated hypertensive men. Arch Intern Med. 2002;162:577-581.

10. Franklin SS, Khan SA, Wong ND, et al. Is pulse pressure useful in predicting risk for coronary heart disease? The Framingham Heart Study. Circulation. 1999;100:354-360.

11. Franklin SS, Jacobs MJ, Wong ND, et al. Predominance of isolated systolic hypertension among middle-aged and elderly US hypertensives: Analysis based on National Health and Nutrition Examination Survey (NHANES) III. Hypertension. 2001;37:869-874.

12. Masuo K, Mikami H, Ogihara T, Tuck ML. Changes in frequency of orthostatic hypotension in elderly hypertensive patients under medications. Am J Hypertens. 1996;9:263-268.

13. Lewington S, Clarke R, Qizilbash N, et al. Age-specific relevance of usual blood pressure to vascular mortality: a meta-analysis of individual data for one million adults in 61 prospective studies. Lancet. 2002; 360:1903-1913.

14. Launer LJ, Ross GW, Petrovitch H, et al. Midlife blood pressure and dementia: The Honolulu-Asia aging study. Neurobiol Aging. 2000; 21:49-55.

15. Stewart R, Xue QL, Masaki K, et al. Change in blood pressure and incident dementia: A 32-year prospective study. Hypertension. 2009;54:233-240.

16. Hajjar I, Lackland DT, Cupples LA, Lipsitz LA. Association between concurrent and remote blood pressure and disability in older adults. Hypertension. 2007;50:1026-1032.

17. Chobanian AV, Bakris GL, Black HR, et al. The Seventh Report of the Joint National Committee on Prevention, Detection, Evaluation, and Treatment of High Blood Pressure: The JNC 7 report. *JAMA.* 2003;289:2560-2572.

18. Gerstein HC, Mann JF, Yi Q, et al. Albuminuria and risk of cardiovascular events, death, and heart failure in diabetic and nondiabetic individuals. *JAMA.* 2001;286:421-426.

19. Hansson L, Zanchetti A, Carruthers SG, et al. Effects of intensive blood-pressure lowering and low-dose aspirin in patients with hypertension: Principal results of the Hypertension Optimal Treatment (HOT) randomised trial. HOT Study Group. *Lancet.* 1998;351:1755-1762.

20. Rochon PA, Gurwitz JH. Prescribing for seniors: Neither too much nor too little. *JAMA.* 1999;282:113-115.

21. The Trials of Hypertension Prevention Collaborative Research Group. Effects of weight loss and sodium reduction intervention on blood pressure and hypertension incidence in overweight people with high-normal blood pressure. The Trials of Hypertension Prevention, phase II. *Arch Intern Med.* 1997;157:657-667.

22. He J, Whelton PK, Appel LJ, et al. Long-term effects of weight loss and dietary sodium reduction on incidence of hypertension. *Hypertension.* 2000;35:544-549.

23. Sacks FM, Svetkey LP, Vollmer WM, et al. Effects on blood pressure of reduced dietary sodium and the Dietary Approaches to Stop Hypertension (DASH) diet. DASH-Sodium Collaborative Research Group. *N Engl J Med.* 2001;344:3-10.

24. Xin X, He J, Frontini MG, et al. Effects of alcohol reduction on blood pressure: A meta-analysis of randomized controlled trials. *Hypertension.* 2001;38:1112-1117.

25. Kelley GA, Kelley KS. Progressive resistance exercise and resting blood pressure: A meta-analysis of randomized controlled trials. *Hypertension.* 2000;35:838-843.

26. Whelton SP, Chin A, Xin X, He J. Effect of aerobic exercise on blood pressure: A meta-analysis of randomized, controlled trials. *Ann Intern Med.* 2002;136:493-503.

27. Appel LJ, Champagne CM, Harsha DW, et al. Effects of comprehensive lifestyle modification on blood pressure control: Main results of the PREMIER clinical trial. *JAMA.* 2003;289:2083-2093.

28. Whelton PK, Appel LJ, Espeland MA, et al. Sodium reduction and weight loss in the treatment of hypertension in older persons: A randomized controlled trial of nonpharmacologic interventions in the elderly (TONE). TONE Collaborative Research Group. *JAMA.* 1998;279:839-846.

29. The ALLHAT Officers and Coordinators for the ALLHAT Collaborative Research Group. Major outcomes in high-risk hypertensive patients randomized to angiotensin-converting enzyme inhibitor or calcium channel blocker vs diuretic: The Antihypertensive and Lipid-Lowering Treatment to Prevent Heart Attack Trial (ALLHAT). *JAMA.* 2002;288:2981-2997.

30. Bolland MJ, Ames RW, Horne AM, et al. The effect of treatment with a thiazide diuretic for 4 years on bone density in normal postmenopausal women. *Osteoporos Int.* 2007;18:479-486.

31. Yusuf S, Teo KK, Pogue J, et al. Telmisartan, ramipril, or both in patients at high risk for vascular events. *N Engl J Med.* 2008;358:1547-1559.

32. Bangalore S, Messerli FH, Kostis JB, Pepine CJ. Cardiovascular protection using beta-blockers: A critical review of the evidence. *J Am Coll Cardiol.* 2007;50:563-572.

33. Carlberg B, Samuelsson O, Lindholm LH. Atenolol in hypertension: Is it a wise choice? *Lancet.* 2004;364:1684-1689.

34. Boutitie F, Gueyffier F, Pocock S, et al. J-shaped relationship between blood pressure and mortality in hypertensive patients: New insights from a meta-analysis of individual-patient data. *Ann Intern Med.* 2002;136:438-448.

35. Fagard RH, Staessen JA, Thijs L, et al. On-treatment diastolic blood pressure and prognosis in systolic hypertension. *Arch Intern Med.* 2007;167:1884-1891.

36. Boshuizen HC, Izaks GJ, van BS, Ligthart GJ. Blood pressure and mortality in elderly people aged 85 and older: Community based study. *BMJ.* 1998;316:1780-1784.

37. Gupta V, Lipsitz LA. Orthostatic hypotension in the elderly: Diagnosis and treatment. *Am J Med.* 2007;120:841-847.

38. Jansen RW, Lipsitz LA. Postprandial hypotension: Epidemiology, pathophysiology, and clinical management. *Ann Intern Med.* 1995;122:286-295.

POST-TEST

1. **Which one of the following statements about hypertension and clinical outcomes is TRUE?**

   A. Hypertension has not been shown to affect functional outcomes in older adults who did not have stroke.

   B. Elevated blood pressure in midlife has been associated with less cognitive decline in late life.

   C. Diastolic pressure is a better predictor of future cardiovascular events than systolic pressure.

   D. Cardiovascular risk roughly doubles for every 20/10 mm Hg increase in blood pressure.

2. **Which one of the following statements is FALSE in evaluating hypertensive elderly patients?**

   A. Exploring the patient's social support system and financial status is important in the treatment decision.

   B. When there is a discrepancy in measured blood pressure between left and right arms, the one with higher pressure should be used for the follow-up measurements.

   C. Osler's maneuver reliably distinguishes true hypertension from pseudohypertension.

   D. Screening for cognitive dysfunction and functional impairment should be a part of routine examination.

3. **Which one of the following statements about the benefits of antihypertensive therapy is TRUE?**
   A. Antihypertensive therapy offers greater benefit in younger adults than in older adults.
   B. Antihypertensive therapy provides mortality reduction even in the very old with stage 2 hypertension.
   C. Selection of antihypertensive agents is more important than achieving a blood pressure target.
   D. Nonpharmacologic treatment has not proven effective in lowering blood pressure in the elderly.

ANSWERS TO PRE-TEST
1. C
2. A
3. C

ANSWERS TO POST-TEST
1. D
2. C
3. B

Index

Page numbers followed by "f" denote figures; "t" denote tables; and "b" denote boxes